Complications of Urologic Surgery

Prevention and Management

SECOND EDITION

Robert B. Smith, M.D.

Professor, Department of Surgery/Urology
University of California School of Medicine
Los Angeles, California

Richard M. Ehrlich, M.D.

Professor, Department of Surgery/Urology
University of California School of Medicine
Los Angeles, California

1990
W.B. SAUNDERS COMPANY
Harcourt Brace Jovanovich, Inc.

Philadelphia London Toronto Montreal Sydney Tokyo

W.B. SAUNDERS COMPANY
Harcourt Brace Jovanovich, Inc.

The Curtis Center
Independence Square West
Philadelphia, PA 19106

Library of Congress Cataloging-in-Publication Data

Complications of urologic surgery: prevention and management /
[edited by] Robert B. Smith, Richard M. Ehrlich.—2nd ed.
p. cm.
Includes bibliographies and index.
ISBN 0-7216-8414-9
1. Genitourinary organs—Surgery—Complications and sequelae.
I. Smith, Robert B., 1939– II. Ehrlich, Richard M. (Richard Michael), 1938–
[DNLM: 1. Genitalia, Male—surgery. 2. Postoperative Complications—prevention & control. 3. Urinary Tract—surgery.
WJ 168 C737]
RD571.C65 1989 617.4'601—dc20
DNLM/DLC 89-6400

Editor: William Lamsback
Designer: Paul Fry
Production Manager: Ken Neimeister
Manuscript Editor: Stephanie Mangum
Illustration Coordinator: Peg Shaw
Indexer: Ruth Low

Complications of Urologic Surgery: Prevention and Management, 2nd edition ISBN 0-7216-8414-9

Printed in the United States of America.

Last digit is the print number: 9 8 7 6 5 4 3 2 1

This book is dedicated to
David Jean deKernion
February 22, 1970–November 7, 1987

A Thought

Why am I
Bound to fly
so high to touch
the morning sky?

The sun shall shine,
to shower my mind
with all the fleeting thoughts
that it may find.

No longer saddened,
my heart rises, becomes gladdened
for it flies high above
The earth, so maddened.

Come the new Morn,
My soul to be reborn,
pain only echoes in the distance,
so dark, so forlorn.

For on this eve,
The moon's glow sheds light—before morn—
Upon the planet's fine weave,
and a child of the sun is born . . .

David deKernion

Contributors

Marvin E. Ament, M.D.
Professor of Pediatrics, UCLA School of Medicine, Los Angeles, California; Chief, Division of Pediatrics, Gastroenterology and Nutrition, and Chief, Hospital Parenteral and Enteral Nutrition, UCLA Medical Center, Los Angeles, California
Total Parenteral Nutrition in the Urologic Surgery Patient

Malcolm A. Bagshaw, M.D.
Professor and Chairman, Department of Radiation Oncology, and Director, Division of Radiation Therapy, Stanford University School of Medicine, Stanford, California; Director, Division of Radiation Therapy, Stanford University Hospital, Stanford, California
Complications Associated with Radiotherapy of Prostate Cancer

Robert R. Bahnson, M.D.
Assistant Professor and Chief of Urologic Oncology, Division of Urologic Surgery and Renal Transplantation, University of Pittsburgh School of Medicine, Pittsburgh, Pennsylvania
Complications of Radical Retropubic Prostatectomy

Zoran L. Barbaric, M.D.
Professor of Radiology, UCLA School of Medicine, Los Angeles, California; Vice Chairman and Chief, Radiological Sciences, Abdominal Division, UCLA Medical Center, Los Angeles, California
Complications of Therapeutic Radiologic Procedures

Paul E. Bellamy, M.D.
Associate Clinical Professor of Medicine, Department of Medicine, UCLA Medical School; Director, UCLA Multi-Campus Critical Care Fellowship Program, UCLA Medical School, Los Angeles, California; Director, Medical Intensive Care Unit, UCLA Medical Center, Los Angeles, California
Pulmonary Complications of Urologic Surgery

William E. Berquist, M.D.
Associate Professor of Pediatrics, UCLA School of Medicine, Los Angeles, California; Attending Staff, UCLA Medical Center, Los Angeles, California
Total Parenteral Nutrition in the Urologic Surgery Patient

Richard Bihrie, M.D.
Assistant Professor, Indiana University Medical School, Indianapolis, Indiana; Attending Staff, Indiana University Hospital, Wishard Memorial Hospital, and Indianapolis VA MBD Center, Indianapolis, Indiana
Complications in Adrenal Surgery

David A. Bloom, M.D.
Associate Professor of Surgery, University of Michigan, Ann Arbor, Michigan; Chief, Pediatric Urology, Mott Children's Hospital, Ann Arbor, Michigan
Complications of Urinary Stomas

Donald R. Bodner, M.D.
Assistant Professor of Surgery/Urology, Case Western Reserve University School of Medicine, Cleveland, Ohio; University Hospitals of Cleveland and Cleveland Veterans Administration Medical Center, Cleveland, Ohio
Complications of Open Renal Stone Surgery

Stuart D. Boyd, M.D.
Associate Professor of Urology, University of Southern California School of Medicine, Los Angeles, California; Attending Urology, Norris Cancer Hospital and Research Institute, Los Angeles, California
The Kock Pouch

William J. Catalona, M.D.
Professor of Surgery (Urology) and Chief, Division of Urologic Surgery, Washington University School of Medicine, St. Louis, Missouri
Complications of Radical Retropubic Prostatectomy

Christian G. Chaussy, M.D.
Professor of Urology, Ludwig-Maximillian University, Munich, West Germany; Permanent Visiting Professor, University of California, Los Angeles; Director, Department of Urology, Krankenhaus München-Harlaching, and Chief of Urologic Service, Krankenhaus München-Neuperlach, Munich, West Germany
Complications of Extracorporeal Shock Wave Lithotripsy (ESWL)

Richard A. Cox, Ph.D.
Radiologic Physics Section/Division of Radiation Therapy, Department of Radiation Oncology, Stanford University School of Medicine, Stanford, California
Complications Associated with Radiotherapy of Prostate Cancer

E. David Crawford, M.D.
Professor and Chairman, Division of Urology, University of Colorado, Denver, Colorado; University Hospital, Denver Veterans Administration, Denver, Colorado
Complications of Retroperitoneal Lymphadenectomy

Gabriel M. Danovitch, M.D.
Associate Professor of Medicine, UCLA School of Medicine, Los Angeles, California; Director of Renal Transplantation, UCLA Medical Center, Los Angeles, California
Metabolic Complications of Urologic Surgery

Richard David, M.D.
Resident in Urology, Division of Urology, Department of Surgery, UCLA Medical Center, Los Angeles, California
Complications of Extracorporeal Shock Wave Lithotripsy (ESWL); Complications of Ureteral Surgery

John P. Donohue, M.D.
Professor and Chairman, Department of Urology, Indiana University Medical Center, Indianapolis, Indiana
Complications in Adrenal Surgery

John W. Duckett, M.D.
Professor of Urology in Surgery, University of Pennsylvania School of Medicine, Philadelphia, Pennsylvania; Director, Division of Pediatric Urology, Children's Hospital of Philadelphia, Philadelphia, Pennsylvania
Complications of Hypospadias Repair

Richard M. Ehrlich, M.D., F.A.C.S., F.A.A.P.
Professor of Surgery and Urology, UCLA School of Medicine, Los Angeles, California
Complications of Ureteral Surgery

Jack S. Elder, M.D.
Associate Professor of Surgery (Urology) and Pediatrics, Case Western Reserve University School of Medicine, Cleveland, Ohio; Director of Pediatric Urology, Rainbow Babies and Children's Hospital, Cleveland, Ohio
Complications of Hypospadias Repair

George R. Fournier, Jr., M.D.
Assistant Professor of Urology, University of California School of Medicine and Veterans Administration Medical Center, San Francisco, California
Complications of Genitourinary Trauma

Alan M. Freedman, M.D.
Clinical Faculty, Harbor-UCLA Medical Center, UCLA School of Medicine, Los Angeles, California; Staff Urologist, Hoag Hospital, Newport Beach, California; Staff Urologist, Fountain Valley Regional Hospital, Fountain Valley, California
Complications of Ureteral Surgery

Anna M. Fuchs, M.D.
Assistant Clinical Professor of Urology/Surgery, UCLA School of Medicine, Los Angeles, California; Fellow in Urology/Lithotripsy, UCLA Stone Treatment Center, Los Angeles, California
Complications of Extracorporeal Shock Wave Lithotripsy (ESWL)

Gerhard J. Fuchs, M.D.
Associate Professor of Surgery/Urology, UCLA School of Medicine, Division of Urology, Los Angeles, California; Director, UCLA-Stone Center, Los Angeles, California
Complications of Extracorporeal Shock Wave Lithotripsy (ESWL)

John P. Gearhart, M.D.
Assistant Director of Pediatric Urology and Assistant Professor of Pediatric Urology, The Johns Hopkins University School of Medicine, Baltimore, Maryland; Division of Pediatric Urology, James Buchanan Brady Urological Institute, The Johns Hopkins Hospital, Baltimore, Maryland
Complications of Exstrophy and Epispadias Surgery

Jacob Golomb, M.D.
Fellow, Department of Surgery, Division of Urology, UCLA School of Medicine, Los Angeles, California
Complications of Bladder Substitution and Continent Urinary Diversion

Thomas M. Grove, M.D., Ph.D.
Clinical Assistant Professor of Anesthesiology, UCLA School of Medicine, Los Angeles, California; Staff Anesthesiologist, UCLA Center for Health Sciences, Los Angeles, California
Anesthetic Complications of Urologic Surgery

Clanton B. Harrison, M.D.
Fellow, Pediatric Urology, Children's Hospital San Diego, San Diego, California; Clinical Instructor, University of California Medical Center, San Diego, Department of Surgery, San Diego, California
Complications of Interstitial Radiotherapy in the Treatment of Carcinoma of the Prostate

Charles M. Haskell, M.D.

Professor of Medicine and Surgery, UCLA School of Medicine, Los Angeles, California; Director, Wadsworth Cancer Center; Chief, Hematology-Oncology Section, Medical and Research Services, West Los Angeles VA Medical Center; Attending Physician, UCLA Center for the Health Sciences, Los Angeles, California
Complications of Chemotherapy in the Urologic Patient

W. Hardy Hendren, M.D., F.A.C.S., F.A.A.P.

Robert E. Gross Professor of Surgery, Harvard Medical School, Cambridge, Massachusetts; Chief of Surgery, Children's Hospital; Visiting Surgeon, Massachusetts General Hospital, Boston, Massachusetts
Complications of Urethral Valve Surgery; Complications of Ureteral Reimplantation and Megaureter Repair

Grace R. Inouye, M.D.

Staff Physician, Hematology/Oncology, Internal Medicine, Kaiser Foundation Hospital, Panorama City, California
Complications of Chemotherapy in the Urologic Patient

Robert D. Jeffs, M.D.

Director of Pediatric Urology, Professor of Pediatric Urology, The Johns Hopkins University School of Medicine, Baltimore, Maryland; Division of Pediatric Urology, James Buchanan Brady Urological Institute, The Johns Hopkins Hospital, Baltimore, Maryland
Complications of Exstrophy and Epispadias Surgery

Aaron Kirkemo, M.D.

Senior Staff Urologist and Director, Female Urology/Urodynamics Laboratory, Henry Ford Hospital, Detroit, Michigan
Complications of Penile Surgery

Carl G. Klutke, M.D.

Fellow, Department of Surgery, Division of Urology, UCLA School of Medicine, Los Angeles, California
Complications of Bladder Substitution and Continent Urinary Diversion

Martin A. Koyle, M.D.

Assistant Professor of Surgery/Urology, UCLA School of Medicine, Los Angeles, California; Sections of Pediatric Urology and Renal Transplantation, Harbor-UCLA Medical Center, Torrance, California; St. Mary Medical Center, Long Beach, California; UCLA Center for the Health Sciences, Los Angeles, California
Complications of Scrotal Surgery

Andrew J. LeRoy, M.D.
Associate Professor of Radiology, Mayo Medical School, Mayo Clinic, Rochester, Minnesota; Staff Consultant at Mayo Clinic, St. Mary's Hospital of Rochester and Rochester Methodist Hospital, Rochester, Minnesota
Complications of Percutaneous Lithotripsy

Michael M. Lieber, M.D.
Professor of Urology, Mayo Medical School, Rochester, Minnesota; Consultant in Urology, Mayo Clinic, Rochester, Minnesota
Complications of Radical Cystectomy

Gary Lieskovsky, M.D.
Associate Professor of Surgery, Department of Urology, University of Southern California Medical Center, Los Angeles, California; Active Staff, Kenneth Norris Jr. Cancer Hospital and Research Institute; Attending Staff, Hospital of the Good Samaritan and Consulting Physician, Huntington Memorial Hospital, Los Angeles, California
The Kock Pouch

J. Keith Light, M.D.
Professor, Department of Urology, Baylor College of Medicine, Houston, Texas; Active Staff, The Methodist Hospital, St. Luke's Episcopal Hospital, Texas Children's Hospital, Institute for Rehabilitation and Research, Houston, Texas
Complications of Surgery for Male Urinary Incontinence

Kevin R. Loughlin, M.D.
Assistant Professor of Surgery (Urology), Harvard Medical School, Cambridge, Massachusetts; Associate Surgeon, Brigham and Women's Hospital, Boston, Massachusetts
Complications of Urinary Conduit Diversion

Andrei N. Lupu, M.D.
Professor of Surgery/Urology, UCLA School of Medicine, Los Angeles, California
Complications of Transabdominal Prostatectomy

Michael T. Macfarlane, M.D.
Assistant Clinical Professor, UCLA Medical Center, Los Angeles, California; Chief of Urology Section, Sepulveda Veterans Administration Hospital, Sepulveda, California
Management of Vascular Complications

Jack W. McAninch, M.D.
Professor and Vice Chairman, Department of Urology, University of California School of Medicine, San Francisco, California; Chief of Urology, San Francisco General Hospital, San Francisco, California
Complications of Genitourinary Trauma

Edward J. McGuire, M.D.
Professor of Surgery (Urology); Head, Section of Urology and Associate Chairman, Department of Surgery, University of Michigan, Ann Arbor, Michigan
Complications of Urinary Stomas

Andrew C. Novick, M.D.
Chairman, Department of Urology, Cleveland Clinic Foundation, Cleveland, Ohio
Complications of Renovascular Surgery

David F. Paulson, M.D.
Professor and Chief of Urology, Duke University Medical Center, Durham, North Carolina
Complications of Perineal Prostatectomy

Jacob Rajfer, M.D.
Associate Professor of Surgery/Urology, UCLA School of Medicine, Los Angeles, California; Chief, Division of Urology, Harbor-UCLA Medical Center, Torrance, California
Complications of Scrotal Surgery

Gordon R. Ray, M.D.
Director, Department of Radiation Oncology, Palo Alto Medical Foundation, Palo Alto, California
Complications Associated with Radiotherapy of Prostate Cancer

Shlomo Raz, M.D.
Professor of Surgery/Urology, UCLA School of Medicine, Los Angeles, California
Complications of Bladder Substitution and Continent Urinary Diversion; Complications of Cystoplasty

Martin I. Resnick, M.D.
Professor and Chairman, Division of Urology, Case Western Reserve University School of Medicine, Cleveland, Ohio; Attending Staff, University Hospitals of Cleveland, Cleveland, Ohio
Complications of Open Renal Stone Surgery

Jerome P. Richie, M.D.
Elliott C. Cutler Professor of Urological Surgery, Harvard Medical School, Cambridge, Massachusetts; Chief Surgeon, Division of Urological Surgery, Brigham and Women's Hospital, Boston, Massachusetts
Complications of Urinary Conduit Diversion

J. T. Rosenthal, M.D.
Assistant Professor, Division of Urology and Department of Surgery, UCLA School of Medicine, Los Angeles, California; Chief, Renal Transplantation, Division of Urology, UCLA Medical Center, Los Angeles, California
Complications of Renal Transplantation and Autotransplantation

Michael H. Rosove, M.D.
Attending Staff, UCLA Medical Center, Los Angeles, California; St. John's Hospital and Medical Center and Santa Monica Hospital, Santa Monica, California
Hematologic Considerations in Urologic Surgery

Peter T. Scardino, M.D.
Professor of Urology, Baylor College of Medicine, Houston, Texas; Attending Urologist, The Methodist Hospital and St. Luke's Episcopal Hospital, Houston, Texas; Consulting Urologist, Veterans Administration Medical Center, and Ben Taub General Hospital, Houston, Texas
Complications of Interstitial Radiotherapy in the Treatment of Carcinoma of the Prostate

Joseph W. Segura, M.D.
Carl Rosen Professor of Urology, Mayo Medical School, Mayo Clinic, Rochester, Minnesota; Staff Consultant at Mayo Clinic, St. Mary's Hospital of Rochester, and Rochester Methodist Hospital, Rochester, Minnesota
Complications of Percutaneous Lithotripsy

Mark B. Sender, M.D.
Clinical Professor of Surgery/Urology, UCLA School of Medicine, Los Angeles, California; Attending in Urology, Harbor-UCLA Medical Center, Torrance, California
Complications of Scrotal Surgery

Donald G. Skinner, M.D.
Professor and Chief, Division of Urology, University of Southern California School of Medicine, Los Angeles, California; Chief of Surgery, Kenneth Norris Jr. Cancer Hospital, Los Angeles, California
The Kock Pouch

Arthur D. Smith, M.D.
Professor of Urologic Surgery, State University of New York at Stony Brook, Stony Brook, Long Island, New York; Chairman, Department of Urology, Long Island Jewish Medical Center, New Hyde Park, New York
Complications of Ureteroscopy

Joseph A. Smith, Jr., M.D.
Professor, Department of Surgery, Division of Urology, University of Utah Health Sciences Center, Salt Lake City, Utah; Director, Urologic Oncology, University of Utah, Salt Lake City, Utah
Complications of Laser Surgery

Robert B. Smith, M.D., F.A.C.S.
Professor of Surgery/Urology, UCLA School of Medicine, Los Angeles, California; Attending Surgeon, UCLA Center for the Health Sciences; Chief, Urology, Wadsworth Veterans Administration Hospital, Los Angeles, California; Attending, Harbor-UCLA Hospital, Torrance, California; Attending, Olive View Medical Center, Van Nuys, California; Attending, Sepulveda Veterans Administration Hospital, Sepulveda, California
Complications of Renal Surgery; Management of Vascular Complications; Complications of Transurethral Surgery

Jeffrey A. Snyder, M.D.
Assistant Professor of Surgery, Division of Urology, University of Colorado Health Sciences Center, Denver, Colorado; Staff, University Hospital, VA Medical Center, Denver, Colorado; Consultant, Mediplex Rehabilitation Hospital, Denver, Colorado
Complications of Cystoplasty

David R. Staskin, M.D.
Assistant Professor of Urology, Boston University Medical Center, Boston, Massachusetts; Director, Continence Center, University Hospital, Boston, Massachusetts
Complications of Female Anti-incontinence Surgery

Jan Tillisch, M.D.
Associate Professor, UCLA School of Medicine, Los Angeles, California; Director, Cardiac Unit, UCLA Medical Center, Los Angeles, California
Cardiac Complications of Urologic Surgery

Richard Turner-Warwick, D.Sc., D.M. (Oxon), M.Ch., F.R.C.P., F.R.C.S., F.A.C.S., F.R.A.C.S. (Hon)
Senior Surgeon, The Middlesex Hospital, London; Senior Consultant, Urological Surgeon, The St. Peters Hospitals; Senior Lecturer, the London University Institute of Urology, London, England
Complications of Urethral Surgery in the Male

Jorge Vargas, M.D.
Assistant Professor of Pediatrics, UCLA School of Medicine, Los Angeles, California; Attending Staff, UCLA Medical Center, Los Angeles, California
Total Parenteral Nutrition in the Urologic Surgery Patient

Jerry J. Weinberg, M.D.
Chief Resident, Department of Urology, Long Island Jewish Medical Center, New Hyde Park, New York
Complications of Ureteroscopy

Steven M. Weiner, M.D.
Assistant Clinical Professor, Division of Urology, University of Colorado, Denver, Colorado
Complications of Retroperitoneal Lymphadenectomy

Alan Wilkinson, M.D.
Visiting Associate Professor of Medicine, UCLA School of Medicine, Los Angeles, California; Director, Clinical Nephrology, UCLA Medical Center, Los Angeles, California
Metabolic Complications of Urologic Surgery

Matthew L. Wilner, M.D.
Senior Resident in Urology, UCLA School of Medicine, Los Angeles, California
Hematologic Considerations in Urologic Surgery

Drew J. Winston, M.D.
Assistant Professor, Department of Hematology/Oncology, UCLA Medical Center, Los Angeles, California
Infectious Complications of Urologic Surgery

Philippe E. Zimmern, M.D.
Urology Staff, Kaiser Foundation Hospital—Sunset, Los Angeles, California
Complications of Transabdominal Prostatectomy

Preface

> "Yes, I have seen this complication many times, but never personally."
>
> Anonymous

It is often said that the surgeon who has patients without complications is no longer operating. Given that fact, for the rest of us mortals, continuing education, postgraduate courses, journal reading, and an inquisitive mind continue to be the backbone of our striving for excellence. This translates into meticulous attention to detail in the operating room, willingness to be open-minded and adaptable, and an ever-expanding search for complication-free surgery and superb patient care.

This volume is a compendium of the experience of well-known authorities in their respective fields who have often written about their subjects of expertise. It is geared to the practicing urologist and the resident in urology as a ready reference for both the prevention and successful treatment of complications of urologic surgery.

As such, it has been our overriding goal to provide up-to-date references and drawings, to include new surgical endeavors such as continent diversion, and to update older techniques.

We are indebted to the many authors for their generous gift of time in the preparation of their manuscripts and to William Lamsback, whose help with this volume has been immeasurable.

ROBERT B. SMITH, M.D.
RICHARD M. EHRLICH, M.D.

Contents

METABOLIC COMPLICATIONS OF UROLOGIC SURGERY

1

Alan Wilkinson • Gabriel M. Danovitch

The medical complications associated with urologic surgery are not unique to this discipline, but particular care needs to be given to a full assessment of renal, cardiovascular, and pulmonary functions. The pulmonary, cardiac, hematologic, and infectious complications are discussed elsewhere, and a full section on parenteral nutrition has been included in this edition. This chapter deals with the management of patients with acute and chronic renal insufficiency, hyperkalemia, hypercalcemia, and diabetes mellitus. Acid-base problems are discussed, and the chapter concludes with a section on the treatment of hypertension.

There are a number of general caveats that apply to patients who most commonly require urologic surgery. These patients are predominantly older males who are predisposed to cardiovascular and pulmonary pathology. Spinal anesthesia now permits operations on previously unacceptable candidates; however, this is not without risks, in particular the risk of hypotension, which may lead to cardiac and renal injury, and adequate preoperative hydration is essential. Although nuclear medicine and ultrasound techniques have decreased the frequency with which intravenous contrast studies are performed, a substantial number of intravenous urograms and arteriograms are still required, and the danger of contrast administration causing a deterioration in renal function in the presence of dehydration, diabetes mellitus, renal insufficiency, or increasing age cannot be overemphasized. Nonsteroidal analgesics are being used increasingly for the treatment of pain, and by virtue of their inhibition of prostaglandin synthesis these may cause rapid deterioration in renal function. This risk increases in the presence of hypercalcemia, which may occur particularly in patients with malignant bone disease.

Postobstructive diuresis, with massive losses of water and electrolytes, has been overemphasized in the past. This complication, unique to urology, will be discussed under salt-and-water homeostasis.

RENAL INSUFFICIENCY

Acute Renal Failure

The causes of acute renal failure (ARF) are conveniently divided into prerenal, renal, and postrenal groups, all of which may be encountered in the course of urologic practice. ARF is characterized by an abrupt deterioration in renal function, with a decline in urine flow to oliguric levels of less than 300 ml/24 hours. The total cessation of urine flow strongly suggests obstruction. In ARF there is a progressive accumulation of urea, creatinine, potassium, phosphorus, sodium, uric acid, and water and the development of a metabolic acidosis and hypocalcemia. If the cause is rapidly reversible, renal function may return soon enough to avoid dialysis, but frequently dialysis will be required until renal function returns. The *oliguric phase* lasts from 2 to 20 days and is followed by the *diuretic phase* in which there is a progressive increase in urine volume. ARF is not always associated with oliguria, and patients may produce as much as 1500 ml urine per day. The prognosis for recovery following renal failure depends on the etiology, and, following established acute tubular necrosis (ATN), rate of recovery is worse with increasing age, pre-existing renal disease, and in the presence of infection or other organ failure. Even with apparent total recovery, the glomerular filtration rate (GFR) is on average only 80 percent of normal at 2 to 3 months after injury.

Prerenal ARF occurs following hypotension (hemorrhage, sepsis, cardiogenic shock) or, more insidiously, with progressive dehydration as a result of vomiting, diarrhea, loss from fistulas or drains, and overenthusiastic diuresis. Insufficient fluid intake in the elderly and ill may also lead to dehydration. Unless damage to the kidneys in the form of ATN has already occurred, there will be evidence of avid retention of salt and water, with a concentrated urine with an extremely low urinary sodium concentration (Table 1–1). This form of renal failure should respond rapidly to rehydration and to an improvement in the systemic blood pressure.

However, if the prerenal factors have been sufficiently severe, a period of ATN in which the small volume of urine will be dilute and the urinary sodium concentration high may follow. Although patients undergoing urologic surgery may have any of the numerous primary renal diseases, the important factor to consider, in addition to ATN secondary to hypoperfusion, is ATN secondary to intravenous dye and nephrotoxic drugs, in particular the aminoglycoside antibiotics and nonsteroidal anti-inflammatory drugs, which should be avoided whenever possible. Acute renal failure may impair the immune response, frequently resulting in severe infections. Many of the organisms will require treatment with aminoglycosides or, in the case of fungal infections, amphotericin. Nephrotoxicity notwithstanding, it is essential to achieve therapeutic serum levels of these drugs while monitoring closely for toxicity. Urinary tract infections occur less frequently if bladder catheters are removed from oliguric patients.

Unless there is only a single functional kidney, postrenal ARF must necessarily involve the obstruction of both kidneys. This most often occurs secondary to bladder outlet obstruction (posterior-urethral valves, prostatic hypertrophy, urethral strictures) or a neurogenic bladder. Bilateral ureteric obstruction may occur with retroperitoneal fibrosis and tumor infiltration. In the presence of a single kidney, ureteric obstruction by a calculus or necrotic papilla may lead to ARF.

The evaluation and management of patients with renal failure is best achieved by following a logical approach to confirm or exclude the causes outlined above. The clinical examination should include an evaluation of the state of hydration, with supine and standing blood pressure, and examination for the presence of a distended bladder. A Foley bladder catheter should be introduced and urine output monitored closely. The intravascular volume and blood pressure should be improved to a level sufficient to maintain glomerular filtration ((mean arterial pressure) [MAP] >80 mm Hg). Urinary electrolyte concentrations and osmolality must be determined before diuretics are given. Thereafter, either mannitol, 25 gm, or furosemide, 40 to 80 mg, is administered intravenously in an attempt to re-establish a urine output above 50 ml/hour, because even if renal function does not recover immediately, it is useful to convert oliguric ATN to the polyuric form. This decreases risks of complications secondary to hyperkalemia, severe acidosis, and water retention and allows more liberal intravenous therapy and nutrition, with less frequent dialysis. If urine output does not improve immediately, ultrasound will exclude the presence of hydronephrosis, but it will not absolutely exclude obstructive uropathy, which can occur without dilatation. It may be necessary to perform a diethylene-triaminepenta-acetic

Table 1–1. URINARY INDICES IN ACUTE RENAL FAILURE

	Prerenal* Azotema	ATN
Urine Osmolality ($mOsm/kgH_2O$)	> 500	< 350
Urine Sodium (mEq/l)	< 20	> 40
Urine to Plasma Creatinine Ratio	> 40	< 20
Fractional Sodium Excretion (100 × [U/P Sodium]/[U/P Creatinine])	< 1	> 2

*Early obstructive uropathy will have similar indices to prerenal azotemia, which will gradually change to resemble those of ATN.

acid (DTPA) technetium 99m (^{99m}Tc) nuclear scan with furosemide washout to confirm obstruction to urine flow. The excretion of ^{99m}Tc DTPA is traced by computer analysis of the radioactivity in the kidney and renal pelvis before and after the administration of 20 to 40 mg of intravenous furosemide in a well-hydrated patient. With dilatation but no obstruction, the isotope is washed out rapidly. If there is obstruction, there is accumulation of isotope in the renal pelvis after administration of the loop diuretic. If there is sufficient pelvic dilatation, anterograde pyelography is the procedure of choice to delineate the site of ureteric obstruction; however, in the absence of dilatation, a high-dose intravenous pyelography (IVP) or retrograde pyelography may be used. Bilateral or unilateral ureteral obstruction is treated by percutaneous nephrostomy drainage and removal of the obstruction where possible.

If it is not possible to restore renal function, management will include fluid and potassium restriction, phosphate binders, antacid therapy, appropriate dietary limitations, and dialysis in order to avoid the complications of uremia. Daily dialysis and ultrafiltration may be necessary to remove sufficient volume in order to allow adequate parenteral feeding. More recently, continuous arteriovenous hemofiltration (CAVH) has been introduced to provide the continuous removal of water and solutes, and, at high blood flow rates, up to 2000 ml/hour can be ultrafiltered, with a clearance of about 10 ml/minute. For CAVH, access to an artery and a vein is required, and filtration is achieved using the systemic arterial pressure and gravity through a hollow fiber coil. In situations in which hemodialysis is hazardous, for example, in the presence of myocardial instability or hypotension, CAVH provides a means of fluid and solute removal with improved cardiovascular stability. Peritoneal dialysis may be used if the peritoneal cavity was not entered during surgery. During the period of ATN, the dosage of renally excreted drugs, including analgesics and magnesium-containing antacids, should be reduced.

Chronic Renal Failure

As kidney function declines, residual functional nephrons are able to maintain normal salt-and-water homeostasis, despite a considerable decrease in the GFR. This progressive adaptation in the function of each single nephron results in an increased fractional clearance of electrolytes and water, which has as its trade-off a number of alterations in the factors controlling renal function. One of these factors, the rise in the serum parathyroid hormone level as the GFR falls below 70 percent of normal, is thought to be involved in a number of the complications of chronic renal failure, such as bone disease, anemia, and impaired cardiac function. An increase in intraglomerular pressure and in the hyperfiltration in each remaining glomerulus is thought to lead to the continuous decline in renal function following the onset of chronic renal failure. Although this adaptation allows the maintenance of homeostasis when a patient is given a normal diet, even with a GFR as low as 10 ml/minute, the ability to compensate for extreme reductions or increases in the intake of salt and water is lost as the kidneys lose their ability to dilute or concentrate the urine or to modulate the excretion of solutes.

The management of chronic renal failure must have as its goals a reduction in the rate of decline in the GFR and, more importantly in the perioperative period, the prevention of further damage. The rate of decline in renal function may be retarded by strict control of hypertension, by a reduction in serum lipids, and by a diet restricted in protein and phosphate. To avoid further renal damage, urinary tract infections must be treated promptly and urethral instrumentation performed only when absolutely indicated. The inability of the kidney to concentrate the urine in these patients means that the patient can become dehydrated rapidly, with a further decline in kidney function, if intake is allowed to fall below 1500 ml/day. Congestive heart failure may impair renal function and should be treated optimally. Nephrotoxic agents must be avoided.

Sodium and water balances are of primary importance. With advanced renal failure and a GFR of 5 ml/minute, a patient may still excrete 120 to 140 mEq of sodium—and thereby remain in sodium balance—on a 5- to 10-gm sodium diet. As a result of nephron adaptation, this solute load will require an obligatory urine volume of 1500 to 2000 ml/24 hours. However, there is a reduced ability to conserve and excrete sodium and these patients may become sodium-depleted if they receive less than 2 gm of sodium per day. Similarly, they are unable to excrete a sodium load of more than 10 to 15 gm per day. Therefore, unless patients are losing sodium as a result of nasogastric suction, vomiting, diarrhea, fistula drainage, or diuretic therapy, they will require 5 to 10 gm of sodium daily either in the diet or intravenously. In the presence of edema or hypertension, this may be reduced to 2 gm, provided care is taken to avoid hyponatremia. Occasionally, patients with interstitial nephritis, medullary cystic disease, or polycystic kidney disease may be "salt-wasters" and require as much as 20 gm of sodium per day if they are not to become dehydrated. The obligatory urine volume of 1500 to 2000 ml/day and the inability to concentrate the urine means that patients will easily become dehydrated if they are too ill to drink or if they are given insufficient intravenous fluid therapy. On the other hand, a water load is well tolerated until renal function has declined to a GFR of less than 10 ml/minute, whereafter infusion or the oral intake of a large volume of water increases sodium losses and results in hyponatremia.

Following the relief of urinary obstruction, there is a salt-and-water diuresis. This is a result not only of the kidney's inability to conserve salt and water but also, frequently, of an accumulated excess of salt and water. The diuresis may also be promoted by the excretion of urea accumulated during the obstruction. Most patients experience only a brief diuresis and rapidly show a return to a normal state of hydration and kidney function appropriate to their degree of irreversible kidney failure. The inability to conserve sodium may be of longer duration, and these patients will need a higher sodium intake. Immediately following the relief of obstruction, strict attention must be paid to the replacement of solute and water losses in sufficient volume to prevent hypotension, a decline in renal function, hyponatremia, hypokalemia, and hypomagnesemia. The diuresis may be prolonged by excessive volume replacement. Urinary losses are usually replaced with 0.45 percent sodium chloride (NaCl) with added sodium bicarbonate ($NaHCO_3$) and potassium chloride (KCl). Magnesium and phosphate may also be required.

Hyperkalemia, as noted in the section on its management, is not usually seen in uncomplicated chronic renal failure unless drugs are given that raise the serum potassium, the ingested potassium load increases suddenly, or there is an abrupt decline in the GFR. A small number of patients may have hyperkalemia in the absence of these factors, and they are often found to have a hyporeninemic-hypoaldosteronemic type IV renal tubular acidosis. This occurs most frequently in older diabetic patients with a GFR below 20 ml/hour and is treated with potassium reduction, by diet, with diuretics and exchange resins, with sodium bicarbonate, and, occasionally, with mineralocorticoids. Mineralocorticoids may lead to volume retention with pulmonary edema and hypertension and should not be used routinely. Hypokalemia occasionally occurs in chronic renal failure as a result of insufficient potassium intake, diuretic use, or hyperaldosteronism secondary to volume depletion, renal artery stenosis, or severe hypertension.

Hypocalcemia and hyperphosphatemia are hallmarks of chronic renal failure once the GFR has fallen below 20 to 25 ml/hour. An increased fractional clearance of phosphate, calcium, and magnesium maintains its balance until then, and only when the GFR is below 5 ml/minute is there a significant rise in serum phosphate. The reduction in tubular phosphate reabsorption is the result of an increase in the parathyroid hormone (PTH) level, which starts to rise even when the GFR is reduced to only 70 percent of normal. Once the serum phosphate level starts to rise, phosphate-binding agents should be prescribed to limit the rise in serum phosphate and reduce its impact on worsening hypocalcemia and further elevations of PTH. Basic aluminum carbonate gel (Basaljel) ($AlCO_3$), aluminum hydroxide gel (Amphojel) ($AlOH_3$), and calcium carbonate are usually given. Recent concern over the accumulation of aluminum in the body has increased the use of calcium carbonate, but this may not always be sufficient. Hypocalcemia, which occurs in spite of a decrease in the absolute excretion of calcium, is a result of decreased intestinal absorption secondary to $1,25(OH)_2$ vitamin D_3 deficiency (which starts to fall when the GFR is below 40 percent of normal), the contributory role of hyperphosphatemia, and decreased bone sensitivity to the action of PTH. The use of calcium carbonate as a phosphate-binding agent will provide calcium; however, symptoms from the hypocalcemia of renal failure are rare, and specific therapy is not usually indicated. Care should be taken not to administer alkali too rapidly to these patients because the rapid pH shift may lower the ionized calicum and precipitate tetany.

When the GFR has fallen below 25 to 30 ml/minute, acidosis invariably develops because patients are now able to excrete only 30 to 40 mEq of hydrogen ions, about 50 percent of the daily acid load generated on a normal diet, and the serum bicarbonate will decrease. This inability to excrete acid results from a reduction in the generation of the ammonia, usually secreted by the renal tubules to buffer the acid load and regenerate serum bicarbonate. The positive hydrogen ion balance is buffered in part by bone salts. Initially, the acidosis will be hyperchloremic with a normal anion gap, but this will progress to an anion-gap acidosis. This acidosis is generally mild, with a pH above 7.35. If the acidosis is symptomatic, it can be treated with either sodium bicarbonate or sodium citrate, 20 to 30 mEq/day. It is not necessary to raise the serum bicarbonate above 16 mEq/l. It is occasionally necessary to treat a severe acidosis (arterial pH below 7.1) with intravenous bicarbonate or dialysis. This correction should bring the pH back to only 7.2 to 7.25 to avoid the complication of decreasing the ionized calcium and precipitating tetany. Although this is still debated, there is also some evidence that increasing the serum bicarbonate too rapidly may, by decreasing ventilation, cause a rise in the carbon dioxide partial pressure (P_{CO_2}) and an increase in the cerebrospinal fluid (CSF) acidosis, altering consciousness.

Anemia affects almost all patients with renal failure. This is usually a normochromic normocytic anemia of chronic disease that fails to respond to iron and vitamin therapy. Repeated blood transfusions increase the risks of virus transmission, hemosiderosis, and sensitization to foreign tissue antigens, which may compromise transplantation. These transfusions, therefore, should be given only to symptomatic patients. Recombinant erythropoietin, currently under investigation for use in end-stage renal disease, will probably also be useful in the treatment of anemia of chronic renal failure. Uremic patients show an increased incidence of gastrointestinal bleeding, and if the hematocrit level falls sharply, this and other factors must be considered.

HYPERKALEMIA

Rapid elevations in the serum potassium usually occur only in the presence of ARF. The rate of rise is influenced by the degree of catabolism, in particular with sepsis or tissue necrosis. Hyperkalemia may also be encountered in patients with a mineral acid metabolic acidosis. Chronic hyperkalemia occurs with adrenal insufficiency or a type IV renal tubular acidosis (hyporeninemic-hypoaldosteronemic RTA) and rises abruptly if these patients receive excess potassium. There are a number of drugs that cause hyperkalemia, including potassium-sparing diuretics, prostaglandin synthetase inhibitors, angiotensin-converting enzyme inhibitors, and cyclosporine.

Chronic renal failure is not usually associated with hyperkalemia in the absence of other factors because adaptive changes maintain a normal serum potassium until renal function is severely impaired. Hyperkalemia may be associated with progressive weakness leading to muscular paralysis and respiratory insufficiency, but frequently it is asymptomatic even when the electrocardiograph (EKG) shows evidence of toxicity. Urgent treatment is essential because death may occur from ventricular asystole. Serial measurements of the serum potassium should be obtained during treatment, and the EKG, a very sensitive indicator of potassium toxicity, should be followed closely. Other electrolyte disturbances, in particular hyponatremia, hypocalcemia, and acidosis, potentiate the adverse effects of hyperkalemia. The cardinal electrocardiographic changes of hyperkalemia are best seen in the precordial leads. Initially, these are tall, peaked T waves, with ST segment depression and a decrease in the R-wave amplitude. This progresses to prolongation of the PR interval and widening of the QRS complex. Therefore the P waves are lost, and there is a sine-wave appearance to the QRS-T wave complex.

The goals of treatment are first, to lower the effective serum potassium concentration and second, to remove the offending cation from the body. Cell stability may be enhanced with intravenous calcium; potassium is shifted from the extracellular to intracellular space by dextrose and insulin and by sodium bicarbonate, which will also raise the serum sodium. Finally, potassium is removed by resins or dialysis. With continuous EKG monitoring, calcium gluconate, 5 to 10 ml of a 10 percent solution, is given intravenously over 2 minutes. This will counter the effects of hyperkalemia for about 1 hour. The dose may be repeated after 10 to 15 minutes if there is no response. Next, sodium bicarbonate, 45 mEq HCO_3 as 7.5 percent $NaHCO_3$, is given intravenously over 5 minutes and is repeated in 10 to 15 minutes if the EKG still shows evidence of potassium toxicity. This is followed by 50 percent glucose (25 gm) with 5 to 10 units of regular insulin given over 5 to 10 minutes. In patients who can tolerate the added volume, the bicarbonate and dextrose can be combined by adding 89 mEq HCO_3 to 1000 ml 10 percent dextrose in water (DW); 300 ml is then given over 30 minutes and the remainder over 2½ to 3 hours. Insulin may be given either subcutaneously (25 square units) or by constant infusion (5 to 10 units/hour), with close monitoring of blood glucose levels.

These measures will provide protection while potassium is removed from the body. This can always be achieved by dialysis, but while dialysis is being organized and when dialysis is considered unnecessary, potassium may be removed by the oral or rectal administration of sodium polystyrene sulfonate (Kayexalate), a polystyrene sulfonate resin, each gram of which will remove 1 mEq of potassium. Fifteen to 30 gm in 30 to 60 ml of 50 percent sorbitol is given orally or 50 to 100 gm in 200 ml of 50 percent sorbitol rectally. In patients with an established venous access, dialysis should be started as soon as possible.

HYPERCALCEMIA AND HYPOCALCEMIA

Causes and Treatment of Hypercalcemia

ARF is usually accompanied by hypocalcemia, for which specific treatment is rarely required. More often, if there has been significant muscle injury, hypercalcemia may occur. The most common causes of hypercalcemia are hyperparathyroidism and malignancy. The former causes hypercalcemia by the effect of PTH on bone resorption and intestinal calcium absorption. Metastases to bone cause bone destruction with the release of calcium, and myeloma and lymphomas may stimulate the release of an osteoclast-activating factor. Several solid tumors are associated with abnormal prostaglandin production and hypercalcemia. Other possible causes of hypercalcemia include immobilization, Paget's disease of bone, tuberculosis, sarcoidosis, thyrotoxicosis, Addison's disease, thiazide diuretics, and vitamin D excess.

The extra serum calcium must be either taken up by bone and tissues or excreted in the urine. It is known that the kidney handles calcium in a manner analogous to the way in which it handles sodium, and treatment is designed to make use of this. Dehydration may result in hypercalcemia, and this should be corrected by giving 1 to 2 liters of normal saline over 1 hour. Adequate hydration can be assessed by measuring the supine and standing blood pressures. Further volume expansion may compromise cardiorespiratory function, and at this stage 40 to 80 mg of furosemide is given intravenously. A bladder catheter is placed, and hourly estimations are made of urine volume and urinary potassium loss. This loss is replaced with normal saline and potassium. Urine output should be maintained at about 300 ml/hour with additional doses of intravenous furosemide. Serum magnesium levels should be checked and magnesium replaced as necessary. Severe hypercalcemia may cause renal failure and neurologic and cardiovascular dysfunction. In this circumstance both calcitonin and mithramycin will lower the serum calcium within several hours. It may also be necessary to use hemodialysis against a calcium-free dialysate if an adequate saline diuresis cannot be obtained. Calcitonin, 4 units/kg intravenously (IV) initially, and 4 units/kg subcutaneously (SC) every 12 to 24 hours, lowers the calcium in 75 to 80 percent of patients. However, even in those who respond initially, resistance to repeated use may develop. This resistance may be partially prevented by steroids. Mithramycin, 25 mg/kg IV, will inhibit bone resorption, and it is used to treat both acute and chronic hypercalcemia.

For the treatment of acute hypercalcemia, the initial dose is repeated daily for 3 days. The calcium concentration should fall within 12 to 24 hours. Repeated use of this drug may be complicated by thrombocytopenia, renal toxicity, and hepatotoxicity. Glucocorticoids may take 2 to 3 days to lower calcium levels, but they are frequently given as part of the initial therapy. They act by decreasing intestinal calcium absorption and by diminishing the hypercalcemic effects of some tumors, in particular myeloma and breast carcinoma. Three to 5 mg/kg/day of hydrocortisone is given initially, followed by lower maintenance doses.

The hypercalcemia associated with malignant disease may also be treated with etidronate disodium, a synthetic diphosphonate. This is a very effective antihypercalcemic agent, an analogue of pyrophosphate, which acts by inhibiting osteoclast-induced resorption of bone. It also reduces the solubility of calcium hydroxyapatite bone crystals. It should be used following, and in combination with, saline hydration and loop diuretics. Some authorities now favor this agent over both calcitonin and mithramycin for the treatment of elevated calcium levels secondary to malignant disease. Etidronate disodium is given initially as a slow infusion, over 1 to 3 hours, diluted in 250 ml of normal saline. The dose is 7.5 mg/kg of body weight per day and is repeated daily for 3 to 7 days. Thereafter, oral treatment can be continued from the day following the last intravenous infusion. The oral dose is 20 mg/kg BW/day for 30 days.

Etidronate disodium is excreted by the kid-

neys, largely in its original form. In occasional patients with mild pre-existing renal dysfunction, etidronate disodium treatment may cause a further depression in renal function. The experience is limited as to the use of etidronate disodium in patients with a serum creatinine level over 2.5 mg/dl, and careful assessment of the overall benefits should be made in this circumstance. *A reduction in dose is advisable.*

Life-threatening hypercalcemia may rarely be treated with the chelating agent ethylene diamine beta-acetic acid (EDTA). This causes an immediate fall in the effective serum calcium concentration by complexing calcium within the blood and thereafter promoting its excretion. The use of EDTA is complicated by severe side effects, not the least of which are nephrotoxicity and hypotension, and its use should be reserved for emergencies. The use of intravenous phosphorus is extremely effective but no longer recommended because it too can cause severe complications including hypotension and extravascular calcification. Oral phosphates are used to reduce intestinal absorption. Elemental phosphorus, 1½ to 3 gm, is given daily. This may be complicated by severe diarrhea. In the presence of renal insufficiency, the serum phosphate concentration should be measured regularly to avoid the risk of extravascular calcification.

Causes and Treatment of Hypocalcemia

Hypocalcemia is rare in the absence of renal failure. Patients who are taking vitamin D supplements following parathyroidectomy can usually go without these supplements in the perioperative period without developing hypocalcemia. Vitamin D deficiency is associated with fat malabsorption following partial gastrectomy, small bowel disease, chronic pancreatitis, intestinal resection, and bypass surgery, and patients on the antiepileptic agents phenobarbital and phenytoin may be hypocalcemic secondary to increased vitamin D metabolism and impaired intestinal absorption of calcium.

Acute hypocalcemia is treated by rapid intravenous infusion of 10 ml of 10 percent calcium chloride (360 mg of elemental calcium) or 20 to 30 ml 10 percent of calcium gluconate (90 mg of elemental calcium per 10 ml). The symptoms of hypocalcemia include tetany, myopathy, impaired mentation, seizures, and extrapyramidal disorders. Hypomagnesemia should be excluded but treated if the serum magnesium level is below 1 mg/dl. Chronic hypocalcemia is treated with supplemental calcium and appropriate vitamin D therapy.

DIABETES MELLITUS

However well controlled diabetes mellitus is under normal circumstances, this common disease will frequently present problems perioperatively, either with increased insulin requirements or with frank diabetic ketoacidosis, as a result of the stress of surgery or the presence of infection. Unrecognized diabetes mellitus may become evident for the first time, and the blood glucose level should always be measured postoperatively. A fasting blood glucose level above 140 mg/dl on more than one occasion signifies glucose intolerance.

Perioperative Management of the Diabetic Patient

All patients must be stable with the disease well controlled, even if this means delaying the time of operation. On the day of surgery, all long-acting and intermediate insulin is discontinued, and control is achieved with regular insulin alone. In the operating room and intensive care setting, insulin can be given by continuous low-dose intravenous infusion, 3 to 5 units/hour, with regular blood glucose monitoring. At the same time 5 percent glucose in water is infused at about 125 ml/hour. An alternative is to add 10 to 20 units of regular insulin to 1000 ml of 5 percent glucose in water and to infuse this at a rate that maintains a normal blood glucose level.

The insulin can also be given subcutaneously, 10 units initially, followed by an infusion of 5 percent glucose in water at 125 ml/hour, with further doses of subcutaneous insulin every 2 to 4 hours according to the blood glucose level. The low-dose infusion method will provide the most precise control. Approximately 50 gm of glucose should be given every 8 hours.

Patients with non–insulin-dependent diabetes mellitus on oral agents will require therapy with insulin only if previous fasting levels of blood glucose on treatment have exceeded 200 mg/dl. If they do require insulin, the schedule is similar to that outlined above for insulin-dependent patients. To prevent hypoglycemia, oral hypoglycemic agents should be discontinued from 24 to 72 hours before surgery, depending on the length of time of their effective half-life.

Management of Diabetic Ketoacidosis

The treatment of diabetic ketoacidosis has been simplified considerably over the last decade, but patients still require meticulous monitoring until the metabolic abnormalities have been corrected. The symptoms of ketoacidosis include thirst, polyuria, confusion, headache, and on examination patients are usually dehydrated and hyperventilating in response to the profound metabolic acidosis. The blood glucose is usually above 300 mg/dl and there is a ketonemia (acetoacetate and beta-hydroxybutyrate) that results in an elevated anion gap acidosis. This state may be precipitated by the stress of surgery, insufficient insulin therapy, and infections, which should be treated promptly. Therapy of diabetic ketoacidosis includes insulin, without which cure is impossible; fluid replacement; electrolyte replacement; and bicarbonate if the acidosis is severe, especially with associated shock or coma.

Insulin is now usually given intravenously. A low-dose constant infusion at a rate of 10 to 15 units/hour (100 units regular insulin in 500 ml of 0.45 percent NaCl) is started and adjusted according to the blood glucose response. Patients may exhibit insulin resistance and may need doses of 50 units/hour to reduce the blood glucose concentration and correct the acidosis. An acceptable rate of response is for the blood glucose to fall at 50 mg/dl/hour. Intramuscular insulin may also be used; however, the titration of the doses is more difficult, and there may be a considerable lag in the response.

Initial fluid management should be tailored according to the estimated volume deficit. In the absence of intravenous pressure monitoring, an accurate record of weights, fluid intake, or urine output, the deficit can be assumed to be 3 to 5 liters. In the presence of hypernatremia, a serum sodium level over 155 mEq of sodium per liter, hypotonic 0.45 percent NaCl should be used as the replacement fluid. In other instances, either 0.9 percent NaCl or Ringer's lactate is used and 1 to 2 l infused over the first hour, followed by 1 l per hour over the next few hours until the extracellular fluid volume deficit is corrected. Once the blood glucose level has fallen to 300 mg/dl, fluid replacement can continue with 5 percent glucose in water. When myocardial infarction, heart failure, or renal failure is thought to have occurred, intravenous pressure monitoring is used to assess the intravascular volume status more accurately.

In the presence of a profound acidosis (arterial pH below 7.1), bicarbonate should be given, especially if there is associated hyperkalemia or shock. There are theoretical dangers in administering too much alkali too rapidly, as this may lead to a rise in P_{CO_2} by inhibiting ventilation. The CO_2 crosses easily into the CSF and exacerbates the acidosis there, which may impair the level of consciousness and potentiate seizures. The real significance of this is not yet established. Alkali therapy may also theoretically impair tissue oxygenation and worsen the lactic acidosis by affecting the release of oxygen from hemoglobin. Tetany may ensue if the ionized calcium falls rapidly. Correction of the hypoglycemia and improved carbohydrate metabolism will of itself generate bicarbonate, and a metabolic alkalosis may result from excessive bicarbonate therapy. The aim of therapy is to raise the pH to 7.2 to 7.25, at which degree of acidosis there should be no complications. Bicarbonate is administered by adding 88 mEq of $NaHCO_3$ per 1000 ml of replacement fluid until the arterial pH reaches 7.2 or the serum bicarbonate is 10 mEq/dl. The serum bicarbonate may be depressed by the chloride infused in the saline, and it is safer to use the arterial pH as a guideline.

The serum potassium concentration is frequently high before treatment is started, but the glucose and insulin and correction of the acidosis will combine to lower the serum potassium rapidly. Patients may also have a significant potassium deficit. If the initial serum potassium is below 4.0 mEq/l, potassium (15 to 20 mEq/hour) is added immediately; otherwise, none is added until the EKG signs of hyperkalemia have been reversed, and the serum level is within the normal range. The rate of potassium infusion is adjusted hourly to maintain a normal value. Although potassium is often given as the chloride salt, patients with diabetic ketoacidosis are often hypophosphatemic, and the use of potassium phosphate in the first hour will restore both electrolytes.

The fall in plasma ketones will lag behind the fall in serum glucose, and insulin and dextrose should be continued until the arterial pH and anion gap have been normalized. The tests for ketones measure only acetoacetate and, as the conversion of beta-hydroxybutyrate to acetoacetate is slower than the metabolism of acetoacetate, the ketone level will initially fall and then later increase again. Frequent monitoring of glucose and electrolytes is essential, and the EKG is useful in following shifts in serum potassium.

After ketoacidosis is corrected, treatment with subcutaneous regular insulin should start immediately. The *nonketotic hyperosmolar* syndrome may also occur, in which hyperglycemia and dehydration occur without an elevation in ketoacids. This is more common in type II diabetics. The treatment is similar to that of ketoacidosis.

HYPOGLYCEMIA

Hypoglycemia can occur as a result of a relative overdose of insulin or when patients miss a meal and are not receiving intravenous glucose. They may initially be irritable, diaphoretic, and confused, and coma or seizures may ensue. Hypoglycemia should be confirmed and treated with oral or intravenous glucose, depending on the circumstances and severity. Glucagon, 1 mg intramuscularly (IM), will raise the blood glucose while an intravenous line is being established. Beta-adrenergic blocking agents may mask the onset of symptoms and should be avoided in labile diabetics.

ACID-BASE DISORDERS

Disorders of the equilibrium of acid and base result from disturbances of metabolic or respiratory functions. Metabolic derangements will alter the plasma bicarbonate concentration ($[HCO_3^-]$), and respiratory dysfunction will alter the arterial carbon dioxide tension (PCO_2). Whether the primary abnormality is metabolic or respiratory, the effect will first be buffered, predominantly by the bicarbonate buffer system, and then the system not responsible for the primary change will attempt to compensate. Thus, metabolic abnormalities result in respiratory compensation and vice versa. The kidneys compensate by adjusting the excretion of bicarbonate, and the lungs compensate by reducing or increasing the excretion of PCO_2. The major buffer pairs are bicarbonate, phosphate, and proteins, mainly hemoglobin. The importance of bicarbonate and PCO_2 is emphasized if the bicarbonate buffer pair in the Henderson-Hasselbalch equation:

$$pH = pK + \log \frac{[HCO_3^-]}{H_2CO_3}$$

is expressed as:

$$pH = pK' + \log \frac{[HCO_3^-]}{S \cdot PCO_2}$$

Table 1–2. ACID-BASE DISORDERS*

	pH†	PCO_2‡	$[HCO_3^-]$§
Metabolic Acidosis	↓	↓	↓
Metabolic Alkalosis	↑	↑	↑
Respiratory Acidosis	↓	↑	↑
Respiratory Alkalosis	↑	↓	↓

*If the PCO_2 and $[HCO_3^-]$ do not change in the same direction, a mixed acid-base disorder is present.
†pH = arterial pH
‡PCO_2 = arterial carbon dioxide tension
§$[HCO_3^-]$ = plasma bicarbonate concentration

where pK′ is the rate constant for bicarbonate and S is the solubility coefficient for CO_2. Acid is generated in two forms, one volatile (CO_2) and one fixed or nonvolatile (sulfuric and phosphoric acids). Nonvolatile acids arise from the catabolism of proteins, at a rate of about 1 mmol/kg/day, are buffered by bicarbonate and then excreted through the kidneys as ammonium salts. The secretion of ammonia results in the generation of bicarbonate by the kidney, and this is returned to the plasma buffer system. Carbon dioxide arises from the metabolism of carbohydrates and lipids (approximately 13,000 mm/day), is buffered by bicarbonate, and is then excreted by the lungs.

There are four primary disorders: (1) metabolic acidosis, (2) metabolic alkalosis, (3) respiratory acidosis, and (4) respiratory alkalosis. The primary changes are detailed in Table 1–2 and discussed briefly below.

Metabolic Acidosis

Metabolic acidosis is characterized by a decrease in the plasma bicarbonate concentration and, therefore, a fall in the arterial pH. A primary reduction in bicarbonate will arise (1) if it is used to buffer a strong acid added to the blood; (2) if bicarbonate is lost through the gastrointestinal tract or kidneys; or (3) by rapid dilution of the plasma by a nonbicarbonate solution. To facilitate understanding and diagnosis, metabolic acidoses are divided into those in which the fall in $[HCO_3^-]$ is matched by a rise in $[Cl^-]$, a hyperchloremic non–anion gap acidosis ($Na^+ = Cl^- + HCO_3^-$), and those in which there is an unmeasured anion (UA^-) and in which the $[Cl^-]$ does not rise ($Na^+ = Cl^- + HCO_3^- + UA^-$), resulting in an increased anion gap acidosis. The common anions that produce an anion gap are lactic acid, ketoacids (acetoacetate and beta-hydroxybutyrate), and toxic substances (salicylates, methanol, ethylene glycol, sulfate, solvents).

The normal anion gap is 12 mEq/l with a range of 8 to 16 mEq/l. Albumin constitutes the majority of the normal anion gap, and this gap falls with hypoproteinemia and rises in hyperproteinemia disorders. The compensatory response to this acidosis is hyperventilation to reduce the P_{CO_2}, followed by renal acid excretion. This is limited in patients with renal failure. In ketoacidosis and lactic acidosis, metabolism of the anions necessitates the utilization of a proton and bicarbonate is regenerated as the primary disorder is corrected. Uremia is also associated with an acidosis and the accumulation of unmeasured anions. These, however, cannot be metabolized to generate bicarbonate.

Hyperchloremic acidosis is associated with a number of conditions, in particular, diarrhea. Other causes include: (1) gastrointestinal bicarbonate loss due to ureterosigmoidostomy, ileal loop conduits, and small bowel or pancreatic fistulas; (2) renal bicarbonate loss associated with a renal tubular acidosis; (3) hyperparathyroidism; (4) hypoaldosteronism; (5) use of carbonic anhydrase inhibitors; and (6) parenteral alimentation acidosis.

Metabolic acidosis is managed by treating the cause of the acidosis. This is particularly true of an anion gap acidosis, which will respond well to reversal of the acid production. If the acidosis is severe, as discussed under the management of diabetic ketoacidosis, bicarbonate may be required to reverse the fall in pH. Because treatment of an anion gap acidosis will generate bicarbonate, only sufficient extrinsic bicarbonate is given to raise the pH to 7.2 or the serum bicarbonate level to 12 mEq/l. In the case of a hyperchloremic acidosis, more bicarbonate will be needed and the amount to be given is calculated so as to reach a target plasma bicarbonate concentration of 18 mEq/l. The amount of bicarbonate required is calculated from the following equation:

$$NaHCO_3 \text{ dose} = (\text{desired } [HCO_3^-] - \text{observed } [HCO_3^-]) \times 0.5 \text{ kg BW}.$$

The correction of a metabolic acidosis should be performed cautiously over 36 to 48 hours, especially after the arterial pH is above 7.2, to avoid the problems outlined in the management of a diabetic ketoacidosis.

Metabolic Alkalosis

A metabolic alkalosis results from a primary increase in the plasma bicarbonate concentration, which leads to a rise in arterial pH. This occurs (1) if there is a loss of protons from the extracellular fluid space, (2) if there is an addition of bicarbonate to the extracellular fluid (ECF) space, or (3) if there is a loss of chloride in excess of bicarbonate. This condition is not uncommon postoperatively as a consequence of nasogastric suction or a deficiency of K^+Cl^-. Loss of protons may be absolute, as in loss through the kidneys or gastrointestinal tract, or relative, when protons shift into cells in response to significant hypokalemia. Chloride loss may be the result of overvigorous use of loop diuretics or of certain forms of diarrhea, e.g., villous adenoma. The lungs will compensate by reducing alveolar ventilation, which will lead to carbon dioxide retention. This compensation will never be complete, as oxygenation will take precedence. Final correction will be provided by the kidney, which will rapidly increase the excretion of bicarbonate, unless factors are present that maintain the alkalosis by impairing bicarbonate excretion. It is therefore useful to approach management in the context of these factors.

There are two forms of metabolic alkalosis: one is sensitive to chloride and volume replacement, and the other is resistant to this therapy. In the first form, the urinary chloride concentration will generally be below 10 mEq/l and there will be a net deficit of sodium chloride and water. This is commonly seen following renal and intestinal loss of salt and water and also in the treatment phase of more chronic forms of hypercapnia, in which chloride deficiency may lead to a metabolic alkalosis. The chloride deficit is important in maintaining this form of alkalosis, as there is insufficient chloride available in the urine for exchange with bicarbonate in the kidney, thus limiting the bicarbonate excretion. Treatment is by the infusion of normal saline to restore the extracellular fluid volume and sodium chloride deficit.

The second form, not sensitive to saline, is in fact often seen in the face of volume expansion. It occurs in states of excessive mineralocorticoid activity, such as in hyperaldosteronism, Bartter's syndrome, Cushing's syndrome, and with an excessive intake of glycyrrhizic acid (glycyrrhizin) by licorice eaters. It may also result from severe potassium depletion. The mineralocorticoid activity leads to sodium retention with volume expansion, which, in turn, decreases sodium reabsorption by the proximal tubule. This results in an increased sodium delivery to the distal tubule for exchange with protons and potassium, leading to loss of these, and a hypokalemic alkalosis. Urinary chloride concentrations are usually higher than 20 mEq/liter. As in all forms of metabolic alkalosis, the potassium deficit must be replaced. On occasion, and particularly in patients with heart failure, acetazolamide, a carbonic anhydrase inhibitor that increases urinary bicarbonate and potassium excretion, may be used, and here too, all potassium loss must be restored. Although a metabolic alkalosis is not usually dangerous, it may on occasion—when pH is above 7.55—depress ventilation or cause confusion. Aggressive therapy using intravenous acid, either as hydrochloric acid (150 mEq/l) or ammonium chloride can then be used. The latter is contraindicated in liver failure, where it may precipitate encephalopathy. Arginine hydrochloride may cause a fatal hyperkalemia and should no longer be used. In patients with renal failure, dialysis against a low bicarbonate dialysate will correct the alkalosis. If there is an added component of respiratory alkalosis, and if provided oxygenation is not compromised, mechanical ventilation against 3 percent CO_2 can be used to induce hypercapnia.

Respiratory Acidosis

A respiratory acidosis will occur following a primary accumulation of carbon dioxide, with a secondary fall in the pH. This is invariably secondary to ineffective alveolar ventilation, with ventilation-perfusion inequality or a decrease in minute ventilation. The rise in carbon dioxide will be buffered by the bicarbonate system, and the kidney will respond to the fall in pH by increasing excretion of protons and the conservation of bicarbonate. There will also be a renal loss of ammonium and chloride ions.

The causes of hypoventilation may be grouped into disorders of the lungs (pneumonia); the airways (obstruction, aspiration, bronchospasm); the thorax (pneumothorax, flail chest); vascular system (massive pulmonary embolus); and inadequate mechanical ventilation. Correction of an acute respiratory acidosis always necessitates correction of its cause and, not infrequently, assisted ventilation. Correction should not be performed too rapidly, particularly if the acidosis is of a few days' duration, as there may be a large accumulation of bicarbonate, and renal excretion of the bicarbonate will be impaired by a relative chloride deficiency. Chronic hypercapnia is seen with chronic obstructive pulmonary disease, limitations of thoracic movement, and neuromuscular disorders. Its main importance is in the treatment of associated hypoxia, in which the respiratory drive may be dependent on a low arterial oxygen tension. Correcting the hypoxemia may cause apnea.

Respiratory Alkalosis

A respiratory alkalosis ensues if there is increased alveolar ventilation with loss of carbon dioxide and a secondary rise in the arterial pH. It is frequently encountered in patients with pain or anxiety. It can also be caused by excessive mechanical ventilation. The fall in carbon dioxide will first be buffered by the bicarbonate system and the release of protons from body buffers, and there will be a fall in the plasma bicarbonate concentration. The kidney will increase the loss of bicarbonate and decrease bicarbonate regeneration. A primary respiratory alkalosis is also seen following salicylate intoxication, with gram-negative bacteremia, hepatic insufficiency, fevers, and with smaller pulmonary emboli, which increase ventilation without causing sufficient ventilation-perfusion inequality to impair carbon dioxide excretion. Treatment is aimed at correcting the cause and is not urgent unless there is evidence of neuromuscular (carpopedal spasm, circumoral tingling) or myocardial irritability.

HYPERTENSION

Systemic arterial hypertension is a common disorder occurring in 15 to 30 percent of the population in the United States. It is found more commonly with increasing age and in males and is thus often encountered by the urologist. The risks of mild to moderate hypertension relate to the duration of the disease, and unless there is evidence of renal or myocardial damage, it is not necessary to institute treatment of hypertension perioperatively. The corollary of this is that it may be possible to taper off the antihypertensive treatment in the weeks prior to surgery in a manner appropriate to each drug. It is far safer for the patient to enter the operating room with a moderately elevated blood pressure than to suffer hemorrhage and hypotension in the presence of full autonomic blockade and with volume depletion secondary to diuretic therapy, with the attendant dangers of acute renal failure, cerebrovascular infarction, and myocardial damage. However, anesthesiologists are now experienced in treating patients who have been taking antihypertensive drugs. Before treatment with any agent is started, it is prudent to review fully the potential side effects, which are discussed briefly here. The perioperative management of patients who cannot take oral medications has been facilitated by the availability of sublingual nifedipine (10 to 20 mg every 30 minutes) and transdermal clonidine patches (0.1 to 0.3 mg/24 hours). This has reduced the need for intramuscular hydralazine or intravenous infusions of other agents.

The most commonly used oral agents are diuretics, anti–alpha- and anti–beta-adrenergic blocking agents, arterial vasodilators, calcium channel blockers, and angiotensin-converting enzyme inhibitors (ACEIs). All of these agents produce side effects that can cause problems at the time of surgery. The diuretics, most commonly thiazides, may lead to a substantial contraction of the ECF volume. Also, in fewer than 10 percent of patients, use of diuretics may result in hypokalemia, with an increased risk of muscle weakness, ileus, and cardiac arrhythmias. Conversely, the potassium-sparing agents—spironolactone, amiloride, and triamterene—may result in hyperkalemia. The arterial vasodilators do not interfere with the sympathetic response to hypotension, and hydralazine and minoxidil are thus safe to use. The remaining agents will all impair the ability of the patient to respond to volume loss. The alpha- and beta-adrenergic blocking agents have a predominantly central action and, in addition, secondary peripheral effects. The alpha-blockers (methyldopa, clonidine, guanficine, prazosin, reserpine) act on the vasomotor center to inhibit the increase in heart rate and vasoconstrictive responses to hypotension. Reserpine alone has a predominantly peripheral action and depletes norepinephrine from adrenergic nerve endings. Clonidine is probably the agent of choice in this group.

In addition to their central action, beta-blockers act by depleting cardiac catecholamines to inhibit increases in the rate and force of myocardial contraction. They are contraindicated in patients with asthma, chronic obstructive pulmonary disease, labile diabetes mellitus, and severe ventricular failure. Other side effects include disturbing dreams, fatigue, and peripheral vasoconstriction. If beta-blockers are used, it is wise to switch from the longer-acting agents such as atenolol and nadolol to shorter-acting agents such as propranolol and metoprolol. Captopril and enalapril, the ACEIs, produce a vasodepressor action. They can cause hyperkalemia and, in the presence of severe renal artery stenosis, may profoundly impair the function of the affected kidney. This will be reflected only by a change in the serum creatinine concentration if there is one functional kidney or if the stenosis is bilateral. The calcium channel-blocking agents act by causing peripheral venous dilatation. Verapamil also acts to delay arteriovenous (A-V) node conduction in the heart, and nifedipine is the agent most frequently used perioperatively.

It should not be forgotten that many of these agents, in particular the calcium channel-blocking agents, ACEIs, vasodilators, and diuretics are also used in the treatment of heart failure and angina by virtue of their effects of preload and afterload reduction. Before these agents are reduced or stopped, this should be taken into consideration.

Accelerated and Malignant Hypertension

The ability of patients to tolerate very high blood pressure varies considerably. Previous enthusiasm for a rapid reduction in the blood pressure in accelerated and malignant hypertension has been tempered by reports of cerebral ischemia and blindness, and it is now recommended that the pressure be reduced more gradually over 24 to 72 hours. Any elevation of the blood pressure to levels of 200/120 should be treated vigorously; however when there is malignant hypertension with encephalopathy (headache, altered vision, confusion, coma, convulsions) or nephropathy, intracranial hemorrhage, aortic dissection, or eclampsia, immediate, urgent treatment is indicated.

As in the case of more moderate hypertension, a stepwise plan has evolved for the therapy of malignant hypertension. In cases of extreme urgency, the patient should be admitted immediately to an intensive care facility and treated with sodium nitroprusside (Nipride), a short-acting arterial vasodilator, with continuous intra-arterial blood pressure monitoring. Nipride has an immediate onset of action, is easily titratable, and its action is very short-lived, with reversal within 2 to 5 minutes after it is discontinued. The usual dose is 0.5 μg/kg/minute (50 μg in 250 ml of 5 percent DW), increasing to an average of 1 to 3 μg/kg/minute. Prolonged therapy (over 24 hours), high doses, and renal insufficiency can result in accumulation of thiocyanate, a toxic metabolite, the serum levels of which should be monitored.

In less urgent situations, treatment can be started with sublingual nifedipine (10 mg), and this can be repeated within 20 to 30 minutes if the initial response does not lower the pressure to the normotensive range. This therapy is safe even in patients who have received a variety of other agents and can be started immediately, as there is no need for intensive monitoring. High-dose oral clonidine loading has also been advocated, with an initial dose of 0.2 mg, followed by 0.1 mg/hour, to a total dose of 0.7 mg. The blood pressure is checked every 15 minutes for the first hour, every 30 minutes over the second hour, and then hourly. Thereafter, regular therapy with a diuretic and clonidine is continued. If oral treatment fails, treatment should be started with nitroprusside or one of the other intravenous agents.

Other agents that may be used include, when not otherwise contraindicated, intravenous beta-blocking agents, e.g., propranolol, metoprolol, and labetalol. Hydralazine, either intramuscularly or intravenously, remains a useful agent except in patients with coronary disease, as it reflexly increases cardiac rate and output. Diazoxide, a direct-acting vasodilator, is again being used either as a continuous infusion, 15 mg/minute, which should produce a steady fall in the blood pressure over 20 to 30 minutes, or in intermittent doses of 1 to 2 mg/kg (not more than 150 mg) every 10 minutes intravenously. The previously advocated method of giving large doses of diazoxide very rapidly may result in profound hypotension with cerebral ischemia and renal failure and should no longer be used. Diazoxide may also cause hyperglycemia, and it invariably causes sodium retention. For this reason, furosemide should be given at the same time. For patients in whom a reflex tachycardia would be dangerous, e.g., post-myocardial infarction or aortic dissection, this drug should not be used without prior beta blockade.

References

Brenner BM, Meyer TW, Hostetter TH: Dietary protein intake and the progressive nature of kidney disease. N Engl J Med 307:652, 1982.

Brezis M, Rosen S, Epstein FH: Acute renal failure. In Brenner BM, Recter FC Jr. eds: The Kidney, 3rd ed. Philadelphia, WB Saunders Co, 1986, p 735.

Bricker NS: On the pathogenesis of the uremic state: an exposition of the "trade-off" hypothesis. N Engl J Med 286:1093, 1972.

Bricker NS, Fine LG, Kaplan M, Epstein M, and Bourgoignie JJ: "Magnification" phenomenon in chronic renal disease. N Engl J Med 299:1287, 1978.

Carroll P, Matz R: Uncontrolled diabetes mellitus in adults: experience in treating diabetic ketoacidosis and hyperosmolar nonketotic coma with low dose insulin and a uniform treatment regimen. Diabetes Care 6:579, 1983.

Cogan MG, Rector FC, Jr: Acid-base disorders. In Brenner BM, Rector FC, Jr eds: The Kidney, 3rd ed. Philadelphia, WB Saunders Co, 1986, p 457.

Cryer PE, Gerich JE: Glucose counterregulation, hyperglycemia, and intensive insulin therapy in diabetes mellitus. N Engl J Med 313:232, 1985.

Haft JI, Lilterer WE: Chewing nifedipine to rapidly treat hypertension. Arch Intern Med 144:2347, 1984.

Kaplan NM: Systemic hypertension therapy. In Braunwald E, ed: Philadelphia, WB Saunders Co, 1984, p 902.

Klahr S: Pathophysiology of obstructive uropathy. Kidney Int 23:414, 1983.

Narins RG: Diagnostic strategies in disorders of fluid electrolytes and acid-base homeostasis. Am J Med 72:496, 1982.

Narins RG, Emmet M: Simple and mixed acid-base disorders: a practical approach. Medicine 59:161, 1980.

Stewart AF: Therapy of malignant hypercalcemia. Am J Med 74:475, 1983.

The 1984 report of the Joint National Committee on Detection, Evaluation and Treatment of High Blood Pressure. Arch Intern Med 144:1045, 1984.

Vandam L: Anesthesia for the hypertensive patient. In Genest J, Kuchel D, Hamet P, Cantin M eds: Hypertension, 2nd ed. New York, McGraw-Hill, 1983, p 1245.

Vidt DG, Gifford RW: A compendium for the treatment of hypertensive emergencies. Cleve Clin Q 51:421, 1984.

PULMONARY COMPLICATIONS OF UROLOGIC SURGERY

2

Paul E. Bellamy

INTRODUCTION

This chapter reviews the common pulmonary complications of urologic surgery. First, there is a discussion of the changes in lung function that occur in the perioperative period as a result of anesthesia and surgery. Then, the various types of pulmonary complications are described, along with pulmonary and nonpulmonary risk factors. Next, given what is known about various predictors, a logical scheme for preoperative evaluation is developed. Finally, preoperative preparation and postoperative treatment regimens are recommended.

PERIOPERATIVE CHANGES IN LUNG FUNCTION

Lung Volume

Before the effects of surgery on lung volumes are discussed, the definitions of the various lung volumes should be reviewed. *Total lung capacity* refers to the volume of air in the lungs after a maximal inspiratory effort. *Residual volume* is the volume that cannot be exhaled even after a maximal expiratory effort. *Vital capacity* is the difference between these two extremes of lung volume, referring to the amount that can be exhaled after a maximal inhalation. *Functional residual capacity* or *end-tidal volume* is the volume of air in the chest when the respiratory muscles are relaxed. It represents a balance of the natural outward recoil of the chest cage and the inward recoil of the lung. Finally, *closing volume* is the lung volume between functional residual capacity and residual volume at which airways in dependent lung zones first begin to close during exhalation. Other lung zones continue to empty below the closing volume until residual volume is reached.

All subdivisions of lung volume, including total lung capacity, decrease after abdominal surgery, but they are not affected by surgery on an extremity.[1–3] Over 50 years ago, Beecher showed that (1) laparotomy led to a 45 percent reduction in vital capacity that gradually returned to normal in 7 to 14 days, and (2) this reduction occurred more often in upper abdominal operations than in lower abdominal surgery.[4,5] Beecher's findings have been confirmed repeatedly by others since.[1–3,6] For example, Tahir and colleagues found significant reductions in postoperative lung function in patients undergoing either upper abdominal surgery or suprapubic prostatectomy.[7] The changes after upper abdominal surgery were much greater than those occurring after prostatectomy.

More recently, Ford and others showed that laparotomy was associated with a significant reduction in diaphragm function that took 7 to 10 days to reverse and essentially paralleled the abnormalities in vital capacity and other pulmonary functions.[8] The diaphragm dysfunction was associated with a shift from predominantly abdominal breathing to rib cage breathing. These investigators thought the diaphragm dysfunction was probably multifactorial but that neural reflexes played a major role. These findings were corroborated by Simonneau and coworkers, who noted no ameliorative effect from pain relief and suspected that gaseous distention and pneumoperitoneum also contributed to the postlaparotomy diaphragm dysfunction.[9] Thus, we now have some basis for explaining the effect of abdominal surgery on lung volumes but probably do not yet fully understand all the mechanisms involved.

The other subdivisions of lung volume are similarly affected, with the exception of the closing volume, which usually increases, setting the stage for airway closure and atelectasis, again primarily at the lung bases.[1] Finally, immersion in water up to the neck, as occurs during extracorporeal shock wave lithotripsy, reduces functional residual capacity from 30 to 36 percent and reduces vital capacity 22 percent.[10] No one has determined how the effect of immersion on lung volumes interacts with the other factors that are operative during lithotripsy, such as anesthesia, age, obesity, underlying lung disease, and so forth.

Breathing Pattern

After abdominal surgery there is a 25 percent increase in respiratory rate, a 20 percent decrease in tidal volume, and a doubling of the sigh frequency.[4] Normally, morphine or other analgesics are given to postoperative patients to reduce pain and to foster cooperation with deep breathing regimens designed to prevent atelectasis. However, when morphine is given after surgery, the frequency of spontaneous sighing is reduced by 75 percent.[11] Since sighing is the body's natural way of reversing atelectasis and stabilizing alveoli through the redistribution of surfactant, it is important to recognize this adverse side effect of narcotic analgesia. Certainly, patients should not be denied pain relief; however, when narcotics are given, every effort must be made to encourage voluntary deep breathing to overcome the adverse effects of the analgesia.

Gas Exchange

In postoperative patients, immobilization in the supine position, diaphragm dysfunction, tight abdominal bandages, and pain all lead to hypoxia. As lung volumes decrease, there is less ventilation than perfusion in areas of airway narrowing and there is frank shunting in areas of atelectasis. Both factors contribute to the widened alveolar-arterial oxygen gradient seen after surgery. George and coworkers demonstrated that in 18 patients, mean arterial P_{O_2} fell from 88 mm Hg before laparotomy to 63 mm Hg after.[12] The usual mild postoperative tachypnea and shallow breathing have little or no effect on arterial P_{CO_2}, but if arterial oxygen desaturation occurs, there will be an additional stimulus to tachypnea, subsequent alveolar hyperventilation, and attendant hypocapnia.[6,12]

Defense Mechanisms

The respiratory system has extensive defense mechanisms to protect itself from insults. Sneezing clears particles from the nasal airway, coughing clears the upper airways, and the mucociliary apparatus clears the lower airways. Alveolar macrophages and pulmonary lymphatics remove materials that reach the alveoli. Cigarette smoking impairs mucociliary function and often stimulates increased production of airway mucus (e.g., as in chronic bronchitis). Gamsu and colleagues used contrast material to show that laparotomy also reduced mucociliary transport.[13] Altered mental status compromises airway protection from aspiration and impairs cooperation with voluntary deep breathing and coughing. Coughing is also inhibited by postoperative pain. Finally, hypoxia can impair phagocyte function.[14] Because different combinations of these factors may be present in postoperative patients, lung defense is compromised to various degrees, setting the stage for aspiration or pneumonia.

PULMONARY COMPLICATIONS

Pulmonary complications arise as an extension of the previously discussed pathophysiologic changes that normally occur in postoperative patients. Throughout the literature, the reported incidences of pulmonary complications differ because of several factors: (1) the underlying condition of the patient population studied, (2) the types of surgery included in the study group, and (3) the definitions of a pulmonary complication. One author may define atelectasis on the basis of chest radiographs alone, whereas another may require clinical concomitants such as hypoxia. However, despite these considerations, certain conclusions can be reached regarding the major pulmonary complications.

Atelectasis

Atelectasis, defined as the collapse of alveoli, is the most common postoperative pulmonary complication. If one accepts microatelectasis as a complication, pulmonary complications are universal after thoracic or abdominal surgery. Microatelectasis is not usually radiographically apparent until it is extensive; then it is manifested by volume loss on the chest radiograph. Macroatelectasis appears as platelike densities, segmental, lobar, or whole lung collapse. Atelectasis results from regional airway closure or narrowing, inadequate sighing, and/or retained secretions. The rapid, shallow breathing pattern of postoperative patients previously mentioned and the effect of analgesia on spontaneous sighing lead to lower lung volumes in most patients, predisposing to atelectasis.

In addition, dependent lung zones tend to have smaller alveoli and less regional ventilation. In such zones, the airways tend to collapse before residual volume is reached, collapsing at the so-called "closing volume." Closing volume is higher in obese patients, smokers, patients with airways disease, the elderly, and postoperative patients.[1–3,15] When these factors cause the closing volume to be higher than the end-tidal volume (functional residual capacity), significant atelectasis will occur. Retained secretions are not a prerequisite for atelectasis but compound the effects of these other mechanisms in patients with hypersecretion of mucus or compromised secretion clearance. In addition, secretions can impair ventilation of well-perfused areas, worsening ventilation-perfusion mismatch and oxygenation.

Pulmonary Infections

Postoperative pulmonary infections run the gamut from bronchitis to pneumonia. Infectious complications are more common in patients with chronic obstructive pulmonary disease, dehydration, diminished cough, atelectasis, and altered lung defenses.[1] Johanson's group showed that respiratory infections developed in 23 percent of patients in whom the airways were colonized with gram-negative bacilli compared with 3 percent of patients in whom the airways were not colonized.[16] In addition to the aforementioned factors that promote infection, conditions that predispose to airway colonization include coma, hypotension, acidosis, and renal insufficiency. Many of these factors are present during the postoperative period, increasing the risk for infection. Working to control such factors as much as possible may reduce the incidence of postoperative infections.

Deep Vein Thrombosis and Pulmonary Embolism

Deep vein thrombosis can be a serious development in any postoperative patient, but it is particularly problematic in patients undergoing urologic surgery. Thrombosis almost invariably occurs in the lower extremities and begins to develop in the operating room as a consequence of venous stasis resulting from immobilization and paralysis.[17,18] The likelihood of venous thrombosis rises as the duration of anesthesia exceeds 1 hour.[19] Other risk factors include advanced age, obesity, malignancy, estrogen use, perioperative immobility, and a history of previous deep vein thrombosis.[17] Unfortunately, the clinical diagnosis can be very difficult because both false-positive examinations and false-negative presentations are as common as true-negatives and true-positives.[20,21]

The only way to establish the incidence of deep vein thrombosis is with prospective studies using sensitive and specific screening tests such as radioactive fibrinogen uptake, impedance plethysmography, or contrast venography. The results of such studies vary widely, but the average incidences of deep vein thrombosis following prostate surgery are 30 to 50 percent after open prostatectomy and 10 to 20 percent after transurethral prostate resection.[17] Clearly, this represents a significant problem for the urologist.

Pulmonary embolism, the most serious complication of deep vein thrombosis, is also prevalent in urologic patients. More than 40 years ago, Colby reported that lethal pulmonary embolism occurred in 2.2 to 8.7 percent of prostate surgery patients, depending upon the operative approach.[22] Since then, others have found that the incidence of lethal pulmonary embolism after urologic surgery ranges from 1.1 to 5.5 percent, whereas that of nonlethal embolism ranges from 3.8 to 22 percent, confirming that embolism is an important contributor to postoperative morbidity and mortality, especially after prostatectomy.[17,20,23] The 22 percent incidence of nonlethal, postoperative embolism is probably the most accurate of the cited figures because it was established with serial lung scans—a more reliable diagnostic method than the clinical judgments used in the other series.[23]

Pulmonary embolism can be as difficult to diagnose with accuracy as is deep vein thrombosis. Routine tests such as electrocardiograms (EKG), arterial blood gases (ABG), and chest radiography are not specific enough to justify a full course of anticoagulant therapy.[24] However, these tests are important in the evaluation of patients in whom pulmonary embolism is suspected, since they may lead to another diagnosis, such as pneumonia or myocardial infarction, which accounts for the patient's presentation, or they may establish an index of suspicion for embolism that leads to further, more specific testing. The best screening test for pulmonary emboli is the perfusion lung scan. If the test result is normal, the physician can safely rule out embolism.[25] If any perfusion defects are present, a ventilation scan should be obtained.

In the appropriate clinical setting, the preservation of ventilation to a lobe or segment that is not perfused (ventilation-perfusion "mismatch") is associated with an 85 to 95 percent chance of pulmonary embolism.[26] Many clinicians are satisfied that this degree of diagnostic confidence justifies anticoagulant therapy, but others cite the very real risks of anticoagulant therapy (a 0.5–1 percent chance of fatal hemorrhage and a 4 to 10 percent chance of significant bleeding) and proceed to more definitive testing, such as pulmonary angiography, before committing themselves and their patients to anticoagulation therapy.[27–29] Considering the risks of bleeding in postoperative patients, the latter approach is generally recommended. An alternative to pulmonary angiography is to document the presence of deep vein thrombosis, since that disease is treated in the same manner as its complication, pulmonary embolism.[27]

Given the incidence of deep vein thrombosis and pulmonary embolism in urologic surgery patients, it is generally recommended that patients undergoing major urologic surgery receive some form of prophylactic treatment. In a comprehensive review, Moser[17] concluded that (1) there were conflicting data regarding the benefits of warfarin and low-dose heparin, (2) there were not enough data to establish the efficacy of dextran infusions, (3) elastic stockings and early ambulation were ineffective, and (4) external mechanical compression of the lower extremities reduced the incidence of thromboembolism in postoperative urologic patients by promoting venous return through pulsatile milking of the calves.[17,30] Thus, he recommended either the application of external mechanical compression devices to the lower extremities during and after surgery until a patient was ambulatory or a transition to low-dose heparin once wound healing was advanced to the point that hemorrhage was unlikely. A joint consensus report by the American College of Chest Physicians and the National Heart, Lung, and Blood Institute (ACCP–NHLBI) concurred with this recommendation.[27]

Once deep vein thrombosis or pulmonary embolism is suspected and the workup is in progress, the surgeon must begin to consider empiric treatment pending outcome of the diagnostic evaluation. Most experts recommend initiation of full-dose heparin during the evaluation unless there is a contraindication, such as a known active bleeding site.[17,27] Although there is some controversy about the routes of administration, dosing strategies, and the need for monitoring of heparin effect, the ACCP–NHLBI report recommended a heparin loading dose of 5000 units followed by continuous intravenous infusion at 1000 units per hour with the infusion adjusted to prolong the activated partial thromboplastin time to 1.5 to 2.0 times normal.[27] Alternatively, the heparin can be administered subcutaneously at 8- to 12-hour intervals, adjusting the dose to achieve the same degree of anticoagulation as with the continuous infusion.

Thrombolytic therapy with either streptokinase or urokinase is an alternative to heparin as initial therapy. However, most experts consider thrombolytic therapy to be contraindicated within 10 days of major surgery, since clots responsible for operative site hemostasis are as vulnerable to thrombolysis as those causing venous thrombosis or pulmonary embolism.[31] After 7 to 10 days of heparin therapy, oral warfarin should be given to patients at doses sufficient to prolong the prothrombin time to 1.2 to 1.5 times control. The ACCP-NHLBI report indicated that greater prolongation adds no further benefit and only serves to increase risk of hemorrhage.[27] The heparin and warfarin courses should overlap for at least 5 days. Warfarin should be continued for 3 months in most patients and indefinitely if the patient remains at continued risk because of such factors as recurrence of thrombosis or embolism, antithrombin III deficiency, protein C deficiency, or malignancy.[17,27]

Surgical interventions, such as inferior vena caval interruption or embolectomy, are rarely indicated. Thrombolytic therapy has generally replaced surgical embolectomy, and inferior vena caval interruption is necessary only when medical treatment has failed. Because heparin inhibits further thrombosis but does not affect embolization of pre-existing thrombi, recurrence of embolization during the first few days of heparin treatment cannot be considered "failure" of medical therapy.[17] Finally, because of the risks of surgical intervention, medical therapy failure must always be confirmed by a definitive test, such as angiography, before surgery is performed.

Respiratory Failure

Respiratory failure is an uncommon postoperative complication that can lead to an unplanned requirement for intubation and mechanical ventilator support. There are two major categories of respiratory failure: (1) hypercapnic with respiratory acidosis, and (2) hypoxic with high inspired oxygen requirements. Hypercapnia develops as a consequence of inadequate alveolar ventilation and inability to eliminate carbon dioxide proportionate to its production by tissue metabolism. The most common etiologies of hypercapnia are (1) diminished central respiratory drive—often due to central nervous system (CNS) depressant drugs, including analgesics; (2) respiratory muscle fatigue and resultant inability to sustain alveolar ventilation; and (3) mechanical defects such as flail chest.

Other mechanical defects can lead to respiratory muscle fatigue by imposing an unsustainably high work of breathing. Examples include the resistive work resulting from bronchospasm and the elastic work associated with pulmonary edema or a stiff chest wall. Treatment for hypercapnic respiratory failure should include measures to (1) reduce work of breathing through the use of bronchodilators, by removal of airway secretions, through reduction of pulmonary edema, and so on; (2) improve respiratory muscle function (correction of hypoxia, hypokalemia, hypophosphatemia); and (3) maintain respiratory drive by reducing the administration of sedative and analgesic drugs. If these measures are not immediately effective, or if significant respiratory acidosis is present, the patient should receive mechanical ventilation until the underlying problems are resolved.

Hypoxic respiratory failure results from such conditions as severe pneumonia, pulmonary edema, excessive mucous plugging, and atelectasis.[32] Supplemental oxygen will often correct the hypoxia while the underlying condition is being treated. However, if patients require 60 percent or more oxygen to correct hypoxia and a diffuse pulmonary process is present, they should be considered candidates for either continuous positive airway pressure (CPAP) by mask or intubation and treatment with positive end-expiratory pressure (PEEP).[33–35] These measures are designed to achieve adequate oxygenation without exposing the patient to the added burden of oxygen toxicity. Adult respiratory distress syndrome (ARDS) or noncardiogenic pulmonary edema is the most serious form of hypoxic respiratory failure and is associated with an overall mortality rate of 50 to 60 percent.[32,36] In surgical patients, ARDS results most commonly from sepsis, hypotension, aspiration pneumonia, trauma, or transfusion reactions (e.g., leukoagglutinating antibodies in the transfused blood product that cause embolization of the pulmonary vascular bed with clumps of activated white blood cells).[36,37]

At the present time, there is no reliable way to prevent the development of ARDS; the evidence regarding prophylactic PEEP is equivocal, and prophylactic steroids have been ineffective.[33,38] Once ARDS has developed, treatment is generally supportive and the primary goal is to achieve optimal arterial oxygenation and systemic oxygen delivery through judicious use of mechanical ventilation, supplemental oxygen, PEEP, and hemodynamic monitoring with a pulmonary artery flotation catheter.[35,39] Because oxygen delivery is defined as the product of arterial oxygen content multiplied by the cardiac output, it takes into account both the beneficial and the adverse effects of PEEP (i.e., increased arterial oxygen content versus decreased cardiac output). Patients with ARDS usually die of complications, such as nosocomial pneumonia, sepsis, or multiple organ system failure, rather than from isolated respiratory failure.[32,36,40] The treating physician must always be vigilant for the earliest sign of complications so that appropriate interventions can be made as soon as possible.

Direct Surgical Complications

Occasionally, urologic surgery leads to thoracic-cavity–related complications that may or may not necessitate consultation with a thoracic surgeon.[41] Each hemidiaphragm separates the superior, lateral, and posterior portions of its ipsilateral kidney from the adjacent pleural space. Thus, it is possible that surgery for renal tumors or trauma could involve the diaphragm, the ipsilateral pleural space, or the lung. Also, given the invasive nature of some renal malignancies, inferior vena caval or cardiac extension is possible. Under these circumstances, pulmonary complications, such as pneumothorax, pleural space hemorrhage, diaphragmatic disruption, and so on, can occur during surgical resection. In addition, because the distal branches of the phrenic nerves are obliquely oriented, radial incisions during diaphragmatic incisions and partial resections must be avoided; otherwise, large areas of the diaphragm may be left denervated and paralyzed.[41] Such paralysis could lead to significant postoperative weaning problems. Further discussion of treatment for these complications is beyond the scope of this chapter.

PULMONARY RISK FACTORS

There is considerable literature examining the various pulmonary function tests as indicators of perioperative risks. Some studies identified patients at high risk for perioperative mortality due to pulmonary complications; others examined the ability to detect patients at risk for perioperative pulmonary morbidity. There are two significant problems with the literature. First, many of the better studies focused upon patients undergoing thoracic surgery; second, there is no clear, reliable way to separate patients into simple categories, such as "safe" and "prohibitive," with respect to risk.

A large part of the problem is due to the great variability of pulmonary function among individuals. There is no single simple test of lung function equivalent to that measuring the serum creatinine. Normal values for pulmonary function tests are predicted by complex regression equations derived from large population studies. In these equations, the major independent variables are age, sex, height, and race.[42] Weight is usually not included in the equations, but its effect is sometimes important for obese individuals. Even after these variables are taken into account, there is still a large variation among individuals (from 20 to 40 percent) who are considered normal. Thus, it should not be surprising that efforts to develop simple classification schemes based on pulmonary function test results almost invariably lead to some degree of risk misclassification.

Table 2–1 summarizes some pulmonary function criteria that predict increased risk for development of postoperative pulmonary complications in patients undergoing abdominal surgery.[43] Most schemes are sensitive but not specific; that is, they can identify those who will develop complications, but they also identify other indistinguishable patients in whom complications do not develop. The surgeon should recognize the limitations of any scheme that purports to easily identify patients who are "safe" for surgery and those who are not. Rather, a continuum of risk should be recognized by both the surgeon and pulmonary consultant. In this process, particularly as it pertains to higher-risk patients, it is often helpful to determine the patient's personal evaluation of risk and benefit. Many patients are able to define how much risk they are willing to take to obtain a given degree of benefit from a procedure.

Under certain conditions, even patients with a 100 percent chance of developing a pulmonary complication could still be reasonable surgical candidates. In other words, a high probability that complications will develop does not preclude surgery for an individual patient, and the risk of postoperative pulmonary complications may even be reduced with meticulous attention to perioperative management. For example, Williams and Brenowitz reported severe obstructive pulmonary disease in a group of 16 patients who would have been considered prohibitive risks by many previous authors.[44] In this group, the major pulmonary complication rate was 19 percent, and only one patient died; however, the death was unrelated to respiratory causes. There are no studies to date that establish pulmonary function criteria that absolutely contraindicate surgery.[1–3,43,44]

NONPULMONARY RISK FACTORS

Important nonpulmonary factors that affect a given patient's risk for perioperative pulmonary complications include general factors, surgical factors, anesthetic factors, and disease-related factors.

General Factors

The most important general factors are age, obesity, and smoking history. Age is associated with increased postoperative morbidity and mortality, probably due in great part to diminished physiologic reserves common to elderly patients.[1,3,45] For example, Mircea and associates found a 50 percent pulmonary complication rate for patients over age 70 years, compared to a 5 percent complication rate for patients younger

Table 2–1. PULMONARY FUNCTION CRITERIA THAT SUGGEST INCREASED RISK FOR POSTOPERATIVE PULMONARY COMPLICATIONS AFTER ABDOMINAL SURGERY*

Forced vital capacity (FVC)	<70% predicted†‡
One-second forced expiratory volume (FEV_1)	<70% predicted
FEV_1/FVC (measures obstruction)	<65% predicted†
$FEF_{25-75\%}$ (measures obstruction)	<50% predicted
Maximal voluntary ventilation	<50% predicted‡

*Adapted from Gass GD, Olsen GN: Preoperative pulmonary function testing to predict postoperative morbidity and mortality. Chest 89:127–135, 1986.[43]

†There is a 100 percent complication rate if both are present.

‡There is prolonged mechanical ventilation postoperatively if both are present and fail to improve after preoperative treatment.

than 40.[45] Elderly patients also have reduced airway protective reflexes, which could impair secretion clearance and even increase the likelihood of aspiration.[1]

Certainly, cigarette smoking can lead to measurable decrements in lung function, which increase perioperative complication rates as discussed earlier, but smoking is also associated with other significant conditions, such as coronary artery disease and peripheral vascular disease, which independently augment perioperative risk by increasing comorbidity.

Obesity can increase the risk of surgical complications in nearly all categories.[1–3,15,45] Those effects that potentially contribute to pulmonary complications are difficult venous access, intubation problems, delayed recovery from lipophilic anesthetic agents, impaired pulmonary mechanics, predisposition to atelectasis and shunt, higher incidence of deep vein thrombosis, more frequent postoperative fevers, and wound complications.[15] For example, Mircea and associates found a 35 percent pulmonary complication rate in obese subjects with gallstones and chronic cholecystitis in contrast to 11 percent in those of normal weight.[45] Thus, obesity augments the pulmonary complication rate for a given surgical procedure.[2,45]

Surgical Factors

The incidence of postoperative pulmonary complications is directly related to the location of the operation. Pulmonary complications are rare (<1 percent) in nonthoracic, nonabdominal surgery, whereas the complication rate for cases of thoracic surgery depends on many factors, including whether or not lung tissue is resected.[1–3,45] For abdominal cases, it is clear that upper abdominal operations are associated with higher pulmonary complication rates than are lower abdominal cases.[1–6,45]

Unfortunately, there is no comprehensive literature addressing these issues as they relate specifically to urologic surgery. However, two interesting studies are applicable. Meyhoff and associates randomized patients in whom moderate benign prostatic hypertrophy was present to undergo either transvesicular (TVP) or transurethral (TURP) prostatectomy.[46] The majority of patients underwent general anesthesia, and there was no operative mortality in either group. Although in the TURP group underlying chronic pulmonary disease was present in twice as many patients, the postoperative pulmonary complication rate was 2 percent compared with 23 percent in the TVP group. In this study, operative approach was a more important risk factor than underlying lung disease.

Heyns and coauthors divided patients with renal stab wounds into two groups based upon the presence or absence of signs of severe blood loss, associated intra-abdominal injury, and gross abnormalities on excretory urography.[47] Patients who had these characteristics went directly to mandatory emergency surgery, whereas the others were randomly selected for either nonmandatory surgery or nonoperative management. Pulmonary complications, defined as pneumonia, bronchitis, iatrogenic pneumothorax, and ARDS, occurred at the following rates: nonmandatory surgery, 33 percent; nonoperative management, 4 percent; and mandatory emergency surgery, 38 percent.

The authors concluded that the rate of probably needless operations in the nonmandatory surgery group was 78 percent. It was clear that apparently unnecessary surgery entailed not only its own inherent risk for morbidity but also morbidity due to postoperative complications that may have otherwise been avoided.

Anesthetic Factors

The expected effects of anesthesia on lung function have been addressed elsewhere in this chapter. By preventing glottic closure, endotracheal intubation interferes with the patient's ability to cough and clear secretions, leaving the patient dependent on the anesthesiologist for pulmonary toilet.[1–3] Most modern inhalation anesthetics are bronchodilators; thus, there is minimal concern about anesthetic-induced bronchospasm; however, endotracheal tubes can precipitate bronchospasm in patients with asthma or other forms of reactive airways disease. Many physicians think that regional anesthesia always carries a lower pulmonary complication rate than does general, but at least one major study has refuted this notion.[45] Spinal anesthesia does not suppress ventilatory drive, but it may affect the respiratory muscles if the level is too high. In addition, its use with sedation may compromise airway control, secretion clearance, and adequate ventilation.[2,45]

Finally, the duration of the operation and anesthetic appears to be related to the incidence of pulmonary complications. For example, Mircea and others found that the rate of pulmonary complications increased geometrically with the duration of surgery, reaching 58 percent for operations lasting more than 4 hours.[45] Similarly, Wightman and coworkers found an increased pulmonary complication rate when operations lasted more than 3 hours.[48]

Comorbidity Factors

Any concurrent disease or comorbid condition will compound the risks inherent in operating on a given patient.[1–3,15] Concurrent diseases also raise two important questions for the surgeon. First, how does the disease affect the expected morbidity and mortality of the proposed operation? Second, how does the comorbid condition affect the patient's prognosis with or without the operation? There may be occasions when the comorbid condition so alters overall prognosis that surgery becomes irrelevant. These considerations may be particularly important when the comorbid condition is an advanced form of chronic, irreversible lung disease and when the risks include a strong possibility of prolonged ventilator support after surgery.[1]

PREOPERATIVE EVALUATION

Preoperative evaluation of all patients should include a complete history and physical examination.[1–3,43] In the process of establishing a sense of pulmonary risk, the history should include questions about smoking; symptoms of lung disease, such as cough, sputum production, wheezing, and dyspnea; and details of any previous surgical or anesthetic experiences. The physical examination should screen for evidence of dyspnea at rest or with minimal activity, orthopnea, signs of increased work of breathing or chronic lung disease, and assessment of the patient's ability to cough. Any significant abnormalities discovered by examination or history should lead to chest radiography, electrocardiography, arterial blood gas analysis, and pulmonary function testing to permit objective assessment of perioperative risk.

Table 2–2. CANDIDATES FOR PREOPERATIVE PULMONARY EVALUATION*

All thoracic surgery patients
All upper abdominal surgery patients
Heavy smokers (present or past)
Morbidly obese patients
Age >70 years
Patients with any chronic lung disease

*Adapted from Tisi GM: Preoperative evaluation of pulmonary function: validity, indications, and benefits. Am Rev Respir Dis 119:293–310, 1979.

Table 2–2 lists patients who should be considered candidates for preoperative pulmonary function evaluation. Depending on the degree of abnormality present, pulmonary consultation may be helpful in further clarifying risks of morbidity and mortality, and recommending perioperative management to reduce these risks as much as possible. (Table 2–1 shows various pulmonary function criteria associated with high risk for perioperative pulmonary problems.)

PROPHYLACTIC MEASURES

Once the preoperative evaluation has identified patients at high risk for the development of pulmonary problems, the surgeon or pulmonary consultant needs to decide what steps to take to reduce those risks. In 1946, Dripps and Deming first reported successful reduction of the incidence of postoperative atelectasis and pneumonia by instituting certain preoperative, intraoperative, and postoperative prophylactic measures.[49] Subsequent sudies by others established an entire armamentarium that can reduce the incidence of perioperative pulmonary complications.[1,43] These steps are listed in Table 2–3. In a report on the preoperative preparation of patients with chronic obstructive pulmonary dis-

Table 2–3. MEASURES TO REDUCE PERIOPERATIVE PULMONARY PROBLEMS*

Preoperative Measures
Smoking cessation
Treatment of ongoing pulmonary infection
Establishment of effective bronchodilator regimen if wheezing
Nutritional optimization and/or weight loss
General education and psychological preparation
Familiarization with deep breathing and respiratory therapy treatments
Intraoperative Measures
Minimize anesthetic time
Airway protection and secretion control
Optimal bronchodilation when indicated
Frequent hyperinflations or sighs
Postoperative Measures
Continue preoperative measures
Minimize narcotic analgesics
Encourage deep breathing, coughing, and secretion clearance
Mobilize and ambulate early
Heparin or other anticoagulant prophylaxis as indicated

*Compiled from Tisi GM: Preoperative evaluation of pulmonary function: validity, indications and benefits. Am Rev Respir Dis 119:293–310, 1979; and Harmon E, Lillington G: Pulmonary risk factors in surgery. Med Clin North Am 63:1289–1298, 1979.

ease, Gracey and colleagues demonstrated not only that the incidence of pulmonary complications varied with the severity of the underlying lung disease, but also that in patients with moderate to severe underlying lung disease the failure to respond or improve with preoperative treatment portended a particularly high probability of serious postoperative pulmonary complications.[50] See Table 2–1.

SUMMARY

Pulmonary complications are major contributors to postoperative morbidity and mortality. Patients at risk for pulmonary complications can be identified by careful history, physical examination, and preoperative laboratory testing. Progress in preoperative pulmonary treatment, anesthetic management, and surgical techniques allows surgical intervention to proceed in patients with significant pulmonary disease who may not have been considered surgical candidates in the past.

References

1. Tisi GM: Preoperative evaluation of pulmonary function: validity, indications and benefits. Am Rev Respir Dis 119:293–310, 1979.
2. Harman E, Lillington G: Pulmonary risk factors in surgery. Med Clin North Am 63:1289–1298, 1979.
3. Gilmour IJ: Perioperative respiratory care. Urol Clin North Am 10:65–76, 1983.
4. Beecher HK: The measured effect of laparotomy on the respiration. J Clin Invest 12:639–650, 1933.
5. Beecher HK: Effect of laparotomy on lung volume: demonstration of a new type of pulmonary collapse. J Clin Invest 12:651–658, 1933.
6. Anscombe AR, Buxton RSJ: Effect of abdominal operations on total lung capacity and its subdivisions. Br Med J 2:84–87, 1958.
7. Tahir AH, George RB, Weill H, Adriani J: Effects of abdominal surgery upon diaphragmatic function and regional ventilation. Int Surg 58:337–340, 1973.
8. Ford GT, Whitelaw WA, Rosenal TW, Cruse PJ, Guenter CA: Diaphragm function after abdominal surgery in humans. Am Rev Respir Dis 127:431–436, 1983.
9. Simonneau G, Vivien A, Sartene R, et al: Diaphragm dysfunction induced by upper abdominal surgery: role of postoperative pain. Am Rev Respir Dis 128:899–903, 1983.
10. London RA, Kudlak T, Riehle RA: Immersion anesthesia for extracorporeal shock wave lithotripsy: review of two hundred twenty treatments. Urology 28:86–94, 1986.
11. Egbert LD, Bendixen HH: Effect of morphine on breathing pattern: a possible factor in atelectasis. JAMA 188:485–488, 1964.
12. George J, Hornum I, Mellemgard K: The mechanism of hypoxemia after laparotomy. Thorax 22:382–386, 1967.
13. Gamsu C, Singer MM, Vincent HH, et al: Postoperative impairment of mucous transport in the lung. Am Rev Respir Dis 114:673–679, 1976
14. Harris SD, Johanson WG, Pierce AK: Bacterial lung clearance in hypoxic mice. Am Rev Respir Dis 111:910, 1975.
15. Pasulka PS, Bistrian BR, Benotti PN, Blackburn GL: The risks of surgery in obese patients. Ann Intern Med 104:540–546, 1986.
16. Johanson WG, Pierce AK, Sanford JP, Thomas SD: Nosocomial respiratory infections with gram-negative bacilli: the significance of colonization of the respiratory tract. Ann Intern Med 77:701–706, 1972.
17. Moser KM: Thromboembolic disease in the patient undergoing urologic surgery. Urol Clin North Amer 10:101–108, 1983.
18. Kakkar VV, Howe CT, Flanc C, et al: Natural history of postoperative deep vein thrombosis. Lancet 2:230–233, 1969.
19. Kakkar VV: Prevention of fatal postoperative pulmonary embolism by low doses of heparin: International Multicentre Trial. Lancet 2:45–51, 1975.
20. Becker J, Borgstrom S, Saltzman GF: Occurrence and course of thrombosis following prostatectomy. Acta Radiol [Diagn] 10:513–533, 1970.
21. Moser KM, Brach B, Dolan GR: Clinically suspected deep venous thrombosis of the lower extremities. JAMA 237:2195–2198, 1977.
22. Colby FH: The prevention of pulmonary emboli after prostatectomy. J Urol 59:920–930, 1945.
23. Allgood RJ, Cook JH, Weedn RJ, et al: Prospective analysis of pulmonary embolism in the postoperative patient. Surgery 68:116–122, 1970.
24. The Urokinase Pulmonary Embolism Trial: A National Cooperative Study. Circulation 47 (Suppl):1–100, 1973.
25. Kipper MS, Moser KM, Kortman KE, Ashburn WL: Longterm follow-up of patients with suspected pulmo-

nary embolism and a normal lung scan. Perfusion scans in embolic suspects. Chest 82:411–415, 1982.
26. Hull RD, Hirsh J, Carter CJ, et al: Diagnostic value of ventilation-perfusion lung scanning in patients with suspected pulmonary embolism. Chest 88:819–828, 1985.
27. Hyers TM, Hull RD, Weg JG: Antithrombotic therapy for venous thromboembolic disease. Chest 89 (Suppl):26–35, 1986.
28. Robin ED: Overdiagnosis and overtreatment of pulmonary embolism: the emperor may have no clothes. Ann Inter Med 87:775–781, 1977.
29. Bellamy PE: Epitomes, important advances in clinical medicine: diagnosing pulmonary embolism. Western J Med 147:322, 1987.
30. Coe NP, Collins REC, Klein LA, et al: Prevention of deep vein thrombosis in urological patients: a controlled randomized trial of low dose heparin and external pneumatic compression boots. Surgery 83:230–234, 1978.
31. Thrombolytic therapy in thrombosis: A National Institutes of Health Consensus Development Conference. Ann Intern Med 93:141–144, 1980.
32. Bartlett RH, Morris AH, Fairley B, et al: A prospective study of acute hypoxic respiratory failure. Chest 89:684–689, 1986.
33. Shapiro BA, Cane RD, Harrison RA: Positive end-expiratory pressure therapy in adults with special reference to acute lung injury: a review of the literature and suggested clinical correlations. Crit Care Med 12:127–141, 1984.
34. Tyler DC: Positive end-expiratory pressure: a review. Crit Care Med 11:300–308, 1983.
35. Hudson LD: Ventilatory management of patients with adult respiratory distress syndrome. Semin Respir Med 2:128–139, 1981.
36. Weideman HP, Matthay MA, Matthay RA: Acute Lung Injury, Vol 2, Philadelphia, Critical Care Clinics, 1986.
37. Dubois M, Lotze MT, Diamond WJ, et al: Pulmonary shunting during leukoagglutinin-induced noncardiac pulmonary edema. JAMA 244:2186–2189, 1980.
38. Wiegelt JA, Norcross JF, Borman KR, Snyder WH: Early steroid therapy for respiratory failure. Arch Surg 120:536–540, 1985.
39. Mohsenifar Z, Goldbach P, Tashkin DP, Campisi DJ: Relationship between O_2 delivery and O_2 consumption in the adult respiratory distress syndrome. Chest 84:267–271, 1983.
40. Montgomery BA, Stager MA, Carrico J, Hudson LD: Causes of mortality in patients with the adult respiratory distress syndrome. Am Rev Respir Dis 132:485–489, 1985.
41. Gill C: The thoracic cavity, a troublesome neighbor: intraoperative consultation by the thoracic surgeon. Urol Clin North Am 12:507–510, 1985.
42. Clausen JL, ed: Pulmonary Function Testing Guidelines and Controversies: Equipment, Methods and Normal Values. New York, Academic Press, 1982.
43. Gass GD, Olsen GN: Preoperative pulmonary function testing to predict postoperative morbidity and mortality. Chest 89:127–135, 1986.
44. Williams CD, Brenowitz JB: Prohibitive lung function and major surgical procedures. Am J Surg 132:763–766, 1976.
45. Mircea N, Constantinescu C, Jianu E, Busu G: Risk of pulmonary complications in surgical patients. Resuscitation 10:33–41, 1982.
46. Meyhoff HH, Nording J, Hald T: Transurethral versus transvesical prostatectomy: physiologic strain. Scand J Urol Nephrol 19:85–91, 1985.
47. Heyns CF, De Klerk DP, De Kock MLS: Nonoperative management of renal stab wounds. J Urol 134:239–242, 1985.
48. Wightman JAK: A prospective survey of the incidence of postoperative pulmonary complications. Br J Surg 55:85–91, 1968.
49. Dripps RD, Deming MVN: Postoperative atelectasis and pneumonia: diagnosis, etiology and management based upon 1240 cases of upper abdominal surgery. Ann Surg 124:94–110, 1946.
50. Gracey DR, Divertie MB, Dider EP: Preoperative pulmonary preparation of patients with chronic obstructive pulmonary disease. Chest 76:123–129, 1979.

INFECTIOUS COMPLICATIONS OF UROLOGIC SURGERY

3

Drew J. Winston

Infections are a common cause of morbidity and mortality in patients undergoing urologic surgery. In addition to the medical consequences of these infections, infectious complications have major economic effects by prolonging hospitalization and increasing the costs of medical care. It has been estimated that a nosocomial, or hospital-acquired, urinary tract infection prolongs hospitalization by 2.5 days and that the average total hospital cost for treatment of this infection is $750 per day.[1] A postoperative wound infection may add several thousand dollars to the cost of hospitalization.[2]

RISK FACTORS FOR INFECTION

There are certain factors that place the urologic patient at risk for infection following surgery (Table 3–1).[3,4] Many patients already have had recurrent urinary tract infections or prostatitis, which may be a source for postoperative infection. These patients usually have structural or functional abnormalities of the urinary tract in the form of bladder outlet obstruction secondary to benign prostatic hyperplasia, a urethral stricture, neuropathic urethers, vesicoureteral reflux, or a neurogenic bladder. Postoperatively, these patients require urinary catheterization. The overall prevalence of bacteriuria during urethral catheterization is approximately 25 percent when the duration of catheterization is 4 to 5 days.[5]

A significant proportion of urologic patients are elderly. Besides the effects of aging itself on host immunity and physiology,[6] older patients commonly have underlying conditions such as obstructive lung disease, diabetes, or malignancy that may enhance their risk for infection. For example, a patient with severe lung disease may be more difficult to extubate and thus be at greater risk for pneumonia, whereas the diabetic patient may have vascular insufficiency, which can impair wound healing and lead to soft-tissue infections. Underlying malignancies and their treatment with chemotherapeutic agents and radiation can cause leukopenia, thrombocytopenia, and other disturbances in host immunity that lead to postoperative infections and bleeding complications.[7] Similarly, renal transplant recipients are given cyclosporine, corticosteroids, immuran, antithymocyte globulin, or other agents that suppress their immunity and predispose them to opportunistic bacterial, fun-

Table 3–1. RISK FACTORS FOR INFECTION AFTER UROLOGIC SURGERY

History of recurrent urinary tract infections or prostatitis
Indwelling catheter
Age (elderly)
Underlying diseases
Obstructive lung-disease
Diabetes
Malignancy
Immunosuppressive therapy (renal transplants)
Malnutrition
Type of surgery
Ileal conduit
Enterocystoplasty
Penile prosthesis
Intraoperative complications
Poor technique
Increased blood loss
Improper drainage
Prolonged operation

gal, and viral infections.[8] Postoperative patients debilitated from these underlying diseases or the surgery itself may have malnutrition, which can increase the risk for infection by causing deleterious effects on cell-mediated immunity, humoral antibody response, and phagocytic function.[9] Finally, certain types of surgery (ileal conduit urinary diversion, enterocystoplasty, or placement of a penile prosthesis) or intraoperative complications (poor technique, prolonged operative time, or increased blood loss) may alter the normal physical barriers to infection. Bacterial colonization of an ileal conduit or enterocystoplasty can be a source of recurrent postoperative bacteremia, and debilitating perineal wound infections and pubic osteomyelitis may complicate penile prosthetic surgery.

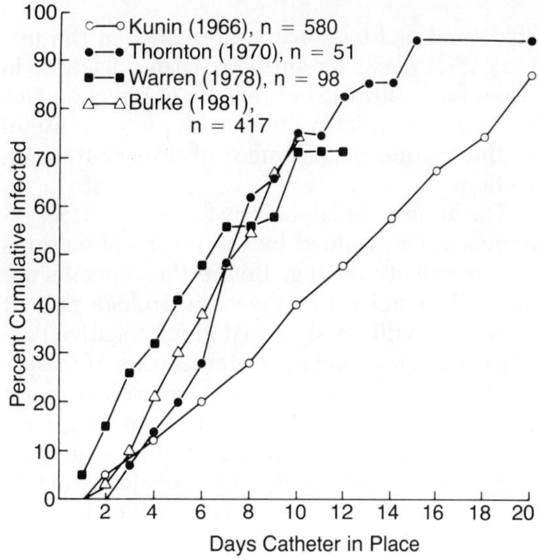

Figure 3–1. Cumulative percent of catheterized patients acquiring urinary infections. (From Fowler JE, Marshall VM: Nosocomial catheter-associated urinary tract infection. Infect Surg 2:43–45, 1983.)

URINARY TRACT INFECTION

The urinary tract is the most common site of nosocomial infection, which accounts for 30 to 40 percent of all hospital-acquired infections.[10,11] The presence of preoperative bacteriuria and an indwelling uretheral catheter are the two most important factors predisposing urologic patients to postoperative urinary tract infections. The duration of catheterization is the most significant risk factor. Whereas the risk of infection is only about 1 to 2 percent with a single ureteral catheterization, the cumulative risk for infection with an indwelling catheter approximates 5 percent per day of catheterization (Fig. 3–1).[12]

Gram-negative enteric bacilli are the most common organisms causing hospital-acquired urinary tract infections. In the National Nosocomial Infection Study Report published by the Centers for Disease Control, the most frequently occurring pathogens were *Escherichia coli*, enterococcus, *Pseudomonas aeruginosa*, *Klebsiella*, *Proteus*, *Candida*, and *Enterobacter*.[11] The gastrointestinal tract is the usual source of urinary tract pathogens, but epidemics of infection have been traced to contaminated antiseptic solutions, irrigation fluids, urine measuring containers, and the hands of medical personnel.[13,14]

Because repeated courses of antibacterial therapy are common in hospitalized patients, antibiotic-resistant isolates may be found.[15] Even fungi such as *Candida* may cause troublesome infection, especially in patients who require chronic indwelling catheters for urinary tract obstruction and who have received extensive antibiotic therapy.

The diagnosis of urinary tract infection is usually made from a combination of the classic clinical manifestations (fever, flank pain, frequency, urgency, and dysuria) and the finding of bacteria in a microscopic examination of the urine sediment or a urine culture. Some patients, especially the elderly, may have atypical symptoms or may be asymptomatic. Most patients with symptomatic urinary tract infection have pyuria; however, the finding of pyuria is nonspecific and its presence or absence may or may not indicate infection. In contrast, the presence of at least one bacterium per oil-immersion field in a clean-catch, gram-stained, uncentrifuged urine specimen correlates strongly with $\geq 10^5$ bacteria/ml of urine.[16] A urine culture showing $\geq 10^5$ bacteria/ml of urine is considered significant and usually indicates infection.[17] However, some urinary tract infections may produce titers of $<10^5$ bacteria/ml and these lower bacterial counts should not always be dismissed in patients with symptoms of infection.[18] Moreover, these criteria apply primarily to gram-negative bacillary organisms and to urines collected by the mid-stream, clean-catch method. Gram-positive cocci and fungi may not reach titers of 10^5/ml in patients with infection.[19] Urines collected by catheterization or suprapubic aspiration may also show counts of $<10^5$ bacteria/ml of urine but yet may be significant. Isolation of more than one bacterial organism from a urine culture usually indicates contamination, except in patients who have a chronic indwelling catheter for a structural or functional abnormality of the urinary tract. Tests for antibody-coated bacteria in urine for localization of the site of infection lack sufficient specificity and sensitivity to be useful in the routine management of urinary tract infections.[20]

The antimicrobial therapy for urinary tract infection is determined by the results of cultures and sensitivity testing. Before these results are available, empiric therapy in the urologic patient needs to be directed against gram-negative bacillary organisms and the enterococcus. If the patient is not critically ill and bacteremia is not an issue, oral therapy with trimethoprim-sulfamethoxazole, a fluorinated quinolone (norfloxacin or ciprofloxacin), or a cephalosporin (cephalexin or cephradine) is reasonable. Empiric therapy with oral ampicillin or amoxacillin is not recommended because of the high frequency of beta-lactamase–producing enteric bacteria in urologic patients that are resistant to these agents. The availability of the broader-spectrum fluorinated quinolones (norfloxacin, ciprofloxacin) has also obviated the use of older agents like nalidixic acid and nitrofurantoin.[21,22] Treatment of urinary tract infection should be given for a minimum of 7 to 10 days. Single-dose therapy, which is effective for uncomplicated urinary tract infections in young females, is generally not appropriate for the complicated infections seen in urologic patients.[10]

In the severely ill patient with possible bacteremia, appropriate empiric therapy is an intravenous aminoglycoside (gentamicin, tobramycin, or amikacin) plus a penicillin (ampicillin, ticarcillin, piperacillin, or mezlocillin). A third-generation cephalosporin (cefotaxime, cefoperazone, or ceftazidine) may be substituted for the aminoglycoside if nephrotoxicity is a concern.[23,24]

Localized noninvasive *Candida* urinary tract infections can be treated with amphotericin B irrigation administered through a catheter or a nephrostomy. A daily irrigation with 50 mg of amphotericin in 1000 ml of sterile water (not saline) is used for 5 to 14 days.[25] If invasive disseminated candidiasis is present, intravenous amphotericin B is required. Oral flucytosine alone is not recommended for fungal infections because of the rapid emergence of resistance during therapy.[26] Oral ketoconazole is not reliable therapy because ketoconazole is primarily excreted in the bile and may not achieve effective concentrations in the urine.[27] Oral fluconazole is a new investigational antifungal agent with a pharmacokinetic prolife that includes both renal excretion and penetration into the central nervous system.[28] When fluconazole becomes available, it may be useful for fungal urinary tract infections as well as central nervous system infections.

Effective antibiotic therapy for a urinary tract infection usually produces symptomatic improvement with negative urine cultures within 48 to 72 hours. Some upper urinary tract infections may take longer to respond, but a delay in clinical improvement beyond 72 hours suggests a need to exclude urinary obstruction, a perinephric abscess, or an intrarenal abscess. Renal ultrasound, computed tomographic (CT) scanning, and magnetic resonance imaging (MRI) are noninvasive studies employed for the diagnosis of obstruction or abscess formation.[29] An intravenous or retrograde urogram and a renal scan may also provide helpful information in certain patients. Diagnostic needle aspiration and percutaneous drainage are effective techniques for the diagnosis and treatment of perinephric or intrarenal abscesses[30]; however, when aspiration or percutaneous drainage fails, open surgical drainage is required. Multiple small abscesses, the need to place multiple catheters, infected tumor, and large blood clots are common causes for failure of percutaneous drainage. Open surgery may also be needed for removal of stones or other obstructing lesions. Percutaneous lithotomy and extracorporeal shock-wave lithotripsy (ESWL) are less invasive approaches for removal of stones.[31]

If a patient with a urinary tract infection relapses after completion of appropriate therapy, a search for a structural or functional abnormality of the urinary tract should be pursued. If no abnormality is found, the relapse may be related to persistent upper urinary tract infection involving the kidneys or to a bacterial prostatitis. A 6-weeks course of oral antibiotic therapy based on results of cultures and sensitivity testing may be curative in a patient who relapses after 1 to 2 weeks of therapy for an upper urinary tract infection.[32] The presence of a bacterial prostatitis is indicated by perineal discomfort, low back pain, and dysuria but the patient is frequently asymptomatic. The cause can be determined by performing quantitative localization cultures before and after prostatic massage.[33] Gram-negative bacilli (*E. coli, Klebsiella, Enterobacter, Proteus*, and *P. aeruginosa*) and the enterococcus are the most common pathogens.[34] Antibiotic therapy for bacterial prostatitis should include the use of drugs that penetrate well into prostatic tissue. The penicillins, cephalosporins,

Table 3–2. SUMMARY OF MAJOR RECOMMENDATIONS FOR PREVENTION OF CATHETER-ASSOCIATED URINARY TRACT INFECTIONS (Center for Disease Control)*

Category I (Strongly Recommended for Adoption)
Educate personnel in correct techniques of catheter insertion and care
Catheterize only when necessary
Emphasize handwashing
Insert catheter using aseptic technique and sterile equipment
Secure catheter properly
Maintain closed sterile drainage
Obtain urine samples aseptically
Maintain unobstructed urine flow
Category II (Moderately Recommended for Adoption)
Periodically reeducate personnel in catheter care
Use smallest suitable bore catheter
Avoid irrigation unless needed to prevent or relieve obstruction
Refrain from daily meatal care
Do not change catheters at arbitrary fixed intervals
Category III (Weakly Recommended for Adoption)
Consider alternative techniques for urinary drainage before using an indwelling urethral catheter
Replace the collecting system when sterile drainage has been violated
Spatially separate infected and uninfected patients with indwelling catheters
Avoid routine bacteriologic monitoring

*From Wong ES: Guideline for prevention of catheter-associated urinary tract infection. Infect Control 2:125–130, 1981.[39]

tetracyclines, and aminoglycosides generally do not, whereas trimethoprim and erythromycin reach high concentrations in prostatic fluid.[35,36] Trimethoprim-sulfamethoxazole or trimethoprim alone is recommended for treatment of bacterial prostatitis. Oral carbenicillin indanyl sodium is also used.[36] Therapy should be continued for several weeks or months to achieve the best results. The quinolones (norfloxacin, ciprofloxacin) are concentrated in prostatic tissue and prostatic fluid, but data on their efficacy for bacterial prostatitis are limited.[37,38]

CARE OF THE INDWELLING URETHRAL CATHETER

The indwelling urethral catheter is one of the most commonly used instruments in hospitals. It is estimated that approximately 10 percent of hospitalized patients receive an indwelling catheter.[10] The recommendations of the Centers for Disease Control for prevention of catheter-associated bacteriuria are summarized in Table 3–2.[39] Maintenance of a closed sterile drainage system is especially important. Meatal care regimens, urethral antibacterial lubricants, antibiotic-impregnated catheters, prophylactic antibiotic bladder irrigation, and instillation of disinfectants into drainage systems have not proved beneficial and are not recommended.[40–42] Routine prophylactic bladder irrigation with a neomycin-polymyxin B solution or the use of prophylactic systemic antibiotics is strongly discouraged because these agents may encourage the emergence of multiresistant strains of gram-negative bacilli and *Candida*. For this same reason, chronic or recurrent asymptomatic bacteriuria in a patient requiring long-term catheterization should not be treated unless the patient becomes symptomatic.

EPIDIDYMITIS

Epididymitis may complicate prostatic surgery, vasectomy, urethral catheterization, or other types of genitourinary instrumentation. Epididymitis is particularly common in patients who undergo urologic surgery or instrumentation while they are bacteriuric. The same organism is frequently isolated from a culture of the semen or an epididymal aspirate and the urine.[43] In contrast to sexually transmitted epididymitis in younger males, most cases of epididymitis after urologic surgery are caused by gram-negative bacilli (*E. coli*, *P. aeruginosa*, *Klebsiella*, *Proteus*, and *Enterobacter*) rather than *Chlamydia* or *Neisseria gonorrhoeae*.[43] Occasionally, enterococcus or *Staphylococcus* is isolated.[44]

Clinically, epididymitis produces unilateral pain, swelling, and tenderness of the scrotum over the epididymis. This painful swelling develops over a 24- to 48-hour period in contrast to the more rapid onset of pain associated with testicular torsion. The swelling and induration are initially limited to the epididymis but may extend to the testis if there is a delay in diagnosis and therapy. Initial empiric treatment with trimethoprim-sulfamethoxazole, trimethoprim alone, tetracycline, or carbenicillin indanyl sodium is appropriate. The choice of antibiotic can then be adjusted when the results of the urine or epididymal aspirate culture become available. Parenteral antibiotic therapy with an aminoglycoside (gentamicin, tobramycin, or amikacin) or third-generation cephalosporin (cefotaxime, cefoperazone, or ceftazidime) may be indicated for more severe cases. If testicular infarction or a scrotal abscess develops, surgical decompression of the epididymis or drainage of the abscess fluid should be performed.[44]

WOUND INFECTION

The overall rate of wound infection in urologic patients has been reported to range from 1.6 to 7.7 percent.[2,45] This rate is highly dependent on the degree of contamination of the wound before surgery. For example, in a 10-year prospective study of 62,939 wounds, the rate of wound infection was only 1.5 percent following clean surgical procedures but increased to 7.7 percent after exposure of a clean operative site to endogenous microflora ("clean-contaminated" surgery) and to 40 percent when pus was encountered at the operative site or a perforated viscus was found ("dirty" surgery).[2] Other factors increasing the rate of wound infection are prolonged hospitalization before the operation, a remote site of infection, and prolonged operative time.[2,4,5,46] The use of razor shaving instead of depilatory cream to remove hair at the operative site causes skin damage and bacterial growth and also prediposes patients to postoperative wound infection.[47]

Most postsurgical wound infections are superficial and involve only the skin and subcutaneous tissues. The usual clinical manifestations are local incisional pain, tenderness, swelling, and erythema. When the infection manifests between the first and second operative days, the causative organism is likely to be *Streptococcus* or *Clostridium* and causes severe systemic toxicity and rapid advance of a cellulitis around the wound.[48] Infections appearing on the third to fourth postoperative day are generally due to *Staphylococcus*. Wound infections caused by gram-negative bacilli usually appear beteen the fifth and fifteenth postoperative days but may occur earlier if the gastrointestinal tract or a contaminated genitourinary tract has been entered.[48] More complicated wound infections with necrosis of soft tissue, fascia, and muscle may occur in diabetic or other immunosuppressed patients (Fig. 3–2).[49] Late complications of wound infection include osteomyelitis (Fig. 3–3).[50]

Effective treatment of a wound infection necessitates the administration of antibiotics as well as appropriate surgical debridement and drainage. For streptococcal or clostridial infection, intravenous penicillin G is the drug of choice. Oxacillin or cefazolin in the penicillin-allergic patient is used for staphylococcal infection. Vancomycin is reserved for treating methicillin-resistant staphylococcal infection and certain penicillin-allergic patients. Gram-negative bacillary wound infections are treated with an aminoglycoside (gentamicin, tobramycin, or amikacin), a cephalosporin (cefazolin, cefoxitin, cefotaxime, cefoperazone, or ceftazidime), or a broad-spectrum penicillin (ticarcillin, piperacillin, or mezlocillin). Clindamycin, metronidazole, and ampicillin/sulbactam are excellent drugs for anaerobic infections.[51]

For severe necrotizing soft-tissue infections, such as Fournier's gangrene, a triple-antibiotic regimen of penicillin G, clindamycin, and an aminoglycoside is recommended to provide therapy for *Clostridium*, other anaerobes, *Staphylococcus*, and gram-negative bacilli.

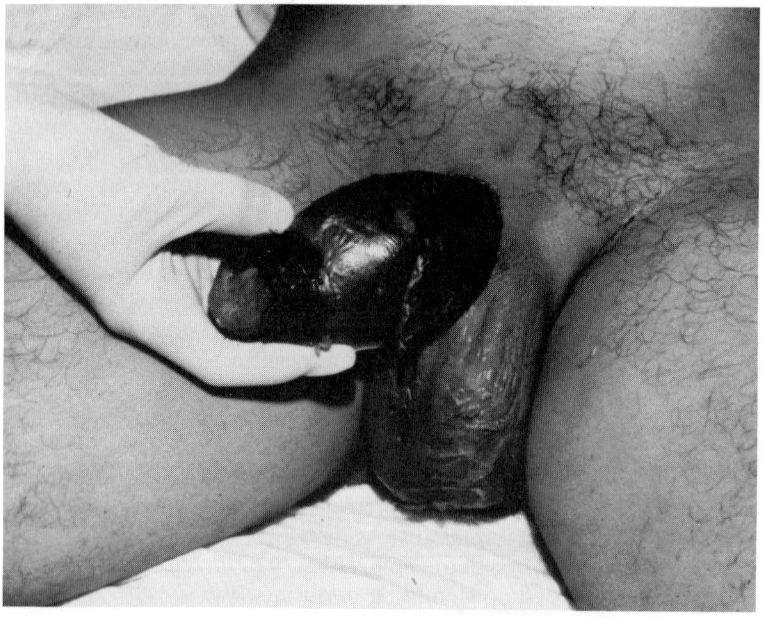

Figure 3–2. *Pseudomonas aeruginosa* cellulitis of the scrotum and penis in a patient with acute leukemia.

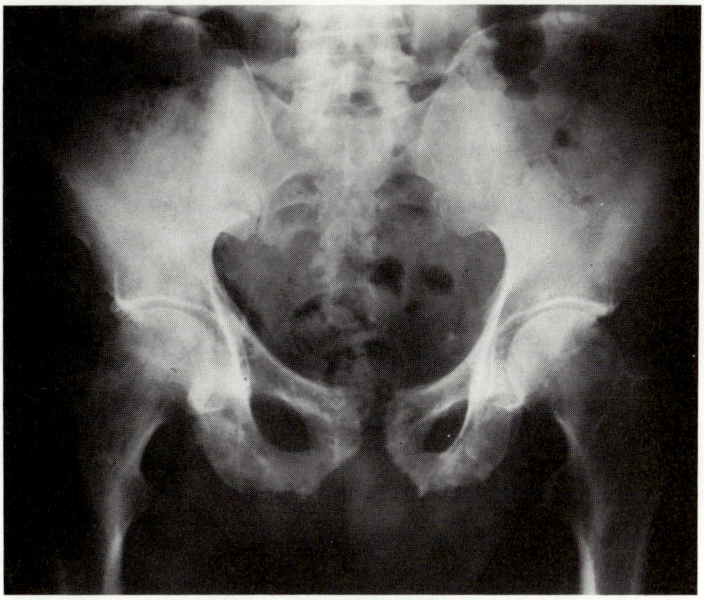

Figure 3–3. *Pseudomonas aeruginosa* osteomyelitis of the pubic rami and symphysis pubis complicating infection of a urinary anti-incontinence device.

Combination therapy with an aminoglycoside plus an antipseudomonal beta-lactam drug is recommended for any severe *P. aeruginosa* infection. If appropriate systemic antibiotics are used, treatment of the wound with topical antibiotics or antibiotic irrigation is unnecessary. A wound infection failing to respond to antibiotic therapy should prompt an evaluation for a deep abscess, a collection of urine, or an underlying osteomyelitis. Removal of foreign materials (such as a prosthesis or catheter) may also be required for complete healing of infected wounds.

BACTEREMIA

The urinary tract is the most frequent source of gram-negative bacteremia in hospitalized patients.[52,53] The risk of bacteremia developing from the urinary tract is about 1.0 percent for all hospitalized patients but is between 8 and 31 percent in patients who undergo manipulation of the urinary tract.[54,55] *E. coli* is the most common cause of gram-negative bacteremia, followed by *Klebsiella, P. aeruginosa, Serratia, Enterobacter,* and *Proteus. P. aeruginosa* is associated with the highest mortality (40 to 70 percent) of all bacteremic infections because of its frequent occurrence in patients with underlying diseases or conditions having a poor prognosis.[52,56]

Urologic patients are also susceptible to gram-positive bacteremias from infected indwelling vascular catheters, wound infections, and urinary tract infections. The increasing use of long-term central intravenous catheters in surgical and other patients has been partially responsible for a growing number of gram-positive bacteremias caused by coagulase-negative staphylococci.[57,58] Enterococcal bacteremia after instrumentation of the urinary tract may be complicated by endocarditis in patients with valvular heart disease.[59] The overall mortality from these gram-positive bacteremias (<10 percent) is significantly lower than the mortality from gram-negative bacteremia (20 to 40 percent).[52,53,56,57] Nonetheless, both gram-positive and gram-negative organisms must be considered in the critically ill urologic patient with suspected bacteremia.

Although there is some evidence that gram-negative and gram-positive bacteremia produce different hemodynamic effects,[60] these differences are relatively small with considerable overlap and cannot be used reliably for making a clinical distinction between gram-negative and gram-positive bacteremia. Most studies of the pathophysiology of bacteremia have concentrated on the bacterial endotoxins (lipopolysaccharides) associated with the cell wall of gram-negative bacilli. Endotoxin or lipopolysaccharide appears to play a role in the activation of Hageman factor (factor XII), which in turn leads to activation of the complement, coagulation, fibrinolytic, and bradykinin systems.[61] Complement activation results in migration of inflammatory cells into tissues, the phagocytosis of bacteria, and the release of vasodilatory anaphylotoxins. Activated Hageman factor initiates the intrinsic clotting cascade and can lead to consumption of clotting factors, e.g., disseminated intravascular coagulation (DIC), and bleeding. At the same time, activation of the fibrinolytic system generates plasmin, which acts to lyse fibrin into fibrin-split products and contributes to bleeding. The effects of endotoxin on the kinin system causes the conversion of kininogen to bradykinin. Bradykinin is a vasoactive peptide that produces vasodilatation and increased vascular permeability.

Evidence has been accumulated that the deleterious effects of endotoxin are mediated by factors produced by macrophages. One of these factors, called *cachectin,* or tumor necrosis factor, is made by endotoxin-stimulated macrophages and causes shock and tissue injury.[62] Passive immunization against cachectin protects mice from the lethal effects of endotoxin.[63] Endogenous opiates and prostaglandins may also participate in the pathophysiology of endotoxinemia. The blockade of opiate receptors with opiate antagonists (naloxone) or the inhibition of prostaglandin synthesis with nonsteroidal anti-inflammatory drugs (ibuprofen) reverses the cardiovascular effects of endotoxin in animals.[64,65]

Diagnosis

The diagnosis of bacteremia is suggested by recognizing the typical clinical manifestations associated with bacteremia and confirmed by isolation of organisms from blood cultures.[66,67] Although the combination of fever, chills, and hypotension following manipulation of the genitourinary tract is almost pathognomonic of bacteremia, this classic presentation is not always seen. In elderly or debilitated patients, fever may be absent or hypothermia may occur. The sudden onset of hyperventilation or a change in mental status may be the initial presentation of bacteremia. Embolic skin lesions characterized by erythematous nodules with a central area of necrosis (ecthyma gangrenosum) may develop. If bacteremic shock develops, initial hemodynamic measurements show a markedly decreased systemic vascular resistance, an increased cardiac output, an increased stroke volume, and a decreased central venous pressure (warm shock). Later findings in bacteremic shock include increased systemic vascular resistance, diminished cardiac output, metabolic acidosis, and anuria (cold shock).[60]

The adult respiratory distress syndrome (ARDS) is another complication of severe bacteremia and is characterized by hyperventilation, hypoxemia, decreased pulmonary compliance, normal pulmonary wedge pressure, a high pulmonary arterial pressure, and extensive bilateral infiltrates.[68] Laboratory abnormalities associated with bacteremia include hyperbilirubinemia, thrombocytopenia, and DIC.[66] Laboratory evidence of DIC includes increased circulating fibrin-split products, hypofibrinogenemia, decreased levels of coagulation factors II, V, VII, and VIII as well as thrombocytopenia.[69] There is no rapid, sensitive, or specific diagnostic test for detection of bacteremia. The limulus test for endotoxemia lacks specificity for clinical usefulness.[70] Two or three sets of blood cultures obtained separately are still required for confirmation of the diagnosis.

Treatment

Initiation of appropriate antibiotic therapy, elimination of the source of infection, and correction of hemodynamic and metabolic abnormalities are the essential keys for the successful treatment of bacteremia. The choice of empiric antibiotic therapy depends on the source of the bacteremia and the underlying condition of the patient. An aminoglycoside (gentamicin, tobramycin, or amikacin) paired with a penicillin (ampicillin, ticarcillin, piperacillin, or mezlocillin) is appropriate when the urinary tract is the source because enterococcus as well as gram-negative bacilli is a more likely pathogen than *Staphylococcus.* If nephrotoxicity is a concern, a third-generation cephalosporin (cefotaxime, cefoperazone, or ceftazidime) instead of an aminoglycoside can be paired with the penicillin drug. For bacteremia from a nonurinary source, oxacillin, cefazolin, or cefoxitin, plus an aminoglycoside or a third-generation cephalosporin alone can be given for staphylococcal as well as gram-negative bacillary infections.

If a central intravenous catheter is the likely source of bacteremia, intravenous vancomycin can be used with an aminoglycoside or third-generation cephalosporin to provide coverage for coagulase-negative *Staphylococcus, Corynebacterium,* and other gram-positive organisms that commonly infect central intravenous catheters. Otherwise, an expensive antibiotic like vancomycin should be reserved for documented methicillin-resistant staphylococcal infections and certain penicillin-allergic patients. A regimen of an aminoglycoside plus an antipseudomonal penicillin or third-generation cephalosporin is recommended for neutropenic patients at high risk for *P. aeruginosa* infection. Final antibiotic selection depends on the results of cultures and sensitivity testing.

Persistence and recurrence of bacteremia despite appropriate antibiotic therapy suggest several possibilities. First, there may be a source of infection that requires removal. In urologic patients, elimination of a source of infection may necessitate drainage of an abscess on an obstructed kidney; removal of an infected urinary catheter, intravascular line, or monitoring device; or the reconstruction of a colonized ileal conduit or enterocytoplasty. Second, serum antibiotic levels may be subinhibitory. This is especially a problem with the aminoglycosides, which have a narrow therapeutic ratio. Third, a superinfection with a resistant bacterial organism or an opportunistic pathogen like *Candida* may have developed.

Insertion of a central venous pressure monitoring device or a Swan-Ganz pulmonary artery catheter is a useful measure to guide the correction of hypotension and other hemodynamic abnormalities in bacteremic patients. Rapid administration of fluid should continue until an increase in central venous pressure or pulmonary artery pressure is observed. If fluid administration fails to restore a normotensive condition in the patient, vasoactive drugs are administered. Dopamine, at doses of 2 to 25 μg/kg/minute is the drug of choice. Dobutamine, isoproterenol, and norepinephrine are also used in special situations. Intravenous infusions of bicarbonate are given to correct severe acidosis, whereas ventilatory assistance is often required when ARDS develops.

The value of corticosteroids in the treatment of bacteremia and septic shock is controversial. However, the weight of available evidence suggests that corticosteroids should not be used. In two multicentered, randomized, double-blinded, placebo-controlled studies of high-dose methylprednisone (30 mg/kg every 6 hours for four doses), it was concluded that high-dose corticosteroids provide no benefit in the treatment of severe sepsis and septic shock and therefore should not be used as adjunctive therapy.[71,72] Moreover, in one study, more deaths related to secondary infections occurred in patients who had renal failure and received corticosteroids.[71] Thus, corticosteroids are not recommended for treatment of septic shock. Similarly, the value of intravenous naloxone, given at doses of 0.4 to 1.2 mg, for treatment of septic shock remains unproven.[73,74]

Evidence from serologic studies in humans and from experimental infections in animals suggests that antibodies directed against a common antigen of the outer cell wall membrane of gram-negative bacilli (core glycolipid) are protective against the biologic effects of endotoxin.[75,76] In one human trial, patients with severe gram-negative bacterial septicemia who were passively immunized with antiserum against the core glycolipid antigen showed improved survival over similar patients not treated with antibody.[77] Trials using a monoclonal antibody directed against the core glycolipid antigen are now in progress.

PNEUMONIA

Obesity, advanced age, and underlying conditions such as chronic lung disease place the surgical patient at increased risk for hospital-acquired or nosocomial pneumonia.[78] In addition, surgical patients are frequently cared for in an intensive care unit or require intubation of the respiratory tract. The incidence of nosocomial pneumonia for intubated patients is four times higher than for nonintubated patients and is even greater after tracheostomy.[79] Residing in an intensive care unit, irrespective of intubation, also increases the risk for pneumonia.[80]

Most nosocomial pneumonias result from aspiration of pathogens that colonize the mucosal surfaces of the upper airway. Colonization by gram-negative bacilli may occur in 30 percent of patients within 48 hours after operation, and in up to 45 percent of intensive care unit patients.[80,81] The patient's own gastrointestinal tract and cross-contamination from other patients by hospital personnel are the most common sources of upper airway colonization.[82,83] Contaminated respiratory therapy equipment and bacteremia from a nonpulmonary site are now infrequent sources of pulmonary pathogens.[79]

The majority of nosocomial pneumonias are caused by gram-negative bacilli (*P. aeruginosa, Klebsiella, Enterobacter, E. coli, Serratia,* and *Proteus*) and *S. aureus*.[11] Oral anaerobic bacteria may be associated with a major aspiration pneumonia. *Acientobacter* and other multiresistant gram-negative bacilli are less frequent but occasional causes of outbreaks of pneumonia in certain hospitals or intenstive care units.[84] Similarly, *Legionella* species is an uncommon pathogen except in hospitals affected by contamination of water supplies.[85] Fungi and viruses should be considered in immunosuppressed patients (*Aspergillus* pneumonia) or pediatric patients (respiratory syncytial virus).[86,87]

The typical clinical findings associated with pneumonia include fever, cough, sputum production, and a new pulmonary infiltrate, but they may not always be present. Moreover, these findings may occur in a patient with atelectasis, pulmonary edema, or infarction rather than in a patient with bacterial pneumonia. There is considerable controversy about the adequacy of sputum or endotracheal cultures for the microbiologic diagnosis of pneumonia because of their frequent contamination with upper airway flora. Nevertheless, Gram stain and culture of an adequate sputum or endotracheal aspirate may be helpful in guiding antibiotic therapy and should be obtained. Transtracheal aspiration or bronchoscopy with a protected brush has been advocated as methods to avoid upper airway contamination, but neither technique may be tolerated by severely ill patients.[89,90] These procedures should be reserved for immunosuppressed patients and patients with more severe complications in whom the etiology of the pneumonia may be obscure. Blood cultures, which are positive in 10 to 20 percent of patients with nosocomial pneumonia, should be performed.[91]

Empiric treatment for a nosocomial pneumonia should provide antibiotic coverage for aerobic gram-negative bacilli and *S. aureus*. Cefoxitin plus an aminoglycoside or clindamycin plus an aminoglycoside is appropriate. These regimens include coverage for mouth anaerobes. If aminoglycoside toxicity is a concern, a third-generation cephalosporin alone (cefotaxime, cefoperazone, or ceftazidime) may be substituted.[23,24] After a pathogen is identified, a specific antibiotic can be selected. In general, a single agent is adequate for treatment of most nosocomial pneumonias. However, for a severe *P. aeruginosa* pneumonia, a two-drug regimen of an aminoglycoside plus an antipseudomonal beta-lactam is recommended. Erythromycin is the drug of choice for suspected or documented *Legionella* pneumonia.[85]

INFECTIONS IN RENAL TRANSPLANTS

Renal transplant recipients are given immunosuppressive drugs, which cause patients to become susceptible not only to the infectious complications associated with other types of urologic surgery but also to certain unique infectious disease syndromes resulting from opportunistic pathogens (Fig. 3–4).[92] A more detailed account of the epidemiology and clinical manifestations of these infections can be found in other references.[8,93,94] A few comments on therapy are made in this chapter.

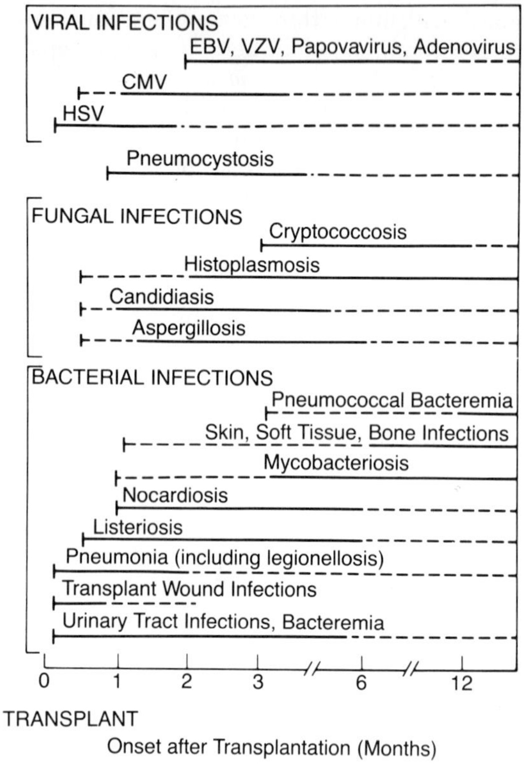

Figure 3–4. Timing of infectious diseases after renal transplantation. Solid lines indicate periods of peak incidence. (From Peterson PK, Simmons RL: Infections in organ transplant recipients. In Mandel GL, Douglas RG, Bennett JE, eds: Principles and Practice in Infectious Diseases, 2nd ed. New York, John Wiley and Sons, 1985, pp 1676–1680.)

During the immediate post-transplant period, oral and genital herpes simplex viral infections are common and are treated with intravenous acyclovir (5 mg/kg every 8 hours for 7 to 10 days) or oral acyclovir (400 mg five times per day for 7 to 10 days).[7] Topical acyclovir is not as effective for the more severe herpes simplex viral infections seen in transplant patients. Localized oral or esophageal candidiasis may also develop. Oral nystatin (10^6 units four times per day), clotrimazole (one troche four times per day), or ketoconazole (400 to 600 mg/day) are used for these localized *Candida* infections but intravenous amphotericin (0.7 to 1.0 mg/kg/day) is necessary when disseminated *Candida* infection occurs.[7] A total dose of 1.0 to 1.5 gm is recommended.

For the patient in whom pneumonia develops between the first and sixth month after transplantation, especially when the pneumonia is a complication of immunosuppressive therapy for graft rejection, *Aspergillus, Pneumocystis carinii, Nocardia,* and cytomegalovirus (CMV), as well as more common bacterial pathogens, need to be considered.[95] Bronchoscopy or an open lung biopsy is usually required to make the diagnosis. Intravenous amphotericin (0.7 to 1.0 mg/kg/day) is the treatment of choice for *Aspergillus,* and a total dose of 1.0 to 2.0 gm is given.[7] Trimethoprim-sulfamethoxazole is used for treatment of *P. carinii* or *Nocardia* pulmonary infection. The dosage of trimethoprim-sulfamethoxazole for *P. carinii* is 20 mg of trimethoprim and 100 mg of sulfamethoxazole/kg/day given in four divided doses for 14 to 21 days.[7] *Nocardia* infections are treated with 160 mg of trimethoprim and 800 mg of sulfamethoxazole three to four times a day for several months.[96] There is no therapy of proven value for (CMV) pneumonia, but ganciclovir is a new antiviral currently being evaluated for treatment of CMV infection.[97] Besides causing pneumonia, CMV may cause persistent fevers, leukopenia, thrombocytopenia, hepatitis, and retinitis. Prophylactic CMV-immune globulin may modify the severity of CMV infection after renal transplantation.[98]

Listeria and *Cryptococcus* are two common pathogens causing central nervous system infections in renal transplant recipients. Symptoms and signs of meningitis may be blunted in many patients. Persistent nonspecific headaches or a slight change in mental status should prompt an analysis and culture of the cerebrospinal fluid. Ampicillin, 2 gm intravenously every 4 hours, is the preferred drug for *Listeria* meningoencephalitis.[99] A combination of intravenous amphotericin (0.3 mg/kg/day) plus oral flucytosine (150 mg/kg/day given in four divided doses) is effective therapy for cryptococcal meningitis.[100]

Opportunistic infections occurring several months after renal transplantation include localized herpes zoster, warts, Epstein-Barr virus (EBV) infection, atypical mycobacterial soft-tissue and bone infections, and pneumococcal bacteremia. Intravenous acyclovir (10 mg/kg every 8 hours) or high doses of oral acyclovir (800 mg five times a day) is the therapy of choice for herpes zoster infection.[7] Cutaneous wart infections due to papillomavirus may be difficult to control by traditional means (cryosurgery with liquid nitrogen, topical podophyllum) unless immunosuppressive therapy is reduced. Similarly, there is no established therapy for EBV infection, which may cause a lymphoproliferative syndrome that resolves only after withdrawal of immunosuppressive therapy.[101] Cultures of an ulcerative, chronically draining skin lesion that are repeatedly negative for common bacterial pathogens and fungi should raise the suspicion of atypical mycobacterial infection.[102] A biopsy specimen for special stains and cultures should be obtained for diagnosis. Since atypical mycobacteria vary in their susceptibility to chemotherapeutic agents, the choice of drugs for treatment needs to be guided by susceptibility tests. Patients who have undergone splenectomy are susceptible to pneumococcal infections. Pneumococcal vaccination of splenectomized patients prior to transplantation may prevent some of these infections.[103]

ANTIBIOTIC THERAPY

There has been a remarkable proliferation in the number of new antimicrobial agents. Table 3–3 summarizes the recommended doses of these agents as well as of older antibiotics commonly used for infections in urologic patients.[104] A comprehensive review of the antibacterial spectrum, pharmacokinetics, and toxicity of these different antibiotics is beyond the scope of this chapter; however, a few comments about the potential advantages and limitations of the newer drugs follow.

When different aminoglycosides are used for treatment of infections caused by susceptible bacteria, the efficacy of these agents is similar. The choice of aminoglycoside is largely dependent upon the resistance pattern of gram-negative bacilli within a specific institution. Because gentamicin is less expensive than tobramycin or amikacin, gentamicin is the preferred aminoglycoside when sensitivity testing shows equivalent susceptibility. Most clinical studies have shown no significant difference in the incidence of nephrotoxicity or ototoxicity associated with the different aminoglycosides.[10]

Among the new penicillins, the ureidopenicillins (piperacillin, mezlocillin) have two potential advantages over the older carboxypenicillins (carbenicillin, ticarcillin). Both piperacillin and mezlocillin have activity for *Klebsiella* organisms, which are resistant to carbenicillin and ticarcillin, whereas piperacillin is significantly more active against *P. aeruginosa.*[105] In addition,

Table 3–3. USUAL ADULT DOSES OF ANTIMICROBIAL AGENTS AND INTERVAL OF ADMINISTRATION*

Drug	Dose†	For Creatinine Clearance (ml/min) >80 (hr)	80–50 (hr)	50–10 (hr)	<10 (hr)	Supplemental Dose After Hemodialysis
Aminoglycosides						
Gentamicin	1–1.5 mg/kg	8	8–12	12–24	24–48	1–1.5 mg/kg
Tobramycin	1–1.5 mg/kg	8	8–12	12–24	24–48	1–1.5 mg/kg
Amikacin	5–7.5 mg/kg	8–12	8–12	12	36–48	2.5–5 mg/kg
Penicillins						
Ampicillin	1–2 gm	4–6	6	8	12	0.5 gm
	0.5–1 gm (p.o.)	6	6	8	12	0.5 gm
Amoxicillin	0.25–0.5 gm (p.o.)	8	8	12	12–24	0.25 gm
Penicillin G	1–3 × 10^6 units	4–6	4–6	4–6	⅓–½ maximum daily dose	0.5 × 10^6 units
Penicillin V	0.25–0.5 gm (p.o.)	6	6	8	12	0.25 gm
Oxacillin	1–2 gm	4–6	4–6	4–6	4–6	—
Dicloxacillin	0.25–0.5 gm (p.o.)	6	6	6	6	—
Carbenicillin	5 gm	4	4	3 gm 6	3 gm 12	2 gm
	1–2 tablets (p.o.)	6	—	—	—	—
Ticarcillin	3 gm	4	4	8	12	2 gm
Piperacillin	3 gm	4	4	8	12	2 gm
Mezlocillin	3 gm	4	4	8	12	2 gm
Amoxacillin/ clavulanic acid	0.25–0.5 gm (p.o.)	8	8	12	—	—
Ticarcillin/ clavulanic acid	3.1 gm	4	4	8	12	3.1 gm
Ampicillin/ sulbactam	3 gm	6	6	8	24	1.5 gm
Cephalosporins						
FIRST-GENERATION						
Cefazolin	1 gm	6	8	12	24	0.5 gm
Cephalexin	0.25–1.0 gm (p.o.)	6	6	12	24	0.25–1.0 gm
Cephradine	0.25–1.0 gm (p.o.)	6	6	8	24	0.25–1.0 gm
Cefadroxil	1 gm (p.o.)	12	12	24	36	1 gm
SECOND-GENERATION						
Cefoxitin	2 gm	6	8	12	24	2 gm
Cefuroxime	0.75–1.5 gm	8	8	12	24	0.75–1.0 gm
Cefotetan	2 gm	12	12	24	48	1 gm
Cefaclor	0.25–0.5 gm (p.o.)	8	8	8	8	0.25–0.5 gm
THIRD-GENERATION						
Cefotaxime	2 gm	8	8	12	12	1 gm
Cefoperazone	2 gm	8–12	8–12	8–12	8–12	—
Ceftazidime	2 gm	8	8	1g q12	1g q24	0.5 gm
Ceftizoxime	2 gm	8	8	1g q12	1g q24	0.5 gm
Ceftriaxone	1–2 gm	12	12	12	12	—
Quinolones						
Norfloxacin	0.4 gm (p.o.)	12	12	24	24	—
Ciprofloxacin	0.5–0.75 gm (p.o.)	12	12	24	24	—
Others						
Trimethoprim-sulfamethoxazole	160 mg TMP/800 mg SM (2 tablets p.o.)	12	12	18	—	—
	4–5 mg/kg (as TMP, IV)	8–12	12	18	—	—
Trimethoprim	0.1–0.2 gm (p.o.)	12	12	24	—	
Tetracycline	0.25–0.5 gm (p.o.)	6	—	—	—	—
Erythromycin	0.5–1.0 gm	6	6	6	6	—
	0.25–0.5 gm (p.o.)	6	6	6	6	—
Vancomycin	0.5 gm	6	12	1g q3–7d	1g q5–7d	—
Clindamycin	0.6 gm	6	6	6	6	—
Metronidazole	7.5 mg/kg	6	6	6	6	—
Imipenem/cilastatin	0.5 gm	6	6–8	12	24	0.5 gm
Aztreonam	2 gm	8	8	12	24	0.25 gm

*Modified from The Medical Letter: Handbook of Antimicrobial Therapy. New York, The Medical Letter Inc, 1986.
†Doses are for moderate to severe infections. Route of administration is intravenous unless otherwise stated. If no dose is given, drug is not usually recommended or supplemental dose is not necessary (hemodialysis).
Abbreviation: p.o. = By mouth.

both piperacillin and mezlocillin contain less sodium than do carbenicillin and ticarcillin, and their administration may be associated with less hypokalemia. Thus, piperacillin or mezlocillin may be advantageous for *Klebsiella* and *P. aeruginosa* infections and for treating patients with fluid and electrolyte disturbances.[7]

Clavulanic acid and sulbactam are beta-lactamase inhibitors that inactivate many of the beta-lactamase enzymes responsible for resistance. They protect amoxacillin, ticarcillin, or ampicillin from degradation by beta-lactamase enzymes and extend their spectrum to include many bacteria normally resistant to these drugs.[106,107] However, the combination of amoxacillin/clavulanic acid, ticarcillin/clavulanic acid, or ampicillin/sulbactam has no major advantages for the urologic patient over older agents or other new antibiotics. Ampicillin/sulbactam has very potent anaerobic activity, which makes it more suitable for intra-abdominal and pelvic infections.[51]

Cefazolin and cefoxitin are the two most frequently used parenteral cephalosporins. The use of cefamandole has declined significantly because of the availability of less expensive, older cephalosporins of equivalent efficacy and of newer cephalosporins with broader antibacterial spectrums. Cefotetan is similar in vitro to cefoxitin but is less active against some anaerobes. Although cefotetan therapy is less expensive than cefoxitin therapy, available data are not adequate to determine whether it is equally effective.[108] The coverage of cefuroxime and cefaclor for *Haemophilus influenzae* is useful in pediatric patients but has no advantages for the urologic patient.

The new third-generation cephalosporins have an extended spectrum of activity against gram-negative bacilli, which allows their use in place of the aminoglycosides in patients for whom nephrotoxicity or ototoxicity is a concern.[23,24] Ceftazidime and cefoperazone are especially active against *P. aeruginosa*. Most of the third-generation cephalosporins also retain some activity against methicillin-sensitive *S. aureus* and other gram-positive bacteria, but they are less active than the first-generation cephalosporins or oxacillin.[109] Cefotaxime, ceftazidime, and ceftriaxone are characterized by excellent penetration into the cerebrospinal fluid and are approved for treatment of patients with certain types of meningitis caused by susceptible organisms. Cefoperazone has the unique pharmacokinetic property of being excreted primarily in the bile, and a dosage adjustment is not required in patients with renal failure. The long half-life of ceftriaxone (8 hours) allows administration of this drug every 12 to 24 hours, which is useful for outpatient therapy of mild to moderate infections caused by sensitive organisms. Hypoprothrombinemia has been associated with the use of cephalosporins possessing a methylthiotetrazole side chain (moxalactam, cefoperazone, cefotetan, cefomandole), and weekly prophylactic vitamin K should be administered to patients receiving these drugs.[110] Coagulation abnormalities and bleeding were reported so frequently with moxalactam that this cephalosporin is now used infrequently.

Norfloxacin and ciprofloxacin are two new oral fluorinated quinolones with a much broader spectrum of antibacterial activity than older quinolones like nalidixic acid, oxalinic acid, and cinoxacin.[21,22] The antibacterial spectrum of norfloxacin and ciprofloxacin covers the common gram-negative bacillary pathogens associated with complicated urinary tract infections, including *P. aeruginosa*, *Serratia*, *Proteus*, and *Providencia*. Oral therapy with norfloxacin or ciprofloxacin is especially useful in place of parenteral antibiotic therapy in outpatients or as follow-up to parenteral therapy in patients ready for discharge from the hospital.

Imipenem is the first of a new class of antibiotics called the *carbapenems*.[111] It is the broadest-spectrum antibiotic commercially available and has potent activity against a wide range of gram-negative, gram-positive, and anaerobic bacteria. Imipenem is administered with cilastatin, a molecule that blocks the metabolism of imipenem by the renal dipeptidase enzyme, dehydropeptidase I. The extreme broad spectrum of imipenem allows this drug to be used for treatment of infections caused by organisms resistant to the penicillins, cephalosporins, and aminoglycosides or as a substitute for combination therapy with the aminoglycosides in patients at risk for nephrotoxicity. Seizures associated with high doses of imipenem have been reported in patients with structural or metabolic abnormalities affecting the central nervous system or with impaired renal function.[111] The administration of imipenem needs to be closely monitored in patients with factors that may predispose them to seizures.

In contrast to imipenem, aztreonam is a new antibiotic with a very narrow antibacterial spectrum confined entirely to gram-negative organisms.[112] Aztreonam belongs to a class of antibiotic called the *monobactams*, which have a unique monocyclic beta-lactam nucleus. Azmonocyclic beta-lactam nucleus. Aztreonam has no major advantages over other new antibiotics for the urologic patient except that its unique structure allows it to be used cautiously in patients allergic to the penicillins and cephalosporins.[113]

Although vancomycin is an older antimicrobial agent, its use has markedly increased because of the growing number of infections caused by methicillin-resistant *S. aureus* and *S. epidermidis*.[57,58] Many of these infections involve central intravenous catheters or dialysis shunts. Vancomycin is a convenient drug for dialysis patients because the drug is not removed by hemodialysis.

Table 3–4 summarizes recommended antibiotics for empiric therapy of common infectious complications of urologic surgery.

PROPHYLACTIC ANTIBIOTICS

The use of antibiotics for the prevention of infections after urologic surgery depends on the preoperative condition of the patient and the type of surgical procedure performed. When the need for prophylaxis is being determined, patients should be placed into one of the following categories: (1) those with preoperative bacteriuria; (2) those with preoperative sterile urine; (3) those undergoing procedures involving entry into the gastrointestinal tract; and (4) those with underlying valvular heart disease.

Patients with documented bacteriuria should clearly receive appropriate *antibiotic therapy* for their infection before instrumentation (cystoscopy, retrograde catheterization, cystography) or surgical manipulation (prostatectomy, urethral dilatation) of the urinary tract. The choice of antibiotic is based on the results of a urine culture and sensitivity testing. If possible, the instrumentation or surgery should be deferred until the urine is sterile. If a delay is not possible, a preoperative dose of an appropriate antibiotic is given at the time of surgery. The *antibiotic treatment* is then continued postoperatively for 7 to 10 days.

The need for antibiotic prophylaxis in patients with sterile preoperative urine is controversial.[4,114–117] Some of the controversy stems from previous trials of antibiotic prophylaxis, which were inconclusive as a result of flaws in design and methodology.[118] Nevertheless, several recent prospective, randomized, controlled studies suggest that antibiotic prophylaxis reduces the incidence of infection in patients whose urine is sterile preoperatively and who are undergoing transurethral resection of the prostate. Based on these results, antibiotic prophylaxis has been recommended by some investigators during transurethral surgery in high-risk patients (debilitated, diabetic, immunosuppressed, and in patients receiving a penile or other prosthetic device).[4,114–116] In most cases, one perioperative dose or a 24-hour perioperative regimen of a parenteral cephalosporin is given. Continued prophylaxis beyond 24 hours has no proven advantages and may increase the risk for a resistant superinfection or an adverse drug reaction.

Table 3–4. EMPIRIC THERAPY FOR INFECTIOUS COMPLICATIONS OF UROLOGIC SURGERY

Infection	Antimicrobial Agent
Urinary tract infection	Trimethoprim-sulfamethoxazole, norfloxacin, ciprofloxacin, or oral cephalosporin
Prostatitis	Trimethoprim-sulfamethoxazole, trimethoprim, or oral carbenicillin indanyl sodium
Epididymitis	Trimethoprim-sulfamethoxazole, trimethoprim, tetracycline, or oral carbenicillin indanyl sodium
Wound infection	
Streptococcus	Penicillin or cephalosporin or vancomycin
Staphylococcus	Oxacillin or cephalosporin
Gram-negative bacilli	Aminoglycoside or cephalosporin
Necrotizing soft-tissue	Penicillin + clindamycin + aminoglycoside
Bacteremia from	
Urinary source	Aminoglycoside or third-generation cephalosporin + ampicillin, piperacillin or mezlocillin
Nonurinary source	Aminoglycoside or third-generation cephalosporin + oxacillin
Central intravenous catheter	Aminoglycoside or third-generation cephalosporin + vancomycin
Neutropenic patient	Aminoglycoside + antipseudomonal penicillin or third-generation cephalosporin
Pneumonia	Cefoxitin or clindamycin + aminoglycoside or a third-generation cephalosporin alone

Patients undergoing ureterointestinal diversion or reconstruction of the urinary tract using intestinal segments (augmentation cystoplasty, ileal ureteral replacement) should receive a preoperative bowel preparation that includes both mechanical cleansing and an oral antibiotic combination effective in suppressing the colonic aerobes and anaerobes. A widely used preoperative regimen consists of a low-residue diet, magnesium sulfate, saline enemas, and a neomycin-erythromycin base.[119] Neomycin and erythromycin are each given at doses of 1.0 gm orally at 1:00 P.M., 2:00 P.M., and 11:00 P.M. on the day before surgery. Whether a parenteral antibiotic (usually a cephalosporin) needs to be combined with the oral antibiotic regimen is controversial, but one study has suggested no benefit.[120]

Prior to instrumentation or surgical manipulation of the urinary tract, patients with suspected or documented valvular heart disease should receive antibiotic prophylaxis for prevention of endocarditis. The prophylaxis should be directed against group D streptococci and gram-negative bacilli.[59,121] A recommended regimen is ampicillin (2 gm intravenously 30 minutes before the procedure) plus gentamicin (1.5 mg/kg intravenously 30 minutes before the procedure).[122] For patients allergic to penicillin, vancomycin (1.0 gm given by slow intravenous infusion 1 hour before the procedure) is substituted for the ampicillin.

References

1. Rutledge KA, McDonald HP: Costs of treating simple nosocomial urinary tract infection. Urology 26:24–26, 1985.
2. Cruse PJE, Foord R: The epidemiology of wound infection: a 10-year prospective study of 62,939 wounds. Surg Clin North Am 60:27–40, 1980.
3. Meares EM: Factors that influence surgical wound infections: role of prophylactic antibiotic therapy. Urology 6:535–545, 1975.
4. Childs SJ: Perioperative prevention of infection in genitourinary surgery. Antibiot Chemother 33:1–29, 1985.
5. Hartstein AI, Garber SB, Ward TT, Jone SR, Morthland VH: Nosocomial urinary infection: a prospective evaluation of 108 catheterized patients. Infect Control 2:380–386, 1981.
6. Saltzman RL, Peterson PK: Immunodeficiency of the elderly. Rev Infect Dis 9:1127–1139, 1987.
7. Ho WG, Winston DJ: Infection and transfusion therapy in acute leukemia. Clin Hematol 15:873–904, 1986.
8. Rubin RH, Wolfson JS, Cosimi AB, Tolkoff-Rubin NE: Infection in the renal transplant recipient. Am J Med 70:405–411, 1981.
9. Gross RL, Newborne PM: Role of nutrition in immunologic functions. Physiol Rev 60:188–302, 1980.
10. Kunin CM: Detection, Prevention and Management of Urinary Tract Infections. 4th ed. Philadelphia, Lea and Febiger, 1987.
11. Horan TC, White JW, Jarvis WL, Emori TG, Culver DH, Munn VP, Thornsberry C, Olson DR, Hughes JM: Nosocomial infection surveillance, 1984. MMWR 35:1755–2955, 1986.
12. Fowler JE, Marshall VM: Nosocomial catheter-associated urinary tract infection. Infect Surg 2:43–45, 1983.
13. Rutala WA, Kennedy VA, Loflin SB, Sarubbi FA: *Serratia marcesens* nosocomial infections of the urinary tract associated with urine measuring containers and urinometers. Am J Med 70:659–663, 1981.
14. Turck M, Stamm WE: Nosocomial infection of the urinary tract. Am J Med 70:651–654, 1981.
15. Schaberg DA, Weinstein RA, Stamm WE: Epidemic of nosocomial urinary tract infection caused by multiple resistant gram-negative bacilli: epidemiology and control. J Infect Dis 133:363–366, 1976.
16. Jenkins RD, Fenn JP, Matsen JM: Review of urine microscopy for bacteriuria. JAMA 255:3397–3403, 1986.
17. Kass EH: Asymptomatic infections of the urinary tract. Trans Assoc Am Physicians 69:56–63, 1986.
18. Stamm WE: Quantitative urine cultures revisited. Eur J Clin Microbiol 3:279–281, 1984.
19. Andriole VT: Diagnosis of urinary tract infection by culture. In Kaye D, ed: Urinary Tract Infection and Its Management. St. Louis, CV Mosby, 1972, pp 28–42.
20. Thomas VL, Forland M: Antibody-coated bacteria in urinary tract infections. Kidney Int 21:1–7, 1982.
21. Wolfson JS, Hooper DC: Fluoroquinolones: structures, mechanisms of action and resistance, and spectra of activity in vitro. Antimicrob Agents Chemother 28:581–586, 1985.
22. Hooper DC, Wolfson JS: The fluoroquinolones: pharmacology, clinical uses, and toxicities. Antimicrob Agents Chemother 28:716–721, 1985.
23. Neu HC: The new beta-lactamase–stable cephalosporins. Ann Intern Med 97:408–419, 1982.
24. Neu HC: Structure-activity relations of new beta-lactam compounds and in vitro activity against common bacteria. Rev Infect Dis 5(Suppl 2):S319–S337, 1983.
25. Wise GJ, Kozinn PJ, Goldberg P: Amphotericin B as a urologic irrigant in the management of noninvasive candiduria. J Urol 128:82–84, 1982.
26. Wise GJ, Kozinn PJ, Goldberg P: Flucytosine in the management of genitourinary candidiasis: 5 years of experience. J Urol 124:70–72, 1980.
27. Graybill JR, Galgiani JN, Jorgensen JH, Strandberg DA: Ketoconazole therapy for fungal urinary tract infections. J Urol 129:68–70, 1983.
28. Humphrey MJ, Jevons S, Tarbit MH: Pharmacokinetic evaluation of fluconazole (UK-49,858), a metabolically stable triazole and antifungal drug. Antimicrob Agents Chemother 28:648–653, 1985.
29. Benson M, Li Puma JP, Resnick MI: The role of imaging studies in urinary tract infection. Urol Clin North Am 14:605–625, 1986.
30. Bernardino ME, Baumgartner BR: Abscess drainage in the genitourinary tract. Intervent Uroradiol 24:539–549, 1986.
31. Shortliffe LMD, Spigelman SS: Infection stones: evaluation and management. Urol Clin North Am 13:717–726, 1986.
32. Turck M, Ronald AR, Petersdorf RG: Relapse and reinfection in chronic bacteriuria. II. The correlation be-

tween site of infection and pattern of recurrence in chronic bacteriuria. N Engl J Med 278:422–427, 1968.
33. Meares EM, Stamey TA: Bacteriologic localization patterns in bacterial prostatitis and urethritis. Invest Urol 5:492–518, 1968.
34. Meares EM: Prostatitis. Ann Rev Med 30:279–288, 1979.
35. Winningham DG, Nemoy NJ, Stamey TA: Diffusion of antibiotics from plasma into prostatic fluid. Nature 219:139–143, 1968.
36. Schaeffer AJ: Pharmacokinetics of antibiotics used in treatment of prostatitis. Urology 24(Suppl):8–9, 1984.
37. Sabbaj J, Hoagland VL, Cook T: Norfloxacin versus cotrimoxazole in the treatment of recurring urinary tract infection in men. Scand J Infect Dis 48(Suppl):48–53, 1986.
38. Childs SJ: Treatment of chronic bacterial prostatitis with ciprofloxacin. Infect Surg 6:649–651, 1987.
39. Wong ES: Guideline for prevention of catheter-associated urinary tract infection. Infect Control 2:125–130, 1981.
40. Burke JP, Garibaldi RA, Britt MR, Jacobson JA, Conti M, Alling DW: Prevention of catheter-associated urinary tract infections: efficacy of daily mental care regimens. Am J Med 70:655–658, 1981.
41. Warren JW, Platt R, Thomas RJ, Rosner B, Kass EH: Antibiotic irrigation and catheter-associated urinary tract infections. N Engl J Med 299:570–573, 1978.
42. Thompson RL, Haley CE, Searcy MA, Guenthner MT, Kaiser DL, Groschel DHM, Gillenwater JY, Wenzel RP: Failure to reduce attack rates of catheter-associated bacteriuria by periodic instillations of a disinfectant into urinary drainage systems. JAMA 251:747–751, 1984.
43. Berger RE, Alexander R, Harnisch JP, Paulsen CA, Monda GD, Ansell J, Holmes KK: Etiology, manifestations and therapy of acute epididymitis: prospective study of 50 cases. J Urol 121:750–754, 1979.
44. Witherington R, Harper WM: The surgical management of acute bacterial epididymitis with emphasis on epididymotomy. J Urol 128:722–725, 1982.
45. Edwards LD: The epidemiology of 2,056 remote-site infections and 1,966 surgical wound infections occurring in 1,865 patients. Ann Surg 184:758–766, 1976.
46. Ad Hoc Committee of the Committee on Trauma, National Research Council Division of National Academy of Sciences: Postoperative wound infections: the influence of ultraviolet irradiation of the operating room and of various other factors. Ann Surg 2(Suppl):1–192, 1964.
47. Seropian R, Reynolds BM: Wound infections after postoperative depilatory versus razor preparation. Am J Surg 121:251–254, 1971.
48. Stone HH: Infection in postoperative patients. Am J Med 81(Suppl 1A):39–44, 1986.
49. Carroll RR, Cattolica EV, Turzan CW, McAninch JW: Necrotizing soft-tissue infections of the perineum and genitalia. West J Med 144:174–178, 1986.
50. Bouza E, Winston DJ, Hewitt WL: Infectious osteitis pubis. Urology 12:663–669, 1978.
51. Reinhardt JF, Johnston L, Ruane P, Johnson CC, Ingram-Drake L, MacDonald K, Ward KW, Mathisen G, George WL, Finegold SM, Mulligan ME: A randomized, double-blind comparison of sulbactam/ampicillin and clindamycin for the treatment of aerobic and aerobic-anaerobic infections. Rev Infect Dis 8(Suppl 5):S569–S575, 1986.
52. Kreger BE, Craven DE, Carling PC, McCabe WR: Gram-negative bacteremia: III. Reassessment of etiology, epidemiology, and ecology in 612 patients. Am J Med 68:332–343, 1980.
53. Fried MA, Vosti KL: The importance of underlying disease in patients with gram-negative bacteremia. Arch Intern Med 121:418–423, 1968.
54. McCabe WR: Incidence of gram-negative rod bacteremia. N Engl J Med 292:111, 1975.
55. Sullivan NM, Sutter VL, Carter WT, Attebery HR, Finegold SM: Bacteremia after genitourinary tract manipulation: bacteriological aspects and evaluation of various blood culture systems. Appl Microbiol 23:1101–1106, 1972.
56. Weinstein MP, Murphy JR, Reller LB, Lichtenstein KA: The clinical significance of positive blood cultures: comprehensive analysis of 500 episodes of bacteremia and fungemia in adults. II. Clinical observations, with special reference to factors influencing prognosis. Rev Infect Dis 5:54–70, 1983.
57. Winston DJ, Dudnick DV, Chapin M, Ho WG, Gale RP, Martin WJ: Coagulase-negative staphylococcal bacteremia in patients receiving immunosuppressive therapy. Arch Intern Med 143:32–36, 1983.
58. Christensen GD, Bisno AL, Paris JT, McLaughin B, Heaster MG, Luther RW: Nosocomial septicemia due to multiple antibiotic-resistant *Staphylococcus epidermidis*. Ann Intern Med 96:1–10, 1982.
59. Mandell GL, Kaye D, Levison ME, Hook EW: Enterococcal endocarditis: an analysis of 38 patients observed at the New York Hospital–Cornell Medical Center. Arch Intern Med 125:258–264, 1970.
60. Gunnar RM, Loeb HS, Winslow EJ, Blain C, Robinson J: Hemodynamic measurements in bacteremia and septic shock in man. J Infect Dis 128(Suppl): S295–S298, 1973.
61. McCabe WR, Olans RN: Shock in gram-negative bacteremia: predisposing factors, pathophysiology, and treatment. In Remington JS, Swartz MN, eds: Current Clinical Topics in Infectious Diseases. New York, McGraw-Hill, Vol. 2, 1981, pp 121–150.
62. Tracey KJ, Beutler B, Lowry SF, Merryweather J, Wolep S, Milsark IW, Hariri RJ, Fahey TJ, Zantella A, Albert JD, Shires GT, Cerami A: Shock and tissue injury induced by recombinant human cachectin. Science 234:470–474, 1986.
63. Beutler B, Milsark IW, Cerami AC: Passive immunization against cachectin/tumor necrosis factor protects mice from lethal effect of endotoxin. Science 229:869–871, 1985.
64. Gurlil NJ, Reynolds PG, Varguish T, Lutz SA, Ganes E: Primate endotoxemic shock reversed by opiate receptor blockage with naloxone. Physiologist 24:118, 1981.
65. Jacobs ER, Soulsby ME, Bone RC, Wilson FJ, Hiller FC: Ibuprofen in canine endotoxin shock. J Clin Invest 70:536–541, 1982.
66. Kreger BE, Craven DE, McCabe WR: Gram-negative bacteremia IV: Re-evaluation of clinical features and treatment in 612 patients. Am J Med 68:344–355, 1980.
67. Sullivan N, Sutter VL, Mims MM, Marsh VH, Finegold SM: Clinical aspects of bacteremia after manipulation of the genitourinary tract. J Infect Dis 120:49–55, 1963.
68. Kaplan RL, Sahn SA, Petty TL: Incidence and outcome of the respiratory distress syndrome in gram-negative sepsis. Arch Intern Med 139:867–869, 1979.
69. Colman RW, Robby SJ, Minnia JD: Disseminated intravascular coagulation: a reappraisal. Ann Rev Med 30:359, 1979.
70. Elin RJ, Robinson RA, Levine AS, Wolff SM: Lack of

clinical usefulness of the limulus test in the diagnosis of endotoxemia. N Engl J Med 293:521–524, 1975.
71. Bove RC, Fisher CJ, Clemmen TP, Slotman GJ, Metz CA, Balk RA: Methylprednisolone Severe Sepsis Study Group: a controlled clinical trial of high-dose methylprednisolone in the treatment of severe sepsis and septic shock. N Engl J Med 317:653–658, 1987.
72. The Veterans Administration Systemic Sepsis Cooperative Study Group: Effect of high-dose glucocorticoid therapy on mortality in patients with clinical signs of systemic sepsis. N Engl J Med 317:659–665, 1987.
73. Peters WP, Johnson MW, Friedman PA, Mitch WE: Pressor effect of naloxone in septic shock. Lancet 1:529–532, 1981.
74. Groeger TS, Grafiano CC, Howland WS: Naloxone in septic shock. Crit Care Med 11:650–654, 1983.
75. McCabe WR, Kreger RB, Johns M: Type-specific and cross reactive antibodies in gram-negative bacteremia. N Engl J Med 287:261–267, 1972.
76. Young LS, Ingram J, Stevens P: Functional role of antibody against core glycolipid of Enterobacteriaceae. J Clin Invest 56:850–861, 1975.
77. Ziegler EJ, McCutchan JA, Fierer J, Glauser MP, Sadoff JC, Douglas H, Braude AI: Treatment of gram-negative bacteremia and shock with human antiserum to a mutant *Escherichia coli.* N Engl J Med 307:1225–1230, 1982.
78. Garibaldi RA, Britt MR, Coleman ML, Reading JC, Pace NL: Risk factors for postoperative pneumonia. Am J Med 70:677–680, 1981.
79. Cross AS, Roup B: Role of respiratory assistance devices in endemic nosocomial pneumonia. Am J Med 70:681–685, 1981.
80. Johnson WG, Pierce AK, Sanford JP, Thomas GO: Nosocomial respiratory infections with gram-negative bacilli. Ann Intern Med 77:701–706, 1972.
81. Johnson WG, Higuchi JH, Chadhur TR, Woods DE: Bacterial adherence to epithelial cells in bacillary colonization of the upper respiratory tract. Am Rev Respir Dis 121:55–63, 1980.
82. Schwartz SN, Dowling JN, Benkovic C, DeQuittner-Buchanan M, Prostko T, Yee RB: Sources of gram-negative bacilli colonizing the tracheae of intubated patients. J Infect Dis 138:227–231, 1978.
83. Maki DG, Alvarado CJ, Hasspman CA, Zilz MA: Relation of the inanimate hospital environment to endemic nosocomial infection. N Engl J Med 307:1562–1566, 1982.
84. Glew RH, Mollering RC, Kunz LJ: Infection with *Acinetobacter calcoaceticus (Herellea vaginicola).* Clinical and laboratory studies. Medicine 56:79–97, 1977.
85. Yu VL: Nosocomial legionellosis: current epidemiological issues. In Remington JS, Swartz MN, eds: Current Clinical Topics: Infectious Disease, Vol 7, New York, McGraw-Hill, 1986, pp 239–253.
86. Meyer RD, Young LS, Armstrong D, Yu B: Aspergillosis complicating neoplastic disease. Am J Med 56:6–15, 1973.
87. Hall CB, Douglas RG, Geiman JM, Messner MK: Nosocomial respiratory syncytial virus infections. N Engl J Med 293:1343–1346, 1975.
88. Murray PR, Washington JA: Microscopic and bacteriologic analysis of expectorated sputum. Mayo Clin Proc 50:339–344, 1975.
89. Bartlett JG: Diagnostic accuracy of transtracheal aspiration bacteriologic studies. Am Rev Respir Dis 115:777–782, 1977.
90. Wimberley NW, Bass JB, Boyd BW, Kirkpatrick MB, Serio RA, Pollock HM: Use of a bronchoscopic protected catheter brush for the diagnosis of pulmonary infections. Chest 80:556–562, 1982.
91. Graybill JR, Marshall LW, Charsche P, Wallace CK, Melvin VB: Nosocomial pneumonia. Am Rev Respir Dis 108:1130–1140, 1973.
92. Peterson PK, Simmons RL: Infections in organ transplant recipients. In Mandel GL, Douglas RG, Bennett JE, eds: Principles and Practice of Infectious Diseases, 2nd ed. New York, John Wiley and Sons, 1985, pp 1676–1680.
93. Peterson PK, Ferguson R, Fryd DS, Balfour HH, Rynasiewicz J, Simmons RL: Infectious diseases in hospitalized renal transplant recipients: a prospective study of a complex and evolving problem. Medicine 61:360–372, 1982.
94. Masur H, Cheigh JS, Stubenbord WT: Infection following renal transplantation: a changing pattern. Rev Infect Dis 4:1208–1219, 1982.
95. Ramsey PG, Rubin RH, Tolkoff-Rubin NE, Cosimi AB, Rusell PS, Greene R: The renal transplant patient with fever and pulmonary infiltrates: etiology, clinical manifestations, and management. Medicine 59:206–222, 1980.
96. Wallace RJ, Septimus EJ, Williams TW, Conklin RH, Satterwhite TK, Bushby MB, Hollowell DC: Use of trimethoprim-sulfamethoxazole for treatment of infections due to nocardia. Rev Infect Dis 4:315–325, 1982.
97. Winston DJ, Ho WG, Bantoni K, Holland GN, Mitsuyasu RT, Gale RP, Busuttil RW, Champlin RE: Ganciclovir therapy of cytomegalovirus infections in bone marrow transplants and other immunosuppressed patients. Rev Infect Dis 10(Suppl 3):S547–S553, 1988.
98. Syndman DR, Werner BG, Heinze-Lacey B, Berardo VP, Tilney NL, Kirkman RL, Milford EL, Cho SI, Bush HL, Levey AS, Strom TB, Carpenter CB, Levey RH, Harman WE, Zimmerman CE, Shapiro ME, Steinman T, LoGerfo F, Idelson B, Schroter GPJ, Levin MJ, McIven J, Leszczynski J, Grady GF: Use of cytomegalovirus immune globulin to prevent cytomegalovirus disease in renal-transplant recipients. N Engl J Med 317:1049–1054, 1987.
99. Stomm AM, Nijmuker WE, Simmons BP, Cobbs CG, Elliott A, Budrich P, Harman J: Listeriosis in renal transplant recipients: report of an outbreak and review of 102 cases. Rev Infect Dis 4:665–682, 1982.
100. Dismukes WE, Cloud G, Gallis HA, Kerkering TM, Medoff G, Craven PC, Kaplowitz LG, Fisher JF, Gregg CR, Bowles CA, Shadomy J, Stamm AM, Dissio RB, Kaufman L, Soong SJ, Blackwelder WC, NIAID Mycoses Study Group: Treatment of cryptococcal meningitis with combination amphotericin and flucytosine for four as compared with six weeks. N Engl J Med 317:334–341, 1987.
101. Hanto DW, Frizzera G, Purtilo DT, Sakamoto K, Sullivan JL, Saemunchson AK, Klein G, Simmons RL, Najarian JS: Clinical spectrum of lymphoproliferative disorders in renal transplant recipients and evidence for the role of Epstein-Barr virus. Cancer Res 41:4253–4261, 1981.
102. Lichtenstein IH, MacGregor RR: Mycobacterial infections in renal transplant recipients: report of five cases and review of the literature. Rev Infect Dis 5:216–226, 1983.
103. Linnemann CC, Finot MR, Schiffman G: Response to pneumococcal vaccine in renal transplant and hemodialysis patients. Arch Intern Med 141:1637–1640, 1981.
104. The Medical Letter: Handbook of Antimicrobial Therapy. New York, The Medical Letter, Inc, 1986.

105. Eliopoulos GM, Mollering RC: Azlocillin, mezlocillin and piperacillin: new broad-spectrum penicillins. Ann Intern Med 97:755–760, 1982.
106. Sutherland R, Beole AS, Boon RJ, Griffin KE, Slocombe B, Stokes DH, White AR: Antibacterial activity of ticarcillin in the presence of clavulanate potassium. Am J Med 79(5B):13–24, 1985.
107. Retsema JA, English AR, Girard A, Lynch JE, Anderson M, Brennan L, Cimochowski C, Faiella J, Norcia W, Sawyer P: Sulbactam/ampicillin: in vitro spectrum, potency, and activity in models of acute infection. Rev Infect Dis 8(Suppl 5):S528–S534, 1986.
108. Cefotetan disodium (cefotan). The Medical Letter 28:70–72, 1986.
109. Thornsberry C: Review of in vitro activity of third-generation cephalosporins and other newer beta-lactam antibiotics against clinically important bacteria. Am J Med 79(Suppl 2A):14–20, 1985.
110. Sattler FR, Weitekamp MR, Ballard JO: Potential for bleeding with the new beta-lactam antibiotics. Ann Intern Med 105:924–931, 1986.
111. Barza M: Imipenem: first of a new class of beta-lactam antibiotics. Ann Intern Med 103:552–560, 1985.
112. Duma RJ: Aztreonam, the first monobactam. Ann Intern Med 106:766–767, 1987.
113. Adkinson NF, Saxon A, Spence MR, Swabb EA: Cross-allergenicity and immunogenicity of aztreonam. Rev Infect Dis 7(Suppl 4):S613–S621, 1985.
114. Madsen PO, Larsen EH, Dorflinger T: The role of antibacterial prophylaxis in urologic surgery. Urology 26(Suppl 1):38–42, 1985.
115. Larsen EH, Gasser TC, Madsen PO: Antimicrobial prophylaxis in urologic surgery. Urol Clin North Am 13:591–604, 1986.
116. Grabe M: Antimicrobial agents in transurethral prostatic resection. J Urol 138:245–252, 1987.
117. Antimicrobial prophylaxis in surgery: The Medical Letter 29:91–94, 1987.
118. Chodak GW, Plaut ME: Systemic antibiotics for prophylaxis in urologic surgery: a critical review. J Urol 121:695–699, 1979.
119. Clarke JS, Condon RE, Bartlett JG, Gorbach SL, Nichols RL, Ochi S: Preoperative oral antibiotics reduce septic complications of colon operations: results of prospective, randomized, double-blind clinical study. Ann Surg 186:251–259, 1977.
120. Condon RE, Bartlett JG, Greenlee H, Schulte WJ, Ochi S, Abbe R, Caruana JA, Gordon E, Horsley JS, Irvin G, Johnson W, Jordan P, Keitzer F, Lempke R, Read RC, Schuman W, Schwartz M, Storm FK, Vetto M: Efficacy of oral and systemic antibiotic prophylaxis in colorectal operations. Arch Surg 118:496–502, 1983.
121. Marrien R, Valenti AJ, Madri JA: Gram-negative endocarditis following cystoscopy. J Urol 119:134–137, 1978.
122. Prevention of bacterial endocarditis. The Medical Letter. 29:109–110, 1987.

HEMATOLOGIC CONSIDERATIONS IN UROLOGIC SURGERY

4

Matthew L. Wilner • Michael H. Rosove

INTRODUCTION

Hematologic disorders may have considerable impact on the patient who is undergoing urologic surgery. The hematologic complications most frequently associated with urologic surgery are hemorrhage and thromboembolic disease. These problems may arise from either coexistent hematologic abnormalities independent of the urologic disease process or hematologic disorders secondary to it.

This chapter reviews (1) the normal hemostatic mechanisms, (2) clinically relevant abnormalities of the cellular and soluble blood components with reference to their preoperative recognition and management, and (3) prophylaxis and treatment for the postoperative hematologic complications encountered in urologic surgery patients.

NORMAL HEMOSTASIS

The mechanism of hemostasis following loss of integrity of a blood vessel involves vasoconstriction, platelet plug formation, and fibrin deposition. Platelets adhere to exposed subendothelial structures such as collagen. The release reaction, in which the platelets extrude the contents of their secretory granules, then takes place. This stimulates further platelet aggregation at the site of injury and is augmented by the metabolism of arachidonic acid by cyclooxygenase to cyclic endoperoxides and thromboxanes.

The coagulation mechanism consists of a series of inactive enzymes that are sequentially activated in a cascade fashion, thus amplifying the initial stimulus and leading to the formation of thrombin, which then generates the insoluble fibrin clot from its precursor fibrinogen (Fig. 4–1). This mechanism can be initiated by the intrinsic pathway, which depends on the surface activation of factor XII, or the extrinsic pathway, which requires tissue thromboplastin released from damaged tissue. Subsequent enzyme complexes are formed in association with phospholipid, which is derived from platelet. Once insoluble fibrin is formed, it is cross-linked into a stable clot by factor XIII.

The activity of the coagulation mechanism is modified by inhibitors and fibrinolytic activity. The major inhibitor is antithrombin III, which inactivates the activated factors XIIA, XIA, IXA, XA, and thrombin. Thrombin itself can inactivate factors V and VIII, which are also inactivated by activated protein C. Fibrinolysis results from conversion by tissue plasminogen activators of plasminogen into plasmin, which digests fibrin into fibrin-degradation products. The entire process evolves in a delicate equilibrium to produce efficient local hemostasis and to allow subsequent tissue repair. Alterations in the concentrations of factors, cofactors, activators, or inhibitors of the coagulation or fibrinolytic process can result in hemorrhagic or thromboembolic complications.[1]

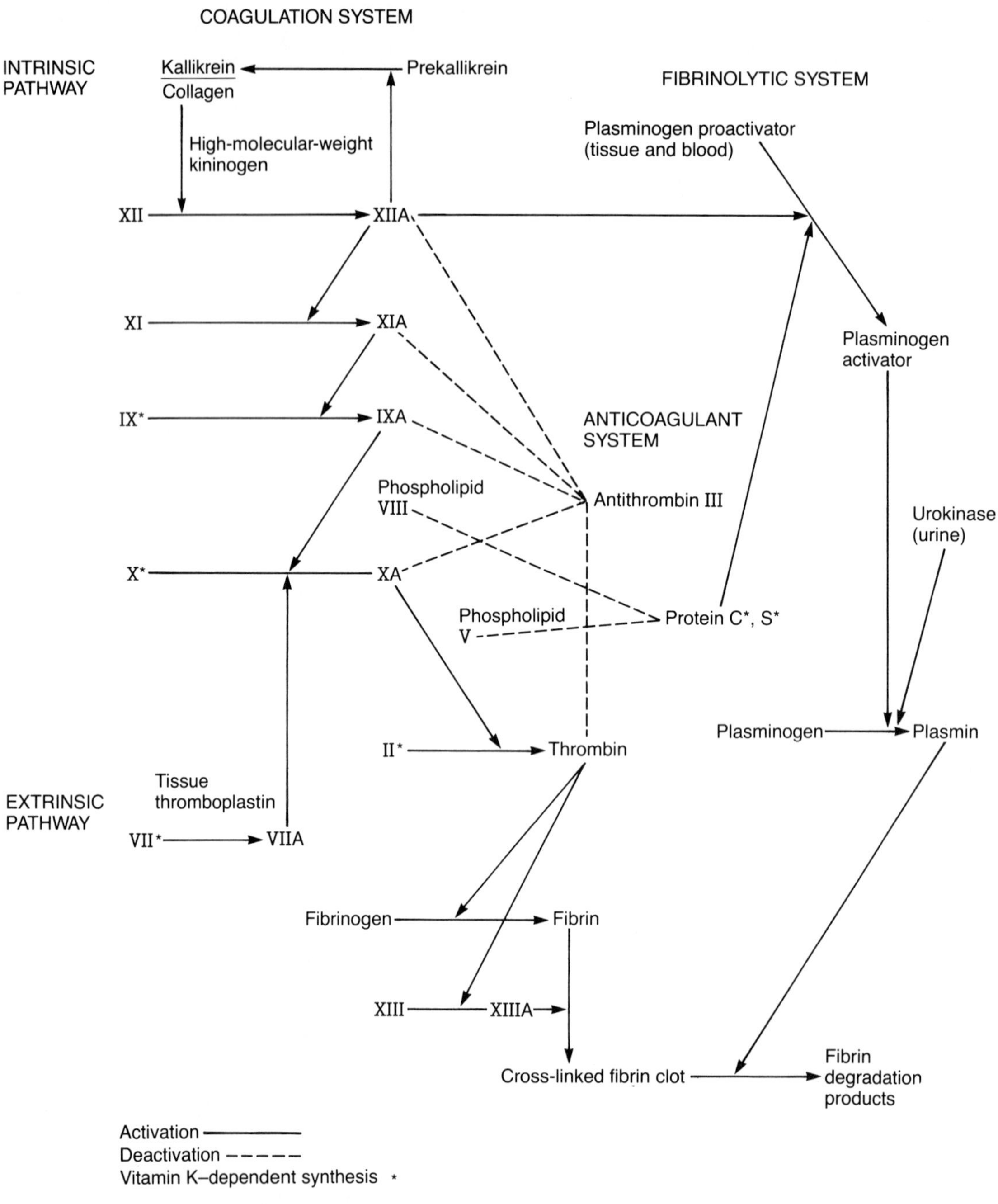

Figure 4–1. Hemostatic cascade.

PREOPERATIVE EVALUATION

The patient with a hemorrhagic diathesis will usually have a history of abnormal bleeding. Specific attention should be directed toward the patient's previous experiences with trauma, dental extractions, and past surgery. Detailed questioning should include whether tendencies toward bruising or prolonged bleeding from minor injury are present and whether previous thromboembolic disease or risk factors exist. Any family history of abnormal bleeding is clearly pertinent. Physical examination is generally unrevealing unless petechiae, purpura, or the stigmata of acquired disease, such as liver failure or uremia, are present. Routine laboratory screening tests should be performed to determine complete blood count, platelet number, prothrombin time (PT), and partial thromboplastin time (PTT). The prothrombin time measures the activity of the extrinsic clotting system, and the partial thromboplastin time measures the intrinsic clotting system. Measurement of the bleeding time is used to identify patients in whom platelet function defects may exist. Further evaluation is not necessary unless history, physical examination, or screening laboratory tests reveal an abnormality.

ABNORMALITIES OF CELLULAR BLOOD COMPONENTS

Anemia

Anemia detected in routine preoperative screening should be approached with respect to two considerations. The first is the functional significance of the anemia with regard to decreased oxygen transport and whether this poses an increased perioperative risk to the patient. The standard preoperative minimum hemoglobin is typically suggested to be 9 to 10 gm%. Lower hemoglobin levels, however, can be tolerated without associated increased morbidity or mortality in some circumstances. In addition to hemoglobin, the delivery of oxygen to body tissues depends on pulmonary gas exchange, the oxygen dissociation curve, and the cardiac output. The minimum acceptable level of hemoglobin in an individual patient must, therefore, take into account the chronicity of the anemia as well as the cardiopulmonary status of the patient.[2]

The second consideration in the evaluation of anemia is the etiology. Anemia may reflect previously unsuspected coexistent disease, which can have a considerable effect on the perioperative course. Understanding the etiology may allow a more precise approach to determining the functional significance of the anemia as well as determining appropriate methods to correct it. Initial diagnostic screening tests include determination of the red blood cell mean corpuscular volume and the reticulocyte count and examination of the appearance of the peripheral blood smear and of the stool for blood. These criteria then direct further investigation.

The anemia may be secondary to the urologic disease. Anemia of chronic disease may accompany chronic renal failure and urologic cancer. Iron deficiency anemia has been associated with renal cell carcinoma when hematuria has been chronic and also may be due to diversion of iron to hemosiderin in the tumor.[3] Direct involvement of the bone marrow by cancer may result in anemia, whereas myelofibrosis may accompany prostate cancer.[4] Radiotherapy for bladder cancer may result in anemia owing to marrow suppression or vitamin B_{12} deficiency as a consequence of radiation-induced damage of the distal ileum.[5] Commonly used antibiotics, including quinolines, nitrofurantoin, and sulfa compounds, can produce hemolytic anemia in patients with glucose-6-phosphate dehydrogenase deficiency.[6] Hemolytic anemia has also been reported in association with renal cell carcinoma and seminoma.[7,8] The thrombotic microangiopathy syndrome of hemolytic anemia and thrombocytopenia has been described in association with prostate cancer, and remission following hormonal therapy for the prostate cancer has occurred.[9] Hematuria itself causes anemia when it is massive or chronic and persistent.

For patients without a correctable underlying cause of anemia and who are judged to be at risk for functional compromise, therapy consists of transfusion with packed red blood cells. Preoperative transfusions should be performed 24 hours in advance to allow for the regeneration of 2,3-diphosphoglycerate, which shifts the oxygen dissociation curve to increase oxygen availability to the tissues. This period allows equilibration of the blood volume following transfusion and permits a better assessment of the change in hemoglobin. Transfusion therapy does have attendant risks of considerable potential morbidity, including hemolytic and allergic reactions and the potential for transmission of viral diseases.

Erythrocytosis

Elevation of the hematocrit level above normal increases blood viscosity and decreases oxygen transport. There is a significant increase in surgical morbidity and mortality, particularly from thromboembolic complications. Erythrocytosis may result from a decrease in plasma volume seen in middle-aged, hypertensive males who smoke. Alternately, erythrocytosis may reflect an increase in red blood cell mass, which is either primary, as in polycythemia vera, or secondary. Secondary erythrocytosis can be a physiologically appropriate response to hypoxic conditions such as severe cardiac and pulmonary disease, high altitude, or hemoglobin abnormalities with increased oxygen affinity.[2] Physiologically inappropriate erythrocytosis may be secondary to neoplasia, such as renal cell carcinoma and Wilms' tumor; other tumors; and possibly from renal cysts and hydronephrosis probably resulting from increased production of erythropoietin.[10–12] Erythrocytosis associated with renal cell carcinoma and Wilms' tumor is resolved following removal of the tumor.[10,12]

It is recommended that patients with polycythemia vera undergo preoperative phlebotomy to lower the hematocrit level to less than 45 percent in order to decrease the risk of thromboembolic complications. In patients with physiologically inappropriate secondary erythrocytosis, the hematocrit level should be lowered to less than 50 percent. When erythrocytosis represents a physiologically appropriate response, the benefits of phlebotomy must be weighed against the risk of decreased oxygen delivery. A hematocrit level between 50 and 60 percent has been recommended in this situation.[2]

Platelet Disorders

A platelet count of greater than 50,000 to 75,000 platelets per microliter (μL) is usually sufficient for adequate surgical hemostasis. Counts less than 50,000 but greater than 20,000 are rarely associated with spontaneous bleeding; however, hemostasis for surgery may be inadequate. Thrombocytopenia is due to decreased production of platelets (primary marrow disorders, alcohol, drugs), increased peripheral destruction of platelets (autoimmune disease, disseminated intravascular coagulation [DIC], sepsis, drugs), sequestration of platelets (splenomegaly, hypothermia), or extracorporeal platelet loss (exsanguination, cardiopulmonary bypass). Rational therapy depends on adequate evaluation. If a treatable underlying cause is not identified, the mainstay of therapy is platelet transfusions. One unit of platelets can be expected to raise the platelet count by 5000 to 10,000. For those patients with increased peripheral destruction or sequestration, there is less response.[13]

Primary thrombocytosis, as with myeloproliferative diseases, can increase the risk for thrombohemorrhagic complications. When the thrombocytosis is secondary to other disease processes, there is no increase in hemorrhagic complications and the potential for thromboembolic events is uncertain.[2,14]

Qualitative platelet disorders are identified by an increased bleeding time despite a normal platelet count. The most common type is von Willebrand's syndrome, which results from the absence of von Willebrand's factor. Wilms' tumor can be associated with acquired von Willebrand's syndrome, which is resolved following removal of the tumor.[15,16]

Inherited intrinsic defects of platelet function are rare. The commonly used drugs, aspirin and non-steroidal anti-inflammatory agents, most often account for acquired intrinsic platelet dysfunction. The effect of aspirin is irreversible inactivation of cyclooxygenase by acetylation and lasts for the life of the platelet. Other drugs, particularly high-dose penicillin derivatives, can cause platelet dysfunction.[17] Platelet dysfunction may also occur in the patient with uremia, hepatic disease, or hypothyroidism. Dipyridimole rarely produces clinically significant bleeding.

Treatment for inherited qualitative platelet defects is with desmopressin (DDAVP), platelet transfusions, or both. For acquired platelet defects, therapy is directed at the underlying etiology. Hypothyroidism should be corrected prior to surgery. Therapy for uremia and hepatic disease are discussed below. In those patients taking aspirin, elective surgery should be postponed for 4 to 5 days after the last dose to allow for the generation of an adequate number of functioning platelets.[18] For emergent surgery, DDAVP may be of benefit.[19] If there is clinically significant bleeding despite DDAVP, platelet transfusion may be considered.

Granulocytosis and Granulocytopenia

White blood cell abnormalities may be the result of primary bone marrow disorders, or they may be secondary to other diseases. The impact on the perioperative period is generally related to the underlying disease. Granulocytopenia, which may be encountered in urologic patients secondary to radiation therapy, chemotherapy, and drugs such as sulfa compounds, may increase the risk of perioperative infection. Elective surgery should be postponed until reversible granulocytopenia is resolved. Idiopathic granulocytopenia, typically seen in black patients, does not predispose to infection.[2]

ABNORMALITIES OF SOLUBLE BLOOD COMPONENTS

Congenital Defects of Coagulation

Inherited hemostatic defects may be due to impaired synthesis of the coagulation factors.

Defective hemostasis will usually be uncovered in the routine preoperative evaluation. The concentration of each factor needed for adequate hemostasis varies with the factor, and the severity of each disorder is dependent upon the degree of decreased synthesis of the factor. The usual treatment is transfusional factor replacement (Table 4–1). Replacement therapy, however, may not achieve the expected level of the circulating factor because of the presence of antibodies. It is essential that factor inhibitory activity be screened preoperatively. Factor replacement is begun prior to surgery so that adequate levels of the deficient factor are maintained throughout the procedure. Replacement therapy is continued through the postoperative period for up to 1 to 2 weeks, depending on the specific setting. As an alternative to replacement therapy for patients with hemophilia A and von Willebrand's disease for whom DDAVP may raise factor levels specifically, DDAVP and/or a fibrinolytic inhibitor (aminocaproic acid or tranexamic acid) may be useful. These agents may obviate the need for replacement therapy in some instances of minor surgery and decrease the patient's exposure to transfusion-related complications.[20,21]

Acquired Defects of Coagulation

Vitamin K Deficiency

A deficiency of vitamin K results in decreased production of factors II, VII, IX, and X and proteins C and S, which all require vitamin K–dependent carboxylation in the liver (Fig. 4–1). This is reflected by a prolonged PT. Primary vitamin K deficiency is extremely rare in healthy people. A wide variety of animal and plant food sources can provide sufficient vitamin K, and the bacterial flora in the intestine are able to synthesize a significant portion of the requirement of dietary vitamin K. Because vitamin K is fat-soluble, adequate bile salt circulation is necessary for absorption. Deficiencies can occur in the following conditions: (1) in the newborn because of poor transfer of vitamin K by the placenta and lack of vitamin K synthesis in the initially sterile intestine; (2) by severe dietary inadequacy, or total parental nutrition; (3) extrahepatic biliary obstruction, and cholestatic syndromes; and (4) in intestinal malabsorption syndromes such as sprue, ileitis, and colitis. Deficiencies can also develop when the intestinal bacteria are significantly reduced with broad-spectrum antibiotics. Coumarin drugs as well as large amounts of salicylates, vitamin A, and vitamin E antagonize the action of vitamin K, resulting in deficiencies of the vitamin K–dependent factors.[22]

Treatment for vitamin K deficiency is replacement, and surgery should be postponed, when possible, until maximal PT correction is obtained. Vitamin K_1 may be given by oral, subcutaneous, intramuscular, or intravenous routes. A single dose of 5 to 10 mg is sufficient in the adult, although larger doses are often needed for complete PT correction in the patient treated excessively with warfarin.

Table 4–1. HEMOSTATIC LEVELS OF COAGULATION FACTORS

Factor	Hemostatic Levels Required for Surgery (Percent)	Usual Replacement Factor
I	100 mg/dl%	Frozen plasma (FFP), cryoprecipitate
II	20–40%	FFP, factor IX concentrate*
V	25–30%	FFP
VII	10–20%	FFP, factor IX concentrate
VIII	40–50%	Cryoprecipitate, factor VIII concentrate
IX	30–50%	FFP, factor IX concentrate
X	20–40%	FFP, factor IX concentrate
XI	15–25%†	FFP
XII, prekallikrein, high-molecular-weight kallikrein	Deficiency not associated with increased bleeding	
XIII	<5%	FFP
von Willebrand's factor	25–50%	FFP, cryoprecipitate

*Factor IX concentrate contains clinically useful amounts of the vitamin K–dependent factors.

†Some patients with factor XI levels as low as 5 percent of normal do not have increased bleeding.

The oral route is unreliable when bile salt deficiency or malabsorption is suspected. PT correction after subcutaneous administration may be delayed for 12 to 36 hours. This route is ideal for prophylaxis in the patient who is taking nothing by mouth (NPO) and is on antibiotics, of which several 5-mg doses per week are sufficient. Correction after intravenous administration is rapid (4 to 8 hours), but this route should be considered only for an emergency patient who is bleeding because of a considerable risk of anaphylaxis. For emergent surgery, replacement therapy with fresh frozen plasma is effective in addition to vitamin K therapy.[22]

Anticoagulation Therapy

Surgical intervention must sometimes be performed in the patient undergoing chronic anticoagulation therapy. The risk of excessive bleeding from anticoagulation must be weighed against the effects of the reversal of anticoagulation, which exposes the patient to a period without protection from the thrombotic events for which he or she is being treated. Surgery in urologic patients who are also undergoing anticoagulation therapy is usually performed after reversal of anticoagulation because of the potential for severe hemorrhagic complications. However, particularly in patients with recurrent thrombotic disease while being anticoagulated, this balance must be carefully examined on an individual basis.

Anticoagulation is achieved with either warfarin or heparin. Warfarin exerts its effect by antagonizing the synthesis of the vitamin K–dependent factors, and its anticoagulant effect is manifested by an elevation of the PT and PTT but not the thrombin time. The PT is used for monitoring. The anticoagulant activity of heparin is due to its ability to facilitate the activity of antithrombin III and results in an elevation of the PTT (Fig. 4–1). The thrombin time is very sensitive and may be markedly prolonged whereas the PT rises at supratherapeutic anticoagulant intensity. The PTT is used for monitoring.

The chronically anticoagulated patient is typically on warfarin therapy. Several management strategies are possible, depending on the need to minimize the period of anticoagulation reversal. The patient can be anticoagulated with heparin while warfarin is withheld for 3 to 5 days prior to surgery. The heparin is discontinued 6 to 12 hours before surgery, and administration is resumed 12 to 24 hours after surgery. When the risk of thrombosis is less likely, warfarin can be discontinued prior to surgery so that coagulation normalizes, and the warfarin is begun again following surgery without the need for heparin anticoagulation. The reversal of the effect of warfarin can be hastened by vitamin K_1 supplementation and with fresh frozen plasma. Doses of vitamin K_1 in excess of 10 mg may make reinstitution of anticoagulation with warfarin more difficult.[23] For the patient undergoing heparin anticoagulation therapy in whom surgery cannot be postponed for at least 6 hours, the heparin can be neutralized by the administration of protamine sulfate. Intravenous heparin is neutralized with 1 mg of protamine sulfate given for every 100 units of heparin received during the prior 4 hours. Hemostatic parameters need to be monitored because a rebound heparin effect can occur as a result of the longer half-life of heparin as compared to that of protamine sulfate.[24]

Liver Disease

Adequate liver function is critical to normal hemostatic mechanisms. The liver is the major source of all coagulation proteins except for factor VIII and von Willebrand's factor, and it is the site of synthesis of plasminogen and the regulatory proteins of coagulation and fibrinolysis. In addition to its role as producer of the components of the hemostatic process, the liver regulates the activity of these components by clearing activated factors of coagulation and fibrinolysis from the blood. These functions can be markedly depressed in hepatocellular disease. Treatment is by transfusion with fresh frozen plasma to replace deficient factors, although this is often limited by the inability of these patients to tolerate large infused volumes.[25]

Altered utilization of vitamin K can occur with chronic liver disease, and vitamin K deficiency may coexist from associated malnutrition or may be secondary to bile salt malabsorption in conditions of obstructive jaundice.[26] Thus, vitamin K therapy should be given empirically to all patients with liver disease.

Chronic liver disease is often associated with thrombocytopenia and platelet dysfunction. Platelet abnormalities can result from the effects of associated splenomegaly, immune reactions, or direct toxic effects of ethanol. When clinical bleeding results, DDAVP and/or platelet transfusions may be considered. Platelet transfusion effectiveness may be diminished, however, by splenic pooling.[19,25]

Low-grade disseminated intravascular coagulation frequently can be detected in patients with liver disease. Alternately, accelerated primary fibrinolysis may exist.[27] Treatment of these conditions is discussed next.

Disseminated Intravascular Coagulation and Systemic Fibrinogenolysis

Disseminated intravascular coagulation develops in association with severe underlying illness. Spontaneous bleeding occurs as a result of the systemic activation of intravascular clotting followed by generalized fibrinolysis resulting in a consumptive coagulopathy. With the consumption of clotting factors, antithrombin III, fibrinogen, plasminogen, and platelets, the PT and PTT become elevated, plasma fibrinogen levels are reduced, circulating fibrin degradation products are increased, and thrombocytopenia develops. Fibrin strands in the microvasculature lead to the fragmentation of red blood cells, which can be seen on the peripheral smear.

The most common settings for the acute form of DIC in urologic patients are sepsis, shock, and prostate cancer. Therapy is directed at the underlying process.[28] Replacement of clotting factors by transfusion may be considered but is of limited benefit because of the consumptive process. The utility of heparin remains controversial.[29–30]

Prostate cancer can be associated with a chronic form of DIC. In this setting, the syndrome may manifest by thromboembolic and/or hemorrhagic events.[31–32] Elevation of fibrin-degradation products has also been noted in bladder cancer and renal cell carcinoma, and their use as tumor markers has been suggested.[33]

Systemic fibrinolysis presents a picture of serious spontaneous bleeding similar to that in DIC. This occurs primarily in urologic patients with prostate cancer.[34,35] The bleeding responds to therapy with antifibrinolytic agents. It is critical to differentiate primary fibrinolysis from DIC because the use of antifibrinolytic agents in the DIC can result in widespread thrombotic complications. The two conditions can appear quite similar; however, because laboratory evidence of a consumptive coagulopathy is present in both, the underlying etiology can be the same and the two syndromes may coexist. A normal platelet count is more suggestive of primary fibrinolysis.[36] Measurement of plasma D-dimer, a thrombin-factor XIIIA–dependent fibrin-degradation product may also be of potential value.

Uremia

Uremia is frequently associated with an abnormal bleeding tendency. A variety of hemostatic disorders can occur, including defective platelet aggregation, decreased platelet factor III, altered levels of factor VIII activity, von Willebrand activity, and factor VIII–related antigen, and increased production of prostacyclin by vessel walls. Clinical bleeding generally correlates with prolongation of the bleeding time. Dialysis is the mainstay of therapy for uremic patients with bleeding; however, this is not uniformly effective. High-dose intravenous conjugated estrogens can significantly improve the bleeding time.[37] DDAVP can transiently improve hemostasis, as can cryoprecipitate.[20,38]

Circulating Anticoagulants

Interruption of the clotting cascade can be due to circulating anticoagulants, which are immunoglobulins directed against one or more coagulation factors. Examples include the lupus anticoagulant, factor VIII antibody in hemophilia A, and, rarely, abnormal immunoglobulins in multiple myeloma. Circulating anticoagulants produce a prolongation of either the PT or PTT. When plasma from the patient is mixed with an equal amount of normal plasma, the circulating anticoagulant activity will be evident because the anticoagulant will prevent the mixture from clotting normally. Lupus anticoagulant and specific factor assays will identify the type of anticoagulant.

Clotting factor inhibitors may cause serious bleeding. Treatments that may be effective include transfusion with large amounts of the target factor, corticosteroids, cyclophosphamide, plasmapheresis, and exchange transfusions. The lupus anticoagulant that prolongs the PTT predisposes to thrombosis rather than to hemorrhage.[39]

Miscellaneous Disorders

Severe hypothyroidism can be accompanied by hemorrhagic complications. Levels of factors VIII, IX, and XI, and the von Willebrand factor may be significantly reduced. Platelet dysfunction and thrombocytopenia can occur.[23] Hemostatic abnormalities may develop in patients with dysproteinemias, such as multiple myeloma, Waldenström's macroglobulinemia, and systemic amyloidosis. Other conditions, including myeloproliferative disorders and primary bone marrow disorders, may also be associated with altered hemostasis.

POSTOPERATIVE COMPLICATIONS

Postprostatectomy Bleeding

Prostatectomy may be accompanied by significant blood loss. The amount of blood loss with transurethral prostatectomy correlates with the weight of tissue resected.[40] Postoperative bleeding is increased by local fibrinolysis as a result of urokinase in the urine and plasminogen activator released from the prostatic bed.[41,42] The use of antifibrinolytic therapy with either aminocaproic acid or tranexamic acid produces effective inhibition of urokinase and tissue plasminogen activator, resulting in less blood loss after transurethral, suprapubic, and retropubic prostatectomy.[43–48] Thromboembolic complications are very uncommon.[49–53] Drug use may result in the formation of obstructing intravesical clot.[54] Addition of furosemide to promote postoperative diuresis to prevent clot retention has been advocated by one author.[55]

Although the toxicity of antifibrinolytic agents is minimal, blood loss in the majority of patients is not serious, and, therefore, routine use of fibrinolytic inhibitors remains controversial. No benefit was demonstrated in a double-blind trial.[56] However, in patients with increased bleeding, antifibrinolytic agents are clearly of value. They can be given by intravenous or oral route. For adult patients, the usual dosage of aminocaproic acid is 12 to 24 gm/day, in divided daily doses, and of tranexamic acid is 3 to 7 gm/day in divided daily doses. For patients with renal insufficiency, the dose should be corrected proportionately to the decrease in glomerular filtration rate. The dosage schedule for tranexamic acid is every 6 to 8 hours, whereas the shorter half-life of aminocaproic acid necessitates a dosage schedule of every 3 to 4 hours or, alternatively, administration by continuous intravenous infusion.

Thromboembolic Disease

Thromboembolic disease is a significant cause of morbidity and mortality in patients undergoing urologic surgery. Death due to postoperative pulmonary embolism has been variably reported to range from 0.5 to 5.5 percent of patients following open urologic surgery.[57–61] Nonfatal pulmonary embolism is more common. Following open prostatectomy, clinical estimates range from 3 to 9 percent, whereas the rate for routine lung perfusion scan has been as high as 22 percent.[57,58,62,63] It is generally accepted that postoperative pulmonary emboli arise from thigh and pelvic deep vein thrombosis.[64]

The incidence of venous thrombosis is high in urologic patients. With the use of sensitive diagnostic techniques, the reported incidence ranges from 28 to 80 percent in patients undergoing open prostatectomy and 7 to 20 percent in transurethral prostatectomy.[59,61,65–67]

Virchow conceptualized three contributing factors in the pathophysiology of deep venous thrombosis: *stasis*, *hypercoagulability*, and *intimal injury*. This concept is evidenced in the currently recognized risk factors for deep venous thrombosis: (1) administration of anesthesia for more than 30 minutes; (2) age over 40 years; (3) previous deep venous thrombosis or pulmonary embolism; (4) prolonged postoperative immobilization; (5) paralysis; (6) malignancy; (7) obesity; (8) estrogen therapy; (9) medical disease leading to venous stasis, such as congestive heart failure; (10) nephrotic syndrome; (11) sepsis; (12) erythrocytosis; (13) lupus anticoagulant; (14) inflammatory bowel disease; and (15) myeloproliferative disorders.

Inherited deficiency of anticoagulant components of the clotting system, including deficiencies of protein C, protein S, plasminogen, antithrombin III, and heparin cofactor II, is an additional risk factor.[68] Evidence suggests that cryoprecipitate coagulum pyelolithotomy increases the risk of pulmonary embolism.[69] The urologic patient, because of age, type of surgery, disease process, and associated illness often has multiple risk factors.

Pulmonary embolism is difficult to diagnose clinically. When signs and symptoms suggest pulmonary embolism, the ventilation-perfusion lung scan is useful. The lung perfusion scan can be used to rule out pulmonary embolism because it reveals areas of decreased perfusion with excellent sensitivity. Areas of decreased perfusion are not necessarily due to emboli, and, therefore, to enhance specificity, a ventilation scan is performed. Segmental areas with poor perfusion combined with good ventilation fulfill the criteria of the ventilation-perfusion mismatch and have a high probability of representing pulmonary emboli. If the areas of decreased perfusion are small or coexist with other pulmonary pathology, the ventilation scan is not discriminatory. For the patient in whom the diagnosis remains uncertain or for whom anticoagulation is associated with high risk, the "gold standard" is pulmonary angiography. The invasive nature and attendant risks limit its clinical utility to these selected cases.[64]

The clinical diagnosis of deep venous thrombosis is also difficult, with estimates of false impressions as high as 50 percent.[64] More accurate diagnoses can be achieved with venography, radiolabeled fibrinogen scanning, impedence plethysmography, and Doppler ultrasonography. Venography remains the definitive test; however, because of its invasive nature with small but potential morbidity, other techniques are often employed. Iodine 125 (^{125}I)–labeled fibrinogen scanning is exquisitely sensitive to formation of distal thrombosis and may give some anatomic venous detail, but it is less useful in identifying proximal vein thrombosis. Because scanning must proceed over several days, this test is less useful clinically when rapid diagnosis is needed; however, it is ideal for prospective screening of patients who are at risk for thrombosis and for whom routine anticoagulant prophylaxis is contraindicated prophylaxis. Impedence plethysmography is noninvasive, very sensitive to proximal vein thrombosis, and relatively insensitive to distal vein thrombosis. By serial testing, both proximal vein thromboses (which progress more proximally) are detected. Because clinically significant pulmonary emboli arise from the thrombi in the proximal veins, this method has proved as reliable as venography in identifying the patients at risk for embolism without the need for invasive testing.[70,71] Doppler ultrasound examination of the thigh veins is similarly noninvasive and sensitive to proximal vein thrombosis; however, this test is subject to greater operator error.[72] The use of the duplex scanner may improve its accuracy.

Perioperative prophylaxis by a variety of methods has proved effective in decreasing the incidence of deep venous thrombosis and pulmonary embolism. Low-dose heparin has been most extensively studied, reducing the incidence of postoperative deep venous thrombosis by 75 percent in large series of mixed patients.[68] The results of low-dose heparin in urologic surgery, including series of open and transurethral prostatectomy, has not been consistent. Many studies support its utility and lack of hemorrhagic complications,[61,65,66,73–76] but others have failed to demonstrate a statistically significant prophylactic effect and have noted increased bleeding.[63,77–79] Heparin-associated thrombocytopenia, which may be accompanied by new thrombotic complications, generally occurs 4 to 14 days after beginning therapy; thus, whereas thrombocytopenia is reported in several percent of all patients treated with heparin, it is seen less often when heparin is used as a prophylactic regimen. The most commonly employed regimen is 5000 units of heparin, given subcutaneously 2 hours before surgery, followed by 5000 units subcutaneously every 12 hours until the patient is ambulatory. The role of venous dilation as a contributor to venous stasis and, hence, thrombosis prompted the use of heparin combined with dihydroergotamine, which increases the tone of venous capacitance vessels. This combination has shown increased efficacy over heparin alone when sensitive diagnostic techniques are used to assess results. However, because there is some increase in arterial resistance, its use is relatively contraindicated in patients with peripheral vascular disease and coronary artery disease.[80,81]

Ergotism, while unusual, can be associated with severe morbidity, and there has been limited overall enthusiasm for the heparin-dihydroergotamine combination. The usual dose is 0.5 mg given subcutaneously with heparin.

The use of oral vitamin K antagonists has been shown to provide effective prophylaxis in orthopedic, gynecologic, and general surgery patients but is consistently associated with a high incidence of bleeding complications.[82] Patients undergoing prostatectomy who are given vitamin K antagonists have shown increased intraoperative and postoperative bleeding.[60] The use of vitamin K antagonists together with aminocaproic acid has been shown to give effective prophylaxis with reduction in hemorrhagic side effects.[83,84]

Low-molecular-weight dextran has been utilized for prophylaxis in general surgery patients. There are no trials in urologic patients. In addition to causing hemorrhage, dextran can result in fluid overload and allergic and renal complications.[64]

Inhibitors of platelet function have been investigated in orthopedic and general surgery patients. Aspirin, hydroxychloroquine, dypyridamole, and sulfinpyrazone have not been consistently effective.[85]

Intermittent external mechanical compression of the legs has been shown to be as efficacious as heparin for thromboembolic prophylaxis in urologic patients.[63] This method offers the advantage of not interfering with the normal hemostatic mechanisms; however, there is some degree of patient discomfort with long-term use.

In summary, prophylaxis against thromboembolic complications is recommended for urologic patients over 40 years of age who are undergoing major surgery and for younger patients with risk factors. Although not all studies of urologic patients have confirmed the efficacy and safety of heparin, the evidence overall from urologic patients supports the data from large collected series of mixed surgical patients that heparin therapy is effective and without major hemorrhagic side effects. Low-dose heparin can be recommended for prophylaxis in urologic surgery.[68] A recommended alternative to heparin is intermittent external mechanical venous compression, although, as yet, its effectiveness has been demonstrated only in small studies.[64,86]

Thromboembolism will occur in some patients despite prophylaxis. Treatment for deep venous thrombosis and for pulmonary embolism is anticoagulation initially by heparin, followed by anticoagulation by warfarin. The most commonly employed regimen is continuous intravenous heparin to maintain the PTT between 1.5 and 2 times the control value. Warfarin overlaps the heparin for 3 to 5 days. Warfarin is adjusted to maintain the PT between 1.2 and 1.5 times the control value.[87]

Experience suggests that warfarin therapy started as early as 1 day following treatment with heparin provides equal therapeutic efficacy with shorter hospitalization.[88] Warfarin is usually continued for 3 months. When heparin is contraindicated or when a patient continues to have pulmonary emboli when the blood is anticoagulated, placement of an intracaval device or surgical vena caval clipping may be indicated.[82]

Thrombolytic agents are useful in the patient with phlegmasia cerulea dolens, massive venous hypertension or massive pulmonary embolism with pulmonary hypertension, or systemic hypotension. Available drugs include streptokinase, urokinase, and tissue plasminogen activator. Relative contraindications include surgery within the preceding 10 days, a cerebrovascular accident within the preceding 2 months, any active intracranial disease process, or any known site of potential bleeding that may have associated morbidity.[89] When a relative contraindication to thrombolytic agents exists, potential benefits of treatment must outweigh risks of therapy. Surgical thrombectomy may be considered in this circumstance.[82]

References

1. Colman RW, Marder VJ, Salzman EW, et al: Overview of hemostasis. In Colman RW, Hirsh J, eds: Hemostasis and Thrombosis: Basic Principles and Clinical Practice. Philadelphia, JB Lippincott Co, 1987, p 3.
2. Fellin F, Murphy S: Hematologic problems in the preoperative patient. Med Clin North Am 71(3):477, 1987.
3. Raphael B, Cooperberg AA, Niloff P: The triad of hemochromatosis, hepatoma and erythrocytosis. Cancer 43:690, 1979.
4. Erf LA, Herbut PA: Primary and secondary myelofibrosis: a clinical and pathologic study of 13 cases of fibrosis of the bone marrow. Ann Intern Med 21:863, 1944.
5. Kinn AC, Lantz B: Vitamin B_{12} deficiency after irradiation for bladder carcinoma. J Urol 131:888, 1984.
6. Rifkind RA, Bank A, Marks PA, et al: Fundamentals of Hematology. Chicago, Year Book Medical Publishers, Inc, 1980, p 77.
7. Spira MA, Lynch EC: Autoimmune hemolytic anemia and carcinoma: an unusual association. Am J Med 67:753, 1979.
8. Canale D, Feldman R, Rosen M, et al: Autoimmune hemolytic anemia associated with seminoma. Urology 5:411, 1975.
9. Antman KH, Skarin AT, Mayer RJ, et al: Microangiopathic hemolytic anemia and cancer: a review. Medicine 58:377, 1979.
10. Hammond D, Winnick S: Paraneoplastic erythrocytosis and ectopic erythropoietins. Ann NY Acad Sci 230:219, 1974.
11. Sufrin G, Mirand EA, Moore RH, et al: Hormones and renal cancer. J Urol 117:433, 1977.
12. Cronin RE, Kaehny WD, Miller PD, et al: Renal cell carcinoma: unusual systematic manifestations. Medicine 55:291, 1976.
13. Eisenstaedt R: Blood component therapy in the treatment of platelet disorders. Semin Hematol 23:1, 1986.
14. Schafer A: Bleeding and thrombosis in myeloproliferative disease. Blood 64:1, 1986.
15. Noronha PA, Hruby MA, Maurer HS: Acquired von Willebrand's disease in a patient with Wilms tumor. J Pediatr 95:997, 1979.
16. Scott JP, Montgomery RR, Tubieger DG, et al: Acquired von Willebrand's disease in association with Wilms' tumor: regression following treatment. Blood 58:665, 1981.
17. Carvalho ACA, Rao AK: Acquired qualitative platelet defects. In Colman RW, and Hirsh J, eds: Hemostasis and Thrombosis: Basic Principles and Clinical Practice. Philadelphia, JB Lippincott Co, 1987, p 750.
18. Salzman EW: Hemostatic problems in surgical patients. In Colman RW, Hirsh J, eds: Hemostasis and Thrombosis: Basic Principles and Clinical Practice. Philadelphia, JB Lippincott Co, 1987, p 920.
19. Mannucci PM, Vicente V, Vianello L, et al: Controlled trial of desmopressin (DDAVP) in liver cirrhosis and other conditions associated with a prolonged bleeding time. Blood 67:1148, 1986.
20. Mannucci PM: Desmopressin (DDAVP) for treatment of disorders of hemostasis. In Coller BS, ed: Progress in Hemostasis and Thrombosis. New York, Grune and Stratton, 1986, p 19.
21. Lusher JM: Hemophilia: desmopressin acetate (DDAVP); its use in disorders of hemostasis. Thromb Haemost 6:385, 1984.
22. Olson RE: Vitamin K. In Colman RW, Hirsh J, eds: Hemostasis and Thrombosis: Basic Principles and Clinical Practice. Philadelphia, JB Lippincott Co, 1987, p 846.
23. Levine MN, Hirsh J, Kelton JG: Hemorrhagic complications of antithrombotic therapy. In Colman RW, Hirsh

J, eds: Hemostasis and Thrombosis: Basic Principles and Clinical Practice. Philadelphia, JB Lippincott Co, 1987, p 873.

24. Ratnoff OD: Some therapeutic agents influencing hemostasis. In Colman RW, Hirsh J, eds: Hemostasis and Thrombosis: Basic Principles and Clinical Practice. Philadelphia, JB Lippincott Co, 1987, p 1026.
25. Kelly DA, Tuddenham EGD: Hemostatic problems in liver diseases. Gut 27:339, 1986.
26. Blanchard RA, Furie BC, Jorgensen BA, et al: Acquired vitamin K–dependent carboxylation deficiency in liver disease. N Engl J Med 305:242, 1981.
27. Francis RB, Feinstein DI: Clinical significance of accelerated fibrinolysis in liver disease. Haemostasis 14:460, 1984.
28. Litt MR, Bell WR, Lepor HA: Disseminated intravascular coagulation in prostatic carcinoma reversed by ketaconazole. JAMA 258(10):1361, 1987.
29. Kursh Ed, Ratnoff OD, Persky L: Current clotting concepts in urology. J Urol 116:214, 1976.
30. Pergament ML, Swaim WR, Blackard CE: Disseminated intravascular coagulation in the urologic patient. J Urol 116:1, 1976.
31. Sack GH, Levin J, Bell WR: Trousseau's syndrome and other manifestations of chronic disseminated coagulopathy in patients with neoplasms: clinical, pathophysiologic, and therapeutic features. Medicine 56:1, 1977.
32. Sanaha RJ, Bruns TNC, Ross GJJ: Chronic intravascular coagulation in metastatic prostate cancer. Arch Surgery 106:295, 1973.
33. Reidmuller H, Thuroff JW, Jacobi GH: Fibrinogen degradation products in urological malignant tumors. Urol Int 39:13, 1984.
34. Tagnon HJ, Whitmore WF, Shulman NR: Fibrinolysis in metastatic cancer of the prostate. Cancer 5:9, 1952.
35. Booth NA, Bennet B: Plasmin-alpha$_2$-antiplasmin complexes in bleeding disorders characterized by primary or secondary fibrinolysis. Br J Haematol 56:545, 1984.
36. Marder VJ, Martin SE, Francis CW, et al: Consumptive thrombohemorrhagic disorders. In Colman RW, Hirsh J, eds: Hemostasis and Thrombosis: Basic Principles and Clinical Practice. Philadelphia, JB Lippincott Co, 1987, p 975.
37. Livio M, Mannucci PMN, Vigano G, et al: Conjugated estrogens for the management of bleeding associated with renal failure. N Engl J Med 315(12):731, 1986.
38. Janson PA, Jubelirer SJ, Weinstein MJ, Deykin D: Treatment of the bleeding tendency in uremia with cryoprecipitate. N Engl J Med 303:1318, 1980.
39. Feinstein DI, Rapaport SI: Acquired inhibition of blood coagulation. In Spaet TH, ed: Progress in Hemostasis and Thrombosis. New York, Grune and Stratton Inc, 1972.
40. Eliot JS, McDonald JK, Fowell AH: Blood loss and fibrinolysin levels during transurethral prostatic resection. J Urol 89:62, 1963.
41. Prentice CRM: Basis of antifibrinolytic therapy. J Clin Pathol 33(Suppl 14):35, 1980.
42. Nilsson IM: Local fibrinolysis as a mechanism for haemorrhage. Thrombos Diathes Haemorrh 34:623, 1975.
43. McNichol GP, Fletcher AP, Alkjaersig N, et al: Impairment of hemostasis in the urinary tract: the role of urokinase. J Lab Clin Med 58:31, 1961.
44. McNicol GP, Fletcher AP, Alkjaersig N, et al: The use of episilon aminocaproic acid, a potent inhibitor of fibrinolytic activity in the management of postoperative hematuria. J Urol 86:829, 1961.
45. Madsen PO, Strauch AE: The effect of aminocaproic acid on bleeding following transurethral prostatectomy. J Urol 96:255, 1966.
46. Hedlund PO: Antifibrinolytic therapy with cyklokapron in connection wth prostatectomy. Scand J Urol Nephrol 3:177, 1969.
47. Sack E, Spaet TH, Gentile RL, et al: Reduction of post-prostatectomy bleeding by epsilon-aminocaproic acid. N Engl J Med 255:541, 1962.
48. Lawrence ACK, Ward-McQuaid JN: The effect of epsilon aminocaproic acid on the blood loss after retropubic prostatectomy. Br J Urology 38:308, 1966.
49. Hedlung PO: Postoperative venous thrombosis in benign prostatic disease: a study of 316 patients with ^{125}I-fibrinogen uptake test. Scand J Urol Nephrol 27(Suppl):1, 1975.
50. Becker J, Borgstrom S: Incidence of thrombosis associated with epsilon-aminocaproic acid administration and with combined epsilon-aminocaproic acid and subcutaneous heparin therapy. Acta Chir Scand 134:343, 1968.
51. Vinnicombe J, Shuttleworth KED: Aminocaproic acid in the control of haemorrhage after prostatectomy. Lancet 1:232, 1966.
52. Sinclair J, Forbes CD, Prentice CRM, et al: The incidence of deep vein thrombosis in prostatectomized patients following the administration of the fibrinolytic inhibitor, aminocaproic acid (EACA). Urol Res 4:129, 1976.
53. Gordon-Smith IC, Hickman JA, el-Masri SH: The effect of the fibrinolytic inhibitor epsilon-aminocaproic acid on the incidence of deep-vein thrombosis after prostatectomy. Br J Surg 95:522, 1972.
54. Ward MG, Richards B: Complications of antifibrinolysis therapy after prostatectomy. Br J Urol 51:211, 1979.
55. Smart CJ, Turnbull AR, Jenkins JD: The use of frusemide and epsilon-amino-caproic-acid in transurethral prostatectomy. Br J Urol 46:521, 1974.
56. Smith RB, Raich P, Kaufman JJ: Epsilon aminocaproic acid and the control of post-prostatectomy bleeding: a prospective double-blind study. J Urol 131:1093, 1984.
57. Allgood RJ, Cook JH, Weedn RJ, et al: Prospective analysis of pulmonary embolism in the postoperative patient. Surgery 68:116, 1970.
58. Antila LE, Markulla H, Iisalv E: Ten-years' experience of geriatric aspects of surgery of patients with benign prostatic hypertrophy. Acta Chir Scand 132:144, 1966.
59. Becker J, Borgstrom S, Saltzman GF: Occurrence and course of thrombosis following prostatectomy. Acta Radiol [Diagn] 10:513, 1970.
60. Holbraad L, Thybo E, Vennits H: A controlled investigation of the value of anticoagulant therapy in cases of prostatectomy. Scand J Urol Nephrol 10:39, 1976.
61. Kakkar VV: International multicentre trial-prevention of fatal post-operative embolism by low doses of heparin. Lancet 2:45, 1975.
62. Colby FH: The prevention of pulmonary emboli after prostatectomy. J Urol 59:920, 1945.
63. Coe ND, Collins REC, Klein LA, et al: Prevention of deep vein thrombosis in urological patients: a controlled, randomized trial of low-dose heparin and external penumatic compression boots. Surgery 83:230, 1978.
64. Moser K: Thromboembolic disease in the patient undergoing urologic surgery. Urol Clin North Am 10(1)101, 1983.
65. Williams HT: Prevention of post-operative deep venous thrombosis with preoperative subcutaneous heparin. Lancet 2:950, 1971.
66. Nicolaides AN, Field ES, Kakkar VV, et al: Prostatec-

tomy and deep-vein thrombosis. Br J Surg 59(6):487, 1972.
67. Mayo ME, Halil T, Browse NL: The incidence of deep venous thrombosis after prostatectomy. Br J Urology 43:738, 1971.
68. NIH Consensus Development Conference: Prevention of venous thrombosis and pulmonary embolism. JAMA 256(6):744, 1986.
69. Pence JR II, Airhart RA, Novicki DE, et al: Pulmonary emboli associated with coagulum pyelolithotomy. J Urol 127:572, 1982.
70. Hull R, Hirsch J, Carter C, et al: Diagnostic efficacy of impedance plethysmography for clinically suspected deep-vein thrombosis: a randomized trial. Ann Intern Med 102:21, 1985.
71. Huisman MV, Büller HR, tenCate JW, et al: Serial impedance plethysmography for suspected deep venous thrombosis in outpatients. N Engl J Med 314:823, 1986.
72. Sigel B, Felix WR, Popky GL, et al: Diagnosis of lower limb venous thrombosis by Doppler ultrasound technique. Arch Surg 104:174, 1972.
73. Kutnowski M, Vandendris M, Steinberger R, et al: Prevention of postoperative deep-vein thrombosis by low-dose heparin in urological surgery. Urol Res 5:123, 1977.
74. Kass EJ, Sonda P, Gershon C, et al: The use of prophylactic low dose heparin in transurethral prostatectomy. J Urol 120:186, 1978.
75. Tscholl R, Straub W, Zingg E: Electroresection of the prostate in patients treated with heparin. J Urol 124:221, 1980.
76. Jasper WS Sr: Anticoagulants in open prostatectomies. J Urol 117:72, 1977.
77. Rosenberg IL, Evans M, Pollock AV: Prophylaxis of postoperative leg vein thrombosis by low dose subcutaneous heparin or preoperative calf muscle stimulation: a controlled clinical trial. Br Med J 1:649, 1975.
78. Sleight MW: The effect of prophylactic subcutaneous heparin on blood loss during and after transurethral prostatectomy. Br J Urol 54:164, 1982.
79. Allen NH, Jenkins JD, Smart CJ: Surgical hemorrhage in patients given subcutaneous heparin as prophylaxis against thromboembolism. Br Med J 1:1326, 1978.
80. Multicenter Trial Committee: Dihydroergotamine-heparin prophylaxis of postoperative deep venous thrombosis: a multicenter trial. JAMA 251:2960, 1984.
81. The Medical Letter 27:45, 1985.
82. Salzman EW, Hirsh J: Prevention of venous thromboembolism. In Colman RW, Hirsh J, eds: Hemostasis and Thrombosis: Basic Principles and Clinical Practice. Philadelphia, JB Lippincott Co, 1987, p 81.
83. Storm O: Suprapubic prostatectomy with pre-operative dicumarol and epsilon-aminocaproic acid prophylaxis. Scand J Urol Nephrol 1:1, 1967.
84. Anderson R, Jensen PB: Prophylactic anticoagulant therapy in prostatic surgery. Acta Chir Scand 132:144, 1966.
85. Hirsch J, Fuster V, Salzman E: Antiplatelet agents: the relationship among dose, side effects and antithrombotic effectiveness. Chest 89(2)Suppl:4S, 1986.
86. Hyers T, Hull RD, Weg JG: Antithrombotic therapy for venous thromboembolic disease. Chest 89(2)Suppl:26S 1986.
87. Hirsch J, Deykon D, Poller L: Therapeutic range for oral anticoagulant therapy. Chest 89(2)Suppl:11S, 1986.
88. Gallus A, Jakamen J, Tillett J, et al: Safety and efficacy of warfarin started early after submassive venous thrombosis or pulmonary embolism. Lancet 2:1293, 1986.
89. NIH Consensus Development Conference: Thrombolytic therapy in thrombosis. Ann Intern Med 93:141, 1980.

CARDIAC COMPLICATIONS OF UROLOGIC SURGERY

5

Jan Tillisch

The origin of perioperative complications of urologic surgery proceeds from the nature of the required procedure with its attendant physiologic stresses and the degree of potential or developed cardiac dysfunction. Tremendous progress has been made over the past decade in reducing the risks of surgical procedures through better anesthesia, improved surgical techniques, more intensive monitoring, and enhanced postoperative care. Where the greatest current and future impact in reducing cardiac complications can be made, however, is in *preoperative* risk assessment and anticipatory therapy to reduce that risk.

To outline the available methods of risk stratification and the appropriate therapeutic responses as well as to describe potential postoperative cardiovascular complications and therapy, the following discussion will focus on broad classes of cardiac disease. It should be recognized that considerable overlap between disease classes occurs; for example, the patient with ischemic heart disease in whom angina may be present preoperatively and in whom congestive heart failure and arrhythmias caused by ischemic injury may be present postoperatively. It is axiomatic that in the patient with the most advanced disease, the greater number of features of that disease will be demonstrated.

ISCHEMIC HEART DISEASE

Ischemic heart disease, generally due to atherosclerotic obstruction of coronary arteries and, less often, to abnormal vasospasm with minimal obstruction or by excessive oxygen demand, may present with angina or myocardial infarction and may be complicated by congestive heart failure or recurrent arrhythmias. The most critical problem in preoperative assessment is determining the degree of potential instability of a given patient's coronary artery disease. Severe but stable coronary atherosclerosis may be less of an operative risk than potentially unstable but less diffuse coronary disease. The degree of potential ischemia is the dominant risk factor leading to perioperative ischemic complications. The method of assessing potential ischemia and, of course, the therapy, differ depending on the manifestation of ischemic heart disease.

Angina

The presence of angina allows risk to be assessed partially by history alone. Stable exertional angina, occurring with above-normal exercise, poses only a relatively modest risk for major surgical procedures. It has been shown by long-term follow-up and angiographic classification that most patients with stable effort angina do not become critically unstable with ischemia in the same vascular distribution. Rather, symptoms become more gradually progressive. This appears to reflect the underlying pathophysiologic difference between progressive but gradual luminal obliteration by a smooth atherosclerotic lesion as contrasted to abrupt thrombosis of a more thrombogenic, but initially less obstructive, lesion.

In contrast, patients with angina at rest may

be of two pathophysiologic types. The first group of patients, usually those who have gone through the stages of effort angina to the point of severity where angina comes at rest, often have severe double or triple vessel disease and are exceedingly high operative risks for urologic surgery without prior mechanical correction of the coronary obstruction.

In the second type of rest angina, the patient generally has less frequent symptoms without accompanying effort angina. These patients appear to have vasomotion (vasoconstriction) in addition to obstructive coronary atherosclerotic lesions. This vasomotion is probably induced by increased alpha sympathetic tone and may occur silently many times a day, even when symptomatic ischemia is infrequent.

True coronary vasopasm (Prinzmetal's angina) is much less common and, in most cases, is characterized by rest angina with relatively modest or no underlying coronary obstruction.

Patients with abrupt transitions from previously stable effort angina to frequent rest angina or those with new onset rest angina generally have superimposed thrombus on a chronic atherosclerotic lesion. These patients are most likely to experience an acute myocardial infarction and require urgent medical and/or surgical intervention.

It can be seen that the anginal history helps to differentiate both the severity and pathophysiologic types of coronary disease. However, more insight into both severity and type of coronary lesion is required for accurate risk assessment and therapeutic planning.

The concern regarding the patient with stable angina is that, although the lesion may not abruptly change, the blood flow requirements during the perioperative period may exceed requirements during normal activity, resulting in ischemia from excessive oxygen demand. Postoperative tachycardia consequent to hypovolemia, excessive venous pooling from anesthetic or analgesic agents, volume redistribution from intra-abdominal fluid shifts, anemia, pain, and anxiety all may be sufficient to induce subendocardial ischemia and injury by increasing myocardial oxygen requirements.

Hypotension accompanying decreased venous return may also compromise available coronary flow; however, hypertension is more likely to cause ischemia through an increase in pressure work of the heart (afterload). The vasoconstrictive and tachycardiac responses to hypovolemia, cold, pain, and respiratory distress induced by either inadequate ventilation or, commonly, by poor tolerance of endotracheal intubation may result in substantial ischemia in a previously stable patient. Additionally, the increased sympathetic tone results not only in the increased oxygen demand outlined above but also in decreased oxygen supply through increased coronary vasoconstriction, a pathophysiologic mechanism previously largely ignored in the genesis of ischemic injury.

Diagnostic Studies

To determine potential tolerance to the rigors of surgical intervention, the standard treadmill stress test has been of use in patients with a history of angina or prior myocardial infarction. Low-workload positive stress tests causing an onset of ischemic manifestations in less than 5 minutes, as well as certain ST configuration patterns, inadequate blood pressure response, or number of leads with ST abnormalities, all predict a high likelihood of triple-vessel- or severe double-vessel-disease. These patients should undergo coronary angiography prior to surgical intervention to determine whether presurgical revascularization should be undertaken.

The addition of thallium isotopic scanning to uncover nonhomogeneous blood flow has improved the sensitivity and specificity of treadmill testing; however, it is not routinely necessary for preoperative risk assessment in patients with angina but without prior myocardial infarction. In patients with prior myocardial infarction, thallium imaging may delineate ischemia remote from prior infarction, thus suggesting multivessel or higher-risk coronary disease.

Examination of ventricular contraction during stress, using gated isotopic blood pool scanning or echocardiography, has a role in assessing severity of coronary disease as well as the functional significance of the ischemia; however, it is of most use in evaluating symptoms of, or potential for, heart failure in patients with ischemic heart disease. Tests to examine ventricular contraction during stress will be more fully discussed subsequently.

Angina Therapy

Patients with effort angina are usually best managed with a combination of a coronary vasodilator (either nitrates or a calcium channel blocker) and beta blockade, if no contraindications to the bradycardiac and contraction depressant aspects of beta-blocker therapy are present. It is particularly important to administer the beta-blocker or calcium channel blocker throughout the perioperative period as long as no adverse side effects, such as excessive heart rate reduction or hypotension, are noted. Abrupt withdrawal of beta blockers has been noted to cause increased angina and occasionally will precipitate myocardial infarction.

In patients with rest angina, nitrates and calcium channel blockers are often used either alone or in combination. In this patient group, abrupt withdrawal of calcium channel blockers may precipitate severe ischemia. Sublingual nifedipine may be used during periods when oral therapy is precluded.

Myocardial Infarction

As alluded to earlier, myocardial infarction may occur through different pathogenetic mechanisms. Q wave infarctions, usually initially heralded by ST segment elevation and formerly called transmural infarcts, are usually associated with thrombotic occlusion of a coronary artery. Postoperative Q wave infarcts can thus best be prevented by (1) preoperative risk assessment and mechanical therapy of highly stenosed coronary vessels (coronary bypass grafting or percutaneous transluminal coronary angioplasty), (2) attempts to ameliorate high sympathetic tone through treatment of causative mechanisms, and (3) possibly, prevention of hypercoagulable postoperative states. This last still-theoretic approach is often in direct opposition to the surgical and postoperative approach to diminish hemorrhagic events. The relative risk-benefit ratio of anticoagulant or antiplatelet therapy after urologic surgery needs to be carefully studied before a recommendation can be made, however compelling the theoretic advantage of antithrombotic therapy.

Non–Q wave infarcts, (formerly called subendocardial infarcts), are usually manifested by ST segment depression and T wave inversion. These infarcts are most often caused by excessive oxygen demands coupled with nonocclusive reduced oxygen flow. They occur more often in the immediate postoperative period when physiologic stresses increase oxygen demand the most. Maintenance of antianginal therapy, aggressive treatment of hypertension, maintenance of hematocrit (Hct) over 30 percent, and avoidance of hypovolemia all may diminish the risk of non–Q wave infarcts. Additionally, particular attention to the treatment of heart failure in patients with ischemic heart disease, discussed below, is critical in avoiding infarction in this patient subset.

Perioperative myocardial infarction is associated with a high in-hospital mortality. Management of each patient is best achieved in a coronary care specialty unit with close interaction between the urologic surgical team and cardiologist, given potentially differing therapeutic goals regarding ambulation, anticoagulation, transfusion, and so on.

Ischemic heart disease may be manifested *only* by acute onset of congestive heart failure; however, generally, this will be heralded by some history of prior myocardial infarction, angina, or symptoms of episodic heart failure. Electrocardiographic abnormalities are common in this group of patients, and such patients are predominantly over 65 years of age. Congestive heart failure will be discussed in detail below.

Fortunately, cardiac rhythm abnormalities as the sole manifestation of ischemia are rare. Generally, serious rhythm abnormalities are associated either with acute myocardial infarction or with advanced left ventricular dysfunction secondary to prior infarcts, and thus patients at risk will be identified in risk assessment for other reasons. Primary cardiac rhythm abnormalities are discussed in this chapter.

Patients with a history of myocardial infarction are often considered to pose a high operative risk. Statistically, the duration of time from the myocardial infarction allows some prediction of risk. It should be stressed, however, that this prediction is based almost exclusively on statistical selection rather than on any pathophysiologic information.

The period of greatest post-infarct risk of a subsequent cardiac event (sudden death, recurrent myocardial infarction, symptomatic angina, or heart failure) is during the first 6 months following the infarct, with the maximum risk period within the first 6 to 12 weeks. Patients who are free of cardiac symptoms at one year following a myocardial infarction have essentially the same mortality rate as an age- and sex-matched patient with no history of infarction. Therefore, if an operation is postponed for 6 months following the infarction, most of the high-risk patients will have died, will have undergone revascularization, or will be a prohibitive operative risk for reasons of heart failure or abnormal cardiac rhythm. This increased operative risk during the first 6 months after infarction has nothing to do with the healing process or recovery from the infarction but is actually a screening period during which high-risk patients are removed from operative consideration.

The corollary of this is that appropriate risk screening during the 6 months following infarction will allow low-risk patients to be operated on safely within that 6-month period and in some cases as early as within 2 to 4 weeks. The same risk screening described above will permit such decisions to be made. The major risk for recurrent cardiac events is the presence of significant multivessel disease, i.e., the infarct-related artery and some additional critical stenosis. In general, treadmill testing with either thallium imaging or some functional assessment (echocardiogram or isotopic ventriculography) will help identify obvious high-risk patients for revascularization, thus removing the cause of their increased operative risk. Those patients whose results are negative and who are without cardiac symptoms of heart failure or cardiac arrhythmias may well be operated on earlier. When the operation planned is major and urgent, coronary angiography will more definitively identify the potential risk of subsequent ischemic events and is recommended.

Patients without evidence of continued postinfarction ischemia, but with either significant left ventricular (LV) dysfunction (ejection fraction less than 30 to 40 percent or symptomatic congestive heart failure) or with recurrent ventricular arrhythmias (usually the same patient population as those with LV dysfunction), can be risk-stratified and treated in the manner described in subsequent sections.

CONGESTIVE HEART FAILURE

Symptoms of pulmonary congestive and peripheral edema have traditionally been ascribed to abnormal cardiac contraction consequent to excessive volume or pressure loading of the heart, as in valvular disease, or to ischemic or post-inflammatory damage to the cardiac muscle. Increasingly, we are seeing patients whose symptoms of "congestion" are due not to abnormal contraction but to impaired relaxation of the heart. This latter condition is often seen in the elderly patient and in those with long histories of hypertension or diabetes.

The importance of this differentiation of the causes of pulmonary and venous congestion is that attempts to improve contraction (as with digitalis, intravenous inotropic agents, or vasodilator "unloading" agents) will benefit the group with impaired contractility but not those with normal contraction but abnormal relaxation.

Physical examination and chest x-ray will often differentiate only the most severely affected of the patients with congestive "heart failure" symptoms. Effective risk assessment necessitates identification of patients in the presymptomatic or early symptomatic phase if effective management is to be achieved during the perioperative period.

Diagnostic Methods

Patients with a history of dyspnea, orthopnea, or unexplained peripheral edema and those asymptomatic patients with physical findings or histories that may be associated with heart failure (severe hypertension, rheumatic or other valvular heart disease, history of myocardial infarction) should undergo assessment of cardiac function, preferably with stress, prior to surgical scheduling.

Echocardiography

Accurate determination of left ventricular function can be obtained with echocardiography. In addition, the degree of valvular incompetence or stenosis can be estimated and approximations of both left ventricular and pulmonary artery pressures can be made. In patients with pulmonary emphysema or extreme obesity, the echocardiogram may be less revealing, although usually satisfactory estimates of ventricular function can be obtained.

Echocardiograms before and after stress can give the physician an idea of the ability of the ventricles to respond to increased load, although the echo may be less accurate than isotopic ventriculography.

Isotopic Ventriculography

This technique, also called gated blood pool imaging, gives an accurate assessment of wall motion and overall left ventricular and right ventricular ejection fraction at rest and with exercise; it can be performed in any patient. Little information about valvular function or left ventricular pressure is obtained, however.

Patients with a history of angina or myocardial infarction and with questionable or real symptoms of congestive heart failure should undergo rest and exercise isotopic ventriculography for preoperative cardiac function assessment. Those with suspected or demonstrable valvular heart disease, possible pulmonary hypertension, systemic hypertension, or suspected congenital heart disease should undergo echocardiography to determine function.

Pulmonary Artery Catheterization

Placement of a pulmonary artery catheter preoperatively should be reserved for patients with demonstrable severe left ventricular dysfunction or pulmonary hypertension. Patients with moderate impairment of ventricular function (ejection fraction greater than 35 to 40 percent and no symptoms of heart failure) in whom pulmonary artery catheterization might be considered are those with severe symptomatic ischemic heart disease in whom revascularization cannot be achieved, either because of emergency urologic procedures or coronary anatomic considerations, and those patients with uncorrected aortic or mitral stenosis.

In patients with severe *symptomatic* heart failure, placement of the pulmonary artery catheter should be performed sufficiently in advance of the urologic procedure to permit optimal adjustment of the hemodynamic state with vasodilators and diuretics. (Usually 12 to 24 hours is sufficient unless no effective therapy for the heart failure has been previously instituted.)

Perioperative determinations of pulmonary artery pressure, pulmonary capillary wedge pressure, and cardiac output permit the anticipation of worsening pulmonary or systemic congestion and allow the physician to determine the causative hemodynamic variable. A falling cardiac output suggests excessive loading of the heart (increasing blood pressure or systemic resistance) or factors depressing cardiac contraction (drugs, ischemia). Increasing wedge and right atrial pressures with initially maintained cardiac output suggest excessive volume administration or fluid shifts into the central vascular space. Attempts to maintain an arbitrary pulmonary wedge or right atrial pressure without consideration of the effects on cardiac output and systemic resistance will result in incomplete therapy.

Therapy of Congestive Heart Failure

The goal of therapy in this setting is to reduce the pulmonary and systemic congestion responsible for the major symptoms of heart failure without compromising the cardiac output.

Diuretic Therapy

Diuretics remain the mainstay of heart failure treatment. However, in the perioperative period, equally important is careful titration of fluid replacement. Accurate assessment of fluid intake and output will only partially reflect vascular volume changes, given changing venomotor tone, fluid shifts, and altered renal water excretion. In the patient who is not undergoing central hemodynamic monitoring, careful examination of the jugular venous pressure, width of the pulse pressure (narrowing of which suggests falling cardiac output and/or systemic vasoconstriction), and heart rate trends are keys to the recognition of hypovolemia. Hypervolemia may be less easily recognized until pulmonary congestion causes rales, reflecting early alveolar edema. This late finding requires diuretic intervention. This can be avoided by limiting fluid intake, again watching for evidence of hypovolemia. In heart failure, hypervolemia is more difficult and dangerous to correct than hypovolemia, despite tradition dictating the opposite.

If hypotension occurs in a patient with a history of congestive heart failure or with severe left ventricular dysfunction, hypovolemia is only one of several possible causes. The judgment as to whether to treat that hypotension with cautious volume repletion must be based on the estimate of fluid loss and shifting—which is often difficult to determine—and on the risk of overhydration. Insertion of a pulmonary artery catheter permits the appropriate therapeutic response and should be considered early in the postoperative course for a patient with complicated fluid management and left ventricular dysfunction.

Loop diuretics (furosemide, bumetanide, ethacrynic acid) are best administered intravenously in the perioperative period so that the duration of response is more easily seen, permitting repeat dosage after 4 to 6 hours if diuresis is suboptimal.

Inotropic Drugs

In general, the need for intravenous inotropic drugs mandates central hemodynamic monitoring and should be reserved for patients with demonstrable depressed cardiac output. The abrupt onset of hypotension unresponsive to volume repletion or in a patient in whom "blind" volume repletion is hazardous mandates the use of dopamine while the pulmonary artery catheter is being placed. Dopamine is chosen because of its inotropic effect without concomitant vasodilatation as may occur with dobutamine or amrinone. Postoperative patients may be excessively vasodilated from sepsis, residual anesthetic, or analgesic therapy, thus making further vasodilatation dangerous. Once the cardiac output and vascular resistance have been determined, the agent can be chosen based on the need or desirability of vasodilatation versus vasoconstriction. Obviously, a low systemic vascular resistance (e.g., less than 1000 dyn-sec cm^{-5}) may be exacerbated by inotropic agents, such as dobutamine or amrinone, which have substantial vasodilating effects. Conversely, systemic vascular resistance greater than 1500 dyn-sec cm^{-5} may benefit by vasodilatation in the presence of heart failure.

Low doses of dopamine offer the additional benefit of renal arterial vasodilatation without substantial systemic vasodilation. However, at these low doses, the inotropic effect is very small. In patients with depressed cardiac output (cardiac index <2.2 L/minute/M^2) and with systemic vasoconstriction, dobutamine would be a preferable agent because impedance to cardiac ejection would be reduced and the increased cardiac output would be more important to renal perfusion than specific renal vasodilatation. Amrinone, a newer non-catecholamine inotropic agent, may be used alternatively. The thrombocytopenia associated with prolonged use and high dosage of this drug is of little concern with short-term use.

Digoxin has little place as an acute inotropic agent. Patients who have a dilated left ventricle and who have been maintained on digoxin may benefit from its continued administration; however, the acute onset of left ventricular contractile failure is better treated with more potent and more easily titrated agents. Digoxin remains a very useful drug in the treatment of atrial arrhythmias, as will be discussed subsequently.

Vasodilator Agents

The use of vasodilator agents to diminish the impedance to left ventricular ejection, and to diminish venous return through direct venodilatation, is often recommended in perioperative treatment of *severe* heart failure. Nitroprusside, administered by experienced nurses and physicians, is the agent of choice in non-ischemic heart failure. The major advantage, apart from its potency, is its short duration of action, permitting accurate titration. Nitroprusside should generally be used with central hemodynamic monitoring except where severe hypertension is being treated, in which case normalization of the blood pressure (140–150/70–80) can be safely achieved without hemodynamic data. More aggressive treatment requires knowledge of the drug's effect on cardiac output, left and right ventricular filling pressures, and systemic vascular resistance.

In patients requiring emergent urologic surgery with ischemic heart failure or who develop postoperative complications of ischemia and heart failure, nitroglycerin is the preferred vasodilator in the nonhypertensive patient. Although nitroglycerin often has been erroneously classified as a venodilator, it is an effective arterial dilator as well, particularly for patients experiencing high vascular resistances. It has the additional advantage of dilating the medium-sized conductance arteries of the heart, including potential collateral blood supply, thus diminishing ischemia by reducing oxygen demand *and* enhancing supply.

Oral vasodilators such as captopril and hydralazine are often substituted as postoperative recovery progresses; these agents are titrated more accurately with ongoing hemodynamic monitoring, although clinical assessment of therapeutic response *may* suffice.

CARDIAC ARRHYTHMIAS

The intraoperative and postoperative periods are notorious for inducing cardiac rhythm disturbances in susceptible patients. Although modern anesthetic agents are only minimally, if at all, arrhythmogenic, the reflex responses of increased adrenergic tone during induction and intubation and during recovery from anesthesia may precipitate both supraventricular and ventricular arrhythmias. Postoperative pain or respiratory distress may have the same effect of increasing catecholamine levels and thus precipitating arrhythmias, as do sympathomimetic agents such as theophylline, inhaled bronchodilators, and inotropic agents. Although sustained ventricular arrhythmias are an uncommon consequence of this phenomenon, they may occur in patients with a prior history of ventricular arrhythmias or in the setting of myocardial ischemia. Supraventricular arrhythmias are particularly common in this setting; for individuals so predisposed (e.g., prior history of supraventricular arrhythmias, age older than 75 years, pulmonary disease) sympathomimetic agents should be prescribed with caution and awareness of the potential risk of inducing atrial fibrillation or flutter.

Electrolyte and acid-base abnormalities, particularly hypokalemia and alkalosis, may induce serious ventricular and, less commonly, atrial arrhythmias. An increase in ventricular ectopy should lead the physician to look for hypokalemia and/or alkalosis as well as to consider causes of heightened adrenergic stimulation. These causes may be remedied without having to resort to antiarrhythmic drug therapy with its attendant complexities and potential toxicity.

Atrial Arrhythmias

Atrial fibrillation and atrial flutter are common postoperative arrhythmias in the elderly patient, particularly in those with hypertension or pulmonary disease. Patients so predisposed have been successfully treated with digitalis prophylactically in several series, thus diminishing the incidence of the arrhythmia. Doses of digoxin, 0.75 mg preoperatively and 0.125 gm/day during the immediate postoperative period, are quite safe and may be effective. Once the arrhythmia has occurred, digoxin will slow the ventricular response and may enhance the chance of conversion to normal sinus rhythm. Incremental doses of 0.25 mg intravenously (IV) every 2 to 4 hours to a total of 1 mg may be employed in patients not already on digoxin. Again, attempts to diminish adrenergic stimulation should be undertaken simultaneously. Beta-blocking drugs will also assist in slowing the rate in patients refractory to digoxin, although beta-blocking drugs are often relatively contraindicated in patients with obstructive pulmonary disease or prior abnormal sinus node function, both types of patients being more susceptible to atrial fibrillation. Intravenous verapamil *transiently* slows the ventricular response to atrial fibrillation but at the risk of inducing hypotension. Its use should be discouraged in this setting in favor of agents with more sustained effectiveness and fewer side effects.

Sick Sinus Syndrome

Sick sinus syndrome, also called brady-tachy syndrome, is characterized by alternating periods of supraventricular tachycardia rhythms such as atrial fibrillation and periods of bradycardia with sinus pauses. It is more commonly seen in the elderly and may be exacerbated by postoperative electrolyte abnormalities, vagal reflex responses, and centrally acting antihypertensives or sedative-tranquilizer drugs.

Attempts to slow the tachycardiac phase may result in worsening of the bradycardiac episodes. Patients with prior history of sinus node disease, particularly in which the inability to effectively raise the heart rate to modest exertional stimuli is present, should have a temporary pacemaker placed preoperatively to permit safe administration of antitachycardiac drugs as well as to provide a backup rate under conditions of postoperative stress.

Atrioventricular (AV) Block and Bundle Branch Block. Patients with asymptomatic Mobitz I AV block (so-called Wenckebach's block) or bundle branch block do not need *prophylactic* pacemaker therapy. For those patients with inadequate heart response or with Mobitz II or complete AV block, a permanent pacemaker should be placed preoperatively unless surgical urgency does not permit. Under these circumstances, a temporary transvenous pacemaker catheter should be employed.

Ventricular Arrhythmias

Although potentially more dangerous, ventricular arrhythmias are often easier and more straightforward to treat in the perioperative period. The major risk of ventricular arrhythmia is a function of the underlying heart disease. Those patients with ongoing ischemia, severe left ventricular dysfunction, and/or progressive cardiac dilatation are at great risk for ventricular arrhythmias. Those with no discernible underlying heart disease are at little or no risk for sustained ventricular tachycardia or fibrillation.

The presence of frequent premature ventricular beats on examination or electrocardiogram at the preoperative evaluation should trigger the search for ischemia or ventricular dysfunction with a treadmill and echocardiogram if history and examination suggest underlying disease.

Under more urgent surgical circumstances, patients with abnormal electrocardiograms, left ventricular enlargement on chest x-ray, cardiac symptoms of angina or heart failure, or prior myocardial infarction who present with frequent premature ventricular beats should be placed on antiarrhythmic therapy prior to surgery to permit some determination of the effect of the chosen drug on the ventricular ectopy. If surgery is imminent, IV therapy is required, recognizing that brief observations may not predict efficacy.

Nonetheless, failure to see suppression of ectopy is prima facie evidence of drug failure and another drug should be tried.

Lidocaine remains the short-term agent of choice primarily because of its limited toxicity when used appropriately. Early lidocaine failure may be due to inadequate blood levels; a double-bolus technique with continued infusion usually prevents subtherapeutic levels early in the therapy.

Procaine amide is an effective agent but with greater hypotensive and proarrhythmic effects. Its empiric use in this setting should be reserved for circumstances in which lidocaine has been ineffective or when both atrial and ventricular arrhythmias are to be treated. A loading dose of 500 to 1000 mg intravenously at a rate not to exceed 50 mg/minute followed by a 2- to 4-mg drip is recommended, with careful monitoring for hypotension, bradycardia, or QT interval prolongation.

Under conditions of sustained ventricular tachycardia, bretylium is considered at least the third-line, if not second-line, agent to prevent recurrence. Its use should be reserved for refractory arrhythmias.

Again, it should be stressed that many perioperative arrhythmias are induced by potentially avoidable factors. Attempts to treat the cause is, of course, preferable to treating the consequence.

HYPERTENSION

The frequency of hypertension in the patient population undergoing urologic surgery is greater than in any of the other complicating cardiac conditions. In contrast to the chronic therapy of hypertension, the perioperative therapy is often directed as much at systolic hypertension as at diastolic hypertension. For patients with a prior history of hypertension who are currently under therapy, antihypertensive agents should be continued through the perioperative period with as short an interruption as possible. The one exception is diuretic therapy. It is often advisable to discontinue diuretics for 1 to 2 days preoperatively to permit potassium repletion and avoid hypovolemia when normal fluid intake is limited prior to surgery.

Patients who have newly discovered severe hypertension or poorly controlled hypertension *and* in whom delay of surgery to permit adequate control of their blood pressure may be dangerous are best controlled with nitroprusside in an appropriate monitoring unit. Nitroprusside is preferable to all other parenteral agents for short-term use because its effect is predictable; rapid in onset and offset, thus allowing for careful titration, and, when used appropriately, produces fewer side effects than IV beta-blocking drugs, ganglionic blockers, or intermittent injectable agents such as hydralazine.

For less urgent circumstances in which oral therapy is appropriate, nifedipine is often effective and is particularly useful when concerns about heart failure or ischemia are present. Clonidine can be administered transcutaneously and may be useful with moderate hypertension in an otherwise stable patient who cannot take oral medications.

Postoperative hypertension should be treated aggressively in patients with cardiac failure or ischemia. As with other cardiac diseases, preoperative control permits better postoperative management, and when possible, surgery should be delayed to permit an adequate drug regimen to be instituted, even though postoperative changes will often need to be made.

The key to avoiding or minimizing cardiac complications of urologic surgery is preoperative risk assessment. Preoperative control of heart failure, angina, cardiac arrhythmis, or hypertension will permit safe surgical intervention even in patients with very complex cardiac conditions. Conversely, unappreciated (and therefore untreated) cardiac risk factors result in the majority of perioperative cardiac complications.

Current cardiac diagnostic methods are reasonably precise in establishing relative risk; application of therapy based on that physiologic determination of cardiac dysfunction will do much to lessen the cardiac impact on the postoperative course of the urologic surgical patient.

ANESTHETIC COMPLICATIONS OF UROLOGIC SURGERY

6

Thomas M. Grove

A variety of anesthetic techniques may be used to allow urologic procedures to be performed. Because of the location of the surgery, many of these procedures are ideally suited for regional anesthesia—spinal, epidural, or caudal. Sometimes, as a result of difficult patient positions or length of the procedure, a regional technique may be combined with a light general anesthetic in order to obtain the benefits of regional anesthesia, such as lower drug requirements, fewer cardiopulmonary depressive effects, and improved postoperative pain relief. Extent of surgery, patient preference, or other factors often preclude the use of regional techniques, and general anesthesia alone may be used.

Urologic patients who require anesthesia are subject to the same risk of anesthetic complications as any patient who is given anesthesia. In addition, specific problems peculiar to some urologic patients and procedures that have significant implications with regard to anesthetic care may exist. The impact of renal failure on the disposition of drugs used during the administration of anesthesia must be carefully considered. Conversely, the effects of anesthetic agents and care on already compromised kidneys or on newly transplanted kidneys must be taken into account when one is dealing with these patients. Extracorporeal shock wave lithotripsy (ESWL) presents special problems for the anesthetist owing to the positioning of the patient in the water bath. Transurethral resection of the prostate also presents peculiar problems related to the use of irrigating fluid and assessment of blood loss. Procedures often necessitate that patients be placed in unusual positions that may interact with the effects of anesthesia to produce cardiovascular instability or respiratory compromise. Surgery for pheochromocytoma presents special problems in terms of managing cardiovascular responses. Despite the many possibilities for complications, the overall risk of serious injury resulting from anesthesia is low.

RISK OF ANESTHESIA

Anesthetic Mortality

The first report of death caused by anesthesia was published by Snow in 1858.[1] Since then, numerous large-scale studies have been published on the mortality and morbidity resulting from anesthesia.[2–9] Older studies,[2–7] as summarized by Tinker and Roberts,[1] found that the incidence of perioperative deaths due primarily to anesthesia was between one in 850 and one in 6000 anesthetics. However, anesthetic practice has changed greatly since these studies were completed.

Large-scale studies, completed in Great Britain and France, give us some idea of modern anesthetic safety. Lunn and associates[8] from Cardiff, Wales, attempted to analyze all in-hospital deaths within 6 days of surgery in five regions of England, Scotland, and Wales in 1980 and 1981. They concluded that only one in 10,000 patients undergoing anesthesia dies solely as a result of the anesthesia. About six in 10,000 die as a result of circumstances that are at least partly attributable to anesthesia.[8]

A prospective survey was carried out in France from 1978 to 1982 in which 198,103 anesthetics were reviewed.[9] The overall incidence of complications related to anesthesia was found to be 13 in 10,000 anesthetics, with eight in 10,000 thought to be totally due to anesthesia. The rate of deaths related to anesthesia was 3.3 in 10,000, with 0.8 in 10,000 totally due to anesthesia. The incidence of death and coma caused solely by anesthesia was found to be 1.3 in 10,000.

Nonfatal Anesthesia-Related Complications

The list of complications that have been related to anesthesia care is long. Circulatory problems that have been reported include cardiac arrest, circulatory collapse, hypotension, hypertension, arrhythmias, acute pulmonary edema, and myocardial infarction (MI). Respiratory problems include aspiration of gastric contents, bronchospasm, airway obstruction and laryngospasm, pneumothorax, atelectasis, and respiratory depression. Neurologic problems include delayed emergence, coma, awareness, postoperative emotional disturbances, and nerve palsies. Disorders of temperature regulation include hypothermia and malignant hyperthermia (MH). Renal problems include fluid and electrolyte disorders, oliguria, polyuria, and urinary retention. Gastrointestinal problems include hepatic injury and nausea and vomiting.

A survey from Canada[13] found that some complication occurred in as many as 17.8 percent of all anesthetics. Although no overall studies of complications allow comparison of incidence based on type of surgery, a follow-up by the Canadian group[14] indicated that renal disease is a very significant factor in increased major cardiovascular complications. Specifically, cardiac arrest was ten times more likely in the recovery room in renal patients than in others. Postoperative myocardial infarction was three times as likely, and the overall incidence of major complications was 2.3 times as likely. These statistics clearly imply that, at least for this group of urologic patients, the chances of significant anesthetic-related complications are markedly increased.

SPECIFIC COMPLICATIONS LEADING TO MORBIDITY AND MORTALITY

Respiratory Complications

Aspiration of gastric contents may occur with obtundation of protective airway reflexes by general anesthesia. Should active vomiting or passive regurgitation of stomach contents occur during a vulnerable period, the likelihood of severe pulmonary damage occurring is high.

In the British survey of Lunn and Mushin[8] and the French survey of Tiret and colleagues,[9] aspiration accounted for 19 and 27 percent, respectively, of the deaths attributed solely to anesthesia. Some studies have indicated that when aspiration is apparent and documented, the overall mortality may be 55 to 70 percent.[12] With such significant mortality, management is focused on preventing its occurrence by utilizing measures such as awake intubation, rapid sequence intravenous inductions with cricoid pressure, or avoidance of general anesthesia by use of regional or local anesthesia.

A retrospective study of incidence of aspiration[11] reported an overall incidence to be 4.7 per 10,000 anesthetics. Of the documented aspirations, 11 percent occurred in urologic patients. Among these was one elderly man who died after vomiting massively while under a spinal anesthetic for cystoscopy. Patients are often nauseated when under spinal anesthesia and may lack the muscular strength to clear the airway if regurgitation should occur. Thus, although spinal anesthesia is usually safer than general anesthesia, when factors predisposing to aspiration are present, careful management of these patients is required.

Control of the airway is essential for maintenance of pulmonary function during general anesthesia. In one study of intraoperative cardiac arrest caused by anesthesia, 12 of 27 arrests were attributed to failure to ventilate.[10] This included such problems as inability to intubate, unrecognized esophageal intubation, unrecognized ventilator disconnection, displaced endotracheal tube, and severe bronchospasm. Johnson and Gold[15] speculated that the release of prostaglandins or other agents from prostatic and surrounding tissues may lead to bronchospasm during prostatectomy. However, in a large-scale retrospective survey, Olsson[16] found no cases of bronchospasm in 672 prostate surgeries, thereby indicating that it is unlikely that such a mechanism is significant.

Another significant respiratory complication is pneumothorax. It may occur as a result of increased airway pressure on a weakened alveolar septum, leading to alveolar rupture, or as a result of a break in the visceral or parietal pleura.[17] Alveolar rupture may occur in any patient, but patients with chronic lung disease are particularly susceptible. Pneumothorax is of particular concern in subdiaphragmatic procedures such as renal biopsy, nephrectomy, and adrenalectomy. It is one of the most frequent complications of donor nephrectomy.[18] Although simple lung collapse may be relatively innocuous, the development of tension pneumothorax may lead to life-threatening circulatory collapse. The well-known effect[19] of nitrous oxide in expanding closed air-containing spaces may prompt the development of tension in an otherwise nonsignificant pneumothorax. Communication between surgeon and anesthetist is essential in preventing this development when diaphragmatic injury is known to have occurred.

Postoperative respiratory depression caused by prolonged effect of anesthetic agents given during surgery, especially narcotic analgesics and muscle relaxants, also leads to morbidity. Indeed, in the French survey,[9] it accounted for more than half of the deaths and comas attributed to respiratory problems.

The use of an endotracheal tube during general anesthesia provides a secure airway for delivery of oxygen and anesthetic agents. A number of complications, usually minor but occasionally serious, have been associated with the placement and use of these tubes. Several authors have reviewed these problems, listing them in logical categories.[32] Briefly, these may include problems occurring at intubation, such as trauma to teeth, lips, tongue, larynx, nose, eye, and cervical spine; consequent retropharyngeal dissection, possibly leading to abscess or mediastinal emphysema; aspiration of gastric contents or foreign bodies; accidental intubation of the esophagus with consequent anoxic brain damage or death if not detected; or misplacement of the tube (e.g., with the tip in the right mainstem bronchus with consequent hypoxia). During the time that the trachea is intubated, problems may occur that are related to obstruction of the airway from kinking of the tube, herniation of the cuff, blockage by blood or secretions, or biting on the tube. At the time of extubation, problems may occur with airway obstruction, tracheal collapse, or aspiration. Complications after extubation include sore throat, glottic edema, vocal cord paralysis, laryngeal ulcers and granulomata, laryngeal or tracheal fibrosis, membranes and webs, or synechiae of vocal cords. None of these complications is specific to patients on the urologic service but may occur.

Cardiovascular Complications

Myocardial Infarction

About 1.13 percent of all patients suffer MI within 5 days after surgery.[13,20] Patients who have suffered previous MI have significantly greater risk of reinfarction, especially when surgery occurs within 6 months of MI. After 6 months, the reinfarction rate seems to stabilize at 2 to 6 percent, but within 6 months the rate is 1.5 to 10 times as great.[21] Mortality from perioperative infarction is especially high. Studies have shown 54 to 87 percent of these patients die as a result of MI.[20] Site of surgery is an important determinant of incidence of MI, being higher for thoracic and upper abdominal operations than for others. In one study,[20] the reinfarction rate was only 4 percent for perineal genitourinary surgery; 6.6 percent for all operations; and 12.2 percent for thoracic and upper abdominal surgeries.

Dysrhythmias

The true incidence of dysrhythmias under anesthesia is difficult to determine because many are benign and transient and are not documented. Studies using continuous tape recording have found the incidence to be as high as 84 percent.[22]

Electrolyte abnormalities may play a role in the development of dysrhythmias. This is an important consideration in patients with poor renal function in whom significant electrolyte abnormalities, particularly hyperkalemia, may be present.[24,25] Succinylcholine is known to cause a mild increase in serum potassium in normal patients. Much larger serum potassium increases leading to serious dysrhythmias occur in patients with burns, massive trauma, tetanus, and neuromuscular diseases.[26,27] There have been reports of cardiac arrest and ventricular tachycardia attributed to succinylcholine-induced hyperkalemia in patients with renal failure.[28,29] Subsequent investigations found that the serum potassium increase after a single dose of succinylcholine was about 0.5 mEq/l (comparable with that in normal patients) but that repeated doses led to further increases.[26,27] Current practice is to avoid succinylcholine in patients in whom preoperative serum potassium concentration is greater than 5.5 mEq/L.[30,31]

Malignant Hyperthermia

Classically, MH is characterized by hypermetabolism and a rapidly increasing temperature during general anesthesia.[33,34] The temperature rise is a result of an acute uncontrolled increase in skeletal muscle metabolism that occurs in susceptible individuals in response to certain triggers. The onset of the hypermetabolic state may be rapid after induction of anesthesia, but the temperature rise may actually be a late sign or may even be absent. The most consistent early sign is tachycardia or rapid ventricular dysrhythmias.[34] Other signs include unstable blood pressure, tachypnea in spontaneously breathing patients (or rising expired carbon dioxide levels in patients on controlled ventilation), and cyanosis. Muscle rigidity may be present, and masseter spasm occuring after a bolus of succinylcholine may be an early sign. Analysis of arterial blood gases demonstrates the presence of severe acidosis, usually metabolic but possibly respiratory as well.

Triggering agents include potent volatile anesthetic agents and succinylcholine, either independently or in combination. Although amide local anesthetics were once suggested as possible triggers, evidence for this is considered weak and amides are probably safe.[34]

The early mortality rate from MH was about 70 percent, but increased vigilance with early diagnosis reduced mortality to 28 percent. The use of dantrolene as a specific treatment for MH in 1979 has reduced mortality to less than 10 percent.[34]

The incidence of reactions in children, adolescents, and young adults is estimated at about one in 15,000 anesthetics; in middle-aged adults, it is at about one in 50,000.[34] Susceptibility is genetically transmitted, although the exact pattern of transmission is not yet clear. Overt reactions are also variable, in that some patients have developed an MH reaction after undergoing previously uneventful anesthesia.[34]

Anesthetic management of patients known or suspected of being susceptible to MH consists primarily of avoiding known triggering agents and being prepared to treat any early signs immediately. Although some pretreat such patients with dantrolene, others prefer to treat only when signs of reaction occur.

Allergic Reactions

Most drugs and blood products administered during anesthesia have been reported to produce life-threatening allergic reactions. A number of these drugs, including morphine, meperidine, D-tubocurarine, metocurine, atracurium, thiopental, and thiamylal are known to cause non-immunologic histamine release in a dose-dependent fashion.[35]

Hepatic Injury

Reports of postoperative hepatitis possibly associated with halothane anesthesia began to appear in 1958, 2 years after its clinical introduction. By 1963, the National Halothane Study was undertaken to look retrospectively for a link between halothane and hepatic injury. Of about 850,000 anesthetics, 82 cases of fatal hepatic necrosis were identified. Twenty-six of these deaths occurred after halothane administration. The overall incidence of death from massive hepatic necrosis after halothane was about one in 10,000. Other causes could be found in all but nine of the 82 cases of massive hepatic necrosis. Seven of these nine cases occurred after halothane—an incidence of one death caused by unexplained massive hepatic necrosis per 35,000 halothane anesthetics. The study concluded that "the possible rare occurrence of halothane-induced hepatic necrosis . . . could not be ruled out."[36] Other studies noted nonfatal hepatitis after halothane in one in 2500 anesthetics and overall mortality of one in 11,000.[37] Since there are a number of other factors that may contribute to perioperative liver dysfunction and because there is no diagnostic test specific for halothane hepatitis, it remains a diagnosis of exclusion. Etiologic factors remain unclear; however, because incidence appears to be higher after a second exposure, an allergic mechanism has been proposed. It has been recommended that halothane anesthesia should not be repeated within a period of 3 to 12 months.[38] Infants and young children seem to be at very low risk, whereas obese, middle-aged patients seem to be at a higher risk.[38]

Complications of Regional Anesthesia

Many urologic procedures are performed using regional anesthesia—usually spinal, epidural, or caudal. Complications resulting from these procedures can be categorized as *drug-related* or *technique-related.*[40]

Drug-Related Complications

Drug-related complications are due to the systemic toxicity of the agents used. Because of the small amount of drug used, systemic toxicity is not a problem with spinal anesthesia. Blood levels of local anesthetic agents with epidural anesthesia are not usually toxic; however, accidental intravascular injection or use of excessive doses can lead to blood levels in the toxic range. Central nervous system (CNS) signs may progress from generalized seizures to generalized depression.[39,40]

Toxic cardiac effects of the local anesthetics usually do not occur until blood levels have exceeded those necessary for CNS effects. Very high drug blood levels may lead to bradycardia, partial or complete atrioventricular dissociation, or sinus arrest. Dose-dependent myocardial depression, which correlates with the anesthetic activity of the agent, also occurs. Cases of sudden irreversible cardiovascular collapse following the use of 0.75 percent bupivicaine have been reported in obstetric patients.[40]

In addition to administration of local anesthetics, the injection of opioids, both epidurally and intrathecally for management of pain in the postoperative period, has gained great popularity. This technique may have advantage for many urologic patients, since it produces excellent relief of pain lasting 12 to 24 hours. There are several significant associated side effects and possible complications.[40] Intense pruritus and nausea and vomiting have been reported in about 10 to 30 percent of these patients. Urinary retention requiring catheterization occurs in 10 to 30 percent of patients. The most serious problem occurring with the use of epidural opioids is that of respiratory arrest. This may occur early, about 1 hour after administration, or late, 6 to 12 hours after administration. Respiratory arrest occurs much less frequently than do the other side effects and appears to be dose-dependent. It also occurs more frequently when epidural narcotics are combined with parenteral narcotics. Naloxone is effective in reversing the respiratory depression as well as the other side effects, but the need for close observation of these patients is obvious.

Technique-Related Complications

A number of side effects and complications of regional anesthesia are related to the specific techniques. Both spinal and epidural anesthesia can have significant cardiovascular effects, primarily as a result of sympathetic blockade. Hypotension may occur as a result of inhibitation of sympathetic arterial and venous vasoconstrictors. With high levels of block, cardiac accelerator fibers are also affected and heart rate may slow markedly. Vasovagal events may occur, precipitating profound bradycardia and hypotension. Rarely, cardiac arrest may ensue.

Nausea and vomiting may occur as a result of the altered balance between parasympathetic and sympathetic gastrointestinal activity.

Motor block, high enough to affect the diaphragm, may occasionally occur following unrecognized dural puncture during epidural anesthesia. Large volumes of anesthetic placed in the subarachnoid space produce high or total spinal blockade. Unconsciousness, respiratory arrest, and severe hypotension may develop, and immediate action is required.

Lumbar puncture headache is a recognized sequela to spinal anesthesia. The incidence, reported to be from less than 1 percent to as high as 30 percent, decreases with increasing age and is more common in women than in men. Smaller needles reduce the incidence of headache. When accidental dural puncture occurs during epidural anesthesia, the incidence of headache may be high owing to the large needle used. A number of other neurologic complications have been reported with spinal and epidural anesthesia, including chronic adhesive arachnoiditis, septic and aseptic meningitis, transverse myelitis, anterior and posterior spinal artery syndromes, direct cord trauma, and epidural hematoma or abscess.[39] Backache may be associated with these techniques, but the incidence is not different from that occurring with general anesthesia.[39]

PROBLEMS IN ANESTHETIC MANAGEMENT OF UROLOGIC PATIENTS

Certain urologic procedures involve problems of special concern to anesthesiologists. In these cases, anesthetic management must be undertaken with the knowledge of these problems in order to reduce the likelihood of significant complication.

Kidney Transplant

These who are to undergo kidney transplant present with a multiplicity of problems related to chronic renal failure, which may have anesthetic implications. Patients may have gastrointestinal disturbances and electrolyte abnormalities, especially hyperkalemia, hyponatremia, and hypocalcemia. Metabolic disturbances may lead to encephalopathy, with implications for altered sensitivity to drugs. The incidence of hypertension and other cardiovascular problems is higher in these patients. Hematologic problems include anemia and coagulopathy. Pharmacokinetic and pharmacodynamic alterations may occur as a result of decreased renal excretion, decreased renal metabolism, changes in protein binding, and possible changes in end organ sensitivity.[18,30,31]

Preoperatively, these patients should undergo hemodialysis to optimize their fluid and electrolyte status. Hypertension should be optimally controlled and antihypertensive medications continued preoperatively.[18] Although control of blood pressure intraoperatively is essential, the use of intra-arterial monitoring is controversial because its use may reduce the availability of vessels needed for dialysis access at a later time. Currently used dialysis sites must be protected and adequate perfusion maintained through them throughout in order to avoid loss of function.

Premedications must be given with care. Uremic patients tend to be more sensitive to all psychotropic drugs.[31] Protein binding of many drugs, including the benzodiozepines diazepam and midozalam, is reduced, and their intensity and duration of activity may be increased.[18,31] Protein binding of morphine is also reduced, and patients may be markedly sensitive.[18] Morphine is not dialyzeable, and respiratory depression as long as 6 days after its administration has been reported.[18] Seizures have been reported after repeated doses of meperidine, apparently as a result of the accumulation of its metabolite normeperidine, which has convulsant properties and is normally excreted in the urine.[31]

Since gastric retention is common in uremic patients, it may be advisable to use metaclopramide and ranitidine or cimetidine preoperatively.[31] Techniques to avoid possible aspiration of gastric contents should be undertaken, especially for those patients undergoing urgent operation for cadaveric transplant who may not have had adequate time for stomach emptying preoperatively.

Both regional and general anesthesia have been used for kidney transplantation. Protein binding of barbiturates is reduced so that initial levels of unbound thiopental reaching the brain may have increased effect during induction of general anesthesia. The distribution and elimination of barbiturates, however, are unchanged.[18,31]

General anesthesia is often maintained with a potent inhalational agent—halothane, enflurane, or isoflurane. Metabolism of enflurane produces free fluoride. Although fluoride levels seen after enflurane anesthesia have not been shown to exceed the usually accepted nephrotoxic threshold, its use in patients with compromised renal function is controversial and is usually avoided.[31] Isoflurane is metabolized to a much smaller extent than is enflurane and produces much lower levels of fluoride. It is currently the most acceptable volatile anesthetic for renal transplant. Narcotics may also be used as part of the anesthetic technique.

Muscle relaxants are an important part of the general anesthetic regimen. Succinylcholine is usually used to facilitate tracheal intubation. As mentioned previously, it brings about release of potassium from skeletal muscle and has been reported to cause cardiac arrest in hyperkalemic patients. Its use is usually restricted to patients in whom serum potassium is less than 5.5 mEq/l. Although pseudocholinesterase levels may be reduced with dialysis, clinically significant increases in duration of action are uncommon.

The duration of action of nondepolarizing muscle relaxants may be significantly altered in renal failure.[18,30,31] Gallamine and metocurine are entirely dependent on kidneys for excretion. While both D-tubocuramine and, to a lesser extent, pancuronium undergo significant elimination via biliary excretion, the duration of action of both is markedly prolonged. Vecuronium elimination is much less dependent on the kidneys and may be used with care as long as hepatic function is maintained. Atracurium undergoes nonenzymatic breakdown (Hofmann elimination) and ester hydrolysis in the blood; hence, it is only minimally affected by both kidney and liver failure. However, it may cause some hypotension with large doses owing to histamine release. Before the advent of vecuronium and atracurium, prolonged muscle paralysis was a fairly common problem in patients with renal failure.

The incidence of cardiac complications is markedly increased in renal failure. These include intraoperative hypotension, severe dysrhythmias, and postoperative MI.

Transurethral Resection of the Prostate

A number of problems associated with transurethral resection of the prostate (TURP) have implications for the anesthesiologist and must be kept in mind during planning and conduct of anesthesia.[41,42] The patients are elderly, a group more likely to have significant cardiovascular and pulmonary disease. During the procedure, the nonelectrolyte irrigating solution may be absorbed in sufficient volume to induce circulatory overload, hyponatremia, and serum hypo-osmolality.

The amount of absorbed fluid depends on the duration of resection, number of open venous sinuses, and hydrostatic pressure of the irrigating solution.[42] Manifestations of the syndrome under regional anesthesia include hypotension; bradycardia; mental changes, such as restlessness and confusion; nausea and vomiting; and cardiovascular symptoms, such as substernal pain, dyspnea, cyanosis, and pulmonary edema.[42] CNS symptoms may be due, in part, to glycine and its metabolite ammonia when glycine is the irrigating solution.[43,44] Under general anesthesia, mental changes cannot be observed and signs of circulatory overload may be masked. The only early sign may be hypertension, which is very nonspecific.

Surgical perforation of the capsule may cause either intraperitoneal or extraperitoneal extravasation of fluid. Intraperitoneal perforation usually causes abdominal rigidity and distension. In the awake patient, referred pain to the shoulder may occur, as may hiccup and shortness of breath. Extraperitoneal perforation usually leads to pain and distension limited to the lower abdomen. Unless extensive extravasation leads to hemodynamic compromise, aggressive treatment is not necessary.

Spinal anesthesia is considered the technique of choice in TURP because the awake patient is able to give early warning of problems of either fluid absorption or perforation.[42,43] General anesthesia may be used for patients unable or unwilling to undergo regional anesthesia. Assessment of blood loss is also very difficult in TURP; however, during procedures lasting less than 1 hour, intraoperative blood replacement is usually not necessary.

Extracorporeal Shock Wave Lithotripsy

For ESWL, anesthesia is required because of the painful stimulus of the shock waves.[45–46] The procedure presents special problems to the anesthetist because the patient is in a sitting position, immersed in a water bath, and relatively inaccessible for airway management or emergency resuscitation. The use of intercostal nerve blocks combined with local infiltration has been reported to be an effective method[51] of achieving analgesia in well-motivated patients not requiring additional urologic procedures. Either general or regional anesthesia with spinal or continuous epidural techniques is used in most centers.[45–48]

Regional anesthesia is stated to offer several advantages. The patient is able to cooperate in movement to and positioning on the suspension apparatus. Many patients require cystoscopy and ureteroscopy before treatment, and, unlike the technique of intercostal nerve block plus local infiltration, epidural anesthesia provides acceptable conditions for both procedures. Spinal anesthesia provides acceptable analgesia, but it may not last long enough when combined procedures are required. Epidural anesthesia with the placement of an indwelling epidural catheter allows for reinjection of local anesthetic should the block begin to wear off. Stone movement with respiratory motion or other patient activity is a disadvantage of regional anesthesia. This problem can be avoided with general anesthesia.[46] High-frequency controlled ventilation with low tidal volumes has been advocated to minimize stone movement and, according to some, to improve the success rate of ESWL.[46,48] Others believe that the problem of stone movement may be overestimated.[50]

Arrhythmias were an early problem seen with ESWL. To minimize their occurrence, the shock waves are triggered by the electrocardiogram to fall in the heart's refractory period.[45,47] Nevertheless, dysrhythmias, including supraventricular tachycardia[49] and ventricular[47] and atrial[46,47] premature contractions, continue to be reported.

London and associates[46] reported hypotension, defined as a fall in blood pressure of greater than 20 percent from baseline, to have occurred in 13 percent of ESWL patients undergoing general anesthesia, in 19 percent of those undergoing epidural anesthesia, and in 26 percent of those undergoing spinal anesthesia. Frank and colleagues[47] reported hypotensive episodes in 46 percent of those with epidural anesthesia. Other complications reported[46,47] include flank pain at site of shock-wave entrance, pain at the exit site of the shock wave when it is above water, apnea, toxic reaction to local anesthetics, hiccups, evidence of histamine release when atracurium is used with general anesthesia, nausea and vomiting, bradycardia, chest pain, and myocardial infarction.

Percutaneous Nephrolithotripsy

Peterson and co-workers[52] reported on 48 cases of percutaneous lithotripsy. Because of the problem of the patient's maintaining a prone oblique position for prolonged periods, general anesthesia with controlled ventilation was thought to be the preferred technique. The authors reported two patients in whom severe metabolic acidosis developed, one of whom proceeded to develop disseminated intravascular coagulation and died. Both patients had suffered rupture of the renal pelvis with instillation of large amounts of fluid into the retroperitoneal space. Other complications considered by this group include hypothermia from the large volumes of irrigating fluid, pneumothorax or hydrothorax, chronic renal failure due to long-standing obstruction with the attendant anesthetic implications, and autonomic hyperreflexia, because many of their patients had high spinal cord transections. Bennett and coauthors[53] reported a case in which a sudden cardiac arrest occurred; in this instance, sterile water irrigation fluid had been used. They speculate that the arrest may have been due to water intoxication.

Adrenalectomy

Adrenalectomy for pheochrocytoma necessitates special consideration for the anesthesiologist because of the potential for marked adrenergic responses during the procedure. Careful preoperative preparation and intensive intraoperative monitoring are essential.

The use of adrenergic receptor blocking drugs in the preoperative period is generally recommended.[21] Mortality associated with pheochromocytoma resection is stated to have been reduced from 40 to 60 percent to 0 to 6 percent with the introduction of preoperative alpha-adrenergic blockade with prazosin or phenoxybenzamine.[21] For patients who have persistent dysrhythmias or tachycardia, beta-adrenergic blockade with propranolol is also recommended. Enough time for preoperative therapy (usually 10 to 14 days) to allow stabilization of blood pressure should be allowed before surgery. Many different anesthetic techniques have been used. All appear to be associated with a high rate of intraoperative dysrhythmias and hypertension requiring vasodilator therapy.[21]

Cystectomy

Radical cystectomy is a major procedure that may be accompanied by massive intraoperative blood loss and a high incidence of perioperative complications. Ryan[54] compared the use of epidural and general anesthesia with fentanyl and relaxant. He found a significantly lower intraoperative blood loss in patients receiving epidural anesthesia, which he attributed to its hypotensive effect. The epidural catheter may also be of significant benefit in management of postoperative pain. Comparing the use of controlled hypotension to normotensive anesthesia in these patients, Ahlering and associates[55] found that this also led to significant reduction in intraoperative blood loss. Although there are potential complications associated with controlled hypotensive anesthesia, including cerebrovascular accident, myocardial infarction, hepatic failure and renal failure, careful use of this technique may confer potential benefits for the patient. The use of controlled hypotension was also reported by Stirt and colleagues[56] to be useful in reducing the intraoperative blood loss during retroperitoneal lymph node dissection for testicular carcinoma.

References

1. Tinker JH, Roberts SL: Anesthesia risk. In Miller RD, ed: Anesthesia. New York, Churchill Livingstone, 1986, pp 359–428.
2. Beecher HK, Todd DP: A study of the deaths associated with anesthesia and surgery. Ann Surg 140:2–34, 1954.
3. Dornette WHL, Orth OS: Death in the operating room. Anesth Analg 35:545–569, 1956.
4. Dripps RDS, Lamont A, Eckenhoff JE: The role of anesthesia in surgical mortality. JAMA 178:261–266, 1961.
5. Clifton BS, Hotten WIT: Deaths associated with anaesthesia. Br J Anaesth 35:250–259, 1963.
6. Memery HN: Anesthesia mortality in private practice: a ten year study. JAMA 194:1185–1188, 1965.
7. Harrison GG: Anaesthetic contributory death: its incidence and causes. Part I: Incidence; Part II: Causes. South Afr Med 42:514, 1968.
8. Lunn JN, Mushin WW: Mortality Associated with Anaesthesia. London, Nuffield Provincial Hospital Trust, 1982.
9. Tiret L, Desmonts JM, Hatton F, Vourc'h G: Complications associated with anaesthesia: a prospective survey in France. Can Anaesth Soc J 33:336–344, 1986.
10. Keenan RL, Boyan P: Cardiac arrest due to anesthesia. JAMA 253:2373–2377, 1985.
11. Olsson GL, Hallen B, Hambraeus-Jonson K: Aspiration during anaesthesia: a computer-aided study of 185,358 anaesthetics. Acta Anaesthesiol Scand 30:84–92, 1986.
12. Kallos T, Lampe KF, Orkin FK: Pulmonary aspiration

of gastric contents. In Orkin FK, Cooperman LH: Complications in Anesthesiology. Philadelphia, JB Lippincott, 1983, pp 752–764.

13. Cohen MM, Duncan PG, Pope WD, Wolkenstein C: A survey of 112,000 anaesthetics at one teaching hospital (1975–83). Can Anaesth Soc J 33:22–31, 1986.
14. Duncan PG, Cohen MM: Postoperative complications: factors of significance to anaesthetic practice. Can Anaesth Soc J 34:2–8, 1987.
15. Johnson EB, Gold MI: Bronchospasm during pelvic surgery: prostaglandin-kinin pathogenesis? Anesth Analg 62:104–108, 1983.
16. Olsson GL: Bronchospasm during anaesthesia. A computer-aided incidence study of 136,929 patients. Acta Anaesthesiol Scand 31:244–252, 1987.
17. Denlinger JK: Pneumothorax. In Orkin FK, Cooperman LH: Complications in Anesthesiology. Philadelphia, JB Lippincott, 1983, pp 173–182.
18. Graybar GB, Tarpey M: Kidney transplantation. In Gelman S, ed: Anesthesia and Organ Transplantation. Philadelphia, WB Saunders Co, 1987, pp 61–110.
19. Eger EI, Saidman LJ: Hazards of nitrous oxide anesthesia in bowel obstruction and pneumothorax. Anesthesiology 26:61–66, 1965.
20. Moffit EA, Harris LK: Perioperative myocardial infarction. In Orkin FK, Cooperman LH, eds: Complications in Anesthesiology. Philadelphia, JB Lippincott, 1983, pp 251–267.
21. Roizen MF: Anesthetic implications of concurrent diseases. In Miller RD, ed: Anesthesia. New York, Churchill Livingstone, 1986, pp 255–357.
22. Kaplan JA, Thuys DM: The electrocardiogram and anesthesia. In Miller RD, ed: Anesthesia. New York, Churchill Livingston, 1986, pp 465–498.
23. Katz RL, Bigger JT: Cardiac arrhythmias during anesthesia and operation. Anesthesiology 33:193–213, 1970.
24. Aldrete JA, Daniel W, O'Higgins JW, et al: Analysis of anesthetic-related morbidity in human recipients of renal homografts. Anesth Analg 50:321–329, 1971.
25. Hirshman CA, Edelstein G: Intraoperative hyperkalemia and cardiac arrest during renal transplantation in an insulin-dependent diabetic patient. Anesthesiology 51:161–162, 1979.
26. Miller RD, Way WL, Hamilton WK, et al: Succinylcholine-induced hyperkalemia in patients with renal failure? Anesthesiology 38:138–141, 1973.
27. Koide M, Waud BE: Serum potassium concentration after succinylcholine in patients with renal failure. Anesthesiology 36:142–145, 1972.
28. Roth F, Wuthrich H: The clinical importance of hyperkalemia following suxamethonium administration. Br J Anaesth 41:311–316, 1969.
29. Powell JN: Suxamethonium-induced hyperkalemia in a uraemic patient. Br J Anaesth 42:806–807, 1970.
30. Marsland AR, Bradley JP: Anaesthesia for renal transplantation: 5 years' experience. Anaesth Intens Care 11:337–344, 1983.
31. Maddern PJ: Anaesthesia for the patient with impaired renal function. Anaesth Intens Care 11:321–332, 1983.
32. Harmer M: Complications of tracheal intubation. In Latto IP, Rosen M, eds: Difficulties in Tracheal Intubation. London, Bailliere Tindall, 1985, pp 36–47.
33. Britt BA: Altered temperature regulation. Section Three: Malignant hyperthermia. In Orkin FK, Cooperman LH, eds: Complications in Anesthesiology. Philadelphia, JB Lippincott, 1983, pp 291–313.
34. Gronert GA: Malignant hyperthermia. In Miller RD, ed: Anesthesia. New York, Churchill Livingstone, 1986, pp 1971–1994.
35. Levy JH: Allergic reactions and anesthesia. In 1986 IARS Review Lectures. International Anesthesia Research Society, 1986, pp 110–114.
36. Bunker JP, Forrest WH, Mosteller M, Vandam LD, eds: The National Halothane Study: A Study of the Possible Association between Halothane Anesthesia and Postoperative Hepatic Necrosis. Bethesda, National Institutes of Health, 1969.
37. Carney FMT, Van Dyke RA: Halothane hepatitis: a critical review. Anesth Analg 51:135–160, 1972.
38. Brown BR, Deha DC: Inhalation anesthetics and hepatic injury. In Orkin FK, Cooperman LM, eds: Complications in Anesthesiology. Philadelphia, JB Lippincott, 1983, pp 436–446.
39. Raj P: Complications due to regional anesthesia. In Raj PP, ed: Handbook of Regional Anesthesia. New York, Churchill Livingstone, 1985, pp 259–273.
40. Covino BG, Scott DB: Handbook of Epidural Anesthesia and Analgesia. Orlando, Grune & Stratton, 1985, pp 131–169.
41. Desmond J: Complications of transurethral prostatic surgery. Can Anaesth Soc J 17:25–36, 1970.
42. Mani M, Keh E, Kartha RK, et al: Transurethral prostatic surgery revisited: a case in point. Anesthesiology Review, 1976, pp 15–19.
43. Alexander JP, Pollard A, Gillespie IA: Glycine and transurethral resection. Anaesthesia 41:1189–1198, 1986.
44. Roesch RP, Stoelting RK, Lingeman JE, et al: Ammonia toxicity resulting from glycine absorption during a transurethral resection of the prostate. Anesthesiology 58:557–559, 1983.
45. Chaussy C, Schmiedt E: Extracorporeal shock wave lithotripsy (ESWL) for kidney stones: alternative to surgery? Urol Radiol 6:80–87, 1984.
46. London RA, Kudlak T, Riehle RA: Immersion anesthesia for extracorporeal shock wave lithotripsy. Ann R Coll Surg Engl 67:341–343, 1986.
47. Frank M, McAteer EJ, Cohen DG, et al: One hundred cases of anaesthesia for extracorporeal shock wave lithotripsy. Ann R Coll Surg Engl 67:341–343, 1985.
48. Riehle RA, Fair WR, Vaughn ED: Extracorporal shock-wave lithotripsy for upper urinary tract calculi. JAMA 255:2043–2048, 1986.
49. Walts LF, Atlee JL: Supraventricular tachycardia associated with extracorporeal shock wave lithotripsy. Anesthesiology 65:521–523, 1986.
50. Perel A, Hoffman B, Podeh D, Davidson JT: High frequency positive pressure ventilation during general anesthesia for extracorporeal shock wave lithotripsy. Anesth Analg 65:1231–1234, 1986.
51. Malhotra V, Long CW, Meister MJ: Intercostal blocks with local infiltration anesthesia for extracorporeal shock wave lithotripsy. Anesth Analg 66:85–88, 1987.
52. Peterson GN, Krieger JN, Glauber DT: Anaesthetic experience with percutaneous lithotripsy. Anaesthesia 40:460–464, 1985.
53. Bennett MJ, Smith RW, Fuchs E: Sudden cardiac arrest during percutaneous ultrasonic nephrostolithotomy. Anesthesiology 60:245–246, 1984.
54. Ryan DW: Anaesthesia for cystectomy. Anaesthesia 37:554–560, 1982.
55. Ahlering TE, Henderson JB, Skinner DG: Controlled hypotensive anesthesia to reduce blood loss in radical cystectomy for bladder cancer. J Urol 129:953–954, 1983.
56. Stirt JA, Korn EL, Reynolds RC: Sodium nitroprusside–induced hypotension in radical thoracoabdominal dissection of retroperitoneal lymph nodes. Br J Anaesth 52:1045–1048, 1980.

TOTAL PARENTERAL NUTRITION IN THE UROLOGIC SURGERY PATIENT

7

Marvin E. Ament • Jorge Vargas • William E. Berquist

Major advances in the surgical management of pediatric and adult urologic patients have occurred during the past two decades. In pediatric patients, operative techniques for reconstruction of the genitourinary tract, and, in adults, surgical treatment of urologic cancer, combined with advances in chemotherapy and radiation therapy, have greatly improved outcome. However, the successful management of such patients has required advances in other areas, such as antibiotics and nutritional support. The success of managing such patients from the outset has required the urologist's recognition of the need for preoperative nutritional assessment and institution of parenteral support in either the immediate preoperative or postoperative period. For many of the patients who now survive, the outcome would not have been successful without the techniques of parenteral support.

Urologists are not unique in their need to be familiar with the importance of and techniques of parenteral nutrition; however, along with abdominal and trauma surgeons, they are among the surgeons who use it most frequently.

Ideally, every hospitalized patient should be screened for nutritional status and, if found to be at high risk for nutritional compromise, should receive a comprehensive nutritional assessment and optimal nutritional support throughout the hospitalization. If the gastrointestinal tract cannot be used, parenteral support should be started as soon as adequate ventilation and hemodynamic homeostasis are established.

NUTRITIONAL ASSESSMENT

Every urologic patient hospitalized for major surgery of the genitourinary tract should be screened for nutritional status. If the patient is found to be nutritionally compromised, nutritional support should be given throughout the hospitalization. If the patient is moderately to severely depleted and surgery can be postponed for 10 to 14 days, nutritional support should be given, as soon as possible, to reverse the nutritional deficit. If surgery cannot be postponed, parenteral support may be started in the immediate postoperative period.

The best way to determine whether a patient is malnourished is to take a complete nutritional history and to perform a thorough physical examination.[1,2] The history and physical examination are the two most important tools an experienced clinician can use in judging whether a patient is malnourished or has a potential for complications that may arise secondary to the nutritional status.[3,4] A limited number of laboratory tests and measurements of body composition are of value in assessing nutritional status.

Height and weight are the two most significant anthropometric measurements of nutritional assessment, for they help to determine whether the patient's weight is ideal for height. Many of the other anthropometric measurements, such as triceps skinfold thickness and mid-arm circumference, are of no great value taken as single determinations; they are of value if measured sequentially. If taken by inexperienced individuals, the measurements are of no value.

ASSESSMENT PARAMETERS

History

The most important question to ask patients is whether they have had a recent change in weight and, if so, how much. Inquiry should be made as to how much weight has been gained or lost during the past month, 6 months, or year and if the weight gain or loss has been voluntary or involuntary. The patient needs to be questioned with regard to the presence or absence of diarrhea, because the latter, if chronic and voluminous, may be associated with major loss of electrolytes and trace metals. Questions should be asked to determine whether there are factors that impair selection, preparation, ingestion, digestion, absorption, and excretion of nutrients in food and liquids. These include chronic diseases affecting nutrient utilization, e.g., diabetes mellitus, pancreatitis, and malabsorption.

The interviewer should determine whether the patient has undergone surgical resection of part or parts of the digestive tract or accessory organs of digestion, such as the pancreas.

A history of any allergies or recognized intolerances to foods should be noted to avoid problems in the postoperative period when feeding is reintroduced. The use of any medications taken should be determined to learn whether they are essential and whether they can be given by the parenteral route. Some medications may cause gastritis and can lead to abdominal pain, nausea, and anorexia. These should be recognized before surgery.

The physician should determine whether there are chewing or swallowing difficulties because this may determine what the patient will be allowed to eat in the postoperative period. The patient's usual bowel habits prior to surgery should be used as a baseline for comparison in the postoperative period.

Physical Examination

Careful observation of the patient's appearance obviously adds to the evaluation of nutritional adequacy.[4] This, however, is in part dependent on the experience and skill of the clinician. The diagnosis of frank malnutrition is often obvious and does not need to be deferred until laboratory tests can confirm it. Some patients present with a skeleton-like appearance of severe protein-calorie malnutrition (marasmus) or with a bloated edematous appearance of kwashiorkor. In such cases, a clinician can easily recognize the presence of the two types of malnutrition. Severe wasting of the subcutaneous fat stores and skeletal protein can be acutely evident. Patients who are very emaciated are deficient in both energy and protein. There are obviously intermediate forms of malnutrition that do occur and are related to inadequate or excessive intake of different nutrients. A review should also be carried out to establish the degree of function of each of the body's systems as it relates to nutritional status.

Anthropometrics

Anthropometry is the science of measurement of body parts. For the clinical urologist, only certain measurements are practical and useful. We will confine our discussion to these.

Height and Weight

The techniques that are used to predict energy and protein needs of the body require data on height and weight in order to be utilized. A history of weight loss is generally considered significant in recovery. Weight loss and body weight are of major importance because they reveal the energy stores and nutrient fuels at a point in time. In patients who lose weight unintentionally, often this is the first sign of an illness or disease. Weight loss diminishes stores of energy, substrates, and other nutrients. A rapid weight loss of 10 percent of usual adult weight is considered significant. A decline of 20 percent is viewed as critical or premorbid, and a weight loss of 30 percent or more is considered near-lethal. Weight loss that occurs rapidly is of much greater immediate importance than weight loss that occurs over a gradual period of time.

There are a number of conditions or disease states that are characterized by abnormalities in body condition. Ascites, pleural effusion, subcutaneous emphysema, and generalized edema may all affect body weight and overall appearance. A body weight that changes by more than 1 pound or 0.5 kg/day indicates fluid shifts, and a 1-liter fluid shift can equal approximately 2 pounds. Patients who suffer severe traumatic injury to the abdomen may require major fluid resuscitation. This can result in invalidation of actual weight information about the patient. On the other hand, traumatic injuries may contraindicate the weighing of the patient. With patients in critical care units, the usual weight and height should be obtained from the patient, family, or friends; the weight can be estimated by physical examination and height by comparing the recumbent length to the known length of the mattress. Awareness of average weight for the patient's height, age, and sex is useful in placing patients on a scale of depletion, adequate nutrition, or obesity.

Table 7–1 compares a commonly used method of calculating desirable or "ideal" body weight with two current reference sets of data on weights of Americans.[5-8] Although assigning an ideal body weight for any person is difficult at best, if not impossible, to do, it is still desirable to view weight in relationship to unusual leanness or notable obesity. Underweight and overweight conditions are defined as weights that are greater or lesser than 10 percent below or above average for height and sex of the individual.

Skinfold Thickness and Arm Circumference

Body stores of fat can be assessed by measuring skinfold thickness. Body stores of protein can be assessed by measuring the mid-upper arm circumference. These measurements are better used for sequential studies than taken as single isolated determinants. They are not commonly used by most people doing practical clin-

Table 7–1. CALCULATED AND PUBLISHED AVERAGE WEIGHTS FOR AMERICANS RELATIVE TO HEIGHT AND SEX

	Weight (kg)		
Height (inches)	*Using Hamwi* Equation*	*1983 Metropolitan Height & Weight Tables†*	*Data from NHANES I and NHANES II‡*
Males			
62	54	61	68
63	56	63	71
64	59	64	71
65	62	65	74
66	65	66	75
67	67	67	77
68	70	68	78
69	73	70	78
70	75	71	81
71	78	73	81
72	81	74	84
73	84	79	85
74	86	81	88
Females			
60	45	54	60
61	48	55	61
62	50	57	61
63	52	58	62
64	55	60	62
65	57	61	63
66	59	62	63
67	61	64	65
68	64	65	67
69	66	66	68
70	68	68	70

*Traditional formula in use within the nutrition community for estimating desirable body weight. Adult women are allotted 100 pounds for the first 5 feet of height plus 5 pounds for each additional inch. Adult men are allotted 106 pounds for the first 5 feet of height plus 6 pounds for each additional inch. A 10 percent adjustment can be made up or down for heavy or light frame.

†Weight averages from ranges for medium-frame individuals based on height, sex, body frame, and lowest mortality from the 1979 Build Study on Americans at ages 25 to 59 years who carried life insurance.

‡Data from a cross-sectional sampling of 21,752 American subjects aged 25 to 74 years from the National Health and Nutrition Examination Surveys I (1971–1974) and II (1976–1980). Weights at 50th percentile, medium frames.

ical nutrition.[9,10] The measurements are of some value in providing a gross analysis of insufficient, adequate, or excessive provision of nutritional support of chronically ill patients who cannot be weighed.

MEASURES OF VISCERAL PROTEIN COMPARTMENT

Four proteins may be evaluated in assessing visceral protein mass and adequacy of protein provision to support necessary hepatic synthesis of circulating proteins: (1) serum albumin, (2) transferrin, (3) thyroxin-binding pre-albumin, and (4) retinol-binding protein.[11–13] Levels of these proteins, as well as total lymphocyte count, have been correlated with morbidity and mortality. Table 7–2 shows the values for albumin, transferrin, pre-albumin, and total lymphocyte count that are used in assessing degrees of malnutrition.

Serum Albumin

A serum albumin level that is low is a frequently cited indication of malnutrition. However, serum albumin can be affected by a number of factors: (1) hydration state or blood loss; (2) albumin infusions; (3) renal or hepatic compromise; (4) ongoing protein losses from wounds, burns, drainage tubes, or the gut; (5) trauma, burns, surgery, or stress; (6) steroid administration; and (7) age.[12]

Low levels of albumin, transferrin, pre-albumin, and other proteins may be related to metabolic changes characteristic of stress and illness as well as to the actual depletion of visceral protein mass or synthesizing ability. Very low albumin levels in reality are recognized to be associated with pronounced malnutrition, in particular marasmus–kwashiorkor, and are therefore of some importance in determining nutritional status. In non-stressed patients, albumin levels may be of greater value in interpreting its significance than when the patient is under stress. Albumin has a half-life of approximately 14 to 19 days. This limits its usefulness in attempting to evaluate response to nutritional therapy. The visceral proteins with shorter half-lives are better markers of the adequacy of nutrient provision.

Transferrin

Transferrin, a circulating protein involved in iron transport, has a half-life of 8 to 10 days and a small extracellular, as opposed to a large body, pool of albumin. Transferrin can be estimated from total iron-binding capacity. However, there are a number of conditions that can affect its level. Elevated levels may be seen in iron deficiency, in acute hepatitis, in pregnancy, or with the use of oral contraceptives. Low levels are found in severe liver disease and protein-losing states. On the other hand, the iron-binding capacity may decrease in marked bacterial infection.[13]

Thyroxin-Binding Pre-albumin and Retinol-Binding Protein

Because of their short half-lives, pre-albumin (1 to 2 days) and retinol-binding protein (10 hours) are much more sensitive indicators of protein synthesis. We believe that pre-albumin is a very useful tool for assessing the body's protein status because it is not affected as much as transferrin by exogenous factors. Within 4 days of repleting the caloric and protein needs of a given patient, the pre-albumin level can show a significant rise. Likewise, if nutritional support is less than adequate, the level may remain the same or may decrease. By obtaining serial pre-albumin levels, the clinician can determine the success or failure of a particular regimen. We typically obtain a baseline pre-albumin value

Table 7–2. DETERMINATION OF PROTEIN-CALORIE MALNUTRITION BY PLASMA VALUES*

Laboratory Data	Normal Values	Degree of Malnutrition: *Moderate*	*Severe*
Serum albumin (gm/dl)	3.5	2.1–3.0	<2.1
Serum transferrin (mg/dl)	180–260	100–150	<100
Total lymphocyte count:			
Per mm^3	1500–4000	800–1200	<800
Percent white blood cells	20%–53%		

*Reproduced by permission from Williams SR: Nutrition and Diet Therapy, 4th ed. St. Louis, Times Mirror Mosby College Publishing, 1981, p 71.

and repeat the procedure 4 days after full caloric and protein support are begun. Adjustments in nutritional support are made, taking into account changes in pre-albumin (Table 1–2). If the level fails to increase, we adjust our caloric support upward by 10 percent. If the pre-albumin level shows an increase, we do not change the degree of support.

IMMUNE RESPONSE AND NUTRITION

Malnourished patients are characterized by increased rates of infection. Immunity develops through the activity of B cells, T cells, other less specific cells, and a group of proteins forming the complement system. When immunity is compromised, there is a reduced response from the complex system designed to aid the body in defending itself against invading organisms. Cutaneous hypersensitivity testing has not been used widely because of the technical, disease-specific, and iatrogenic factors that can alter the cutaneous response to the test antigens[14]; however, immune response is apt to be changed by nutrient adequacy. Zinc, riboflavin, thiamine, and vitamin B_6 are all known to be involved in the immune function. Energy calories and protein are among the factors necessary for the activity of cell-mediated immunity. Estimating the optimal operation of this function is difficult at present and beyond the scope of just doing simple skin recall tests. Total lymphocyte counts may be used to indicate the body's ability to combat invasive organisms as a means of assessing adequacy of protein provided. This may be of value in screening nonseptic patients; however, because the counts are so radically altered in a septic patient or those treated with adrenocorticosteroids or chemotherapeutic agents, their usefulness has been questioned. We advise following the lymphocyte count in the nonseptic patient as a sign of the adequacy of parenteral support. Lymphocyte count increases or decreases, depending on the nutritional status of the patient. If anabolic, it increases; if catabolic, it decreases.

MEASUREMENT OF SOMATIC PROTEINS

Nitrogen balance and creatinine height index are two techniques that have been used to determine adequacy of protein supply and maintenance of lean body mass. Of the two techniques, the nitrogen balance index is the superior. Nitrogen balance is defined as the state of equilibrium that occurs when the intake and excretion of nitrogen are equal. If more nitrogen is taken in than is excreted, nitrogen balance is said to be *positive* and an *anabolic* state can exist. When more nitrogen is excreted than is taken in, nitrogen balance is said to be *negative* and a *catabolic*, or starvation, state exists. Nitrogen losses occur through the urine, with a small, constant amount lost via the skin and feces.

The estimation of nitrogen balance can be made by deducting the quantity of urea nitrogen loss daily in the urine and the nitrogen intake from enteral and/or parenteral sources. Calculations are as follows:

$$\text{nitrogen balance} = \text{nitrogen intake} - \text{nitrogen excretion}$$

which equals the protein intake divided by 6.25 minus the 24-hour urine urea nitrogen plus estimated loss in stool.

The accuracy of such studies depends a great deal on the completeness of urine collections as well as on a careful measurement of the protein being administered. As a practical measure, we rarely perform such a study because of difficulties encountered in doing 24-hour urine collection. If necessary, these studies can be done if the nurses are informed of the critical need and the necessity to collect all urine. Following the pre-albumin levels serially is easier and gives similar information.

DETERMINATION OF NUTRIENT NEEDS

Before specialized nutritional support through either an enteral or a parenteral route is started, the clinician must determine (1) the total energy needs of the patient; (2) the distribution of kilocalories (Kcal) from carbohydrate, protein, and fat; and (3) the requirement for fluids, vitamins, minerals, and trace minerals. Decisions with regard to the support are based on the knowledge of the patient's prior nutritional status, requirements during the critical period, and awareness of the special changes caused by the illness. In the immediate postoperative period, patients are in a physiologic state of stress as a result of surgery. The body's reactions to stress are regulated by the central nervous system and are sympathetically mediated. Elevations in antidiuretic hormone, adrenocorticotropic hormone, catecholamines, insulin, and growth hormones have been reported. The level of stress can be categorized by defining the severity of surgery and by stratifying the metabolic aberrations in response to stress.[15] Such an outline for clinical use has been established.[16] It is based on urea nitrogen loss, plasma glucagon, glucose, and various plasma organic acids. In starvation, the metabolic rate decreases the carbohydrate reserves, which are minimal and present in the form of glycogen in the liver. They are used first as the preferred energy source and are usually depleted within 24 hours. Gluconeogenesis is activated simultaneously with body stores of fat and protein providing supplies of nutrients for energy production during early starvation. After several weeks of starvation, adaptation to this state occurs and the brain utilizes increasing quantities of ketones for energy. The transition from protein catabolism to lipid catabolism follows with resulting sparing of protein breakdown.

By contrast, with the stress that follows surgery, metabolic rate increases; hyperglycemia develops, although usage of glucose for energy is impaired. Endogenous fat deposits are not used in early or mild stress. Protein catabolism occurs and is a major source of energy. Protein from lean body mass, and eventually from the viscera, becomes a significant energy substrate. Protein is depleted both indirectly, via gluconeogenesis, and directly, as peripheral muscle stores of the branch chain amino acids are converted to energy sources.[17–19] The classic signs of the surgical patient in the immediate postoperative period are hypermetabolism, hypercatabolism with negative nitrogen balance, hyperglycemia, and altered energy substrate utilization with increased usage of the branch chain amino acids from the muscles.

ENERGY REQUIREMENTS (Table 7–3)

Energy expenditure is relative to age, sex, body size, and activity level. Sufficient energy must be provided to maintain physiologic processes, to ensure repair and growth of the organism, to sustain physical movement, and to maintain body temperature even in a state of health. Following illness or surgery, energy needs may be further increased as the metabolic rate may be driven upward by the response to stress. Energy requirements are assessed in a variety of ways. Indirect or direct calorimetry has been used as a means to determine energy consumption.[20] If such sophisticated tools are not available, we have to make use of other means and the experience of others to accurately predict the energy requirements of the patient. In practice it is commonest to estimate, rather than measure, energy requirements following surgery.

Predicted Energy Requirements

The current practice is to provide adequate calories to meet energy needs during the critical period at a level that facilitates maintenance of actual body weight and lean body mass. Repletion to previous usual weight (if weight loss has occurred) or weight loss (in the overweight patient) is deferred until after the resolution of the critical period. Overfeeding, with its associated complication of fluid overload, increased carbon dioxide (CO_2) production, and aberrations of hepatic enzyme function, should be avoided. In the critically ill patient, the goal should be to provide sufficient energy to maintain weight and optimal metabolic function without overshooting or undershooting the goal.

The energy required to fuel basic life functions—respiration, circulation, and other physiologic processes in a normal, healthy individual at rest in a neutral thermoenvironment, 10 or more hours after eating—is defined as the basal energy expenditure (BEE). The resting energy expenditure (REE), which is approximately 5 percent greater than BEE, also includes energy expenditure for digestion, absorption, and utilization of nutrients (the specific dynamics action of food). Studies have shown that the BEE and REE measured in healthy and injured individuals varied by less than 5 percent. In the clinical situation, they should be considered equivalent.

$$\text{BEE (male)} = 66.47 + 13.75\,W + 5.0\,H - 6.76\,A$$

$$\text{BEE (female)} = 655.1 + 9.56\,W + 1.85\,H - 4.68\,A$$

where W equals weight in kilograms, H equals height in centimeters, and A equals age in years.

The physician must also consider the energy needs that go beyond basal or resting needs. Our estimation of energy needs must be increased to reflect the energy required for physical activ-

Table 7–3. CALORIE AND PROTEIN NEEDS IN STRESS*

Stress Level	Clinical Setting	Estimated kcal Need—Total Kcal/Kg/day	NPC:N†	AA gm/kg/day	AA‡	Percentage of Total Kcal CHO§	Fat
0	Simple starvation	28	150:1	1.0	15	60	25
1	Elective surgery	32	100:1	1.5	20	50	30
2	Polytrauma	40	100:1	2.0	25	40	35
3	Sepsis	50	80:1	2.5	30	70	0

*Adapted with permission from Nutritional Support Services 5(1):26–27, 1985. Copyright © January 1985, Creative Age Publications.

†Non-protein calorie to nitrogen ratio.

‡Amino acids.

§Carbohydrates.

ity and any anticipated hypermetabolic response to illness or injury. A set of factors have been used in the Harris Benedict equation to predict the increased percentage of energy needs required in various activities and degree of injury. These factors are included in the correction of the Harris Benedict equation in the following manner:

$$\text{BEE} \times (\text{activity factor}) \times (\text{injury factor}) = \text{TEE}^*$$

The factors for *activity* are suggested to be 1.2 for the bedridden patient and 1.3 for the ambulatory, hospitalized patient. Injury factors for surgery (minor) are 1.2; for trauma (skeletal or blood), 1.35; for sepsis (severe), 1.6; and for burns, 2.1. The duration of elevation of energy needs is greatest for patients with thermal (burn) injuries. Metabolic rate can also be elevated by the presence of fever, with an approximately 7 percent increase in energy expenditure per degree of temperature elevation from normal in Fahrenheit or 13 percent per degree of temperature elevation from normal in Celsius. For the typical surgical patient, we estimate needs to be in the range of 40 to 45 Kcal/kg of body weight/day. This includes the basal requirement plus that required to meet the needs of surgical recovery.

Measured Energy Expenditure

The goal of measurements of energy expenditure in critically ill patients is to determine the REE.[20] Investigators have recorded the energy expenditure during seven basic activities in intensive care units. The highest oxygen consumption is recorded during chest physical therapy, these values being 32 percent above REE values. The lowest values for oxygen consumption occur during sleep and are 9 percent lower than REE values.[21]

Indirect calorimetry is a technique that can be used both with the critically and noncritically ill patient to determine energy expenditure by the measurement of respiratory gas exchange. It is based on the fact that oxygen consumption (V_{O_2}) and CO_2 production (V_{CO_2}) represent intracellular metabolism. Indirect calorimetry is attractive because it (1) is noninvasive, (2) is portable, (3) can be used on spontaneously breathing or mechanically ventilated patients requiring elevated inspired oxygen concentration (F_{IO_1}), and (4) compares favorably with direct calorimetric techniques. By utilizing this technique, physicians can determine not only the energy consumed but also the proportion of protein, fat, and carbohydrate providing the fuel for energy expenditure. In order to do the latter, one must collect urine for 24 hours to determine nitrogen excretion.[22] The utilization of indirect calorimetry mechanically in the ventilated patient depends in part on having the adaptors necessary to connect the calorimeter to the airway.

The measurement of mechanically ventilated patients is the most difficult of all. The accurate measurement of REE and respiratory quotient (RQ) in mechanically ventilated patients can be used to monitor nutritional support and facilitate weaning. Indirect calorimetric measurements, combined with urinary nitrogen values, can be used to adjust nutritional support, to provide adequate kilocalories, and to determine what part each of the nutrients—carbohydrate, fat, and protein—are being used.[22] Overfeeding in terms of kilocalories per day and/or percent of carbohydrates has been implicated in precipitating respiratory failure and prolonged weaning in those on ventilators, because of the factor of excessive CO_2 production resulting from the

*Total energy expenditure.

high RQ of carbohydrates.[23] Additionally, excessive kilocalories may result in lipogenesis, which is also associated with an increase in CO_2 production.[24,25] Calories provided in excess of 30 percent predicted from the Harris Benedict equation are adequate to meet the metabolic needs of most stressed patients. It is prudent to provide caloric intake of 10 to 30 percent above REE to all but the paralyzed or comatose patient. In critically ill patients with CO_2 retention on or off the ventilator, it is wise not to provide excess calories and to use as much fat as is tolerated as an energy source.[26]

Carbohydrate

Energy can be derived in humans from carbohydrate, protein, or fat, but the preferred energy source is carbohydrate. In the oral diet, this energy substrate is plentiful and represents an efficient source of energy; it is also a regulator of protein and fat metabolism. When carbohydrate is present in adequate quantity to meet normal energy needs, it both results in protein-sparing and is antiketogenic. The body requires 100 to 150 gm of carbohydrate per day to achieve protein-sparing and to prevent ketosis.

In stress, carbohydrate metabolism is dramatically changed. Hyperglycemia is one of the responses of stress. Primary utilization of glucose as an energy substrate changes to catabolism of peripheral muscle, with subsequent increased usage of the branch chain amino acids for energy. In very severe stress, lipolysis occurs with mobilization of triglycerides as potential energy substrates via ketone production. Despite very high levels of circulating glucose, the RQs of severely injured or traumatized patients suggest the dependence on fat, not carbohydrate, as the major energy substrate.[27] However, in prolonged periods of stress, energy derived from fat is also impaired. Proteolysis, therefore, begins to occur with severe and often catastrophic results. Under normal circumstances, the body can oxidize glucose at the rate of 2 to 4 mg/kg/minute. This rate is independent of elevations of serum levels of either glucose or insulin. One cannot enhance the oxidation and utilization of glucose for energy by providing either excessive quantities of glucose or insulin. Even in severe stress, the oxidation rate of glucose is only slightly greater at 3 to 5 mg/kg/minute. Administration of glucose in excess of 4 to 5 mg/kg/minute exceeds the body's ability to oxidize and use it as an energy source. Conversion of fat from unused glucose may increase CO_2 production, impairing the process of weaning of patients if they are ventilator-dependent. The provision of energy in excess of need may actually cause a rise in energy expenditure of 1 Kcal for every 5 Kcal beyond requirements.

D-Glucose is the most common form of carbohydrate used for intravenous infusion. D-glucose monohydrate, when in solution, has a caloric value of 3.4 Kcal/gm. Other carbohydrate sources for intravenous use include glycerol, sorbitol, maltose, fructose, and xylitol. They are rarely used. Glycerol is used to reduce the osmolarity in intravenous fat emulsion. In central venous total parenteral nutrition (TPN), dextrose concentrations from 10 to 35 percent may be used. In peripheral TPN, dextrose concentration is limited to 10 percent.

Protein

Protein is required for growth, for maintenance and repair of tissue, and for structural inclusion in enzymes, hormones, and carrier or transport molecules. There is 1 gm of nitrogen available in each 6.25 gm of protein. Nitrogen balance is achieved when protein synthesis and breakdown are in equilibrium.

In the average American diet, percentage of kilocalories derived from protein varies, generally from about 10 to 15 percent. In some segments of the American population, this may be as high as 20 percent, although this percentage is in excess of need, is costly, and is energy-inefficient.

Dietary protein contains 20 common amino acids. Of these, nine amino acids found in protein are considered essential to humans. These are histidine, isoleucine, leucine, lysine, methionine, phenylalanine, tryptophan, and valine.

The recommended dietary allowance (RDA) of protein for an adult who is not pregnant or lactating is 0.8 gm/kg/day. This figure provides a margin of safety, assuming that dietary intake can be of mixed origin (animal and vegetable). Protein needs in critical care are somewhat different. High-biologic-value protein is the one of choice for hospitalized patients. In critical illness, after trauma, or in the postoperative period, protein requirements for humans are increased. Some additional protein is needed for synthesis of acute phase proteins within the body, for wound repair, or for replacing protein loss in drainage or exudate. Protein metabolism also occurs as peripheral role energy needs are met by utilization of branch chain amino acids from skeletal muscles. Urinary nitrogen increases in the stressed or postoperative state. Hence, protein needs are elevated both because of increased losses and increased usage for synthesis, repair, and energy.

Recommendations for the quantity of protein to be provided in critical illness or postoperatively vary rather widely. A range of 1.2 to 1.5 gm/kg/day, with ongoing monitoring of urinary nitrogen and nitrogen balance for assessment of tolerance and adequacy is typically used. In healthy individuals, 0.4/kg/day is the minimal amount of protein necessary to sustain positive nitrogen balance; 0.8 to 1.0/kg/day is more than adequate in most patients.[28] In a study by Cerra and colleagues, the estimate of proteins in stress is 2 gm/kg in polytrauma and 2.5 gm/kg in sepsis. In such patients with sepsis, they do not recommend any fat as an energy source.[29] In the seriously ill patient, it is necessary to match energy and protein requirements as accurately as possible. Alterations in the ratio of non-protein calories to grams of nitrogen to lower levels have been suggested. Some investigators have suggested ratios of 80:1 to 100:1 in severe stress.[26,27] A typical difficulty in periods of severe stress is that multiple organ failure occurs with renal compromise. This often prevents the administration of the necessary amount of grams of protein. High protein intake has been observed to cause an elevated ventilatory response to CO_2. Respiratory failure of patients in severe stress may impair the high caloric intake with a high percentage of kilocalories from carbohydrate recommended. High branch chain amino acid solutions appear to be superior for the management of patients with moderate to severe stress because of their sparing of breakdown of muscle protein (Table 7–3).

Fat

Fat is required in the diet of humans because it functions as the carrier for fat-soluble vitamins and provides essential fatty acids. It is needed as a constituent of cell membranes, as an insulating agent, as padding around vital organs, and as a rich source of energy. As 40 to 50 percent of calories in the Western diet come from fat, this quantity far exceeds needs. Current recommendations of the desirable intake of fat do not exceed 35 percent of the energy intake, especially for populations at high risk for coronary artery disease or hyperlipidemia. Two polyunsaturated fatty acids (linoleic and linolenic acid) are thought to be essential for humans. Linoleic acid can be converted into another important fatty acid, *arachidonic* acid. One to 2 percent of caloric intake provided by linoleic acid is usually adequate to prevent essential fatty acid deficiency (EFAD).[30,31] The deficiency of linoleic acid manifests itself in three major ways:

1. Growth retardation in infants and children.
2. A scaly dermatitis in adults and children.
3. Alteration of the normal triene:tetraene ratio, which derives its diagnostic value from the altered metabolic pathways activated in states of normal and inadequate fat intake.

Linoleic acid, when present in sufficient amounts, is in a different manner desaturated and elongated into arachidonic acid, a tetraene. In linoleic deficiency, linoleic acid that is present is converted to *oleic acid,* an atriene. A ratio of 0.4 or greater is indicative of EFAD. In adults who have received parenteral dextrose and amino acids but no fat source, biochemical EFAD developed by the end of the second week. By the end of the seventh week, all patients documented had clinical EFAD. If parenteral nutrition solutions containing only dextrose and amino acids are administered, fatty liver, cholestasis, and increased CO_2 production typically ensue.

Intravenous lipid emulsions have been used increasingly to replace some of the carbohydrate kilocalories. The lipid emulsions currently available are primarily from vegetable oils, generally soy or a combination of soy and safflower, and are composed for the most part of long-chain triglycerides (LCTs). Of concern are complications from the use of intravenous long-chain triglyceride infusions, which include hyperlipidemia, rarely impaired alveolar diffusion capacity, and rarely reduced function of the reticuloendothelial system. Intravenous fat emulsion can be used to provide either calories or essential fatty acids or may be provided in a small volume to prevent only EFAD. If peripheral parenteral nutrition is used, these lipid emulsions should be used to the maximum allowable to ensure that the patient's energy requirements are being met.

Vitamins and Minerals (Table 7–4)

In regard to the needs for nutrients by critical care patients receiving only parenteral support, common sense dictates that the known needs be

Table 7–4. RECOMMENDATIONS FOR PARENTERAL VITAMIN FORMULATIONS*

Vitamins	Adults		Children 11 Years and Under
	Intravenous	*Intramuscular*	
A (retinol), mg	1.0		0.7
D (ergocalciferol), μg	5.0		10.0
E (dl-alpha tocopheryl), mg	10.0		7.0
B_1 (thiamine), mg	3.0	3.0	1.2
B_2 (riboflavin), mg	3.6	3.6	1.4
Nicotinic acid, mg	40.0	40.0	17.0
Pantothenic acid, mg	15.0	15.0	5.0
B_6 (pyridoxine), mg	4.0	4.0	1.0
C (ascorbic acid), mg	100.0	100.0	80.0
Folic acid, μg	400.0	400.0	140.0
B_{12} (cyanocobalamin), μg	5.0	5.0	1.0
Biotin, μg	60.0	60.0	20.0
Phytonadione (vitamin K_1), μg			200.0

*Adapted with permission from "Multivitamin Preparations for Parenteral Use. A Statement by the Nutrition Advisory Group" by American Medical Association, Department of Foods and Nutrition. JPEN 3:260, 1979. Copyright © 1979, American Society of Parenteral and Enteral Nutrition.

considered first and recommendations for unusual requirements be considered second. The RDAs do not take into account elevated requirements that may occur as a result of sepsis, injury, surgery, or trauma. However, when enteral support is used, selected products can be evaluated for quantity required to meet the RDA. This evaluation can then serve as a starting point for determining whether further supplementation is indicated.

Water-soluble vitamins are stored in limited quantities in the body and must be replenished regularly.[32] Because the vitamins can be excreted in the urine, toxicity is infrequent, even when large doses are administered; however, it can occur. Fat-soluble vitamins are stored within the body, and excessive provision can result in toxicity, especially hypervitaminosis A and D. Care should be taken not to exceed the published guidelines for administration of this group of vitamins.

The goal of nutritional support is to provide quantities of vitamins and minerals that at least meet recommendations for maintenance. Beyond maintenance requirements, little of a definitive nature is known regarding the need for increased amounts of either vitamins or minerals during critical illness or injury, except for those nutrients involved in wound repair. *Major minerals* (calcium, phosphorus, magnesium) are present in the body in significant quantities. They are typically provided in standard parenteral preparations, as are the *electrolytes* sodium, potassium, and chloride. *Trace elements* include iron (Fe), zinc (Zn), copper (Cu), manganese (Mn), chromium (Cr), iodine (I), selenium (Se), and molybdenum (Mb). (See also "Trace Elements and Vitamins" later in this chapter.) Deficiency states for these trace elements are unlikely to occur during illnesses of brief duration unless conditions exist in which stores are readily depleted, such as in severe malnutrition or chronic malabsorption syndromes.[33,34] Deficiency states can develop in patients receiving long-term parenteral support. Trace elements can also be toxic in excess, and care is required in making certain that patients are neither underdosed nor overdosed (Table 7–5).

Fluids

Many factors affect fluid balance. Equilibrium is achieved between intake and output when an awareness of all sources of intake (oral, enteral, intravenous fluid/medications, and parenteral infusions) and of all losses (in urine and stool; from drainages, fistulas, and emesis; and from

Table 7–5. RECOMMENDED DOSES OF PARENTERAL TRACE ELEMENTS

	Daily Requirement	Deficiency
Zinc	2–4 mg + 17.1 mg (stool) + 12.2 mg (fistula)	Acrodermatitis enteropathica
Copper	0.5–1.5 mg	Anemia, neutropenia
Chromium	20 μg	Hyperglycemia
Manganese	1–3 mg	Impaired growth, skeletal abnormalities, ataxia, convulsions
Selenium	40–120 μg	Muscle weakness, diffuse cardiomyopathy, macrocytosis, loss of skin and hair color

Table 7–6. INDICATIONS FOR TPN IN THE UROLOGIC SURGERY PATIENT

Preoperatively

Elective surgery: Moderate to severe malnutrition in which the digestive tract cannot be used:
1. Secondary to fistulas.
2. Short bowel syndrome.
3. Obstruction.
4. Chronic diarrhea.

Postoperatively
1. Mild to moderate to severely malnourished patients who require immediate surgery and in whom the digestive tract cannot be used for more than 7 days.
2. Prolonged ileus, secondary to:
   a. Sepsis.
   b. Electrolyte imbalance.
   c. Postsurgical.
   d. Chemotherapy and radiation therapy.
3. Fistula formation.
4. Bowel resection and reanastomoses.
5. Bowel obstruction.

respiratory, expiratory, and evaporative losses) is required. Generally, under normal circumstances, an estimate of fluid needs for an adult is expressed as 1 ml/Kcal. Renal compromise, congestive heart failure, and progression of ascites are a few of the conditions that demand careful monitoring of fluid status and the restriction of intake. Third spacing of fluid is common in the critically ill patient and makes estimates of weight and fluid balances difficult. Fluid management must be responsive to electrolyte balance, hemodynamic variables, and optimal functioning of all organs and systems. It is critically important that for each day a patient receives parenteral support, intake and output be added and subtracted from one another and insensible losses be calculated to determine whether the patient is in fluid balance.

INDICATIONS FOR PARENTERAL NUTRITION (Table 7–6)

The enteral route of administration of nutrients is always preferred. The parenteral route is indicated when the enteral route is inadequate, because of short bowel syndrome, malabsorption syndromes, long bone fractures, or major burns. Enteral nutrition should be avoided in cases of enterocutaneous fistulas (unless the fistula is distal in the small bowel), severe pancreatitis, acute inflammatory bowel disease with severe diarrhea, gastrointestinal obstruction, paralytic ileus, short bowel syndrome, and severe malabsorption. Enteral nutrition may be hazardous in patients with inadequate gag reflex and in bowel intubation if an enteric tube cannot be passed beyond the pylorus because the risk of reflux and aspiration in this situation is high.

Conditions for which parenteral nutrition is commonly required at some time during the course of illness include:

1. Gastrointestinal (GI) dysmotility syndromes.
2. Crohn's disease, chronic pancreatitis with ileus, hemorrhagic pancreatitis.
3. Complications of GI surgery, such as fistulas, paralytic ileus, abdominal abscess, peritonitis, and gastric outlet obstruction.
4. Oncologic and immunologic therapy, such as bone marrow transplantation.
5. Critical illness, such as sepsis, respiratory failure, trauma, acute renal failure, liver failure, and pulmonary disease requiring ventilation.
6. Complications of thoracic or pleural vascular surgeries affecting GI function.

In urologic surgery patients, parenteral nutrition is commonly used for patients in whom postoperative fistulas, prolonged ileus, and chronic diarrhea develop secondary to bowel resection with reanastomoses and radiation therapy.

ESTABLISHING THERAPEUTIC OBJECTIVES

The objective of nutritional support is to maintain or replete lean body mass, thereby avoiding consequences of malnutrition. It is important to the clinician to promote wound healing, to reduce susceptibility to infection, and to reduce duration of hospitalization and convalescence from illness. There are times when the treatment of the critical condition takes priority over nutritional support. In cases such as this, it is probably wisest to hold nutritional support until the acute episode is corrected, because provision of complicated therapy—when the utilization of exogenous nutrients is hindered by the hormonal milieu, as in acute injury—may do more harm than benefit. The priorities in acute situations are, first, to moderate the injury component of acute illness; second, to temper the endocrinologic response to injury so that the patient's tolerance and utilization of exogenous nutrients is improved; and third, to provide substrate required for energy. In some patients, it may be appropriate to accept suboptimal nutrition. There may be patients whose tolerance or utilization of nutrients is unpredictable but is likely to be impaired, and very low dosages or restricted quantities of certain nutrients may be prescribed, with dosage to tolerance being the plan for therapy.

PARENTERAL NUTRITION REQUIREMENTS

Nutritional requirements are the net sum of (1) normal requirements in health as defined by the minimal daily requirements and the recommended daily allowance for all nutrients, (2) correction of pre-existing deficits occurring as a result of disease or lack of adequate intake, and (3) planned replacement of continuous extraneous losses.

Calories

The sources of energy calories include carbohydrate and fat. Protein is not usually considered a source of energy calories. Caloric requirements should be based on the Harris Benedict equation for basal energy expenditure, with consideration of energy and activity by using factors for varying patient conditions to increase the BEE.

The usual energy requirements for a typical adult are in the range of 2000 to 2500 Kcal/day or between 30 and 35 Kcal/kg of body weight/day. Generally, the actual body weight is used for this calculation, except in cases of morbid obesity. To avoid complications of refeeding, patients with severe malnutrition should not be dosed at any more than the BEE or 20 to 25 Kcal/kg of body weight/day initially, with a consideration for increases of nutrients made on a less frequent than daily basis. At the point of body mass depletion and a reduced vital organ function, pre-existing nutrient deficiency impairs the body's ability to tolerate the work of metabolism.

Protein is essential for tissue synthesis in repair, transport of nutrients and waste, and maintenance of immune function. Normally, the diet consists of a total calorie-to-nitrogen ratio of 120:1, with adjustments in this recommendation made for the critically ill patient to 80–100:1. In conditions of renal or hepatic failure, an increased calorie-to-nitrogen ratio is indicated to ensure optimal utilization in tolerance of administered dose of protein.

Protein

Recommended doses for the hospitalized patient are in the range of 1 to 1.5 gm/kg of body weight/day. Some authors have recommended a dose of 2 to 2.5 gm/kg/day for those patients with severe illness, but this may not be possible in some because of the impairment of organ function. Depending on the patient's underlying clinical condition, certain types or classes of amino acids may play a significant role in metabolism. High branch chain amino acids should be considered in cases of high stress and sepsis. For patients with hepatic encephalopathy, those solutions that are high in branch chain but low in aromatic amino acids should be considered. In patients in renal failure, a mixed solution of essential and nonessential amino acids has been shown to be as good as or better than using just essential amino acids. The number of grams of protein per kilocalorie to be put in the solution depends, in part, on the volume of solution that can be administered as well as on the amount of calories that are required.

Fat

The main purpose of including fat in parenteral nutrition is to prevent development of EFAD. The dose of intravenous fat to prevent deficiency is 4 percent of total calories as lipid emulsion. Because it is costly to administer partial bottles of the intravenous fat, it is typical practice to prescribe a 500- or 250-ml bottle of 10 or 20 percent lipid emulsion, respectively. However, the infrequency of this administration may predispose the patient to biochemical abnormalities consistent with subclinical deficiency. It may be more prudent to administer the dose in a smaller volume more frequently. When fat is used as an energy source, as it must be in peripheral parenteral nutrition, part of the non-protein calories is still proved by carbohydrate, although at a lower level. It is recommended by some that the dose of calories for intravenous (IV) fat be 60 percent of total non-protein calories if it is given peripherally. Caloric doses of fat in excess of 60 percent may exceed the patient's metabolic capacity for safe removal in the oxidation of fat and may impair nitrogen retention. Intravenous fat emulsions should be administered over as long a time as possible to give the body a chance to optimally metabolize it, to decrease the osmolarity of the solutions being infused intravenously, and to optimize the utilization of the nutrient mixture.

Electrolytes

The management of fluid and electrolyte status is extremely important in parenteral nutrition. It is important to use a logical approach to prescribing both fluids and electrolytes. Electrolyte requirements are based on three conditions: (1) replacement of deficit, (2) nutritional needs, and (3) recognition of the appropriate replacement of extraneous fluid losses.

In states of malnutrition, deficits may be intracellular and may not be indicated by low or altered serum chemistries. For such electrolytes as magnesium, body depletion may be present without any deviation in serum magnesium levels from normal. The optimal ratios of electrolytes per gram of nitrogen administered that promote appropriate repletion of lean body mass are phosphorus, 0.8 gm; sodium, 3.9 mEq; potassium, 3 mEq; chloride, 2.5 mEq; and calcium, 1.2 mEq. When these ratios are not maintained, either negative nitrogen balance persists or weight is gained as fat during repletion of malnourished subjects.

Large deficits in fluid and electrolyte balance may occur in critically ill patients. In most cases, when drainage exceeds 500 ml/day, IV electrolyte replacement of that fluid by a parenteral fluid with similar electrolyte content to that being lost is indicated. Draining 1000 ml of nasogastric fluid per day may be predicted to result in acquired loss of 140 mEq/l, and replacement would be adequately provided by an equivalent volume of 0.9 percent sodium chloride solution. An electrolyte replacement solution of extraneous fluid losses may be accomplished by the addition of extra electrolytes to the parenteral nutrition solution; fluctuations of fluid volume in electrolyte content usually lead to frequent changes in total parenteral nutrition electrolyte content, a technique that causes excessive waste and increases the cost of providing therapy. More frequent laboratory monitoring may also be necessary at increased cost to the patients. Fluid and electrolyte deficits must be corrected before the initiation of parenteral nutrition. Infusion is then initiated with an optimal electrolyte content per gram of nitrogen dose for lean body mass repletion.

Finally, extraneous losses should be recognized and parenteral replacement fluid prescribed with equal amounts of fluid and electrolyte. When fluid needs to be restricted, the electrolyte content of the replacement fluid may be modified to concentrate the electrolyte content, and the replacement may be decreased fractionally until the desired fluid restriction is accomplished.

Trace Elements and Vitamins

Trace elements are substances that are present in human tissue in minute amounts, micrograms and picograms of weight per organ weight. Metallic trace elements have several important biologic functions, especially as metalloenzymes. Trace elements participate in protein and organic acid synthesis, membrane transport, mitochondrial function, nerve conduction, and muscle contraction. Essential trace elements for human existence are iron, iodine, cobalt, zinc, and copper. Three additional elements—chromium, manganese, and selenium—are most likely essential as well.[35]

When studies of trace metals are ordered, one has to consider whether or not the patient has a condition that has predisposed to the deficiency state. Second, the deficiency may not be manifested by clinical symptomatology until the patient is fed. Third, the dosage of trace elements may have to replace individual deficits of a trace element as well as provide maintenance dosages required to support the metabolism of nutrients. Excessive replacement of trace metals in patients with organ dysfunction, such as of the kidney or liver, can lead to toxicity. Diagnosis of trace element deficiency is difficult because plasma levels do not correlate to total body quantities of these elements and may be altered by the patient's clinical state. Individual requirements for trace elements are provided in Table 7–5.

Vitamin recommendations of the American Medical Association are listed in Table 7–4. As a general rule, we do not use additional vitamins in our parenteral nutrition solutions. Vitamins are added to the solution just before they are to be administered.

Water

Minimal requirements for water are 1.5 liters/M^2. Special consideration is required for patients with severe edema or conditions of impaired water metabolism, as occurs in renal or liver failure. When appropriate, water restriction may be accomplished by limiting the volume of drug infusions and IV replacement in maintaining peripheral maintenance infusion with heparin lock rather than with a continuous

IV solution. In this manner, fluid for nutrient administration may be spared and overzealous use of diuretics may be avoided.

Peripheral Versus Central TPN

In designing the parenteral nutrition formulation, the clinician must decide whether the peripheral or the central venous TPN route will be used. When peripheral parenteral nutrition is used, maximal utilization of lipids should be done to ensure that maintenance calories are provided. Sixty percent of the total calories may be administered in the form of lipid emulsion. By using the 20 percent concentration of emulsion, the maximal number of calories can be given peripherally. In most adults, maintenance calorie levels up to 2200 to 2300 Kcal/day may be provided. Peripheral parenteral nutrition can be used when parenteral needs are for a period not to exceed 2 weeks. Beyond this point, venous access becomes increasingly difficult and necessitates the use of a central venous line.

Therefore, the first decision has to be whether a peripheral or central TPN route is to be used. Once the decision is made, the physician must obtain baseline laboratory data to determine whether there are any major electrolyte deficits. If these are present, they should first be corrected before parenteral nutrition is ordered. The solutions are then formulated based on the volume to be administered, the calories to be given, and the proportions to be provided between carbohydrate and fat. Patients who receive central venous parenteral nutrition obviously can be provided with concentrations of dextrose in excess of 10 percent. Concentrations of dextrose of up to 35 percent can be safely used by the central route. This will provide up to 1.2 calories/ml for 35 percent dextrose solution. Twenty percent lipid emulsions can be used either centrally or peripherally. Their advantage is that they provide concentrated calories in a smaller volume of solution. For patients with limitations on volumes of fluid tolerated, the more concentrated dextrose and lipid emulsions should always be used. The amino acids required should be given in such a concentration that they will provide for adequate protein synthesis. Their concentration in the final solution will depend, in part, on the volume that is permissible to administer. Parenteral nutrition solutions should contain quantities of electrolytes in order to provide for maintenance values. Ongoing losses can be provided for by simultaneously infusing replacement solutions. Whereas peripheral parenteral nutrition can be started at maximal rates of infusion the first day, patients for whom the central venous route is selected cannot immediately be administered the more concentrated solutions of dextrose because they might not be able to tolerate the osmolar load acutely.

MONITORING THE PATIENT

Patients receiving TPN should be weighed on a daily basis, when possible, with accurate recording of their intake and output charted. All intake, as well as output, should be recorded regardless of source. At the end of each day, these numbers should be added and it should be determined from them whether or not the patient is receiving an excessive amount of fluid and is receiving the calories ordered. Daily calories should be calculated from intake and protein should be determined to establish whether patients are receiving optimal nutrition. Laboratory tests to establish the adequacy of the support should be done. Serum levels of electrolytes, calcium, magnesium, and phosphorus should be determined on the first day to establish adequacy of the mineral support. Then, if stable, the patients should be rechecked in the same manner on the second and third days. If the electrolytes are stable by the third day, the patient may then be checked every other day for the following week. Following the second week on parenteral support, patients need to be checked only weekly. A complete blood count (CBC) may be done on a once-a-week or twice-a-week basis.

PROGRAM FOR ASSESSING AND ESTABLISHING A PATIENT ON TPN

Perform a nutritional assessment.

1. Measure height and weigh the patient.
2. Examine the patient carefully for signs of nutritional deficiencies.
3. Measure the serum albumin.
4. Measure either transferrin or pre-albumin.
5. Measure the absolute lymphocyte count.

Determine the patient's ideal weight for height and sex, and calculate the percentage of ideal body weight (IBW) as follows:

$$\%\ \text{IBW} = \frac{\text{current weight}}{\text{IBW}} \times 100$$

where >90% <110% = normal; 80–89% =

mild malnutrition; 70–79% = moderate malnutrition; 60–69% = severe malnutrition; and <60% = very severe malnutrition.

Calculate the caloric needs for IBW with the Harris Benedict equation.

$$\text{BEE (males)} = 66.47 + 13.75W + 5.0H - 6.76A$$

$$\text{BEE (females)} = 655.1 + 9.56W + 1.85H - 4.68A$$

where W = weight in kg; H = height in cm; and A = age in years.

Now calculate total energy needs:

$$\text{TEE} = \text{BEE} \times (\text{activity factor}) \times (\text{injury factor})$$

Activity factors = 1.2, bedridden patient; 1.3, ambulatory, hospitalized patient.

Injury factors = 1.2, minor surgery; 1.35, trauma; 1.60, severe sepsis; 2.10, burns.

Temperature = 7 percent increase for each degree Fahrenheit; 13 percent increase for each degree Celsius.

Once the energy needs are calculated, determine whether support is to be parenteral (central venous line, peripheral venous support) or enteral. Also determine whether there are any factors that may limit volume of parenteral support administered, i.e., cardiac, pulmonary, or renal disease.

If peripheral TPN is to be utilized, use the maximal amount of 20 percent fat emulsion allowed, up to 60 percent of total energy calories. The remainder of calories are to be given as 10 percent dextrose.

If central venous TPN is utilized, use 25 to 30 percent of calories from lipid emulsion and the remainder from concentrated dextrose. Concentration of dextrose used depends on whether there is any restriction of fluid volume.

Protein needs may be met for most clinical situations by providing 1.5 gm/kg/day of a balanced amino acid solution. The amino acid solutions are available in concentrations of 10 and 8.5 percent and are diluted with concentrated dextrose and water to provide the appropriate final concentration. Most of the concentrated amino acid preparations are available either with or without electrolytes and phosphate to provide for normal maintenance requirements. The electrolyte free solutions are utilized for patients who require fewer electrolytes than are provided for in the standard solutions. If extra electrolytes are needed, they may be added to the final solution or given as a separate infusion. Both electrolyte-containing solutions and electrolyte free amino acid solutions are calcium-free.

Give multiple vitamin infusions daily. Most available preparations are complete and provide necessary requirements.

Provide trace elements to prevent trace metal deficiency and to correct it in those individuals who are deficient. For routine TPN usage, trace metal solutions are available either as a combination of four agents or as single agents.

Before starting TPN, make certain that fluid and electrolyte deficits are corrected. Obtain weight daily, and keep intake and output records correctly. Monitor blood chemistry as follows:

1. Daily for the first 3 days—electrolytes, blood urea nitrogen (BUN), creatinine.
2. If stable, every second day for 4 days.
3. If stable at end of 1 week, check twice a week.
4. Baseline liver function tests and lipid profile (triglyceride and cholesterol level); repeat liver profile after 2 weeks.
5. Triglycerides and cholesterol after 3 days and weekly thereafter to make certain the lipid emulsion is being effectively cleared from the plasma.

If central venous TPN is used, administer the most concentrated dextrose solutions from the beginning, but keep the rate of administration low to avoid hyperglycemia. Advance the rate slowly hour by hour, carefully monitoring blood glucose to keep it below 200 mg/dl until the full rate is reached. As an alternative, use more dilute dextrose solutions and raise their concentration daily until the final concentration is reached.

Duration of TPN depends on the condition being treated *and* the goals of treatment. Most postoperative fistulas close within 4 weeks of initiation of TPN. If there has not been a reduction of 50 percent or more in fistula drainage after 5 weeks, it is unlikely that the fistula will heal. If the fistula does stop draining, TPN should be continued for 7 more days before feeding is reintroduced. If TPN is done to ensure healing following intestinal resection and reanastomosis, a minimum of 7 days of full support should allow for proper healing of anastomoses. For postoperative ileus, TPN should be continued until normal bowel sounds recur and nasogastric drainage becomes minimal. In hemorrhagic pancreatitis, TPN is utilized until pain ceases, ascites clears, and ileus disappears.

CANCER IN THE UROLOGIC PATIENT

There is nothing unique, as far as we know, about the malnutrition that may develop in urologic patients with cancer. Anorexia is a common symptom in these patients and determines who will develop cachexia.

Loss of appetite, with secondary loss of weight, and early satiety are typical symptoms and signs of cancer cachexia, but they are not unique to any one type of tumor. They may be seen with a variety of tumors that are unrelated to the GI tract. Anemia and weakness secondary to chronically poor intake of nutrients are other manifestations of cancer cachexia.

Why Do These Patients Become Malnourished?

The reason these patients become malnourished is secondary to impaired or inadequate food intake, impaired digestion, external nutrient loss, tumor host competition for nutrients, and increased energy expenditures of the host. The decreased appetite characterizing cancer patients may be secondary to:

1. Tumor variables (site, size, and growth rate of primary tumor).
2. Presence of metastatic tumor.
3. Host variables, including premorbid conditions, effects of decreased caloric intake, patient responses to illness (including psychologic), abnormalities in taste sensation, and metabolic changes.

Changes Associated with Starvation

All nutrient and energy systems are involved in the metabolic changes that arise from malnutrition in cancer patients. The human body stores the majority of excess calories as fat (9.4 kcal/gm). A smaller amount of calories is stored as a protein (4.0 kcal/gm), and only a small fraction of total body calories is carbohydrate (3.4 kcal/gm). In starvation, circulating carbohydrate is adequate for fuel for only 24 to 48 hours. Within 24 hours, the fat and protein stores begin to break down, with fat supplying two thirds and protein one third of the body's basic energy requirements. The proteins are broken down into amino acids that enter the gluconeogenic system. The fat is metabolized to triglycerides. The latter, in turn, are metabolized further into glycerol and free fatty acids, which form ketones used for energy by peripheral muscle.

Adaptation continues to take place as starvation persists. Over a month to 6 weeks, more of the energy needs are met by mobilization of triglycerides and their breakdown to ketones.

Metabolic Changes Specific to Cancer Patients

The metabolic alterations in cancer patients are not necessarily unique to the starvation that a cancer may cause. Some cancer patients may manifest an increased glucose turnover, glucose oxidation, and total caloric expenditure. Liver glycogen becomes depleted, and there is decreased glycogen response to glucagon. Body lipids may become depleted as mobilization of free fatty acids proceeds. If this deficit cannot be met, protein breakdown begins to play a larger role in supplying energy.

Protein Metabolism

Negative nitrogen balance develops as skeletal muscle mass is lost secondary to cachexia. Skeletal muscle converts primarily high branch chain amino acids to glucose, which releases aromatic amino acids into the circulation. The stress of cancer typically results in a rate of breakdown of body protein that is three to four times greater than occurs in simple starvation.

COMPLICATIONS

Complications from parenteral nutrition are not common; they fall into three categories:

1. Mechanical problems relating to placement of the central venous catheter when one is used.
2. Septic complications relating to contamination of the catheter itself.
3. Metabolic and nutritional complications relating to the administration of the solutions themselves.

The complication rates are inversely proportional to the care and attention provided in maintaining catheters and peripheral lines and to the time spent ensuring that nutritional requirements are being provided.

Catheter Placement and Contamination

The most serious and frequent complication of TPN is catheter-related sepsis. *Catheter sepsis* is defined as a septic episode in which no other site of infection is found, cultures from the catheter and peripheral blood yield the same organism, and treatment of the catheter with antibiotics or removal of the catheter results in resolution of the fever. The incidence may be as high as one episode in 60 days of usage to one episode in 1700 days. The occurrence of catheter sepsis may be minimized by proper care of the catheter site and strict cleaning procedures for separating the catheter from the intravenous tubing. Each time a catheter is opened, it should be carefully cleaned. The more carefully this is done, the lower the risk. Solutions themselves seldom become contaminated, but it can occur.

If the patient who is receiving TPN becomes febrile, the following plan should be followed:

1. Examine the patient for obvious sources of infection.
2. Culture the blood from the central line and a peripheral vein.
3. Culture urine, sputum, and other appropriate sites for bacteria and fungi.
4. Continue TPN if no recognized break in catheter care technique has occurred.
5. Begin antibiotics empirically if the patient appears septic.
6. If fever persists and the condition deteriorates despite use of antibiotics, remove the catheter.

Nutritional Complications

Nutritional complications are uncommon when sufficient calories, protein, essential fat, vitamins, trace metals, and minerals are provided. Nutrient toxicity usually results from long-term accumulation of fat-soluble vitamins or trace metals; the latter occurs when there is either excessive intake or impaired elimination.

References

1. Pettigrew RA, Charlesworth PM, Farmilo RW, et al: Assessment of nutritional depletion and immune competence: a comparison of clinical examination and objective measurements. JPEN 8:21, 1984.
2. Detsky AS, Bauer JP, Mendelson RA, et al: Evaluating the accuracy of nutritional assessment techniques applied to hospitalized patients: methodology and comparisons. JPEN 8:153, 1984.
3. Buzby GP, Mullen JL: Nutritional assessment. In Rombeau JL, Caldwell MD, eds: Enteral and Tube Feeding. Philadelphia, WB Saunders Co, 1984, pp 127–147.
4. Bauer JP, Detsky AS, Wesson DE, et al: Nutritional assessment: a comparison of clinical judgment and objective measurement. N Engl J Med 16:969, 1982.
5. Hamwi GJ: Therapy, 1964: changing dietary concepts. In Donowski B, ed: Diabetes Mellitus: Diagnosis and Treatment. New York, American Diabetes Association, Inc, pp 73–78.
6. Gray GL, Gray LK: Anthropometric measurements and their interpretation: principles, practices and problems. J Am Dietet Assoc 77:534, 1980.
7. Weigley ES: Average? Ideal? Desirable? A brief overview of height-weight tables in the United States. J. Am Dietet Assoc 84:417, 1984.
8. Frisancho AR: New standards of weight and body composition by frame size and height for assessment of nutritional status of adults and the elderly. Am J Clin Nutr 40:808, 1984.
9. Grant JP: Nutritional assessment in clinical practice. Nutr Clin Pract 1:3, 1986.
10. Frisancho AR: Triceps skin fold and upper arm muscle size norms for assessment of nutritional status. Am J Clin Nutr 27:1052, 1974.
11. Burritt MF, Anderson CF: Laboratory assessment of nutritional status. Human Pathol 15:130, 1984.
12. Forse AR, Shizgal HM: Serum albumin and nutritional status. JPEN 4:450, 1980.
13. Roza AM, Tuitt D, Shizgal HM: Transferrin—a poor measure of nutritional status. JPEN 8:523, 1984.
14. Twomey P, Ziegler D, Rombeau J: Utility of skin testing in nutritional assessment: a critical review. JPEN 6:50, 1982.
15. Fischer JE: Nutritional support in the seriously ill patient. Curr Probl Surg 17:465, 1980.
16. Hassett J, Cerra F, Siegel J, et al: Multiple system organ failure: mechanism and therapy. Surg Ann 14:27, 1982.
17. Cerra FB, Upson D, Angelico R, et al: Branched chains support postoperative protein synthesis. Surgery 92:192, 1982.
18. Hill GL, Church J: Energy and protein requirements of general surgical patients requiring intravenous nutrition. Br J Surg 71:1, 1984.
19. Kinney JM, Elwyn DH: Protein metabolism and injury. Ann Rev Nutr 3:433, 1983.
20. Weissman C, Kemper M, Askanazi J, et al: Resting metabolic rate of the critically ill patient: measured versus predicted. J Anesthesiol 64:673, 1986.
21. Weissman C, Kemper M, Damask MC, et al: Effect of routine intensive care interactions on metabolic rate. Chest 86:815, 1984.
22. Weir JB: New methods for calculating metabolic rate with special reference to protein metabolism. J Physiol 109:1, 1949.
23. Goldstein S, Askanazi J, Thomashow B, et al: Metabolic demand, ventilation and muscle function during repletion of malnourished COPD and surgical patients. Anesthesiology 63:A276, 1985.
24. Askanazi J, Weissman C, LaSala PA, et al: Effect of protein intake on ventilatory drive. Anesthesiology 60:106, 1984.
25. Dark DS, Pingleton SK, Kerby GR: Hypercapnea during weaning: a complication of nutritional support. Chest 88:141, 1985.
26. Baker JP, Detsky AS, Steward S, et al: Randomized trial of total parenteral nutrition in critically ill patients: metabolic effects of varying glucose-lipid ratios as the energy source. Gastroenterology 87:53, 1984.
27. Elwyn DH: Nutritional requirements of adult surgical patients. Crit Care Med 8:9, 1980.
28. Anderson GH, Patel DG, Jeejeebhoy KN: Design and evaluation of nitrogen balance and blood aminograms of an amino acid mixture for total parenteral nutrition of adults with gastrointestinal disease. J Clin Invest 53:904, 1974.
29. Cerra FB, Cheung NK, Fischer JE, et al: Disease-specific amino acid infusion (F080) in hepatic encephalopathy: a prospective, randomized, double-blind trial. JPEN 9:288, 1985.

30. Holman RT: The ratio of trienoic:tetraenoic acids in tissue lipids as a measure of essential fatty acid deficiency. J Nutr 70:405, 1960.
31. Wene JD, Connor WE, BenBesten L: The development of essential fatty acid deficiency in healthy men fed fat-free diets intravenously and orally. J Clin Invest 56:127, 1975.
32. American Medical Association Department of Foods and Nutrition: Multivitamin preparations for parenteral use: a statement by the Nutrition Advisory Group. JPEN 3:258, 1979.
33. American Medical Association Department of Foods and Nutrition: Guidelines for essential trace element preparations for parenteral use. JAMA 241:2051, 1979.
34. Antonenko DR: Vitamins and minerals. In Kirkpatrick JR, ed: Nutrition and Metabolism in the Surgical Patient. Mt. Kisco, New York, Futura Publishing Co, 1983, pp 163–197.
35. Triplett WC: Clinical aspects of zinc, copper, manganese, chromium and selenium metabolism. Nutr Int 1:60, 1985.

COMPLICATIONS ASSOCIATED WITH RADIOTHERAPY OF PROSTATE CANCER

8

Malcolm A. Bagshaw • Gordon R. Ray • Richard A. Cox

INTRODUCTION

Systematic external beam radiation therapy for carcinoma of the prostate was introduced in the mid-1950s, when post–World War II megavoltage radiation therapy devices (^{60}cobalt units, linear accelerators, and betatrons) made it possible to treat deep-seated neoplasms.[1–5] Even though the prostate is shielded by the bones of the pelvic girdle, the relative lack of absorption by bone and the improved soft tissue penetration of these high energy x-ray or gamma-ray beams effectively opened up the pelvis to this form of treatment. There was then, and continues to be now, a concern about the radiation tolerance of adjacent organs and normal tissues. Originally, treatment was limited to the prostate and the immediate periprostatic region. Since most of these tissues were inferior to the peritoneal reflections, the prostatic region was irradiated without exposing the small bowel and most of the urinary bladder to radiation. It was necessary, however, to treat that part of the rectum that is directly posterior to the prostate. Initially, rotational moving beam therapy seemed a reasonable choice for treating the prostate, which is centrally located within a symmetric ellipsoid cross-section of the pelvis. The development of the rotational or moving beam arc technique was the central theme at Stanford University, although others used parallel opposed anteroposterior radiation beams, postero-anterior radiation beams, perineal applications, and other techniques.

In the late 1960s and early 1970s, there was sufficient evidence for control of prostatic cancer at the primary site to shift the focus in treatment strategy to include treatment of the primary-echelon lymphatics of the prostate in addition to the prostate.[6] The primary-echelon lymph nodes include the internal iliac, external iliac, and common iliac as well as the presacral lymph nodes, which ultimately join to ascend in the para-aortic chains. At that time, the significance of lymph node involvement was being clarified by staging laparotomy, which demonstrated the step-wise progression of lymph node involvement from the obturator nodes to the external iliacs, to the common iliacs, and then to the para-aortic lymph nodes. Parallel involvement included the internal iliac and presacral nodes. In order to encompass both the primary site and the potential lymphadenopathy, treatment programs were expanded to include not only the prostate but also its primary-echelon lymphatic drainage. This necessitated full pelvic irradiation to the level of the sacral promontory and, in some series, even farther to include the para-aortic lymph nodes to the level of the diaphragm. Although indirect evidence exists that suggests a survival advantage in treating involved lymph nodes,[7–9] the efficacy of preventing further spread and improving survival by treating the regional adenopathy has not been established by properly randomized prospective clinical trials.[10,11] Along with the expansion of the radiation treatment volume to include at least the pelvic lymphatics, the introduction of computed tomography (CT) controlled treatment planning suggested that in some instances, the seminal vesicles were not always included appropriately in the treatment volume.[12,13]

Thus, since the introduction of irradiation of prostatic adenocarcinoma, the target volume has expanded from the prostate and the immediate periprostatic region to include the entire contents of the pelvis, and even in some instances, the para-aortic region; this makes it possible to adequately treat the first- and second-echelon prostatic lymphatics. Radiation volumes have been devised that range from fields measured at isocenter as small as 6 × 6 cm or 8 × 8 cm, restricted to the prostate only, to radiation fields as large as 22 × 16 cm to include the entire pelvic region, and even in some cases to 6 or 8 × 20 cm extensions to permit inclusion of the para-aortic region. Within this enormous variation in treatment volume and attendant normal tissues at risk, there was often simultaneous use of lymph node dissection, making it extremely difficult to document the pattern of radiation complications.

TRANSIENT REACTIONS

Acute Reactions During Radiation Treatment

During irradiation, patients may experience increased fatigue, diarrhea, proctalgia or dysuria manifest as burning on urination, frequency, or nocturia. Usually these symptoms commence between one third and one half of the way through the treatment program.

In the Stanford experience, 750 transient symptoms requiring medication for symptomatic relief, or requiring less than 1 week of interruption in therapy and requiring no pain medication, occurred in 503 of the 914 patients. A tabulation of the most frequently encountered symptoms (9 or more) that occurred during treatment is presented in Table 8–1. Usually, mild medication or dietary management alleviated acute reactions during treatment. For example, regulation of fluid intake by increasing fluids during the day and refraining from them after 6 P.M. and by eliminating coffee, usually relieved urinary burning. Occasionally, medications such as phenazopyridine hydrochloride (Pyridium) or flavoxate hydrochlorine (Urispas) or a few days' interruption of radiation treatment were required to quiet the acute symptoms.

Diarrhea was reasonably controlled with a low-residue diet and by avoiding excessively spicy or irritating food such as strong alcoholic beverages and exotic and hot spices such as those in Mexican and Szechuan cuisine. Diphenosylate hydrochloride with atropine sulfate (Lomotil) or loperamide hydrochloride (Imodium) in modest doses usually controlled diarrhea. Mild anorexia was encountered, but nausea was rare and vomiting did not occur. Hemoglobin, white blood cell counts, and platelet counts were monitored weekly, but a lowering of blood elements sufficient to interrupt therapy was not encountered.

Table 8–1. NUMBER OF ACUTE REACTIONS DURING IRRADIATION

Urinary		Intestinal	
Burning	112	Diarrhea	304
Frequency	59	Cramps	56
Obstruction	17	Proctitis	38
Hematuria	13		
Retention	12		
Cystitis	9		

Symptoms recorded 9 or more times were tabulated.
Seven hundred fifty transient symptoms were recorded in 503 of the 914 patients at Stanford University (1956–1985).

Properly fractionated treatment with modern megavoltage radiotherapy equipment, e.g., linear accelerators, using multiple beams, shaped to maximize protection of normal structures, is well tolerated. It is usually conducted on an outpatient basis. Although many patients notice increased fatigue during therapy, most who are regularly employed find that they are able to continue working during the course of treatment. More severe or intractable symptoms during treatment are usually related to tumor progression or intercurrent illness and require more serious intervention. Severe symptoms occurring months to years following irradiation suggest serious organ dysfunction.

Irradiation Technique (Stanford University)

The basic technique includes three steps: (1) tumor localization, (2) treatment planning, and (3) therapy. Orthogonal radiographs are obtained with the patient in the treatment position, using contrast medium in the rectum and urethra for precise delineation of anatomy. These localization films are supplemented by CT scans with the patient in treatment position and, more recently, by magnetic resonance imaging. In the 4-field technique, the corners of the anterior and posterior fields are trimmed to minimize target

Table 8–2. STATUS OF 914 PATIENTS WITH PROSTATE CANCER TREATED WITH EXTERNAL BEAM IRRADIATION AT STANFORD

	5 Years	10 Years	15 Years
Nominal stages A & B	80	60	35
Nominal stage C	60	36	18

Percent survival at 5-year intervals calculated by Kaplan-Meier method. One hundred one patients have survived beyond 15 years.

volume, and the left and right lateral fields are shaped to the individual's anatomy by the preparation of customized collimators for precise beam definition to minimize irradiation of the rectum, anus, and proximal urethra.

Two general radiation therapy routines have been utilized.* The original routine, applied in the first 300 patients treated, included irradiation to the prostate and the prostatic region only, with either a 360-degree rotational or a bilateral (left and right) 120-degree moving beam arc technique. In that technique, 7600 rad were delivered to the prostatic region in 7½ weeks at the rate of 200 to 225 rad per day calculated to a volume of tissue of 6 to 8 cm in diameter. In more recent years, first-echelon lymph nodes and, occasionally, second-echelon lymph nodes have been included in the treatment plan, necessitating a 4-field box technique. In some instances, para-aortic lymph nodes were treated as well. When the pelvic adenopathy was treated, the box technique was used first to approximately 2600 rad in 13 treatments, at which point a coned-down booster dose was delivered to the prostate for only 2000 rad in 10 treatments, using left and right 120° moving beam arc therapy. Then the treatment program was expanded to the original 4-field box to include the entire pelvic first-echelon lymphatic drainage system. This program delivers 7000 rad in 7 weeks to the prostate and 5000 rad in 7 weeks to the first-echelon adenopathy. When the para-aortic lymph nodes were also included, 5000 rad were delivered to the para-aortic lymph nodes. This program has been extremely well tolerated, with only rare instances of prolonged urinary discomfort or morbidity, usually associated with pretherapeutic transurethral resection. More explicit technical detail has been published previously.[8,11,14] The overall treatment results are summarized in Table 8–2.

*Linear accelerators with photon energies of approximately 4 megavolts (Mv) at 80 cm source to axis (SAD) distance, and 5 and 6 Mv at 100 SAD have been used exclusively in this study.

Timing of Radiation Following Surgery

Transrectal or Transperineal Needle Biopsy. Usually, no particular precautions or delays in starting radiation therapy following either transperineal or transrectal needle biopsy are required. Aside from the rare incidence of a biopsy-induced hematoma, there was no morbidity in this study attributed to needle biopsy.

Post-transurethral Resection. A 6- to 12-week delay following transurethral resection is recommended before starting radiation treatment. The precise timing depends on the extent of the transurethral resection, the pace of convalescence, and the histopathology. In patients who have undergone a modest transurethral resection and who are convalescing well, radiation treatment may be started relatively early, i.e., at 6 weeks. Also, early treatment is preferred in patients with tumor of high histologic grade, such as a Gleason pattern score of 8 or greater. In patients with an extensive transurethral resection and some postsurgical morbidity, radiation treatment should be delayed for 8 to 12 weeks.

Post-prostatectomy. Patients should be past the period of convalescence and essentially leading normal lives before postoperative irradiation is instituted following radical perineal or retropubic prostatectomy or suprapubic prostatectomy. This may require 3 to 6 months. However, it is not necessary to await complete return of continence, which may even improve during or soon after completion of the radiation treatment. As is the case following transurethral resection, it may be prudent to start radiation treatment earlier if the malignancy is of high grade. In patients requiring postoperative irradiation because of transected tumor margins, lymph node metastases have been usually ruled out by appropriate node sampling. Therefore, the treatment volume is limited to the prostatic bed but with a liberal margin extending beyond the vesiculourethral anastomosis. In patients with overt recurrence, usually several years post radical prostatectomy, the irradiated volume usually includes the primary-echelon lymphatics as well as the recurrent neoplasm.

PERSISTENT SEQUELAE

Tissues At Risk

The significant tissues at risk in the treatment of prostatic carcinoma include the prostatic ure-

Table 8–3. RTOG* MORBIDITY GRADING SYSTEM

Grade 1	Minor symptoms requiring no treatment
Grade 2	Symptoms responding to simple outpatient management, lifestyle (performance status) not affected
Grade 3	Distressing symptoms altering patients' lifestyle (performance status). Hospitalization for diagnosis or minor surgical intervention (such as urethral dilation) may be required
Grade 4	Major surgical intervention (such as laparotomy, colostomy, cystectomy) or prolonged hospitalization required
Grade 5	Fatal complications

Four hundred twenty-four of 611 patients were not scored as to source of complications; of those scored, about one half (73) were attributed to x-ray technician (XRT).

*Radiation Therapy Oncology Group. From Pilepich MV, Krall JM, Sause WT, et al: Correlation of radiotherapeutic parameters and treatment related morbidity in carcinoma of the prostate: analysis of RTOG study 75-06. Int J Radiat Oncol Biol Phys 13:351–357, 1987.

thra and urinary bladder, the rectum, the rectosigmoid, and the small bowel. The pelvic lymphatics are rarely obstructed by irradiation alone, but the combination of extensive lymphadenectomy and irradiation may be followed by debilitating genital and/or lower-extremity edema.[15,16] Subcutaneous fibrosis and either pubic or femoral osteonecrosis are seldom encountered, particularly with modern multifield techniques. Ureteral damage is also rare.[17] The vascular supply to the corpora may be compromised by irradiation, and this may be the pathogenesis of radiation-induced erectile impotence.[18] The nerves of the lumbosacral plexes, and in the case of para-aortic treatment, the nerves of the distal cord, are irradiated, but neither nerve nor spinal cord damage has been encountered.

Morbidity Grading Systems

The evaluation of the morbidity in prostatic cancer is hampered by the lack of a well-defined and universally accepted categorization of radiation injury. The Radiation Therapy Oncology Group (RTOG) has developed a classification of radiation injury that has been applied in the studies of that organization (Table 8–3).[19,20] This morbidity grading system was derived from a system previously reported by Pilepich and associates from the Division of Radiation Oncology, Washington University School of Medicine.[15] In that study of 267 patients, the following 4 grades of morbidity were described: Grade 1—minor or transient symptoms responding to simple outpatient management; Grade 2—distressing, persistent, or recurring symptoms occasionally requiring brief hospitalization and/or minor surgical intervention; Grade 3—complications requiring major surgery or prolonged hospitalization; and Grade 4—fatal complications. A system employing a nearly identical 4-grade categorization was adopted by a French consortium of five centers that reported an analysis of complications in 597 patients.[21]

In the present RTOG system, 5 grades of morbidity are enumerated (Table 8–3). Grades 1 and 2 represent minor symptoms requiring no treatment or symptoms responding to simple outpatient management. Grade 3 includes distressing symptoms altering lifestyle or requiring hospitalization for diagnosis or minor surgical intervention, and Grade 4 includes symptoms requiring major surgical intervention or prolonged hospitalization. This gradation appears comparable to that described by Hanks in the Patterns of Care Study (PCS), in which a major complication was defined as requiring admission to the hospital for diagnosis or management.[22] This was later revised to include a Grade 5, defined as admitted to hospital for surgical management.[23]

In both the RTOG and the PCS studies, there were 2 deaths attributed to a complication of radiation therapy, and these were assigned Grade 5 in the RTOG study and Grade 6 in the latest PCS description.[23] A summary of treatment-related morbidity in the RTOG study is presented in Table 8–4. Although complications in the Stanford system were scored differently, it was possible to retrieve data on the basis of RTOG Grades 3, 4, and 5 morbidity. Table 8–5 presents an overview of equivalent grades used in these major studies as referenced to the RTOG system, which is given in Table 8–3. Table 8–6 summarizes the data on severe and major complications derived from these four large studies and also includes new data from the Stanford experience. It is not meant to present a comparison among the institutions listed but to give the reader an overview of the incidence and severity of complications based on a large experience in different environments.

Overview of Severe Complications

Reference to Table 8–6 demonstrates reasonably close agreement among the Stanford University, Washington University, and French

Table 8–4. TREATMENT-RELATED MORBIDITY (RTOG)*

	Grade 1	2	3	4	5	Total (%)
Diarrhea	26	40	1	0	0	67 (12.7)
Proctitis	19	27	5	1	0	52 (9.9)
Cystitis	36	16	6	2	0	60 (11.4)
Hematuria	11	6	12	1	0	30 (5.7)
Rectal bleeding	30	11	3	1	1	46 (8.7)
Rectal-anal stricture	17	5	1	0	0	23 (4.4)
Urethral stricture	1	2	11	1	0	15 (2.9)
Rectal ulcer	0	4	1	1	0	6 (1.1)
Bowel obstruction	0	0	0	2	1	3 (0.6)

*Radiation Therapy Oncology Group. From Pilepich MV, Krall JM, Sause WT, et al: Correlation of radiotherapeutic parameters and treatment related morbidity in carcinoma of the prostate: analysis of RTOG study 75-06. Int J Radiat Oncol Biol Phys 13:351–357, 1987.
(See Table 8–3 for grade designation.)

Table 8–5. EQUIVALENT MORBIDITY GRADES

Group	Moderate Grade	Severe Grade	Death Grade
Washington U.	2	3	4
French	2	3	4
RTOG	3	4	5
PCS	2, 4	5	6
Stanford U.	2, 3, 4	5	6

data when adjusted for overall numbers, whereas a somewhat lower incidence of moderately severe complications is revealed in the PCS and RTOG studies in the severe category. However, this may be because the criteria for severe complications, which include admission to hospital for major surgical interventions, are considerably less ambiguous than are the criteria for moderately severe complications, which include "distressing symptoms altering patient life-styles." Also, it should be noted that in both the Stanford University and the Washington University series, an earlier period in the treatment of prostatic cancer is represented, a period during which techniques were being developed and dose ranges established. Also, both the Washington University and the Stanford University series are single data bases, which were more consistently managed in a single institution.

In the Stanford study, other criteria were also used to provide an opportunity to develop a broader view of treatment-related morbidity. The complications or conditions summarized in the Stanford study and presented in Table 8–1 were also categorized as either transient or persistent, that is, of being either less or more than 2 years' duration. Also, in the original Stanford grading system, 3 levels of severity were enumerated. These have been expanded to 6 grades in order to more closely approximate the RTOG and PCS grading systems. The current severity scale for the Stanford data is presented in Table 8–7.

The data from the Stanford study differ from the two national cooperative efforts in that the Stanford data have been collected at a single site by a single observer and also over a much longer time and by periodic and repeated patient assessment. Approximately two thirds of the patients have been followed in-house, and the remainder of the data is continually updated by interviewing both the patient and the patient's follow-up physician at least annually. Because of this serialization of the data on each individual,

Table 8–6. SUMMARY OF MODERATE AND SEVERE COMPLICATIONS IN 5 MAJOR STUDIES

Group	Period	Total Number of Cases	Number with Complications: *Moderate*	*Severe*	*Death*
Washington U.	1967–1978	267	66	5	1
French	1975–1982	597	373/144*	17/16*	4
RTOG	1976–1983	526	40	9 + 11**	2
PCS	1973–1975	662	17	14	2
Stanford U.	1956–1985	914	106	22	3

*Complications/Patients
**11 patients were arbitrarily excluded from the tally for no apparent reason. These included 3 with bladder neck contractures, 3 with contracted bladders, 1 with a urethral ulcer, 1 with a colocutaneous fistula, 3 with gastric ulcers.

Table 8–7. CURRENT STANFORD MORBIDITY GRADING SYSTEM

Grade	
1	Mild (responding to medications for control)
2	Moderate (failure to respond to medications after 3 months)
3	Symptoms altering lifestyle (includes dilation)
4	Hospitalization for diagnosis or minor surgery (e.g., TURP)
5	Major surgical intervention (e.g., colostomy, prolonged hospital stay)
6	Death from complications

there is an opportunity to develop the long-term natural history for each individual and to identify and examine cofactors in the induction of treatment-related morbidity. These include the impact of surgical staging, the influence of transurethral resection, particularly on the development of incontinence, and the influence of the evolution of treatment techniques.

Surgical Staging Effects on Morbidity

Table 8–8 demonstrates that patients who underwent surgical staging prior to radiation treatment were at significantly increased risk for gastrointestinal, urologic, and other morbidity. In fact, surgical staging was the single most significant cofactor that contributed to parairradiation morbidity in this series. Moderate and severe complications were 3.4 times more frequent in the staged patients. Intestinal complications, commonly small bowel obstruction, were 3.7 times more prevalent, and genital and lower extremity edema were 10 times more prevalent. Urinary complications, on the other hand, were less affected by staging procedures and were only 1.4 times more frequent in the staged patients. Note that staged and unstaged patients were drawn from approximately the same time period so that other factors, such as technique, were more likely to have been equally distributed between the 2 groups. In some patients, a transperitoneal exploration was used to evaluate metastatic disease in the para-aortic lymph nodes. This was soon perceived to be an ill-advised approach that was abandoned because 60 percent of the complications that developed in the staged patients occurred in this group. Nevertheless, even the retroperitoneal approach was not without substantial complications, 40 percent occurring in these patients. Fortunately, the data provided for the first time the knowledge that retroperitoneal pararenal adenopathy was present in at least 20 percent of the investigated patients with prostate cancer.[6]

Effect of Transurethral Resection on Radiation Morbidity

Perhaps less dramatic but equally conclusive was the observation that pararadiotherapeutic or postradiotherapeutic incontinence was usually linked to transurethral resection. Table 8–9 demonstrates clearly that transurethral resection, whether before, during, or after radiotherapy, or multiple transurethral resections of the prostate (TURP), increased the likelihood of incontinence. This is not to condemn transurethral resection, which is often vitally necessary in this group of patients, but to point out that the incontinence that occurs is a consequence of the overall treatment and not necessarily of one specific modality. From the point of view of

Table 8–8. COMPLICATIONS ATTRIBUTED TO RADIATION THERAPY IN SURGICALLY STAGED PATIENTS VS. UNSTAGED PATIENTS, FEBRUARY 1970–JUNE 1978

		Staged		Unstaged	
Treatment Profile		47:57:42*		37:126:23*	
Complications		*Number*	%	*Number*	%
Persistent (Gr. 2–6)†	GI	16	(11)	5	(3)
	GU	2	(1)	4	(2)
	Other	11	(8)	1	(1)
	Total	29	(20)	10	(6)
Transient (Gr. 2–6)†	GI	13	(9)	5	(3)
	GU	8	(6)	5	(3)
	Other	5	(3)	1	(1)
	Total	26	(18)	9	(7)

*Numbers of patients treated to: *Prostate: Prostate and Pelvic Nodes: Prostate and Pelvic Nodes and Para-aortic Nodes*
All patients treated with similar technique.
†See Table 8–7 (Current Stanford Morbidity Grading System).
Chi Square P = 0.00003

Table 8–9. URINARY INCONTINENCE VS PRE AND/OR POST XRT TURP (1956–1984)

	Number of Patients	Number with Persistent Incontinence n = 39
TURP	394	34* (8.6%)
No TURP	499	5* (1.0%)
Total	893	39 (4.4%)

*P = <0.01

radiotherapy, it is better to try to execute the radiotherapy without transurethral resection, even though the patient may suffer from modest obstructive symptoms.

Green and coworkers also noted severe para-radiotherapeutic complications in 3 of 5 patients who underwent TURP and 5 of 10 patients who had prostatectomies.[24] They advocated the avoidance of urologic instrumentation and catheterization in conjunction with radiation whenever possible, preferring instead a preradiotherapeutic trial of estrogen therapy to relieve obstructive uropathy. Maneuvers such as prescribing phenoxybenzamine to aid micturition or employing either diethylstilbestrol or a luteinizing hormone-releasing hormone (LHRH) prior to and/or during irradiation are often successful in forestalling the need for transurethral resection during radiation therapy. It has been our impression that if prolonged bladder drainage is required, a percutaneous suprapubic tube is superior to an indwelling urethral catheter during the course of irradiation. It appears to be important to minimize even the slight trauma of an indwelling catheter to the prostatic urethra during radiation treatment.

Other Complications

Although observed rarely, a patient with unilateral ureteral stenosis following irradiation (6000 rad in 6 weeks with 360-degree rotation) was the subject of a case report.[17] In this patient, the stenotic segment of ureter was excised and a successful ureteroneocystostomy was performed. One Stanford patient died at home of uremia that was attributed to bilateral ureteral stenosis, although there was no objective evidence to support ureteral damage. Ureteral obstruction can occur as a consequence of direct extension of the tumor into or around the ureters as they pass through the bladder wall.

Severe prostatic calcification was noted after radiation therapy in three patients.[25] In each of these cases, the stones developed following external beam irradiation carried out relatively soon after transurethral resection. The authors suggested that the stones might have been avoided if an interval of at least 6 weeks was allowed between transurethral resection and the radiation therapy. As discussed elsewhere, incontinence is also associated with too short an interval between TURP and irradiation. Unless there are extenuating circumstances such as bleeding or a histopathologically highly aggressive tumor, an interval of 6 weeks should be considered the minimum.

Potency

Radiation-associated impotence (RAI), according to Goldstein and colleagues, has been reported in from 22 to 84 percent of patients receiving radiation treatment for prostatic cancer.[18] They suggest that the etiology is secondary to radiation-induced endarteritis of the branches of the internal pudendal and penile arteries, which course lateral to the prostate, and they have demonstrated obstruction of these by dissection and arteriography. This is an attractive hypothesis. Perez cites the possible causes as (1) hormonal—decreased T and DHT; (2) mechanical—fibrosis, decreased external glandular secretions; (3) neurologic—pudendal nerve injury; and (4) psychological.[26] Goldstein and colleagues, however, in an elegant series of clinical studies, present compelling evidence implicating radiation-induced vascular insufficiency of the internal pudendal and penile arteries as the major contributing factor.[18] They could demonstrate neither significant hormonal deficiency nor neurologic defects in patients who complained of RAI. On the other hand, they demonstrated substantial vascular deficiency in the hypogastric-cavernous arterial bed by penile Doppler ultrasonography. In addition, they demonstrated abnormal nocturnal penile tumescence (NPT) and tortuosity and narrowing of the internal pudendal arteries by pudendal arteriography. Progressive obliterative endarteritis is a well-known late effect of radiation that occurs in virtually every organ system subjected to direct irradiation.

The influence of radiation on erectile potency was recently restudied in the Stanford series. Figure 8–1 demonstrates the postirradiation status of potency in 434 patients in the Stanford series who claimed erectile potency (about 50 percent) prior to irradiation. Whereas 86 per-

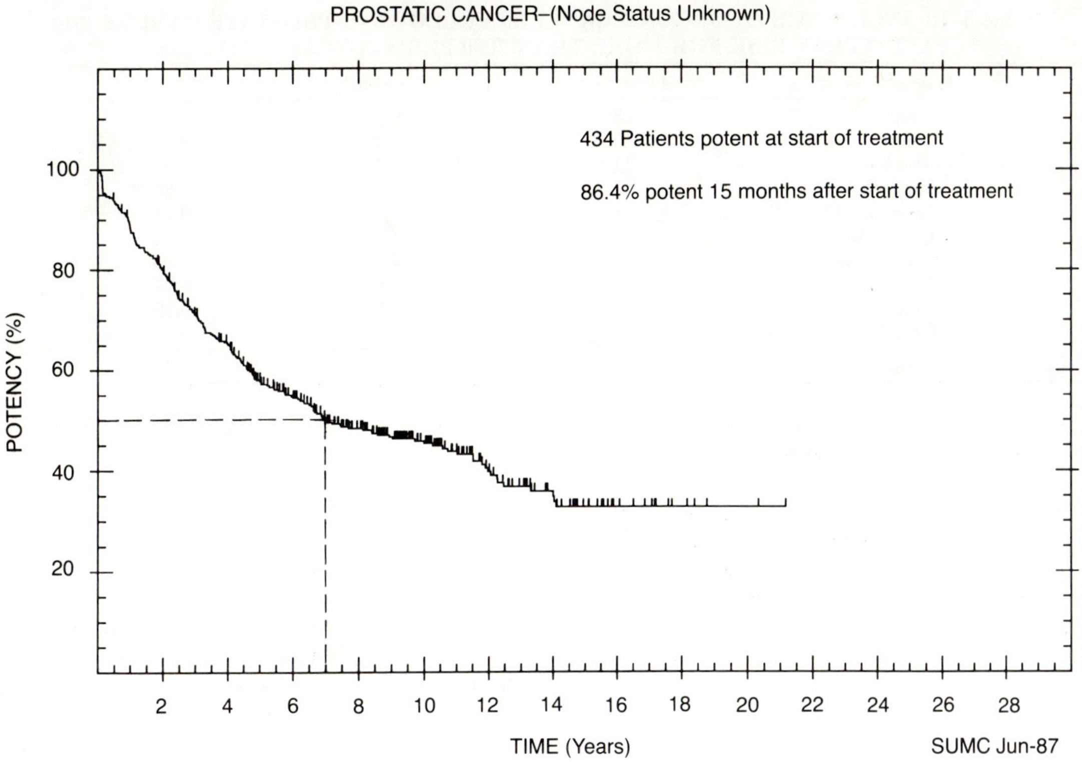

Figure 8–1. Status of erectile potency after external beam irradiation.

cent of the patients remained potent at 15 months post treatment, the median potency period was 7 years, and approximately 30 percent of the patients maintained erectile potency until death. Although the normal gradual decline of erectile potency with advancing age has not been corrected for in Figure 8–1, the pattern of decay in erectile potency following irradiation is compatible with, and inversely proportional to, the slow progression of radiation-induced vascular injury. The recognition that this disability is vascular in nature suggests the possibility for the development of a vascular bypass procedure or some other protective or corrective measure.

Incidence of Secondary Neoplasms

There was no increase in the incidence of second cancers observed in the 914 Stanford patients compared with the expected incidence calculated from the Surveillance, Epidemiology, and End Results (SEER) program data for San Francisco Bay Area white males (Table 8–10).[27] Note the remarkable agreement between the observed and expected incidence rates. There was no evidence to suggest that the radiation treatment of prostatic cancer played a systematic role in the induction of second neoplasms in these patients.

REDUCTION OF IATROGENIC DISEASE

Target Volume

Table 8–11 demonstrates a trend toward reduction in complication rates during the period 1968 through 1985. Although there was no change in complication rates between the period 1968 through 1971 and 1972 through 1977, from the standpoint of treatment strategy, there was a substantial increase in the radiation volume that might have been expected to increase complication rates. During the period 1968 through 1971, 171 patients underwent prostate treatment only; 14 underwent treatment to the prostate plus the pelvic lymph nodes, i.e., treatment volume extending from the ischial tuberosities to the 5th lumbar vertebral body; and in 5 additional patients, para-aortic fields were also treated. During the period 1972 through 1977, the patient mix was 37 with treatment to the

Table 8–10. INCIDENCE OF SECOND CANCERS FOLLOWING PROSTATE CANCER (914 PATIENTS AT RISK FOR MORE THAN 7000 PERSON-YEARS) (1956–1985)

Type of Cancer	Observed	Expected	P-Value
Lung	28	29.3	0.81
Colon	15	15.2	0.96
Bladder	11	10.2	0.80
Stomach	6	5.4	0.80
Rectum	4	7.4	0.21
Leukemia	4	3.8	0.92
Lymphoma	3	4.1	0.65
Pancreas	3	4.6	0.27
Kidney	1	2.9	0.26
Other	24	(24.0)	—
Total	99 (10.8%)	106.9	0.48

NIH Publ 85–1837, 1984.

Observed second cancers vs. expected incidence as calculated by the method of Monson from SEER Program data for San Francisco Bay Area white males.

prostate only, 126 to the entire pelvis, and 23 to the para-aortic region as well. Although the patient mix stayed about the same from 1978 to 1985, i.e., 35 prostate, 138 pelvis, and 17 para-aortic, the overall complication rate was reduced by more than half, from 11.3 to 4.2 percent. This included reduction of intestinal complications from 5.4 to 2.1 percent, urinary complications from 4.9 to 2.2 percent, and other complications, mainly edema of the genitals or lower extremities, from 1 percent to 0. Note that the surgically staged patients were excluded from this analysis as were patients in whom the complications were attributed to progression of cancer.

In order to protect the bladder during the boost part of the treatment, part of the bladder can be moved out of the target volume by instructing patients to allow urine to accumulate so that they are treated with a full bladder. In the mid-1970s, the lateral pelvic fields for the 4-field box technique were modified to stress protection of the posterior rectal wall. This technique was further refined in 1980 by individualizing the lateral pelvic fields by the preparation of customized Cerrobend collimators in which the posterior margins of the lateral field would follow the course of the mid-lumen of the presacral sweep of the rectum, thus protecting the entire posterior rectal wall during exposure through the lateral fields. This is, in essence, a form of conformational treatment in which the treatment volume is tailor-made to conform to the target volume.

Radiation Dose, Technique, and Fractionation

There are data which indicate that when the tumor dose exceeds 7000 rad given over 7

Table 8–11. OVERALL GASTROINTESTINAL AND GENITOURINARY COMPLICATION RATE FOR UNSTAGED PATIENTS

		Small Field 1968–1971		Extended Field 1972–1977		Extended Field 1978–1985	
Treatment Profile*		171:14:5*		37:126:23*		35:138:17*	
Complications		*Number*	*%*	*Number*	*%*	*Number*	*%*
Persistent (Gr. 2–6)†	GI	6	(3.2)	5	(2.7)	3	(1.6)
	GU	6	(3.2)	4	(2.2)	2	(1.1)
	Other	1	(0.5)	1	(0.5)	0	(0.0)
Transient (Gr. 2–6)†	GI	2	(1.1)	5	(2.7)	1	(0.5)
	GU	6	(3.2)	5	(2.7)	2	(1.1)
	Other	1	(0.5)	1	(0.5)	0	(0.0)
	Total	22	(11.7)	21	(11.3)	8	(4.3)

*Number of patients treated to:
Prostate: Prostate and Pelvic Nodes: Prostate and Pelvic Nodes and Para-aortic Nodes
All patients treated with similar technique.

†See Table 8–7 (Current Stanford Morbidity Grading System)

This reduction in serious sequelae, although not strictly statistically significant, demonstrates a trend toward overall reduction in complications.

weeks, there is an unacceptable increase in moderate and severe complications. Neglia and coworkers noted 11 major complications, usually requiring diverting colostomies, in 110 patients treated to 7000 rad or more, but complications in only one in 44 patients receiving 6750 rad or less.[28] Similarly, Hanks noted that the severe complication rate increased from 3.5 percent below 7000 rad to 6.9 percent when 7000 rad was exceeded.[22] In the RTOG study, diarrhea was significantly increased when the prostatic *boost* was carried to 7000 rad and beyond.[20] The RTOG study also showed a significant increase in diarrhea when the radiation dose was boosted with either lateral fields only or perineal fields only. Interestingly, bladder complications were not significantly increased with doses of 7000 rad to the prostate.

In an earlier series, a higher incidence of rectal and subcutaneous tissue injury was reported in patients treated with parallel opposed fields using ^{60}Co.[29] A higher incidence of complications was also found in the PCS study with the use of parallel opposed anteroposterior-posteroanterior fields when only 1 field per day was treated.[30] Early in the development of the technique for prostatic irradiation, some therapists treated only 1 field per day. This was a common practice with ^{60}Co treatment, no doubt encouraged by the generally longer treatment times. Although Rounseville and associates worked with a 25 megaelectron volt (MeV) betatron, their study clearly demonstrated that 100 percent of the complications requiring major surgical correction (Grade 3) or resulting in a fatality (Grade 4) occurred when only one field each day was treated.[31] When all fields were treated every day, Grades 3 and 4 complications were not encountered. A reduction in radiation treatment–related morbidity has been attributed to a split-course technique in which 4500 rad are delivered to the midplane with 180 rad fractions, followed by a 2-week rest, after which the course is completed with a reduced prostatic tumor volume to a total dose of 6500 rad.[32,33] The overall gastrointestinal and genitourinary severe complication rate of 3 percent is essentially the same as seen in the most recently treated group in the Stanford series (Table 8–11), in which a form of split-course therapy was also utilized (see section on Technique).

Other factors that may have contributed to reduction in morbidity include more careful patient selection, the adoption of a modified split-course technique, more attention to dietary regulation during treatment, and more liberal use of supportive medications, such as Anusol with hydrocortisone suppositories, stool softeners when needed, or diphenoxylate hydrochloride and atropine (Lomotil), and other supportive care during therapy. It is our opinion that the individualized lateral fields, the introduction of the booster dose midway through the full pelvic treatment plan, and the insistence on treatment to every field every day, are the most important technical advances. During the past decade, it has been rare to interrupt the treatment because of either urinary or intestinal side effects. In fact, the best illustration of patient tolerance during external beam irradiation of prostatic cancer in 1988 is our assurance that he is unlikely to miss a day's work during the 7-week course of external beam irradiation.

SUMMARY

Comparison of various studies indicates that there are specific treatment techniques that tend to reduce therapeutic morbidity. Given a daily fraction dose of 180 to 200 rad per day, 5 days per week, delivered to the intersection of the central axes of the various treatment fields or the 100 percent isodose contour, one may observe the following: (1) Morbidity increases significantly as the total radiation dose of 7000 rad delivered to the isocenter point is exceeded. (2) Irrespective of the radiation field arrangement, morbidity is significantly reduced if all fields bearing on a single target volume are treated every day. Although often unavoidable, pelvic and abdominal surgery and radiation therapy do not mix from the standpoint of morbidity. Any type of surgical intervention for staging or resection appears to increase morbidity when the primary therapeutic approach is external beam irradiation. This may not be true when external beam irradiation is used judiciously as a supplement to surgery in the event that the tumor has not been completely resected. (3) It appears that there is a trend toward the diminution of morbidity with linear accelerators as opposed to ^{60}Co units.[24]

In summary, morbidity may be reduced by

1. Avoiding abdominal or pelvic exploration in conjunction with radiotherapy, particularly if a transperitoneal surgical approach is employed
2. Avoiding TURP whenever possible
3. Avoiding an external beam dose in excess of 7000 rad in 7 weeks to the target volume with present techniques delivered by external beam irradiation

4. Tailoring the radiation fields to conform to the target volume by minimizing the small bowel, rectal, and anal radiation doses

5. Delivering the dose homogeneously to the target volume on each treatment day. A single-field daily treatment to a complicated treatment volume should be avoided

6. Careful attention to supportive care during treatment such as fluid-intake control, dietary management, and administration of appropriate medication such as Anusol HC suppositories, phenoxybenzamine, Lomotil or ibuprofen (Motrin), Urispas, ditropan or Pyridium, or antibiotics.

References

1. Budhraja SN, Anderson JC: An assessment of the value of radiotherapy in the management of carcinoma of the prostate. Br J Urol 36:535–540, 1964.
2. Bagshaw MA, Kaplan HS, Sagerman RH: Linear accelerator supervoltage radiotherapy. VII. Carcinoma of the prostate. Radiology 85:121–129, 1965.
3. George FW, Carlton CE Jr, Dykhuizen RF, Dillon JR: Cobalt-60 telecurietherapy in the definitive treatment of carcinoma of the prostate: a preliminary report. J Urol 93:102–109, 1965.
4. Del Regato JA: Radiotherapy in the conservative treatment of operable and locally inoperable carcinoma of the prostate. Radiology 88:761–766, 1967.
5. Ray GR, Cassady JR, Bagshaw MA: Definitive radiation therapy of carcinoma of the prostate: a report of 15 years' experience. Radiology 106:409–418, 1973.
6. Pistenma DA, Bagshaw MA, Freiha FS: Extended-field radiation therapy for prostatic adenocarcinoma: status report of a limited prospective trial. In Johnson DE, Samuels ML, eds: Cancer of the Genitourinary Tract. New York, Raven Press, 1979, p 229.
7. McGowan DG: The value of extended field radiation therapy in carcinoma of the prostate. Int J Radiat Oncol Biol Phys 7:1333–1339, 1981.
8. Bagshaw MA: Current conflicts in the management of prostatic cancer. 1985 ASTRO Gold Medal Address. Int J Radiat Oncol Biol Phys 12:17–23, 1985.
9. Ploysongsang S, Aron BS, Shehata WM, Jazy FK, Scott RM, Ho PY, Morand TM: Comparison of whole pelvis versus small-field radiation therapy for carcinoma of prostate. Urology 27:10–16, 1986.
10. Pilepich MV, Krall JM, Johnson RJ, Sause WT, Perez CA, Zinninger M, Martz K: Extended field (periaortic) irradiation in carcinoma of the prostate: analysis of RTOG 75-06. Int J Radiat Oncol Biol Phys 12:345–351, 1986.
11. Bagshaw MA: Radiotherapeutic treatment of prostatic carcinoma with pelvic node involvement. Urol Clin North Am 11:297–304, 1984.
12. Asbell SO, Schlager BA, Baker AS: Revision of treatment planning for carcinoma of the prostate. Int J Radiat Oncol Biol Phys 6:861–865, 1980.
13. Pilepich MV, Prasad SC, Perez CA: Computed tomography in definitive radiotherapy of prostatic carcinoma, Part 2: definition of target volume. Int J Radiat Oncol Biol Phys 8:235–240, 1982.
14. Bagshaw MA: External radiation therapy of carcinoma of the prostate. Cancer 45:1912–1921, 1980.
15. Pilepich MV, Perez CA, Walz BJ, Zivnuska FR: Complications of definitive radiotherapy for carcinoma of the prostate. Int J Radiat Oncol Biol Phys 7:1341–1348, 1981.
16. Freiha FS, Pistenma DA, Bagshaw MA: Pelvic lymphadenectomy for staging prostatic carcinoma: is it always necessary? J Urol 122:176–177, 1979.
17. Jacobs JA, Rosenthal RS, Shaw JL: Localized ureteral fibrosis: an unrecognized complication of radiation therapy for prostatic carcinoma. J Urol 115:610–611, 1976.
18. Goldstein I, Feldman MI, Declose PJ, Babayan RK, Krane RJ: Radiation-associated impotence. JAMA 251(7):903–910, 1984.
19. Pilepich MV, Krall J, George FW, Asbell SO, Plenk HD, Johnson RJ, Stetz J, Zinniger M, Walz BJ: Treatment-related morbidity in phase III RTOG studies of extended-field irradiation for carcinoma of the prostate. Int J Radiat Oncol Biol Phys 10:1861–1867, 1984.
20. Pilepich MV, Krall JM, Sause WT, Johnson RJ, Russ HH, Hanks GE, Perez CA, Zinninger M, Martz KL, Gardner P: Correlation of radiotherapeutic parameters and treatment related morbidity in carcinoma of the prostate: analysis of RTOG study 75-06. Int J Radiat Oncol Biol Phys 13:351–357, 1987.
21. Douchez J, Allain YM, Cellier P, Fenton J, Fregevu Y, Hay M, Le Bourgeois JP, Vincent F: Cancer de la prostate: intolérance et morbidité de la radiothérapie externe. Bull Cancer (Paris) 72:6:573–577, 1985.
22. Hanks GE: Optimizing the radiation treatment and outcome of prostate cancer. 1984 ASTRO Presidential Address. Int J Radiat Oncol Biol Phys 11:1235–1245, 1985.
23. Hanks GE, Diamond JJ, Krall JM, Martz KL, Kramer S: A ten-year follow-up of 682 patients treated for prostate cancer with radiation therapy in the United States. Int J Radiat Oncol Biol Phys 13:499–505, 1987.
24. Green N, Melbye RW, George FW III, Morrow J: Radiation therapy of inoperable localized prostatic carcinoma: an assessment of tumor response and complications. J Urol 111:662–664, 1974.
25. Jones WA, Miller EV, Sullivan LD, Chapman WH: Severe prostatic calcification after radiation therapy for cancer. J Urol 121:828–830, 1979.
26. Perez CA: Carcinoma of the prostate, a vexing biological and clinical enigma. Presidential address of the 24th annual meeting of the American Society of Therapeutic Radiologists. Int J Radiat Oncol Biol Phys 9:1427–1438, 1983.
27. National Institutes of Health: SEER Program: Cancer Incidence and Mortality in the United States 1973–1981. NIH Publication No. 85-1837, Washington, DC, Public Health Service, U.S. Dept of Health and Human Services, 1984.
28. Neglia WJ, Hussey DH, Johnson DE: Megavoltage radiation therapy for carcinoma of the prostate. Int J Radiat Oncol Biol Phys 2:873–882, 1977.
29. Hill DR, Crews QE, Walsh PC: Prostate carcinoma: radiation treatment of the primary and regional lymphatics. Cancer 34:156–160, 1974.
30. Leibel SA, Hanks GE, Kramer S: Patterns of care outcome studies: results of the national practice in adenocarcinoma of the prostate. Int J Radiat Oncol Biol Phys 10:401–409, 1984.
31. Rounsaville MC, Green JP, Vaeth JM, Purdon RP, Heltzel MM: Prostatic carcinoma: limited field irradiation. Int J Radiat Oncol Biol Phys 13:1013–1020, 1987.
32. Pino y Torres JL, Lee DJ, Leibel SA, Wharam MD, Cantrell BB, Bross DS, Order SE: Local control and

reduced complications in split course irradiation of prostatic cancer. Int J Radiat Oncol Biol Phys 7:43–47, 1981.
33. Forman JD, Zinreich E, Lee DJ, Wharam MD, Baumgardner RA, Order SE: Improving the therapeutic ratio of external beam irradiation for carcinoma of the prostate. Int J Radiat Oncol Biol Phys 11:2073–2080, 1985.

Acknowledgment

The authors wish to acknowledge the assistance of Joyce Ramback and the Friends of Radiology in the preparation of this work.

COMPLICATIONS OF CHEMOTHERAPY IN THE UROLOGIC PATIENT

9

Grace R. Inouye • Charles M. Haskell

INTRODUCTION

In the last two decades, the field of cancer chemotherapy has expanded rapidly and continues to grow increasingly complex. This chapter acquaints the urologist with commonly used chemotherapeutic drugs and their toxicities. Because chemotherapeutic agents have a very narrow therapeutic index, any decision to initiate treatment should be carefully considered in terms of the natural history of the disease, expected benefits of therapy, and side effects. Certainly, these drugs should only be used when the diagnosis of a malignancy has been histologically established. Occasionally, a physician may be strongly tempted to initiate a "therapeutic trial" of chemotherapy in a patient with strong circumstantial evidence for cancer but without a tissue diagnosis. However, this urge should be repressed because neither the patient nor the physician benefits if the diagnosis is incorrect.

The ultimate goal of chemotherapy can be defined as curative or palliative. In this respect, it is helpful to classify cancer into one of three categories. In the first category, a malignancy is potentially curable with chemotherapy alone or in combination with surgery or radiation. Examples include gestational trophoblastic neoplasia, testicular carcinoma, and lymphoma. A patient with a testicular tumor would be strongly supported in continuing chemotherapy, even in the face of significant toxicity, with the ultimate goal of cure. Conversely, a decision not to treat a patient with a potentially curable tumor would require careful consideration.

In the second category, the cancer may not be curable, but significant palliation of symptoms and increased survival may be accomplished with chemotherapy. For example, hormonal manipulation for metastatic prostate cancer does not prolong overall survival, but it can produce significant symptomatic control for months to years.

In the final category, which, unfortunately comprises most neoplasms, chemotherapy is given only with the hope for palliation, and cure is not a realistic endpoint. Included in this group are colorectal, lung, head and neck, renal, and bladder carcinomas. Here chemotherapy has infrequently cured the patient of cancer, and other factors need to be considered, such as the expected palliation of symptoms weighed against the toxicity of the treatment. The patient's performance status, age, general health, and psychological makeup must be taken into consideration.

Because treatment produces significant side effects, it is essential to follow objective parameters of response. Changes in therapy should be guided by whether the disease has responded, remained stable, or progressed according to serum markers, radiographs, nuclear scans, or other measurable tests. Finally, modern medical facilities should be available to monitor and treat any side effects of the chemotherapy.

PHARMACOLOGIC FACTORS

Most chemotherapeutic agents exert their action by inhibition of an enzyme or substrate involved in deoxyribonucleic acid (DNA) synthesis in the normal, as well as in the malignant, cell. Although malignant cells appear to bear the brunt of damage, some degree of injury occurs to normal tissues during the course of treatment. The tissues with the highest proliferative capacity, i.e., bone marrow, gastrointestinal epithelium, and hair follicles, are commonly affected.

Many factors can modify the toxicity of chemotherapy. They include (1) drug bioavailability, (2) drug excretion and metabolism, and (3) interactions with other drugs. An example of the first situation occurs when the bioavailability of methotrexate (MTX) is altered in a patient who has a third-space collection, such as ascites or a pleural effusion. Normally, MTX is distributed to all body water and is cleared by the kidney in 8 to 12 hours. However, in the presence of a pleural effusion, the drug enters the pleural space as well as the plasma volume. This site can serve as a depot for a prolonged release of MTX into the bloodstream, producing persistent levels of the drug, severe mucositis, and profound pancytopenia.[1]

The kidney and liver are the most common routes of excretion of chemotherapeutic agents. When there is renal or hepatic insufficiency, the toxicity of certain drugs can be potentiated. Methotrexate and bleomycin are of particular importance in patients with renal insufficiency because these agents are primarily excreted by the kidneys and cannot be removed by dialysis. Because doxorubicin and vinblastine are excreted primarily in the bile, patients with jaundice from cirrhosis or biliary obstruction can experience severe myelosuppression when given a standard dose of these drugs. Guidelines for dose reduction in renal and hepatic dysfunction are listed in Tables 9–1 and 9–2.[2,3]

Drug interactions are also important because they may not only antagonize a desired antitumor effect but can result in increased toxicity. For example, aspirin, sulfonamides, phenylbutazone, and probenecid can all potentiate MTX toxicity and should not be used while the patient is receiving this drug.[4]

COMMON SIDE EFFECTS

Hematologic

The most frequent dose-limiting toxicity of chemotherapy is bone marrow suppression. In general, the leukocytes are the most sensitive to chemotherapy, followed by the platelets, and then by the erythrocytes. The absolute granulocyte count is more important than the total white blood cell count. An absolute granulocyte count below 500 to 1000/μl is associated with an increased incidence of serious infections and bacteremia. Concomitant thrombocytopenia is usually not associated with hemorrhage unless the platelet count falls below 20,000/μl. Patients with thrombocytopenia should be cautioned to avoid aspirin, nonsteroidal anti-inflammatory agents, and anticoagulants, all of which can exacerbate bleeding. Occasionally, a patient with active bleeding and thrombocytopenia will reqire platelet transfusions. Patients who have undergone extensive pelvic irradiation or skeletal metastases are at higher risk of severe bone marrow depression. In these situations, starting the drug at 75 percent of the calculated dose is prudent. With the exception of steroids and hormones, very few drugs are truly bone marrow–sparing. However, vincristine and bleomycin generally do not cause significant myelosuppression.

Gastrointestinal

Nausea and vomiting are the most common acute manifestations of chemotherapy toxicity and may result in dehydration, azotemia, hypokalemia, metabolic alkalosis, and weight loss. In elderly or debilitated patients, this additional insult may be sufficient to cause a major deterioration.

The emetogenic potential of antineoplastic drugs is variable. Certain drugs, such as cisplatin, produce severe vomiting in virtually all patients. Standard antiemetics alone are generally ineffective for this, and the addition of high-dose metoclopramide is necessary. Doxorubicin, intravenous cyclophosphamide, and etoposide can cause mild to moderate nausea and vomiting, which can be controlled with standard antiemetics. Conventional doses of MTX (30 to 60 mg/m^2) and 5-fluorouracil usually cause only mild nausea.

Nausea and vomiting can be managed in several ways.[5] First, antiemetics are given prior to chemotherapy rather than after vomiting has supervened. Second, the route of administration is adjusted to ensure adequate absorption of the medication. Most of the phenothiazines can be given parenterally or as a suppository. Finally, some patients develop a conditioned response to the mere thought of chemotherapy. Even walking into the clinic or seeing the chemo-

Table 9–1. DOSE MODIFICATION WITH RENAL DYSFUNCTION*

Drug	Percent of Usual Dose to Administer If		
	GFR ≥ 50 ml/minute	*10–50 ml/minute*	*< 10 ml/minute*
Bleomycin	100%	75%	50%
Doxorubicin	100%	100%	100%
Cisplatin†	100%	50%	Omit
Cyclophosphamide	100%	100%	50%
5-Fluorouracil	100%	100%	100%
Melphalan	100%	100%	100%
Methotrexate‡	100%	50%	Omit
Mithramycin	100%	75%	50%
Nitrosoureas (BCNU, CCNU)	100%	Omit	Omit
Vincristine	100%	100%	100%
Vinblastine	100%	100%	100%

*Reprinted from Schilsky RL: Renal and metabolic toxicities of cancer treatment. In Perry MC, Yarbro JW, eds: Toxicity of Chemotherapy. Orlando, Grune and Stratton, Inc, 1984, p 332.

†May give full doses if renal dysfunction is due to ureteral obstruction by cisplatin-sensitive tumor.

‡Omit for glomerular filtration rate (GFR) 10–50 ml/minute if renal dysfunction due to methotrexate or if high dose methotrexate is to be given.

therapy nurse can provoke nausea and vomiting. Often, a short-acting sedative, such as lorazepam, is effective for anticipatory nausea.

Table 9–3 lists some of the more commonly used antiemetics.[6] Phenothiazines, such as prochlorperazine (Compazine) and thiethyperazine (Torecan), are frequently used. For cisplatin, metoclopramide, 1 to 2 mg/kg given every 2 hours, is usually effective prophylaxis. Acute dystonic reactions can occur with high doses of metoclopramide, and they respond to diphenhydramine (Benadryl), 25 to 50 mg intravenously. Delta-9-tetrahydrocannabinol (Dronabinol) is the principal psychoactive substance present in marijuana. It has recently become available for the treatment of nausea and vomiting that has failed to respond to conventional antiemetics. The usual starting dose is 5 mg/m^2 given every 2 to 4 hours. Frequent side effects with higher doses include disturbing central nervous system symptoms such as drowsiness, muddled thinking, elation, and dizziness.[7]

Chemotherapy also produces oral ulcerations, cheilosis, glossitis, and esophagitis. Typically, the patient first exeriences a burning sensation in the mouth about 1 week after treatment. This is followed by erythema and discrete ulcerations that may become confluent. The lesions usually last for 10 to 14 days and tend to recur unless doses are reduced. Aside from the discomfort, mucositis can compromise oral intake and also can become superinfected with *Candida*. Treatment is primarily symptomatic, consisting of topical anesthetics. Nystatin suspension or clotrimazole troches are used for oral candidiasis. Patients may require blenderized foods, soups, and supplemental liquid diets until the lesions have resolved.

Drug Extravasation

Even with meticulous attention to detail by an experienced physician or nurse, extravasation

Table 9–2. DOSE MODIFICATION WITH HEPATIC DYSFUNCTION*

Drug	Percent of Usual Dose to Administer			
	Bili < 1.5 mg % and SGOT < 60 IU	*Bili = 1.5–3.0 mg % or SGOT = 60–180 IU*	*Bili = 3.1–5.0 mg % or SGOT > 180 IU*	*Bili > 5.0 mg %*
5-Fluorouracil	100%	100%	100%	Omit
Cyclophosphamide	100%	100%	75%	Omit
Methotrexate	100%	Use with caution in any patient with hepatic dysfunction		
Daunorubicin	100%	75%	50%	Omit
Doxorubicin	100%	50%	25%	Omit
Vinblastine Vincristine Etoposide	100%	50%	Omit	Omit

*Reprinted from Perry MC: Hepatotoxicity of chemotherapeutic agents. In Perry MC, Yarbro JW, eds: Toxicity of Chemotherapy. Orlando, Grune and Stratton, Inc, 1984, p 307.

Abbreviations: Bili = bilirubin; SGOT = serum glutamic-oxaloacetic transaminase.

Table 9–3. ANTIEMETICS*

Name	Generic Name	Dosage and Administration
Compazine	Prochlorperazine	5–10 mg p.o. q 4–6 hr 5–10 mg IM q 3–4 hr 25 mg suppository q 4 hr
Torecan	Thiethylperazine	10 mg p.o. q 4–6 hr 10 mg IM q 3–4 hr 10 mg suppository q 4 hr
Thorazine	Chlorpromazine	10–20 mg p.o. q 4–6 hr 25–50 mg IM q 3–4 hr 50–100 mg suppository q 6–8 hr
Haldol	Haloperidol	1–2 mg p.o. q 4–6 hr
Benadryl	Diphenhydramine	25–50 mg p.o. or IV q 6 hr
Reglan	Metoclopramide	1–2 mg/kg IV q 2–3 hr
Ativan	Lorazepam	0.04 mg/kg IV q 4–6 hr
Marinol	Dronabinol	5 mg/m^2 q 2–4 hr, may increase by 2.5 mg/m^2 to maximum 15 mg/m^2
Decadron	Dexamethasone	10–20 mg p.o. or IV q 4–6 hr

*Reprinted with permission from Mitchell EP, Schein PS: In Perry MC, Yarbro JW, eds: Toxicity of Chemotherapy. Orlando, Grune and Stratton, Inc, 1984, p 275.

Abbreviations: p.o. = By mouth; IV = intravenous; IM = intramuscular.

of chemotherapy occurs in about 2 to 5 percent of venipunctures. Certain chemotherapeutic agents are vesicants, and when extravasated into tissue, they produce changes from mild induration and erythema to severe necrosis and sloughing of the dermis and the underlying structures. Drugs that are known vesicants are doxorubicin, daunorubicin, nitrogen mustard, mithramycin, mitomycin-C, actinomycin D, and streptozocin.[8]

Clearly, administration of chemotherapy should be undertaken only by individuals thoroughly familiar with its toxic effects. To our knowledge, no controlled studies have determined the best method for treatment of extravasation; however, the following conservative steps have been proposed:[9]

1. Stop the injection immediately, and do not remove the needle.
2. With the needle in place, withdraw 3 to 5 ml of blood and any drug remaining in the tubing.
3. If there is an obvious bleb of extravasated drug, aspirate as much of the remaining solution as possible with a 25-gauge needle.
4. A potential antidote, if appropriate, can be injected through the needle. Various purported antidotes have been tested in animal models and in case reports; however, their efficacy has not been established conclusively.[9]
5. An ice pack should be applied immediately to produce local vasoconstriction and to decrease drug absorption.
6. The extremity should be placed in a sling or should be elevated to minimize edema. The patient should be instructed to apply ice packs for 20 minutes four times a day for 72 hours.
7. Recording of events should include the approximate amount of extravasated drug, time to intervention, type of intervention, and measurement of any lesions with a photograph if possible.
8. The patient should be referred to a plastic surgeon within 72 hours.

Using a similar protocol except for the omission of antidotes, Larson[10] was able to manage 75 percent of extravasations with conservative treatment. Twenty-five percent of patients required surgical intervention, which consisted of a wide local excision and split-thickness skin graft.

Metabolic Complications

Uric acid nephropathy and acute tumor lysis syndrome are two well-known complications in patients with non-urologic neoplasms. Hyperuricemia is common in the myeloproliferative disorders (polycythemia rubra vera, chronic myelogenous leukemia, myelofibrosis with myeloid metaplasia), acute leukemias, and lymphomas due to increased cell turnover of the neoplastic tissues. It can occur as an incidental finding or can be precipitated by chemotherapy or radiotherapy of the underlying disorder. Long-standing hyperuricemia, especially in patients with myeloproliferative disease, can lead to gout, urate nephrolithiasis, and chronic renal insufficiency. Thus, in patients with myeloproliferative diseases, prophylactic and chronic administration of allopurinol for hyperuricemia seems indicated. In patients with bulky lymphomas and acute leukemias, alkaline diuresis, in addition to allopurinol, should be instituted.

Certain tumors with rapid growth rates are extremely sensitive to antineoplastic drugs and may respond dramatically within days of instituting chemotherapy. The massive release of tumor cell contents can result in life-threatening hyperuricemia, hyperkalemia, hyperphosphatemia, and hypocalcemia several hours or days after the institution of chemotherapy. The most common neoplasms associated with the tumor lysis syndrome are the high-grade non-Hodgkin's lymphomas and the acute leukemias.[11] Less commonly, intermediate and low-grade non-Hodgkin's lymphomas, accelerated-phase chronic myelogenous leukemia, and small cell carcinoma have been reported as causes of tumor lysis syndrome.[12,13]

In patients with acute leukemia or bulky, high-grade lymphoma who are at greatest risk for tumor lysis syndrome, prophylactic measures *prior* to the initiation of chemotherapy are mandatory. A high pretreatment serum lactate dehydrogenase (LDH), (>1500 IU/L) and baseline renal insufficiency can also identify the high-risk patient. Proper measures include (1) adequate prehydration, (2) prophylactic allopurinol, and (3) alkaline diuresis. Specifically, intravenous hydration at 300 ml/m^2 body surface area per day (BSA/day) to maintain urine flow at 100 ml/hour can prevent the supersaturation of urate crystals in the distal renal tubule. Allopurinol, 500 mg/m^2 on the first 2 days, followed by 200 mg/m^2/day, is effective in lowering the serum uric acid concentration through inhibition of uric acid synthesis. Alkaline diuresis, achieved by intravenous infusion of 50 to 100 mEq/L of sodium bicarbonate to maintain the urine pH > 7.0, increases the solubility of urate crystals. Patients undergoing this treatment require careful monitoring of serum electrolytes, blood urea nitrogen (BUN), creatinine, phosphate, calcium, magnesium, and uric acid, initially every 6 to 8 hours for the first 24 to 48 hours. The abrupt onset of oliguria and rising creatinine in a high-risk patient soon after chemotherapy strongly suggests the diagnosis of acute tumor lysis syndrome. Management should be directed toward excluding treatable causes of renal failure, such as hypovolemia, obstruction, hypercalcemia, both contrast-related and drug-induced. Patients developing severe hyperkalemia (>6 mEq/L), hyperphosphatemia (>10 mg/dl), azotemia, or fluid overload require dialysis.[3]

Gonadal Dysfunction

The treatment of urologic malignancy can interfere profoundly with normal sexual and reproductive functions. Erectile impotence following standard radical prostatectomy is almost inevitable, and ejaculatory impotence occurs in a high percentage of patients undergoing retroperitoneal lymph node dissection for testicular cancer.

Testicular function is highly susceptible to injury by many chemotherapeutic agents. The damage varies with the drug and total dose adminstered as well as with the patient's age and pubertal status. Histologically, this results in a progressive, dose-related depletion of the germinal epithelium lining the seminiferous tubules. In the extreme state of germinal aplasia, all spermatogonia are depleted and only the Sertoli cells lining the tubules remain. Patients experience marked reduction in testicular volume, oligospermia, or azoospermia, and become infertile.[14]

Alkylating agents are clearly associated with germinal depletion. Cyclophosphamide, chlorambucil, nitrogen mustard, busulfan, procarbazine, lomustine (CCNU), and carmustine (BCNU) all have been associated with infertility.[15] Combination chemotherapy may produce even more profound effects. Studies of male patients receiving MOPP (nitrogen mustard, vincristine, procarbazine, prednisone) show a greater than 80 percent incidence of long-term germinal aplasia.[16,17]

A prospective study of patients with advanced testicular cancer reported a high incidence of oligospermia and azoospermia even prior to chemotherapy; only 6 percent of patients could meet criteria for pretreatment sperm banking.[18] All patients were rendered azoospermic with cisplatin-based chemotherapy. However, the recovery for patients with spermatogenesis was more encouraging than recovery for patients with Hodgkin's disease. Recovery of sperm counts occurred at 1.5 to 2 years, and about half of the patients had normal sperm counts (i.e., $>20 \times 10^6$/ml).

Second Malignancies

Unfortunately, many of the commonly employed antineoplastic drugs are potentially carcinogenic and leukemogenic. This problem was first noted in long-term survivors of Hodgkin's disease who had been treated with MOPP and radiation therapy. In these patients, the actuarial risk of acute leukemia approached 5 to 10 percent at 10 years.[19] The consensus today is that alkylating agents (melphalan, cyclophosphamide, chlorambucil), procarbazine, azathioprine, and methyl-CCNU are leukemogenic in humans.[20,21] In contrast to de novo acute leukemias, treatment-related leukemias tend to occur after a latent period lasting several years, which is often preceded by a preleukemic phase of pancytopenia. Absence or deletion of chromosomes 5 and 7 is frequently seen, and patients respond poorly to standard antileukemic therapy. Survival is generally 1 to 4 months.[19]

At least 19 cases of leukemia have been reported in patients with testicular cancer who were treated with either radiation alone or in combination with chemotherapy. The cumulative probability of leukemia developing at 10 years was 1.3 percent.[22]

CHEMOTHERAPEUTIC DRUGS IN UROLOGIC ONCOLOGY

The following section reviews the pharmacology and toxicity of individual chemotherapeutic drugs in more detail. Each of the drugs has been selected for one of the following reasons: (1) it has major genitourinary toxicity, (2) its safe use is dependent on intact renal function, or (3) it has an important role in the treatment of urologic cancer. Other drugs are referred to in Tables 9–1 and 9–4.

Actinomycin D

Actinomycin D is one of a large group of related antibiotic drugs that have either been chemically synthesized or have been derived from extracts of *Streptomyces parvulus*. At low concentrations, actinomycin D inhibits ribonucleic acid (RNA) synthesis by intercalating with the double-stranded DNA template. At higher concentrations, it inhibits both DNA and RNA synthesis.[23]

The drug has major clinical value in the treatment of Wilms' tumor, Ewing's sarcoma, rhabdomyosarcoma, and gestational trophoblastic neoplasia. In testicular carcinoma, actinomycin D is part of combination therapy in the VAB-6 protocol.[24] The antibiotic has a long plasma half-life of 36 hours because it is slowly released from tissue stores, where it is extensively bound. Most of the drug is excreted unchanged in the bile and urine. The most common schedule is 0.15 mcg/kg intravenously (not to exceed a single dose of 0.5 mg) each day for 5 days. The course is repeated every 3 to 4 weeks.[25] Lower doses may be used for patients with limited bone marrow reserve. An alternate regimen based on the long plasma half-life is a single dose of 2 mg/m^2 every 4 weeks. It is no more toxic, and at least as effective, as the traditional 5-day program.[26]

Myelosuppression is the dose-limiting toxicity, but gastrointestinal side effects can be quite significant. The nadir granulocyte count occurs at 8 to 14 days. Gastrointestinal side effects include nausea, vomiting, stomatitis, gastritis, and diarrhea. Alopecia is common, and acneiform skin eruptions can occur. Actinomycin D is highly toxic, and its extravasation may result in severe ulceration and necrosis of tissue. Like doxorubicin, actinomycin D acts as a radiation sensitizer when given with concurrent radiation treatment. One theory for this is that actinomycin D interferes with the cellular process of DNA repair. It can also produce a radiation recall phenomenon, in which patients develop a severe inflammatory reaction in areas of previous radiation months to years after radiation has been completed.[23]

Bleomycin

Bleomycin (Blenoxane) is an antibiotic complex that was isolated in 1962 from a strain of *Streptomyces verticillus*. The primary action of bleomycin is to produce single-stranded and double-stranded breaks in DNA.[27] This drug is an important part of combination chemotherapy regimens for patients with testicular carcinoma, such as the Einhorn regimen[28] and the newer cisplatin-bleomycin-etoposide (BEP) program.[29] Cure rates for patients with metastatic germ cell tumors treated with either regimen range from 70 to 85 percent.

As a single agent, bleomycin is given 10 to 20 U/M^2/week as a subcutaneous, intramuscular, or intravenous dose. Bleomycin is cleared primarily by the kidney. Its clearance is markedly diminished in renal failure, and, as a rule, the bleomycin dose should be reduced by 50 percent when the creatinine clearance is $<$10 ml/minute.[3]

Unlike most antitumor agents, bleomycin produces little bone marrow toxicity. Its principal

Table 9–4. GENITOURINARY TOXICITY OF CHEMOTHERAPEUTIC AGENTS*

	Glomerular	Tubular	Ureters/Bladder	Testis
Cisplatin		Proximal and distal tubular necrosis; azotemia		Probably oligospermia or azoospermia
Streptozotocin		Tubulo-interstitial nephritis; proximal renal tubular acidosis; Fanconi's syndrome; proteinuria		
Cyclophosphamide		Hyponatremia	Hemorrhagic cystitis Delayed urothelial cancers	Oligospermia or azoospermia
High-dose Methotrexate		Tubular precipitation of hydroxy-methotrexate; azotemia		
Nitrosoureas (methyl-CCNU, CCNU, BCNU)	Focal glomerular sclerosis	Interstitial nephritis with tubular atrophy; azotemia		Oligospermia or azoospermia
Mitomycin-C	Hemolytic uremic syndrome			
Mithramycin		Tubular necrosis; azotemia		
Alkylating Agents (chlorambucil, nitrogen mustard, busulfan)				Oligospermia and azoospermia
Procarbazine				Oligospermia and azoospermia

*Modified from Schilsky RL: In Perry MC, Yarbro JW, eds: Toxicity of Chemotherapy. Orlando, Grune and Stratton, Inc, 1984, p. 317.

toxicity occurs in the lung and skin. The reason for these organ system specificities is presumably because the degradation of bleomycin is mediated by bleomycin hydrolase, an enzyme that is present in tumor cells, and in the kidney and liver, but is notably absent in the skin and lung.

A subacute or chronic pneumonitis may develop in patients that can progress to pulmonary fibrosis. The overall incidence of pulmonary toxicity is about 10 percent. Several large studies estimate the incidence of pulmonary fibrosis at 2 to 3 percent, with an additional 1 to 2 percent of patients experiencing fatal pulmonary toxicity.[30] The first signs are cough, dyspnea, and bibasilar rales. Chest x-rays reveal bibasilar interstitial infiltrates. Pulmonary function studies usually show a restrictive pattern with an abnormal carbon monoxide diffusing capacity (DLCO).[27] These findings may be difficult to distinguish from other pulmonary syndromes in patients with cancer, such as lymphangitic metastasis and radiation injury, and in patients with infections such as those due to cytomegalovirus or *Pneumocystis carinii.* An open lung biopsy may be necessary to establish the correct diagnosis and treatment. In bleomycin interstitial pneumonitis, the lung biopsy shows interstitial edema, intra-alveolar hyaline membrane formation, hyperplasia of type II alveolar macrophages, and collagen deposition.[31]

The incidence of pulmonary damage is clearly related to the total dose of bleomycin. At total doses under 400 units (U), there is a constant sporadic incidence of pulmonary toxicity that increases markedly (>10 percent) above a threshold cumulative dose of 450 to 500 U (Fig. 9–1).[30] Other factors that have been associated with a greater risk of pulmonary fibrosis include (1) age over 70, (2) prior or concurrent radiation to the mediastinum and lungs,[32] (3) high-dose oxygen during anesthesia,[33] and (4) the use of bleomycin in combination chemotherapy programs.[34]

The outcome of pulmonary toxicity depends on the severity of damage upon diagnosis, but

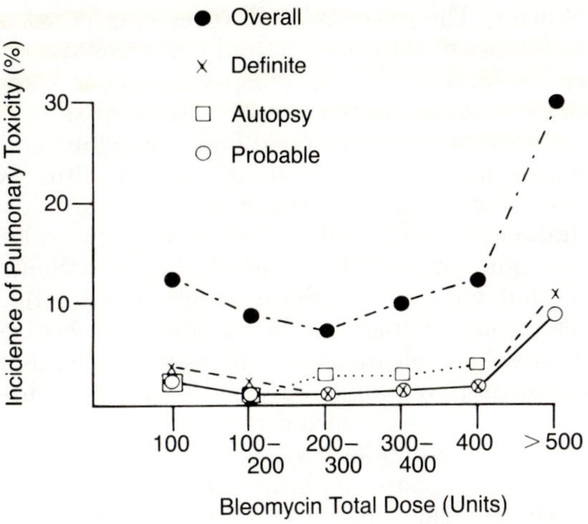

Figure 9–1. The relationship between pulmonary toxicity and the total cumulative bleomycin dose. (Reproduced, with permission, from Ginsberg SL, Comis RL: The pulmonary toxicity of antineoplastic agents. Semin Oncol 9:35, 1982. Copyright, Grune & Stratton.)

the mortality has been reported to be as high as 50 percent. Although steroids have been tried, there is no effective therapy other than discontinuation of the drug as soon as the problem is recognized. Some guidelines for monitoring bleomycin therapy are:

1. Obtain a baseline chest x-ray and pulmonary function tests, including DLCO.
2. Follow serial pulmonary function, and consider discontinuation of bleomycin for a DLCO <40 percent of the pretreatment value, a forced vital capacity (FVC) <25 percent of baseline, or a clinical picture compatible with bleomycin pneumonitis.
3. Do not exceed a cumulative bleomycin dose of 350 to 400 U.
4. During anesthesia, use the minimal concentration of oxygen necessary and only modest fluid replacement.

Finally, there is a much rarer hypersensitivity pneumonitis associated with bleomycin that is different from the interstitial fibrosis. It typically presents with fever, diffuse infiltrates, and eosinophilia, and it appears to respond to steroid therapy.[35]

Up to 50 percent of patients experience skin reactions that are commonly manifested as erythema, induration, thickening, and eventual peeling on the fingers, palms, and interphalangeal joints. Hyperpigmentation of the skin creases and a general darkening of the skin develop in many patients. Bleomycin often causes edema and skin changes leading to fibrosis. Indurated plaques and sclerodactyly may progress to ulceration and gangrene of fingertips.[36] Partial alopecia occurs in about one third of patients and is dose-related.[37]

Vogelzang and associates[38] described Raynaud's phenomenon in 37% of patients with testicular cancer who received bleomycin and vinblastine with or without cisplatin. Digital ischemia developed in 21 percent of patients treated only with bleomycin and vinblastine and in 41 percent of patients treated with cisplatin plus the other two drugs. The symptoms generally developed 10 months after the start of chemotherapy and persisted for up to 18 months in half of the patients.[38] Of note is that in every reported case of patients experiencing chemotherapy-related Raynaud's phenomenon, each had received bleomycin, either alone or in combination with a *Vinca* alkaloid or cisplatin. This suggests that bleomycin may be the primary offending drug and that there is synergistic toxicity with the addition of vinblastine and cisplatin.[39]

Hyperpyrexia, as high as 40° C, has been noted in 25 percent of patients, and it is occasionally fatal. An uncommon fulminant reaction with hyperpyrexia, hypotension, diaphoresis, and cardiopulmonary arrest has been reported, predominantly occurring in patients with lymphoma.[40,41] The actual incidence of fulminant reaction has been reported at 1 to 8 percent and can occur with doses as small as 1 unit.

Cisplatin

Cisplatin (*cis*-diamminedichloroplatinum II, CDDP [Platinol]) is the first heavy metal coordination compound to have antineoplastic activity.[42] It has become a first-line drug in the treatment of testicular neoplasms, ovarian carcinoma, and small cell carcinoma of the lung. In three generations of studies of nearly 300 patients with disseminated testicular cancer treated with cisplatin-based regimens, such as the Einhorn regimen or VAB-IV, approximately 70 percent are free of disease. Nearly all patients with stage A or B disease are curable with appropriate surgery and chemotherapy, and over 80 percent of stage C patients will achieve a complete response with combined modality therapy.[18]

In other tumors of the genitourinary system, cisplatin has moderate activity. Several investigators have demonstrated responses ranging from 20 to 43 percent in patients with metastatic bladder carcinoma. However, these responses are usually partial, and the median duration of response is only 4 to 6 months. Newer, multidrug, cisplatin-based protocols for transitional cell carcinoma, reported by Sternberg and associates[43] and Harker and associates,[44] have demonstrated even higher total response rates (57 to 70 percent), and complete response rates of 30 to 50 percent. Whether these improved response rates will ultimately translate into improved survival is too early to answer. In prostate cancer, because of the limitations of assessing disease progression, the response rates with cisplatin have ranged from 6 to 31 percent.[45] Cisplatin is also reported to be effective in metastatic squamous cell carcinoma of the penis, with three out of six patients achieving a partial response.[46] Like most chemotherapeutic agents, cisplatin is inactive in the treatment of renal cell carcinoma.

The exact mechanism of action of cisplatin is unclear. It appears to bind DNA, producing interstrand and intrastrand cross-linking between guanine residues. Cisplatin produces synergistic antitumor effects with radiation, etoposide, 5-fluorouracil, and cytarabine. Cisplatin should not come in contact with aluminum needles because a brown precipitate will form. Other metal components, such as stainless steel needles, do not elicit an observable reaction.

Cisplatin is administered intravenously over 4 to 6 hours in doses of 50 to 120 mg/m^2, either as a single infusion or in divided doses over 5 days. The treatment is repeated every 3 to 4 weeks. The unbound, active cisplatin is rapidly cleared from the plasma and has a half-life of 40 to 48 hours. The principal route of excretion is through the kidney.[25]

The most common side effects are severe nausea and vomiting, nephrotoxicity, otoxicity, peripheral neuropathy, and bone marrow suppression. Gastrointestinal side effects are universal and are best treated with multiple antiemetics. An effective regimen consists of (1) metoclopramide, 1 to 2 mg/kg IV 30 minutes prior to cisplatin and every 2 hours for five total doses, (2) diphenhydramine, 25 to 50 mg IV with each dose of metoclopramide; (3) dexamethasone, 10 mg IV every 4 hours; (4) and lorazepam, 1 to 2 mg IV.

Early studies of cisplatin described renal dysfunction in 26 to 37 percent of patients, manifested by a rising BUN and creatinine levels.[47] Histologically, extensive proximal and distal tubular necrosis was seen, without prominent glomerular damage. However, nephrotoxicity is usually preventable by the use of hydration that produces a brisk diuresis of at least 100 ml/hour of urine. The patient should receive at least 1.5 to 2 liters of intravenous fluid prior to cisplatin and at least 1 to 1.5 L after the infusion. Mannitol is given concurrently with cisplatin to maintain good urine flow, and potassium and magnesium are replaced as needed. Studies have demonstrated that even with aggressive hydration, a subclinical reduction in glomerular filtration rate (GFR) occurs.[48] In 24 patients treated with the Einhorn regimen (cisplatin, bleomycin, vinblastine), a 23 percent decrease in creatinine clearance was measured, although the serum creatinine was unchanged. Concurrent use of antihypertensive agents or aminoglycoside antibiotics may also have a synergistic effect on cisplatin nephrotoxicity.[45,49]

Hypomagnesemia and hypokalemia due to renal tubular wasting is a frequent complication. When hypomagnesemia occurs, it is best managed by parenteral replacement with magnesium sulfate. The use of oral magnesium is not recommended because large doses can produce significant diarrhea. Hypocalcemia as a result of hypomagnesemia is unresponsive to calcium replacement alone and can be corrected with magnesium replacement.[50]

Ototoxicity occurs in as many as 50 percent of patients who have received a mean cumulative dose of 203 mg/m^2.[51] Ototoxicity presents as tinnitus and high-frequency hearing loss in the 4.0 to 8.0 kHz range and is usually irreversible. Otalgia, acute deafness, and vestibular symptoms are uncommon.

Peripheral neuropathy similar to other heavy metal intoxications leads to paresthesias in a stocking-and-glove distribution, loss of proprioception and vibratory sense and, rarely, motor dysfunction.[52] Myelosuppression is generally not a significant problem, but mild suppression of all hematopoietic cell lines may occur and appears to be dose-related. In addition, a few cases of hemolytic anemia have been described.[53] Hypersensitivity reactions ranging from a skin rash to anaphylaxis (facial flushing, angioneurotic edema, wheezing, hypotension) have been reported. The National Cancer Institute noted only four cases of serious anaphylactic reactions in 267 consecutive courses, and no deaths have been directly related to this complication.[54] The incidence of this problem ranges from a low rate (1 to 5 percent) when cisplatin is given alone, to a higher rate (14 to 25 percent) when it is given in combination with bleomycin and vinblastine.[55]

Cyclophosphamide

Cyclophosphamide (Cytoxan), discovered in 1958, is the most widely used alkylating agent.

It is used in the treatment of leukemias, lymphomas, sarcomas, and various carcinomas. In patients with prostate cancer who have failed to respond to hormonal therapy, it has produced a response rate of 38 percent.[56] Cyclophosphamide exerts some activity in transitional cell carcinoma of the bladder, yielding a 25 to 30 percent response in metastatic disease.

Cyclophosphamide is usually given as an intermittent, intravenous bolus of 30 to 40 mg/kg every 3 to 4 weeks or as a daily dose of 1.0 to 2.5 mg/kg orally. It is well absorbed and must undergo activation in the liver.[25] Aldophosphamide, a metabolite produced by the hepatic microsomal system, is then converted in the tumor cells to the final metabolites acrolein and phosphoramide mustard. Phosphoramide mustard is thought to be the active antitumor product. Acrolein is an inactive metabolite that may be the major agent responsible for hemorrhagic cystitis.[57] About 90 percent of the metabolites are excreted in the kidney, and in patients with a creatinine clearance <25 ml/minute, the dose should be reduced by 50 percent.[3]

Marrow suppression is the major dose-limiting side effect. Delayed nausea and vomiting are common. Alopecia is also a frequent side effect. Cyclophosphamide is a potent suppressor of both humoral and cellular immunity. It is carcinogenic in animals and leukemogenic in man.[19] As of 1983, 32 cases of bladder carcinoma had been described in patients receiving cyclophosphamide, including 22 cases of transitional cell carcinoma; six cases of squamous carcinoma; and one case each of adenocarcinoma, undifferentiated, mixed, and fibrosarcoma.[58,59] In addition, two cases of transitional cell and one case of squamous cell carcinoma of the renal pelvis had also been described.[60]

Water intoxication resulting from a direct antidiuretic effect on the renal tubules has occurred.[61] This usually develops with large doses of cyclophosphamide (>50 mg/kg) and can be overlooked, especially while the patient is being vigorously hydrated to prevent cystitis. Hyponatremia, seizures, and death have resulted.[62] Cyclophosphamide has rarely caused pulmonary interstitial fibrosis similar to bleomycin. In very high doses, such as used in bone marrow transplantation (>180 mg/kg), acute myocardial necrosis and pulmonary edema have led to a fatal outcome.[63]

As previously mentioned, acrolein can produce a severe chemical cystitis by direct contact with the bladder mucosa. It produces mucosal edema, hemorrhage, ulceration, and telangiectasia. In severe cases, fibrosis of the detrusor muscle can lead to a permanently contracted bladder. The incidence varies between 2 and 40 percent, and risk increases with higher doses.[25] Although the hemorrhage is usually mild and controlled by withdrawal of the drug, it can be severe, protracted, and life-threatening. The most important prophylactic measure is vigorous hydration with frequent voiding in an attempt to dilute the toxic metabolite and to minimize the time of contact with the bladder mucosa.[58,64] In patients receiving high-dose cyclophosphamide, the administration of sulfhydryl-group–containing agents, such as sodium-2-mercaptoethane sulfonate (MESNA) and N-acetylcysteine, has been effective in reducing the occurrence of hematuria without interfering with the antitumor effect.[65,66] However, MESNA is available only as an investigational drug in the United States.

The urologic management of moderate to severe hemorrhagic cystitis is initially conservative, with discontinuation of the drug, maintenance of adequate hydration, and good urine output. The use of continuous bladder irrigation is controversial but, presumably, allows for bladder rest and minimizes toxic exposure to the mucosa. Cystoscopy is performed with electrocautery of any discrete bleeding sites, but frequently the bleeding is diffuse. With severe uncontrollable hemorrhage, more invasive methods include the instillation of silver nitrate, phenol, or formalin into the bladder.[67,68] In refractory cases, urinary diversion, with or without cystectomy or ligation of the hypogastric arteries, has been performed. The intravesical instillation of 1 to 4 percent formalin has been proposed by Fair as a safe approach to massive bleeding from the urinary tract.[69] In a review of 106 patients treated with formalin, Fair reported that 86 percent achieved cessation of bleeding after only one treatment. However, serious complications, including ureterovesical obstruction with hydronephrosis, papillary necrosis, ureterofibrosis, and intraperitoneal extravasation, have been reported.[69]

Doxorubicin

Doxorubicin (Adriamycin) is an anthracycline antibiotic derived from the soil fungus *Streptomyces.* Its mechanism of action is by intercalation into the DNA double helix and possibly by the generation of free radicals or divalent cation chelation.

When used as a single agent, the drug is given as a 60-mg/m^2 dose infused over 5 minutes, and it is repeated every 3 weeks. Reduced doses (20 to 40 mg/m^2) are administered to patients receiving doxorubicin as part of a combination regimen who have had extensive prior chemotherapy or significant radiation to bone marrow–producing sites. Because doxorubicin is excreted primarily in the bile, dose reduction is mandatory in patients with jaundice or hepatic dysfunction. In general, when the bilirubin level is 1.2 to 3.0 mg/dl, the dose should be decreased by 50 percent, and if the bilirubin exceeds 3 mg/dl, only 25 percent of the calculated dose should be given.[2]

Doxorubicin is a highly toxic drug. Although the major dose-limiting toxicity is cardiac damage, the drug also causes a high incidence of nausea and vomiting (21 to 55 percent), myelosuppression (60 to 84 percent), and alopecia (85 to 100 percent).[70,71] Bone marrow suppression is dose-related and primarily manifested as neutropenia. It is greater when the drug is part of a multiple-drug regimen. Alopecia is virtually inevitable with doxorubicin, but it is reversible with discontinuation of chemotherapy. Patients should also be warned that the drug will temporarily turn the urine red.

Doxorubicin extravasation can cause severe tissue necrosis and may ultimately require surgical debridement with skin grafting. Although various animal models suggest the efficacy of subcutaneous hydrocortisone, local intravenous sodium bicarbonate, and topical dimethyl sulfoxide (DMSO) for extravasations, none has been tested in clinical studies in a comparative, prospective manner.[8]

Doxorubicin is not immunosuppressive, but it is potentially mutagenic, teratogenic, and carcinogenic. It is a radiosensitizer, and great caution should be exercised when both modalities are combined simultaneously. This effect can be manifested as an increased immediate toxicity (e.g., radiation dermatitis occurring at a lower-than-usual dose of radiation) or as a recall phenomenon when doxorubicin is administered long after previous radiation therapy. Although these reactions are difficult to quantify, Mayer suggests that when the two modalities are used concurrently, a full course of doxorubicin is equivalent to approximately 1000 rad.[72]

Doxorubicin can produce two forms of cardiac toxicity. First, acute changes can occur a few hours to days after any dosage. They are unrelated to the cumulative dose and usually manifested as nonspecific ST-T wave changes, conduction disturbances, and almost any type of arrhythmia. The acute changes are reversible and are not related to the development of congestive cardiomyopathy.[73] Very rarely, an acute myopericarditis syndrome occurs and is often fatal. The second form of cardiac injury is a congestive cardiomyopathy that is usually delayed, dose-related, and irreversible. The mortality rate is as high as 61 percent.[74] The most significant risk factor for development of cardiomyopathy is the lifetime cumulative dose of doxorubicin expressed as mg/m^2.

There is no totally safe dose of doxorubicin below which cardiotoxicity is absent. However, clinically apparent toxicity is rare under cumulative lifetime doses of 400 mg/m^2 (Fig. 9–2). In several studies, the incidence of heart failure in patients receiving less than 550 mg/m^2 ranged from 0.1 to 1.2 percent, in contrast to patients receiving doses greater than 550 mg/m^2 when the incidence was 30 percent.[75] Advanced age has also been associated with an increase in cardiac toxicity. Based on these clinical experiences, the general recommendation is that doxorubicin be discontinued when a cumulative dose of 550 mg/m^2 is reached. Furthermore, patients who may be at higher risk, such as those over age 70, with previous mediastinal and cardiac radiation, with concurrent treatment with cyclophosphamide, and with preexisting coronary, valvular or myocardial disease should only receive a cumulative dose of 450 mg/m^2.[25,76]

Presently, the best non-invasive technique for monitoring cardiac performance is the radionuclide ejection fraction. Patients who are at high risk for cardiotoxicity should undergo an initial baseline scan, another scan when receiving 300 mg/m^2, and a scan at every 100 mg/m^2 increment thereafter. In general, if the ejection fraction is less than 45 percent or is reduced by 10 percent from the baseline scan, doxorubicin should not be continued. The physical examination, chest x-ray, and symptoms are not adequate means of assessing toxicity because they are abnormal only when the cardiomyopathy is well established. Other than conventional methods for managing congestive heart failure, there is no specific treatment available.[77]

Etoposide

Etoposide (VP-16, VePesid) is a semisynthetic derivative of podophyllum extract. It was first synthesized in 1973 and, since then, has become an important drug in the treatment of metastatic

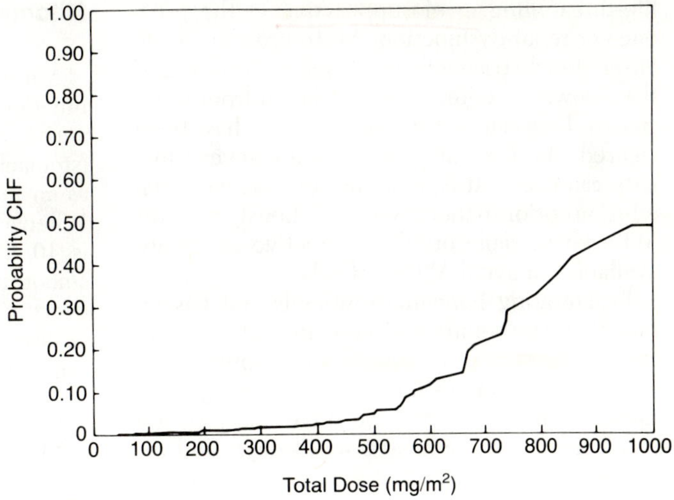

Figure 9–2. Cumulative probability of developing congestive heart failure versus total cumulative dose of doxorubicin in all patients receiving the drug (88 cases of congestive heart failure in 3941 patients). (Reprinted, with permission, from Von Hoff DD, Layard MW, Basa P *et al:* Risk factors for doxorubicin-induced congestive heart failure. Ann Intern Med 91:710, 1979.)

testicular carcinoma. Early studies demonstrated that etoposide had a major role in the salvage treatment of patients with advanced testicular tumors who failed to respond to first-line therapy with cisplatin, vinblastine, and bleomycin. In refractory patients or in those experiencing relapse, the single-agent response rate of etoposide was 34 percent,[77] and when it was used in salvage regimens consisting of etoposide, cisplatin, and bleomycin, 38 to 42 percent achieved disease-free status.[78,79] The substitution of etoposide for vinblastine in the widely used Einhorn regimen has also proved to be an effective first-line therapy for advanced testicular cancer, with comparable response rates.

Etoposide appears to induce breaks in single-stranded DNA. It has specificity for the late S phase and early G_2 phase of the cell cycle, and it is considered a schedule-dependent drug. Preliminary data suggest that etoposide acts synergistically with cisplatin. Renal excretion accounts for approximately 40 percent of its clearance, suggesting that dosages should be attenuated in severe renal insufficiency. However, up to 16 percent of a dose is excreted in the bile. The majority of clinical studies recommend dose reduction in the presence of severe hepatic dysfunction; a conservative reduction is 50 percent of the calculated dose for a bilirubin level >3 mg/dl.[80]

As a single agent, etoposide is given as 300 to 600 mg/m² divided over 3 to 5 days and is repeated every 3 to 4 weeks. Myelosuppression is the usual dose-limiting side effect, with a nadir in the white blood cells occurring on days 10 to 14 and recovery by days 16 to 21. Previous chemotherapy or radiation can increase the incidence of neutropenia and may be an indication to start at a lower dose.[25] Other toxicities that occur less than 50 percent of the time include moderate nausea and vomiting, alopecia, and stomatitis. Hypotension invariably occurs if the drug is infused too rapidly; the standard infusion time is from 30 to 60 minutes.[81,82] Twelve cases of hypersensitivity reactions have been described, with an estimated incidence of 2 percent.[55] Peripheral neuropathy and radiation recall reactions are uncommon side effects.

Methotrexate

Methotrexate, a folic acid antagonist, is one of the oldest and most widely used chemotherapeutic agents today. In urologic oncology, methotrexate has a limited role in the management of metastatic prostate cancer and advanced transitional cell carcinoma of the bladder. Methotrexate works by competitively binding to the enzyme dihydrofolate reductase, which ultimately leads to inhibition of the synthesis of thymidylate, purine nucleotides, and DNA.[83]

Methotrexate is given in conventional doses of 25 to 75 mg/m² once a week. Doses in this range produce peak plasma levels of 1×10^{-5} M to 1×10^{-6} M, whereas the concentration required to inhibit DNA synthesis is 1×10^{-7} M to 1×10^{-8} M. Tissue damage and toxicity are related both to the MTX concentration and the duration of exposure to the drug. Its clearance is reasonably complete in 1 to 2 days, except in the presence of renal insufficiency or third-space effusions. Since the drug is dependent on renal excretion, the BUN and creatinine levels should be followed frequently during treatment. Even small doses of MTX may cause life-threatening myelosuppression in the presence of renal dysfunction. Methotrexate slowly enters third-space effusions such as ascites, and then slowly re-enters the circulation from these spaces long after the initial dose has been cleared. As a result, unexpectedly severe toxicity can occur. It is advisable to evacuate such effusions prior to therapy and cautiously monitor MTX levels daily or, if other active drugs are available, to avoid MTX entirely.[1]

Proliferating bone marrow cells and gastrointestinal epithelium are the principal organs of toxicity. Mucositis and diarrhea are common side effects and are indications for interrupting treatment. Both mucositis and myelosuppression reach their maximums at 5 to 14 days, and recovery soon follows.

Renal toxicity is rare with standard doses of MTX. However, high dose therapy (>1 gm/m^2) without adequate hydration or alkalinization is associated with a 10 percent incidence of acute renal insufficiency. Extremely toxic plasma levels of MTX can result from the combination of a huge dose of MTX and the inability to rapidly excrete the drug. Furthermore, dialysis is ineffective for the removal of MTX in these patients.[1]

Methotrexate can produce acute hepatocellular injury, usually with the high-dose therapy. Long-term oral maintenance MTX is associated with a 30 percent incidence of hepatic fibrosis. A more serious complication—cirrhosis—has been reported in up to 24 percent of patients receiving daily oral MTX.[2]

Less commonly, MTX can produce three types of pulmonary complications: (1) noncardiogenic pulmonary edema, (2) an acute syndrome of pleuritic chest pain, and (3) interstitial pneumonitis similar to bleomycin.[30] Other side effects are osteoporotic fractures, immunosuppression, congenital malformations, and immune hemolytic anemia. Methotrexate does not appear to be carcinogenic.

The bone marrow and gastrointestinal toxicity of MTX can be prevented by the timely administration of exogenous reduced folate. The most widely used rescue agent is folinic acid (N5-formyltetrahydrofolate, leucovorin, citrovorum factor). Leucovorin is generally not necessary with conventional doses of MTX, except if there is previous bone marrow dysfunction, unexpected pharmakokinetics resulting in increased MTX plasma levels, or renal insufficiency. The leucovorin dose ranges from 10 to 100 mg/m^2 every 6 hours until the MTX level is less than 5×10^{-8} M.[4]

Mitomycin-C

Mitomycin-C is an antitumor antibiotic that functions as an alkylating agent. It is moderately active against a variety of adenocarcinomas (stomach, pancreas, colon, breast) and is used as an intravesical agent for bladder carcinoma. When administered systemically, the usual dose is 10 to 20 mg/m^2, slowly pushed through a smoothly running IV line. The dose is repeated every 6 to 8 weeks. Mitomycin-C is a severe vesicant and, when inadvertently extravasated, can produce chronic, progressive, and deep ulcers similar to those caused by doxorubicin.[84]

Side effects of systemic mitomycin include mild anorexia, nausea, and vomiting. An idiosyncratic interstitial pneumonitis is a rare complication and may respond to corticosteroid administration. Myelosuppression is the major dose-limiting side effect, and it is usually delayed and cumulative. The white blood cell count nadir occurs at 3 to 4 weeks, with recovery by 8 weeks. Renal toxicity may be an isolated event, but more frequently it occurs as a microangiopathic hemolytic anemia with thrombocytopenia and renal failure. Pathologic examination demonstrates fibrin thrombi in the afferent arterioles and glomerular capillary loops, with glomerular necrosis.[85] Unfortunately, many patients experience progressive renal failure despite plasmapheresis, immunosuppressive drugs, and antiplatelet agents. Although this syndrome occurs in the majority of patients after 6 to 12 months of mitomycin therapy, it can occur after only one dose or even after discontinuation of the medication.

Intravesical mitomycin is used for the treatment and prophylaxis of superficial bladder tumors and for carcinoma in situ of the bladder. Several studies involving over 400 patients who received mitomycin for superficial bladder tumors report a complete response rate of 47 percent and a partial response rate of 28 percent.[43] The usual dose is 20 to 60 mg instilled intravesically every week for 8 weeks. Myelosuppression is rare because the antibiotic is poorly absorbed. Local toxicity, such as cystitis, occurs in 6 to 32 percent of the cases. Perineal rashes and palmar desquamation have also been reported.[86]

Thiotepa

Thiotepa (N, N′, N″-triethylenethiophosphoramide) is a polyfunctional alkylating agent that has a spectrum of toxicity and clinical use similar to that of nitrogen mustard. Intravesical administration of thiotepa is indicated for the treatment of superficial bladder cancer and prophylaxis of recurrent superficial bladder tumors. In patients with established lesions, approximately 30 percent of patients achieve a complete response and 26 percent, a partial response.[87] Randomized controlled studies with prophylactic intravesical thiotepa have also demonstrated about 20 percent reduction in the number of recurrences at 1 year.[88] For carcinoma in situ, thiotepa has not proved to be as effective.

The usual dose of thiotepa is 30 to 60 mg in 10 to 60 ml of sterile water instilled into the bladder for 1 to 2 hours a week for 4 weeks, then at monthly intervals. Toxicity consists of severe bladder irritation, urinary tract infections, and myelosuppression. The incidence of myelosuppression ranges from 18 to 40 percent[89] and is due primarily to the low molecular weight (M.W.) of thiotepa of 189, which permits systemic absorption. Since thiotepa absorption is also related to the integrity of the bladder epithelium, some urologists delay intravesical treatment for 1 week after tumor resection to allow for healing to occur.

Vinca Alkaloids

Two of the most useful antineoplastic agents, vincristine and vinblastine, are alkaloids extracted from the periwinkle plant. The *Vinca* alkaloids are large and complex molecules, differing from each other only on the side chains of the parent molecule. Both agents exert their major antitumor effect by binding to microtubule proteins and interfering with the formation of the mitotic spindle in dividing cells. Despite their structural similarity, vincristine and vinblastine have entirely different spectrums of activity and toxicity, and they are not cross-resistant.[25]

Vinblastine

Vinblastine is an important drug used in combination chemotherapy for testicular tumors and is also associated with rare benefit in the palliative treatment of renal carcinoma. The usual dose is 0.1 to 0.15 mg/kg once a week until the desired antitumor effect is achieved or until bone marrow toxicity precludes further treatment. As part of the regimen of Einhorn and Donohue, it is given as a dose of 0.15 mg/kg/day on days 1 and 2 of each 3-week cycle.[28]

The drug is excreted primarily in the bile as biodegraded products, but about 20 percent of the drug is excreted unchanged in the urine. A 50 percent dose reduction is advised for patients with a bilirubin greater than 3 mg/dl.[2] No dose attenuation is needed for renal insufficiency.

Granulocytopenia is the most frequent and dangerous toxic effect. The nadir occurs within 5 to 9 days after a dose and resolves within 14 to 21 days. Other less common side effects include nausea, vomiting, mucositis, alopecia, malaise, weakness, skin vesiculation and, rarely, neurotoxicity. The neurologic toxicities are reportedly similar to vincristine but less severe. Vinblastine is minimally immunosuppressive. It is a vesicant and can cause severe local tissue damage if extravasation has occurred.[1]

References

Cited References

1. Chabner BA, Myers CE: Clinical pharmacology of cancer chemotherapy. In DeVita VT Jr, Hellman S, Rosenberg SA, eds: Cancer: Principles and Practice of Oncology. Philadelphia, JB Lippincott Co, 1985.
2. Perry MC: Hepatotoxicity of chemotherapeutic agents. Semin Oncol 9:65, 1982.
3. Schilsky RL: Renal and metabolic toxicities of cancer chemotherapy. Semin Oncol 9:75, 1982.
4. Bleyer WA: The clinical pharmacology of methotrexate: new applications of an old drug. Cancer 41:36, 1978.
5. Seigel LJ, Longo DL: The control of chemotherapy-induced emesis. Ann Intern Med 95:352, 1981.
6. Mitchell EP, Schein PS: Gastrointestinal toxicity of chemotherapeutic agents. Semin Oncol 9:52, 1982.
7. Sweet DL: Delta-9-tetrahydrocannabinol as an antiemetic for patients receiving cancer chemotherapy: a pilot study. J Clin Pharmacol 21:705, 1981.
8. Harwood KV, Aisner J: Treatment of chemotherapy extravasation: current status. Cancer Treat Rev 68:939, 1984.
9. Ignoffo RJ, Friedman MA: Therapy of local toxicities caused by extravasation of cancer chemotherapeutic drugs. Cancer Treat Rev 7:17, 1980.
10. Larson DL: Treatment of tissue extravasation by antitumor agents. Cancer 49:1796, 1982.
11. Tsokos GC, Balow JE, Spiegel RJ, Magrath IT: Renal and metabolic complications of undifferentiated and lymphoblastic lymphomas. Medicine 60:218, 1981.
12. Cervantes F, Ribera JM, Granena A, Montserrat E, Rozman C: Tumor lysis syndrome with hypocalcemia in accelerated chronic granulocytic leukemia. Acta Hematol 68:157, 1982.
13. Vogelzang NJ, Nelimark RA, Nath KA: Tumor lysis syndrome after induction chemotherapy of small cell bronchogenic carcinoma. JAMA 249:513, 1983.
14. Thachil JV, Jewett MAS, Rider WD: The effects of cancer and cancer therapy on male fertility. J Urol 126:141, 1981.
15. Schilsky RL, Sherins RJ: Gonadal dysfunction. In DeVita VT Jr, Hellman S, Rosenberg SA, eds: Cancer: Principles and Practice of Oncology. Philadelphia, JB Lippincott Co, 1985.

16. Cunningham J, Mauch P, Rosenthal DS, Canellos GP: Long-term complications of MOPP chemotherapy in patients with Hodgkin's Disease. Cancer Treat Rep 66:1015, 1982.
17. Whitehead E, Shalet SM, Blackledge G, Todd I, Crowther D, Beardwell CG: The effects of Hodgkin's disease and combination chemotherapy on gonadal function in the adult male. Cancer 49:418, 1982.
18. Drasga RE, Einhorn LH, Williams SD, Patel DN, Stevens EE: Fertility after chemotherapy for testicular cancer. J Clin Oncol 1:179, 1983.
19. Li FP: Second Cancers. In DeVita VT Jr, Hellman S, Rosenberg SA, eds: Cancer, Principles and Practice of Oncology. Philadelphia, JB Lippincott Co, 1985.
20. Canellos GP: Therapy-related leukemia: a necessary complication of successful systemic chemotherapy? J Clin Oncol 2:1077, 1984.
21. Haskell CM: Principles of cancer chemotherapy. In Haskell CM, ed: Cancer Treatment. Philadelphia, WB Saunders Co, 1985a.
22. Redman JR, Vugrin D, Arlin ZA, Gee TS, Kempin SJ, Godbold JH, Schottenfeld D, and Clarkson BD: Leukemia following treatment of germ cell tumors in men. J Clin Oncol 2:1080, 1984.
23. Glaubiger D, Ramu A: Antitumor antibiotics. In Chabner B, ed: Pharmacologic Principles of Cancer Treatment. Philadelphia, WB Saunders Co, 1982.
24. Vugrin D, Herr HW, Whitmore WF, Sogani PC, Golbey RB: VAB-6 combination chemotherapy in disseminated cancer of the testis. Ann Intern Med 95:59, 1981.
25. Haskell CM: Drugs used in cancer chemotherapy. In Haskell CM, ed: Cancer Treatment. Philadelphia, WB Saunders Co, 1985b.
26. Blatt J, Trigg ME, Pizzo PA, and Glaubiger D: Tolerance to single-dose dactinomycin in combination chemotherapy for solid tumors. Cancer Treat Rep 65:145, 1981.
27. Chabner BA: Bleomycin. In Chabner BA, ed: Pharmacologic Principles of Cancer Treatment. Philadelphia, WB Saunders Co, 1982.
28. Einhorn LH, Donohue JD: Cis-diamminedichloroplatinum, vinblastine, and bleomycin combination chemotherapy in disseminated testicular cancer. Ann Intern Med 87:293, 1977.
29. Peckham MJ, Barrett A, Liew KH, Horwich A, Robinson B, Dobbs HJ, McElwain TJ, Hendry WF: The treatment of metastatic germ-cell testicular tumors with bleomycin, etoposide, and cis-platin. Br J Cancer 47:613, 1983.
30. Ginsberg SL, Comis RL: The pulmonary toxicity of antineoplastic agents. Semin Oncol 9:34, 1982.
31. Bedrossian CW, Luna MA, Mackay B, Lichtiger B: Ultrastructure of pulmonary bleomycin toxicity. Cancer 32:44, 1973.
32. Samuels ML, Johnson DE, Holoye PY, Lanzotti VJ: Large dose bleomycin pulmonary toxicity: a possible role of prior radiotherapy. JAMA 235:1117, 1976.
33. Goldiner PL, Carlon GC, Cvitkovic E, Schweizer O, Howland WS: Factors influencing postoperative morbidity and mortality in patients treated with bleomycin. Br Med J 1:1664, 1978.
34. Schein, PS, DeVita VT, Hubbard S, Chabner BA, Canellos GP, Berard C, Young RC: Bleomycin, adriamycin, cyclophosphamide, vincristine, and prednisone (BACOP) combination chemotherapy in the treatment of advanced diffuse histiocytic lymphoma. Ann Intern Med 85:417, 1976.
35. Holoye PY, Luna MA, MacKay B, Bedrossian CW: Bleomycin hypersensitivity pneumonitis. Ann Intern Med 88:47, 1978.
36. Cohen IS, Mosher MB, O'Keefe EJ, Klaus SN, DeConti RC: Cutaneous toxicity of bleomycin therapy. Arch Dermatol 107:553, 1973.
37. Yagoda A, Mukherji B, Young C, Etcubanas E, Lamonte C, Smith JR, Tan CTC, Drakoff IH: Bleomycin, an antitumor antibiotic: clinical experience in 274 patients. Ann Intern Med 77:861, 1972.
38. Vogelzang NJ, Bosl GJ, Johnson K, Kennedy BJ: Raynaud's phenomenon: a common toxicity after combination chemotherapy for testicular cancer. Ann Intern Med 95:288, 1981.
39. Vogelzang NJ: Raynaud's phenomenon and cancer chemotherapy (letter). Ann Intern Med 96:256, 1982.
40. Carter JJ, McLaughlin ML, Bern MM: Bleomycin-induced fatal hyperpyrexia. Am J Med 74:523, 1983.
41. Ma DDF, Isbister JP: Cytotoxic-induced fulminant hyperpyrexia. Cancer 45:2249, 1980.
42. Zwelling LA, Kohn KW: In Pharmacologic Principles of Cancer Treatment. Chabner BA (ed), Philadelphia, WB Saunders Co, p. 309, 1982.
43. Sternberg CN, Yagoda A, Scher HI, Watson RC, Ahmed T, Weiselberg LR, Geller N, Hollander PS, Herr HW, Sogani PR, Morse MJ, Whitmore WF: Preliminary results of M-VAC (methotrexate, vinblastine, doxorubicin, and cisplatin) for transitional cell carcinoma of the urothelium. J Urol 133:403, 1985.
44. Harker WG, Meyers FJ, Freiha FS, Palmer JM, Shortliffe LD, Hannigan JF, McWhirter KM, Torti FM: Cisplatin, methotrexate, and vinblastine (CMV): an effective chemotherapy regimen for metastatic transitional cell carcinoma of the urinary tract: a Northern California Oncology Group study. J Clin Oncol 3:1463, 1985.
45. Loehrer PJ, Einhorn LH: Diagnosis and treatment: cisplatin. Ann Intern Med 100:704, 1984.
46. Sklaroff RB, Yagoda A: Cis-diamminedichloride platinum II (DDP) in the treatment of penile carcinoma. Cancer 44:1563, 1979.
47. Finley RS, Fortner CL, Grover WR: Cisplatin nephrotoxicity: a summary of preventative interventions. Drug Intell Clin Pharm 19:362, 1985.
48. Meijer S, Sleijfer DT, Muldur NH, Sluiter WJ, Marrink J, Koops HS, Brouwers TM, Oldhoff J, Van Der Hem, GK, Mandema E: Some effects of combination chemotherapy with cis-platinum on renal function in patients with nonseminomatous testicular carcinoma. Cancer 51:2035, 1983.
49. Markman M: Nephrotoxicity with cisplatin and antihypertensive medications (letter). Ann Intern Med 96:257, 1982.
50. Blachley JD, Hill JB: Renal and electrolyte disturbances associated with cisplatin. Ann Intern Med 95:628, 1981.
51. Reddel RR, Kefford RF, Grant JM, Coates AS, Fox RM, Tattersall HN: Ototoxicity in patients receiving cisplatin: importance of dose and method of drug administration. Cancer Treat Rep 66:19, 1982.
52. Hadley D, Herr HW: Peripheral neuropathy associated with cis-dichlorodiammineplatinum (II) treatment. Cancer 44:2026, 1979.
53. Getaz EP, Beckley S, Fitzpatrick J, Bozier A: Cisplatin-induced hemolysis. N Engl J Med 302:334, 1980.
54. Von Hoff DD, Schilsky R, Reichert CM: Toxic effects of cis-dichlorodiammineplatinum (II) in man. Cancer Treat Rep 63:1527, 1979.
55. Weiss RB, Bruno S: Hypersensitivity reactions to cancer chemotherapeutic agents. Ann Intern Med 94:66, 1981.
56. Perez CA, Fair WR, Ihde DC, Labrie F: Cancer of the prostate. In DeVita VT Jr, Hellman S, Rosenberg SA,

eds: Cancer: Principles and Practice of Oncology. Philadelphia, JB Lippincott Co, 1985.
57. Cox PJ: Cyclophosphamide cystitis: identification of acrolein as the causative agent. Biochem Pharmacol 28:2045, 1979.
58. Klein FA, Smith MJ: Urinary complications of cyclophosphamide therapy: etiology, prevention, and management. South J Med 76:1413, 1983.
59. Wall RL, Clausen KP: Carcinoma of the urinary bladder in patients receiving cyclophosphamide. N Engl J Med 293:271, 1975.
60. Fuchs EF, Kay R, Poole R, Barry JM, Pearse HD: Uroepithelial carcinoma in association with cyclophosphamide ingestion. J Urol 126:544, 1981.
61. DeFronzo RA, Braine H, Colvin OM, Davis PJ: Water intoxication in man after cyclophosphamide therapy: time course and relation to drug activation. Ann Intern Med 78:861, 1973.
62. Harlow PJ, DeClerck YA, Shore NA, Ortega JA, Carranza A, Heuser E: A fatal case of inappropriate ADH secretion induced by cyclophosphamide therapy. Cancer 44:896, 1979.
63. Gottdiener JS, Applebaum FR, Ferrans VF, Deisseroth A, Ziegler J: Cardiotoxicity associated with high-dose cyclophosphamide therapy. Arch Intern Med 141:758, 1981.
64. Droller JJ, Saral R, Santos G: Prevention of cyclophosphamide-induced hemorrhagic cystitis. Urology 20:256, 1982.
65. Scheef W, Klein HO, Brock N, Burkert H, Gunther U, Hoefer-Janker H, Mitrenga D, Schnitker J, Voigtmann R: Controlled clinical studies with an antidote against the urotoxicity of oxazaphosphorines: preliminary results. Cancer Treat Rep 63:501, 1979.
66. Burkert H: Clinical overview of Mesna. Cancer Treat Rev 10 (Suppl A):175, 1983.
67. Shrom SH, Donaldson MH, Duckett JW Jr, Wein AJ: Formalin treatment for intractable hemorrhagic cystitis: a review of the literature with 16 additional cases. Cancer 38:1785, 1976.
68. Fair WR: Formalin in the treatment of massive bladder hemorrhage: Techniques, results, and complications. Urology 3:573, 1974.
69. Fair WR: Urologic emergencies. In DeVita VT Jr, Hellman S, Rosenberg SA, eds: Cancer: Principles and Practice of Oncology. Philadelphia, JB Lippincott Co, 1985.
70. Blum RH, Carter SK: Adriamycin; a new anticancer drug with significant clinical activity. Ann Intern Med 80:249, 1974.
71. Young RC, Ozols RF, Myers CE: The anthracycline antineoplastic drugs. N Engl J Med 305:139, 1981.
72. Mayer EG, Poulter XA, Aristizabal SA: Complications of irradiation related to apparent drug potentiation by adriamycin. Int J Radiat Oncol Biol Phys 1:1179, 1976.
73. Unverferth DV, Magorien RD, Leier CV, Balcerzak SP: Doxorubicin cardiotoxicity. Cancer Treat Rev 9:149, 1982.
74. Von Hoff DD, Piccart M: The cardiotoxicity of anticancer agents. Semin Oncol 9:23, 1982.
75. Von Hoff DD, Layard MW, Basa P, Davis HL Jr, Von Hoff AL, Rozencweig M, Muggia FM: Risk factors for doxorubicin-induced congestive heart failure. Ann Intern Med 91:710, 1979.
76. Bristow MR, Mason JW, Minningham ME, Daniels JR: Doxorubicin cardiomyopathy: evaluation by phonocardiography, endomyocardial biopsy, and cardiac catheterization. Ann Intern Med 88:168, 1978.
77. Goorin AM, Borow KM, Goldman A, Williams RG, Henderson IC, Sallan SE, Cohen H, Jaffe N: Congestive heart failure due to adriamycin cardiotoxicity: its natural history in children. Cancer 47:2810, 1981.
78. Williams SD, Einhorn LH: Etoposide salvage therapy for refractory germ cell tumors: an update. Cancer Treat Rev 9 (Suppl A):67, 1982.
79. Lederman GS, Garnick MB, Canellos GP, Richie JP: Chemotherapy of refractory germ cell cancer with etoposide. J Clin Oncol 1:706, 1983.
80. Arbuck SG, Douglass HO, Crom WR, Goodwin P, Silk Y, Cooper C, Evans WE: Etoposide pharmacokinetics in patients with normal and abnormal organ function. J Clin Oncol 4:1690, 1986.
81. Issell BF, Crooke ST: Etoposide (VP-16-312). Cancer Treat Rev 6:107, 1979.
82. O'Dwyer PJ, Leyland-Jones B, Alonso MT, Marsoni S, Wittes RE: Etoposide (VP-16-213). Current status of an active anticancer drug. N Engl J Med 312:692, 1985.
83. Jolivet J, Cowan KH, Curt GA, Clendeninn NJ, Chabner BA: The pharmacology and clinical use of Methotrexate. N Engl J Med 309:1094, 1983.
84. Argenta LC, Manders EK: Mitomycin C extravasation injuries. Cancer 51:1080, 1983.
85. Cantrell JE, Phillips TM, Schein PS: Carcinoma-associated hemolytic-uremic syndrome: a complication of Mitomycin C chemotherapy. J Clin Oncol 3:723, 1985.
86. Nissenkorn I, Herrod H, Soloway MS: Side effects associated with intravesical mitomycin C. J Urol 126:596, 1981.
87. Scher HI, Sternberg CN: Chemotherapy of urologic malignancies. Semin Urol 3:239, 1985.
88. Koontz WW, Prout GR, Smith W, Frable WJ, Minnis JE: The use of intravesical thiotepa in the management of non-invasive carcinoma of the bladder. J Urol 125:307, 1981.
89. Hollister D, Coleman M: Hematologic effect of intravesicular thiotepa therapy for bladder cancer. JAMA 244:2065, 1980.

Uncited References

Doll DC, List AF, Greco FA, Hainsworth JD, Hande KR, Johnson DH: Acute vascular ischemic events after cisplatin-based combination chemotherapy for germ-cell tumors of the testis. Ann Intern Med 105:48, 1986.

Drasga RE, Einhorn LH, Williams SD: The chemotherapy of testicular cancer. CA 32:66, 1982.

Solberg LA Jr, Wick MR, Bruckman JE: Doxorubicin-enhanced skin reaction after whole body electron-beam irradiation for leukemia cutis. Mayo Clin Proc 55:711, 1980.

COMPLICATIONS IN ADRENAL SURGERY

10

Richard Bihrle • John P. Donohue

Surgery performed on the adrenal glands varies significantly in accordance with the underlying disease process. Complications of adrenal surgery are often encountered because the initial surgical approach has not been optimal. In a discussion of surgical complications of adrenal surgery, it should be recognized that the surgical approach and exposure to the adrenal gland will be tailored to the underlying disease process. It is equally important to recognize that most adrenal surgery involves metabolically reactive disease processes that necessitate special preoperative, intraoperative, and postoperative precautions.

This chapter reviews the anatomy of the adrenal glands as well as the technical aspects of the *transabdominal* and *dorsal* surgical approaches to the gland. An overview of the more common adrenal diseases, and the technical surgical complications and metabolic complications peculiar to each of these disease entities, will be discussed.

ANATOMY OF THE ADRENAL GLAND AND ITS CONTIGUOUS STRUCTURES

The adrenals are two small flattened glands residing in the retroperitoneal space, lying just superior and anterior to each kidney. The right adrenal gland is slightly smaller than the left and is more triangular in shape, as opposed to the half-moon shape of the left adrenal gland. The right adrenal gland rests on the right crus of the diaphragm and the anterosuperior surface of the right kidney. Anteriorly, it is covered by a portion of the liver and at times may even be found to be embedded within the liver parenchyma. Medially, the suprarenal portion of the inferior vena cava is in close proximity to the adrenal gland, and in many cases, the vena cava will actually cover the anterior medial aspect of the adrenal gland. Inferiorly, the right adrenal gland is bordered by the right renal vein and right renal artery. This close proximity to the vena cava, along with a short right adrenal vein that enters directly into the vena cava as a high insertion beneath the liver, makes surgical exposure of the right adrenal gland more difficult than the left.

The major portion of the arterial supply to the right adrenal gland comes from the inferior adrenal artery, which is the first branch off the right renal artery. The right adrenal gland also obtains blood supply from the middle adrenal artery, which is a branch directly off the aorta. The middle adrenal courses behind the vena cava and branches early into several tributaries that supply the medial portion of the gland. The superior adrenal artery is a branch off the inferior phrenic and supplies the apex of the adrenal gland, usually as one or two tributaries.

The left adrenal gland is slightly larger than the right and is more semilunar in shape. Much like its counterpart, it is bordered posteriorly by the crus of the diaphragm and the anteromedial aspect of the upper pole of the kidney. Anteriorly, it is crossed by the tail of the pancreas and the splenic artery. The spleen is often intimately involved with the anterior lateral aspect of the adrenal gland. Medial to the left adrenal lies the aorta, but this is usually not closely involved with the adrenal. Inferiorly, it is bordered by the left renal artery and renal vein.

The major arterial supply to the left adrenal gland is via the middle adrenal artery, which arises from the lateral aspect of the aorta and enters the adrenal medially. The left adrenal gland also obtains blood supply from a smaller inferior adrenal artery that courses up from the renal artery, and a small superior adrenal artery that courses downward from the inferior phrenic. The venous drainage of the gland is through the left adrenal vein, which enters directly into the left renal vein just lateral to the aorta.

The sessile covering of both adrenal glands is provided by a superior extension of Gerota's fascia. The anterior and posterior leaflets of Gerota's fascia, which surround the kidney, fuse superiorly at the kidney's upper pole to become a common sheath. The fascia then divides into anterior and posterior leaflets once again to surround the adrenal glands. This unique relationship provided by Gerota's fascia allows the adrenal gland to be separated easily and cleanly from the kidney during an adrenalectomy or a simple nephrectomy. It also allows the adrenal gland to be retracted downward by gently retracting the kidney downward. This is a key maneuver that is used in the surgical exposure of the adrenal gland.

ALDOSTERONISM

Although primary aldosteronism may be the result of bilateral, micronodular hyperplasia of zona glomerulosa cells, it is usually associated with a discrete adenoma involving the zona glomerulosa. The resulting syndrome is characterized by slowly progressive benign hypertension and hypokalemic alkalosis secondary to the inappropriate and excessive production of aldosterone. In addition, the unprovoked release of aldosterone results in suppression of the plasma renin level.

Major clinical features are benign hypertension, usually in the absence of severe vascular disease. The patient may also present with complaints of muscular weakness, polydipsia and polyuria. Urinary aldosterone and potassium excretion are elevated; likewise, plasma aldosterone is elevated, but serum potassium is decreased. Although relative hypervolemia exists, hypernatremia is only mild and metabolic alkalosis is usually not severe.

The key to establishing a diagnosis is to determine the presence of elevated urinary and plasma aldosterone levels, together with unprovoked hypokalemia. The second major criterion for establishing a diagnosis is to establish whether suppression of renal renin production exists. The two most reliable tests for diagnosing primary aldosteronism are:

1. Failure to suppress aldosterone during sodium loading. An aldosterone excretion ratio of greater than 14.0 μg/24 hours after 3 days of salt loading (negative saline suppression test) is diagnostic.
2. Failure to stimulate plasma renin activity during sodium deprivation (negative Lasix stimulation test).

Once the diagnosis of primary aldosteronism has been established by a negative saline (aldosterone) suppression test and a negative lasix (renin) stimulation test, the next major step is to determine localization of the disease. The tumors are classically small, measuring less than 1 or 2 cm in diameter. Localization is therefore difficult. Selective catheterization for adrenal venous aldosterone, in addition to venographic demonstration of the tumor, can be most helpful. The radioisotope iodocholesterol scan and, more recently, the new imaging isotope I-131-I-6B-iodomethyl-19-norcholesterol scan have made localization slightly more simple.

Treatment

Surgical treatment is best reserved for those patients diagnosed as having unilateral disease. Patients with bilateral hyperplasia (excessive aldosterone production from both adrenals in the absence of any adenoma imaged on venography, isotope scan, or computed tomographic [CT] scan) or who are poor surgical risks should be treated medically with oral spironolactone. Total bilateral adrenalectomy should never be performed for the treatment of aldosteronism because the morbidity of adrenal insufficiency and corticosteroid replacement is greater than that of the benign hypertension of aldosteronism.

Surgery for Aldosteronism: The Dorsal Approach

A dorsal incision is best employed while the patient is in the prone position. The radiologic studies are reviewed, and the suitable rib is chosen for subperiosteal excision; usually this is a

12th or 11th rib in the larger patient. The rib is removed as proximal as possible to its articulation to facilitate exposure. A supracostal incision may be used if one chooses to spare the rib. Whether the subdiaphragmatic retroperitoneal rib-excision approach or the supracostal incision is used, care must be taken to remain extrapleural and extraperitoneal.

If the pleural cavity is entered, we do not routinely leave a chest tube in place. At the end of the procedure, a red rubber catheter is placed through the pleural opening, and the pleural opening is closed with nonabsorbable sutures. The air is removed from the pleural space, with the anesthesiologist maintaining positive pressure ventilation as the red rubber catheter is placed under a water seal.

A major point in the exposure of the adrenal gland through the dorsal route is caudad and lateral mobilization of the adrenal gland within the contents of Gerota's fascia. This is done by placing gentle postcaudad and lateral traction on the kidney with either a sponge stick or the hand. On the right side, such posterolateral retraction of the kidney will allow separation of the superior aspect of the adrenal gland from the diaphragm and hepatic structures. The gland must be carefully freed from the surface of the liver, particularly in cases in which the adrenal gland is embedded within the lower parenchyma. If an inadvertent laceration of the liver occurs, most small lacerations can be closed with 3–0 or 2–0 chromic catgut interrupted sutures. If necessary, a plug of gelatinous sponge (Gelfoam) or murofibrillar collagen hemostat (Avitene) can be used as well.

With the gland retracted caudad, its anterior and posterior aspects can be freed from surrounding structures by both blunt and sharp dissection. The middle and inferior adrenal arteries cross superficially to the vena cava before entering the adrenal gland. Care must be taken to locate these arteries and to divide them to permit better lateral mobilization of the gland. We usually ligate with 2–0 black silk on the proximal side of the gland, and use vascular clips on the body wall or renal side. This allows us to use the silk sutures as traction sutures to avoid repeated and excessive manipulation of the gland itself. Any rough movements can cause swelling or bleeding within the gland and subsequent difficulty in identifying adenomas. Gentle lateral traction on the mobilized gland will expose the short right adrenal vein as it enters the inferior vena cava. The short right adrenal vein usually enters higher than expected on the vena cava, and it is often obscured by the overlying liver.

Excessive lateral traction on the gland may cause inadvertent avulsion of the vein and uncontrollable hemorrhage, which are the most common surgical complications encountered in the dorsal approach of the right adrenal gland. If the vein is avulsed from the vena cava, it should be secured with Allis forceps to bring the edges of the vena cava together to control the hemorrhage. The cavotomy can then be closed with 5–0 Prolene vascular sutures. Once the adrenal vein has been ligated, the gland can be easily detached from the upper pole of the kidney and removed.

On the left side, the kidney and adrenal gland should be retracted downward, gently mobilizing the plane just anterior and posterior to the adrenal gland. The apical ligaments can then be palpated and these ligaments should be secured with silver clips or 3–0 silk ties.

The apical ligaments contain vessels arising from the inferior phrenic arteries. Dissection is carried medially to identify and transect the middle adrenal and the inferior adrenal artery. The aorta, which lies medially, is usually not intimately involved with the adrenal gland and does not pose any particular problem. The adrenal vein arises from the renal vein and courses upward to the adrenal gland, running just lateral to the inferior adrenal artery. When dissection is performed anterior to the adrenal gland, great care must be taken not to injure the tail of the pancreas or splenic artery. Injury to the tail of the pancreas may occur during left adrenalectomy through the dorsal approach; if a small injury does occur, simple suturing of the injury is usually sufficient. In injuries to the pancreas, particularly the tail, an attempt should be made to identify the pancreatic duct so that the duct can be suture-ligated separately using 3–0 silk suture. Interrupted 3–0 silk sutures are then used to close the pancreatic defect and to approximate the substance of the gland. If a more significant injury to the pancreas has occurred, the gland should be cleanly transected and the pancreatic duct identified and suture-ligated with 3–0 silk suture. The substance of the pancreas can then be closed with interrupted 3–0 silk suture as well. In all cases, after pancreatic injury, a drain should be left to the repaired pancreas. However, most pancreatic injuries are simple contusions and retractor-related and should be recognized clinically as postoperative "chemical pancreatitis," which resolves spontaneously.

In summary, the major adrenal surgical complications in the dorsal approach are right renal vein avulsion on the right side and pancreatic injury on the left side. In addition, a possible postoperative metabolic complication can result from failure to recognize transient hyperkalemia, which may occur in the first few days after surgery. The contralateral adrenal gland's zona glomerulosa may be so suppressed that normal endogenous production of aldosterone is inadequate; however, this is relatively infrequent and transient. Potassium levels should be checked routinely and frequently in the immediate postoperative period. If hyperkalemia is encountered, aggressive therapy should be employed.

PHEOCHROMOCYTOMA

Pheochromocytoma accounts for less than 1 percent of all cases of hypertension, but its potentially lethal nature makes early diagnosis and prompt surgical therapy paramount. Surgeons are often the first to diagnose pheochromocytoma because it often presents as a sudden hypertensive crisis during induction of anesthesia or as unexplained, profound hypotension following surgery. Delay in diagnosis is the chief cause of mortality, accounting for nearly 800 deaths per year. Recognizing the typical signs and symptoms of pheochromocytoma and employing early and proper surgical management are essential to reducing the mortality and morbidity associated with this disease.

The variable complex of symptoms experienced by patients with pheochromocytoma probably reflects the relative proportion of norepinephrine to epinephrine secreted. Symptoms stem more from the secretion of epinephrine, whereas norepinephrine determines the extent of hypertension. Most patients experience headaches and excessive sweating. Other symptoms that may be seen include palpitations, anxiety, pallor, flushing, weakness, nausea, tremor, chest pain, shortness of breath, and abdominal cramps.

It is well recognized that any one patient's symptom complex may occur in "spells," which may or may not be associated with precipitating events such as smoking, sexual intercourse, micturition, defecation, or pressure placed on the abdomen. Hypertension is a consistent finding in pheochromocytoma. Although the hypertension is well known for its paroxysmal nature, nearly 50 percent of patients have sustained hypertension. An orthostatic decrease in blood pressure in a patient who has not been treated for hypertension suggests the presence of pheochromocytoma. (This finding is also suggestive of primary aldosteronism.) In many cases, the single clue to the existence of a pheochromocytoma is a hypertensive crisis associated with pregnancy, anesthesia, surgery, or the use of certain drugs. Drugs such as morphine, ACTH, parenteral guanethidine, or parenteral methyldopa may release catecholamines, whereas propranolol may increase the pressor response to epinephrine.

Diagnosis

The suggested presence of pheochromocytoma is best confirmed by measurement of plasma catecholamines using the catechol-O-methyltransferase method. This technique has proved nearly 100 percent effective in distinguishing patients with pheochromocytoma from other hypertensive patients. The clonidine suppression test may be employed as an adjunctive test in differentiating patients with pheochromocytoma from the subset of patients with essential hypertension in whom catecholamine levels are elevated.

When a diagnosis of pheochromocytoma is firmly established, it is important to localize the extent of the tumor prior to surgical exploration. Initial localization is best achieved by CT. Over 90 percent of cases can be correctly localized by a CT scan alone. Despite recent improvements in CT sector scanning, multiple, asymptomatic, or metastatic pheochromocytoma has remained difficult to locate because prior imaging techniques were nonspecific. The advent of the radiopharmaceutical agent, 131-I meta-iodobenzylguanidine (131-M1BG), permits scintigraphic localization based on functional principles. This agent resembles norepinephrine in molecular structure and is thought to enter adrenergic tissue by the same mechanism as the hormone itself. Incorporation in medullary tissue metabolic pathways localizes the isotope effectively for scanning. It is particularly valuable in localizing multiple, metastatic, or asymptomatic tumors.

Treatment

Prompt surgical removal of the tumor is the only effective treatment for pheochromocytoma.

The hypertensive crisis precipitated by anesthetic induction or surgical manipulation, as well as profound, postoperative shock secondary to hypovolemia, are potential complications peculiar to pheochromocytoma. In an effort to reduce the possibility of these complications and their attendant sequelae of cerebrovascular accident, myocardial infarction, or death, several preoperative and intraoperative recommendations are made.

Preoperative medical therapy may be useful to control hypertension and to prevent arrhythmias in patients with severe crisis. Preoperative treatment with phenoxybenzamine dampens or may even abolish the hypertensive episodes that can be associated with induction of anesthesia and with handling of the tumor. It is the authors' view that alpha adrenergic blockade is indicated in all cases to control blood pressure, relax the vascular tree, and thus increase blood volume. This effectively decreases hypertensive episodes during surgery and nearly eliminates potential for severe hypotension postoperatively.

Some workers avoid preoperative blockade, preferring to transfuse patients with whole blood preoperatively and to use volume expanders and blood intraoperatively as needed. Their rationale is that the palpation for other tumors is more effective in the patient who has not undergone blockade. However, because multiplicity occurs in only 10 percent of cases, and CT and isotopic scanning is highly effective in localizing retroperitoneal tumors, we have avoided the uncertainties of this approach with its attendant risks of hepatitis and blood pressure swings.

Intraoperatively, it is important to have an experienced anesthetic team in attendance. Constant blood pressure monitoring through an arterial line, along with easy, quick access of pharmacologic and anesthetic agents through intravenous lines, is mandatory. Anesthesia is usually induced with thiopental (Pentothal) and maintained with nitrous oxide. Halothane anesthetics are absolutely contraindicated because of the increased risk of ventricular arrhythmias. Hypertensive crisis and arrhythmias are promptly controlled with appropriate agents. Regitine is usually used for hypertensive crisis, while sodium nitroprusside is employed for persistent hypertension. Propranolol is most often used for arrhythmias.

Postoperative considerations include careful monitoring of the central venous blood pressure. We prefer a Swan-Ganz catheter for optimal central wedge pressure monitoring, and also use intra-arterial lines from the moment of surgical induction to 1 or 2 days postoperatively. Hypotension is exceedingly rare since we routinely use dibenzyline blockade for 1 to 2 weeks preoperatively.

Finally, a team approach cannot be overemphasized. Internists, anesthesiologists, and urologic surgeons—all with a background in endocrinology and experience in the field—are the ideal combination for patient management, preoperatively and postoperatively.

Surgical Approach for Pheochromocytoma: Transabdominal Approach

Our preference is a high abdominal transverse incision, extending bilaterally from the tip of the 12th rib and up along the costal margins. Bilateral adrenal exposure as well as paravertebral examination will be obtained with this approach (Fig. 10–1).

To explore the right adrenal gland, the liver and gallbladder are retracted cephalad, the right colon is reflected medially, and the stomach and duodenum are drawn medially (Fig. 10–2). Care must be taken when mobilizing the duodenum off the kidney and adrenal, especially if a large tumor mass is encountered. In the case of malignancy, if the tumor mass directly invades the duodenum, it is permissible to resect a small segment of the duodenum to totally excise the invading tumor.

If a wedge incision of the lateral wall of the duodenum is performed, the defect can be closed in two layers. It is best to close the mucosa and submucosa with a continuous suture of 3–0 chromic catgut using the Connell technique. The seromuscular layer can be closed with interrupted 3–0 silk suture using the Lembert technique.

If the duodenum defect cannot be closed primarily, a Roux-en-Y jejunal segment should be mobilized and brought up to close the defect. Drainage of the duodenum is not required if either the primary closure or Roux-en-Y is employed.

Once the adrenal has been adequately exposed, it is important to gently draw the kidney caudad and to develop and retract the inferior vena cava medially to obtain control of the right adrenal vein. In the care of pheochromocytoma, early ligation of the vein should be performed prior to manipulation of the adrenal. Precaution should be taken when securing the high-lying right adrenal vein. If inadvertent avulsion from

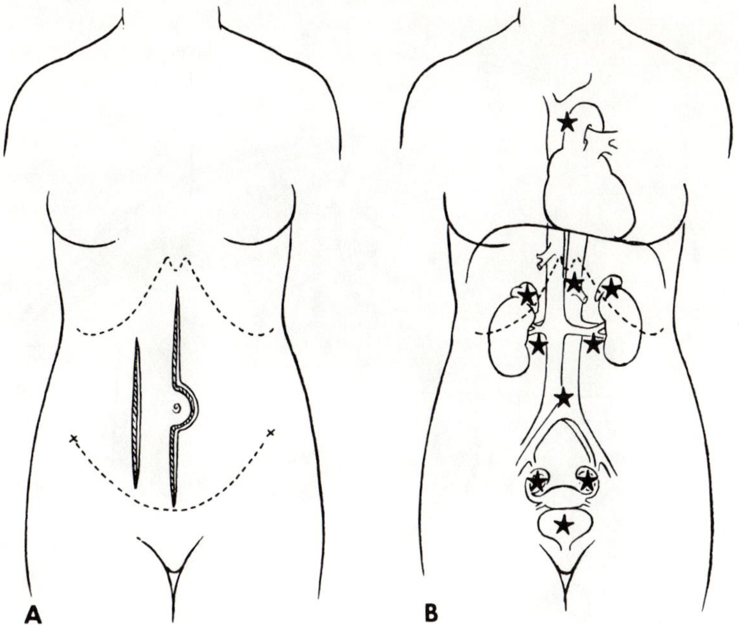

Figure 10–1. A schematic approach for pheochromocytoma is noted. The stars represent areas of special interest. An anterior approach is required for contralateral glandular checking as well as for checking the ganglia in the paravertebral area. A thoracic aspect of this incision is very useful in large tumors. In smaller tumors, however, the incision can be basically transabdominal and transverse with the approaches noted earlier. (From Glenn JF: Adrenal surgery. In Glenn JF, ed: Urologic Surgery. New York, Harper & Row, 1975, pp 1–30.)

the vena cava occurs, the defect should be handled as previously described.

The left adrenal gland may be exposed in the event of a small tumor by incising the posterior peritoneum and ligament of Treitz, and by ligating the inferior mesenteric vein and dividing it. This allows cephalad retraction of the body of the pancreas in a deep Harrington-Pemberton retractor. The adrenal will be easily visualized just lateral to the superior mesenteric artery and medial to the upper pole of the left kidney. In most instances, the left adrenal vein is easily secured through this approach (Fig. 10–3). If the left adrenal tumor is large, most physicians prefer to incise the mesocolon and divide the lienocolic and lienorenal attachments and again mobilize the pancreas cephalad (Fig. 10–4). If the left adrenal tumor is quite large, it is sometimes best to continue the incision of the mesocolon cephalad to include the lienophrenic attachments. Furthermore, exposure is facilitated by continuing the posterior peritoneal incision above the spleen to the gastroesophageal hiatus. Then the spleen and pancreas can be mobilized in continuity cephalad and medially, thus exposing the entire upper retroperitoneal space. Occasionally, division of the short gastric vessels may be necessary to mobilize the adrenal completely out of the left upper quadrant (Fig. 10–5).

Mobilization of the spleen, left colon, and pancreas en bloc permits better exposure of the adrenal gland when larger tumors are present. This will reduce the occurrence of injury to the pancreas or spleen. If, despite good technique, an injury to the spleen occurs, splenorrhaphy should be attempted.

During the past two decades, the occurrence of sepsis after splenectomy has been increasingly recognized, especially in children under the age of 5. The incidence of postsplenectomy sepsis in young children is between 2 and 5 percent. The incidence drops to 0.2 to 1 percent in older children and young adults; it drops again to 0.1 to 0.5 percent in adults. Despite its infrequent occurrence, when postsplenectomy sepsis occurs, it can be a disastrous problem involving pneumococcal meningitis, pneumonia, and death. Although, the need for splenectomy still exists in cases of uncontrollable bleeding or tumor invasion into the spleen, splenic suture repair should be attempted whenever possible.

Splenic repair can be accomplished by compressing the splenic pedicle, cauterizing the capsular edge of the spleen, and suturing the splenic defect with interrupted 3–0 chromic catgut or silk suture. Occasionally, the entire lower pole of the spleen can be resected and the defect sutured for hemostasis.

Additional measures to provide hemostasis when suturing the spleen include (1) Gelfoam pledgets, (2) suturing over Gelfoam plugs, (3) suturing omentum into the defects, or (4) applying Avitene liberally to the splenic defect.

When splenorrhagia is not possible, because of a major splenic injury, invasion by tumor, or

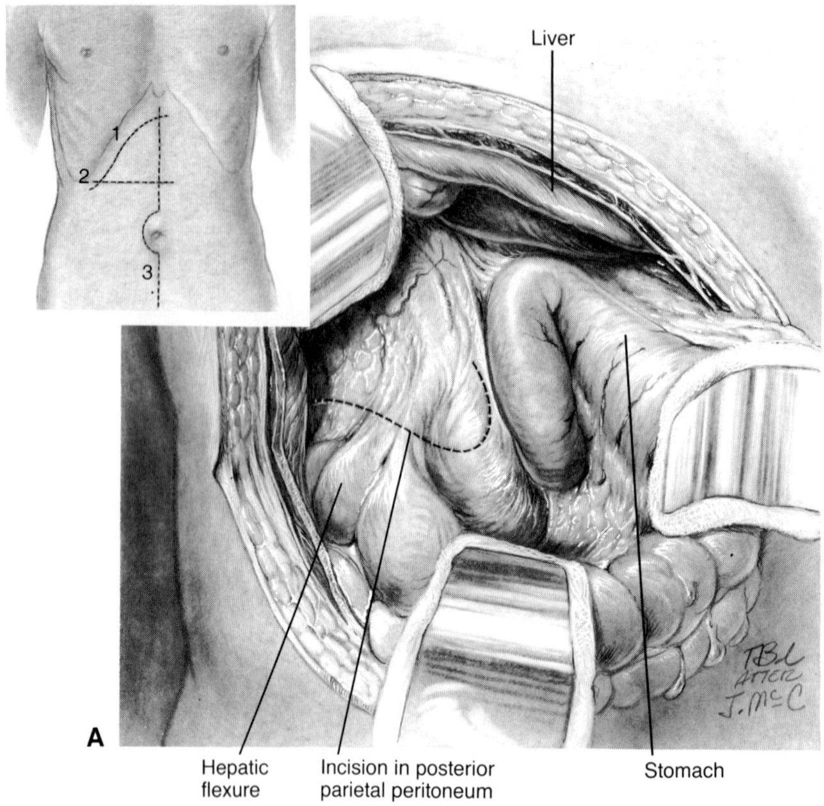

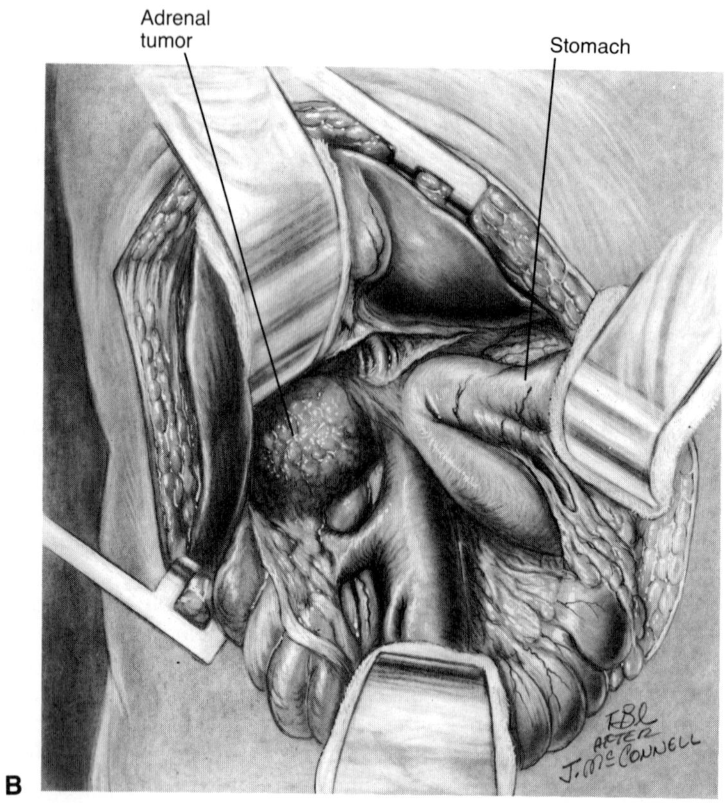

Figure 10–2. The right-sided approach is shown. Division of the colonic mesentery and right hepatocolic attachments allows the Kocher maneuver to expose the cava below the duodenum and head of the pancreas, which are placed in laparotomy pads; retraction is medial and cephalad. (From Graham JB: Renal malignancies. In Glenn JF, ed: Urologic Surgery. New York, Harper & Row, 1975, pp 73–85.)

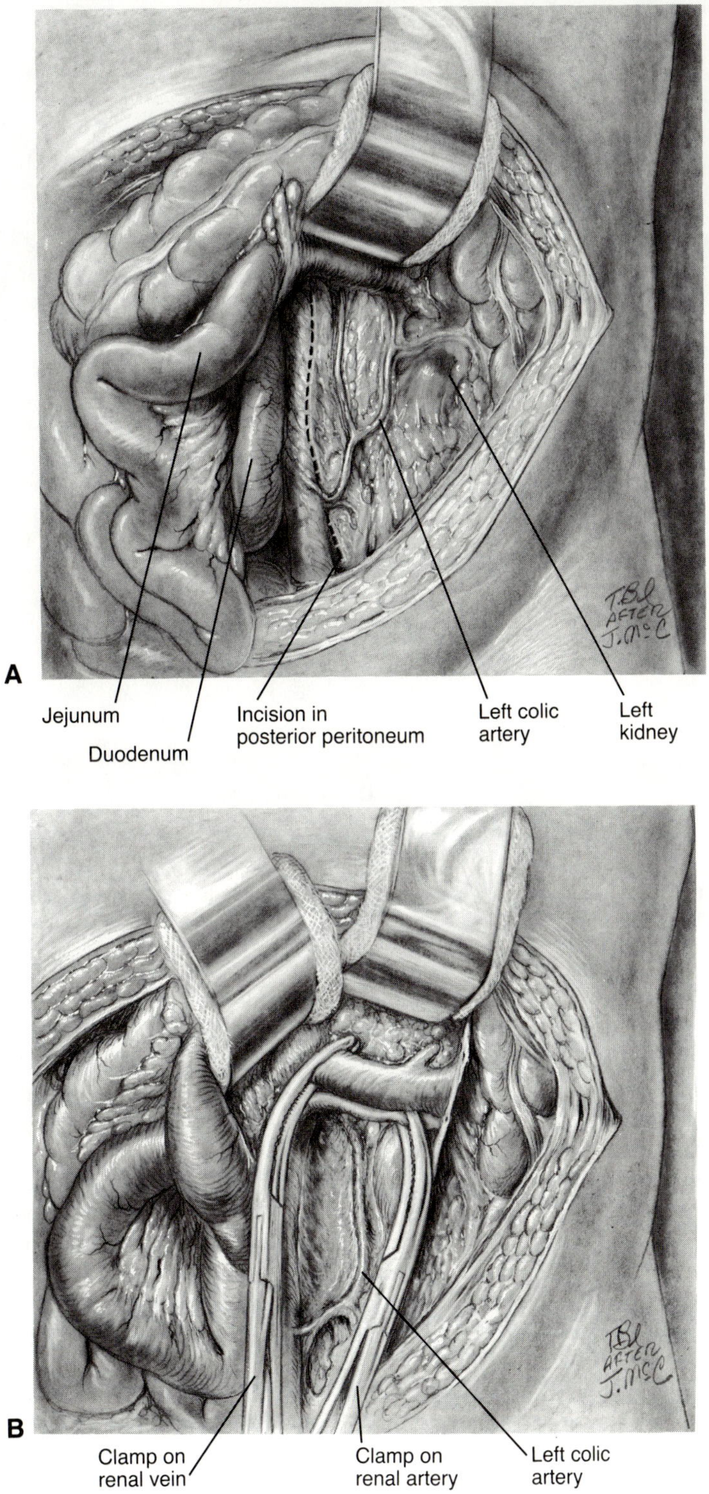

Figure 10–3. The transmesenteric approach to the adrenal gland is here shown for left-sided lesions. The root of the small bowel is divided, the inferior mesenteric vein is divided between silk ligatures, and a posterior incision below the pancreas mesentery is performed to elevate the pancreas and expose the left renal vein and the adrenal vein. This is a practical approach, particularly for small adrenal tumors of the left that are approached transabdominally. (From Graham JB: Renal malignancies. In Glenn JF, ed: Urologic Surgery. New York, Harper & Row, 1975, pp 73–85.)

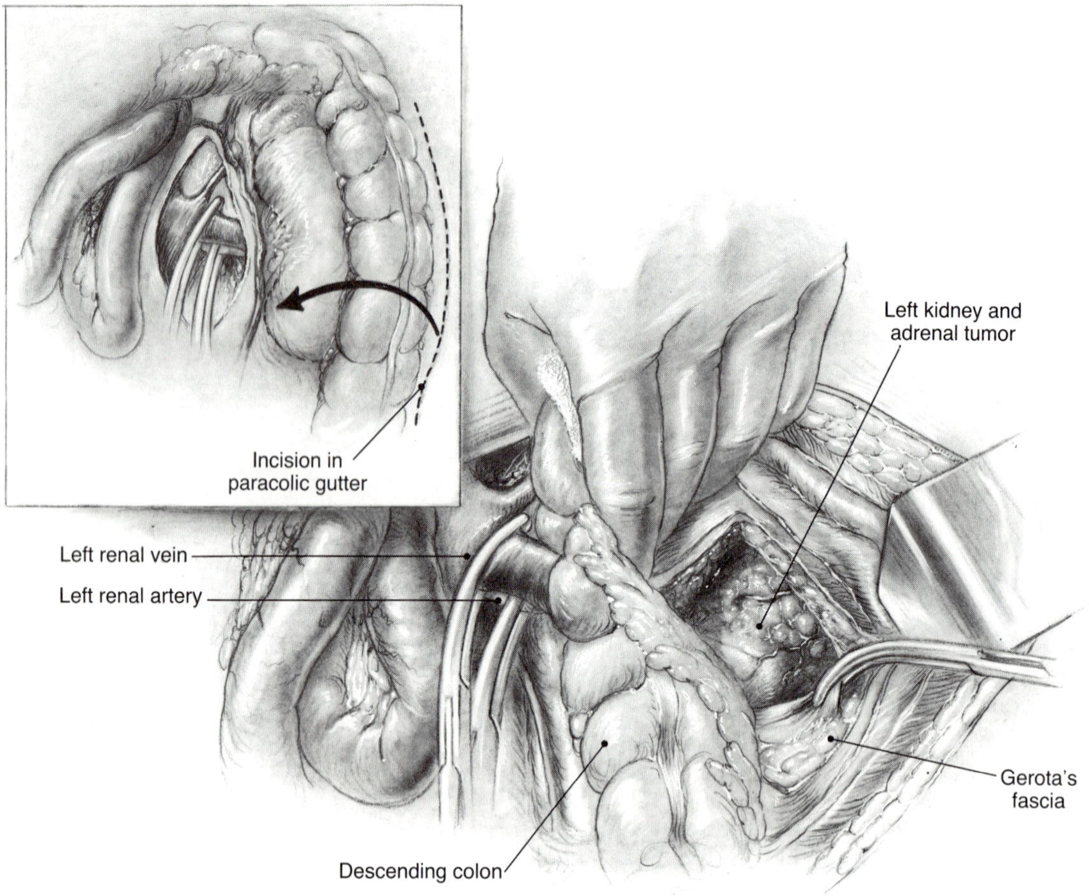

Figure 10–4. For left-sided tumors, the colon is reflected medially by dividing the left mesocolon and the lienocolic attachments. This is a standard anterior approach to both the kidney and adrenal gland and is useful, for example, in donor nephrectomy.

the need to minimize operative time, splenectomy is indicated. If good hemostasis is achieved after splenectomy, left upper quadrant, subdiaphragmatic drainage is not required.

If a pancreatic injury has been sustained, repair should be performed as described for pancreatic injuries in the section on primary aldosteronism (above).

Once exposed, the tumor is removed with great care to minimize manual pressure on the tumor itself. Ligatures and clips are preferred, if at all possible, with gentle traction on proximal ligatures providing elevation of the tumor mass. With preoperative alpha blockade using Dibenzyline, this maneuver is somewhat less critical than it was in the past. Nonetheless, it is a very important consideration and one that will ensure stable blood pressure throughout the operation. Every effort is made to tie the adrenal vein first. Opportunities to clip and divide small adrenal artery branches early in the angle between the crus of the diaphragm and the renal artery should be encouraged. Once the essential vascular tributaries are divided and ligated, the tumor is gently elevated out of the wound. Every effort should be made to stay wide around the tumor capsule, even excising adjacent nodes and fat to a moderate degree. Because 10 percent of these lesions are malignant, we feel wide excision is better than capsular or subcapsular enucleation.

Although preoperative alpha blockade and volume expansion have significantly reduced the risk of hypotension following removal of a pheochromocytoma, this potentially disastrous complication cannot be overlooked. If hypotension occurs, appropriate volume expanders should be administered. Central venous pressure monitoring should be used throughout the operative procedure in order to prevent overtransfusion,

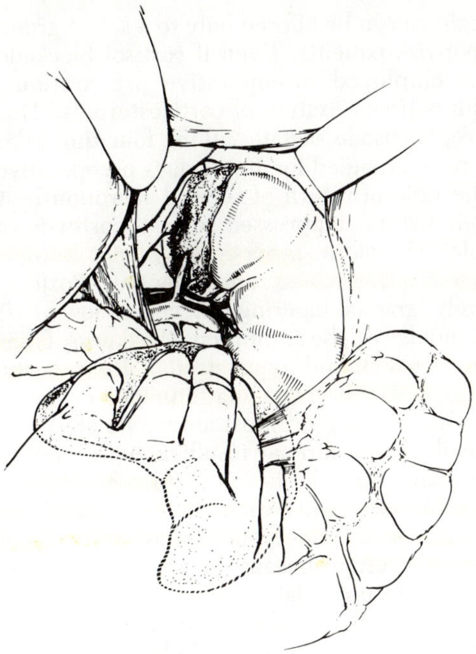

Figure 10–5. Enlarged left-sided lesions, requiring special exposure, with visualization of the celiac axis, superior mesenteric artery, and upper aorta, demands additional incision beyond the mesocolon to include the lienophrenic attachments extending even to the gastroesophageal hiatus in the diaphragm and will allow mobilization of the stomach, spleen, and pancreas medially (indeed, placement in the right side). (From Glenn JF, Peterson RE, Mannix H Jr: Surgery of the Adrenal Gland. New York, Macmillan, 1968, p 158.)

with the resultant sequelae of congestive heart failure, pulmonary edema, and myocardial infarct. When blood products are being used, the potential complications of hepatitis or acquired immune deficiency syndrome (AIDS) must always be considered.

CUSHING'S SYNDROME

Cushing's syndrome is a general term referring to the clinical presentation of corticosteroid excess. This can be produced by administration of glucocorticoid or may occur naturally from several pathologic dysfunctional states. Most commonly, the syndrome is due to Cushing's disease, with the primary focus being a basophilic, corticosteroid-producing adenoma demonstrable on CT scan. A much smaller group, accounting for fewer than 5 percent of patients, is due to ectopic production of ACTH from extra-adrenal tumors. The most common malignant tumors producing ectopic ACTH are oat cell bronchogenic carcinomas, thymic tumors, and islet cell tumors of the pancreas. The third major group causing Cushing's syndrome, comprising between 20 and 35 percent of cases, is that of primary adrenal cortical adenomas or adenocarcinomas.

The clinical presentation of Cushing's syndrome is classic. Prominent findings are truncal obesity with peripheral extremity muscle wasting. Plethora, hypertension, and increased bruising and striae are also prominent features. In the female, amenorrhea and hirsutism may also be seen. On physical examination, the moon facies and buffalo hump are nearly always present.

Diagnosis

In all patients with Cushing's syndrome, serum cortisol levels are elevated. In addition, the normal circadian rhythm, which normally produces peak cortisol levels upon awakening in the morning and trough levels at night, is generally lost. Low-dose dexamethasone administration will usually suppress cortisol levels in the normal patient, whereas it will not usually suppress cortisol in the normal patient with Cushing's syndrome. Low-dose dexamethasone is therefore a good screening test for Cushing's syndrome.

High-dose dexamethasone, 2 mg four times a day for 48 hours, will suppress cortisol levels in patients with bilateral adrenal hyperplasia secondary to a pituitary basophilic adenoma. Those patients whose cortisol levels are not suppressed with high-dose dexamethasone will either have a primary adrenal tumor or an ACTH-producing extra-adrenal tumor. If the serum ACTH levels are low, this indicates suppression by cortisol levels secreted independently from a primary adrenal tumor. If ACTH levels are elevated, independent production of ACTH from an ectopic ACTH-producing malignancy is likely.

It is important to localize adrenal tumors causing Cushing's syndrome because of the surgical implication. CT scanning has been an extremely reliable method of imaging the adenomata. Also, isotopic scanning with iodine 125 (^{125}I) cholesterol and venography, arteriography, and adrenal venous sampling can be done but are usually clinically unnecessary if the CT scan results are definitely positive.

Treatment

The treatment of Cushing's syndrome is directed toward the primary dysfunction. Adrenalectomy is indicated in the 20 to 35 percent of patients in whom the syndrome is caused by primary adrenal tumors. The nearly 60 percent of cases attributable to pituitary adenoma is best treated by transsphenoidal hypophysectomy. In the rare patient with Cushing's disease who does not respond to hypophysectomy, bilateral adrenalectomy through a posterior retroperitoneal approach should be performed.

The small adrenal adenoma producing Cushing's syndrome can be treated by the dorsal approach as described earlier for primary aldosteronism. However, larger tumors, if localized to one side, are best approached through a transverse upper abdominal or thoracoabdominal incision. If malignancy is suspected, wide excision including nephrectomy and regional lymphadenectomy should be performed. In all cases of adrenalectomy for Cushing's syndrome, whether unilateral for adenoma or bilateral for adrenal hyperplasia, the adrenalectomy should be complete because partial adrenalectomy results in many recurrences that necessitates a second operation and further increases the operative risk.

Complications

When an adrenalectomy for a small adenoma or bilateral adrenal hyperplasia is performed through the posterior approach, the patient is subject to all the potential complications discussed in the section on surgery for aldosteronism. Likewise, when the transabdominal approach is used for large tumors that produce Cushing's syndrome, the same complications as previously discussed for the transabdominal approach may be encountered.

Because of the ranges of their primary disease, patients with Cushing's disease are at increased risk for several complications peculiar to Cushing's disease. In extremely poor-risk patients, improvement in their general physical condition can be achieved by completely blocking the synthesis of cortisol at various levels in the adrenal gland, thus completely reversing the metabolically adverse effects of the hyperfunctioning gland. This blockade can best be implemented with the administration of metyrapone, 250 mg four times daily, and aminoglutethimide, 250 mg four times daily. Maintenance therapy with dexamethasone, 0.5 mg three times daily, must be given to prevent adrenal insufficiency.

Because of the expense and undesirable side effects of long-term medical therapy, this drug regimen can be offered only to a select group of poor-risk patients. Even if cortisol blockade is not employed, preoperative preparation requires tissue fixation of corticosteroids. Therefore, cortisone acetate, 50 mg four times daily, is recommended for 1 or 2 days preoperatively. The ratio of return of adrenal secretion by the contralateral suppressed adrenal cortex is variable. Therefore, intraoperative and postoperative corticosterones are essential. Postoperatively, gradual tapering to levels as low as 10 to 15 mg/day can be attempted. Weakness, fatigue, hypotension, and hyponatremia are indications that replacement is inadequate. Postoperatively, the surgeon must always be alert to the possibility of adrenal insufficiency. Even after discharge from the hospital, if nausea and vomiting develop, the patient should always be admitted on an emergency basis for parenteral steroid therapy because acute adrenal insufficiency can prove fatal.

Intraoperative and postoperative bleeding can complicate surgery of any kind or degree. However, the easy friability of tissue makes bleeding a particular problem in patients with Cushing's syndrome. Meticulous hemostasis must be achieved throughout surgery for these patients.

Infection is the most serious postoperative complication, and the signs can be masked by steroid therapy. If unexplained fever, malaise, or ileus develops postoperatively, the patient should be thoroughly examined for a deep wound infection or subphrenic abscess. The failure to diagnose and properly treat either of these complications could prove fatal to the patient.

Wound separation, dehiscence, and evisceration is also more prevalent because of the generally poor tissues and compromised healing capabilities of these patients. Although the authors prefer a transverse transabdominal incision, if one chooses to use a midline transperitoneal approach, strong consideration to a retention suture closure should be given.

Persistent or recurrent hyperadrenocorticism following adrenal surgery for Cushing's syndrome indicates that functional adrenocortical tissue remains, either ectopic or as a result of normotropic adrenal remnants. If this is the case, re-exploration to excise residual functioning tissue is required. Usually, a different approach than that originally utilized should be performed.

References

Donohue JP: Primary aldosteronism. In Kaufman JJ, ed: Current Urologic Therapy, Philadelphia, WB Saunders Co, 1980, p 6.

Egdahl RH: Surgery of the adrenal gland. N Engl J Med 278:939–949, 1968.

Ganguly A, Henry D, Yune HY, Pratt JH, Grim CE, Donohue JP, Weinberger MH: Diagnosis and localization of pheochromocytoma. Am J Med 67:21, 1979.

Glenn JF, Peterson RE, Mannix H Jr: Surgery of the Adrenal Gland. New York, Macmillan Publishing Co, 1968.

Hunt TK, Schambelan M, Biglieri EG: Selection of patients and operative approach in primary aldosteronism. Am Surg 182:353–360, 1975.

Kay R: Intraoperative consultations. Urol Clin North Am 12(3):417–419, 1985.

Liddle GW: Tests of pituitary-adrenal suppressibility in the diagnosis of Cushing's syndrome. J Clin Endocrinol Metab 20:1539–1560, 1960.

Scott HW Jr, Liddle GW, Mulherin JL Jr, et al.: Surgical experience with Cushing's disease. Ann Surg 185:524–534, 1977.

Stephen CR: Anesthesia for adrenal surgery. In Glenn JF, ed: Urol Clin North Am 4:319–328, 1977.

Weinberger MH, Grim CE, Donohue JP, et al.: Primary aldosteronism: diagnosis, localization and treatment. Am Intern Med 90:386, 1979.

COMPLICATIONS OF RENAL SURGERY

11

Robert B. Smith

Complications related to renal surgery can be considered from many different perspectives. Complications, a number of which are common to many urologic procedures, can arise in regard to the general status of the patient. A few of these, however, are more important and need to be emphasized in the management of patients undergoing renal surgery. Also, complications exist relative to the surgical approach to the kidney (including those involving the type of incision used) and to the mobilization of the kidney to perform the desired operation. There are also complications, both intraoperative and postoperative, that are related to each specific operative procedure performed on the kidney as well as those that are related to wound closure. These are considered within the context of this chapter.

PREOPERATIVE EVALUATION OF PATIENT STATUS

Medical complications are discussed quite completely in other chapters, including the metabolic, pulmonary, infectious, hematologic, cardiac, and anesthetic complications detailed in Chapters 1 through 6. In addition, there is a very complete discussion of the nutritional status of the urologic patient in Chapter 7. The material presented in these chapters cannot be overemphasized because the average patient undergoing renal operations is in the older age group.

The patient should enter the operating room well hydrated and in optimal nutritional condition. When a prolonged postoperative period is expected and the patient may not be able to tolerate oral food intake, strong consideration should be given to preoperative hyperalimentation. In patients with a documented preoperative infectious process, culture-specific antibiotics with therapeutic blood levels should be available at the time of surgery. Patients with a strong likelihood of bowel involvement in the disease process (e.g., large renal tumors, multiple prior surgeries, or severe infectious processes) should undergo meticulous preoperative bowel preparation.

The kidney is an extremely vascular organ and because of the chance of significant blood loss with any renal procedures, the coagulation status of the patient must be evaluated in detail. Minimal evaluations include a prothrombin time, partial thromboplastin time, platelet count, and bleeding time. Any abnormality must be identified preoperatively and corrected if possible. Arrangements should be made for the collection of autologous blood in most cases of renal surgery. In addition, all necessary diagnostic tests must be performed to make certain that the procedure can be performed as safely as possible. Preoperative diagnostic tests that are specific for the individual operative procedures are discussed later.

SURGICAL APPROACH TO THE KIDNEY

The surgical approaches to the kidney are many and varied. The incision utilized depends largely on the renal pathology and on the scope of the planned procedure. Also, the location of the kidney varies in individuals, which must be taken into consideration along with consideration of the body habitus.

Each type of incision has advantages and disadvantages as well as variations in the morbidity associated with it. The choice of incisions is left to the discretion of the surgeon, based on his operative experience and expertise. Inadequate incision, regardless of the approach, is responsible for many intraoperative misadventures; a generous incision is desirable in most instances.

Standard Flank Incision

The various flank incisions are still the most widely utilized today for renal surgery. The approach is direct, and the peritoneal cavity is not violated. By avoiding entry into the peritoneal cavity, the introduction of infected drainage material and urine into it is prevented, and the postoperative complications of intestinal adhesions and possible small bowel obstruction are obviated. The incision is particularly suitable for obese patients because the large panniculus in these patients will fall forward, away from the flank area. "Rarely does the fat person have a fat flank."

The disadvantages of flank incisions are that the renal vasculature is not accessible as with anterior approaches and that patients experience increased postoperative pain. Postoperative pain from flank incisions can be alleviated with bupivacaine hydrochloride injections. Also, the incidence of atelectasis and pulmonary complications may be slightly higher in patients with flank incisions. The increased postoperative pain makes deep breathing more difficult, which leads to atelectasis. In addition, with flank incisions, there is a higher chance of pleural entry, causing pneumothorax. If recognized, however, this causes only minimal morbidity.

Flank incisions may not be the best choice in young children because the space between the lower rib and the iliac crest is very small. Also, patients with severe cardiopulmonary compromise may not be able to tolerate the lateral position, especially when the table is flexed. Venous return from the lower extremities can be reduced, and the central venous pressure may fall. In these instances, the patient should be placed in the supine position, hydrated further, and another attempt made to position him. Often there is a fine line between properly hydrating these patients to tolerate the flank position and placing them in fluid overload. Clearly, if a patient cannot tolerate the lateral position, either the procedure should be terminated until the patient's medical condition improves or an alternative anterior approach should be made. In rare instances, disease of the thoracic or lumbar spine (unstable lesions) will contraindicate the flank incision.

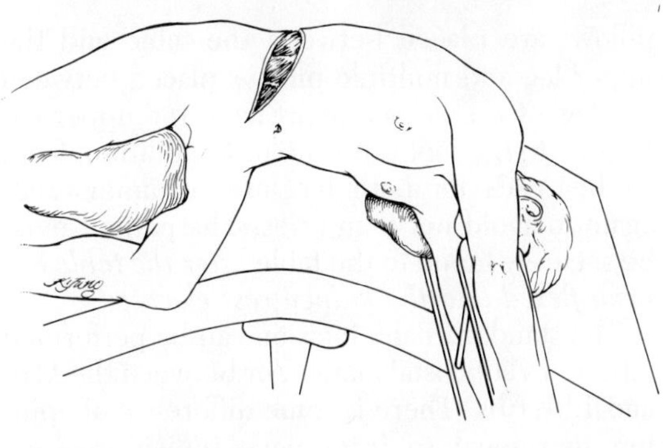

Figure 11–1. Right flank position. The upper extremities are completely supported on a double arm board with an axillary bolster to guard against brachial plexus palsy. (An IV bag is ideal for this use.) A pillow is placed between the lower extremity with the limb closest to the table flexed at the hip and knee. The upper leg is extended at the hip and knee. The patient is then securely taped to the table *after the table has been flexed and the kidney rest elevated.*

Proper positioning of the patient is essential to reducing complications related to flank incisions. Although the anesthesia team and nursing staff participate in the positioning of the patient, the ultimate responsibility is with the surgeon. Figure 11–1 demonstrates the correct flank position for a right flank incision. The patient is placed so that the break in the table is located at the iliac crest. When the table is flexed, there is maximal separation between the iliac crest and the lower rib. A pad is placed under the lowermost axilla to avoid excessive pressure on the brachial plexus, which can result in a severe palsy involving the nerves of the brachial plexus and which can be a basis for litigation postoperatively. Nerve injuries such as this can take a long time to heal and may require extensive postoperative physical therapy. A soft rolled towel is suitable for padding; more recently, a 1-L IV bag has been used with good results.

The patient's upper arm is supported on an "airplane" arm support, which has multiple joints to allow ideal placement of this extremity. The support should also be well padded to prevent any nerve injury. The elbow of the lower arm should be flexed gently, taking care that the lower extremity does not rest on any of the upper extremity supports, again to avoid nerve injury. The leg closest to the table is flexed and multiple pillows are placed between the table and the upper leg and multiple pillows placed between the legs. Complete support from the upper extremity to the foot is essential. In addition, foam rubber pads for both feet are recommended, again to avoid nerve injuries. The patient must be securely taped to the table *after the table has been flexed and the kidney rest elevated.*

The standard flank incision can be performed either in a subcostal manner or between the 11th and 12th ribs. There is some difference of opinion in regard to interspace incisions, i.e., whether it is more advisable to resect a rib and go through the bed of the 11th or 12th rib. In my experience, rib resection is rarely necessary because I feel that the excision of a rib does not improve exposure, and that it *does* increase postoperative pain. (In the late 1960s, an operative procedure was designed to control male incontinence in which a fifth anterior rib was resected subperiosteally for implantation across the pubic arch to provide urethral compression. Whereas the result of this operation was only briefly successful and was thus abandoned, I was very startled in regard to the increased postoperative pain these patients experienced simply from a subperiosteal rib resection.)

Use of the flank incision should be determined by the position of the patient's kidney and by the operation to be performed. It is my feeling that when doubt exists, the higher level should be used because one is rarely compromised by coming in too high on the kidney, whereas a lower than ideal approach can make the operative procedure much more difficult. In all flank approaches, the appropriate intercostal nerve is encountered, and it is a nuisance to the operating surgeon. Although some surgeons simply sacrifice this nerve, I believe that all attempts should be made to preserve it, since transection of the intercostal nerve results in a paresthesia anterior to the incision and in decreased muscle tone in the flank, giving rise to an incisional bulge, which can be confused with an incisional hernia. This bulge can be extremely bothersome to the patient and is a source of much postoperative pain.

The intercostal nerve lies between the internal oblique muscle and the transversus abdominis muscle. On occasion, one can find an apparently significant nerve between the external and internal oblique muscle layers. This nerve can be sacrificed with minimal consequences. If the nerve is inadvertently damaged during the resection, it is probably best to completely transect it. Otherwise, a potentially painful neuritis in the distribution of the nerve may result.

If an incision is to be made through the bed of the 11th or 12th rib in place of a true interspace incision, subperiosteal resection of the rib is preferred. The incision is carried down through the periosteum of the rib, and the periosteal elevator is used to strip the periosteum and its attachments, including the intercostal muscle, from the rib (Fig. 11–2,*A*). The periosteum is more easily stripped away from the rib by pushing the periosteal elevator *down* in the direction of the umbilicus toward the upper side of the rib and upward toward the posterior aspect of the wound on the downside of the rib. The phrase "above forward, below backward" has been used for years to help residents and physicians remember this technique. Alexander periosteal elevators are especially useful during this portion of the procedure.

A Doyen periosteal elevator is employed, moving from the upper aspect of the rib down toward the distal tip of the rib (Fig. 11–2,*B*). Care must be taken in initially passing the Doyen elevator to prevent perforation of the periosteum and entry into the pleural cavity. After the rib has been freed by the Doyen elevator, the posterior aspect of the rib is resected (Fig. 11–2,*C*) with a cutter, and the edges of the rib are then trimmed with a rongeur to remove any sharp, bony spicules that may cause pleural perforation.

As mentioned in the foregoing discussion, in my experience, resection of the rib is not necessary, and totally comparable exposure can be achieved with the simple intercostal incision. The pleura, of course, must be swept superiorly and should be in view at all times. One should not rush this portion of the procedure lest the pleura be entered.

In order to gain exposure with the intercostal approach, the costovertebral ligament must be taken down (Fig. 11–3*A*,*B*). This is felt as a very sharp edge at the posterior aspect of the incision and should be taken down sharply. This maneuver can result in pleural entry if the pleura has not been elevated properly away from the costalvertebral ligament. The use of a Kitner dissector is particularly useful for pushing the pleura away from the chest wall. If incision has been completed and the pleura properly moved away, mobilization begins, and if appropriate, depending upon the procedure, Gerota's fascia is opened. At this time the pleura can be deceivingly adherent to what one thinks is Gerota's fascia at the superior aspect of the incision, and care must

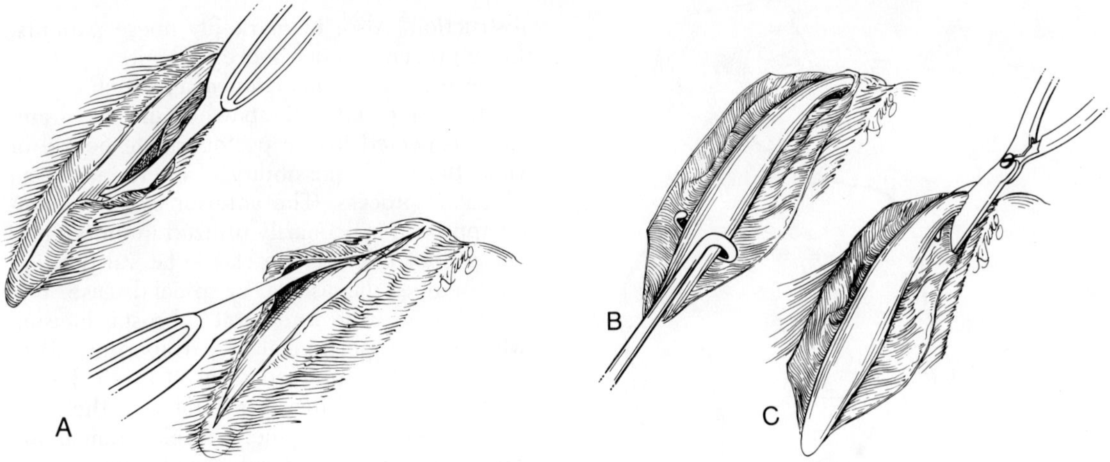

Figure 11–2. *A*, Subperiosteal rib resection. A Doyen periosteal elevator is used to strip the periosteum and muscle attachments from the ribs. On the upper side of the rib, the elevator is employed toward the umbilicus; on the lower side of the rib, it is employed toward the spine of the patient ("above, forward; below, backward"). *B*, The medial aspect is freed, moving from the upper aspect of the rib down toward the distal tip of the rib. Care must be taken initially in passing the Doyen elevator to prevent perforation of the pleura. The elevator is brought out just below the rib to avoid injury to the intercostal nerve. *C*, After the rib has been freed by the Doyen elevator, the posterior aspect of the rib is resected with the cutter. The edges of the rib should then be trimmed with the rongeur to remove any sharp, bony spicules.

be taken not to enter the pleura through a rather cavalier incision in Gerota's fascia.

In closing the flank incision, care must be taken not to include the intercostal nerve in the suture line. In the lower interspace incisions (10th interspace, 11th interspace extrapleural), rib approximation is not necessary. Reapproximation of the anterior and posterior muscles (external and internal obliques, latissimus dorsi, and posterior serratus) will bring ribs together. Unnecessary pericostal sutures may entrap the intercostal nerve and cause postoperative pain.

The choice of sutures to close the incision is left to the surgeon; however, my usual plan is to close the posterior musculature with individual figure-of-eight sutures of 0 polyglactin 910 (Vicryl) in one layer, to close the anterior aspect of the wound in two layers using a running 0 Vicryl suture for the internal oblique and transversus abdominis muscles, and to close the external oblique musculature with interrupted figure-of-eight sutures. In the absence of infection, flank hernia should be a rare consequence of this incision. Marcaine injection in the intercostal

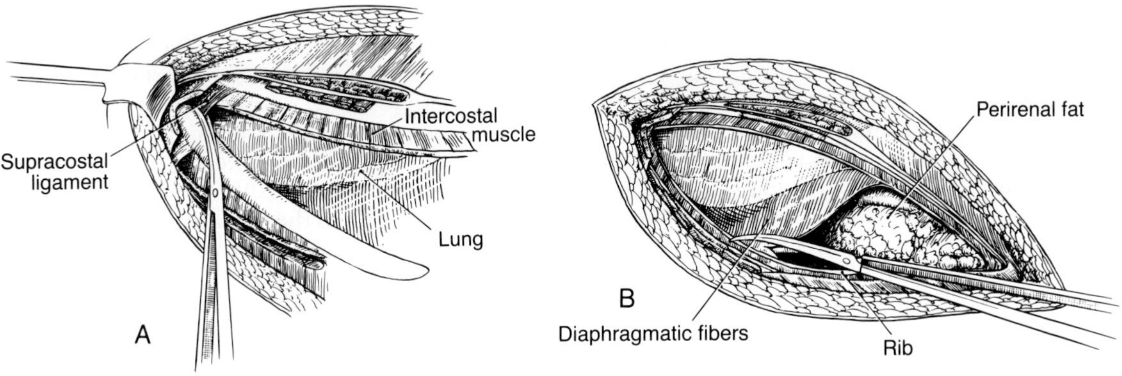

Figure 11–3. *A*, With the intercostal approach, the supracostal ligament must be taken down to allow the inferior rib to hinge downward to avoid fracture. This costovertebral ligament is felt as a very sharp edge at the posterior aspect of the incision and should be taken down sharply. The area of the costovertebral ligament is another potential site of pleural entry if the pleura has not been properly elevated away from the structure. The use of the Kitner dissector is particularly useful for pushing pleura away from the chest wall. *B*, The diaphragmatic fibers, which insert on the underside of the rib, are sharply incised, allowing exposure of the entire field of dissection. Pleura may be deceivingly adherent to what one thinks is Gerota's fascia at the superior aspect of the incision, and care must be taken not to enter the pleura during incision of Gerota's fascia. (From deKernion JB: Radical nephrectomy. In Ehrlich R, ed: Modern Techniques in Surgery. Mt Kisco, NY, Futura Publishing Co, 1980.)

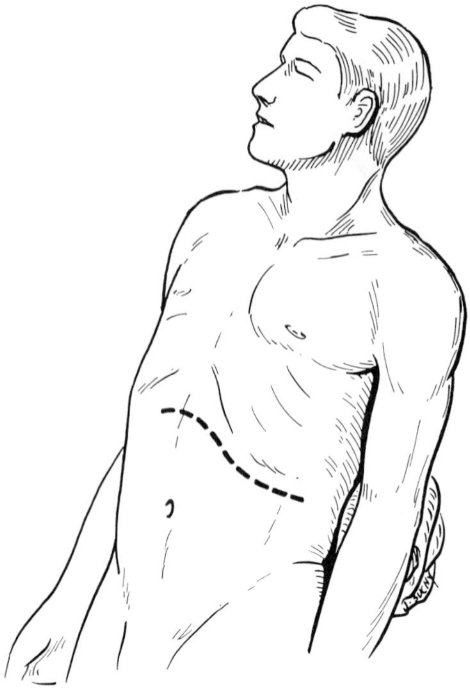

Figure 11–4. Left unilateral subcostal transperitoneal incision. A sheet is rolled beneath the upper lumbar spine, which produces a forward arching of the abdominal wall. The incision obviously can be extended bilaterally to make a classic "chevron" incision.

nerve can lessen postoperative pain considerably.

Anterior Transperitoneal Approach

The principal advantage of this operative approach is that it provides excellent exposure of the vascular structures associated with renal surgery.[1] The vena cava and aortorenal artery and vein can be approached easily before the kidney is manipulated. In addition, the supine position is easily tolerated by most patients. The actual incision used can be a unilateral subcostal incision (Fig. 11–4), a bilateral "chevron" subcostal incision, or a midline transabdominal incision.[2] The incision utilized depends upon the experience of the surgeon and on the procedure to be performed.

The abdominal approach also allows for exploration of the peritoneal contents, which permits the surgeon to perform a combined procedure (e.g., cholecystectomy and renal exploration) in selected patients with associated disease of intra-abdominal organs. The disadvantage of this approach is the formation of adhesions with the potential for future small bowel obstruction. Also, in markedly obese patients, this approach is much more difficult.

The anterior *extraperitoneal* approach is preferable in selected patients when urinary drainage is expected in the postoperative period or when there is a possibility of operating on an infectious process. The anterior *extra-abdominal* approach is primarily utilized in individuals who cannot tolerate the classic lateral position because of cardiovascular or spinal disease. It is helpful to use the unilateral subcostal incision (whether intraperitoneal or extraperitoneal) to pull the patient upward to a 30 to 45 degree angle with a mild flex in the table at the level of the upper lumbar spine. This elevation allows extension of the incision upward between the 11th and 12th ribs if problems of exposure are encountered. The incision begins anteriorly below the costal margin and extends laterally toward the anterior axillary line. As mentioned previously, this can be extended upward as far back as the midline or even the posterior axillary line if necessary. The incision can be extended across the midline into the contralateral rectus sheath and muscle, if needed, to obtain adequate exposure. Medial extension of this incision can affect exposure in the area containing the great vessels.

Thoracoabdominal Incision

The thoracoabdominal incision is preferred by many surgeons for adrenal surgery and radical nephrectomies.[3,4] The exposure of the upper pole of the kidney is unparalleled compared with other incisions. This incision also facilitates the regional lymphadenectomy, which many surgeons feel to be important to perform along with radical nephrectomy.

The thoracoabdominal incision can be performed through the 9th interspace or through the bed of the 9th or 10th rib. The pleura is formally opened and the diaphragm incised. The phrenic nerve should be avoided when the diaphragmatic incision is made. Superior exposure afforded by this incision is counterbalanced by the increased operative time necessary to close it and by the need for a chest tube in the postoperative period. However, an additional advantage is the potential to palpate the ipsilateral lung in selected patients.

It is necessary to perform a very careful closure of this diaphragm (the methods of which can be varied and are up to the individual surgeon) to prevent a diaphragmatic hernia. A rib approximator as well as pericostal sutures with 2–0 chromic catgut must be utilized to approximate the ribs. A chest tube is brought out through a separate stab wound. The chest tube should be placed to Pleurovac suction for the initial 24 to 48 hours and then placed under water seal for at least an additional 24 hours until the drainage has decreased. It is my practice to leave a chest tube in place until the amount of fluid produced is less than 100 ml/day. It is rarely necessary to replace a chest tube or to perform thoracentesis if these guidelines are followed.

Posterior Approach

The posterior approach to the kidney has been popularized by Vernet, but in my experience, it is used only on rare occasions. The main advantage of this incision is that it causes less morbidity from incisional pain, but this is at a cost of decreased surgical exposure. This approach, of course, is an excellent incision for the patient in the prone position who requires bilateral adrenal exploration. When it is used for renal surgery, I feel that the patient should rarely be placed in the prone position because the kidney usually falls away from the surgeon. The incision, however, can be made with the patient in a straight lateral position that does not require flexing of the operative table as required in the standard flank incision.

The exposure of the great vessels and renal artery and vein is limited by this incision, and it may be very difficult to control inadvertent damage to these vessels, which may result in significant hemorrhage. There have been instances in which it has been necessary to securely pack the wound posteriorly and to immediately turn the patient over for exploration either through the flank or transabdominally to gain control of the hemorrhage sites.

ABDOMINAL EXPLORATION

In transabdominal cases, after the peritoneal cavity has been entered, a thorough exploration of the abdomen is performed. When the right kidney is to be exposed, the ascending colon and hepatic flexure of the colon are taken down, beginning with an incision along the white line of Toldt. The colon is reflected medially. The second portion of the duodenum comes into view, and this is reflected medially (as with the Koher maneuver) by incising the posterior peritoneum

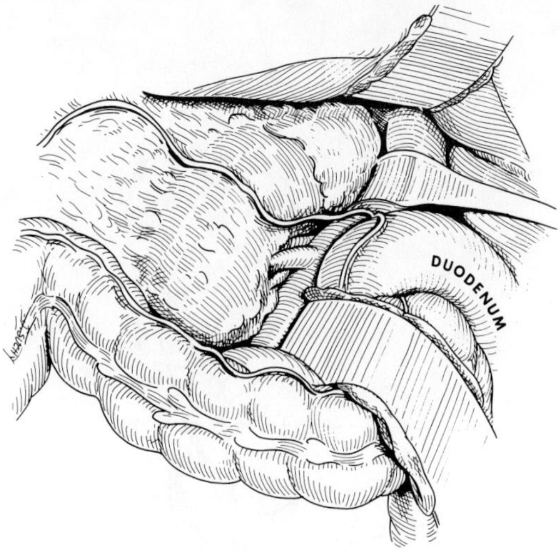

Figure 11–5. Mobilization of the right colon and retroperitoneal portion of the duodenum. After the posterior peritoneum has been incised along the white line of Toldt, the colon is reflected medially. The second portion of the duodenum comes into view and is reflected medially as with the Kocher maneuver by gently dissecting the second portion of the duodenum off the vena cava.

parallel to the duodenum and by gently dissecting the second portion of the duodenum off the vena cava (Fig. 11–5).

Care should be taken during this portion of the procedure not to injure the duodenum. If entry is made in the duodenum, this should be closed very carefully in at least two layers, utilizing an inverting type of suture for the outer seromuscular layer. It is also wise to wrap omentum around this area at the end of the procedure. Hematomas of the duodenum, if enlarging, should be incised and the bleeding sites identified and controlled. The serosa should be reapproximated in a manner similar to the procedure used for closure of the duodenum, and omental tissue should be wrapped around this area as well.

The left kidney is approached by mobilization of the descending colon medially and by the taking down of the splenic flexure (Fig. 11–6). This incision is also made in the peritoneum lateral to the colon along the white line of Toldt. The incision is then carried up the splenic flexure, making certain that the entire splenocolic ligament is taken down. Subsequent traction on the spleen may cause a capsular tear, and the spleen should be carefully inspected at the end of the procedure to ensure that injury has not occurred.

It may be difficult to get into the plane between the mesentery of the descending colon

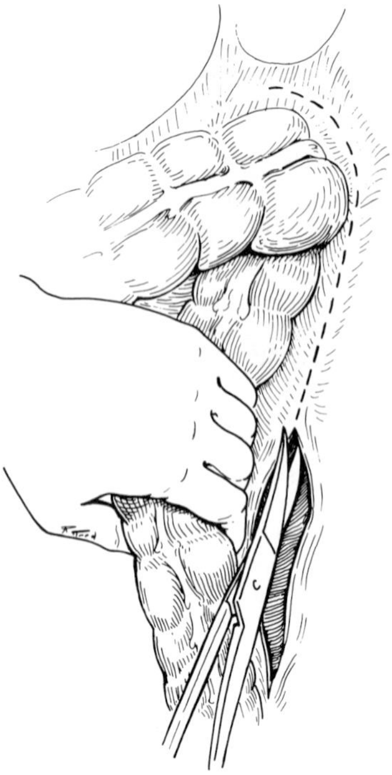

Figure 11–6. The left kidney is approached by mobilization of the descending colon medially and taking down the splenic flexure. The renocolic ligament is divided. All attachments between the colon and spleen must be completely divided to prevent inadvertent splenic injury from traction on the spleen. The spleen should be carefully inspected at the end of the case to ensure that inadvertent injury has not occurred.

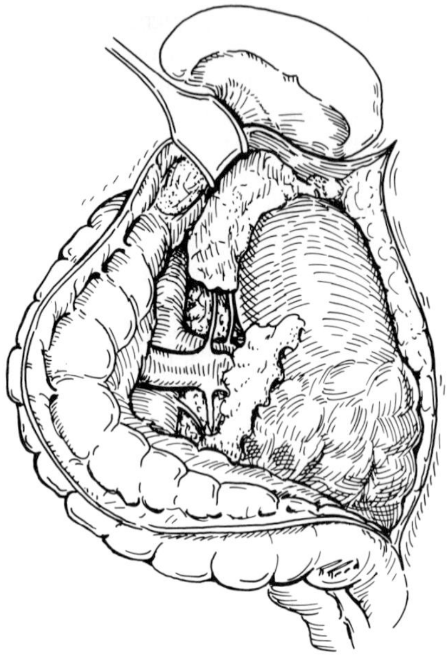

Figure 11–7. The colon is mobilized medially after the splenic flexure has been taken down. Special care should be taken to keep the proper plane between the mesocolon and the anterior aspect of Gerota's fascia. Mesenteric injuries can occur during this phase of the procedure. If the major vessel of the mesentery is injured and if ligation is necessary, careful inspection of the colon in regard to viability must be made.

and Gerota's fascia (Fig. 11–7). Mesenteric injuries can occur during this portion of the procedure. If a major vessel of the mesentery is injured and if ligation is necessary, careful inspection of the colon in regard to viability must be performed. If any question of colon viability is present, I believe that considering the possibility of litigation, a general surgeon should be called in for consultation.

Mesenteric damage occurs primarily in patients with large renal cancers or inflammatory disease of the kidney. Such patients should have a meticulous preoperative bowel preparation, which will facilitate correction of the colon problem should this occur. Defects within the colon mesentery must be closed to prevent subsequent herniation.

COMPLICATIONS OF RENAL EXPOSURE

Pneumothorax

Pneumothorax may occur with any flank exposure involving an interspace or rib resection. Strict attention to detail will minimize this possibility. It is certainly not of major importance to enter the pleura, but obviously recognition is essential. Small tears in the pleura may not be noted intraoperatively, and to guard against postoperative problems, all patients who have had flank incisions should undergo routine chest x-ray in the recovery room. If a pneumothorax exceeding 15 percent is found, needle aspiration via the anterior 4th or 5th interspace usually will resolve the problem. Rarely is it necessary to insert a chest tube in these patients. Patients without respiratory distress or mediastinal shift and with a pneumothorax of less than 15 percent can be followed expectantly. This air is rapidly absorbed and is of no consequence. On occasion, mediastinal or subcutaneous air can be seen on this postoperative chest x-ray and is no cause for alarm.

Small tears can be noted intraoperatively if the wound is filled with saline and if the anesthesiologist is instructed to give a deep inspiration by hand. This is also helpful after closing recognized pleural tears to make certain that the closure has been adequate. If the pleura is opened, it should be closed utilizing 3–0 or 4–0 chromic catgut sutures, leaving a Robinson catheter in place at one extremity of the pleural closure. A pursestring suture is then placed around the Robinson catheter, and the air is evacuated from the pleural cavity either by suction on the catheter or by placing this under water seal. Using negative pressure, the tube is rapidly removed and the pursestring suture simultaneously tied.

Rarely is it necessary to leave a chest tube in place in these individuals unless a formal thoracoabdominal incision has been performed. A follow-up chest x-ray in the recovery room is, of course, mandatory to make certain that the pneumothorax has been corrected. The same criteria of aspiration apply as with the undetected tears.

Splenic Injuries

Injury can occur with any exposure of the left kidney, but splenic injury is the most common intraoperative complication during left radical nephrectomy.[5] This complication is reported as being as high as 12 percent of patients who undergo radical nephrectomy. If splenic tear has occurred, the entire spleen should be thoroughly inspected. One should attempt to salvage the spleen if possible. Certainly, mild or even moderate splenic lacerations can be treated conservatively without splenectomy.

Avitene is of great help in managing splenic injury; closure of the spleen is done with bolsters of Surgicel in addition to Avitene. Minor lacerations need no closure; Avitene application alone can control the majority of these. Severe lacerations of the spleen mandate splenectomy. In patients experiencing severe hemorrhage from the spleen, bleeding can be controlled by compressing the splenic artery and vein. The sac is opened, and the tail of the pancreas is pressed between the thumb and forefinger to compress these structures.

If splenectomy is mandated, the attachments from the colon and kidney should be taken down as well as the lateral peritoneal attachments and the attachments to the diaphragm. This allows the spleen to be delivered into the center of the wound. The tail of the pancreas is identified in the hilum of the spleen and sharply dissected away, which is facilitated by dividing the short gastric vessels. The splenic artery and vein can then be identified and ligated and transected. The tail of the pancreas must be carefully inspected to make sure that no damage has occurred to this structure.

Patients who have undergone splenectomy have reduced resistance to bacteria that have a polysaccharide capsule. These bacteria include pneumococcal organisms as well as species of *Streptococcus, E. coli, Staphylococcus aureus*, and *Haemophilus influenzae*. These patients should receive Pneumovax therapy on a periodic basis and should be given prophylactic penicillin for dental work or other procedures that have an inherent risk of bacteremia.[6–8]

Pancreatic Injuries

Pancreatic mobilization is often necessary for renal surgery, particularly in the treatment of left-sided lesions, which are approached anterotransabdominally. Any pancreatic mobilization carries the risk of the patient developing pancreatitis. Patients should be monitored in the postoperative period for chemical pancreatitis to determine serum amylase and urinary diastase levels. Patients with chemical pancreatitis are probably best managed with delayed feeding and prolonged nasogastric drainage because premature feeding can result in a more serious pancreatic complication.

In patients with a persistently elevated amylase, computed tomography (CT) scans should be performed to check for pancreatic edema or fluid collection in or around the pancreas. Any fluid that accumulates should be aspirated and checked for pH concentration and amylase content. Characteristically, pancreatic fluid is alkaline, with a pH concentration in a 7.0 to 8.5 range. If a leak of pancreatic fluid is found, drainage is mandatory.

The pancreas is at its greatest risk of injury during dissection of the superior medial aspect of the left kidney. It is also at risk during manipulation of the second portion of the duodenum during the Kocher maneuver and during exposure of the right renal hilum. It is especially important to use a well-padded retractor during retraction of the head of the pancreas. Lacerations or tears in this area are rare, but contusions are not uncommon if retraction is traumatic. Pancreatic lacerations occur mainly with left renal procedures associated with mobilization of the tail and mid-portion of the pancreas. These injuries need to be carefully evaluated to see if the pancreatic duct is injured or whether the tear is strictly into the pancreatic parenchyma. Laceration of the parenchyma, as long as the duct is intact, can be repaired simply by closing the pancreatic capsule with nonabsorbable suture material. The pancreatic enzyme can cause premature disintegration of absorbable sutures before the healing is complete. It is essential that all tears, whether or not they involve the ducts, be accompanied by some drainage, with the drain exiting through the retroperitoneal space.

If injury to the pancreatic duct is not recognized, there is a tremendous increase in morbidity and mortality associated with this injury. Injuries involving the distal two thirds of the pancreas with ductal injuries can be managed by resection of the distal portion of the pancreas with a suture ligation of the duct and closure of the pancreatic capsule of the respective end. If possible, general surgical consultation should be requested. It is rarely indicated to reanastomose the transected duct because of the prohibitive risk of postoperative complications. This is especially applicable if the renal collecting system has been opened and repaired during the renal portion of the operation.

Patients who develop a pancreatic fistula need not be re-explored. They should be treated with long-term parenteral hyperalimentation until spontaneous healing of the fistula has occurred. Rarely is surgical closure of the fistula necessary.

Liver Injuries

Injuries to the liver are generally related to rough surgical technique. These obviously occur more commonly with right-sided renal surgery. Retractors must be well padded to prevent injury. Liver lacerations are the most common injury and may simply be repaired with horizontal mattress sutures utilizing a Surgicel bolster. Direct involvement of the liver by renal pathology is exceedingly rare; often a CT scan overestimates the potential for hepatic involvement with renal pathology.

Deep lacerations of the liver, which may involve a bile leak, should be drained. Deep lacerations or avulsion injuries to the liver that are associated with troublesome hemorrhage may require cross clamping of the porta hepatis (Pringle maneuver) until the patient can be stabilized. On occasions when there is direct involvement of the liver by a renal process, partial hepatectomy may be necessary. Major resections should be performed by a general surgical team.

Duodenal Injuries

Injuries to the duodenum most commonly involve the second portion and occur during mobilization for exposure of the right renal hilum. Duodenal lacerations should be closed in multiple layers with interrupted sutures, utilizing nonabsorbable sutures for the serosa layer. Omental wrap and prolonged nasogastric drainage are helpful in preventing subsequent duodenal fistulas.

Duodenal hematomas must be observed closely. If they increase in size, they must be opened to identify and control the bleeding site. Subsequent closure of the serosa is performed with omental wrap, as discussed in the foregoing section. General surgical consultation, of course, should be sought for severe injuries.

Colonic Injuries

Injury to the colon itself should be rare. Patients in whom there is high index of suspicion of colon involvement by a primary renal pathology (large renal cell carcinomas, xanthogranulomatous pyelonephritis) should undergo meticulous bowel preparation. In such patients, segmental colonic resection is straightforward with reanastomosis. If mesenteric vascular damage occurs and there is some question about viability of the colon, exteriorization of the colon should be performed with secondary reoperation to restore the continuity of the colon. Again, general surgical consultation is advisable. Colonic mesenteric defects should be closed to prevent subsequent internal herniation.

Adrenal Injuries

Injury to the ipsilateral adrenal gland is not uncommon in difficult mobilizations of the kidney associated with infectious processes or prior surgery. Tears in the adrenal can cause significant bleeding that is usually venous in origin. A torn adrenal gland may be oversewn with running 4–0 absorbable sutures, which is, to my mind, preferable to the indiscriminate application of hemostatic clips.

In patients in whom a contralateral adrenal is present, resection of the remaining portion of the gland may be the most expeditious way to control this hemorrhage. The right renal vein is particularly susceptible to injury because of its short course and direct insertion into the vena cava, which is rather inflexible in this area. Avulsion of the adrenal vein can cause rather impressive hemorrhage. Initial control with pressure is applied until adequate suction can be obtained to find the site of evulsion. This is nicely controlled with Allis clamps until the cavotomy can be closed with running 5–0 vascular sutures.

CONSIDERATIONS RELATED TO SPECIFIC RENAL OPERATIVE PROCEDURES

Radical Nephrectomy

Radical nephrectomy continues to be the recommended surgical treatment for renal cell carcinoma, although recent evidence suggests that this may not be mandatory in all patients with renal cell carcinoma. The term radical nephrectomy suggests control of the renovasculature before significant manipulation of the kidney is performed. It also includes removal of Gerota's fascia and the ipsilateral adrenal gland, and it generally includes a regional lymphadenectomy. Diagnostic techniques, including renal ultrasonography, CT imaging, magnetic resonance imaging (MRI), and angiography, generally characterize most lesions, making exploration of most symptomatic renal masses rarely necessary. With increased use of ultrasonography and CT imaging, many incidental renal masses are identified. At times it is more difficult to characterize these, and many of these lesions need to be explored, which is discussed in a subsequent section.

The preoperative work-up for patients with renal cell carcinoma includes accurate staging of the local lesions as well as evaluations to exclude metastatic disease. Tumor thrombus extending from the renal vein into the vena cava occurs in from 4 to 10 percent of patients.[9–12] It is essential to make a preoperative diagnosis because the surgical procedure and approach to the kidney may have to be changed dramatically should this exist.

Tumor thrombi of the vena cava can be diagnosed with the aid of inferior venacavography, selective renal venography, and CT scanning techniques. More recent use of MRI has been a great aid in determining the extent of involvement of the vena cava and in some cases gives better imaging than the venacavography. It is essential to know the upward extent of the tumor, and in some instances a superior right heart catheter, permitting visualization of the right atrium and the superior portion of the inferior vena cava, is necessary. However, radical nephrectomy is currently the most effective method of management of localized renal cell carcinoma. Excision of Gerota's fascia and its contents is logically the most effective method of controlling local disease. The biologic potential of this malignancy may, in fact, be a more important predictor in regard to clinical outcome than the actual surgical procedure performed.

The addition of regional lymphadenectomy and its importance is still debatable. Surgeons who favor regional lymphadenectomy point to the occasional patient with positive nodes who can be cured and also emphasize the fact that a regional lymphadenectomy adds little to the morbidity associated with radical nephrectomy and adds little increase in operative time. Prognostic information is also gathered by lymphadenectomy to help the patient plan his personal affairs in the future.

People who do not favor routine lymphadenectomy point out the poor survival rate for patients with positive nodes (5 to 10 percent in 5 years)[13] and also the fact that lymphatic drainage from a renal cell tumor occurs in a very haphazard fashion when the hilar lymphatics have been occluded by tumor cells. Therefore, the primary site of lymph node metastasis may not be near the hilum at all and lymph nodes throughout the peritoneal cavity may be involved. Also, they point out that blood flow spread from renal cell carcinoma is at least as common as lymphatic metastases. Nevertheless, it is my position to perform regional lymphadenectomy because valuable staging information is obtained and the addition of a limited lymphadenectomy does not increase morbidity.

Preoperative embolization of the renal artery is rarely used in my experience because the expense of and complications associated with the procedure, including fever, nausea, vomiting, and pain, outweigh the benefits. When a CT scan indicates possible extensive hilar involvement of lymph nodes in tumor in which access to the renal artery may be difficult, preoperative embolization may have a place and has been used in my experience. This will help to reduce blood loss during nephrectomy.

The choice of incision is left primarily to the surgeon, but it also depends on the anticipated pathology. Radical nephrectomy can be equally well accomplished by a transperitoneal approach, through a standard flank incision at the 10th or 11th interspace or at the 11th or 12th rib, or through a true thoracoabdominal incision. Each method has its virtues, which have been discussed previously. The worst possible scenario is to have an incision that is too low to gain adequate control of a lesion involving the upper pole. It is my feeling that an extraperitoneal approach is never indicated for renal carcinoma surgery because it is essential to perform intraperitoneal exploration to detect unsuspected metastasis. (Tumor involvement of the vena cava involves different considerations and is discussed later.)

Radical nephrectomy involves early control of the renal vasculature and excision of the kidney and ipsilateral adrenal gland, including all of Gerota's fascia and perinephric fat. In my opinion, the procedure should include a regional lymphadenectomy. In a transabdominal approach, the midline incision is the most commonly used. However, in obese patients, an upper chevron incision is helpful, especially in those who have had prior lower abdominal surgery. In extremely obese patients or in patients with lesions that are very high, the thoracoabdominal approach is preferred. In left-sided tumors, the descending colon is mobilized medially, and the attachment of the spleen to the kidney is taken down carefully as outlined in the aforementioned discussion in the splenic injury section.

Direct invasion of the spleen is a rare event, but splenic injury is very common in radical nephrectomy. Often the spleen has been displaced upward by the renal neoplasm, making exposure of this area difficult. Also, with large lesions, the spleen often has been displaced anteriorly and may lie directly over the hilum, thus affecting exposure.

Complete splenic mobilization facilitates radical nephrectomy. In performing this mobilization, obviously one must be careful in handling the pancreas to avoid pancreatic injuries, which are perhaps more frequent in radical nephrectomies than in any other renal operation. The initial part of the procedure should be to identify and isolate the renal artery and vein. Extreme care must be exercised during this portion of the procedure, especially with large left-sided lesions. I have seen other vessels, including the celiac axis, superior mesenteric artery, and contralateral renal artery, misidentified as renal arteries. The chance of confusing these vessels, especially the contralateral renal artery, is exaggerated when the patient is in the lateral position.

The left and right renal arteries are very close together in the lateral position when one considers anteroposterior relationship. Often one can slide over the aorta without knowing it and identify the contralateral renal artery as the ipsilateral renal artery. Absolute certainty regarding the identification of these vessels is mandatory before transection can be performed. If major vessels are transected and the transection is identified, reanastomosis should be performed expeditiously. For vessels that have been simply ligated but not transected, simple deligation can suffice. However, one must make sure that reflow in the involved vessel has been established and continues throughout the operation. The obvious risk of ligation injury is an intimal disruption with dissection and thrombosis.

Injury to these aforementioned vessels is much more common with left radical nephrectomy than with right radical nephrectomy. (In fact, I have never seen these structures injured during the course of a right radical nephrectomy.) In the abdominal approach, the best way to reach the left renal hilum is to follow the inferior mesenteric vein up toward the splenic vein. It is then isolated, ligated, and divided. This immediately exposes the left renal vein and the underlying left renal artery. The left renal arteries should be ligated before the vein to prevent congestion of the kidney. Division of the artery is generally deferred until the vein has been ligated and transected because this is more easily accomplished after the vein has been divided.

Generally the hilar structures are doubly ligated with heavy silk and reinforced with a large Liga clip. After securing the renal hilum, the left colon is reflected medially along the white line of Toldt (see Fig. 11–6). The splenocolic ligament is divided as well to avoid splenic injury. The left colon and splenic flexure are retracted, also to avoid injury.

In patients with large renal cell carcinomas, on occasion the colon or its mesentery can be involved with tumor and may be difficult to resect. Those patients should undergo a meticulous preoperative bowel preparation so that colon resection can be accomplished with reanastomosis in the usual fashion.

After the kidney has been mobilized and removed, a unilateral lymphadenectomy is performed as part of nephrectomy, isolating lymph nodes along the aorta, going no farther distal than the mesenteric artery and working superiorly to the level of the superior mesenteric artery. Lymph nodes from the medial aspect of the aorta to the sympathetic chain are removed during this dissection. In patients with tumors that invade the body wall, it is appropriate to take body wall musculature with the specimen. We have been gratified to see a low incidence of local recurrence in such patients. One should be especially cognizant of the fact that there is a left lumbar vein, which often drains into the renal vein, that can be avulsed during this procedure. If this occurs, it often retracts backward into the posterior paraspinus muscles and must be controlled with pressure. Deep suture ligatures of nonabsorbable 3–0 to 4–0 material will then control this hemorrhage.

Because of the collateral blood flow to large renal cell carcinomas, blood loss can be considerable and the anesthesiologist should be forewarned of this possibility. Adequate units should be typed and crossmatched, and two intravenous lines should be available for rapid blood replacement, should this become necessary. If the patient becomes hypotensive from blood loss during the procedure, the bleeding can always be controlled by packing the wound, allowing the anesthesiologist to "catch up."

Right radical nephrectomy is associated with the aforementioned potential liver and duodenal injuries. The duodenum must be carefully mobilized and retractors carefully padded to prevent injuries to this structure as well as to the head of the pancreas. Direct invasion of the liver by a right renal cell carcinoma is rare, but when noted, appropriate liver resection should be accomplished. If major lobectomy is required, a general surgeon should be present at the procedure.

Liver lacerations and duodenal injuries are reviewed in the foregoing discussion. It is well known to all urologists that the involvement of the vena cava with tumor is much more common with right-sided tumors. Every patient with right-sided renal cell carcinoma *must* undergo preoperative investigation of the vena cava by the aforementioned method. (The management of vena caval tumor thrombi is discussed later.)

In patients with large right-sided renal tumors or in patients in whom a large tumor thrombus involves the renal vein, it is often easier and more expeditious to obtain control of the renal artery as it exits from the aorta. This is accomplished by mobilizing the vena cava laterally to expose the right renal artery at its takeoff. However, large lumbar veins can be avulsed in this process, and these must be identified and individually ligated to prevent this complication. As noted, these vessels often retract and require deep suture ligation to control.

The adrenal gland is of special concern in right radical nephrectomy because of the short adrenal vein that inserts directly into the vena cava. Avulsion injuries can occur with large renal tumors. A thoracoabdominal incision is especially advantageous for large upper pole tumors, and it is my incisional choice for these types of tumors. It obviously has the additional advantage of permitting exploration of the ipsilateral lung and mediastinum in patients in whom possible metastatic disease exists.

If a solitary metastasis is found and it is resectable, it is possible to obtain long-term survival in these patients (up to 25 percent at 5 years), and one should proceed with the operation.[14] A finding of multiple metastatic lesions or the involvement of the liver with metastatic disease should persuade the surgeon to terminate the nephrectomy unless the patient is symptomatic from the primary lesion or is involved in an investigative protocol with immune manipulation. Most studies indicate that the response rate to immune manipulation is greater in those patients with a reduced tumor burden.

The closure of a thoracoabdominal incision is more difficult and more time consuming than that of the midline inferior abdominal incision. Careful diaphragmatic closure must be performed to guard against diaphragmatic hernia formation. A chest tube is required.

Tumor extension from the renal vein into the inferior vena cava occurs in up to 10 percent of patients with renal cell carcinoma. The surgical approach (i.e., type of incision used) is greatly affected by the superior limit of the tumor extension into the vena cava as well as by the laterality of the tumor. It is mandatory in the preoperative evaluation of such patients to assess the superior extent of this tumor thrombus. The MRI scan is a superior tool in this regard and may, in fact, be superior to venacavography.

Often patients with renal cell carcinoma and tumor extension have undergone a myriad of diagnostic studies that involve the injection of contrast material. It is not uncommon for a patient to rapidly undergo an evaluation with intravenous pyelography (IVP), CT scan with contrast, renal angiography, inferior venacavography, and right heart catheterization. This contrast load exposes the patient to potential nephrotoxicity, which may be exceedingly important in the postoperative period. If these studies are performed on the patient preoperatively, enough time should elapse to make certain that nephrotoxicity has not occurred in the kidney that is to remain.

The MRI scan to evaluate the caval thrombus yields information that equals, if not surpasses, that gained from inferior venacavography and combined right heart catheterization and, of course, involves no additional contrast agent with its inherent toxicity. In fact, I have seen patients in whom the MRI scan has picked up extension of tumor beyond what was thought to exist on inferior venacavography. In the vast majority of patients with conditions involving the vena cava, the tumor originates from the right side. Left-sided renal cell carcinomas with caval extension present an extraordinary operative problem.

Usually extension involves a simple protrusion of tumor thrombus from the renal vein into the vena cava of only a few centimeters. Those tumors that are confined below the hepatic veins can be managed in a rather straightforward fashion through the aforementioned standard techniques. It is, nevertheless, my preference to approach these patients with a right thoracoabdominal incision just in case the superior extent of the tumor has been underestimated. With the use of the thoracoabdominal incision, the mobilization of the liver is facilitated, and division of the triangular and hepatic coronary ligaments can be performed much more easily than through the anterior approach, permitting the surgeon to gain suprahepatic control of the vena cava if necessary.

In patients with renal vein and venous involvement, I generally approach the renal vein and vena caval thrombus as the last portion of the procedure. Initially the renal artery is ligated after exposure by gentle deflection of the renal vein or from a posterior approach to the hilum. On occasion, the tumor thrombus within the renal vein is so bulky that one fears manipulation of the renal vein may cause the tumor thrombus to fragment, allowing it to dislodge and flow into the atrium. In such patients, it is far better to mobilize the vena cava laterally, taking down the necessary lumbar vessels to gain exposure of the right renal artery at its takeoff and at the aorta. It is then ligated in this position.

After the tumor has been mobilized circumferentially by the aforementioned techniques, attention is given to the transection of the renal vein with extraction of the tumor thrombus. At this point in the procedure, it is vitally important that the patient's blood has been adequately replaced and that the patient is not in a precarious state as a result of fluid depletion. If problems exist, this portion of the operation should be delayed to allow the anesthesiologist to correct such problems.

Patients with caval thrombus should have at least two large-caliber venous lines as well as a central venous line or a Swan-Ganz monitor. The vena cava is mobilized distal to the tumor thrombus. The entire vena cava is also mobilized proximal to the superior aspect of the thrombus, taking down the necessary lumbar veins. The left renal vein is also isolated and encircled with tape. Tumors that extend up into the intrahepatic portions of the vena cava can be approached by taking down the first or second hepatic vein to allow the vascular clamp to be placed across the vena cava at this point. Tumors that extend beyond this region require complete mobilization of the liver to expose the suprahepatic subdiaphragmatic portion of the vena cava. For tumors that extend beyond the diaphragm, it is important to have a cardiac team available to place the patient on cardiopulmonary bypass if necessary. Also, a median sternotomy incision is probably preferable to a lateral approach in this situation. We have, on occasion, used bypass and dealt with these lesions from the lateral position, and it can indeed be accomplished.

The vena cava below the tumor thrombus is occluded first and a few seconds allowed to pass to see what hemodynamic effect this has on the patient. The renal vein is then occluded and if one anticipates a prolonged time to extract the tumor from the vena cava, i.e., if there is some evidence of possible tumor adherence to the wall and invasion, and if the tumor is at the level of the hepatic veins, the porta hepatis should be occluded as well to decrease venous return from the hepatic vessels (Pringle maneuver). As mentioned previously, most of the lumbar veins have been controlled during the mobilization with the vena cava. If a vascular clamp can be placed proximal to the tumor thrombus, it is occluded before the vena cava is opened (Fig. 11–8). If the tumor is situated just superior to where the clamp can be placed, an alternative approach to complete the mobilization of the vena cava up to the diaphragm would be to place the clamp around the vena cava but not to occlude it until after the tumor thrombus has been pulled down below this level during the extraction. Rapid occlusion is then performed.

An incision is made around the renal vein as it enters the vena cava, extending it superiorly, if necessary (Fig. 11–9), and then extracting the tumor from the vena cava. This lessens the likelihood of caval narrowing for bulky thrombi. If the tumor adheres to the vena cava, it can be removed in a piecemeal fashion, apparently without affecting curability. It is of utmost importance in patients undergoing such procedures to have complete visualization of the vena

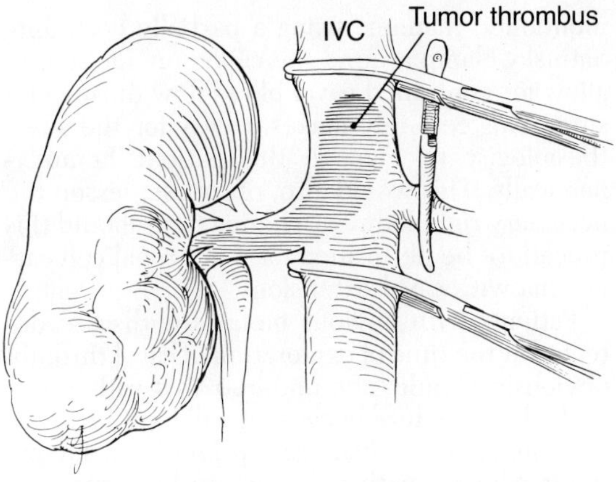

Figure 11–8. Infradiaphragmatic extension of tumor thrombus into the inferior vena cava. The lumbar veins have been ligated to allow total mobilization of the cava. If the tumor extends above the level of the first hepatic vein, complete mobilization of the liver may be necessary. The renal vein must be temporarily occluded during the process. Because of collateral venous outflow from the left kidney, control of the left renal artery is not necessary. Clamps are placed proximal and distal to the thrombus before the cava is opened. (From deKernion JB, Smith RB: The kidney and adrenal glands. In Paulson D, ed: Genitourinary Surgery. New York, Churchill Livingstone Publishers, 1984.)

cava, which requires control of all vessels in this area. In higher lesions, this should be done with the aid of cardiopulmonary bypass with exsanguination to allow complete inspection of the vena cava in a controlled situation.

When excising the renal vein from the vena cava, one must be careful not to incise too far into the vena cava on the posterior aspect. Unnecessary narrowing of the vena cava can result in complications of lower venous hypertension and thrombosis of the cava. I have seen one patient with caval thrombosis in whom simple thrombectomy and anticoagulation did not suffice, and the patient subsequently had to undergo reconstruction of the caval wall with a vena caval graft of Goretex. Pericardium has also been used for this purpose.

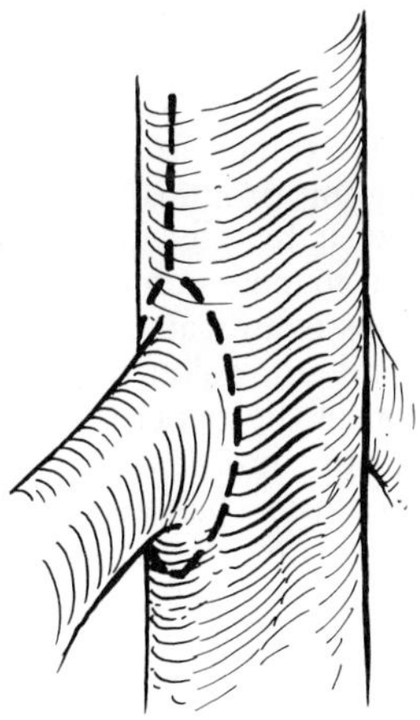

Figure 11–9. Caval incision. An incision is made around the renal vein and the vena cava, extended superiorly if necessary. Large elliptical incisions can unnecessarily narrow the cava, causing increased thrombotic complications. If, on the other hand, the cava is invaded by tumor, resection of the involved cava is necessary with ligation of the uninvolved parts. (See discussion in this chapter and in Chapter 17.)

Salvage of the vena cava, of course, is not necessary in a right-sided tumor because the left renal vein can be occluded at the vena cava, and the left renal function can be preserved by collateral flow via the left gonadal and adrenal veins. For left-sided tumors, it is far better to preserve the vena cava, and if this is not possible, the right renal vein must be anastomosed to the portal vein or the kidney autotransplanted to the iliac fossa with the vein being anastomosed to the common iliac system for drainage. The aid of a Foley catheter to extract the tumor thrombus has been mentioned by many surgeons, but it is rarely used in our experience. If there is a hint of invasion of the vena cava, caval resection is indicated and is well tolerated.

Patients who have had prior total caval occlusion experience few postoperative problems from this. In patients without caval obstruction, transient lower extremity pain or edema can result until paravertebral collaterals have been established. Patients with thrombosis of the vena cava following thrombectomy and cavotomy should undergo thrombectomy if they are symptomatic, and one should then consider anticoagulation and/or placement of a vena caval clip to prevent subsequent pulmonary emboli. Patients with tumor thrombi advancing into the supradiaphragmatic region but below the atrium can be managed without cardiopulmonary bypass. The plans for this eventuality, however, should be made and a cardiac team should be available.

One has to weigh the risks inherent in cardiopulmonary bypass versus the improved visibility and exposure in the patient experiencing exsanguination. The pericardium must be opened to expose the subatrial portion of the inferior vena cava. I have seen patients in whom right-sided tumor thrombi have extended into, and indeed invaded, the left renal vein. Although we have no cures for this situation, there have been long-term survivors with appropriate palliation.

Left-sided renal cell carcinomas with caval extension should *never* be approached via the left thoracoabdominal incision. Patients who have extension of tumor thrombus in the infrahepatic area are best approached anterotransabdominally, with the chevron incision being favored. Adequate mobilization of the vena cava is quite possible via this approach. Patients with higher extension of the tumor into the intrahepatic area but below the diaphragmatic portion of the vena cava are approached through a right thoracoabdominal incision, which affords adequate exposure to perform the left nephrectomy and, of course, gives all the advantages of complete visualization of the vena cava with proper mobilization of the liver. Patients with the possibility of hilar adenopathy or perhaps tumor thrombus involving the lumbar vein of the left kidney should not be treated with the right thoracoabdominal approach and should be approached in an anterior fashion with the possibility of extension of the incision upward into a medial sternotomy, if necessary. For the left-sided tumors extending into the vena cava, control of the vena cava is done in a similar way as for right-sided tumors. However, the right renal vein should not be occluded; instead, the right renal artery should be occluded. This prevents congestion of the remaining right kidney, which can be a cause of temporary renal failure in the postoperative period.

On occasion, there is some collateral blood flow to the right kidney, and the right renal vein may have to be occluded to improve intracaval visualization and to decrease blood loss, but this is not usually necessary. In patients in whom tumor has been extracted from the vena cava, the inferior clamp should be released first, prior to completion of the suture line, so that possible air within the vena cava can be extracted, thus preventing potentially fatal air embolization.

It goes without saying that patients with atrial extension and indeed those with extension into the supradiaphragmatic area of the vena cava should be treated from the anterior approach, utilizing median sternotomy and midline incision and with a cardiopulmonary bypass team in attendance. If caval resection is necessary, the vena cava should be transected flush with the remaining renal vein. Allowing a segment of vena cava to remain below the renal vein can present a potential source of thrombus formation in the future with the attendant risk of subsequent pulmonary embolization or more generalized caval thrombosis. Sutures of 5–0 cardiovascular silk are generally used to close the cavotomy. It is our practice, when the integrity of the vena cava has been preserved, to remove the cross clamps on the vena cava in the aforementioned manner, using a partially occluding Satinsky clamp around the cavotomy incision to allow for continued caval blood flow during closure. This certainly makes it easy for the anesthesiologist to manage the patient hemodynamically. This would also, of course, lessen the necessary right kidney ischemia time should this procedure be performed for a left renal cell carcinoma with caval extension.

Patients with obvious metastatic disease detected at the time of exploration of caval thrombi obviously should not undergo this rather formidable procedure because it will have little impact on their survival. Exceptions exist for patients who are with pain, severe hematuria, or untreatable endocrinopathy related to the renal cell tumor from the local lesion or patients who are experiencing recurrent pulmonary emboli. Patients with atrial extension of the tumor have a poor prognosis. Nevertheless, it is worth the rather extreme combined operative efforts of the urologic and cardiac teams because no other therapeutic alternative is available. Whereas the prognosis for patients with atrial extension is far worse than for those with simple vena caval involvement, long-term survival has occurred.

Acute renal failure has been reported postoperatively after the left renal vein has been ligated in conjunction with right radical nephrectomy and cavectomy.[15,16] Indeed it has also been reported with temporary occlusion of the left renal vein.[17] This renal failure is most likely due to venous hypertension in the remaining kidney and generally resolves in time as collateral flow is established. On occasion, interval dialysis is necessary. The chance of renal failure in this patient population should encourage the surgeon to maintain the integrity of drainage of the left renal vein into the vena cava if possible.

Locally invasive renal carcinoma occurs rarely and carries a poor prognosis. Again, because there is little else to offer these patients, aggressive surgical management in the absence of metastatic lesions is indicated. On occasion, resection of the spleen, colon, duodenum, liver, or distal portion of the pancreas may be necessary. Treatment of these lesions presents a tremendous therapeutic challenge, but the occasional disease-free survivor does occur, and it is extremely rewarding. If effective immune modulation therapy becomes available, extensive debulking of such tumors will make immune manipulation more effective.

NEPHROURETERECTOMY

Patients with urothelial tumors involving the upper urinary collecting system should undergo

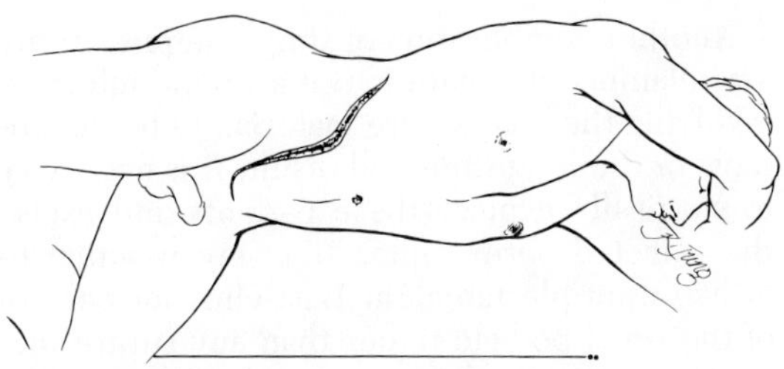

Figure 11–10. Flank incision for nephroureterectomy. The patient is placed in a modified flank position with a slight torque. The incision is usually started from the tip of the 12th rib, extending above and below the 12th rib as necessary. The incision is then carried down, using a modified Pfannenstiel incision.

total nephroureterectomy with a cuff of bladder. Whereas subtotal ureteral resections have been performed in patients with low-grade tumors, the multifocal nature of this neoplasm mandates close follow-up. Nephroureterectomy can be performed through a flank incision extending into a modified Pfannenstiel incision, utilizing the torque flank position (Fig. 11–10), through two separate incisions (flank and midline suprapubic), or through a single transabdominal midline incision (xiphoid to pubis). The patient's body habitus has some impact on the selection of the incision. In patients who are thin, a single incision can be easily accomplished, but obese patients would perhaps be better managed with a standard flank incision followed by a separate lower abdominal incision. In patients in whom two incisions are used, the mobilized kidney is simply placed down into the lower limits of the wound and removed intact with the ureter during the lower portion of the procedure.

The procedure should be a *radical* nephrectomy, and it is my feeling that a regional lymph node dissection should be performed. Long-term survival in patients with positive nodes has been recorded with current neoadjuvant and adjuvant chemotherapy for transitional cell cancer. During the nephrectomy phase of the procedure, the dissection of the ureter is carried as far distal as possible, and then the kidney and ureter are passed downward to be delivered through the lower incision. The dissection of the ureter continues to the intervesical wall. I feel that it is essential to make a cystotomy incision to complete the bladder cuff portion of the operation. Extravesical removal of the "intramural ureter" runs a risk of including the contralateral ureteral orifice, giving rise to obstruction.

With the exception of damage to the contralateral orifice, complications of nephroureterectomy are not different from those with radical nephrectomy and should indeed be less severe because the renal portion of the procedure is usually quite straightforward. I must emphasize that it is essential to remove the entire cuff of the ureter and bladder since a ureteral recurrence rate as high as 20 to 30 percent has been reported.[18,19]

SIMPLE NEPHRECTOMY

Simple nephrectomy should be a straightforward procedure, and any variety of the aforementioned incisions can be utilized. In certain patients, nephrectomy is performed because the kidneys have been destroyed by other disease processes, including infection, trauma, or calculous disease, with or without obstruction. Often many of these patients have had prior kidney surgeries. It is the perinephric inflammation and scar tissue from prior surgery that can make simple nephrectomy difficult. Obviously it is important that patients who perhaps have an infectious process have an extraperitoneal and extrapleural approach if possible. My preferred approach is an 11th interspace extrapleural incision. In most of these patients, rarely should an anterotransabdominal incision be made.

The performance of a subcapsular nephrectomy may considerably facilitate a nephrectomy and decrease operating time. In a subcapsular nephrectomy, the hilum of the renal capsule should be circumcised to approach the renal vessels. Often in such patients, the renal vessels are taken up well within the hilum, and multiple branches of the renal artery and vein may be encountered and may need to be controlled. In patients undergoing subcapsular nephrectomy, after the kidney has been removed, an attempt should be made to remove as much renal capsule as possible to prevent a subsequent focus for infection, and adequate drains should be placed in the renal fossa. Wound irrigation with dilute povidone-iodine (Betadine) solution may in fact be indicated in such patients. In other patients in whom the renal artery and vein cannot be safely dissected separately, mass ligation of the pedicle can be performed (Fig. 11–11). Also one must emphasize that in difficult right nephrectomies, prior surgery, or infection, care must be taken in approaching the hilum from the standpoint of duodenal mobilization. In addition, on left-sided lesions, especially in such disease processes as xanthogranulomatous pyelonephritis, special care must be taken to prevent splenic injury, as is mentioned in the radical nephrec-

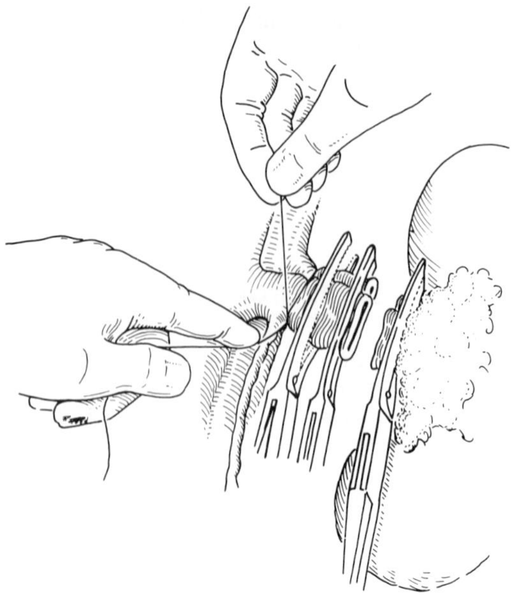

Figure 11–11. In cases in which the renal artery and vein cannot be safely dissected separately, mass ligation of the pedicle can be performed. This procedure should be used only as a last resort. Often a simple suture, as shown, can be reinforced by large Liga clips being placed above or below the suture. Often suture ligatures are preferable to mass ligation but may increase the incidence of arteriovenous fistulas, which are a complication of mass ligation of the renal pedicle.

tomy section. If in controlling the pedicle, one of these vessels is lost, initial severe intraoperative hemorrhage can be controlled by compression of the pedicle against the vertebral bodies until adequate suction devices are available and the anesthesiologist is able to stabilize the patient with adequate volume expanders, should they be needed. In placing a clamp across the entire renal pedicle, special care must be taken not to include the duodenum in this clamp. Duodenal injury and/or fistula has ben reported with mass ligation of the pedicle. The management of such complications is discussed in the section on duodenal injuries.

Arteriovenous (AV) fistulas are another complication of mass ligation of the pedicle and can be very difficult to fix. Arteriovenous fistulas cause complications such as high cardiac output failure and must be explored and corrected. This is exceedingly dangerous surgery. The transabdominal approach to patients requiring such repair is essential. For right-sided AV fistulas, ligation of the right renal artery between the vena cava and aorta often will solve the situation. Left-sided AV fistulas are more difficult to manage because often the left arterial stump is quite short.

Another complication of simple nephrectomy for inflammatory conditions is a wound infection involving the hilar suture material. Often an abscess or draining sinus will result. It is necessary to surgically explore these patients and excise the infected suture line. It is my practice to utilize multiple tantalum Liga clips for control of the renal pedicle rather than any suture material in patients with a high risk of developing infection. Should sutures be used, they should be of monofilament material. I have had experience with infections of the vena caval suture line following right nephrectomy. The infected subsuture line was excised and the vena cava closed successfully with chromic catgut suture (4–0 material).

Simple nephrectomy performed for the very large, nonfunctioning hydronephrotic kidney can be facilitated with decompression by making a small nephrotomy incision and removing the excess urine. This procedure compresses the hydronephrotic kidney, thus facilitating its mobilization.

Nephrectomy for polycystic kidney disease is performed much less commonly than in the past. There was a time when the removal of polycystic kidneys was thought to be required before renal transplantation could be carried out. Morbidity from this procedure was indeed extreme, with many severe complications including hemorrhage, retroperitoneal hematomas, and sepsis. Clearly, nephrectomy of polycystic kidneys in the end-stage renal patient should be carried out only if specific indications exist, such as uncontrolled hypertension, kidneys that are so large that there is no room for the transplant, history of infected cysts, or history of perinephric bleeding.

On occasion, patients with polycystic kidneys will require urgent surgery. Polycystic kidney disease is a cause of spontaneous hemorrhage, and I have seen patients who experienced exsanguinating hemorrhage from polycystic renal disease and required nephrectomy. Prior to submitting the patients to surgery for this problem, renal angiograms should be performed with attempted control through embolization techniques. This has not been uniformly successful, however. Patients with a history of sepsis and infected cysts, of course, must undergo drainage and treatment in a similar manner as patients with cortical abscess or perinephric abscess.

In such patients, however, it is essential to expose the entire kidney because multiple infected cysts may be present, and simply finding one infected cyst does not guarantee that the entire disease process has been controlled. In patients with infected cysts, the extraperitoneal incisional approach is mandatory. In doing nephrectomy or surgery on polycystic disease for other reasons, I feel that the transabdominal approach is better because of the superior exposure it provides. On occasion, there will be cysts that obstruct the collecting system, and patients can benefit from decompression of selected cysts causing this obstruction. There is no place for simple decompression of multiple cysts to reduce the bulk of the polycystic kidney as had been advocated many years ago.

LIVING DONOR NEPHRECTOMY

Special consideration needs to be given to living related donor nephrectomy in regard to the surgical approach and the avoidance of complications. Meticulous care to prevent complications in these "normal patients" is essential. It is my feeling that this procedure should be done through a flank approach, utilizing the 11th intercostal space; the incidence of incidental splenectomy, postoperative ileus, and subsequent bowel obstruction is higher when a transabdominal transperitoneal approach is used.

It is essential in the preoperative work-up that good quality angiograms be performed to ensure that all polar vessels are identified. To overlook such a vessel dramatically complicates implantation, and disastrous side effects can occur. I believe that there is some risk in performing digital subtraction angiography in this regard, and it is my feeling that good quality standard selective angiography is important in the donor evaluation. The left kidney is preferred as the donor source when one has a choice because of its longer renal vein. Obviously, if a double renal artery is present on the left side, a right donor nephrectomy is performed. A right donor nephrectomy should include removal of the renal vein to the vena cava, which generally requires closure of the vena cava with a running 5–0 vascular suture.

A larger than normal incision is needed for a donor nephrectomy because superior exposure to the hilum is essential to a safe, effective donor nephrectomy. Meticulous dissection must be performed, dissecting the renal artery and vein with minimal damage to the other hilar structures. This dissection should be done well away from the renal pelvis, and special care must be taken not to damage the arterial branches from the renal artery that give rise to the ureteral blood supply.

Ureteral fistula formation secondary to a necrotic ureter is the most common technical complication in living related donor transplants. The incidence is in fact higher in living related donor transplants than in cadaveric transplants. It is essential in performing a donor nephrectomy that the ureter be dissected out sharply, leaving the ureteral adventitia intact. Mobilization of the ureter should be done sharply, staying well away from the ureter to preserve the periureteral arterials arising from the renal artery.

Multiple renal vessels are not a contraindication to donor nephrectomy. When a donor nephrectomy has to be performed on a kidney with two arteries, the risk of ureteral ischemia and its attendant complications are increased. Multiple arteries can be conjoined in any number of ways prior to implantation in the recipient. Unrecognized polar vessels that have been transected so that they are too short to be anastomosed to the renal artery represent a special problem. The amount of parenchyma supplied by this polar vessel must be assessed. If it supplies a portion of the parenchyma larger than the size of a quarter, this ischemic portion of the kidney is of sufficient size that necrosis may occur into the collecting system, and a caliceal cutaneous fistula may result. The saphenous vein could be utilized to revascularize this artery. Otherwise, the segment of kidney supplied by this vessel should be excised to prevent subsequent necrosis and fistula formation.

When performing left donor nephrectomy, care must be taken not to be too enthusiastic about obtaining the longest possible piece of artery for the recipient surgeon. One must leave an adequate stump of renal artery to allow for safe ligation. I have witnessed a disaster when the suture came off a very short stump of renal artery, resulting in a near-fatal exsanguinating hemorrhage in the postoperative period.

PARTIAL NEPHRECTOMY

Partial nephrectomy has been utilized for years for calculous disease, especially in patients with distorted lower-pole calices, segmental obstruction (duplicated collecting systems), caliceal diverticula, renal trauma, infectious processes, and vascular lesions involving a branch renal artery. Partial nephrectomy in cases of renal cell carcinoma has also been used to treat bilateral renal cell carcinoma or carcinoma in a solitary kidney, but its use for carcinoma is expanding with the presence of a contralateral kidney. It is my feeling that the state-of-the-art approach in patients with renal cell carcinoma who have some potential compromise of the contralateral kidney and who have a polar lesion less than 4 cm in size (which appears to be encapsulated on CT scan) is partial nephrectomy. This has been further supported by the comparison of stage-for-stage survival statistics of patients treated with partial nephrectomy for renal cell carcinoma in solitary kidneys and bilateral renal cell carcinoma with patients treated with radical nephrectomies. In addition, an ever-increasing number of incidental renal masses are being noted on routine abdominal ultrasound and CT scan procedures performed for other reasons. While many renal masses can be detected by these modern scanning techniques, the nature of many of these renal masses remains in question and demands exploration.

To perform radical nephrectomy in these individuals would involve the removal of a tremendous number of kidneys for benign disease. Simple exploration is unreliable in ruling out cases of cystic renal cell carcinoma. Even frozen-section biopsies are frequently incorrect, and cancer has been diagnosed on permanent-section biopsies. It is very difficult to assess the whole periphery of a spherical cystic lesion on frozen section. Clearly, lesions that are not compatible with simple cysts on scanning techniques should be explored and excised with a rim of normal renal parenchyma. Enucleation procedures should not be attempted in this instance.

In patients with other than simple lower-polar lesions, I feel that preoperative angiography is essential to provide a vascular map to help with the operative procedure. Small, peripheral lesions in any location of the kidney, of course, would not require this preoperative study. Patients with renal carcinoma should undergo renal venography to check venous drainage of the salvageable portion of the kidney, especially in large central lesions or in lesions that occupy most of the parenchyma. The IVP should show the entire internal collecting system. If this is not conclusive, retrograde pyelography is an important preoperative test that should be performed. It is obvious that in order to save a portion of parenchyma, one must have a supplying artery, a draining vein, and a portion of the collecting system that can be reconstructed in such a way as to drain to the bladder.

The surgical approach for partial nephrectomy is generally via the flank, utilizing a standard extrapleural, extraperitoneal technique. When one is treating a malignant condition of the kidney, I believe that it is important to do transperitoneal exploration to rule out other sites of metastatic disease.

If ex vivo surgery with autotransplantation is indicated, it is my preference to have the patient in a supine position and to use a midline transabdominal incision. Cystic polar lesions of questionable diagnostic etiology are best managed by a straightforward partial excision of the parenchyma with a margin of normal tissue. We have not had any patients who have had a positive margin in this procedure. Even when a frozen-section diagnosis is reversed and a malignant process confirmed in a patient thought to have benign disease, it is not our policy to go back to complete a radical nephrectomy when good margins have been obtained. On occasion, this policy has been mandated by the wishes of the patient, but in no instance have we found residual carcinoma. One caution is that patients with multiple cystic renal carcinomas may well have other undetected lesions.[20] If this is a unilateral lesion, consideration should be given to radical nephrectomy. The obvious exception to this is the patient with von Hippel–Lindau disease.

It is my feeling that the renal artery and vein should be isolated, even in straightforward polar resections, in case severe hemorrhage occurs. Manual compression of the parenchyma usually suffices, and rarely is it necessary to include the renal pedicle. Once the offending tissue has been removed, the parenchymal vessels should be controlled by individual suture ligatures of 4–0 chromic catgut. The use of large mattress sutures should be discouraged because of possible necrosis. It is also wise to place perinephric fat or omentum in the defect created by the partial nephrectomy.

When it is necessary to occlude the renal hilum during the course of partial nephrectomy, one must occlude the artery carefully to avoid intimal damage with possible resection and thrombosis. Schwartz clips are particularly useful in this regard. The encirclement technique accomplished with Meditapes also can be used and is atraumatic. (We have seen intimal damage to vessels with a standard Rummel tourniquet.)

Any time up to 30 minutes for occlusion is well tolerated. All patients undergoing such a resection should be well hydrated preoperatively, and if the pedicle is to be occluded, mannitol should be administered before the hilum is occluded. It is known that mannitol does have a protective effect against ischemic damage of the kidney. It is also of special benefit if cooling of the kidney is needed in conjunction with the vascular occlusion.

If ischemia times exceed 30 minutes, renal damage can occur and cooling is mandatory. Administration of mannitol before pedicle occlusion and cooling increases the osmolarity of the glomerular filtrate and decreases the hazard of ice crystallization within the renal tissue during the cooling process. Also, the osmotic effect of mannitol helps promote a diuresis once the renal pedicle has been released. If it is to be cooled, usually a rubber dam is utilized to help contain the ice in and around the kidney. Renal core temperatures in the 14 to 16° C range are ideal. Ischemia can be safely prolonged for 60 to 90 minutes with this technique without danger of permanent loss of renal function.

Almost all malignant lesions of the kidney can be removed by in situ partial nephrectomy. Only rarely should it be necessary to resort to ex vivo resection. We have had to perform ex vivo resection in less than 10 percent of patients undergoing nephron-salvage surgery for renal cell carcinoma. Nonetheless, with large central lesions, preparation should be made for this possibility by placing the patient in the aforementioned midline position and by having Collins' solution available. It should be emphasized that enucleation of renal cell carcinoma should never be performed because it is exceedingly common that renal tumors invade a so-called pseudocapsule.[21,22]

In our series of over 50 patients with renal cell carcinoma in solitary kidneys, the only three local recurrences that occurred were in patients who underwent enucleation procedures. In no instance have we seen recurrence when a margin of normal parenchyma had been taken. If partial nephrectomy is performed for hemostasis, one must be very careful to close the collecting system. This can be accomplished by injection of a dilute solution of methylene blue or indigo carmine into the renal pelvis to indicate leaks. If a collecting system has been opened, an internal stent can be passed down to the bladder and left in place during the postoperative period to decompress the upper tract. Administration of furosemide (Lasix) appears to be of value in improving renal perfusion after ischemic injury to the kidney. Lasix appears to increase the renal blood flow by stimulating the release of intrarenal prostaglandin E_1, which is a potent vasodilator. The use of intra-arterial papaverine hydrochloride is useful for patients whose kidneys have had the vascular supply occluded, causing vasospasm to occur.

Increased intraoperative bleeding is a common complication of partial nephrectomy. If one cannot occlude bleeding sites with sutures, prolonged manual compression of the parenchyma may help control these smaller vessels. Combining this technique with occlusion of the pedicle for 5 minutes will help in difficult cases. Delayed bleeding is also a complication of partial nephrectomy. These patients must be treated with bed rest and serial hematocrit determinations. If bleeding continues or is severe, an angiogram should be performed to try to find the bleeding source, and if feasible, percutaneous embolization should be performed. One must be careful not to embolize too large a branch vessel because necrosis of the tissue supplied by this vessel will occur, with potential involvement of the collecting system and resulting caliceal fistula and urinoma. Caliceal fistulas are another recognized complication of partial nephrectomy. Patients undergoing partial nephrectomy should be well catheterized with Penrose drains. I believe that suction catheters (Jackson-Pratt and similar devices) should not be used, since a suction drain can perpetuate a fistula.

Excess wound draining following partial nephrectomy can be confirmed to be urine either by the intravenous injection of indigo carmine, noting the blue stain on the dressings, or by the collection of the drainage fluid with determination of its creatinine level. A ureteral stent should be placed, if not already employed, to decompress the upper tract to facilitate spontaneous fistula healing. An indwelling catheter should also be left in the bladder to prevent reflux up the stent when the patient voids (which may delay closure of the fistula) until the output from the fistula has dropped considerably.

When partial nephrectomy is done for benign disease, such as lower-pole nephrectomy for stone or segmental inflammatory disease, the capsule of the kidney should be stripped back before the parenchyma is incised. This is later used to facilitate closure of the exposed parenchyma. This procedure cannot be done in patients with carcinoma. (The adjoining perinephric fat and capsule should be removed over a carcinomatous lesion.)

Surgery for Benign Renal Cysts

In the past, simple renal cysts in adults were operated on except in rare instances. However, with the advent of modern radiographic imaging techniques and the development of safe methods of percutaneous puncture, most cysts can be diagnosed without renal exploration.[23] It is my current feeling that if a mass lesion of the kidney is clearly determined to be cystic on ultrasound, CT scan, and/or MRI imaging, observation can be a reasonable alternative to needle aspiration. I also feel that if there are any characteristics that are not totally compatible with a benign cyst on any of the imaging studies, at the minimum, needle aspiration is mandatory. If examination of the cyst fluid raises any question in regard to cytology, if the lipid content is increased, or if the fluid shows signs of old or fresh hemorrhage, exploration with excision is mandated. If the cyst appears complex, has a reading on MRI that deviates from classic fluid content (black on T_1 weighted images and gray/white on T_2 weighted images), or is calcified, exploration and excisional biopsy with a margin of parenchyma is indicated (Fig. 11–12).

When one is removing a cystic lesion from the kidney, special care must be taken to ensure that this cyst does not represent a caliceal diverticulum. If any question exists regarding communication with the collecting system, the entire base should be widely fulgurated, even if communication cannot be demonstrated intraoperatively.

Surgery for Peripelvic Cysts

Peripelvic cysts are usually of lymphatic origin and, of course, by the nature of their descriptive name, occur in the hilum of the kidney. Often these cysts distort the pelvis and collecting system and can cause obstruction (Fig. 11–13). They are often more difficult to differentiate from a simple renal cyst, and more commonly, peripelvic cysts are explored.

For exploration of a peripelvic cyst, a classic flank incision or an anterior extra-abdominal in-

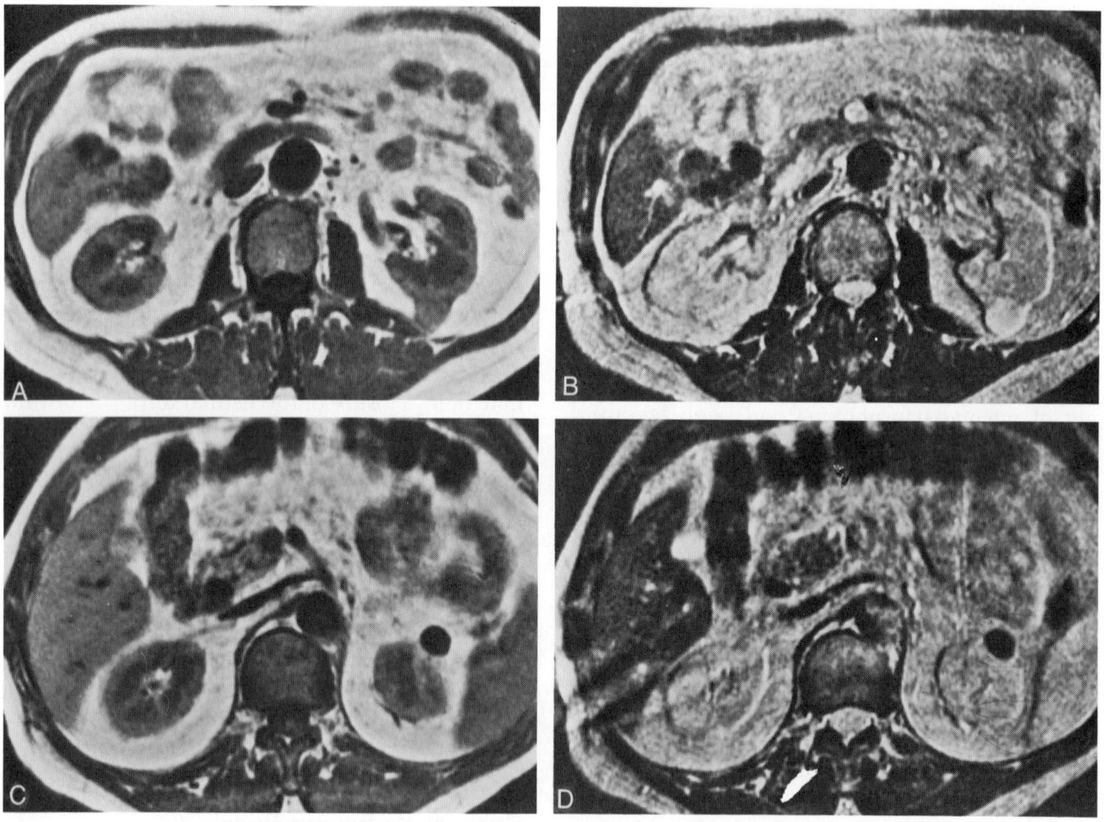

Figure 11–12. Incidentally found masses on CT scan, both of which appeared to be cystic. Please note the MRI scan in which the appearance of these lesions deviates from the classic simple cyst fluid content (black on T_1 weighted images and gray-white on T_2 weighted images). One can conclude from the MRI scan that these do not represent simple cysts and that exploration is mandated. The kidney was explored and these masses proved to be cystic renal cell carcinomas. (*A*, *C*, T_1 weighted image; *B*, *D*, T_2 weighted image.)

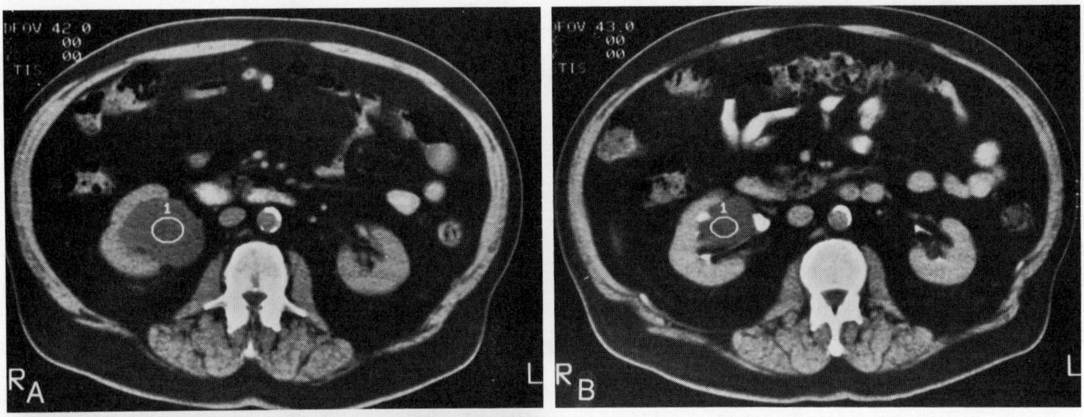

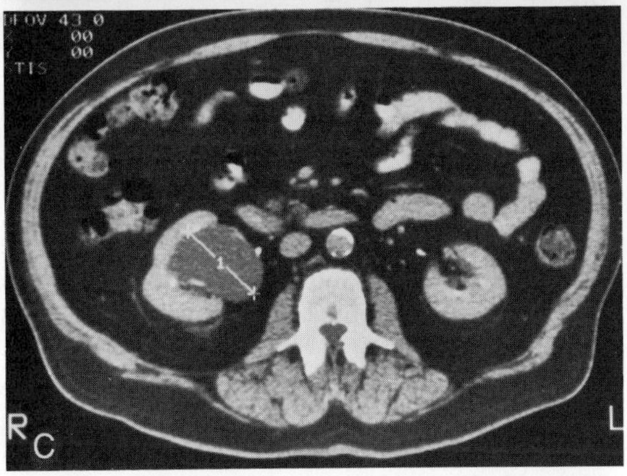

Figure 11–13. Classic peripelvic cyst. *A*, Note CT scan without contrast. This could easily be interpreted as a hydronephrotic renal pelvis. *B*, *C*, Contrast has been injected, which clearly outlines this large peripelvic cystic mass.

cision may be used. I feel that this procedure should not be done transabdominally in case a collecting system is opened during the dissection. Exploration of peripelvic cysts requires a thorough dissection of the renal hilum including the renal artery, vein, and pelvis. Special care must be taken to identify the renal artery and its branches, tagging each with a vessel loop for easy access and identification. Gilvernet retractors are especially useful for elevating the parenchyma off these peripelvic cysts. Lymphatic vessels in the area should be occluded with small Liga clips to prevent any lymphatic leak. It is my opinion that patients with these lesions should have a retroperitoneal drain in place. The drain should be removed in 48 hours if drainage is insignificant.

PYELOPLASTY

Before pyeloplasty is performed, one must prove that an apparent obstruction is functionally significant. One should be careful not simply to "treat x-rays" (apparent obstruction). A thorough knowledge of the pathogenesis of ureteropelvic junction (UPJ) obstruction is critical to a satisfactory surgical result. Congenital intrinsic obstruction is responsible in most patients for UPJ obstruction. Histologic evaluation of the intrinsic obstructive area demonstrates dysplasia of the smooth muscle as well as an increase in the amount of collagen and intracellular ground substance.[24,25] Arteries and veins coursing aberrantly to the lower pole are also a common cause of obstruction. In addition, kinks and ureteral bands may cause obstruction.

High insertion of the ureter in the pelvis is the most common cause of UPJ obstruction in ectopic kidneys. Causes of UPJ obstruction also include ureteral polyps or valves.[26] The functional significance of UPJ obstruction needs to be confirmed with more than a renal ultrasound study or excretory urography. A voiding cystourethrogram should be performed to rule out reflux, which can aggravate UPJ obstruction, interfere with the success of repair, and indeed even be a primary cause of the secondary UPJ obstruction. Diethylenetriamine penta-acetic acid (DPTA) diuretic renography is also useful to monitor renal emptying. An IVP done with and without Lasix can also give valuable functional information. If there is question of the functional significance of the lesion, a percutaneous antegrade pyelogram should be performed, with pressures being measured simultaneously in the renal pelvis and bladder.[27] (The so-called Whitaker test beautifully elaborates on the details of this study.)

In patients who have a kidney that is nonfunctional on IVP or has poor uptake on renal scan, a percutaneous nephrostomy should be performed to allow for decompression of the kidney. Serial creatinine clearances from this organ should be monitored. Patients presenting with septic complications from an infected hydronephrosis should have a percutaneous nephrostomy performed for decompression and systemic antibodies administered. Repair is undertaken after the patient has been stabilized and achieved defervescence. The amount of renal function remaining in this obstructed kidney sufficient to justify repair depends on multiple factors, e.g., age of the patient, status of the contralateral kidney, anatomy of the obstructing lesion, and general status of the patient. Obviously in an adult patient with a normal contralateral kidney, one must think twice about performing a reconstructive procedure on a kidney with borderline renal function. It is my feeling that the obstructed kidney in an adult should contribute at least 20 percent to the overall renal function to justify repair. In children, I believe that any functional unit should be conserved.

If reflux exists, one must be certain that the reflux is not causing or aggravating the UPJ obstruction. When a mild degree of reflux exists with a UPJ obstruction, the ureteropelvic pathology is usually primary, and therapy should be directed to this problem. When severe degrees of reflux are present, UPJ obstruction is often secondary to increased tortuosity and kinking of the upper ureter secondary to the reflux. It is my feeling that in patients in whom the reflux is thought to be the cause of the UPJ obstruction, the reflux should be corrected initially by stenting the UPJ obstruction. In most patients, the UPJ obstruction will resolve spontaneously. On the other hand, when UPJ obstruction is severe and does coexist with massive degrees of reflux, it is my feeling that pyeloplasty should be performed. Pyeloplasty should be the preliminary procedure in these cases with correction of reflux to be performed 2 to 3 months later.

The traditional incision for renal pelvic surgery is through the flank, utilizing any of the aforementioned flank incisions depending upon the location of the kidney. In young patients, the flank approach does not offer the exposure that can be achieved through an anterior extraperitoneal incision, especially on the right side, where the kidney is lower than on the left. If possible, the transperitoneal approach should be avoided and indeed *must* be avoided in cases of UPJ obstruction complicated by infection. It is not necessary to mobilize the kidney to perform pyeloplasty. Only the necessary portion of the renal pelvis and upper ureter are mobilized routinely.

The full procedures have been described to correct UPJ obstruction, including the dismembered Hines-Anderson pyeloureteroplasty, the dismembered Foley Y–V pyeloplasty, Culp-Scardino flap pyeloplasties, vertical flap pyeloplasty, spiral flap pyeloplasty, and Foley Y–V pyeloplasty. While all of these operative approaches can be and usually are successful, it is my feeling that a resident surgeon needs to be familiar only with the dismembered technique, with and without pelvic resection, and the Foley Y–V pyeloplasty. These two procedures will suffice for any ureteropelvic pathology. In patients with UPJ obstruction secondary to aberrant lower-pole vessel, a pyelopyelostomy is the procedure of choice. In this approach, one brings the ureter and renal pelvis around the offending vessel and reanastomoses the pelvis together (Fig. 11–14).

The dismembered pyeloplasty is used most commonly in my experience and is the most versatile of all procedures. It can be employed in nearly every patient experiencing UPJ obstruction, from either intrinsic or extrinsic causes. It can also be used when the ureter is inserted high in the renal pelvis.

My preferred procedure, however, in regard to UPJ obstruction is the Foley Y–V pyeloplasty. (As mentioned earlier, this condition is seen generally in ectopic kidneys and is further discussed under that heading.) In performing the dismembered pyeloplasty (Fig. 11–15), the ureter is generally transected transversely, making certain that this transection is below the level of obstruction. An oblique incision is made in the renal pelvis, and if excess renal pelvis exists, this is resected. Special care must be taken not to resect too much of the lower portion of the renal pelvis, which can compromise the lower infundibulum. The ureter is then spatulated and anastomosed to the renal pelvis. It is my general practice to utilize a Y–V plasty with this repair, making a V out of the lower portion of the renal pelvis and inlaying this V in the spatulated portion of the ureter.

Blood supply is most precarious at the tip of

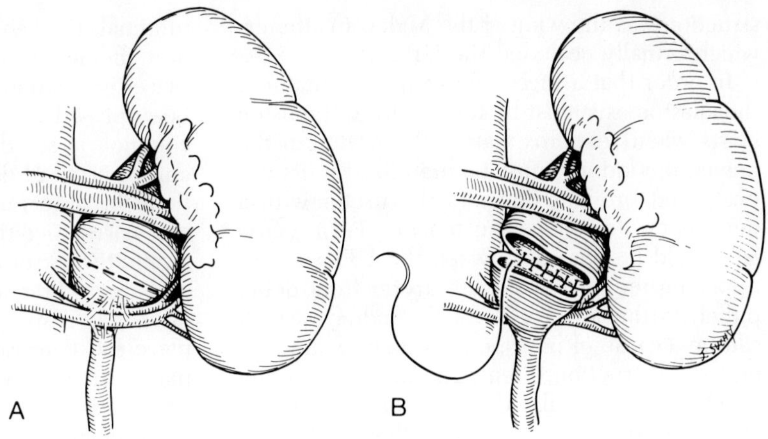

Figure 11–14. Pyelopyelostomy is the procedure of choice to treat ureteropelvic junction obstruction secondary to an aberrant lower-pole vessel. *A*, The pelvis is transected well above the ureteropelvic junction. *B*, The ureter, with a cuff of renal pelvis, is then placed in front of the aberrant renal vessel, and anastomosis is completed along the original lines of incision in the renal pelvis.

this V, and it is my feeling that interrupted sutures of 5–0 catgut or polyglycolic acid (Dexon) should be used for the first two to three sutures on either side in order to lessen the chance of impairing its blood supply. The remainder of the suture line can be completed in a running fashion. It is essential to handle these tissues delicately with the use of Jerrel forceps, manipulating the pelvic flap and ureter as little as possible. The anastomosis is generally done over an internal stent. Nephrostomy drainage is rarely employed. Under no circumstances should a nephrostomy tube be used to drain a kidney with UPJ obstruction without leaving a stent through the anastomosis. "Something" must go through the UPJ in the early postoperative period, whether it be a stent or urine. In straightforward cases involving patients with a delicate ureter and a renal pelvis in which the repair is ideal, stenting is not mandatory. In all patients, of course, the ureter should be drained through the flank. It is my preference to use small Penrose drains because I believe that suction drainage systems can perpetuate a urinary leak although it is not uncommon to have a temporary urinary leak via the flank. Prolonged drainage, however, is a cause for concern. When nephrostomy tubes were used more frequently in conjunction with pyeloplasty, the common cause of increased drainage of persistent ob-

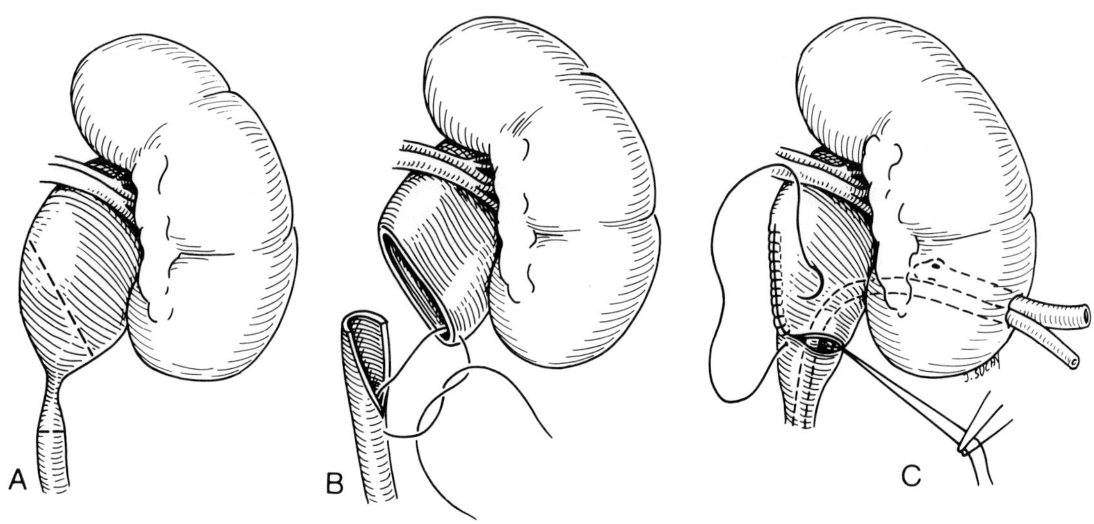

Figure 11–15. Dismembered pyeloplasty. *A*, The ureter is transected below the level of obstruction. The pelvis is then transected obliquely above the level of obstruction. *B*, The ureter is spatulated and the apex is anastomosed to the most dependent opening in the pelvis. At the discretion of the surgeon, a V may be formed at the most dependent portion of the pelvis to inlay within the apex of the spatulated ureter (dismembered Foley Y–V plasty). The back wall of the anastomosis is usually completed first. *C*, After completion, the front wall of the anastomosis is completed and the remainder is closed. This is covered with a nephrostomy tube or internal stent, at the discretion of the surgeon.

struction was the wing of the Malecot catheter, which actually occluded the UPJ.

In order that a successful result be obtained, the anastomosis must be tension free. If tension exists when reapproximating the ureter to the pelvis, the kidney must be mobilized in its entirety and brought down to the ureter with a nephropexy to relieve this tension. Perinephric fat should be placed between the UPJ and the upper ureter to prevent the ureter from being pulled to the lower pole of the kidney, which can be a cause of postoperative failure and secondary obstruction. Stents and/or nephrostomy tubes should be utilized whenever the repair is compromised by any of the following factors: significant inflammatory changes in renal pelvis or upper ureter or surrounding tissue; previous failed pyeloplasty; thickened renal pelvic tissue; and if the surgeon has any concern regarding the technical success of the repair. External stents should be left a minimum of 10 to 14 days. If stents are placed internally, one can easily leave them for 1 to 2 months, removing them after a pyelogram has been performed to check on the postoperative result. It is my practice to repeat a pyelogram 1 to 2 months following stent removal and then to generally follow these patients with ultrasonography, obtaining the final pyelogram at 1 year following surgery. I feel that flap pyeloplasties are technically difficult for the neophyte surgeon to understand and do not offer any advantage with regard to successful outcome over the standard dismembered pyeloplasty. I do feel, however, that the Foley Y–V plasty has a place in the ectopic kidney with a high UPJ, but that the Davis intubated ureterostomy is inappropriate. Even long strictures involving the UPJ can be handled with ureteral and renal mobilization.

The Penrose drain should be brought out through a posterolateral position, taking care that the patient will not be lying on the drain. Although some surgeons advocate placing a stoma appliance over a drain if considerable urinary drainage occurs, I have seen infectious complications related to this. It is absolutely impossible to keep a drainage bag over a Penrose drain sterile. The infected urine in this bag can certainly run backward down the Penrose drain almost as easily as urine can exit from the wound to the outside. It is preferable and safer in my opinion to have the nursing staff perform frequent dressing changes, even though this may be a nuisance to the nursing staff.

I believe that a drain should be left in place for a minimum of 5 days, even if drainage is minimal. If, of course, the drainage is excessive, one should make certain that the stent (if in place) is functioning properly. If a stent has not been placed, one should be used. It is not uncommon to see drainage from a pyeloplasty occur for up to 21 days. If drainage persists longer than this interval, consideration to reoperation and correcting the drainage should be given. Again, the use of suction drains such as Hemovac or Jackson-Pratt drains can perpetuate urinary drainage. Also, one should be careful not to place the Penrose drain too close to the pyeloplasty. If urinary drainage is occurring, ultrasonography should be peformed to ensure that the drainage is adequate and that a urinoma is not forming around the site of repair. A urinoma can be the source of an intense inflammatory reaction, with a subsequent secondary fibrosis of the UPJ repair. Additional percutaneous drains should be placed if this is found.

Patients who require pyelopyelostomy in cases of aberrant lower-pole vessels should be investigated carefully during surgery to make certain that a significant intrinsic UPJ obstruction does not exist. On several occasions, I have seen patients in whom initial exploration suggested the presence of lower-pole vessels that at the outset appeared to be the source of the UPJ obstruction. When the pelvis was opened in order to perform the pyelostomy, intrinsic ureteral obstruction was found and was deemed to be the most significant cause of this obstruction. In such patients, a standard dismembered pyeloplasty was performed, resecting the UPJ obstruction, rather than a pyelopyelostomy. This must be carefully looked for in such patients.

In performing pyeloplasty, one must be certain that the blood supply of the ureter is intact. When the ureteral vascularity is in question, fluorescein should be injected intravenously by the anesthesiologist and a Wood's lamp used to check on ureteral blood supply.

The place of endourologic techniques in the management of UPJ obstruction remains undetermined. Whereas encouraging early results by Smith and colleagues (see Chapter 21) have been achieved, long-term results are not available. Nevertheless, it certainly is an interesting approach to this problem, and this therapeutic option must be presented to the patient for fully informed consent.

SURGICAL NEPHROSTOMY

Nephrostomy drainage is utilized for short- and long-term drainage of the upper urinary tract following many procedures. The use of percutaneous techniques has actually reduced the need for open surgical nephrostomy for drainage purposes. Nevertheless, in conjunction with such procedures as ileal ureter and pyeloplasty, open surgical placement of a nephrostomy tube is necessary. When properly placed, excellent decompression can be accomplished with minimal morbidity.

Choice of size and type of tube for nephrostomy drainage depends on the preference of the surgeon and on the configuration of the renal pelvis. In patients with a small renal pelvis, a Foley catheter should not be used because the balloon may obstruct the UPJ. A Malecot catheter has certain advantages over the Foley catheter in that the lumen of the Malecot catheter is larger for a given external diameter, and is maintained in position without the need for a balloon, which can obscure the UPJ. When a Malecot catheter is used, it is wise to cut off two of the four wings to lessen their irritation of the renal pelvis. The disadvantage of the Malecot catheter is that it is harder to change than the Foley catheter. Most commonly, open surgical nephrostomy tubes are utilized for brief periods of healing following major reconstructive renal operations.

Technique

The renal pelvis needs to be exposed for placement of the surgical nephrostomy tube. A curved clamp is directed through a very small pyelotomy of the lower-pole calyx until it can be palpated on the surface of the kidney (Fig. 11–16,*A*). It is then passed through the parenchyma at the tip of the calix, and a No. 18 Fr. or No. 20 Fr. red Robinson catheter is sutured to the eye of the Randallstone forceps (Fig. 11–16,*B*). The site of the exit of the nephrostomy tube should be in a dependent portion of the kidney, with the calyx having the least amount of overlying cortex. The Robinson catheter is then secured to the eye of the clamp with a suture, and the catheter is drawn back through the kidney and out the pyelostomy incision and is disconnected from the Randallstone forceps (Fig. 11–17). The distal end of a No. 24 to 26 Fr. Malecot catheter is sutured to the red Robinson catheter, which is then used to bring the Malecot catheter through the renal parenchyma (Fig. 11–18). This obviates the need to bring the wings of the catheter through the cortex of the kidney, which may cause a tear in the parenchyma and result in troublesome bleeding. Again, two of the four wings of the Malecot catheter are removed to lessen pelvic irritation and to reduce the chance for pelvic junction obstruction. The Malecot catheter is then carefully situated in the lower-pole calyx and the pyelotomy closed with interrupted 4–0 chromic catgut sutures. The larger sized Malecot catheter (compared with the No. 18 or 20 Fr. Robinson catheter) usually will tamponade the nephrostomy tract, and thus persistent bleeding from the kidney will seldom be a problem. An incision in the abdominal wall is then made in such a position to allow as direct a passage as possible of the tube from the kidney to the outside without undue bending or kinking. Also, it is essential to place the site of the nephrostomy tube so that the patient will not be lying on the tube in the supine position. The tube should be securely attached to the skin with nonabsorbable suture material and a sterile dressing placed around the nephrostomy tube.

Complications of Nephrostomy

If significant bleeding should occur through the nephrostomy tube at the time of placement,

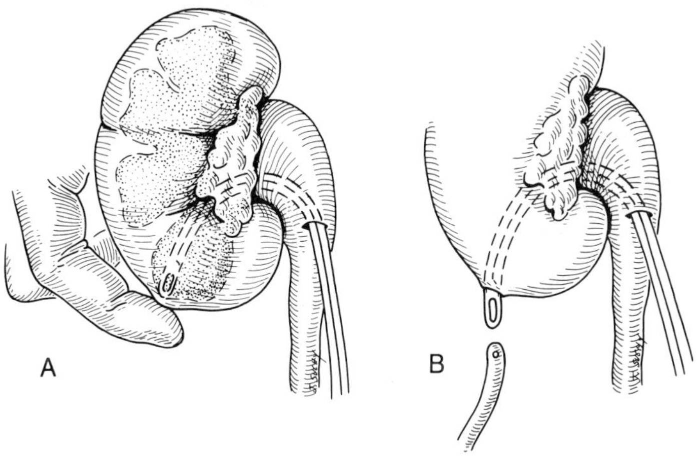

Figure 11–16. Surgical nephrostomy. *A*, A clamp is directed through a very small pyelotomy to the lower-pole calix until it can be palpated on the surface of the kidney. *B*, The clamp is used to grasp an 18 or 20 Fr. red Robinson catheter (usually secured with a suture).

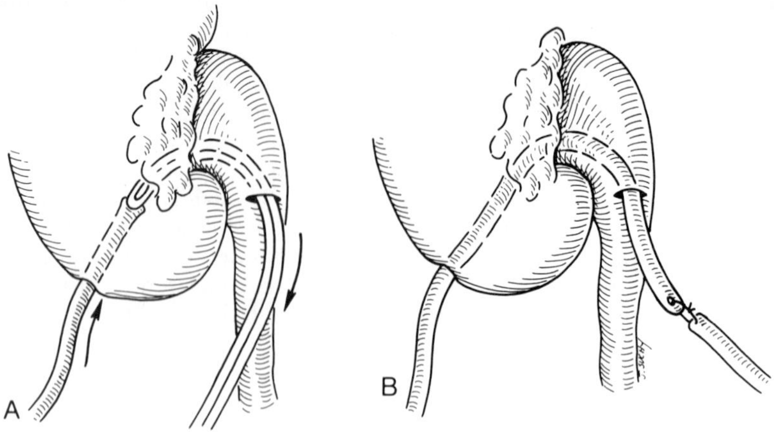

Figure 11–17. Surgical nephrostomy. The catheter is drawn *A*, *B*, through the kidney and out the pyelostomy incision where it is sutured to the end of a Malecot catheter.

the nephrostomy catheter should be occluded and left in place. This will ordinarily result in tamponade of the bleeding site. Undue surgical hemorrhage can be controlled by occluding the renal artery for 5 minutes with a Schwartz clip (or other atraumatic occlusion mechanism) and by manually compressing the kidney at the site of the nephrostomy tract. This will almost always stop significant intraoperative hemorrhage. If significant postoperative hemorrhage occurs, the nephrostomy catheter should be plugged and left in place. This will ordinarily tamponade the bleeding. Generally, clots that form do not need to be removed by irrigation because the production of urokinase will generally result in dissolution of these clots.

If accidental removal of the nephrostomy tube occurs in the immediate postoperative period, it is worth an attempt to replace the tube under fluoroscopic control. In most cases, however, this will not be successful. For such patients, it would be necessary to establish a second percutaneous tract with percutaneous replacement of the nephrostomy tube. (See Chapter 16.)

If a nephrostomy tube fails to drain in the immediate postoperative period, gentle irrigation should be performed by the physician. If this does not accomplish drainage, a gravity nephrostogram should be performed to check on tube placement. It will also give information as to whether there are clots within the renal pelvis causing the drainage problem.

Subsequent change of an established nephrostomy tube should be easily performed. The initial change is generally best done under fluoroscopic control. If an established tube has become dislodged, it is often helpful to have the patient bring the tube with him at the time of the replacement. It is essential that the patient come in immediately for the replacement, since the nephrostomy tract can rapidly decrease in size, and delay can make replacement much more difficult.

The dislodged tube often undergoes a color change at the skin level that gives the urologist some idea of its length from the skin level to the renal pelvis. The corresponding length can be marked on the new catheter to help with depth control during replacement. On occasion, it may be difficult to place the Malecot catheter because this requires a guide. It would be better to replace the Malecot catheter with a Foley

Figure 11–18. Surgical nephrostomy. *A*, *B*, The red rubber Robinson catheter is sutured to the end of a large Malecot catheter to bring it through the renal parenchyma. This obviates the need to bring the wings of the Malecot catheter through the cortex, which may cause a tear in the parenchyma and result in troubling hemorrhage. The larger size of the Malecot catheter tamponades the red Robinson tract.

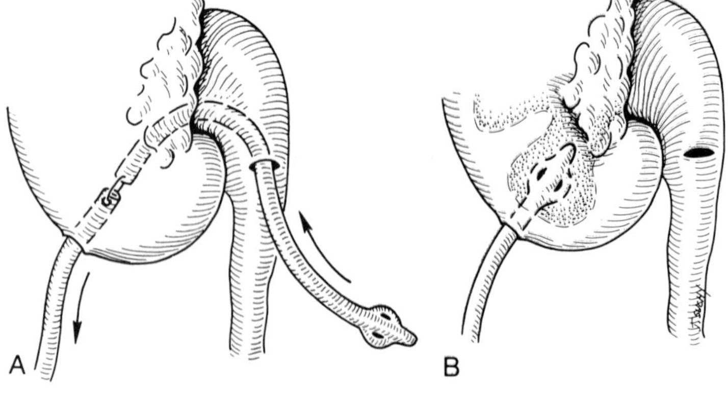

catheter at this time and when the good tract has been re-established. If the tube appears to be in the correct position, a gentle gravity nephrostogram should be performed to ensure that the nephrostomy tube is in the renal pelvis and that there is no extravasation of contrast material. If desired, an existing nephrostomy tract can be dilated by using sequentially larger catheters at each change.

PERINEPHRIC ABSCESS

Perinephric abscess is a potentially fatal disease entity. These patients are usually gravely ill, but no patient with this suspected diagnosis is too ill to withstand a drainage procedure. Rarely will a patient improve with conservative therapy alone. Perinephric infections usually arise from rupture of a renal abscess but may also be secondary to pyelonephritis or hematologic dissemination or bacteremia. The sooner the abscess is drained, the sooner the patient will begin to recover.

When the diagnosis is made, immediate broad-spectrum antibacterial therapy is desirable prior to performing the drainage procedure. Evidence confirmed by CT scan or ultrasonography is advisable. In the poor-risk patient, percutaneous drainage with ultrasound control represents an attractive alternative to open surgical drainage. If adequate drainage cannot be accomplished this way, the patient should undergo adequate open surgical excision and drainage.

Surgical excision should be done through the flank position. If the diagnosis is in doubt, a large spinal needle may be inserted into the retroperitoneal space to determine if purulent material can be obtained. A small flank incision is made in the subcostal area, taking care not to enter the pleural cavity. Also, the peritoneal cavity should be carefully avoided. Rarely should a definitive surgical procedure be performed acutely because of the excessive risk to the patient. It is better to return another day to treat the causative problem. Patients with perinephric abscess associated with obstruction should also have the obstruction relieved by placement of an internal stent transurethrally, by a percutaneous nephrostomy, or by surgical nephrostomy drainage.

The clinical presentation of perinephric abscess is flank pain and fever. Often, these patients suffer from severe diabetes or have a history of recurrent urinary tract infection, pyelonephritis, or stone disease. Blood and urine cultures should be performed; in a series by Sanford, blood cultures were positive in 40 percent of patients, and urine cultures were positive in 80 percent.[28] Organisms responsible for perinephric abscess are predominantly *Proteus*, *Escherichia coli*, and *Staphylococcus aureus*. *Enterobacter*, *Serratia*, *Pseudomonas*, and *Klebsiella* are less common causes.

Cultures should be obtained for aerobic and anaerobic organisms, and the wound should be irrigated with saline copiously, followed by irrigation with 1 percent neomycin solution. Several large Penrose drains should be left with the open surgical drainage and should be brought out through a separate stab incision. The fascia and muscles should be closed with interrupted absorbable sutures. Even with the use of absorbable sutures, there is a chance of suture abscess, which can cause a persistent problem in the postoperative period. The skin and subcutaneous tissues are best left open and then closed from 5 to 9 days after initial incision and drainage. The Penrose drains should be left in place until all significant drainage has stopped. It may be necessary to leave such drains for many weeks. Slow advancement of the drains is preferable to rapid removal. Gradual removal is less likely to allow pockets of infected material to remain, causing recurrent perinephric infectious process.

RENAL BIOPSIES

Percutaneous needle biopsies of the kidney should be performed in preference to surgical renal biopsy except when the former is contraindicated. Contraindications to percutaneous renal biopsies generally include bleeding disorders, uncontrolled hypertension, sepsis secondary to infection in the kidney, presence of severe renal insufficiency with small kidneys, and solitary kidney.

Computed tomography and ultrasonography control for percutaneous needle biopsies have dramatically reduced the complications from these procedures. When open renal biopsy is indicated for parenchymal renal disease, generally the right kidney is approached because of its lower position. A small muscle-splitting subcostal incision is used. An anteroextraperitoneal approach can also be used in relatively thin individuals and in children. In some, the posterior approach is satisfactory, but this should be done in the lateral position so that the kidney does not fall away from the surgeon. A generous wedge biopsy should be taken through the capsule of the kidney, producing a good piece of parenchyma for evaluation, including tissue for standard hematoxylin and eosin (H&E) sectioning, immunofluorescence, and electron microscopic investigation. Generally a piece approximating 3 × 1 × 1 cm is sufficient. The wedge is cut with a knife, and small scissors are used to complete the dissection, cutting across the bottom of the edge. The scissors are employed to lift the wedge of tissue out so that it is not handled by crushing forceps.

In patients in whom there has been severe perinephric inflammation, the capsule may be thickened and mistaken for cortex. A frozen section should be made in such patients to make certain that adequate parenchymal tissue has been obtained to allow a diagnosis to be made.

Bleeding is controlled by placement of parallel sutures of 2–0 or 3–0 chromic catgut before the wedge biopsy is performed. This allows rapid approximation of these sutures after biopsy material has been removed to lessen hemorrhage. The individual ends of these two separate sutures are then tied together to make a mattress suture. This is generally tied over a bolster of perinephric fat or over a Surgicel/Avitene "sandwich." If troublesome bleeding persists following placement of this suture, usually compression of the biopsy site for 5 minutes will suffice. If this does not, the renal artery should be occluded for 5 minutes, along with manual compression of the biopsy site, to cause large venules and arterioles to occlude.

Complications of wedge or percutaneous renal biopsy include arteriovenous (AV) fistulas, which occasionally can be of functional significance or can cause hematuria. Arterial embolization of the feeding vessel can solve this problem. On occasion, secondary exploration or partial nephrectomy may be necessary.

Gerota's fascia should be reapproximated in case postoperative bleeding occurs; tamponade of the bleeding site may be facilitated by Gerota's fascia closure. Rarely is renal exploration required for bleeding.

SURGERY OF ECTOPIC AND HORSESHOE KIDNEYS

Patients with fused or ectopic kidneys are especially vulnerable to infection, calculus formation, and hydronephrosis. The urologist needs to focus special attention on these kidneys because of surgical considerations caused by their malposition, malrotation, and variable vascular supply. The incidence of surgical complications resulting from these anomalies is usually increased when compared with surgery on a normally positioned kidney. The hallmarks of ectopic fused organs are a low position; multiple, varied arterial supply; and malrotation with anterior positioning of the renal pelvis.

A horseshoe kidney is by far the most common of the fusion anomalies, occurring in 1:400 to 500 people. This is second only to duplication anomalies in occurrence. Other fusion anomalies are much rarer and include the so-called pancake fused pelvic kidney, cross-fused ectopia, simple pelvic kidney, and sigmoid kidney.

Horseshoe Kidney

Horseshoe kidneys are typically fused at the lower pole. The connecting isthmus can be fibrous and thin or can contain a great deal of functioning nephrogenic tissue. The isthmus generally is located anterior to the great vessels, but on occasion it has been reported posterior to the great vessels. Pain is the chief presenting symptom in patients with horseshoe kidney, with urinary tract infection being the second most common presenting symptom.

The problem associated with horseshoe kidney is stasis of urine, leading to possible infection and calculus formation. The malrotation of the kidney and the extreme anterior position of the renal pelvis account for the stasis as well as a high insertion of the ureter in the renal pelvis, which is usually the case. A bulky isthmus can also cause accentuation of the obstruction. This, however, is not as important as was thought many years ago. A common surgery required for horseshoe kidney is for correction of these obstructive lesions, with or without removal of renal calculi. Rovsing's syndrome with nausea, vomiting, and abdominal pain, which is aggravated by hyperextension of lumbar spine, may be considered an indication for operative intervention in the absence of obstruction. This indication for surgery has been rare in my experience.

Because the pelvis of horseshoe kidneys may have an ectatic appearance and because of a tendency of the renal pelvis and infundibulum to be extrarenal, retrograde pyelography should be performed, obtaining late draining films to document the significance of apparent stasis and obstruction. A Lasix intravenous pyelogram or Lasix renal scan will also help confirm the obstruction. It is somewhat more difficult to perform a Whitaker test in ectopic and horseshoe kidneys, but in questionable cases this could be done with ultrasonography or CT control.

If surgery on a horseshoe kidney is contemplated, a preoperative study of the blood supply to the kidney is recommended. Either a preoperative renal angiogram or, in selected instances, an MRI study may give information regarding the vascular supply of the kidney. With the variable blood supply going to these kidneys, which is often multiple, a renal artery supplying a significant portion of the parenchyma can be damaged during mobilization of the horseshoe kidney if the location of these vessels is not known preoperatively. Also, often the isthmus is supplied by a Y branch coming off either the common iliac artery or the base of the aorta, which makes division of the isthmus with lateral pexy of the lower poles difficult.

The surgical approach to a horseshoe kidney can be either through an anterior abdominal incision (exterior or interperitoneal) or through a lateral flank incision. In my view, the lateral flank incision jeopardizes one's flexibility with surgery. Often in performing the "simplest" of horseshoe kidney operations (i.e., nephrectomy), it is necessary to have access to the other side in order to resect all potentially devitalized tissues and to close collecting systems properly. With the utilization of an anterior incision, all options are available to the surgeon. When a unilateral procedure is contemplated, it is often possible with an anterior incision to stay extraperitoneal. If a bilateral procedure is contemplated, generally a transperitoneal approach is best.

In the past, there was little question in regard to whether the isthmus of a horseshoe kidney should be routinely divided when a pyeloplasty or pyelolithotomy was performed. More recently, many surgeons have questioned the need for isthmus division and lateral nephropexy. In my view, if one is operating on a horseshoe kidney, it is generally so easy to perform division of the isthmus with lateral nephropexy that I see little reason not to do so. In the rare patient whose functioning parenchyma may have to be resected in order to achieve these ends (i.e., when there is a single artery from the base of the aorta supplying both sides of the isthmus), division may not be indicated. In these patients if the surgeon does not feel that the isthmus is causing significant obstruction, the transection is not warranted.

Surgical exposure of the renal pelvis for pyelolithotomy and pyeloplasty is often easier for horseshoe and ectopic kidneys than for normally placed kidneys because the renal pelvis is anterior and often extrarenal in position. The most common cause of UPJ obstruction is a high insertion of the ureter on the renal pelvis. A Foley Y–V pyeloplasty is ideal for correction of this anatomic lesion. If the isthmus is to be divided, a simple placement of mattress sutures at each end of the divided isthmus will control the bleeding. In patients in whom a bulky isthmus is present where functioning parenchyma must be divided, special care must be taken to ensure that the inferior medial calyx has not been entered with this transection. The development of fistulas is one of the most common complications of isthmus division. Urinary fistulas can also occur if one fails to resect all functioning parenchyma on the removed side (in cases of nephrectomy).

Complications of urinary fistula formation and hemorrhage occur much more frequently with horseshoe or ectopic renal surgery than with standard urologic surgery. Other complications seem to occur at the same rate. Inadvertent damage to renal artery or veins is also a cause of increased complications in horseshoe or ectopic renal surgery.

On occasion, the horseshoe or ectopic kidney is encountered incidentally in the performance of major vascular procedures. The major concern in these situations is the origin of the renal vasculature. If arteriography has not been performed preoperatively, intraoperative angiography should be performed. On occasion, it may be necessary to perform resection of portions of a horseshoe or ectopic kidney in order to correct a vascular anomaly, especially in resections of rapidly enlarging or ruptured aortic aneurysms.

Because the synthetic vascular graft is often necessary in these procedures, careful closure of the collecting system is essential to prevent the formation of urinary fistulas and urinomas in association with a synthetic graft. If possible, omentum or peritoneum should be interposed between the graft and the exposed renal surface.

COMPLICATIONS OF FLANK WOUND CLOSURE

Complications related to flank incision involve hernia formation, a flank bulge secondary to denervation of the intercostal nerve by transection, and nerve entrapment. Occasionally with transthoracic intercostal incisions, suture abscesses can occur in and around large pericostal sutures. These sutures always should be absorbable, and expectant therapy with incision and drainage as necessary usually suffices. On occasion, the suture itself should be removed even though it is theoretically absorbable. It can take several months to absorb and thus perpetuate the local abscess.

Whenever possible, the intercostal nerve of the involved interspace should be spared. Paresthesias that result can be annoying to the patient, and a significant flank bulge develops from denervation of the flank musculature. This can simulate a flank hernia. In most patients, this, of course, requires no treatment. Occasionally patients may experience some discomfort from the bulge, which can be relieved by support with a corset.

In patients who have severe distortion of the abdominal wall and are bothered by this because of its appearance or discomfort, plication of the flank musculature can improve the appearance. This is accomplished by separating the various layers in the flank and plicating this in multiple layers to double the thickness of the flank in the involved area. When the nerve is entrapped in scar tissue and neuritis-like symptoms occur with pain and/or dysesthesia, neurolysis with the combination of steroid injection and long-acting Marcaine can help alleviate this process. Usually reassurance and time will allow the problems to resolve. In mild cases, neurolysis is rarely necessary.

FLANK HERNIA

Hernias of the flank should be rare and occur more commonly in patients who are obese or who have been on immunosuppression medication and as a complication of wound infection. As mentioned in the foregoing discussion, flank hernia can often be confused with a flank bulge secondary to denervation of the flank musculature. Careful examination will reveal a fascial defect in patients with flank hernia.

The repair of flank hernias can be difficult indeed. Usually it is best to free up all fascial tissues and to mobilize tissues widely. The flank fascia and musculature should remain close in multiple layers using a "vest over pants" technique with nonabsorbable sutures. In selected patients, Marlex may be necessary to achieve repair. Marlex should never be used at a potentially infected site.

References

1. Poutasse EF: Anterior approach to the upper urinary tract surgery. J Urol 85:199, 1961.
2. Chute R, et al: The transverse upper abdominal chevron incision in urologic surgery. J Urol 99:528, 1968.
3. Chute R: Value of thoracoabdominal incision in removal of kidney tumors. N Engl J Med 241:951, 1949.
4. Robson CJ: Radical nephrectomy for renal cell carcinoma. J Urol 89:37, 1963.
5. Swanson DA, Borges PM: Complications of transabdominal radical nephrectomy for renal cell carcinoma. J Urol 129:704, 1983.
6. Gopal D, Bisno AL: Fulminate pneumococcal infections in "normal" asplenic hosts. Arch Intern Med 137:1526, 1977.
7. Stollerman GH: Pneumococcal vaccine (Letter). JAMA 247:1809, 1982.
8. Dickerman JD: Splenectomy and sepsis: a warning. Pediatrics 63:938, 1979.
9. Waters WB, Richie JP: Aggressive surgical approach to renal cell carcinoma: review of 130 cases. J Urol 122:306, 1979.
10. Scheff TP, Novick AC, Straffon RA, Stewart B, et al: Surgery for renal cell carcinoma extending into the inferior vena cava. J Urol 120:28, 1978.
11. Siminovitch JNP, Montie JE, Straffon RA: Inferior vena cavography in the preoperative assessment of renal adenocarcinoma. J Urol 128:908, 1982.
12. Clayman RV, Gonzalez R, Fraley EE: Renal cell cancer invading the inferior vena cava: clinical review and anatomical approach. J Urol 123:157, 1983.
13. Cherrie RJ, Goldman DG, Lindner A, et al: Prognostic implications of vena caval extension of renal cell carcinoma. J Urol 128:910, 1982.
14. deKernion JB, Ramming K, Smith RB, et al: Natural history of metastatic renal cell carcinoma: computer analysis. J Urol 120:148, 1978.
15. Clark CD: Survival after excision of a kidney, segmental resection of the vena cava, division of the opposite renal vein. Lancet 2:1015, 1961.
16. Pathak IC: Survival after right nephrectomy, excision of infrahepatic vena cava and ligation of left renal vein: a case report. J Urol 106:599, 1971.
17. Marshall VF, Middleton RG, Holswade GR, et al.: Surgery for renal cell carcinoma in the vena cava. J Urol 103:414, 1970.
18. Bloom NA, Vidone RA, Lytton B: Primary carcinoma of the ureter: a report of 102 new cases. J Urol 103:590, 1970.
19. Strong DW, Pearse HD: Recurrent urothelial tumors following surgery for transitional cell carcinoma of the upper urinary tract. Cancer 38:2178, 1976.
20. Mukamel E, Konickezky M, Engelstein D, et al: Incidental small renal tumors accompanying clinically overt renal cell carcinoma. J Urol 140:22, 1988.
21. Blackley SK, Ladaga LL, Woolfitt RA, et al: Ex-situ study of effectiveness of enucleation in patients with renal cell carcinoma. J Urol 140:6, 1988.
22. Rosenthal CL: Organ preserving surgery in renal cell carcinoma: tumor enucleation vs partial kidney resection. Eur Urol 10:222, 1984.
23. Lang K: Diagnosis of renal parenchymal tumors. In Skinner DG, deKernion JB, eds: Genitourinary Cancer. Philadelphia, WB Saunders Co, 1978, p 40.
24. Hanna MK, Jeffs RD, Sturgess LM, et al: Congenital ureteropelvic junction obstruction and primary obstructive megaureter. Part II. J Urol 116:725, 1976.
25. Gosling JA, Dixon JS: Functional obstruction of the ure-

ter or renal pelvis: the histologic and electron microscopic study. Br J Urol 50:145, 1978.
26. Kelalis PP: Ureterovesical junction. In Kelalis PP, King LR, eds: Clinical Pediatric Urology. Philadelphia, WB Saunders Co, 1976, p 239.
27. Whitaker RH: The Whitaker test. Urol Clin North Am, 6(3):529, 1979.
28. Sanford JP: Perinephric abscess. In Harrison JH, Gittes R, Perlmutter A, Stamey T, Walsh P, eds: Urology, Vol 1. Philadelphia, WB Saunders Co, 1978, p 708.

COMPLICATIONS OF OPEN RENAL STONE SURGERY

12

Donald R. Bodner • Martin I. Resnick

There has recently been much interest in "noninvasive" or "nonsurgical" techniques to remove or break up renal stones. Although most calculi are small and pass spontaneously, a select minority are too large and become lodged in the renal pelvis, calyx, infundibulum, or ureter. Currently, most of these are managed with extracorporeal shock wave lithotripsy or percutaneous nephrostolithotomy, and understandably there is a tendency to forget the significant improvements that have occurred in open renal surgery over the past several years. Because urology residents have limited experience with open renal techniques they probably will not be proficient when open procedures on the kidney are required. Although it is apparent that the role of open renal surgery will not be as prominent in the future as it once was, urologists must maintain proficiency and knowledge of a variety of open renal techniques. Traditional surgery will most likely continue for management of complete staghorn calculi associated with intrarenal scarring and associated infundibular and calyceal stenosis, a condition in which intrarenal reconstruction is required. Similarly, other open procedures, such as partial nephrectomy, will at times also be necessary. The clinical urologist must be adept not only at the performance of these procedures but also at the appropriate preoperative and postoperative management of patients.

The complications that occur secondary to open renal surgery are directly related to the particular procedure and the surgical technique employed. It must also be remembered and emphasized that the goal of any procedure for stone removal—invasive, noninvasive, or surgical—is to remove all stone fragments and preserve maximal renal function. In this chapter, we review the techniques involved in the various open renal stone procedures and discuss the specific complications that occur with them.

HISTORY OF OPEN RENAL SURGERY

Hippocrates is credited with performing the first operation on the kidney. In his time, it was common practice to drain renal and perirenal abscesses; on occasion, the collecting system of the kidney was entered and the stone extruded either at the time of surgery or during the postoperative period. Celcus, Galen, and other early physicians mentioned kidney stones in their writings, but none believed extraction to be safe or feasible. In 1501, Cardan, of Milan, described removing 18 stones when a renal abscess was drained. Hevin, in 1775, is credited with first using the term nephrolithotomy.[1]

European surgeons, in the 1700s and early 1800s, limited the use of nephrotomies to obstructed, infected kidneys; if the stone could not readily be removed, it was left to pass spontaneously through the fistulous tract. Prior to the late 1800s, nephrolithotomy remained an imprecise operation usually performed inadvertently in association with drainage of renal and perirenal abscesses. Intrarenal hemorrhage was a major problem, because when specifically performed for removal of intrarenal stones, knowledge of intrarenal anatomy was limited. The gradual evolution of modern nephrolithotomy in the 1960s closely followed research on intrarenal anatomy, physiology, renal preservation, and perioperative techniques.

Dr. William Ingalls is credited with performing the first deliberate nephrolithotomy in the United States at the Boston City Hospital in 1872 in a patient in whom he had previously drained a perinephric abscess.[2] In 1880, Henry Morris, an English surgeon, performed the first nephrolithotomy on an apparently healthy kidney with no associated abscess.[3] He subsequently described his initial experience with 34 nephrolithotomies with 33 recoveries and one death. His results established that nephrolithotomy was a safe surgical procedure and refuted the previous teachings that renal stones should be removed only from an abscess cavity.[4]

Surgeons practicing in the early 1900s had an excellent understanding of the gross renal anatomy, but it was not until the studies of Josef Hyrtl, a 19th century Viennese anatomist, that the intrarenal vasculature was defined.[5] He described a relatively avascular plane between the anterior and posterior segments of the renal artery. *The Intrinsic Blood Vessels of the Kidney and Their Significance in Nephrotomy* was then published by Max Brodel, a medical artist at the Johns Hopkins Medical School.[6] In this classic report, he accurately described the branching of the main renal artery and its lack of free anastomosis between segmental branches. The relatively avascular plane between the anterior and posterior arterial segments, known as "Brodel's line," was also noted. Cullen and Derge in 1909 suggested that nephrotomy incision be made with a thin silver wire passed between arterial branches from within outward.[7] They recommended an L-shaped nephrotomy incision to avoid ischemic infarction of the papillary tips. In the late 1920s, after studying the effect on the kidney of different incisions, Deming concluded that the best nephrotomy incision was a longitudinal one through the avascular plane described by Hyrtl and Brodel.[8,9] Smith and Boyce then combined this incision with intrarenal reconstruction of the collecting system to remove staghorn calculi to improve renal drainage.[10]

Improvements in intraoperative stone localization with radiography and hypothermia to preserve renal function deserve special mention. Robson was the first to suggest the use of intraoperative x-rays to localize renal stones.[11] Refinements in radiography and development of ultrasonography helped to diagnose renal stones more accurately not only preoperatively but also intraoperatively. Subsequently, intraoperative x-rays and ultrasonography, along with the use of direct palpation and needles for localization, have helped to further define the exact location of the stone.

A significant advance to open renal surgery occurred when it was learned that the adverse effects of ischemia could be prevented by *hypothermia.* It was known as early as 1880 that ischemia resulted in damage to the kidney. Litten[12] noted histologic damage to the epithelium of the proximal tubule when the kidney was made ischemic; other investigators also noted ischemic changes when the total warm ischemic time was 30 minutes and was reversible only when it was less than 1 hour.[13–15]

Renal cooling reduces cellular metabolic activity and consequently protects the proximal tubule from ischemic damage. The optimal temperature to which kidney must be cooled is controversial, but temperatures of 15 to 20° C appear to be most effective. There are numerous methods to cool the kidney, and there appears to be little practical difference between them.[16–22] Hypothermia, by whichever method, is an important tool in open renal surgery and should be considered when the renal artery is clamped for any prolonged period of time.

RENAL ANATOMY

To better understand the principles of open renal surgery, the intrarenal arterial anatomy and associated collecting structures are first reviewed. In 70 to 80 percent of kidneys, the main renal artery branches in the distal third of the vessel prior to entering the renal hilum into the anterior and posterior segment arteries, each of which is an end artery with no collateral circulation (Fig. 12–1). Further branching continues in an orderly manner, with eight to 12 interlobar arteries coursing along opposite sides of the infundibulum toward the papilla. The interlobar arteries then branch into the transmedullary arteries, which form near the renal parenchyma and enter at the caliceal cup. They are paired and pass into the medulla through the interpapillary spaces to reach the cortex, and some continue as the arcuate arteries (Fig. 12–2).

The kidney is divided into four surgical segments by division of the renal artery. They include the superior, inferior, anterior, and posterior segments (Fig. 12–3). In about 50 percent of patients, the first division of the main renal artery is the posterior segment, which supplies

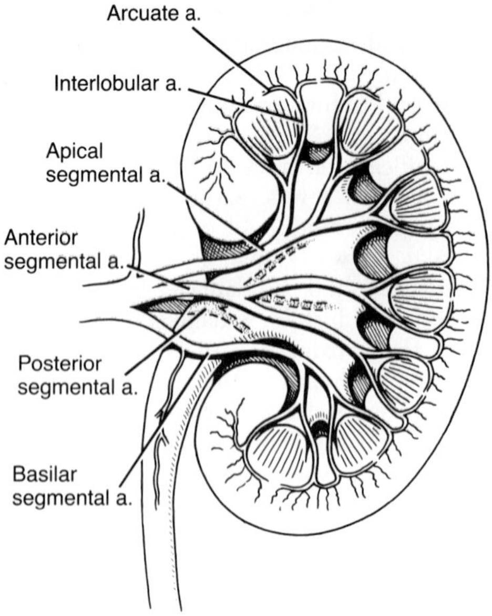

Figure 12–1. Anatomy of the renal artery.

the posterior portion of the kidney; however, in a third of patients, the first branch supplies the inferior pole. The posterior branch continues without division to supply the posterior segment of the kidney. The anterior segmental artery is the larger division and divides into three or four branches, as it is the continuation of the main renal artery. The anterior division typically supplies the superior, inferior, and anterior segments. The artery to the inferior segment enters

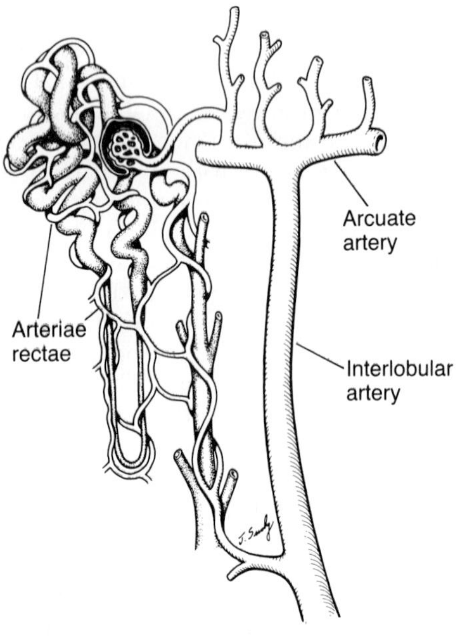

Figure 12–2. Intrarenal continuation of the renal artery.

the renal hilum, descends obliquely to its lower border, and then crosses the renal pelvis and divides into anterior and posterior divisions.

The exact number and distribution of the calyces constitute the most variable parts of renal anatomy (Fig. 12–4). The ureter generally is a direct continuation of the renal pelvis. In most kidneys, the pelvis divides within the substance of the kidney into two or three main sections known as infundibula, or *major calyces.* These divide into secondary and tertiary sections known as the *minor calyces.* The calyces are well-defined units that can be simple and drain one papilla or can be complex and drain multiple papillae. Polar calyces are the most variable and are frequently complex. The total number of calyces averages eight but ranges from four to 12. The calyx from the most superior division is most often complex. The remainder of the calyces are paired anterior and posterior to an imaginary line that divides the kidney longitudinally. The anterior calyces are irregularly arranged at an angle of 70° to 75° from the frontal plane, whereas the posterior calyces are more regularly arranged at a 20° angle from the frontal plane.

PREOPERATIVE CONSIDERATIONS

Approximately 15 to 20 percent of all urinary calculi are struvite or "infection" stones in nature. They occur more frequently in females than in males (2:1) and often form a staghorn configuration in the kidney. Infection stones occur more frequently in patients with neurogenic bladders and recurrent urinary tract infections as well as in patients with chronic indwelling catheters and external urinary diversions. Typically, the infection is caused by a urease-producing bacterium, which includes *Proteus mirabilis, Providencia, Klebsiella,* and, occasionally, *Pseudomonas.* Strains of *Pseudomonas* appear the most difficult to eradicate and are consequently associated with the highest incidence of stone recurrence.[23] *Escherichia coli* is not a urea splitter, and infections associated with *E. coli* should be suspected of being superinfections and not associated with the formation or growth of the stone.

It is mandatory to treat all urinary tract infections adequately prior to open renal surgery to prevent the postoperative complications of sepsis, abscess formation, and wound infection. It is often difficult to totally eliminate the bacteria in the presence of an infection stone, infundibular or intracalyceal scarring, and a kidney

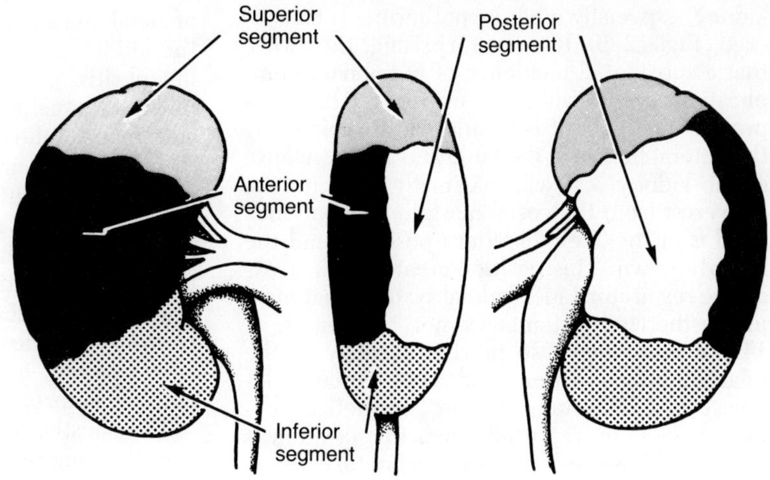

Figure 12–3. Vascular segments as determined by distribution of the renal artery.

with areas of "patchy pyelonephritis."[24] The presence of retained bacteria is likely in these kidneys despite negative bladder urine cultures.

Preoperative infections should be treated for a minimum of 24 to 48 hours with an appropriate antibiotic, the selection of which is based upon in vitro culture and sensitivity studies. Semisynthetic penicillins and cephalosporins should be used when appropriate. Aminoglycosides and other nephrotoxic agents should be reserved for patients with resistant infections with sensitivities. When required, peak and trough levels of the antibiotic should be obtained to ensure appropriate dosages of the medication, and serial renal function studies should be obtained routinely. It is advisable to repeat urine cultures once the antibiotics have been discontinued to ensure that the infection is completely resolved.

At the time of surgery, cultures of any mucinous material in an obstructed calyx and of stone fragments removed from the kidney should be obtained. These cultures are helpful in the selection of postoperative antibiotics, for it has been shown that the bacteriology of the stone may differ greatly from the preoperative urine cultures.[25] Intravenous antibiotics begun preoperatively should be continued both perioperatively and postoperatively. The exact duration is controversial, but a 2- to 4-week course of antibiotic suppression is not unreasonable. Urine cultures should be repeated after the antibiotics have been discontinued. If the infection stone is removed completely at surgery, if urine cultures are monitored closely postoperatively, and if all recurrent infections are promptly treated, recurrent stone formation can be markedly diminished.[26] The main cause of recurrent stone formation is residual stone fragments left at the time of surgery. It is well recognized that systemic antibiotics sterilize only the surface of the stone and that bacteria remain harbored deep within the interstices.[27] Removing all the stone fragments, therefore, becomes very important.

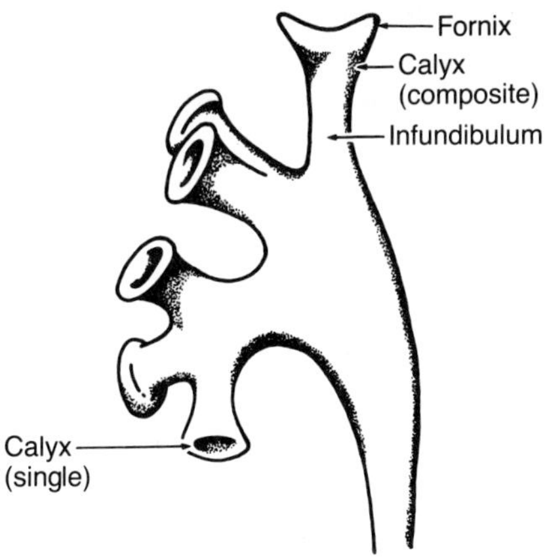

Figure 12–4. The renal calyces are shown. Their exact number and configuration are variable.

INTRAOPERATIVE AND POSTOPERATIVE COMPLICATIONS

Pulmonary Dysfunction

Pulmonary dysfunction is perhaps the most common postoperative complication occurring in 5 to 10 percent of all patients undergoing open renal surgery.[27] Birch and Mims reviewed their experience with patients undergoing anatrophic nephrolithotomy and found an incidence of pulmonary complications in 37 percent, with atelectasis being the greatest.[16] The lateral, or flank, position is most frequently used to enter the kidney, especially when hypothermia is considered (Fig. 12–5). It is not surprising, therefore, that a substantial incidence of pulmonary complications occurs when one utilizes the flank approach. The patient is positioned in such a way that lateral flexion of the table and additional use of the kidney rest will maximally separate the iliac crest from the costal margin. The patient's head is in the Trendelenburg position, and the feet are down. This position creates such stress on the respiratory and skeletal systems that most unanesthetized patients cannot tolerate it. A 14.5 percent decrease in vital capacity in the unanesthetized patient and a 14 percent decrease in tidal volume in the anesthetized patient have been reported when this position is used.[28,29] These reductions in respiratory capacity are due to direct restriction of the chest wall in all directions, with excursion most limited laterally.[30]

There has been concern that the down lung may be at increased risk for pulmonary complications secondary to venous congestion and inability to expand fully; however, clinical experience has shown that these complications occur with equal frequency in both lung fields.[16] Postoperative pulmonary problems are complicated by the position of the patient's wound. Deep breathing and coughing are extremely important but painful. Occasional use of a pillow on the abdomen or an abdominal binder may be of help. Pulmonary physiotherapy should be instituted preoperatively and continued well into the postoperative period. The routine use of incentive spirometry appears to be of value in all patients. Ultrasonic aerosols may also be of help, but whether they should be used routinely is debatable. Early ambulation is of great importance to minimize postoperative complications and should be emphasized.

Pneumothorax

Pneumothorax occurs in fewer than 5 percent of patients undergoing open surgery for removal of renal stones. Patients with prior surgery on the kidney and patients with a history of pyelonephritis are at higher risk for sustaining a pneumothorax. In these patients, there is often adherence of the upper pole of the kidney to the diaphragm and attached pleura, making inadvertent entry into the chest more common. Pleural injury is also more frequent when the 11th or 12th interspace is used for the incision than when a 12th rib or subcostal incision is used. This is because of the attachment of the pleura to the ribs. When a small pleural entry is recognized, it can be closed with a running chromic suture.

The anesthesiologist is instructed to fully inflate the lung prior to completing the closure of the pleura to ensure that no air remains. If there is concern that the pleural incision is not adequately closed, use of a small chest tube is appropriate. The tube can generally be removed 48 hours postoperatively. A portable chest x-ray should be obtained in the recovery room if a pleural repair has been performed or if a pneumothorax is suspected. If a pneumothorax is confirmed on this film, a chest tube should be considered and follow-up chest x-rays are essential.

Pulmonary Emboli

Pulmonary emboli can occur after any surgical procedure, and specific techniques to prevent them are controversial. Early ambulation is important, and perhaps thigh-high elastic stockings or sequential venous compression stockings should be considered in the high-risk patient. Boyce reported three fatal (0.3 percent) and nine (0.9 percent) pulmonary emboli in his series of 951 patients undergoing anatrophic nephrolithotomy, for a total incidence of just over 1 percent.[31]

A fatal pulmonary embolism was also reported

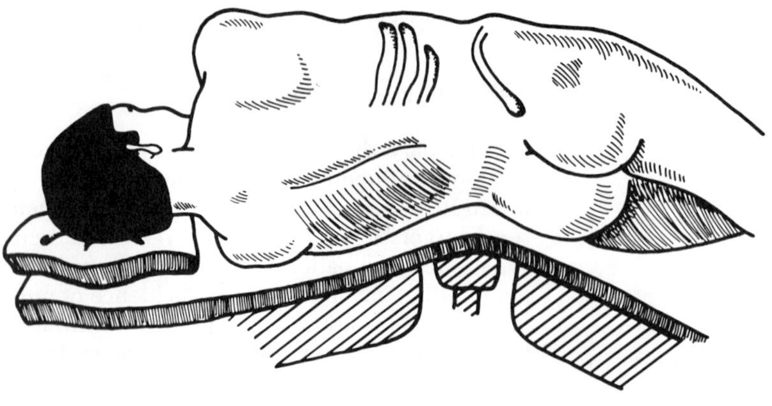

Figure 12–5. Flank position. Table flexion and use of the kidney rest provide optimal exposure to the kidney.

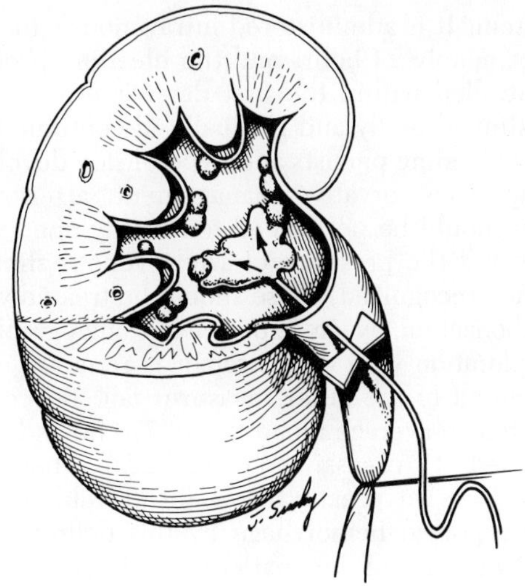

Figure 12–6. Coagulum pyelolithotomy. The ureter is occluded and the coagulum injected.

in association with coagulum pyelolithotomy (Figs. 12–6 and 12–7).[32] It is believed in this instance that the embolus occurred secondary to overfilling of the renal pelvis and subsequent pyelovenous backflow with intravascular leakage of the coagulum, which is composed of thrombin, calcium chloride ($CaCl_2$), and cryoprecipitate. Figure 12–6 illustrates a coagulum pyelolithotomy in which a mixture of thrombin, $CaCl_2$, and cryoprecipitate is injected into the pelvis to form a coagulum to remove all the stones.

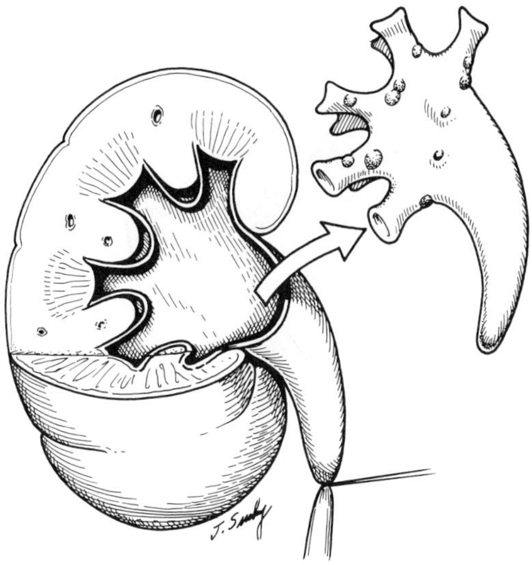

Figure 12–7. The coagulum is a cast of the renal pelvis and calyces containing all the stone fragments.

Table 12–1. ANATROPHIC NEPHROLITHOTOMY 1963–1982: MORTALITY*†

	No. of Patients
Myocardial infarction	1
Pulmonary embolus	3

*Modified from Boyce WH: Surgery of urinary calculi in perspective. Urol Clin North Am 10:585–594, 1983.
†Mortality = 0.42 percent in less than 3 months.

Cardiovascular Complications

In addition to pulmonary complications from open renal surgery, cardiovascular changes should be considered as well. In the flank position, decreased venous return is the rule and hypotension may be encountered. It is important to gradually add flexion and raise the kidney rest while continually monitoring blood pressure. Mediastinal shifting and displacement of the liver have been implicated in the hypotension, and the use of elastic stockings may improve venous return.[33] In his series of 951 patients undergoing anatrophic nephrolithotomy, Boyce[31] reported one myocardial infarction for an incidence of just over 0.1 percent and accounting for one death (Table 12–1).

Hemorrhage

Significant postoperative renal hemorrhage occurs in less than 10 percent of open renal surgical procedures.[34] The urologist's ability to operate on the kidney with minimal blood loss and preservation of renal function is directly related to knowledge of the intrarenal arterial anatomy and the various vascular segments (see Figs. 12–1 and 12–3). The avascular plane between the anterior and posterior branches of the renal artery must be identified in each kidney to place intersegmental nephrostomy incisions without resulting in massive hemorrhage. The kidney is completely mobilized, and the main renal artery is dissected. The posterior segment can be clamped and methylene blue injected intravenously if an anatrophic nephrolithotomy is considered (Fig. 12–8). The avascular plane can be easily differentiated from Brodel's line (Fig. 12–9).

As noted, to minimize hemorrhage, the kidney can be cooled and the renal artery clamped. Precise closure of the collecting system with repair of the intrarenal vessels and careful closure of the renal capsule will minimize subsequent postoperative hemorrhage (Fig. 12–10). When

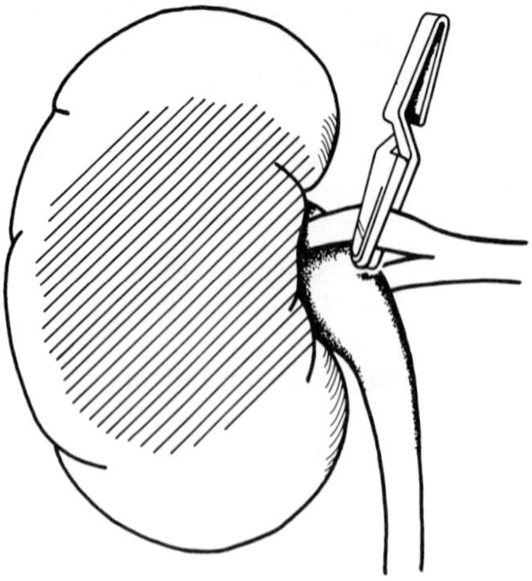

Figure 12–8. The posterior segment of the renal artery is occluded, and methylene blue is then given to define the avascular plane.

bleeding is encountered, it is frequently intrapelvic and occurs spontaneously 1 to 2 weeks postoperatively. The bleeding often results from inadequately closed intrarenal vessels, and expectant treatment is generally sufficient. Blood transfusions, intravenous fluids, and bed rest often stabilize the patient.

The administration of aminocaproic acid (Amicar) may also be of benefit when hemorrhage does not immediately subside.[35] Amicar is an antifibrinolytic agent and is helpful in association with the high levels of urokinase in the urinary system. It is administered intravenously for approximately 24 hours and the bleeding is often controlled within the first day. Amicar can be continued orally and gradually discontinued.

If bleeding persists and hypotension develops despite conservative management, arteriography should be performed to identify open vessels and the presence of arteriovenous shunts. When recognized, these should be treated with embolization by an experienced angiographer. Exploration with direct repair is required only when all of the other measures fail. Boyce reported an average blood loss of 778 ml and considered it "excessive hemorrhage" when the blood loss was greater than 1000 ml (Table 12–2). He reported hemorrhage by this definition in 6.8 percent of his patients undergoing anatrophic nephrolithotomy.[31]

Complications Associated with Vascular Manipulation

When extensive nephrotomies are required, it is often advantageous to clamp the main renal artery. This helps not only in reducing intraoperative blood loss but also in diminishing kidney turgor, which permits easier localization of stone fragments and entry into the collecting system. Clamps can damage the vessel to which they are applied; therefore, atraumatic clamps should be utilized and placed meticulously. Care

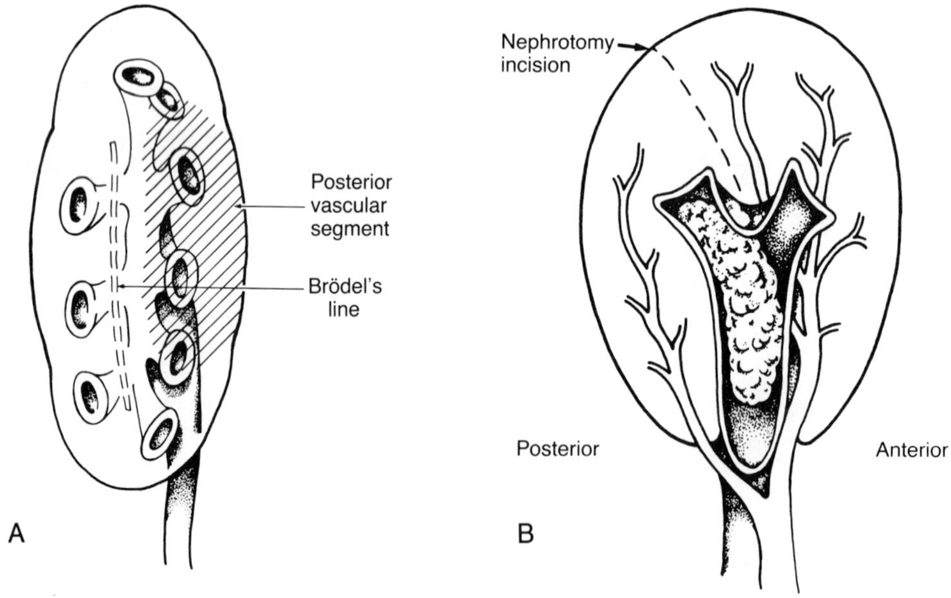

Figure 12–9. *A*,*B*, The nephrotomy incision will be made after the avascular plane is defined.

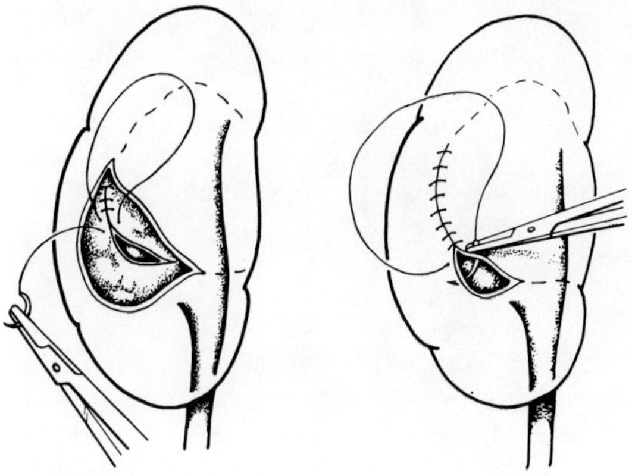

Figure 12–10. Careful closure of the collecting system and renal capsule will minimize subsequent bleeding.

should be exercised in dissection of the renal artery prior to placement of the clamp; to reduce injury to the vessel, the adventia and small vessels about the artery should be preserved. In Boyce's large series of anatrophic nephrolithotomies, he reported no instance of either acute or delayed injury to the renal artery.[31] Once the vascular clamp is removed, the vessel should be inspected for injury to the renal artery or one of its segments; this can easily be recognized, and, if present, it can be repaired (Fig. 12–11).

Renal vein injuries are extremely rare because the renal vein is not clamped during periods of hypothermia. It is also important not to clamp the renal vein during the hilar dissection because this can lead to venous thrombosis and subsequent renal infarction.

Once the renal artery is carefully dissected, it is important to be sure that the patient is well hydrated and that there are no hypotensive episodes. Increased amounts of intravenous fluids

Table 12–2. ANATROPHIC NEPHROLITHOTOMY 1963–1982: MORBIDITY (COMPLICATIONS WITH RECOVERY IN 951 PATIENTS)*

	No. of Patients (Percent)
Hemorrhage > 1000 ml (reoperation 3)	65 (6.8%)
Arteriovenous fistulas reoperated	4 (0.4%)
Atelectasis, any degree, by x-ray	232 (24.4%)
Pneumothorax	36 (3.8%)
Pulmonary embolus	9 (0.9%)
All others, including temperature greater than 100° F, gastrointestinal bleeding, etc.	153 (16.1%)

*Modified from Boyce WH: Surgery of urinary calculi in perspective. Urol Clin North Am 10:585–594, 1983.

should be administered, and mannitol may also be of value in both increasing the renal plasma flow and decreasing intrarenal vascular resistance. Mannitol should be administered 5 to 10 minutes prior to clamping of the renal artery.[36,37] In addition to increasing renal plasma flow, mannitol also increases the osmolarity of the tubular fluid, which helps to protect the kidney from hypothermic injury during periods of surface cooling. The kidney can be cooled by a multitude of techniques, all of which are effective in preventing post-ischemic renal failure.[16–22] Direct surface cooling with ice is as effective as other methods. The kidney is surrounded by a rubber dam, and the main renal artery is occluded. An ice slush is then placed in direct contact with the kidney (Fig. 12–12) and kept in contact with the kidney until the procedure is completed and the vascular clamp removed. The kidney suffers ischemic injury when the warm ischemic time exceeds 30 minutes.[16–22]

Stone Migration

Migration of the stone during intraoperative manipulation of the kidney with the resultant inability to localize it is a serious problem when encountered. When a pyelolithotomy is being performed, the renal pelvis should be opened directly over the stone after the ureter distal to the stone is secured with a vascular loop. It is important that the incision be made in a transverse direction as far away from the ureteropelvic junction as possible. An incision at this location is least likely to tear into the ureteropelvic junction (Fig. 12–13). Extension is also possible along each calyx when needed. Securing the ureter distal to the stone will prevent the stone from passing into the ureter. If, however, this occurs and is not recognized, it can cause acute urinary obstruction resulting in postoperative flank pain and urosepsis. These complications necessitate the performance of an emergency secondary procedure, either placement of a percutaneous nephrostomy or the passage of a ureteral stent. When anatrophic nephrolithotomy is performed, a Silastic stent should be passed down the ureter from the renal pelvis into the bladder. The stent usually passes spontaneously postoperatively and protects the kidney from obstruction secondary to passage of small stone fragments. If the stent does not pass spontaneously, it can be removed cystoscopically on the seventh postoperative day.

For branched calculi that are difficult to re-

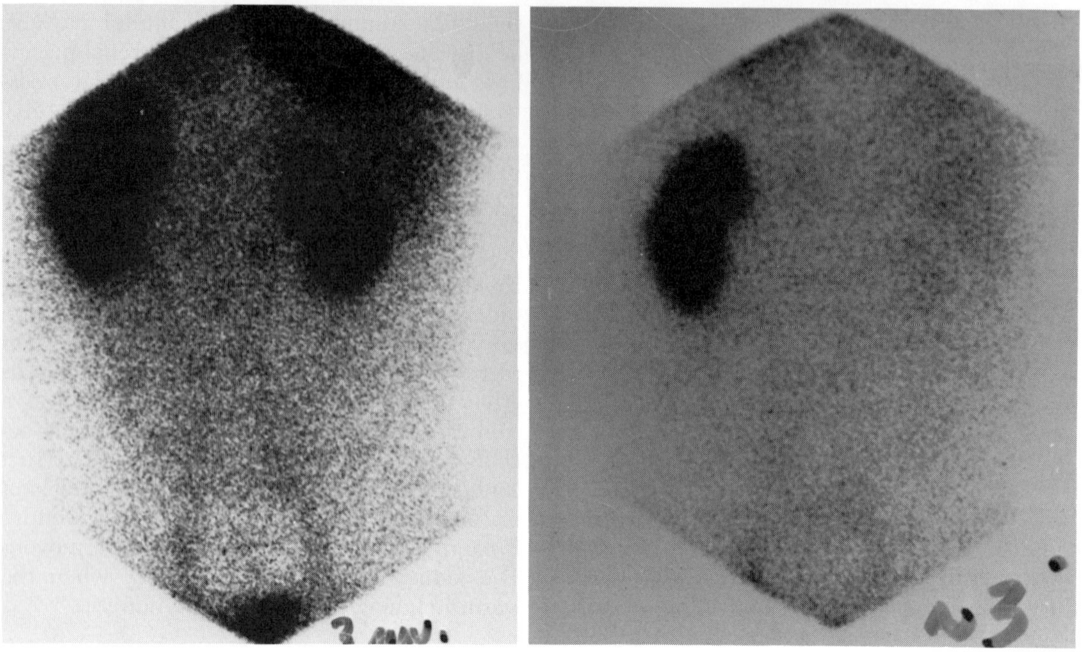

Figure 12–11. Preoperative and postoperative renal scans from a patient referred after renal artery injury during anatrophic nephrolithotomy. Note the absence of function postoperatively.

move with *simple* pyelolithotomy, *extended* pyelolithotomy should be considered. The renal pelvis is dissected free of peripelvic fat, and the posterior edge of the renal sinus is completely exposed. A pyeloinfundibular incision is made to conform with the location of the calculi, and the stone is then delivered.

Radial nephrotomy is also of benefit in removing renal stones. Following the clamping of the main renal artery and application of hypothermia, parenchymal incisions can be made that parallel the course of the intrarenal vessels (Fig. 12–14). This prevents transection of these vessels, lessens bleeding, and minimizes parenchymal destruction. Stone localization is facilitated by intraoperative x-rays obtained prior to making the incision. Whenever possible, radial nephrotomies should be made on the posterior convexity of the kidney to avoid the large venous branches on the anterior surface of the kidney.

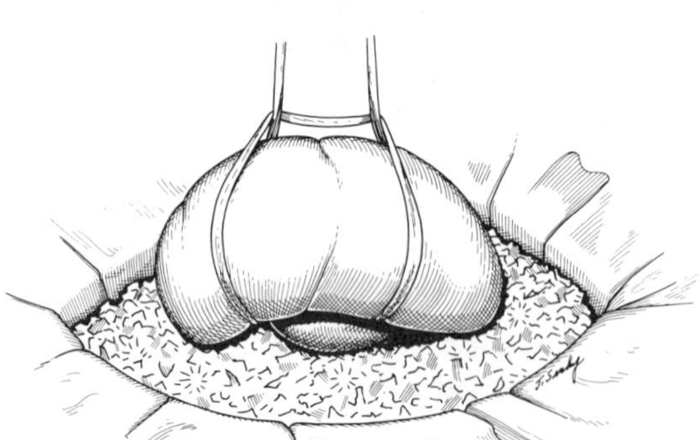

Figure 12–12. An ice slush solution is placed in direct contact with the kidney after the renal artery is first clamped. A rubber dam keeps the ice in contact with the kidney.

Retained Stone Fragments

Retained stones represent a major concern in terms of a nidus for further calculus formation and is reported to have an incidence of 5 to 30 percent (Table 12–3).[30,38–40] Residual stone fragments are probably of less concern for calcium oxalate, cystine, and uric acid stones than for struvite stones. Stones of these compositions may grow in size but are influenced by the concentration of the active products in urine and

Table 12–3. ANATROPHIC NEPHROLITHOTOMY 1963–1982

Final Intraoperative X-ray	Percent
No calculi or calcification	79.5%
Papillary calcification	5.0%
Parenchymal calcification	15.5%

Modified from Boyce WH: Surgery of urinary calculi in perspective. Urol Clin North Am 10:585, 1983.

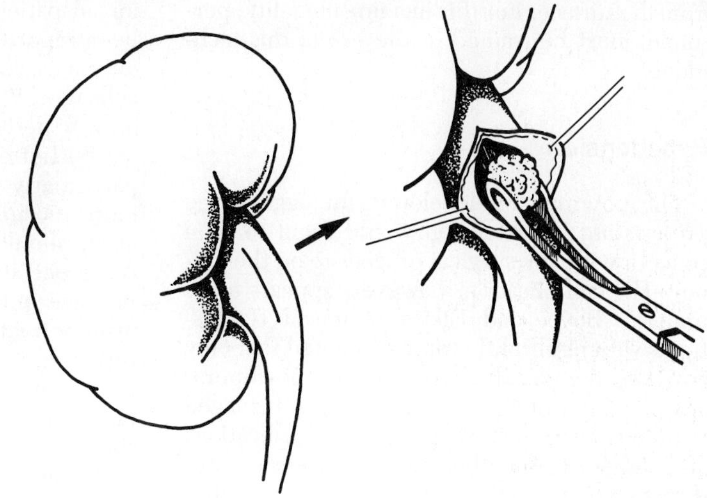

Figure 12–13. Simple pyelolithotomy performed improperly. An incorrect incision is made over the renal pelvis in a vertical direction. With this incision, tearing into the ureteropelvic junction and subsequent complication are likely.

the formation product of these substances and not the presence of the stone fragment.[41] Sleight and Wickham reported that 70 percent of retained infected stones increased in size but only 30 per cent of uninfected stones did so.[42]

The intersegmental nephrotomy is indicated for full staghorn calculi and branched calculi with infundibular stenosis. This technique provides maximal exposure to the renal collecting system. Prior to making the nephrotomy incision, intraoperative x-rays should be obtained to define the extent of the stone (Fig. 12–15). Once the bulk is removed, further films are obtained to identify remaining fragments. Needles can be placed to help localize the stone, and final films should confirm the absence of residual fragments. If stone fragments cannot be localized, intraoperative nephroscopy may be helpful. Intraoperative ultrasonography can also be employed to localize remaining fragments 2 to 3 mm in diameter.[43] Ultrasonography offers the distinct advantage in identifying radiolucent calculi and also in quantitating the depth and angle

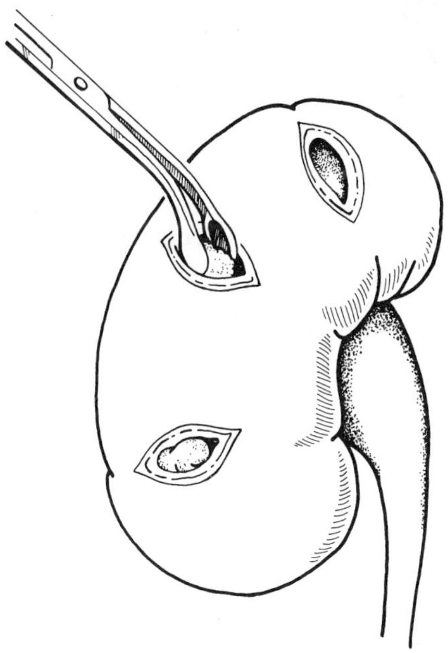

Figure 12–14. Multiple radial nephrotomies are made after the renal artery is clamped and after hypothermia is begun. The incisions should parallel the course of the intrarenal vessels.

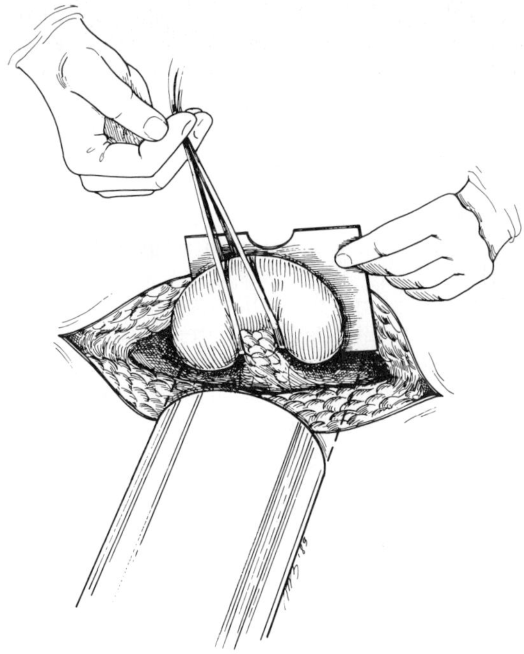

Figure 12–15. Sterilized x-ray films can be placed in direct contact with the kidney and can accurately assess residual fragments.

from the surface. For this imaging modality, personnel must be trained in the use of this technique.

Hypertension

The potential of developing or aggravating pre-existing hypertension would seem to be a concern with any surgical procedure on the kidney. The complication, however, appears to be unusual. Boyce and Elkins reviewed 100 patients with nephrolithotomy and noted that only two became mildly hypertensive postoperatively.[38] Both of these patients were managed with low doses of antihypertensive medications and did well. Whether the hypertension was directly related to the surgical procedure rather than a natural occurrence could also be debated. By careful dissection of the renal artery, accurately mapping the avascular plane, and by use of hypothermia, ischemic injuries to the kidney can be minimized.

Decreased Renal Function

Despite following all the techniques to preserve renal function as previously described, trauma to the renal parenchyma can still occur and some patients will demonstrate diminished renal function postoperatively. Boyce and Elkins noted that of 100 patients undergoing nephrolithotomy, only two showed a decrease in renal function postoperatively and one of the patients subsequently required a nephrectomy.[38] Experience with anatrophic nephrotomy in patients with a solitary kidney also reveals that the average preoperative renal function equals the average postoperative function. Although diminution in function was noted in some patients, a marked improvement was noted in others. In this latter group, the relief of obstruction and resolution of infection associated with stone removal likely contributed to the result.[44,45] The general principles of careful dissection of the renal artery, atraumatic clamping of the artery, the use of methylene blue to help identify the avascular plane between the anterior and posterior renal segments, and hypothermia enable one to approach the excellent results reported by Boyce and Elkins.

Stone Recurrence

After eradication of all stone fragments, subsequent stone recurrence is a potential problem for all patients. The stone recurrence rate has been reported to be between 20 and 30 percent over a period of 6 to 10 years.[46,47] Russell and colleagues[47] noted that the recurrence rate was only 9 percent in females but 43 percent in males. Better control of urinary tract infections, particularly the *Pseudomonas* strains with the more recently available broad-spectrum antibiotics, should be very helpful in lowering the recurrent stone rate. Appropriate use of suppressive antibiotics in patients with recurrent urinary tract infection may also be of benefit in reducing recurrent stones. Acetohydroxamic acid, a urease inhibitor, may also be of benefit in slowing infection stone enlargement and possibly recurrence.

Probably the most important aspect of reducing the recurrence rate relates to identifying and treating metabolic problems as they relate to stone formation. In Boyce's experience, many of the patients who developed recurrent stones had unrecognized metabolic problems, and with a better understanding of the pathogenesis of the disease as exists now, this recurrence rate should be markedly reduced.

Chemolysis

Because a retained stone fragment can be a nidus for further infection stone formation, every effort should be made to remove all stone fragments at the time of the surgical procedure. However, when it is impossible to accomplish this, a nephrostomy tube and a ureteral stent can be left in place.

Approximately 5 to 7 days into the postoperative period, direct irrigation with hemiacidrin (Renacidin), a 10 percent solution of citric acid, D-gluconic acid, magnesium hydroxycarbonate, magnesium adic citrate, calcium carbonate, and water at a pH of 4, is begun. Because struvite stones are soluble in acid, 73 to 100 percent of struvite stones can be effectively dissolved with this approach (Fig. 12–16).[48–51] When irrigation is being performed with Renacidin, the urine must first be sterile. During irrigation, the intrapelvic pressure must be maintained below 20 to 25 cm water.[49] A manometer with a pop-off valve is required to prevent introduction of the agent at a high pressure. Because the solution contains large amounts of magnesium, hypermagnesemia may result if the intrapelvic pressure is high; therefore, serial magnesium levels must be obtained. When the urine is sterile, irrigation is begun with sterile

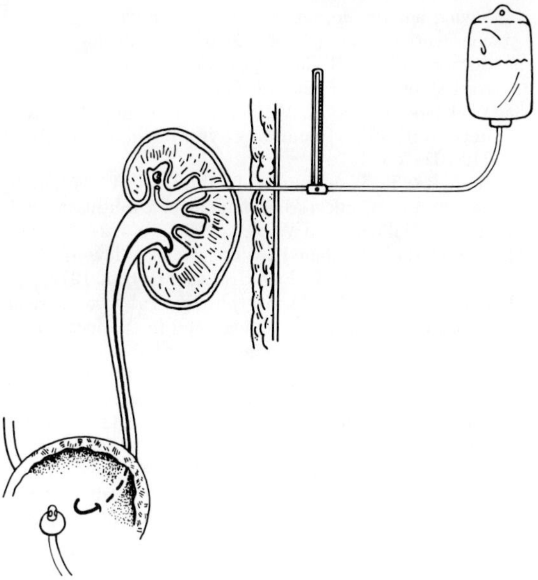

Figure 12–16. Irrigation set-up for dissolving residual stone fragments with hemiacidrin (Renacidin). A nephrostomy tube, ureteral stent, and Foley catheter are all required.

saline for 24 to 48 hours. The rate of irrigation with Renacidin can then slowly be increased but should not exceed 120 ml per hour.

The intact nature of the collecting system free of extravasation should be established by nephrostogram prior to beginning the irrigation. The treatment should be discontinued if the patient experiences severe flank pain or fever or if a urine culture becomes positive during the period of treatment.

Urinary Leakage

Pyelocutaneous fistulas producing prolonged urinary leakage represent another complication associated with renal surgery. Distal ureteral obstruction, infection, and foreign bodies are the main causes and generally resolve spontaneously within 2 to 3 weeks postoperatively. Intervention is rarely required; however, when necessary, placement of an indwelling ureteral stent will suffice. Routine placement of a ureteral stent is suggested following anatrophic nephrolithotomies and procedures requiring extensive dissection of the renal collecting system or in the presence of infection.

Urinoma formation is a rare complication resulting from premature removal of operative drains. In the presence of urinary infection, sepsis can result. Placement of a ureteral stent is helpful in managing this problem, and percutaneous or formal drainage may be required.

References

1. Hevin P: Recherches historiques et critiques sur la nephrotomie, ou Taille du Rein. Mem Acad Roy Chir 3:238, 1778.
2. Bundy FE, Ingalls WM: Nephro-lithotomy: recovery of comparatively good and continuous health during the past eight years. Boston Med Surg J 106:483–486, May 25, 1882.
3. Morris H: A case of nephro-lithotomy or the extraction of a calculus from an undilated kidney. Trans Clin Soc Lond 14:31, 1881.
4. Morris H: Quoted in History of Urology, vol 2. Baltimore, The Williams and Wilkins Co, 1933, p 17.
5. Hyrtl J: Handbuch der Topographischen Anatomie, Vol 1. Vienna, Braumuller, 1882.
6. Brodel M: The intrinsic blood vessels of the kidney and their significance in nephrotomy. Bull Johns Hopkins Hosp 12:10–13, 1901.
7. Cullen EK, Derge HF: The use of silver wire in opening the kidney: preliminary report. Bull Johns Hopkins Hosp 20:350–352, 1909.
8. Deming CL: Renal circulation following various types of nephrotomies. Am J Surg 4:424–431, 1928.
9. Deming CL: Renal circulation following various types of elongations of pyelotomy incisions. J Urol 20:713–723, 1928.
10. Smith MJ, Boyce WH: Anatrophic nephrotomy and plastic calyorrhaphy. Trans Am Assoc Genitourinary Surg 59:18–24, 1967.
11. Robson AWM: A method of exposing and operating on the kidney without division of muscles, vessels or nerves. Lancet 1:1315–1317, 1898.
12. Litten M: Untersuchungen Uber den Haemorrhageschen Infarct and uber die Einwirkung arterieller Anaemie auf lebende Gewebe. Z Klin Med 1:131, 1880.
13. Badenoch AW, Darmady EM: The effects of temporary occlusion of the renal artery in rabbits and its relationship to traumatic uraemia. J Pathol Bacteriol 59:70–92, 1947.
14. Eisendrath F, Strauss DC: The effects on the kidney of temporary compression of its vessels. JAMA 55:2286–2289, 1910.
15. Koletsky S: Effects of temporary interruption of renal circulation in rats. Arch Pathol 58:592–603, 1954.
16. Birch AA, Mims GR: Anesthesia considerations during nephrolithotomy with slush. J Urol 113:433–435, 1975.
17. Farcon EM, Moarces P, Al-Askari S: In vivo hypothermia perfusion during renal surgery. Urology 3:414–420, 1974.
18. Marburger M, Gunther R, Mayer, EJ, et al: A simple method for in situ preservation of the ischemic kidney during renal surgery. Invest Urol 14:191–193, 1976.
19. Marshall VF, Blandy J: Simple renal hypothermia. Br J Urol 46:253–256, 1974.
20. Shioshvili TI: Results of the clinical use of a "dry" kidney's hypothermia. Eur Urol 3:154–158, 1977.
21. Newman H: Renal hypothermia produced by the direct application of ice. South Med J 56:849–852, 1963.
22. Wichelm E, Schrott KM, Kroner E, et al: Transvenous perfusion cooling of the kidney: a new technique of local renal hypothermia. Invest Urol 16:87–90, 1978.
23. Resnick MI, Boyce WH: Bilateral staghorn calculi: pa-

tient evaluation and management. J Urol 123:338–341, 1980.
24. Boyce WH, Harrison LH: Complications of renal stone surgery. In Smith RM, Skinner DG, eds: Complications of Urologic Surgery: Prevention and Management. Philadelphia, W.B. Saunders Co, 1976, pp 87–105.
25. Fowler JE: Bacteriology of branched renal calculi and accompanying urinary tract infection. J Urol 131:213–215, 1984.
26. Silverman DE, Stamey TA: Management of infection stones: the Stanford experience. Medicine 62:44–51, 1983.
27. Nemoy NJ, Stamey TA: Surgical, bacteriological and biochemical management of infection stones. JAMA 215:1470–1476, 1971.
28. Case EW, Stiles JA: The effect of various surgical positions on vital capacity. Anesthesiology 7:29–31, 1946.
29. Jones JR, Jacoby J: The effect of surgical positions on respiration. Surg Forum 5:686–691, 1955.
30. Welborn SG: Anesthesiologic considerations: urology. In Martin JT, ed: Positioning in Anesthesia and Surgery. Philadelphia, WB Saunders Co, 1978, pp 170–174.
31. Boyce WH: Surgery of urinary calculi in perspective. Urol Clin North Am 10:585–594, 1983.
32. Pence JR II, Airhart RA, Novicki DE, et al: Pulmonary emboli associated with coagulum pyelolithotomy. J Urol 127:572–573, 1982.
33. Kropp KA: Surgical requirements. In Martin JA, ed: Positioning in Anesthesia and Surgery. Philadelphia, WB Saunders Co, 1978, pp 162–170.
34. Spirnak JP, Resnick MI: Anatrophic nephrolithotomy. Urol Clin North Am 10:665–675, 1983.
35. Juengst KN, Kursh ED: Pyelolithotomy: Urol Clin North Am 10:649–658, 1983.
36. Collins GM, Green RD, Boyer P, et al: Protection of the kidneys from warm ischemic injury: dosage and timing of mannitol administration. Transplantation 29:83–84, 1980.
37. Nosowsky EE, Kaufman JJ: The protective action of mannitol in renal artery occlusion. J Urol 89:295–299, 1983.
38. Boyce WH, Elkins IB: Reconstructive renal surgery following anatrophic nephrolithotomy: Follow-up of 100 consecutive cases. J Urol 111:307–312, 1974.
39. Sutherland JW: Residual postoperative upper urinary tract stone. J Urol 126:573–575, 1981.
40. Wickham JP, Coe N, Ward JP: One hundred cases of nephrolithotomy under hypothermia. J Urol 112:702–705, 1974.
41. Roth RA: Residual stones. In Roth RA, Finlayson B, eds: Stones: Clinical Management of Urolithiasis. Baltimore, Williams and Wilkins, 1983, pp 422–439.
42. Sleight MW, Wickham JEA: Long-term follow-up of 100 cases of renal calculi. Br J Urol 49:601–604, 1977.
43. Marshall FF, Smith NA, Murphy JB, et al: A comparison of ultrasonography and radiography in the localization of renal calculi: experimental and operative experience. J Urol 126:576–580, 1981.
44. Stubbs AJ, Resnick MI, Boyce WH: Anatrophic nephrolithotomy in the solitary kidney. J Urol 119:457–460, 1978.
45. Thomas R, Lewis RW, Roberts JA: The renal quantitative scintillation camera study for determination of renal function after anatrophic nephrolithotomy. J Urol 125:287–288, 1981.
46. Griffith DP: Infection induced stones. In Coe FL, ed: Nephrolithiasis, Pathogenesis and Treatment. Chicago, Year Book Medical Publishers, 1978.
47. Russell JM, Webb RT, Harrison, LH, et al: Long-term follow-up of 100 anatrophic nephrolithotomies. Presentation, International Urinary Stone Conference, Perth, Australia, August 4–8, 1979.
48. Fam B, Rossier AB, Yalla S, et al: The role of hemiacidrin in the management of renal stones in spinal cord injury patients. J Urol 116:696, 1976.
49. Blaivas JG, Pais VM, Spellman RM: Chemolysis of residual stone fragments after extensive surgery for staghorn calculi. Urology 6:680–686, 1975.
50. Royle G, Smith JC: Recurrence of infection calculi following postoperative renal irrigation with stone solvent. Br J Urol 48:531–537, 1976.
51. Sant GR, Blaives JG, Meares EM: Hemiacidrin irrigation in the management of struvite calculi: long-term results. J Urol 130:1048–1050, 1983.

COMPLICATIONS OF PERCUTANEOUS LITHOTRIPSY

13

Joseph W. Segura • Andrew J. LeRoy

Percutaneous methods of renal stone removal have become standard procedure in the urologic armamentarium in the last few years.[1–5] Although these procedures are considerably less invasive than open operations for stone removal, some of the characteristics of open surgery as well as some of the features found in other endoscopic procedures still exist. Because the methods are invasive, there is risk of bleeding and damage to the kidney and adjacent organs. Because of their endoscopic nature, the procedures feature much of the precision required for transurethral operations but without the relatively wide margin of error that can occur when these latter procedures are performed in the bladder and on the prostate. Furthermore, most of the simpler, smaller stones are removed preferentially by extracorporeal shock wave lithotripsy today. This has left large, more complicated stones to be treated with percutaneous lithotripsy, and it is in this group that complications are most likely to occur.[6]

Problems and complications may occur at any point in the percutaneous removal of a stone. As with other open surgical methods, knowledge of what complications may occur will assist in their prevention and awareness of how to manage such complications will minimize their impact.

Percutaneous stone removal is performed in slightly different ways by different physicians. Such differences are usually not significant, and it is possible to divide the procedure into two parts: (1) percutaneous access and (2) the process of stone removal. The exact temporal relationship of these two events, who performs them, and precisely how the stone is removed usually have little relation to the final result. However, this division does provide a framework with which to discuss the complications and problems that may occur during percutaneous stone removal.

COMPLICATIONS RELATED TO ACCESS

Access to the renal stone may be achieved using either fluoroscopic control or ultrasonic guidance. Most American radiologists have preferred the former method because of the image quality and the precision available with current equipment. In Europe, ultrasound is the standard method of acquiring access. As long as the operator is experienced with the method, it should make little difference which technique is employed.

Inadequate Access

It is a truism that the most important part of the procedure is accurate and adequate access. Proper percutaneous tract placement will simplify a difficult situation and reduce the risk of complications. A tract that allows access to the collecting system but only permits the stone to be removed with difficulty will precipitate a complication. When tract placement is recognized to be suboptimal, the surgeon should consider using another, more appropriate tract.

This is particularly true with ureteropelvic

junction (UPJ) and upper ureteral stones. Removal of such stones is best accomplished if the kidney is approached laterally or from the upper pole. When the goal is removal of a stone in a specific calyx or, more commonly today, removal of a stone in a diverticulum, access must be achieved directly into the calyx or failure will result (Fig. 13–1).

Trauma

Percutaneous access may be very difficult in patients with abnormal anatomic configurations or in those who are morbidly obese. Indeed, a first step in avoiding complications is to make an accurate assessment of the ability to achieve access in a given circumstance. Variations in anatomic configurations may reduce or eliminate the retroperitoneal "window" through which safe access is achieved. These factors, as well as errors in technique, may result in damage to the kidney or to adjacent organs.

Kidney

The "ideal" nephrostomy tube placement is through a posterior calyx. Such a position ensures that an adequate amount of renal parenchyma is present so that the parenchyma will not tear when it is dilated. If the approach is too lateral or too medial, the kidney may tear as successively larger dilators are inserted (Fig. 13–2). A caliceal approach, in which the guide wire passes through the infundibulum into the renal pelvis, will also minimize the risk of damage to intrarenal blood vessels. These vessels are smallest toward the periphery and become successively larger near the hilus.

Because of the limitations of fluoroscopic and ultrasonic guidance systems and variations in normal anatomy, on occasion, a significant blood vessel may be injured. Nevertheless, none of the approximately 1500 patients at the Mayo Clinic who underwent percutaneous nephrostomy tube placement (PNTP) for renal stone removal bled as a result of this procedure to the extent that transfusion was necessary.

Damage to the renal pedicle from an improperly placed needle or guide wire can occur and significant bleeding may ensue if the trauma is caused by a needle larger than 22 gauge. Whether surgical repair is indicated or not depends on the particular circumstance.

If the surgeon suspects that significant arterial injury has occurred, arteriography may be indicated to further define the situation. On the other hand, if the episode of acute bleeding has passed and the patient is stable, the patient may be studied more leisurely without emergency

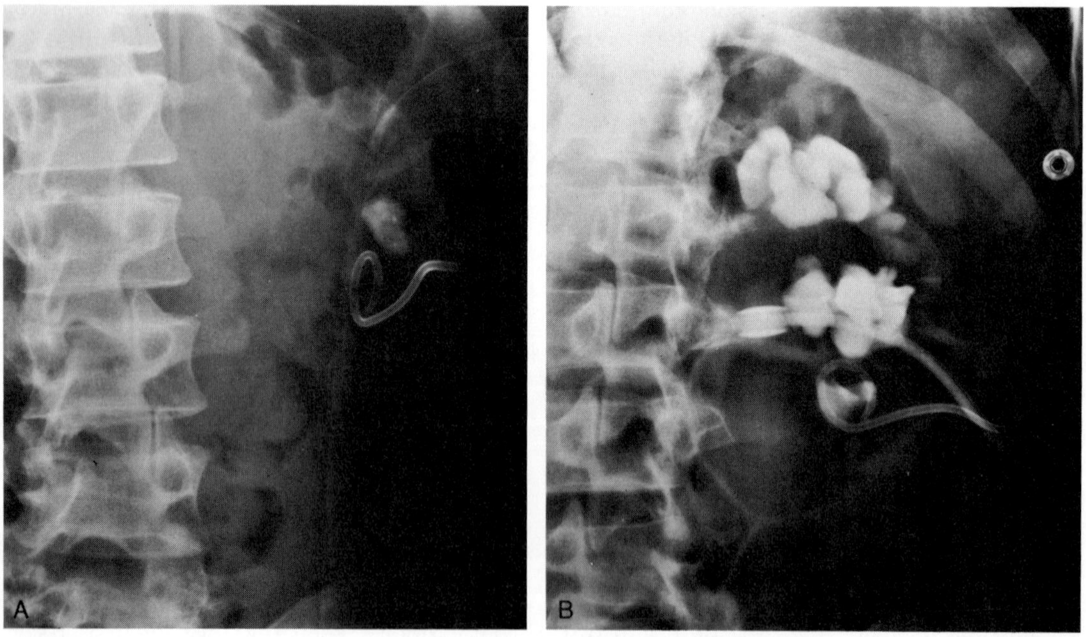

Figure 13–1. A stone is in an enlarged calyx in a patient with intrarenal calicectasis. *A*, The nephrostomy tube missed the appropriate calyx and was placed in an adjacent calyx. *B*, Access through the true calyx resulted in successful removal of the stone.

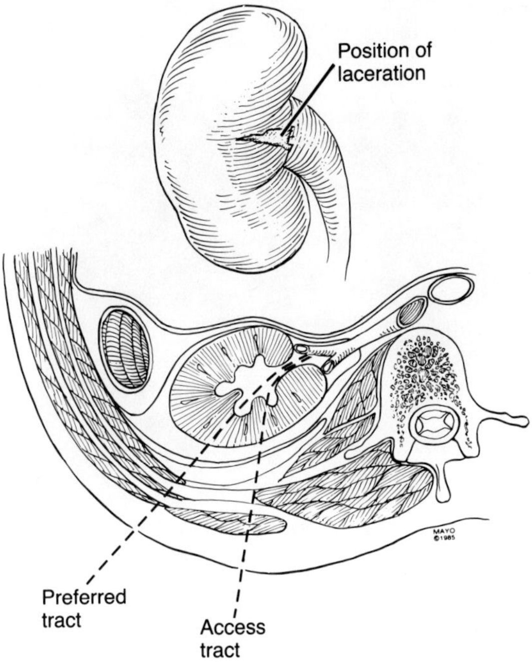

Figure 13–2. The preferred tract should go through a substantial amount of parenchyma. In this case, the actual tract was too lateral and the parenchyma tore as the larger dilators were inserted. (From Segura JW, Patterson DE, LeRoy AJ, et al: Percutaneous removal of kidney stones: review of 1,000 cases. J Urol 134:1077, 1985.)

measures. In our experience, most significant bleeding, when it occurs, accompanies tract dilatation or stone removal.

Spleen

If the spleen is of normal size, damage to it is unlikely when access is through a typical sub–12th rib approach. Splenomegaly may be present to such a degree that PNTP is dangerous or impossible. Such situations may be suggested by review of the plain film, and doubtful cases may be clarified by computed tomography (CT) scan. Indeed, CT guidance may be necessary for safe nephrostomy tube placement. Certainly, if the spleen is injured, significant bleeding will take place and will necessitate emergency surgery and, likely, splenectomy.

Liver

Hepatomegaly occurring to such a degree as to pose risk of injury during routine PNTP must be rare. We have not identified such a patient among those who were candidates for stone removal. Review of the plain film should identify patients who are at risk, and questionable situations should be evaluated by CT scan.

Pleura

Pleural injury is a function of several variables, including the location of the kidney relative to the pleura, the downward extent of the pleural cavity, and, most important, the frequency of upper-pole approaches to the kidney. The risk of pleural injury is slight when the kidney is in normal position and when the approach is through the lower pole.

We have had two known cases of pleural injury. In the first, an upper-pole approach was chosen to optimize conditions for the removal of a struvite stone from a composite upper-pole calyx (Fig. 13–3). The patient was symptomatic and the 15 percent pneumothorax was not discovered on routine postoperative nephrostogram until the third day. The pneumothorax resolved spontaneously without a chest tube.

The second case involved a 10-kg, 2½-year-old with a similar upper-pole stone. The transgression of the pleural cavity was recognized as we were attempting to remove the stone. Because irrigating fluid was entering the pleural cavity, and because we were having difficulty identifying the stone, a chest tube was placed and the procedure completed without difficulty 5 days later after the tract had matured. Other cases may have occurred but may have not been recognized because the patients were asymptomatic.

Colon

Normally, the colon lies anterior and slightly medial to the kidney but may extend to the lateral aspect of the kidney. If the colon is enlarged, it may wrap itself around the kidney and interfere with proper percutaneous access. This may be more likely at the splenic flexure and descending colon. Some patients who have undergone a jejunoileal bypass for chronic morbid obesity have an enlarged colon, possibly because of the large volumes of water that must be processed. In an occasional normal patient, the colon seems to wrap around the kidney, but it does not seem possible to predict in whom this may occur. A CT scan may be useful in situations when significant colonic enlargement is suspected.

We have had two cases of colon injury in the 1500 patients who have undergone percutaneous stone removal. In one of these patients, the

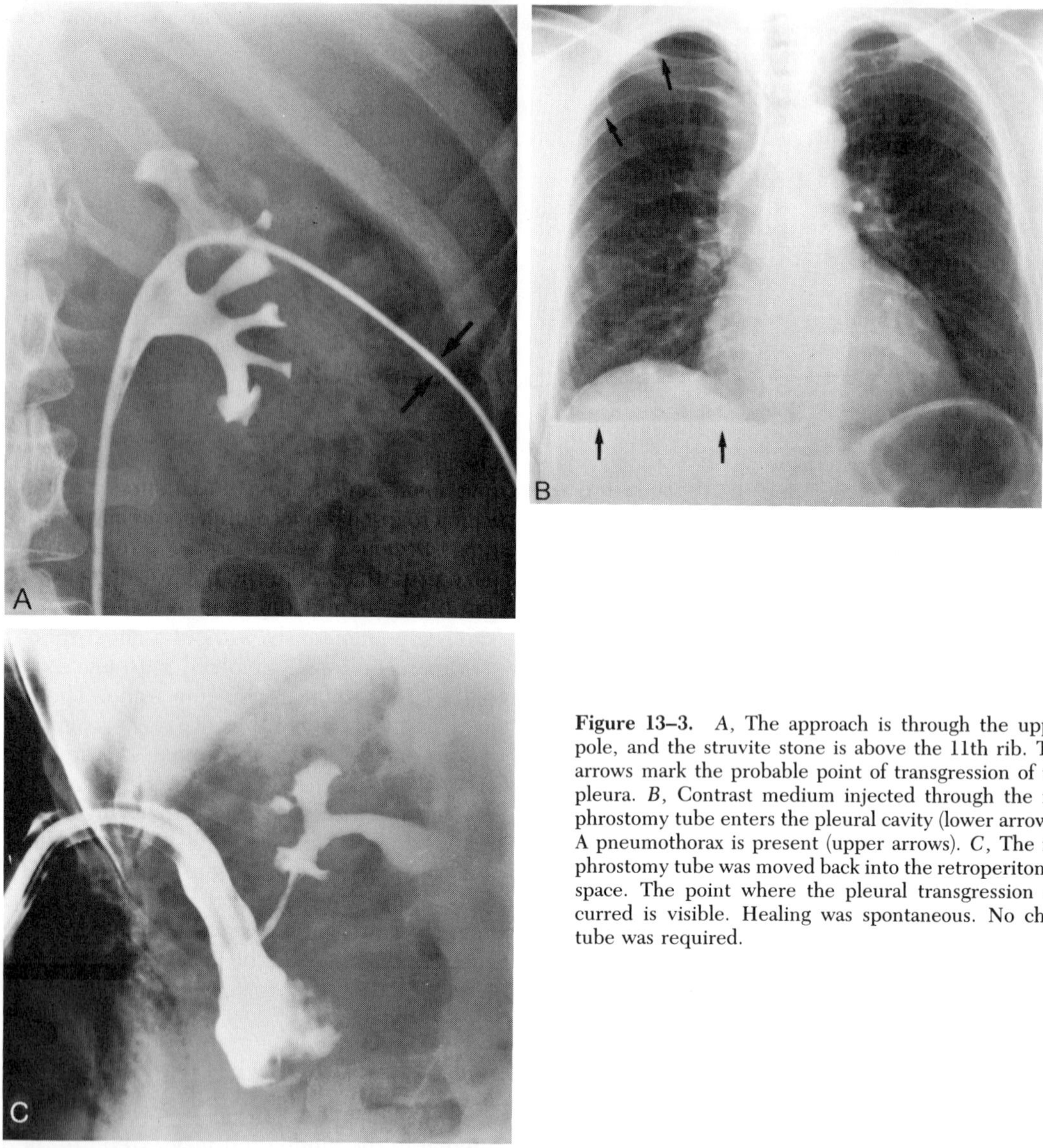

Figure 13–3. *A*, The approach is through the upper pole, and the struvite stone is above the 11th rib. The arrows mark the probable point of transgression of the pleura. *B*, Contrast medium injected through the nephrostomy tube enters the pleural cavity (lower arrows). A pneumothorax is present (upper arrows). *C*, The nephrostomy tube was moved back into the retroperitoneal space. The point where the pleural transgression occurred is visible. Healing was spontaneous. No chest tube was required.

lithotripsy was proceeding well, but the procedure was stopped somewhat before all of the stone was removed because of discrepancies between the input and output of the irrigating fluid. A nephrostomy tube was placed, and the patient remained asymptomatic. A routine nephrostogram performed 48 hours later revealed contrast medium entering the descending colon.

The situation was managed by pulling the nephrostomy tube back into the colon and inserting a double-J stent for internal urinary diversion. After several days, contrast placed in the nephrostomy tube no longer went into the kidney, and the "colostomy" tube was removed. The tract into the colon then sealed spontaneously.

LeRoy and coworkers[7] discussed this case and a second case in more detail. Lange[8] also reported success in conservative management of a similar problem. Neustein and colleagues[8] were similarly successful with the colonic fistula responding to nonoperative measures, but surgery was required to remove the stone. Vallancien and associates[9] reported a more significant injury, for which open surgical management was required.

Duodenum

The duodenum lies medial to the right kidney and may occasionally be subject to injury. This usually happens during the access procedure, when needles or guide wires are pushed through the renal pelvis and penetrate the duodenum. With careful fluoroscopic monitoring of the PNTP, the incidence of duodenal injury should be minimal. If damage is suspected, a nasogastric tube should be placed, the patient should receive nothing by mouth, and management should otherwise be conservative.

COMPLICATIONS RELATED TO STONE REMOVAL

In our practice, the tract is almost always dilated at the same time that the stone is removed. Although it may be difficult to separate entirely problems associated with the dilatation from those related to the lithotripsy, some events are clearly related to dilating.

The most vexing problem that occurs at this step is loss of the guide wire. The operator may be forced to go back to the beginning to reestablish the tract in a situation now complicated by bleeding and, possibly, by extravasated contrast medium. A reserve or safety wire should be placed as soon as possible to facilitate reaccess, should the original wire be lost. Placement of the wire down the ureter and coiling it in the bladder will minimize the risk of inadvertent removal. Also, the wire may bend or kink; if this happens, the wire should be replaced because such kinks will complicate all other succeeding steps in the procedure.

The dilator may be pushed through the wall of the renal pelvis with surprising ease, even if the guide wire is oriented down the ureter. This complication is minimized by remembering where the medial wall of the renal pelvis is located and by being certain to push in the point of the dilator no farther than this. Managing this step is a relatively straightforward procedure when flexible dilators are used. These tend to curve and follow the course of the guide wire, and there is a lesser risk of perforation than occurs with the more rigid dilators. When the stone fills most of the collecting system, the dilator should be passed no farther than the stone because the collecting system may not accommodate both stone and dilator.

Bleeding

The only absolute contraindication to a percutaneous procedure is an uncorrected bleeding diathesis. Dipyridamole (Persantine) should be discontinued at least 24 hours before the procedure, and, ideally, aspirin should be stopped for 5 to 7 days before. The effects of warfarin may be followed by measurement of the prothrombin time.

Bleeding occurs to a greater or lesser extent at every step in the procedure. Occasionally, during the dilatation the blood may seem to "gush" from the tract. A characteristic of tract bleeding is that it always tamponades when a dilator is in place. Such bleeding is usually parenchymal in origin, and it is also tamponaded when the nephroscope sheath or Amplatz sheath is inserted.

As the process of stone removal progresses, bleeding will gradually increase, much as occurs in a transurethral resection (TUR), and may increase to the point that the rate of stone removal is significantly compromised. When this occurs, it is usually best to insert a nephrostomy tube and continue the procedure 24 to 48 hours later. Bleeding may be aggravated by up-and-down, side-to-side movement of the nephroscope, and it is usually true that simpler stones should be removed first, followed by calculi where access is difficult to achieve.

Occasionally, at the end of the procedure, a marked amount of venous blood will be obvious, particularly when the irrigating fluid is turned off. Injected contrast medium will often be seen in the renal vein and inferior vena cava. When the nephrostomy tube is in place, venous blood may flow out the nephrostomy tube as if there were a direct connection to the venous system. If this occurs, the nephrostomy tube should be plugged for 45 minutes and a diuretic administered. This has the effect of tamponading the collecting system; shortly the kidney will begin to produce urine and the bleeding will have stopped. We have performed this maneuver many times, and the venous bleeding has always ceased.

The most significant complication the surgeon may face is tract bleeding from arteriovenous fistula formation. We have had seven definite cases in some 1500 procedures (0.5%), a rate similar to that in other large series.[10,11] Precisely how and when this problem occurs is not always clear. Nephrostomy tube placement may damage a peripheral artery, the process of dilatation may tear a vessel, or there may be a combination of these. Several of our cases were clearly associated with trauma. One patient began to bleed when he pulled his nephrostomy tube out with the balloon inflated. In two patients, the ultrasonic probe was blindly pushed through parenchyma in an attempt to access fragments. For other patients, there was no record of trauma at all. The exact incidence is unknown because subclinical cases may resolve spontaneously. Patterson and associates has discussed our patients in detail.[12]

These patients may bleed at any time, although in most cases bleeding begins shortly after the stone has been removed. Bleeding occurs at an impressive rate and is clearly urgent in nature. Curiously, in some people the bleeding stops and then starts again spontaneously. In two patients, bleeding was delayed 7 to 10 days after the procedure.

Treatment is straightforward. The patients should undergo arteriography with embolization of the damaged peripheral vessel. This is the most conservative, parenchyma-sparing procedure possible, and it is preferred to surgery, in which the most optimistic result will likely be a partial nephrectomy.

We type and screen blood but do not crossmatch it because the overall transfusion rate is only 3 percent, with most of the transfusions administered in patients with staghorn calculi.

Extravasation

Because vision through the endoscope is often obscured by blood and debris, continuous irrigation is necessary to maintain clarity. Normal saline is the preferred medium; water or glycine should never be used. The use of saline as an irrigating fluid will ensure that if extravasation of significant amounts of irrigation fluid occurs, its effects will be manageable. The situation is very much comparable to that which appears with a TUR. Significant overload of water will precipitate a "TUR syndrome" in which the patient may experience alterations in serum electrolytes and symptoms of water intoxication.

Extravasation at the time of PNTP is almost always of no significance, particularly if access is successful and if the PNTP provides good internal drainage. Extravasation during the process of stone removal is more likely to occur if a sealed system is employed—as we commonly use in working through the nephroscope sheath—or if the Ruttner sheath is used. It is less likely to occur when working through an Amplatz system because the irrigating fluid flows out freely. The circulating nurse should measure the amount of fluid found in the drains and catheter output and compare this to the amount of irrigating fluid used.

It is difficult to say how much fluid can be extravasated before it becomes significant, because this judgment will depend on the patient's cardiovascular status, size, and general condition. As a rule, we feel that if discrepancies of 500 ml between the amounts of input and output cannot be accounted for by spillage, collection in the bladder, and so on, the surgeon should consider stopping the procedure. It may be apparent that the fluid is leaking through a hole in the pelvis, and it may be possible to complete the procedure without much additional fluid loss. However, if the leakage is intravascular, the lithotripsy should be stopped immediately because the patient may be rapidly absorbing large volumes of irrigating fluid.

Retroperitoneal extravasation owing to a defect in the collecting system is not usually serious, but it must be recognized. The treatment is straightforward; a nephrostomy tube is left indwelling and the procedure continued 24 to 48 hours later. It is of interest that such holes close off within hours as long as there is internal drainage via the nephrostomy tube. Intravascular extravasation is best managed by the administration of diuretics and measurement of serum electrolytes, and it also ceases after a short period of time.

Intraperitoneal extravasation is rare. We have had two cases in the days before input and output were routinely measured. In both patients, about 5000 ml of 0.9 percent saline were absorbed. Diuretics were administered, and the fluid mobilized over the succeeding few days. Carson and Nesbitt[13] reported two cases managed by peritoneal taps, which resulted in immediate relief of abdominal distention.

Retained Fragments

The incidence of retained stone fragments is a function of various factors, including the mix of patients in one's practice, the kind of stone treated, and the effort the patient and physician are willing to expend to remove the stones. Among our best-selected patients—the first 200 we treated—the retained fragment rate was 3 percent. Overall, the rate was 8.0 percent.

A retained fragment is a complication if it is composed of struvite or if it is of such a size that it cannot reasonably be expected to pass in the urine without symptoms. These should be identified before the nephrostomy tube is removed so that an effort can be made to remove the stones through the existing tract. If a stone enters the ureter in the few days after nephrostomy tube removal, it may cause the tract to reopen and to drain urine until the ureteral stone passes.

If the residual stone is in such a position that access is considered impossible or dangerous, shock wave lithotripsy of the fragment should be considered.

The significance of non-obstructive, non-infected, "non-surgical" fragments is unknown. No increase in stone formation was found by Marberger[14] or Segura[15] and their colleagues in patients followed from 1 to 4 years following percutaneous stone removal. It seems likely that the more important factors are the underlying metabolic and/or anatomic abnormalities predisposing the patient to new stone formation. Still, some feel[16] that residual fragments may provide nidi for new stone growth.

Fragments sometimes exit through holes made in the collecting system. No special effort should be made to remove these stones.

Sepsis

Sepsis may occur at any point in the procedure. A temperature rise is common after PNTP and also after stone removal, despite routine use of preoperative antibiotics. We have seen two patients go into septic shock immediately after lithotripsy. These patients had infected stones, and we believe intravascular extravasation occurred, resulting in overwhelming stress on defensive systems. Both patients were treated immediately, vigorously, and successfully.

MISCELLANEOUS COMPLICATIONS

We have continued to be impressed by the lack of "general medical" complications. Only two patients have experienced venous thrombosis, one of whom turned out to have a hypercoagulable state secondary to carcinoma of the pancreas. One patient suffered a postoperative myocardial infarction, and one had a pulmonary embolus from which he recovered. One death occurred. A 65-year-old woman with bilateral staghorn calculi underwent percutaneous removal of both stones 1 week apart without difficulty. The morning after the second procedure, she was removed from bed to be weighed and suffered a cardiac arrest. Efforts to resuscitate her were unsuccessful. The likely cause of death was arrhythmia secondary to myocardial infarction. At autopsy, she was found to have suffered previous myocardial infarctions, as well as other significant pathology. However, her kidneys were normal.

LONG-TERM COMPLICATIONS

The incidence of long-term complications after percutaneous procedures is unknown. Marberger and colleagues[15] studied 82 patients in detail up to four years post procedure and found nothing untoward. We have identified two patients with mild postprocedural ureteropelvic junction obstruction. One did not require treatment. There was no pyelectasis present in the second patient, but he began to form uric acid stones, whereas previously the stones had been composed of calcium oxalate. The exact incidence of this problem is unknown because many patients have not had postoperative urography. Still, typically, urograms in the usual postoperative patient are normal.

The risk of long-term complication in patients who have had some short-term problem remains a subject for future investigation.

References

1. Segura JW, Patterson DE, LeRoy AJ, et al: Percutaneous removal of kidney stones: preliminary report. Mayo Clinic Proc 57:615, 1982.
2. White EC, Smith AD: Percutaneous stone extraction from 200 patients. J Urol 132:437, 1984.
3. Clayman RV, Surya V, Miller RP, et al: Percutaneous nephrolithotomy: extraction of renal and ureteral calculi from 100 patients. J Urol 131:868, 1984.
4. Brannen GE, Bush WH, Correa RJ, et al: Kidney stone removal: percutaneous versus surgical lithotomy. J Urol 133:6, 1985.
5. Wickam JEA, Kellet MJ, Miller RA: Elective percutaneous nephrolithotomy in 50 patients in an analysis of the technique results in complications. J Urol 129:904, 1983.
6. Segura JW, Patterson, DE, LeRoy AJ, et al: Percutaneous removal of kidney stones: review of 1,000 cases. J Urol 134:1077, 1985.
7. LeRoy AJ, Williams HJ, Jr, Bender CE, et al: Colon perforation following percutaneous nephrostomy and renal calculus removal. Radiology 155:83, 1985.
8. Neustein P, Barbaric ZL, Cossomen J: Nephrocolic fistula: a complication of percutaneous nephrostolithotomy. J Urol 135:571, 1986.
9. Vallancien G, Capdeville R, Veillon B, Charton M, Brisset JM: Colonic perforation during percutaneous nephrolithotomy: case report. J Urol 134:1185, 1985.
10. Lalude AO, Conroy RM: Vascular complication of percutaneously placed pigtail ureteral stent. J Urol 130:553, 1983.
11. Cope C, Zight RN: Pseudoaneurysms after a nephrostomy. Am J Radiol 139:255, 1982.

12. Patterson DE, Segura JW, LeRoy AJ, et al: The etiology and treatment of delayed bleeding following percutaneous lithotripsy. J Urol 133:447, 1985.
13. Carson CC, Nesbitt JA: Peritoneal extravasation during percutaneous lithotripsy. J Urol 134:725, 1985.
14. Marberger M, Stackl W, Hruby W, et al: Late sequelae of ultrasonic lithotripsy of renal calculi. J Urol 133:170, 1984.
15. Segura JW, Patterson DE, LeRoy AJ et al: Percutaneous removal of kidney and ureteral stones. Abstract 579. J Urol 131:248, 1984.
16. Smith LH: Personal communication, 1988.

COMPLICATIONS OF EXTRACORPOREAL SHOCK WAVE LITHOTRIPSY (ESWL)

14

Gerhard J. Fuchs • Richard D. David • Anna M. Fuchs • Christian G. Chaussy

INTRODUCTION

Since its clinical introduction in West Germany in 1980, extracorporeal shock wave lithotripsy (ESWL) has revolutionized the treatment of urinary stones. The underlying principle of using shock waves to pulverize urinary stones involves (1) generation of a high-energy shock wave at the source; (2) focusing the shock wave at a distant point; (3) coupling the shock wave to the body; and (4) localization of the target (stone) and positioning of the target in the distant focal zone of the focusing device.[1–3]

After extensive testing showed it to be feasible and safe in an animal model, ESWL was introduced clinically at the University of Munich in 1980. Owing to the high success rates and virtual absence of complications, its application as the first noninvasive method of treating upper urinary stones spread rapidly. In 1984, the United States Food and Drug Administration (FDA) approved the original device, the Dornier HM3 lithotripter, for the treatment of human kidney and upper ureteral stones. Since then, more than 300 lithotripters have been operational, with approximately 1,500,000 treatments having been performed worldwide. Recently, two additional machines, the Siemens Lithostar and the Medstone 1050 lithotripters, have received FDA premarket approval. In addition, approximately ten new machines are being tested clinically.[4,5] The mode of action of these new devices is similar to that of the original device, so that for the purpose of this chapter, the technical data of the original device are used as the reference.

The unprecedented effectiveness and ease of handling of this new device, along with a relatively low complication rate, have led many users to believe that the use of high-energy shock waves on human tissues is safe regardless of the amount of energy delivered. In the wake of this notion, we have become aware of an increasing number of complications. It has become evident, however, that many of these complications stem from inappropriate indication for ESWL, imprudent use of the shock wave energy, insufficient follow-up, and/or unfamiliarity with endourologic auxiliary procedures.

This chapter describes the potential risks to the patient undergoing ESWL therapy, the management of complications after they have occurred, future recommendations based on the empirical clinical use of ESWL, and the use of high-energy shock waves in various experimental settings. These recommendations are based on 9 years of clinical experience and have enabled the authors to keep their rate of complications to a minimum without sacrificing the efficacy of the method to eradicate stone disease.

PREVENTION OF COMPLICATIONS

Patient Selection

Initially, in the United States, ESWL was approved for the treatment of upper ureteral and kidney stones; however, because of its high success rate and patient acceptance, the method was expanded to encompass most urinary stones.[6–9,13,55] Evaluation and treatment of a large number of patients have led to the formulation of several determinants of success including (1) overall stone burden; (2) anatomy of the renal collecting system (renal stones) and upper urinary tract; (3) stone composition; (4) functional status of the upper urinary tract; and (5) patient compliance.[11]

It has become obvious that as the stone size increases, the amount of energy required to sufficiently fragment the stone likewise increases. Clear-cut safety margins for this increased energy requirement have not yet been established. The original FDA approval recommended a maximum of 2000 shock waves per treatment session; however, questions still remain regarding the maximum energy per session, the necessity for a renal recovery period between subsequent sessions, and the overall maximum energy delivered to a renal unit. Our experience, based on approximately 1000 patients requiring multiple treatment sessions, has shown that 2400 shock waves delivered at an average energy of 21 kV at 2-day intervals did not lead to any measurable energy-related complications.[12] When more than two sessions became necessary to treat the stone, the following sessions were performed at least 2 weeks after the initial treatments.

At this time, controversy still exists regarding the treatment approach for staghorn stones. Accordingly, different treatment strategies have evolved, such as ESWL monotherapy with placement of a double pigtail catheter versus percutaneous stone debulking followed by ESWL. Staghorn stone treatment with ESWL monotherapy has found its limitations because it requires additional ESWL sessions and auxiliary procedures. In fact, stones greater than 3.5 cm and staghorn stones filling a dilated renal collecting system have required auxiliary procedures in more than 60 percent of cases, which have exposed the patient to an increased risk of complications.[8,9,11] Therefore, large stones are best managed by a planned percutaneous endoscopic surgical procedure that can then be followed by ESWL as necessary. Regardless of the treatment modality, however, the basic intent remains to render the patient stone-free with a minimum of invasiveness and complications.

ESWL treatment of stones in a collecting system with distal obstruction or anatomic alteration has produced less than satisfactory results.[8] If the obstruction is amenable to minimally invasive endoscopic surgery, such as an endoscopically controlled incision of ureteropelvic junction obstruction or ureteral strictures, the patient would be better served in a center with appropriate experience in endoscopic renal and ureteral surgery.

Excessive use of energy has been reported in the treatment of impacted stones situated in the ureter. ESWL monotherapy of ureteral stones that cannot be repositioned in a retrograde or antegrade manner has a success rate of no more than 50 percent for a single session. Similarly, the use of excessive energy in this situation cannot be condoned, since its effects on the ureter and adjacent organs are not yet known. These stones are therefore better accessed with ureteroscopic direct-contact lithotripsy. To minimize complications in these complex situations, endourologic experience is of utmost importance (Table 14–1).

Less than 5 percent of patients are excluded from treatment with ESWL because of technical reasons or increased risk of periprocedural complications.[13] Among the high-risk patients, those with bleeding disorders or severe heart conditions have been treated successfully; however, these conditions require careful preoperative evaluation and preparation, which frequently involves the participation of specialty consultants.

Bleeding time, prothrombin time, partial thromboplastin time, and platelet counts must be within normal limits. Aspirin (acetylsalicylic acid), aspirin-containing medications, and nonsteroidal anti-inflammatory drugs must be discontinued for at least 10 days prior to the ESWL treatment. Patients requiring continuous anticoagulation are converted to intravenous heparin sulfate prior to the procedure. The infusion is discontinued 4 to 6 hours prior to ESWL and restarted 6 hours following treatment.

Patients with cardiac pacemakers have been treated safely, provided that certain precautions are taken. Individuals with single-chamber devices usually require no pacing adjustment; however, for patients with dual-chamber pacemakers, pacing in the atrium should be reprogrammed to the ventricular mode during ESWL. If the mechanism is implanted in the abdomen, however, ESWL treatment is contraindicated.[14] We routinely have all our patients with pacemakers undergo a preoperative cardiology evaluation of their cardiac status and pacemaker function. The first ten patients with cardiac pacemakers were treated with a cardiologist in attendance. Having had no pacing problems, we now simply notify the cardiologist when the treatment commences.

Table 14–1. PREVENTION OF COMPLICATIONS OF ESWL (PATIENT SELECTION)

Stones	Limitation	Possible Complications from Treatment of Larger Stones
Renal	Size >2.5 cm	More energy necessary More auxiliary procedures Higher rehospitalization rate Prolonged stone elimination Higher risk of loss of renal function Lower stone-free rate Higher incidence of recurrence
	Obstruction distal to stone	Insufficient fragment elimination More energy used More auxiliary procedures
Ureteral	Degree of impaction	Lower success of fragmentation Higher energy requirement Ureteral injury (during retrograde manipulation) Unpredictable outcome

Calcifications of the ipsilateral renal artery or the aorta are considered only relative contraindications.[13] Experimental studies performed at UCSF exposed calcified cadaveric aortas to extracorporeal shock wave energy, and no disruption of the plaques was noted. Likewise, surgical clips in the treatment area are at no risk of being dislodged, as further UCSF studies in a cadaveric model have shown.[15] Abdominal aortic aneurysms, especially those measuring greater than 6 cm in diameter, are a contraindication, as with other surgical procedures, since their risk of rupture increases exponentially with size. Also, patients unfit for anesthesia in general are not candidates for ESWL treatment on currently available machines that require anesthesia.

Finally, certain technical limitations exist. For example, the Dornier HM3 cannot support patients weighing more than 300 lb, nor can patients over 6 feet 8 inches tall be accommodated. Patients with spinal or developmental deformities can present problems with stone localization and can be at increased risk of damage to adjacent organs. Similar body limitations exist with the newer lithotripsy devices.

Prevention of Energy-Related Complications

The impressively low incidence of immediate complications related to the energy of the shock wave has led many users to believe that the amount of energy used per treatment session and the treatment intervals could be determined arbitrarily. However, recent clinical studies have shown short-term renal changes related to the use of high-energy shock waves.[16–22] Initial animal experiments with extracorporeal shock waves indicated minimal damage to living bodily tissues, with the exception of lung tissue.[23–27] These experiments, however, were conducted at less than clinically applied energy levels. More recent animal studies revealed renal injury secondary to shock wave energy when higher than clinically recommended energy levels were used. These injuries include disruption of renal vessels, damage to tubular epithelium, and eventual formation of focal and segmental interstitial fibrosis.[28–30] The underlying injury pattern can be described as the result of acoustic cavitation, which the lithotripters have been shown to generate in their focusing field.[31–33] Studies on canine kidneys after exposure to 500 to 8000 shock waves revealed modest to large hematomas and/or interstitial hemorrhage in all kidneys. The severity and extent of damage were dose- and pressure-dependent. Unless exceedingly high levels of energy were used, however, the shock wave–induced morphologic changes were found to be transient (Table 14–2).[21]

Prevention of Potential Cardiovascular Complications

The potential for induction of cardiac arrhythmias secondary to the shock wave exists; however, effective prevention is achieved by coupling the shock wave discharge to the electrocardiogram. Lithotripters operating on a spark electrode discharge are gated to discharge the shock only after the R wave during the refractory period of the cardiac cycle.[34] Because

Table 14–2. SHOCKWAVE–INDUCED MORPHOLOGIC CHANGES

Acute Changes
Clinically Detectable
Hematuria (transient, usually subsides within 24 hr)
Subcapsular or perirenal hematomas in 0.1–0.66% (risk factors: existing hypertension, bleeding disorder)
Shockwave–dependent arrhythmias (rare)
Gastric and duodenal erosion (rare)
Pancreatitis (rare)
Hematochezia secondary to colon injury (rare)
Other Detectable Changes of Questionable Significance
Low–signal-intensity changes in perinephric fat on magnetic resonance imaging (MRI)
Loss of corticomedullary demarcation (MRI)
Perirenal or capsular fluid (MRI)
Partial to total ureteral obstruction
Delayed to complete loss of contrast excretion with or without ureteral obstruction
Enlargement of kidney (excretory urography)
Cystic hemorrhage
Decrease in effective plasma flow in treated kidney
Marked congestion of kidney with mild tubular degeneration
Rupture and congestion of perirenal capillaries
Disruption and edema of urothelium
Increased N-acetylglucosaminidase
Increased beta-galactosidase
Increased bilirubin, lactic dehydrogenase
Increased serum glutamic transaminase and creatine phosphokinase
Chronic Changes
New onset of hypertension
Perirenal fibrosis
Patchy fibrosis of ureter
Loss of renal function

shock wave delivery of the Dornier HM3 has been triggered by the ECG, we have not seen any severe arrhythmias in our accumulated series of more than 7000 patients. Piezoelectric lithotripters have not been found to generate cardiac arrhythmias.

Prevention of Complications of Immersion

A second possible complication is relative to the Dornier HM3 and involves immersion of the patient in warm water. Immersion leads to peripheral vasodilatation and sequestration of fluid into the pulmonary vascular bed, which can be of consequence in patients with compromised cardiac output. These problems can be avoided by careful preoperative evaluation, liberal use of intracardiac pressure monitoring (i.e., via Swan-Ganz catheterization), and minimal immersion by keeping the water level just above the skin entry site (skin exit site in thin patients).[35]

Prevention of Damage to Adjacent Organs

Damage to nearby organs is a very infrequent complication. Pulmonary contusions can occur during treatment of an upper-pole renal stone in a patient who is breathing heavily. Good anesthesia technique and careful positioning can minimize these problems. Lung injuries can be significant in the small (pediatric) or deformed patient, and protection of the lung fields with a Styrofoam pad in these patients is advocated. Isolated cases of acute pancreatitis, with elevations in serum amylase as well as increased amylase in the absence of symptoms, have been reported. Gastric or duodenal erosions have been detected after ESWL in a few cases. Mucosal erosion of the colon with hematochezia has been reported in the literature. Transient elevations of hepatic enzymes have also been noted following lithotripsy. All of these changes, however, have proved to be transient and have not had significant clinical consequences.[36]

Management of ESWL-Induced Bleeding

Transient macroscopic hematuria occurs in most patients regardless of the energy source used (first- or second-generation lithotripter). However, clinically significant hematuria or bleeding with the development of a perirenal hematoma is a rare occurrence (0.1 to 0.66 percent).[36,37] With the advent of more sensitive imaging modalities, immediate changes in renal morphology have been described following shock wave treatment for renal stones.[38,39] Subcapsular bleeding, perirenal fluid collections, and loss of corticomedullary differentiation have been detected by magnetic resonance imaging (MRI) in as many as 63 percent of patients.[40] Knapp and associates reviewed the incidence of perinephric hematomas and found that patients with existing uncontrolled hypertension were more likely to develop this complication.[37] In this regard, it is important to monitor postoperative pain because severe continuous pain can herald bleeding around the kidney. Subcapsular blood or fluid usually is reabsorbed within 6 weeks, but it may persist up to 6 months. In our experience, in the rare patient developing a perirenal hematoma, blood transfusions were necessary for 50 percent of patients with clinically significant bleeding. No open surgical intervention was required, however. Four of nine patients in our series who developed clinically significant perirenal bleeding had an underlying bleeding disorder that had been corrected medically prior to their ESWL treatment.

Management of Post-ESWL Ureteral Obstruction

The most common complication after ESWL relates to problems of passage of fragments, namely, ureteral colic or ureteral obstruction (Table 14–3). The incidence of postprocedural complications during the elimination of gravel and the length of elimination time are directly related to the initial stone mass. Stones less than 2.5 cm in size require endourologic auxiliary procedures (percutaneous nephrostomy, ureteroscopy) in approximately 10 percent of patients after ESWL. With larger stones, however, the rate of auxiliary procedures increases to 60 percent.[11] To reduce the incidence of post-ESWL complications in this latter group, we frequently place double J stents prior to ESWL.[41]

Steinstrasse presents as ureteral columnization with stone gravel with or without ureteral obstruction and hydronephrosis. In the case of smaller stones, the Steinstrasse usually resolves within days without any clinical problems other than occasional pain. In cases of prolonged obstruction, however, frequent and compulsive monitoring is mandatory. In cases of obstructive pyelonephritis or asymptomatic obstruction of over 4 weeks' duration, percutaneous drainage is required. The authors believe in the liberal use of percutaneous nephrostomy tubes because they prevent loss of renal function and urosepsis, aid in stone passage from the obstructed adynamic ureter by restoring its normal peristaltic activity, and provide information on the functional parameters of the kidney. If ureteral debris does not pass within 8 weeks despite percutaneous decompression, we perform antegrade or retrograde ureteroscopy to disintegrate and remove the remaining stone fragments.

Table 14–3. ROUTINE FOLLOW-UP PROTOCOL FOR ESWL PATIENTS AT UCLA

Immediate Inpatient Aftercare
On return to the ward
IV to heplock
Continue IV antibiotics
Patient mobilized
Oral fluid intake 2–3 L/day
Examinations
Ultrasound to exclude perirenal fluid collections and monitor hydronephrosis
KUB and ultrasound to assess degree of stone disintegration and monitor stone passage
Discharge instruction
Fluid intake of 200 ml/hr
Physical activity as tolerated
Return to clinic in 2 weeks
For PRN colicky pain not responsive to oral pain medication, persistent pain, temperature > 38.5, prolonged bleeding
Discharge medication: oral antibiotic for 5 days for patients who had instrumentation
Oral pain medication PRN pain q 4–6 (# 20)
Outpatient Follow-up
High fluid intake continued
Physical activity
Examinations
2-week follow-up for KUB, ultrasound, urinalysis, blood pressure
If stone-free at 2 weeks, 3-month follow-up for KUB, ultrasound, urinalysis, urine culture, blood pressure, metabolic evaluation
If not stone-free at 2 weeks, additional check-ups at 2- to 4-week intervals depending on amount of residual debris and presence of ureteral obstruction
If Steinstrasse and hydronephrosis persist, insertion of percutaneous nephrostomy tube after 4 weeks (maximum)
Further checks at 2-week intervals until stone-free or auxiliary procedure (PCNL and URSL) when ureteral debris does not clear within 8 weeks

Prevention and Management of Infection

To minimize septic complications after ESWL, all patients have a urinalysis and urine culture performed prior to admission. Patients with infection or pyuria undergo 2 days of oral antibiotic therapy prior to treatment. Immunocompromised or chronically ill patients receive intravenous antibiotics. During stone disintegration, bacteria can be liberated from the stone. Additionally, shock waves may create local tissue trauma and increase the permeability of bacteria into the bloodstream.[42] Twenty-four hours of perioperative intravenous antibiotics are given and patients are discharged with a 7-day course of oral antibiotics. With this approach, our incidence of serious infections and sepsis has been extremely low (<2 percent).

LONG-TERM BIOEFFECTS OF ESWL

The impressively low incidence of immediate complications from ESWL has led to the belief that there are no significant long-term effects related to the shock wave energy. Recent reports in the literature now have challenged this belief. Although preliminary studies found no change in creatinine clearance or other crude measures of renal function after lithotripsy, Bomanji and coworkers found significant decreases in glomerular filtration rate (GFR) immediately following ESWL. These changes returned to baseline within 3 weeks following treatment.[43] To date, no significant long-term adverse effect on kidney function has been described, even in patients who have undergone multiple treatments.

In the last 2 years, various retrospective studies reported an incidence of new onset of hypertension of up to 8 percent within a 2-year period following extracorporeal lithotripsy.[44–49] However, these figures were obtained retrospectively and have yet to be reproduced in prospective studies. New data from the group at Methodist Hospital in Indianapolis have also shown that patients who form stones have a higher rate of de novo hypertension even if not treated for their stones.[50] Many animal and clinical studies are under way to define and quantify these risks.

In view of the aforementioned incidence of intrarenal and perirenal hematomas detected, a presumed mechanism for the hypertension may be the formation of a Page kidney.[51–53] In this model, hematoma leads to fibrosis formation, which in turn causes renal compression and decreased perfusion resulting in increased renin release and subsequent hypertension. Animal studies have shown that higher accelerating voltage is associated with an increased incidence of hematoma and fibrosis formation.[54] It would seem prudent at the present time, then, to use as low an accelerating voltage as is necessary to fragment the targeted stone. Therefore, the authors would recommend limiting the treatment voltage to less than 21 kV until the hypertension issue has been resolved.

CONCLUSIONS

ESWL has evolved as the primary treatment for kidney stones. Slow and careful expansion of the indications and careful patient selection, combined with large patient demand and satisfaction, have been the driving forces behind the success of this method. ESWL is safe, and the clinical experience has borne this out when the energy is used with caution. Although there is a low rate of reported complications associated with the lesser amount of energy and the passage of fragments, there appears to be an increasing number of patients who experience complications from too liberal use of energy and the lack of follow-up. It has always been our philosophy that the best management of complications is prevention. Therefore, again, a word of caution in patient selection, the use of energy, and the need for careful, thorough postoperative follow-up is appropriate. ESWL is certainly a technology that is here to stay, although the long-term implications of the use of high-energy shock waves on tissue are not yet fully appreciated.

References

1. Chaussy C, Eisenberger F, Wanner K, et al: The use of shock waves for destruction of renal calculi without direct contact. Urol Res 4:175, 1976.
2. Chaussy C, Brendel W, Schmiedt E: Extracorporeally induced destruction of kidney stones by shock waves. Lancet 13:1265–1268, 1980.
3. Chaussy C, Schmiedt E, Jocham D: First clinical experience with extracorporeally induced destruction of kidney stones by shock waves. J Urol 127:417–420, 1982.
4. Fuchs G, Chaussy C: Extracorporeal shock wave lithotripsy: an update. Endourology 2:1, 1987.
5. Rassweiler J, Westhauser A, Bub P, et al: Second generation lithotripters: a comparison study. In Lingeman J, Newman D, eds: Shock Wave Lithotripsy: State of the Art. New York and London, Plenum Press, 1989.
6. Fuchs G, Chaussy C, Stenzl A: Current management concepts in the treatment of ureteral stones. J Endourol 2:117–122, 1988.
7. Chaussy C, Fuchs G: Extracorporeal shock wave lithotripsy. Monogr Urol 8(4):80, 1987.
8. Winfield H, Clayman R, Chaussy C, et al: Monotherapy of staghorn renal calculi: a comparative study between percutaneous nephrolithotomy and ESWL. J Urol 139:895, 1988.
9. Fuchs G, Fuchs A, Royce P, et al: Staghorn stone treatment with extracorporeal shock wave lithotripsy (ESWL): the fate of residual stones. In Lingeman J, Newman D, eds: Shock Wave Lithotripsy: State of the Art. New York and London, Plenum Press, 1989.
10. Gleeson M, Shabsigh R, Griffith D: Outcome of ESWL in patients with multiple renal and ureteral calculi based on stone burden and location. In Lingeman J, Newman D, eds: Shock Wave Lithotripsy: State of the Art. New York and London, Plenum Press, 1989.
11. Fuchs G, Chaussy C, Fuchs A: Management of post ESWL complications: Steinstrasse. In Lingeman J, Newman D, eds: Shock Wave Lithotripsy: State of the Art. New York and London, Plenum Press, 1989.
12. Fuchs G: Unpublished data, 1989.
13. Chaussy C, Fuchs G: Extracorporeal Shock Wave Lith-

otripsy: New Aspects in the Treatment of Kidney Stone Disease. New York, S Karger Publ, Inc. (in press).
14. Littleton R, Webb C, Lynch J, et al: Effects of Extracorporeal Shockwave Lithotripsy on Cardiac Pacemakers. 5th Symposium on Shock Wave Lithotripsy: Urinary and Biliary. Indianapolis, Indiana, March 1989.
15. Abber J, Thuroff J: Personal communication, 1987.
16. Thomas R, Roberts J: Effect of extracorporeal shock wave lithotripsy on renal function. In Lingeman J, Newman D, eds: Shock Wave Lithotripsy: State of the Art. New York and London, Plenum Press, 1989.
17. Begun F, Lawson R: Renal injury resulting from focused electrohydraulic shock waves, Part 2. J Urol 139(4):323A, 1988.
18. Krongrad A, Saltzman B, Tannenbaum M, et al: Enzymuria following extracorporeal shock wave lithotripsy (ESWL), Part 2. J Urol 139(4):324A, 1988.
19. Abrahams C, Lipson S, Ross L: The effects of shock wave lithotripsy (ESWL) on canine kidneys, Part 2. J Urol 139(4):324A, 1988.
20. Das G, Wickham J: Enzymuria as a marker of tubular recovery after extracorporeal shock wave lithotripsy and extracorporeal piezoelectric lithotripsy. In Lingeman J, Newman D, eds: Shock Wave Lithotripsy: State of the Art. New York and London, Plenum Press, 1989.
21. McCullough D, Yeaman L: Experimental effects of extracorporeal shock waves on the rat ovary and fetus. In Lingeman J, Newman D, eds: Shock Wave Lithotripsy: State of the Art. New York and London, Plenum Press, 1989.
22. Jaeger P, Redha F, Hauri D: Morphologic changes after shock wave treatment of canine kidneys. In Lingeman J, Newman D, eds: Shock Wave Lithotripsy: State of the Art. New York and London, Plenum Press, 1989.
23. Delius M, Enders G, Heine G: Biological effects of shock waves: lung hemorrhage by shock waves in dogs—pressure dependent. Ultrasound Med Biol 13:61, 1987.
24. Delius M, Enders G, Xuan Z: Biological effects of shock waves: kidney damage by shock waves in dogs—dose dependent. Ultrasound Med Biol 14:117, 1988.
25. Chinn S, Michaels E, Fowler J, et al.: Hemodynamic and adrenal response to shock wave energy, Part 2. J Urol 139(4):324A, 1988.
26. Yeaman L, McCullough LD, Jerome C: Effects of extracorporeal shock waves on immature bone growth of the rat, Part 2. J Urol 139(4):324A, 1988.
27. Kurzweil S, Smith J, Van Arsdalen K: Effects of extracorporeal shock waves on renal growth in the infant rabbit. Part 2. J Urol 139(4):325A, 1988.
28. Donovan J, Drach G: Effect of extracorporeal shock waves on structure and function of normal rabbit kidneys. In Lingeman J, Newman D, eds: Shock Wave Lithotripsy: State of the Art. New York and London, Plenum Press, 1989.
29. Newman R, et al: Pathologic effects of ESWL on canine renal tissue. Urology 29:194, 1987.
30. Gunasekaran S, Drach G: Effect of extracorporeal shock wave lithotripsy (ESWL) on the structure and function of rabbit kidney. J Urol 141:1250, 1989.
31. Coleman A, Saunders J: Acoustic cavitation generated by extracorporeal shock wave lithotripsy. Ultrasound Med Biol 13:69, 1987.
32. Fischer N, Muller H, Gulhan A, et al: Cavitation effects: a possible cause of tissue injury during extracorporeal shock wave lithotripsy. In Lingeman J, Newman D, eds: Shock Wave Lithotripsy: State of the Art. New York and London, Plenum Press, 1989.
33. Delius M, Muller M, et al: Shock waves and cavitation. In Ferrucci J, Delius M, Burhenne HJ, eds: Biliary Lithotripsy. Chicago, Year Book Publ, 1989.
34. Carlson C, Gravenstein J, Gravenstein A: Ventricular tachycardia during ESWL: etiology, treatment, and prevention. In Gravenstein J, Peter K: Extracorporeal Shock Wave Lithotripsy for Renal Stone Disease: Technical and Clinical Aspects. Stoneham, MA, Butterworth Publ, 1986, p 119.
35. Weber W, Madler C, Keil B: Cardiovascular effects of ESWL. In Gravenstein J, Peter K: Extracorporeal Shock Wave Lithotripsy for Renal Stone Disease: Technical and Clinical Aspects. Stoneham, MA, Butterworth Publ, 1986, p 101.
36. Lingeman J, Evan A: Bioeffects of ESWL. J Endourol 1:89, 1987.
37. Knapp P, Lingeman J: ESW-induced perirenal hematomas. J Urol 139:700, 1988.
38. Grote VR, Dohring W, Aeikens B: CT and sonographic demonstration of renal and perirenal changes following extracorporeal lithotripsy. Fortschr Rontgenther 144(4):434, 1986.
39. Kaude J, et al: Renal morphology and function immediately after extracorporeal shock wave lithotripsy. Am J Radiol 145:305, 1985.
40. Baumgartner BR, Dickey KW, et al: Kidney changes after extracorporeal shock wave lithotripsy: appearance on MR imaging. Radiology 163:531, 1987.
41. Pryor J, Jenkins A: Use of double-pigtail stents in extracorporeal shock wave lithotripsy (ESWL), Part 2. J Urol 139(4):291A, 1988.
42. Zink R, Frohmueller J, Eberhardt J, et al.: Urosepsis following ESWL, Part 2. J Urol 139(4):265A, 1988.
43. Bomanji J, Boddy SAM, et al: Radionuclide evaluation pre- and postextracorporeal shock wave lithotripsy for renal calculi. J Nucl Med 28:1284, 1987.
44. Lingeman J, Kulb T: Hypertension following ESWL. J Urol 137:142A, 1987.
45. Williams C, et al: Extracorporeal shock wave lithotripsy: long-term complications. Am J Radiol 150:311, 1988.
46. Lingeman J, et al: Hypertension following extracorporeal shock wave lithotripsy. J Urol 137:14A, 1987.
47. Williams C, Newman R: ESWL: long-term complications. Am J Radiol 150:311, 1988.
48. Mulley A, Dretler S: ESWL: Slam–bang effects, silent side effects? Am J Radiol 150:316, 1988.
49. Lingeman J, Evan A, Wood J, et al: The bioeffects of shock wave and the risk of hypertension following ESWL, Part 2. J Urol 139(4):291A, 1988.
50. Lingeman J, Newman D, et al.: The Risk of Hypertension Following Various Forms of Treatment for Urolithiasis. 5th Symposium on Shock Wave Lithotripsy: Urinary and Biliary. Indianapolis, Indiana, March 1989.
51. Page I: The production of persistent arterial hypertension by cellophane perinephritis. JAMA 113:2046, 1939.
52. Page I, et al: A crystalline pressor substance (angiotonin) resulting from the reaction between renin and renin-activator. J Exp Med 71:29, 1940.
53. Goldblatt J, et al: Studies on experimental hypertension I: the production of persistent elevation of systolic blood pressure by means of renal ischemia. J Exp Med 59:347, 1934.
54. Fuchs A, Fuchs G: Morphological effects of high energy shock waves on the rabbit kidney and ureter. J Endourol 2(4):341, 1988.
55. Chaussy C, Fuchs G: Current state and future developments of noninvasive treatment of human urinary stones with ESWL. J Urol 141:3, 1989.

COMPLICATIONS OF RENOVASCULAR SURGERY

15

Andrew C. Novick

INTRODUCTION

There are two main categories of renal artery disease, atherosclerosis and fibrous dysplasia, which account for approximately 60 and 40 percent of all such lesions, respectively. Other unusual causes of renal artery disease include an arterial aneurysm, arteriovenous fistula, neurofibromatosis, extrinsic obstruction of the renal artery, the middle aortic syndrome, and renal artery thrombosis or embolism. Intervention may be indicated in these disorders to treat associated hypertension, to preserve renal function, or to prevent rupture of an arterial aneurysm.[1]

There are presently two interventive therapeutic approaches for patients with significant renal artery disease, namely percutaneous transluminal angioplasty (PTA) and surgical revascularization. The role of surgical therapy in the management of these patients has changed in recent years for several reasons.[2] These include the advent of PTA as an alternate effective form of treatment for certain patients, the development of new and more effective techniques for surgical revascularization, and an enhanced appreciation of advanced atherosclerotic renal artery disease as a correctable cause of renal failure. At present, PTA is the preferred initial therapeutic approach for patients with main renal artery stenosis that is due to fibrous dysplasia or a non-ostial atherosclerotic plaque.[3,4]

Surgical revascularization remains the treatment of choice for patients with branch renal artery disease, with an ostial atherosclerotic lesion, with an arterial aneurysm, and in whom PTA has been unsuccessful. Surgical revascularization continues to provide excellent long-term results in properly selected patients with renal artery disease, as shown in a study of 361 cases from the Cleveland Clinic.[2]

SURGICAL TECHNIQUES FOR RENAL REVASCULARIZATION

In patients who require surgical treatment for renal artery disease, total or partial nephrectomy is rarely done today because it is now possible to achieve successful vascular reconstruction in most cases. These operations are occasionally indicated in patients with renal infarction, severe arteriolar nephrosclerosis, severe renal atrophy, and noncorrectable renovascular lesions. Nephrectomy may also be indicated in the elderly poor-risk surgical patient with a normal contralateral kidney or following a failed revascularization procedure.

A variety of renal revascularization techniques are available, and these are all performed transabdominally, through either a bilateral subcostal or midline incision. Aortorenal bypass with an autogenous vascular graft (Fig. 15–1) remains the preferred approach for most patients.[5,6] This operation can be modified to allow in situ repair of extrahilar branch renal artery lesions.[7] In some patients, severe atherosclerosis or a previous operation on the abdominal aorta may preclude safe performance of an aortorenal bypass. In such cases, alternate techniques allow revascularization to be accomplished more safely and effectively. These include a splenorenal bypass

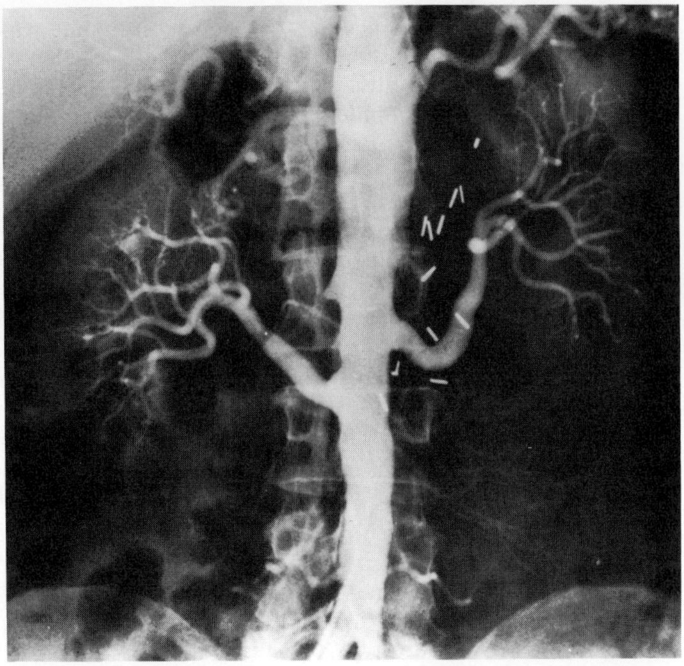

Figure 15–1. Aortogram 7 years following bilateral aortorenal saphenous vein bypass shows patent grafts to both kidneys.

for left renal revascularization,[8] a hepatorenal bypass for right renal revascularization,[9] a mesenterorenal bypass,[10] and a ileorenal bypass.[11] Patients with complex branch renal artery disese are managed with extracorporeal microvascular reconstruction and autotransplantation.[12]

OPERATIVE MORTALITY

Most patients with non-atherosclerotic lesions, such as fibrous dysplasia or an aneurysm, are young and otherwise healthy. Therefore, the risk of operative death in this group is minimal. However, several studies during the 1970s indicated significant operative mortality rates of 6 to 10 percent in patients with atherosclerotic renal artery disease.[13] These patients compose an older group and often have associated coronary, cerebrovascular, and/or peripheral vascular disease. In the National Cooperative Study, coronary artery disease was the leading cause of operative mortality following surgical treatment for atherosclerotic renal artery disease.[14] Other significant risk factors include the magnitude of the operation performed and the presence of extracranial cerebrovascular disease.

At the Cleveland Clinic, several policies have been adopted to reduce operative mortality following surgical revascularization in patients with atherosclerotic renal artery disease. These include preliminary screening and correction of existing coronary or cerebrovascular occlusive disease, avoidance of bilateral simultaneous renal operations, and reliance upon methods of revascularization that avoid operation on a badly diseased aorta. We evaluated the impact of these policies in 100 consecutive patients with atherosclerotic renovascular disease who underwent revascularization from 1974 to 1980.[13] These patients constituted a high-risk group for surgical therapy in view of the large number with extrarenal atherosclerosis (83 percent), azotemia (31 percent), bilateral renovascular disease (61 percent), or a solitary kidney (24 percent). There were only two operative deaths (2 percent) in this group of 100 patients.

In a more recent review, we reported our experience with surgical revascularization for renal artery disease in 361 patients from 1975 to 1984.[2] The cause of renal artery disease was atherosclerosis in 241 patients and fibrous dysplasia or an arterial aneurysm in 120 patients. The operative mortality rate was 2.1 and 0 percent in the former and latter groups, respectively. These data indicate that when appropriate measures are taken, the risk of operative mortality following renal revascularization is small even in older patients with generalized atherosclerosis.

SURGICAL COMPLICATIONS

In patients who undergo renal revascularization, general complications associated with any type of major intra-abdominal surgery can develop postoperatively. These include wound hematoma or infection, pleural effusion, atelectasis, pneumonia, thrombophlebitis, pulmonary embolism, paralytic ileus, mechanical bowel obstruction, cerebrovascular accident, or myocardial infarction. Occurrence of the latter two complications can be minimized by preoperative screening for coronary and cerebrovascular disease, as outlined above. Complications that relate specifically to the performance of renovascular surgery are reviewed in the remainder of this chapter.

Hypertension

Hypertension following renal revascularization may be due to stenosis or thrombosis of the repaired renal artery but, more commonly, is a transient phenomenon that is due to a variety of factors. These include hypervolemia, intraoperative renal ischemia, incisional pain, or vasoconstriction from total body hypothermia. An elevated blood pressure due to any or all of the latter causes can persist for several days, and, in fact, this occurs in approximately 50 percent of patients who are ultimately cured of hypertension by renal revascularization. Adequate blood pressure control immediately after surgery is essential because an elevated blood pressure can cause hemorrhage from fresh vascular anastomoses.

At our center, patients are initially placed in an intensive care unit, where the diastolic blood pressure is maintained at 90 to 100 mm Hg to ensure satisfactory renal perfusion. Hypertensive episodes are managed initially with a continuous intravenous infusion of sodium nitroprusside and, subsequently, with conventional maintenance therapeutic agents as necessary. When hypertension persists following renal revascularization, patency of the repaired renal artery must be evaluated with digital subtraction or conventional angiography.[15]

Post-ischemic Renal Failure

Because all renal revascularization operations necessitate temporary occlusion of the renal artery, acute renal failure induced by ischemia is a potential complication. There are several general measures that are helpful in limiting the occurrence of this complication. These include liberal preoperative and intraoperative hydration, avoidance of excessive manipulation or traction on the renal artery, prevention of perioperative hypotension, systemic or regional heparinization prior to renal arterial occlusion, continuous rather than intermittent clamping of the renal artery,[16] and intraoperative administration of mannitol.[17] These measures help to limit post-ischemic renal injury by ensuring optimal cortical perfusion at the time of arterial occlusion and restoration of blood flow throughout the kidney when the renal artery is unclamped.

In general, the kidney can sustain 30 minutes of warm renal ischemia in situ before permanent damage occurs.[16] When surgery on a solitary kidney or a kidney with extensive collateral arterial supply is being performed, a longer period of ischemia may be safely tolerated. In situ renal revascularization is generally performed by placing a bypass graft to the kidney from the aorta, hepatic, splenic, iliac, or mesenteric arteries. In all of these operations, the period of renal ischemia is limited to the time required for performing a single (usually end-to-end) vascular anastomosis, which is well under 30 minutes. If it is anticipated that the period of in situ renal arterial occlusion will exceed 30 minutes, or if extracorporeal revascularization or autotransplantation is done, additional specific measures to protect against post-ischemic renal injury are necessary. These techniques are reviewed elsewhere and generally involve surface renal hypothermia with or without intra-arterial flushing using a cold electrolyte solution.[16]

Post-ischemic acute renal failure following revascularization is generally manifested by a rise in the serum creatinine level with oliguria or anuria; occasionally, non-oliguric renal failure may be present. If the repaired renal artery is patent, an isotope renal scan will demonstrate continued perfusion of the revascularized kidney with evidence of diminished function. The cornerstone of treatment for acute renal failure in such cases is proper fluid management to ensure normal extracellular volume and sodium content. Administration of diuretic and vasoactive drugs may also be helpful, particularly during the period immediately following ischemic renal injury.

Hemorrhage

Acute hemorrhage following surgical revascularization of the kidney is an infrequent complication. When this occurs, it is generally due to technical factors, such as inadequate hemostasis of the operative field, an unsecured branch of a saphenous vein bypass graft, or vascular anastomotic bleeding caused by improper suture placement or tension at the site of anastomosis. Other factors that may predispose to early postoperative hemorrhage include hypertension, unrecognized coagulopathy, or incomplete reversal of systemic heparinization.

When there is mild postoperative hemorrhage in an asymptomatic patient, surgical re-exploration is not required because small hematomas generally undergo complete reabsorption without sequelae. With severe or uncontrolled bleeding, immediate reoperation is necessary to evacuate the hematoma and to secure hemostasis. In unusual cases, late hemorrhage may occur months or years following renal revascularization as a result of an infected vascular suture line,[18] rupture of a false anastomotic aneurysm,[19] or prosthetic graft erosion into an adjacent organ.[20]

Renal Artery Thrombosis or Stenosis

Postoperative thrombosis or stenosis of the repaired renal artery occurs in fewer than 5 percent of patients undergoing revascularization.[2] The causes include postoperative hypotension; a hypercoagulable state; hypovolemia; severe intrarenal arteriolar nephrosclerosis; incomplete excision of primary vascular disease; faulty suture technique; injury to the bypass graft during procurement; trauma from vascular clamps; wide disparity in vessel size; dissection of a distal intimal flap created at surgery; recurrent primary vascular disease; and torsion, angulation, or kinking of the anastomosed vessels. Figures 15–2 and 15–3 illustrate the most common errors in the positioning of an aortorenal bypass graft that can lead to thrombosis or stenosis.

Arterial thrombosis generally occurs within the first few days of surgery, and the diagnosis must be established immediately in order for salvage of the kidney to be possible. The most helpful clinical clues are persistent or sudden hypertension and an elevated serum creatinine level. In the event of either of these findings, isotope renography, arteriography, or both should be done to verify arterial patency. The treatment for postoperative arterial thrombosis is emergency surgical re-exploration with thrombectomy and/or graft revision if the kidney is viable. Unfortunately, in most cases, the kidney is no longer viable and a nephrectomy is done. Systemic anticoagulation is not effective as primary therapy for this problem but is a useful adjunctive measure following surgical thrombectomy.

Stenosis of a surgically repaired renal artery can occur weeks, months, or even years following revascularization. For this reason, all patients are followed at yearly intervals postoperatively with blood pressure measurements, assessment of renal function, and isotope renography. Recurrent functionally significant (>70 percent) renal artery stenosis is generally accompanied by an elevated blood pressure and/or evidence of deteriorating renal function. If either of these conditions is present, or if there is isotope renographic evidence of diminished renal perfusion, angiography should be performed. The most common location for recurrent arterial stenosis is at a vascular suture line, but this may occur anywhere along the course of the repaired renal artery (Fig. 15–4). When intervention is indicated, the therapeutic options are a secondary operation or PTA. Since secondary surgical revascularization is difficult in such cases, it is reasonable to attempt PTA initially if this is technically feasible.

Renal Artery Aneurysm

Postoperative graft dilatation has been observed upon long-term angiographic study of patients who have undergone an aortorenal saphenous vein bypass operation. In two studies,[21,22] the incidence of this complication ranged from 25 to 52 percent with frank aneurysm formation occurring in 5 to 8 percent of patients. The clinical significance of these abnormal-appearing vein grafts remains uncertain because many of these patients remain normotensive with excellent renal function. In some cases, graft dilatation has been associated with a distal anastomotic stenosis (Fig. 15–5), suggesting the latter as a possible etiologic factor. However, in other cases, similar dilatation has been found with no evidence of stenosis (Fig. 15–6). This problem thus far has not been observed with arterial autografts. In patients with aneurysmal dilatation of the repaired renal artery, secondary surgical revascularization may be indicated if such dilatation is either progressive or associated with recurrent hypertension.

Following renal revascularization, a false aneurysm may develop at a vascular anastomotic site months or years later. Mycotic false aneurysms are caused by deep wound infection in-

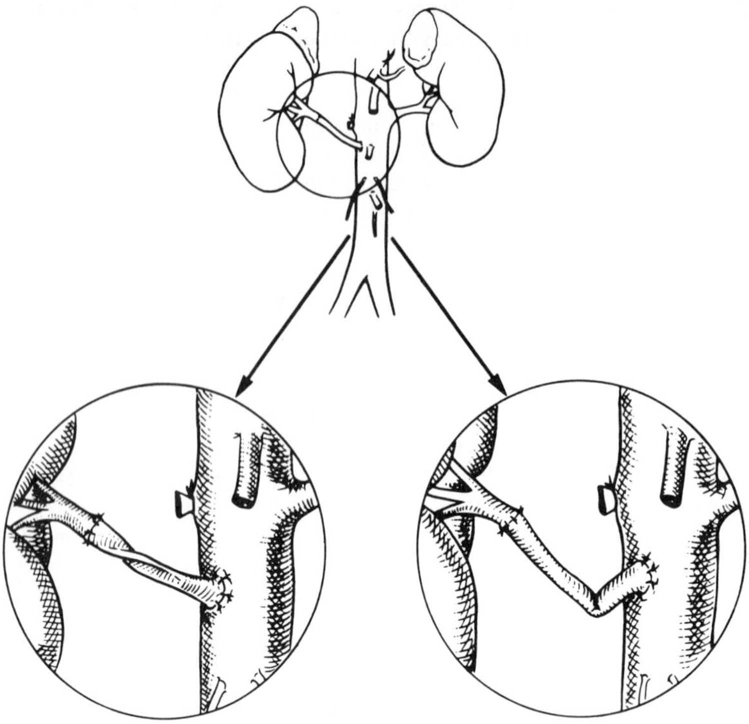

Figure 15–2. Sketch illustrating improper placement of an aortorenal bypass graft with longitudinal torsion (left) or angulation (right) that can lead to postoperative thrombosis or stenosis. (Reproduced with permission from Marshall F, ed: Urologic Complications. Chicago, Year Book Medical Publishers, 1987.)

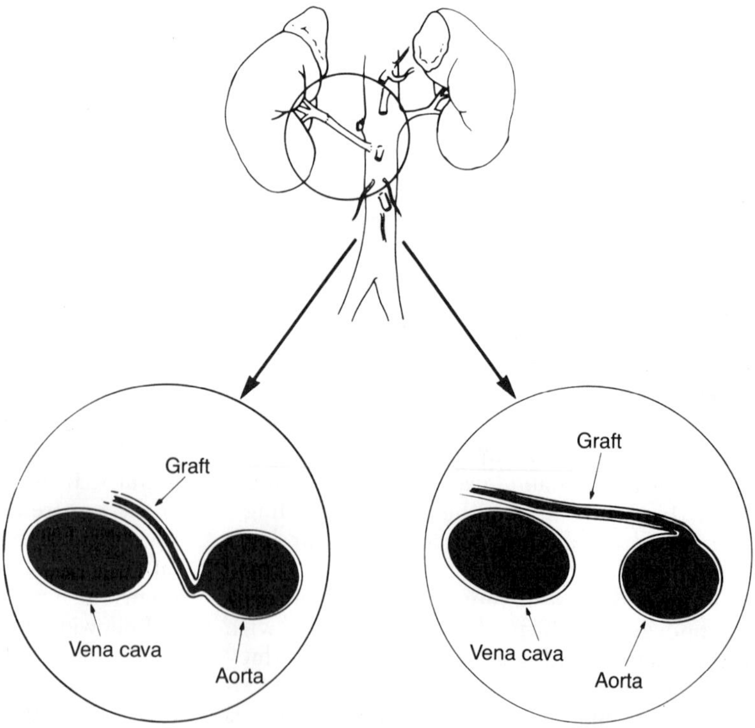

Figure 15–3. When an aortorenal bypass is being performed, the graft must be brought off the anterolateral aspect of the aorta. If the graft originates too far posteriorly (left) or anteriorly (right), this can predispose to postoperative thrombosis or stenosis at the origin of the graft. (Reproduced with permission from Marshall F, ed: Urologic Complications. Chicago, Year Book Medical Publishers, 1987.)

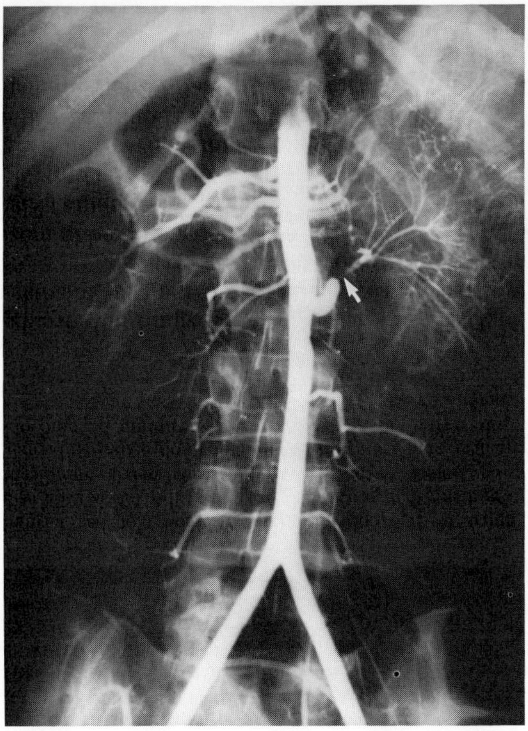

Figure 15–4. Postoperative aortogram after left aortorenal bypass shows stenosis of the renal artery beyond the distal anastomosis (arrow).

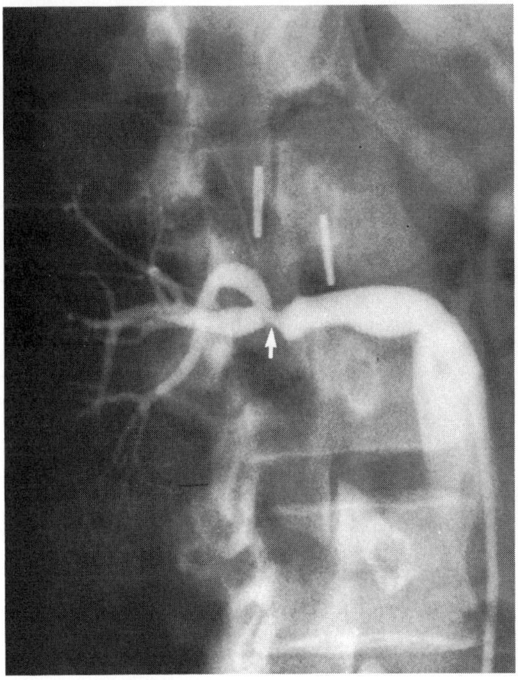

Figure 15–5. Right renal arteriogram following aortorenal saphenous vein bypass shows dilatation of the graft with a distal anastomotic stenosis (arrow).

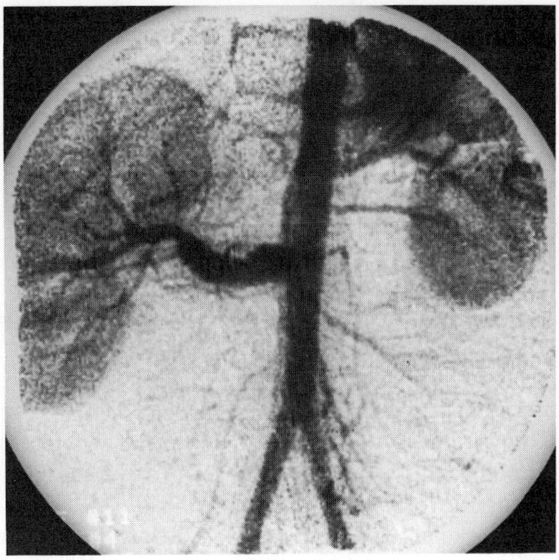

Figure 15–6. Digital subtraction angiogram following right aortorenal bypass shows aneurysmal dilatation of the bypass graft with no evidence of stenosis.

volving a vascular suture line.[23] Noninfected false aneurysms have been associated with the use of synthetic bypass grafts.[19] All false anastomotic aneurysms necessitate immediate surgical repair to obviate the risk of spontaneous rupture.

Injury to Donor Vessels or Organs

All renal revascularization operations involve the use of another major vessel with uncompromised arterial flow as a new source of blood for the kidney. As such, complications may develop in relation to the donor vessel, adjacent structures, or other vital organs that it supplies.

Aortorenal Bypass

During an aortorenal bypass operation, clamping and unclamping of the abdominal aorta are performed. When the aorta is involved with atherosclerosis, this maneuver can cause dislodgment of plaque resulting in aortic thrombosis, dissection, or distal embolization. These problems can be minimized by using a healthy portion of the abdominal aorta or, if such an area is not available, by using alternate techniques such as splenorenal or hepatorenal bypass.

Splenorenal Bypass

When a splenorenal bypass is being performed, there is no need to remove the spleen, which remains viable as a result of collateral vascular supply from the short gastric and gastroepiploic arteries. Nevertheless, a retractor-induced splenic laceration may occur during this operation, which necessitates performance of an incidental splenectomy.[8] Other potential complications associated with a splenorenal bypass include an inadvertent laceration of the splenic vein or injury to the pancreas with resulting pancreatitis or pseudocyst formation.

Hepatorenal Bypass

The common hepatic artery and its major branches must be carefully mobilized to avoid damaging the portal vein or common bile duct. Hepatorenal bypass is usually performed by end-to-end anastomosis of an interposition saphenous vein graft to the common hepatic artery, which preserves distal hepatic arterial flow and obviates ischemic complications.[9] However, occasionally, a direct end-to-end anastomosis of the hepatic and right renal arteries is done and produces a complete interruption of hepatic arterial flow.[24] This condition is well tolerated by the liver but not by the gallbladder, which may undergo ischemic necrosis following deprivation of its blood supply from the hepatic artery. This problem can be avoided by performing an adjunctive cholecystectomy when complete hepatic dearterialization is produced.

References

1. Novick AC: Renovascular hypertension. In Kendall R, Karaffin L, eds: Practice of Surgery. New York, Harper & Row, 1983.
2. Novick AC, Ziegelbaum M, Vidt DG, Gifford RW, Pohl MA, Goormastic M: Trends in surgical revascularization for renal artery disease: ten years' experience. JAMA 257:498, 1987.
3. Flechner SM: Percutaneous transluminal dilatation: a realistic appraisal in patients with stenosing lesions of the renal artery. Urol Clin North Am 11:515, 1984.
4. Council on Scientific Affairs: Percutaneous transluminal angioplasty. JAMA 251:764, 1984.
5. Novick AC, Stewart BH, Straffon RA: Autogenous arterial grafts in the treatment of renal artery stenosis. J Urol 118:919, 1977.
6. Straffon RA, Siegel DF: Saphenous vein bypass graft in the treatment of renovascular hypertension. Urol Clin North Am 2:337, 1975.
7. Streem SB, Novick AC: Aortorenal bypass with a branched saphenous vein graft for in situ repair of multiple segmental renal arteries. Surg Gynecol Obstet 155:885, 1982.
8. Khauli R, Novick AC, Ziegelbaum W: Splenorenal bypass in the treatment of renal artery stenosis: experience with 69 cases. J Vasc Surg 2:547, 1985.
9. Chibaro EA, Libertino JA, Novick AC: Use of the hepatic circulation for renal revascularization. Ann Surg 199:406, 1984.
10. Khauli R, Novick AC, Coseriu G: Superior mesenterorenal bypass for renal revascularization in patients with infrarenal aortic occlusion. J Urol 133:188, 1985.
11. Novick AC, Banowsky LH: Ilial-renal saphenous vein by pass: alternative for renal revascularization in patients with surgically difficult aorta. J Urol 122:243, 1979.
12. Novick AC: Management of intrarenal branch arterial lesions with extracorporeal microvascular reconstruction and autotransplantation. J Urol 126:150, 1981.
13. Novick AC, Straffon RA, Stewart BH, Gifford RW, Vidt DG: Diminished operative morbidity and mortality in renal revascularization. JAMA 246:749, 1981.
14. Franklin SS, Young JD, Maxwell MH, et al: Operative morbidity and mortality in renovascular disease. JAMA 231:1148, 1975.
15. Zabbo A, Novick AC: Digital subtraction angiography for non-invasive imaging of the renal artery. Urol Clin North Am 11:409, 1984.
16. Novick AC: Renal hypothermia: in vivo and ex vivo. Urol Clin North Am 10:637, 1983.
17. Collins GM, Green RD, Boyer D, et al.: Protection of kidneys from warm ischemic injury: dosage and timing of mannitol administration. Transplantation 29:83, 1980.
18. Szilagy DE, Smith RF, Elliot JP, et al: Infection in arterial reconstruction with synthetic grafts. Ann Surg 176:321, 1972.
19. Moore WS, Hall DD: Late suture failure in the pathogenesis of anastomotic false aneurysms. Ann Surg 172:1064, 1970.
20. Cerny JC, Fry WJ, Gambee J, et al: Aortoduodenal fistula. J Urol 107:12, 1972.
21. Dean RH, Wilson JP, Burko H, et al: Saphenous vein aortorenal bypass grafts: serial arteriographic study. Ann Surg 469:180, 1974.
22. Stanley JC, Ernst CB, Fry WJ: Fate of 100 aortorenal vein grafts: characteristics of late graft expansion, aneurysmal dilatation and stenosis. Surgery 74:931, 1974.
23. Nerstrom B, Engell HC: Operative treatment of renovascular hypertension: a study of 60 consecutive patients with follow-up findings between 1 and 7 years postoperatively. Ann Surg 176:590, 1972.
24. McElroy J, Novick AC: Renal revascularization by end-to-end anastomosis of the hepatic and renal arteries. J Urol 134:1089, 1985.

COMPLICATIONS OF THERAPEUTIC RADIOLOGIC PROCEDURES

16

Zoran L. Barbaric

INTRODUCTION

The past decade has seen several radical changes in the practice of urology in the United States. Most of the changes have had to do with improvements in radiologic imaging, which now provide for earlier and more specific diagnosis. Advances in imaging have also played a crucial role in the development of interventional radiology and endourology and in many ways have been pivotal in the design and development of modern-day lithotriptors. Improvement in catheter technology has provided another impetus, as better nephrostomy catheters, lithotripsy sets, stents, and angiographic and balloon catheters reached the market.

The boom in interventional radiology (and endourology) was accompanied by the inevitable complications and iatrogenic injuries. To some degree, these were related to the relative inexperience of the performing radiologist (or urologist) and reflected a learning curve. Some interventionalists have gained considerable experience, and their complication rate is minimal. Others may never become proficient because of insufficient training in the available imaging and interventional techniques or because of sporadic practice of interventional procedures. It is important for urologists to become familiar with the range of complications that they will surely encounter in practice, either as a consultant or as a primary care physician.

Interventional procedures in or around the urinary tract may be classified as percutaneous or vascular.

PERCUTANEOUS TECHNIQUES

When a percutaneous procedure is being planned, blood clotting parameters should be checked and corrected if they are abnormal to minimize potential for bleeding. The puncture site must be carefully chosen so that other organs or cavities are not along the intended needle pathway. For instance, pneumothorax may be caused by an intercostal needle approach to an upper-pole cyst or upper-pole calyx, or the ascending and descending colon may be transversed by a percutaneous nephrostomy tube.

Cyst Puncture/Ablation

Cyst puncture, aspiration, and subsequent contrast (or double-contrast) examination constitute perhaps the oldest diagnostic interventional technique.[1,2] The purpose is to obtain renal cyst fluid; analyze it for possible presence of malignant cells, blood, or infection; and examine the inner walls of the cyst for irregularities or protrusions that may suggest a tumor.

Complications of renal cyst puncture are rare,[3–6] with transient hematuria and mild associated pain being the most common. More severe and lasting hematuria may be due to traumatic arteriovenous fistula. This, in turn, may necessitate selective renal angiography for diagnosis and even definitive treatment using transcatheter embolization techniques.

Retroperitoneal hematoma is rare and, if suspected, is easily diagnosed with computed tomography (CT) or, with somewhat greater difficulty, by ultrasound. If normal sterile precautions are exercised, the introduction of bacterial infection into the cyst is extremely uncommon.

The rarest complications are the most feared: pneumothorax of a magnitude requiring a chest tube and splenic laceration necessitating splenectomy. Mortality is extremely rare and could be the result of one of the complications described above, particularly if it remains unrecognized during or after the procedure. We like to keep the patient in the department for observation for several hours after the procedure and leave a specific set of instructions on steps to be taken should any symptoms appear.

Renal cyst ablation is performed by installing ethanol into the symptomatic renal cyst.[7] The ethanol is removed after a period of 10 to 15 minutes. Potential complications include ethanol extravasation into the retroperitoneum and ureteral stricture if the cyst is in close proximity to the ureter.

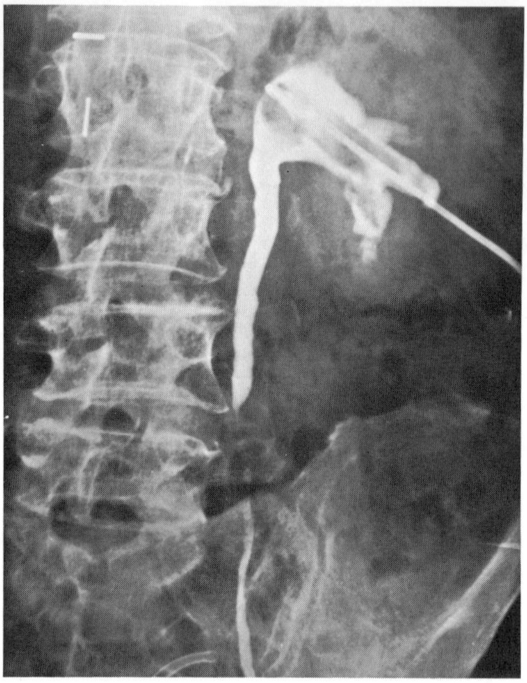

Figure 16–1. Nephrostogram. A blood clot has formed around the shaft of the nephrostomy tube and is seen as a "filling defect" in the contrast-filled renal pelvis. Significant impairment of urine flow through the nephrostomy tube may result as the side holes and catheter lumen become obstructed.

Antegrade Pyelography

Antegrade pyelography is a diagnostic procedure in which contrast is introduced into the collecting system via a percutaneously placed needle.[8–10] In addition to yielding radiographic diagnostic information, it can be used for more sophisticated procedures, such as flow pressure measurements (Whittaker test) or as a prelude to nephrostomy tube placement. Complications are identical to those related to renal cyst puncture (see above).

Percutaneous Nephrostomy

Percutaneous nephrostomy is perhaps the most widely used percutaneous procedure in interventional radiology.[11–14] It provides for temporary or permanent supravesical urinary tract diversion, usually in patients too ill to undergo surgery, chemotherapy, or radiation therapy. The severity of the patient's underlying illness, complicated and aggravated by the obstruction, places many patients undergoing this procedure at risk.

If the obstruction is complicated by infection, one should expect septicemia following percutaneous tube placement and the patient should be started on appropriate antibiotics ahead of time. Shaking chills, hypotension, and circulatory collapse may occur and may be misdiagnosed as post-procedural hemorrhage.

Some degree of hematuria is expected in most patients and usually clears within 24 hours (Fig. 16–1). Obstruction by the blood clot is possible (Fig. 16–2). Persistent hematuria requiring blood replacement is rare but should raise the possibility of arteriovenous fistula, and angiography and embolization may be necessary. If such is the case, the old nephrostomy should be pulled out during the embolization procedure and a fresh nephrostomy inserted at a different site. To minimize the risk of hemorrhage, a detailed knowledge of renal vascular anatomy and its relation to the collecting system is mandatory.

Transcolonic placement has been reported. In some instances, the tract was dilated to 30 Fr. and the draining catheter left in place, unrecognized, without serious consequences.[15]

The catheter may be placed through the collecting system and then inadvertently looped either in the renal sinus or perinephric space (Fig. 16–3). This is a consequence of utilizing a single fluoroscopic projection during nephrostomy placement. Such a misplacement may re-

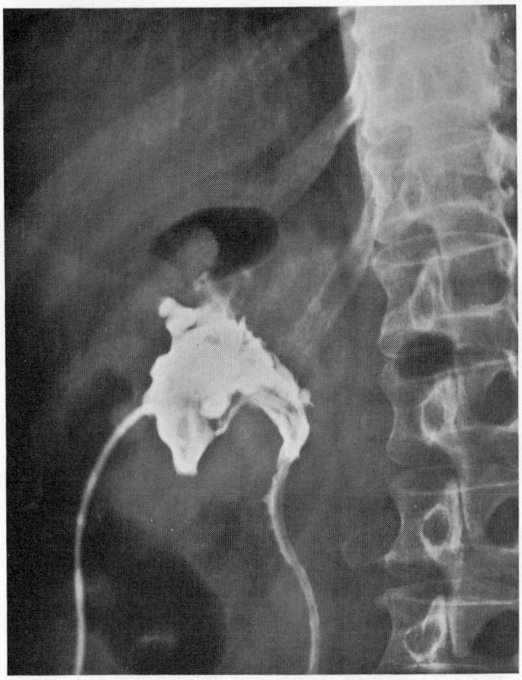

Figure 16–2. Nephrostogram. The entire lumen of the right renal pelvis is filled with a blood clot. Irregular appearance of the contrast along the medial aspect of renal pelvis suggests that some contrast is outside the renal pelvis and that perforation may be present. Ureteral stent is in place, apparently filled with clot and afunctional. Within 24 hours, most blood clots will lyse and disappear.

main unrecognized for long periods of time, even if only one side hole is within the collecting system and continues to drain (Fig. 16–4). To position the nephrostomy tube properly, a transparenchymal approach is required. On occasion, the catheter will be introduced through the extrarenal pelvis. This is likely to result in discomfort and chronic pain (Fig. 16–5). Rarely will the entire kidney be missed and the catheter inadvertently placed into or through the proximal ureter. This, in turn, may eventually lead to ureteral stricture formation.

The most frustrating complication is that of total or partial catheter dislodgment following a difficult placement (Fig. 16–6). The new catheters, such as those configured with the Cope loop, are a marked improvement in this regard. However, if the catheter is to remain for any prolonged period of time, the larger sizes (12 Fr. and 14 Fr.) should be used. Since these catheters are self-retaining, skin suture becomes unnecessary except on very uncooperative patients. This reduces complications associated with skin sutures, e.g., infection, granuloma, and abscess. It is possible for the catheter to break at skin level and migrate under the skin. This is usually an annoying problem, and biplane fluoroscopy may be needed to locate the lost end and retrieve it with forceps.

Self-retaining catheters have caused yet another set of complications. House staff is usually unfamiliar with catheter design and will on occasion successfully pull (discontinue) the catheter in its locked position from the kidney. Hemorrhage and pain may result (Fig. 16–7).

Last, prolonged catheter drainage produces copious epithelial debris, which may eventually clog the catheter. A catheter flush may have to be employed, but caution should be exercised to avoid excessive pressure and introduction of infection.

Antegrade Stent Placement

Excellent antegrade stent catheters are now available. Generally, complications involving

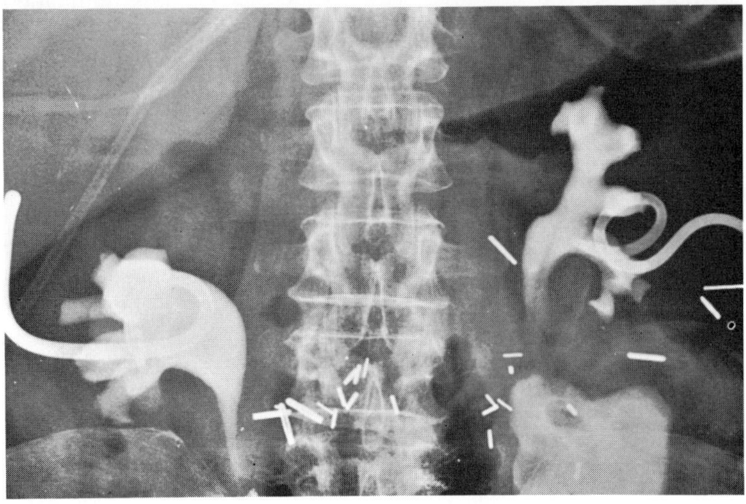

Figure 16–3. Bilateral nephrostogram. Improper placement of nephrostomy tube (elsewhere) is clearly seen on frontal projection. Only the very tip of the left nephrostomy tube is in the renal pelvis. The rest of the coil is probably in the peripelvic space.

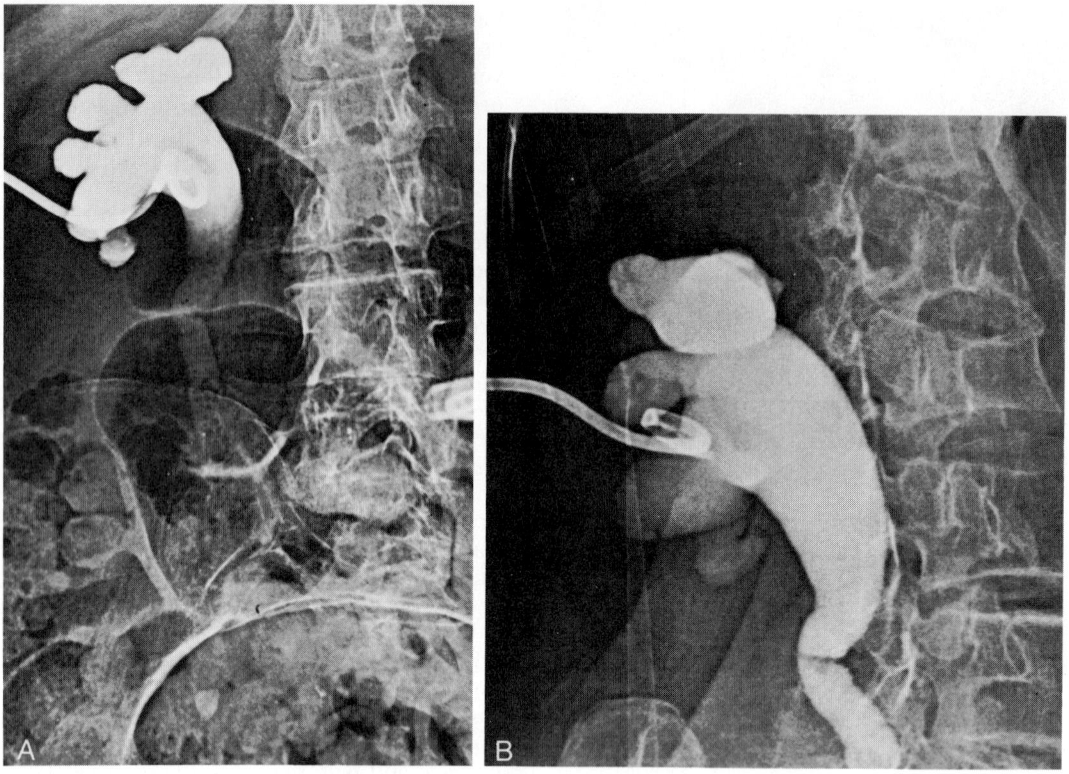

Figure 16–4. Nephrostogram. *A*, At first glance, the nephrostomy tube appears to be adequately placed and coiled within the renal pelvis. Obstruction is caused by a distal ureteral calculus seen toward the bottom of the image. *B*, Same patient. On left posterior oblique (LPO) projection, the nephrostomy tube is out of the renal pelvis and only the tip is communicating with the lumen.

this procedure are similar to those of percutaneous nephrostomy and, indeed, the two procedures are frequently performed at the same time.[16,17] Stiff wires may have to be used with some force to transverse the area of the obstruction. This may result in ureteral perforation. However, if nephrostomy drainage continues uninterrupted, no serious consequences are expected.

Common complications include (1) placement of too long a stent, causing bladder irritation and discomfort and (2) losing control of the stent before it reaches the bladder. A lost stent is a major problem if it cannot be reached from the bladder or through the ureter by retrograde ureteroscopy (Fig. 16–8). Lost stents (antegrade or retrograde) may be retrieved percutaneously using a special grasping forceps through a 12 Fr. polytef (Teflon) sheet. If this is unsuccessful, the tract must be dilated to at least 24 Fr. to accommodate a sheet and an endoscope.[18,19]

Tract Dilatation

Dilatation of the nephrostomy tract is used in conjunction with almost any nephrostomy tube placement. This is accomplished by exchanging increasingly larger stiff dilators over a guide wire or by using a balloon to dilate the tract to 30 Fr. and then using only one dilator for placement of the Teflon sleeve. If, for instance, the tract is readied for percutaneous nephrolithotripsy, dilatation to 30 Fr. is common and considerably less traumatic if the balloon technique is used. During the dilator exchange over the guide wire, the contents of the collecting system may spill into the perinephric and posterior paranephric space. In the presence of infection, perinephric abscess may develop, and eventually a separate draining catheter may be required.

Significant hemorrhaging may occur during exchange of the larger dilators. Tamponade caused by final catheter placement usually brings bleeding under control. Occasionally, a major hemorrhage may occur after a large catheter is discontinued, even after a prolonged period of time. Reinserting the catheter or tamponade with a special balloon catheter and/or immediate angiography and embolization of the bleeding site may be indicated.

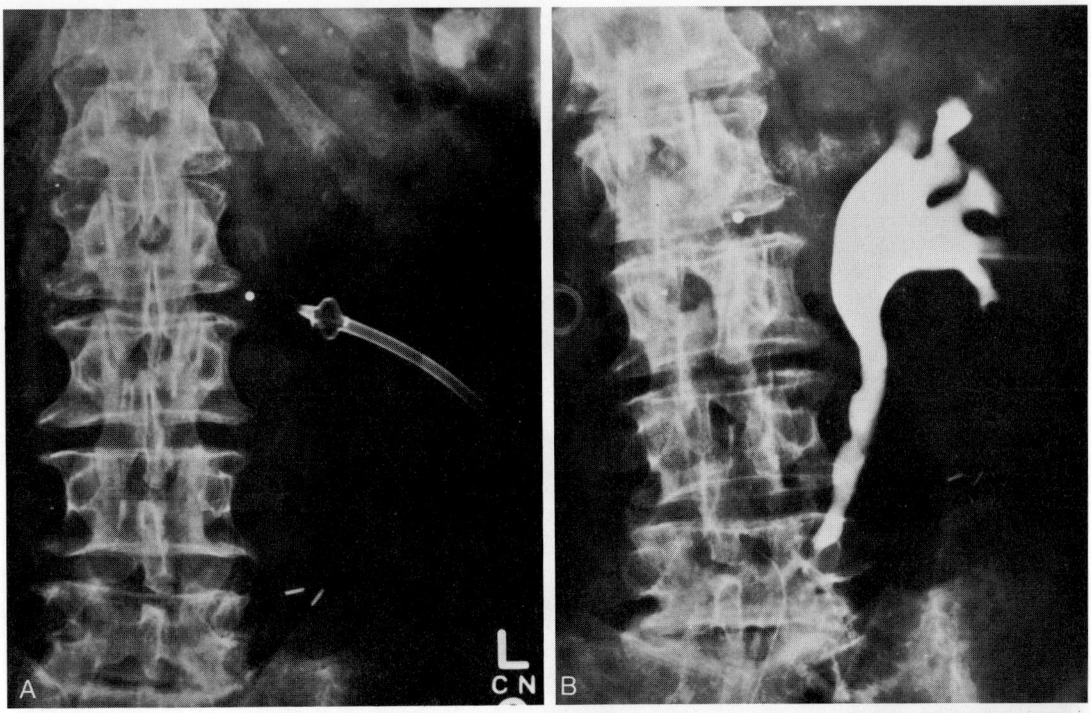

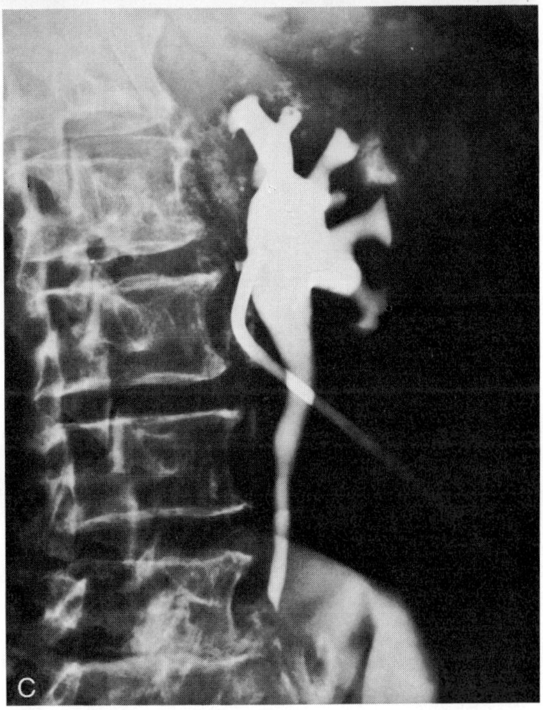

Figure 16–5. *A*, Abdominal radiograph. Left Malecot-type percutaneous nephrostomy tube is in place, apparently in excellent position. *B*, Nephrostogram in same patient as in *A*. On anteroposterior (AP) projection, the nephrostomy tube appears to be in excellent position. The entrance point appears to be through the lower caliceal group and the flare in the middle of the renal pelvis. *C*, Nephrostogram in same patient. On left posterior oblique (LPO) projection, the nephrostomy tube has not entered through the lower pole caliceal group but, rather, through the renal parenchyma and posterior wall of the renal pelvis. Also, one of the retaining flares is clearly outside of the renal pelvis. Unsuspected malplacement, such as this, may be very dangerous if dilatation to large sizes is attempted, such as in percutaneous lithotripsy.

Percutaneous Nephrostolithotomy

In addition to the complications described for percutaneous nephrostomy and tract dilatation, other complications are associated with percutaneous stone manipulation.[20–23] This procedure is now reserved mainly for staghorn and other large or very dense calculi. Exact catheter and guide wire placement is of the utmost importance for successful dilatation and complete stone fragmentation and extraction.

Because most of the collecting system may be occupied by the calculus, dilatation to a large French size could result in a pelvicaliceal system rupture and significant retroperitoneal extrava-

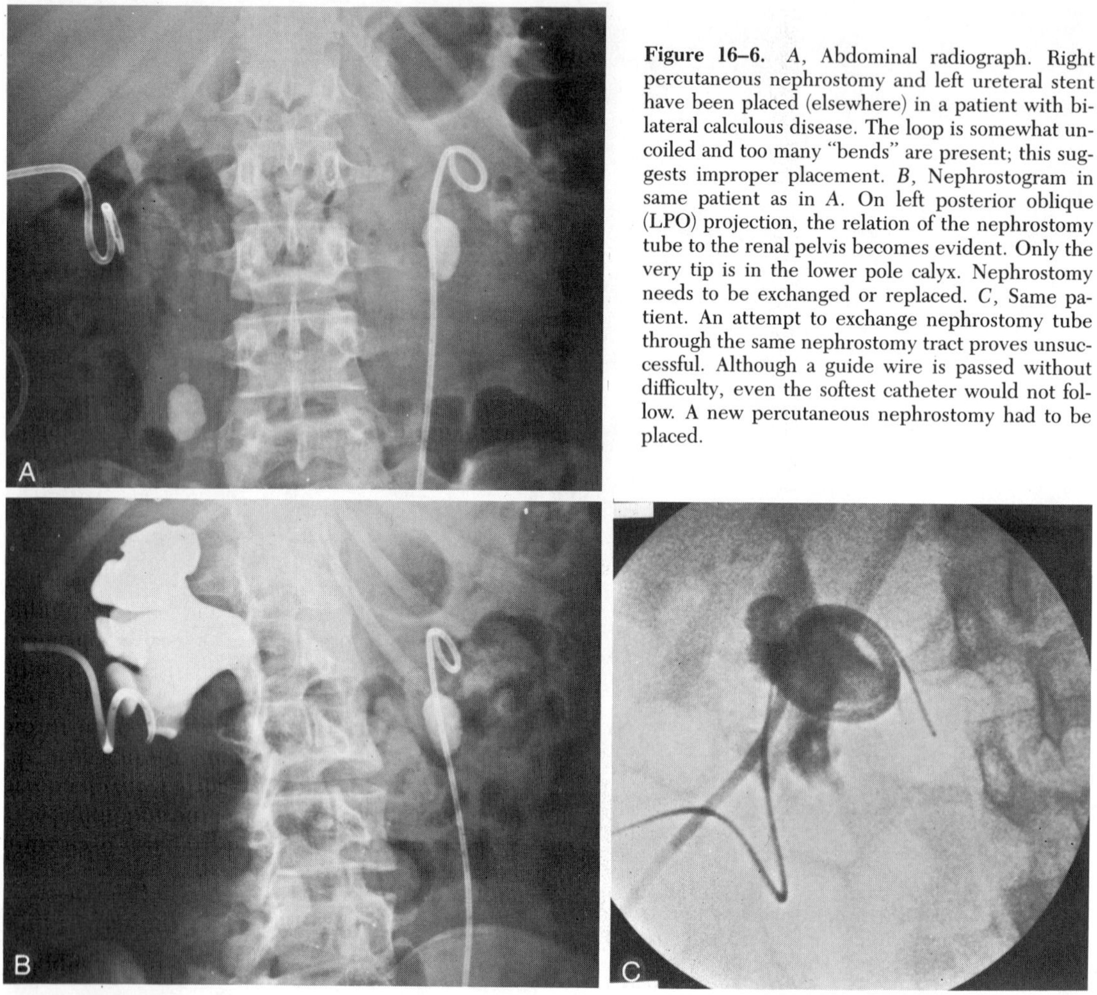

Figure 16–6. *A*, Abdominal radiograph. Right percutaneous nephrostomy and left ureteral stent have been placed (elsewhere) in a patient with bilateral calculous disease. The loop is somewhat uncoiled and too many "bends" are present; this suggests improper placement. *B*, Nephrostogram in same patient as in *A*. On left posterior oblique (LPO) projection, the relation of the nephrostomy tube to the renal pelvis becomes evident. Only the very tip is in the lower pole calyx. Nephrostomy needs to be exchanged or replaced. *C*, Same patient. An attempt to exchange nephrostomy tube through the same nephrostomy tract proves unsuccessful. Although a guide wire is passed without difficulty, even the softest catheter would not follow. A new percutaneous nephrostomy had to be placed.

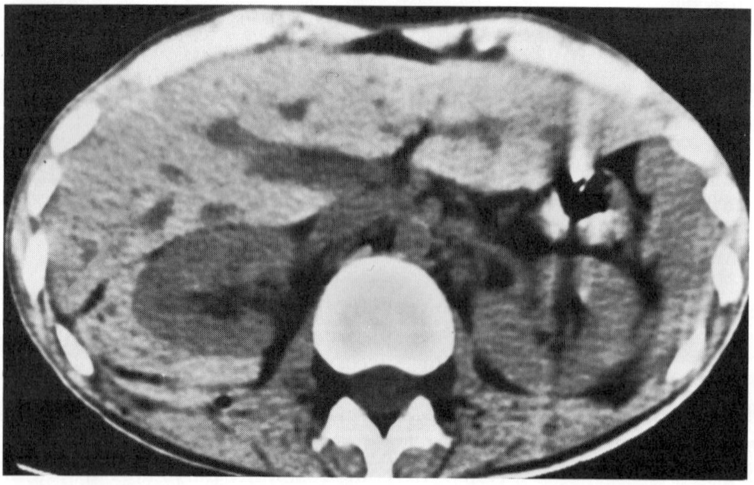

Figure 16–7. CT without contrast. The examination is obtained several hours after a failed attempt in right percutaneous nephrostomy tube placement. The failure rate is higher if the collecting system is not appreciably dilated, as in this patient. The "liver window" is used to amplify soft tissue attenuation differences. Kidney is less radiodense than liver. Fresh perinephric hematoma is clearly seen posterior and lateral to the right kidney, obliterating perirenal fat and exhibiting x-ray attenuation similar to that of the liver.

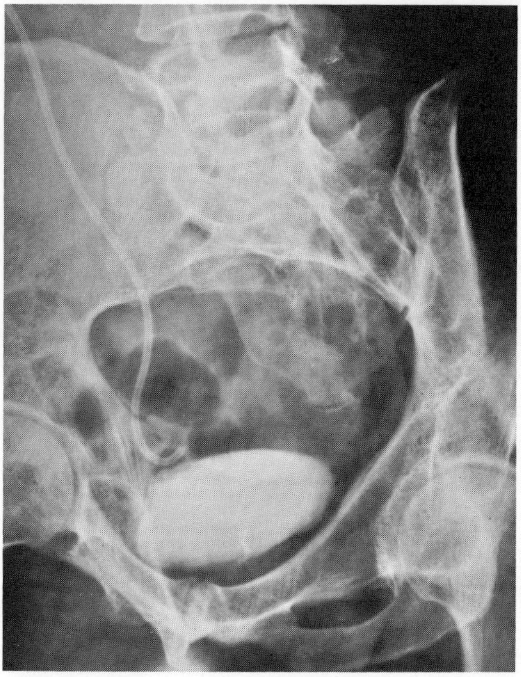

Figure 16–8. Excretory urogram. The distal end of a ureteral stent is "lost" for retrieval by simple cystoscopy. The tip is clearly outside the bladder, and the tensile force of the distal coil is deforming the distal ureter. Retrieval is usually accomplished through a ureteroscopic approach, or, if unsuccessful, by percutaneous techniques.

sation and hemorrhage. Because copious amounts of irrigating solution are used, the unrecognized rupture may lead to large retroperitoneal fluid collections.

Perforation of the ureter may occur during manipulation and guide wire introduction. Rigid ureteroscope, various baskets, retrieving forceps, and graspers may all injure the pelvis, renal parenchyma, and ureter. Ureteral stricture may be the final result.

Complications may also be caused by the patient's being in a prolonged prone position under general anesthesia. Improper positioning of the endotracheal tube, restricted ventilation caused by retroperitoneal fluid accumulation, or obesity may cause atelectasis, post-procedural pneumonia, and so on. Pneumothorax or hemopneumothorax may occur if an intercostal approach is used.

Ureteral Occlusion

On rare occasions, occluding the ureter above a ureteral fistula, either permanently or temporarily, is desirable. This can be achieved by using a balloon catheter, detachable vascular balloons, or a specially designed clip placed using a percutaneous approach. Detachable balloons may deflate or migrate back into the kidney, allowing the fistulous tract to reopen.

Abscess Drainage

Percutaneous drainage of intra-abdominal[24–27] and intrathoracic abscesses is now commonly practiced even in the smallest hospitals throughout the country. Exact placement of large draining catheters and sump catheters is achieved with relative ease. Even deep intra-abdominal abscesses, such as those in the pancreatic bed or deep in the pelvis, are approachable. If the abscess or fluid collection is compartmentalized, multiple draining catheters may be placed.[28–30]

Anticipated complications are bacteremia and septicemia due to manipulation during the procedure. Septic shock and circulatory collapse have been described. Many of these patients are usually already seriously ill and poor candidates for surgery.

VASCULAR PROCEDURES

Renal Artery Embolization

Renal artery embolization or ablation may be employed in preoperative or palliative management of renal neoplasms and in the management of many benign renal diseases such as acute hemorrhage, hypertension, or proteinuria.[31–37]

An expected complication is post-infarction syndrome, which is characterized by fever, flank pain, leukocytosis, and elevated serum enzymes. The severity and duration of the symptoms depend on the volume of infarcted tissues. A supraselective embolization of a small bleeding artery or ethanol ablation of a 3-cm small kidney will be almost symptomless. Ablation of normal-size kidneys (nephrotic syndrome) or a large renal carcinoma would almost certainly be very symptomatic. Heavy analgesia is desirable for these patients. One should be aware of temperature elevation and leukocytosis and should not confuse these symptoms with those of acute pyelonephritis.

Particulate material, e.g., polyvinyl alcohol (Ivalon) and absorbable gelatinous sponge (Gelfoam), or Gienturico coils and intra-arterial balloons may inadvertently be lost in the aorta and may migrate distally into another vessel, such as the contralateral renal artery, the inferior mesenteric artery, or the arteries of pelvis or limb.[31] This may necessitate a major surgical procedure.

Ethanol or other sclerosing liquid materials may spill in a retrograde fashion into the aorta or may reach splanchnic circulation via renal capsular arteries.[35–36] It is important to use a catheter with an occlusive balloon at the tip to prevent such a spill and to infuse a sclerosing agent distal to recurrent capsular arteries. There have been a few isolated reports of colon necrosis and one case of spinal cord infarction.[32]

Embolization of a kidney that may harbor infection is contraindicated. There have been a few isolated instances of development of renal and perirenal abscesses,[33] one of which resulted in a nephrocolic fistula.

Finally, there has been at least one death reported during renal ablation performed using general anesthesia on a child with end-stage renal disease. The cause of death remains uncertain and may not have been related to the sclerosing agent (ethanol).[37]

Hypogastric Artery Embolization

Embolization of hypogastric artery branches is indicated in cases of severe or chronic hemorrhage caused by trauma or infiltrating pelvic neoplasm.[38–41] In the elderly, or in patients with somewhat compromised circulation, one should attempt to perform supraselective embolization of the bleeding artery when possible. Necrosis of the skin over the buttocks has been described in such patients.

Renal Artery Angioplasty

The treatment of renovascular hypertension has undergone drastic changes in the past decade. Complications of transluminal renal artery angioplasty may occur during attempts to cross the stenosis, during active dilatation, or following technically successful dilatation.[42–47]

A tight stenosis, multiple stenotic areas (such as in fibromuscular dysplasia), long stenotic segment, and a tortuous vessel may all prevent the radiologist from successfully crossing the stenosis. During the attempt, however, an intimal flap may be raised, the artery may be temporarily occluded, or the intima may be damaged sufficiently for thrombosis to occur. The diagnosis may be immediately evident from a follow-

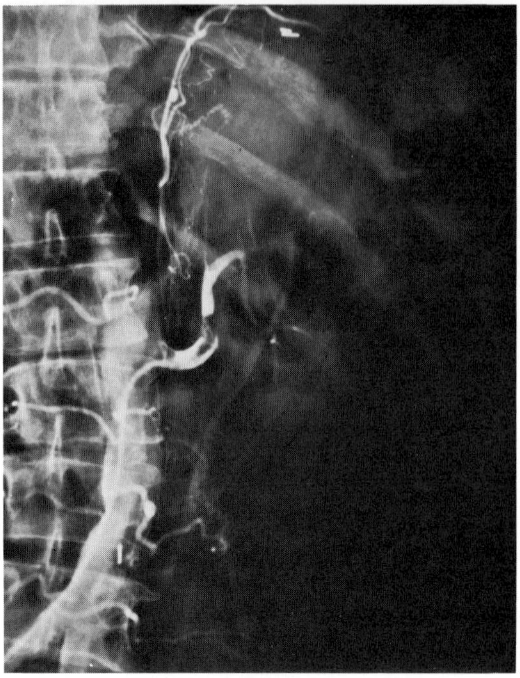

Figure 16–9. Selective left renal arteriogram. Inadvertent renal artery dissection occurred during angiography. Angiography was performed as a prelude to a preoperative left renal artery embolization for a moderate-sized left renal carcinoma, and no permanent harm was done. The unusual upward curve of the renal artery probably contributed to the subintimal injection of some radiographic contrast and cessation of antegrade flow.

up angiogram, or complete occlusion may be delayed even after 24 hours. If there is any clinical suspicion, a renal blood flow scan should be obtained immediately and, if clinically indicated, an aortorenal bypass graft performed.

Usually, significant intimal damage appears following successful angioplasty. The lumen remains open because the media has been overstretched and has therefore lost much of its elasticity. Irregularity at the dilatation site is usually unimportant and probably represents damaged intima. If the lumen is open and the blood flow normal, this irregularity will likely disappear in time.[44,47] It is possible, however, to disrupt the intima so that subintimal dissection occurs. Small dissections are probably unimportant as long as there is adequate blood flow on follow-up angiogram. However, a dissection may also progress and cause complete or partial renal artery occlusion (Fig. 16–9). Renal artery rupture and significant retroperitoneal hemorrhage rarely occur. For this reason, a renal artery angioplasty should not be attempted without a competent surgeon in attendance.

Delayed renal artery occlusion caused by

thrombosis or dissection following a technically successful angioplasty is rare.[47] Symptoms include flank pain and sometimes fever. Delays in diagnosis and surgical intervention may result in loss of the kidney.

Spermatic Vein Occlusion

Spermatic vein occlusion is an interventional procedure that is gaining in popularity in Europe and is likely to gain a foothold in United States as well.[48–51] There are two distinct techniques. The first involves placing one or more detachable balloons in the spermatic vein at levels determined most appropriate by selective spermatic vein venography.[48] Migration of the silicone balloon and asymptomatic embolization of the lung occurred in 6 percent of the procedures undertaken during the development of this technique. As a result of improved methods, this migration no longer occurs.[51]

The second technique involves the introduction of sclerosing agents into the spermatic vein, causing thrombosis and fibrosis and eventually complete occlusion of the vessel. This technique is a very exacting one, providing the sclerosing agent does not reach plexus panpiniformis. If it does, there could be some swelling and pain, usually self-limiting. Otherwise, the procedure is safe and is performed on an outpatient basis.[49]

Angiography in General

Complications associated with general angiography, whether it is used for interventional or diagnostic purposes, include hematoma and arteriovenous fistula at the puncture site, peripheral embolization resulting from dislodged atheroma or blood clots, reaction to contrast or other medications used in the course of the examination, and oliguric renal failure caused by the nephrotoxic effect of contrast material on some patients. The latter is addressed in the next section.

MISCELLANEOUS

Prostatic Balloon Dilatation

There is renewed interest in dilatation of the prostate for treatment of outflow bladder obstruction that is due to benign prostatic hypertrophy. A balloon 2 cm in diameter is inflated above the external sphincter. Apparently, the prostatic capsule is overstretched, explaining partially, at least, the successful abatement of outflow obstruction symptoms. The only complication reported was some incontinence, which occurred when the balloon was inflated at the level of the external sphincter.[52–55]

Biopsies

Thin-needle aspiration biopsy is now liberally used for diagnostic purposes. Because exact needle placement is possible under CT, ultrasound, and fluoroscopy, transversing other organs can be avoided. Complications are extremely rare and include hemorrhage, pneumothorax, and seeding along the needle tract.[56–58]

Intravenous Contrast

Complications related to intravenous or intraarterial administration of the contrast may be idiopathic, allergic, or nephrotoxic.[59,60]

Hypotension following administration of contrast material may be due to anaphylactic reaction, unknown causes (idiopathic), or vasovagal reaction. A vasovagal reaction may be recognized if bradycardia is detected, and it should be treated accordingly. If tachycardia is present, one should assume that the patient is having an allergic reaction and institute appropriate treatment. Death may occur in one out of 100,000 cases.[59]

Other uncommon reactions to contrast material include laryngospasm, bronchospasm, seizures, angioneurotic edema, and fever. Common reactions are nausea, vomiting, and urticaria.

Although the administration of contrast material does not influence renal function in a majority of patients, renal function may be adversely affected in a high-risk group of patients. These are patients with already compromised renal function from age, diabetes, atherosclerosis, multiple myeloma, and so on, in whom contrast may induce oliguric renal failure (which, although usually reversible, may in some instances be irreversible). This is believed to be the result of the direct nephrotoxic effect of contrast upon tubular cells. The total amount of contrast injected also seems to be a factor. Therefore, alternative imaging methods should be utilized for this group of patients.

Low-osmolar non-ionic contrast has become

available and should be the only type used for this particular group of patients when intravascular contrast examination is unavoidable.[61–66] The high price of non-ionic contrast is offset by reducing possible complications and the medical cost associated with them. It is expected that prices may drop substantially in the future and that non-ionic contrast will benefit patients with normal renal function as well.

Radiation Exposure

It is worthwhile remembering that exposure from 15 to 20 seconds of fluoroscopy equals that of a radiograph of the same area. Some complicated interventional procedures, such as percutaneous nephrostolithotripsy, may go on for several hours with intermittent use of fluoroscopy. Therefore, significant radiation exposure to the patient, and indeed to the operator and other personnel, is possible. Caution should be exercised by using the smallest field size and by using fluoroscopy for the shortest period of time possible.

References

Cyst Puncture

1. Dean AL: Treatment of solitary cyst of kidney by aspiration. Trans Am Assoc Genitourin Surg 32:91, 1939.
2. Lindblom K: Diagnostic kidney puncture in cysts and tumors. AJR 68:209–215, 1952.
3. Branitz BH, Schlossberg IR, Ereed SZ: Complications of renal cyst puncture. Urology 7:578–580, 1976.
4. Lang EK: Renal cyst puncture and aspiration: a survey of complications. AJR 128:723–727, 1977.
5. Wayman PJ, McClennan BL, Lee JKT, et al: CT of calcified renal masses. AJR 138:1095–1099, 1982.
6. Bosniak MA: The current radiological approach to renal cysts. Radiology 158:1–10, 1986.
7. Bean WJ: Renal cysts: Treatment with alcohol. Radiology 138:329–331, 1981.

Antegrade Pyelography

8. Lieberman RP, Kearney G, Helfrich W, et al: Fine needle antegrade pyelography in the renal transplant. J Urol 126:155–158, 1981.
9. Whitaker RH: Methods of assessing obstruction in dilated ureters. J Urol 45:15–22, 1973.
10. Pfister RC, Newhouse JH, Hendren WH: Percutaneous pyeloureteral urodynamics. Urol Clin North Am 9:41–49, 1982.

Nephrostomy

11. Goodwin WE, Casey WC, Woolf W: Percutaneous trocar (needle) nephrostomy in hydronephrosis. JAMA 157:891–894, 1955.
12. Stables DP, Ginsberg NJ, Johnson ML: Percutaneous nephrostomy: a series and review of the literature. AJR 130:75–82, 1978.
13. Lang EK, Price ET: Redefinitions of indications for percutaneous nephrostomy. Radiology 147:419–426, 1983.
14. Pollack HM, Banner MP: Percutaneous nephrostomy and related pyeloureteral manipulative techniques. Urol Radiol 2:147–154, 1981.
15. Neustein P, Barbaric ZL, Kaufman JJ: Nephrocolic fistula: a complication of percutaneous nephrostolithotomy. J Urol 135:571–573, 1986.

Stent Removal

16. Bigongiari LR, Lee KR, Moffat RE, et al: Percutaneous ureteral stent placement for stricture management and internal urinary drainage. AJR 133:865–868, 1979.
17. Lang EK: Diagnosis and management of ureteral fistulas by percutaneous nephrostomy and antegrade stent catheter. Radiology 138:311–317, 1981.
18. Boren SR, Dotter CT, McKinney M, Rosch J: Percutaneous removal of ureteral stents. Radiology 152:230–231, 1984.
19. LeRoy AJ, Williams HJ, Segura JW, et al: Indwelling ureteral stents: percutaneous management of complications. Radiology 158:219–222, 1986.

Nephrostolithotomy

20. Castaneda-Zuniga WR, Clayman R, Smith A, et al: Nephrostolithotomy: percutaneous techniques for urinary calculus removal. AJR 139:721–726, 1982.
21. LeRoy AJ, May GR, Bender CE, et al: Percutaneous nephrostomy for stone removal. Radiology 151:607–612, 1984.
22. Dunnick NR, Carson CC, Braun SD, et al: Complications of percutaneous nephrostolithotomy. Radiology 157:51–55, 1985.
23. Lang EK: Percutaneous nephrostolithotomy and lithotripsy: a multi-institutional survey of complications. Radiology 162:25–30, 1987.

Abscess

24. Gerzof SG: Percutaneous drainage of renal and perinephric abscess. Urol Radiol 2:171–179, 1981.
25. Caldamone AA, Frank IN: Percutaneous aspiration in the treatment of renal abscesses. J Urol 123:92–93, 1980.
26. Gerzof SG, Robbins AH, Johnson WC, et al: Percutaneous catheter drainage of abdominal abscesses: a five-year experience. N Engl J Med 305:653–657, 1981.
27. Cronan JJ, Amis ES Jr, Dorfman GS: Percutaneous drainage of renal abscesses. AJR 142:351–354, 1984.
28. vanSonnenberg E, Mueller PR, Ferrucci JT Jr, et al: Percutaneous drainage of abdominal abscesses and fluid collections in 250 cases. Part I. Results, failures and complications. Radiology 151:337–341, 1984.
29. Butch RJ, Mueller PR, Ferrucci JT Jr et al: Drainage of pelvic abscesses through the greater sciatic foramen. Radiology 158:487–491, 1986.
30. Lang EK, Springer RM, Glorioso LW, Cammarata CA: Abdominal abscess drainage under radiologic guidance: causes of failure. Radiology 159:329–336, 1986.

Renal Artery Embolization

31. Woodside J, Schwarz H, Bergreen P: Peripheral embolization complicating bilateral renal infarction with Gelfoam. AJR 126:1033–1034, 1976.
32. Gang DL, Dole KB, Adelman LS: Spinal cord infarction following therapeutic renal artery embolization. JAMA 237:2841–2842, 1977.
33. Tupper TB, Cronan JJ, Wald LM, Dorfman GS: Renal abscess: a complication of ethanol embolization. Radiology 161:35–36, 1986.
34. Rankin RN: Gas formation after renal tumor embolization without abscess: a benign occurrence. Radiology 130:317–320, 1979.
35. Cox GG, Lee KR, Price HI, et al: Colonic infarction following ethanol embolization of renal cell carcinoma. Radiology 145:343–345, 1982.
36. Mulligan BD, Espinosa GA: Bowel infarction: complication of ethanol ablation of a renal tumor. Cardiovasc Intervent Radiol 6:55–57, 1983.
37. Garel L, Mareschal JL, Gagnadoux MF, et al: Fatal outcome after ethanol renal ablation in child with end-stage renal disease. AJR 146:593–594, 1986.

Hypogastric Artery Embolization

38. Athanasoulis CA, Waltman AC, Barnes AB, et al: Angiographic control of pelvic bleeding from treated carcinoma of the cervix. Gynecol Oncol 4:144–145, 1976.
39. Mitchell ME, Waltman AC, Athanasoulis CA: Control of massive prostatic bleeding with angiographic techniques. J Urol 115:692–694, 1976.
40. Kobayashi T, Shohichi K, Takasi M: Selective embolization of the vesical artery in the management of massive bladder hemorrhage. Radiology 136:345–346, 1980.
41. Matalan TSA, Athanasoulis CA, Margolies MN, et al: Hemorrhage with the pelvic fractures: efficacy of transcatheter embolization. AJR 133:859–862, 1979.

Renal Artery Angioplasty

42. Schwarten DE: Transluminal angioplasty of renal artery stenosis: 70 experiences. AJR 135:969–974, 1980.
43. Sos TA, Pickering TG, Sniderman K, et al: Percutaneous transluminal renal angioplasty in renovascular hypertension due to atheroma or fibromuscular dysplasia. N Engl J Med 309:274–279, 1983.
44. Puijlaert CBAJ, Boomsma JBH, Ruys JHJ, et al: Transluminal renal artery dilatation in hypertension: technique, results and complications in 60 cases. Urol Radiol 2:201–210, 1981.
45. Tegtmeyer CJ, Kofler TJ, Ayers CA: Renal angioplasty: current status. AJR 142:17–21, 1984.
46. Puijlaert CBAJ, Mali WP, Rosenbusch G, et al: Delayed rupture of renal artery after renal percutaneous transluminal angioplasty. Radiology 159:635–637, 1986.
47. Gardiner GA, Meyerovitz MF, Stokes KR: Complications of transluminal angioplasty. Radiology 159:201–208, 1986.

Spermatic Vein Embolization

48. White RI Jr, Kaufman SL, Barth KH, et al: Occlusion of varicoceles with detachable balloons. Radiology 139:327–334, 1981.
49. Saeyferth W, Jecht E, Zeitter E: Percutaneous sclerotherapy of varicocele. Radiology 139:335–340, 1981.
50. Morag B, Rubinstein ZJ, Goldwasser B, et al: Percutaneous venography and occlusion in the management of spermatic varicoceles. AJR 143:635–640, 1984.
51. Shuman L, White RI Jr, Mitchell SE, et al: Right-sided varicocele: technique and clinical results of balloon embolotherapy from the femoral approach. Radiology 158:787–791, 1986.

Prostate and Urethra

52. Burhenne HJ, Chisholm RJ, Quenville NF: Prostatic hyperplasia: radiological intervention. Radiology 152:655–657, 1984.
53. Quinn SF, Dyer R, Smathers R, et al: Balloon dilatation of the prostatic urethra. Radiology 157:57–58, 1985.
54. Hare WS, McOmish D, Nunn IN: Percutaneous transvesical antegrade passage of urethral strictures. Urol Radiol 3:107–112, 1981.
55. Russinovich NA, Lloyd LK, Griggs WP, Jander HP: Balloon dilatation of urethral strictures. Urol Radiol 2:33–37, 1980.

Fine-Needle Aspiration Biopsy

56. Ferrucci JT Jr, Wittenberg J, Mueller RP, et al: Diagnosis of abdominal malignancy by radiologic fine needle aspiration biopsy. AJR 141:29–32, 1980.
57. Bret PM, Fond A, Casola G, et al: Abdominal lesions: a prospective study of clinical efficacy of percutaneous fine-needle biopsy. Radiology 159:345–346, 1986.
58. Reading CC, Charboneau JW, Felmlee JP, James EM: US-guided percutaneous biopsy: use of a screw biopsy stylet to aid needle detection. Radiology 163:280–281, 1987.

Radiographic Contrast

59. Shehadi WH, Toniolo G: Adverse reactions to contrast media: a report from the Committee on Safety of Contrast Media of the International Society of Radiology. Radiology 137:299–302, 1980.
60. Ansell G, Tweedie MCK, West CR, Evans P, Couch L: The current status of reactions to intravenous contrast media. Invest Radiol (Suppl) 15:S32–S39, 1980.
61. Spataro RF, Fisher HW, Boylan L: Urography with low-osmolality contrast media: comparative urinary excretion of iopamidol, hexabrix and diatrizoate. Invest Radiol 17:494–500, 1982.
62. Dawson P, Heron C, Marshall J: Intravenous urography with low osmolality contrast agents: theoretical considerations and clinical findings. Clin Radiol 35:173–175, 1984.
63. Foord KD, Kaye B, Howard J, Cumberland DC: Comparison of the side-effects of low-osmolar contrast media in intravenous urography. Clin Radiol 36:379–380, 1985.
64. Loughran CF: Clinical intravenous urography: comparative trial of ioxaglate and iopamidol. Radiology 161:455–458, 1986.
65. Thompson WM, Foster WL, Halvorsen RN, Dunnick NR, et al: Iopamidol: new nonionic contrast agent for excretory urography. AJR 142:329–332, 1984.
66. Dalla Palma L, Rossi M, Stacul F, Agostini R: Iopamidol in urography: comparison between ionic and nonionic contrast media in patients with normal and impaired renal function. Urol Radiol 4:1–3, 1982.

MANAGEMENT OF VASCULAR COMPLICATIONS

17

Michael T. Macfarlane • Robert B. Smith

INSTRUMENTATION

In order to reduce the incidence of vascular complications in urology and to perform successful repairs, a full array of vascular instruments should be available for every major urologic procedure. These instruments include the following:

1. Vascular forceps with jaws of fine interdigitating teeth or serrations for delicate handling of the vessel without crushing the wall
2. Fine Metzenbaum scissors for use in routine dissection around the vessels
3. Forty-five and 90-degree angle Pott's-Smith scissors for spatulating a vessel or extending an incision in a vessel wall
4. Vascular needle holders with fine tips and diamond jaws for control in grasping the fine needles without damaging them
5. Vascular clamps to provide temporary occlusion without crushing or damaging the vessel walls.

The jaws of vascular clamps must have atraumatic interdigitation with serrations capable of securely grasping the vessel without damaging it. Totally occlusive clamps come in various sizes, shapes, and angles for larger vessels, whereas smaller vessels are best controlled with spring-loaded bulldog clamps, which have no handles to get in the way. Schwartz clips are particularly valuable for control of small vessels, including the renal artery and its branches. Partially occluding C-shaped clamps allow one to grasp the side walls of the aorta or vena cava without completely stopping flow of the vessel. These are especially helpful at the takeoff of the renal pedicle. Jaws with interdigitating teeth are used on the aorta, and serrated jaws are best utilized on the vena cava. The Poutasse clamp is of particular use for partial aortic occlusion. Allis's clamps are of great use in helping to control vena caval or lumbar vein hemorrhage.

SUTURES

Suture material of cardiovascular silk, Tevdek, or monofilament polypropylene (Prolene) should be used at the discretion of the surgeon. Silk is easier to handle and tie; however, monofilament Prolene produces less inflammatory response and has significantly less potential for becoming infected, has a higher tensile strength with minimal degradation over time, and slides more easily through delicate vascular tissue. More knots must be used when dealing with Prolene. A personal preference of most physicians making routine vascular suture lines is Tevdek, which is also non-reactive and ties better than Prolene.

A synthetic material should always be chosen when suturing a synthetic vascular graft. These anastomoses never heal and rely on suture material for their strength. The higher risk of infective complications associated with synthetic grafts also demands that monofilament sutures be used. Silk should never be used in potentially infected suture lines. Suture sizes ranging from 2–0 to 7–0 should be available (Table 17–1).

Table 17–1. SUTURE SIZE RECOMMENDATIONS FOR VARIOUS VESSELS ENCOUNTERED IN UROLOGIC SURGERY

Vessel	Suture Size
Vena cava	4–0
Aorta	3–0 or 4–0
Renal vein/branches	5–0 or 6–0
Renal artery/branches	6–0 or 7–0

VASCULAR GRAFTS

Experimental data of vascular prostheses have demonstrated that early patency is dependent on the thrombogenic potential of the vascular replacement (i.e., the chemical composition, the surface charge, and the material used). A long-term patency requires formation and adherence of a neo-intima, which is dependent upon high porosity of the graft material.

The autogenous saphenous vein remains the most consistently suitable substitute for the renal artery. It has a good long-term patency rate; adequate lengths are readily available; and its caliber usually approximates that of the main renal artery. Aneurysmal dilation, however, can be expected to occur in up to 40 percent of patients, and preservation of the saphenous vein for coronary bypass surgery must be considered.[1–5]

Free grafts of autogenous artery, most commonly the hypogastric artery, are also highly suitable and are used for renal artery replacement when available. However, obtaining an adequate length of suitable nonatherosclerotic artery is often a limiting factor.[6,7]

Knitted Dacron or expanded polytetrafluoroethylene (PTFE-Gore-Tex) grafts are commonly used for renal artery replacement. The high porosity of knitted Dacron grafts can lead to significant blood loss if the graft is not preclotted. Gore-Tex, in particular, allows excellent tissue ingrowth and can be easily trimmed to the correct length. When the rare occasion arises when replacement of a section of inferior vena cava is necessary, Gore-Tex can be used successfully. On occasion, the creation of a temporary arteriovenous (AV) fistula to increase graft flow may be necessary. If patch grafts are necessary for vein or artery, Gore-Tex is the preferred synthetic material.

SURGICAL TECHNIQUES

The primary goal of all vascular repairs is the maintenance of normal flow and the restoration of intimal continuity. The reapproximation of the intima with fine suture material minimizes the risk of early thrombosis by limiting platelet access to the thrombogenic subintima during the healing process. Within 2 weeks, the anastomotic line will be covered with a continuous layer of antithrombogenic neo-intima. To restore normal blood flow, one must avoid reduction in luminal diameter and minimize turbulence. Flow rate is directly proportional to the radius of the vessel raised to the fourth power. Turbulence is produced by any irregular or sharp edge and by changes in flow direction.

ARTERIAL PROBLEMS

Repair of Lacerations

The most important aspect of repairing vascular lacerations is to not alter the caliber of the vessel. A narrow vessel will have reduced flow and be at increased risk of thrombosis. Larger vessels can be closed with a continuous suture. Medium and small vessels, however, should be closed with interrupted sutures with the aid of a vein or Gore-Tex patch graft. An elliptical piece of vein or Gore-Tex is fashioned to fill the longitudinal defect. Synthetic continuous sutures of suitable caliber are utilized for the involved vessel.

Arterial Transection

When performing a vascular anastomosis, factors that would create turbulence must be avoided because of adverse effects on flow. End-to-end anastomosis with vessels should be utilized whenever possible. End-to-side anastomosis is the next best alternative. Turbulence can be minimized by creating an elliptical ostium in the recipient vessel, spatulating the smaller vessel, and reducing the change in flow direction by making an acute angle of the anastomosis. Again, every effort must be made not to leave a constriction at the suture line.

A careful and precise technique is required for successful vascular surgery. Proximal and distal control of the major vessels must be secured prior to undertaking repair. Forceps should be used to expose the lumen and to stabilize the vessel without grasping the intima. After carefully removing the vascular adventitia from around the lumen where the anastomosis will take place, double-armed corner sutures are placed 180 degrees apart and tied. Sutures are then placed, beginning at the corners and working toward the middle.

In an end-to-side anastomosis, the suturing should begin with the corner suture at the heel of the anastomosis. The vessel should be flushed with dilute heparin solution at the beginning of the procedure and just prior to placing the final suture to lessen the likelihood of air emboli. This is especially important in renal artery repairs.

After re-establishing flow, small leaks from the needle holes can usually be stopped with light pressure. Larger leaks will require placing some additional sutures. Systemic or regional heparinization is not necessary for most renovascular repairs. Systemic heparinization should be considered if arterial flow to the lower extremity is to be totally occluded for a prolonged period during repair of a vascular injury.

The most disastrous vascular transections occur during left radical nephrectomy for large left renal tumors. We have personally seen the celiac axis, the superior mesenteric artery, and the contralateral renal artery transected during the resection of a large left renal cell carcinoma or a large retroperitoneal sarcoma.

Renal Artery Occlusion

Primary occlusion of the renal artery can occur either by embolic phenomenon or by thrombotic phenomenon. Iatrogenic occlusion occurs primarily following angiography or angioplasty or from atherosclerotic emboli after surgical manipulation of the aorta. Renal artery occlusion can result from intimal rupture and dissection, most commonly seen with rough handling of arteries during open surgery, and with angiography or balloon angioplasty.

Embolization most commonly involves secondary or peripheral branches of the renal vasculature, with infarcts involving less than half the kidney.[8] Emboli can also develop as a result of mitral valvular disease, atrial fibrillation and myocardial infarction, ventricular aneurysms, atherosclerotic disease of the aorta, and renal artery aneurysms. Acute renal artery thrombosis can occur secondary to surgical trauma with a vascular clamp or to spontaneous intimal dissection or can develop superimposed on an atherosclerotic plaque.

Rough technique in retracting and handling the renal artery can cause intimal disruption, intimal dissection, and thrombosis. Intimal dissection can also occur if improper technique is used to occlude the renal artery in the course of renal surgery. The Schwartz clip is an especially gentle way of controlling the renal artery. We have seen intimal dissection and thrombosis of the renal artery and common iliac artery associated with the Rumel tourniquet technique. We rarely use this technique now.

Intimal Dissection and Thrombosis

If intimal dissection has occurred and thrombosis is present in the patient, the artery must be opened and explored. Since intimal dissection of the renal artery often is extensive because of its high flow rate, it frequently involves the branch vessels. Renal cooling should be instituted as soon as the complication is noted. Even if it is a minimal injury, a simple thrombectomy will not suffice; the disrupted intima must be tacked down to the arterial wall.

Often it is best to resect the involved area of the renal artery and to do an end-to-end anastomosis, which will automatically repair the intima. At times, an interposition graft of hypogastric artery, synthetic vein, or Gore-Tex must be utilized. The needle should always be passed from the inside out on the side distal to the injury to guard against further intimal disruption. (Vascular sutures should always be passed in the direction of flow, if at all possible, to lessen the likelihood of intimal elevation.)

If the dissection has extended into the branch vessels, a nephrectomy should be performed and ex vivo repair of the branch vessels attempted. Rarely, however, can this be accomplished. It is the most common disaster we have seen following percutaneous angioplasty of the renal artery. The saphenous vein or hypogastric artery with its branches is necessary for this type of repair. The kidney is then autotransplanted back to the iliac fossa, using standard transplantation technique. (We have never personally been able to salvage a kidney with dissection extending into the branch vessels secondary to percutaneous angioplasty.)

Renal Artery Emboli

Patients with primary occlusion of the renal artery by thrombosis or emboli present with flank or upper abdominal pain, usually associated with hematuria. The "colicky" nature of the pain often leads to confusion with other etiologies including ureteral stone passage. Patients will often have fever, vomiting, and an elevated white blood cell count, sedimentation rate, and serum lactate dehydrogenase. Selective renal angiography is the definitive diagnostic study.

Conservative management is generally recommended for unilateral renal artery embolic occlusion by either anticoagulant therapy or percutaneous transcatheter thromboembolectomy or thrombolysis. Kidneys can often be salvaged despite angiographic evidence of total occlusion for up to 2 months, if prior occlusive disease is present, and if collateral channels have formed.[9,10] Management with supportive hemodialysis may be necessary initially for bilateral embolization or for occlusion in a solitary kidney. Delayed surgical revascularization with aortorenal bypass should be employed if conservative therapy is not effective within 5 to 7 days and if at the time of exploration there is good back bleeding noted in the renal artery. Anticoagulation should be maintained both intraoperatively and postoperatively.

Arteriovenous Fistulas

Arteriovenous fistulas are abnormal communications between adjacent arteries and veins. On angiography, AV renal fistulas of congenital type have a characteristic angiomatous configuration of multiple tortuous coiled vessels in a cluster. Congenital AV fistulas account for less than 25 percent of all cases; most renal AV fistulas are acquired as complications of surgery, trauma, inflammation, or cancer. Acquired AV fistula most commonly results from needle biopsy of the kidney.[11] Surgical causes include mass ligation of the renal pedicle, packing of the renal bed, infection, and recurrent tumor.[12–14]

Most patients with AV fistulas will have a loud, high-pitched, continuous abdominal bruit. Diastolic hypertension with congestive heart failure and cardiomegaly occurs frequently, and angiography confirms the diagnosis. Acquired AV fistulas generally have identifiable entering and exiting vessels with decreased vascularity distal to the shunt.

As noted in the foregoing discussion, renal AV fistulas that develop following needle biopsy are by far the most common type.[11] Fortunately, the majority of these (up to 70 percent) will close spontaneously within 18 months.[15] Observation is also appropriate for most traumatic fistulas—at least initially—because many of these can be expected to spontaneously resolve or improve. Indications for surgical treatment include hypertension, high-output heart failure, progressive renal failure or rupture, and severe hematuria. Transcatheter angiographic embolization has been successfully employed in treating smaller fistulas such as those that occur after needle biopsy.

Most congenital renal AV fistulas have been managed by partial or total nephrectomy. More recently, parenchyma-sparing procedures, utilizing microvascular techniques, have been performed in situ and extracorporeally with success.

Arteriovenous fistulas involving the renal pedicle that has been mass ligated present a particularly challenging problem. Typical situations that require the pedicle to be mass ligated in the first place make the repair of this problem exceedingly hazardous. Usually mass ligatures are done in patients who have undergone multiple prior surgeries or have experienced a severe inflammatory process (e.g., infected hydronephrosis, xanthogranulomatous pyelonephritis, or perinephric abscess). Mass ligations of the pedicle should never be performed unless absolutely necessary.

It is much easier to treat an AV fistula involving a mass ligation of the right renal pedicle than of the left. Control of the right renal artery can be obtained far away from the site of the AV fistula and can be relatively easy to control by mobilizing the vena cava laterally to expose the takeoff of the right renal artery. Simple ligation of the proximal right renal artery will solve the problem.

The approach to a right renal artery fistula should be made through an anterior transabdominal transperitoneal incision. The peritoneum is opened, beginning at the cecum, and carried superiorly to the ligament of Treitz. The inferior mesenteric vein will lead the surgeon to the left renal vein, which directly overlies the origin of the right renal artery.

Left-sided AV fistulas should also be approached with a similar incision; the aorta should be mobilized proximal and distal to the renal pedicle to gain control. This dissection can be extremely tedious. Usually the medial aspect of the aorta will be less involved in reactive tissue, and it will be easier to establish the proper plane on the aortic adventitia in this area. Once this plane has been identified, the reactive tissue can be further separated from the aorta with blunt dissection, using a tonsil or right-angle clamp and incising the elevated tissue with scissors or the electrocautery. The inferior mesenteric vein can also be helpful in identifying the left renal vein, which can be incredibly enlarged by the high flow of the AV fistula. This must be mobilized with extreme care because inadvertent entry can be "exciting."

Approaching the left renal vein initially near the vena cava is usually recommended because reaction in this area may not be as severe. One can get above the renal vein and dissect the medial aspect of the aorta to begin to gain proximal control of the aorta. A Satinsky clamp should be placed around the aorta at this point but not secured. A vascular tape can also be placed around the aorta distal to the renal pedicle to allow rapid control if necessary. Meticulous dissection of the renal pedicle is then carried out, isolating the left renal artery near its takeoff. Once isolated, it is ligated and the problem solved.

Infected Vascular Sutures

When an infected vascular suture line is present, it can be manifested by a fistula to the skin or by recurrent septic episodes. Positive blood cultures without other sources (e.g., valvular heart disease) should suggest this diagnosis. Infected arterial suture lines should be excised. If the aorta is involved, the infected suture line is excised along with a "rim" of aortic tissue. After copious specific antibacterial irrigation, this can usually be re-closed using monofilament synthetic suture material without significant narrowing of the aorta. Broad-spectrum systemic antibiotics should be administered in full therapeutic doses, preoperatively, intraoperatively, and for at least 7 days postoperatively. External suction drainage should also be employed.

Infected arterial suture lines that involve smaller vessels where the lumen would be compromised require a patch of autologous material (usually saphenous vein), using monofilament synthetic suture material. In no instance should a synthetic patch graft be used.

Infected sutures that involve small veins can usually be managed by excision of the suture line and ligation of the vein. If the renal vein is involved and simple excision and closure of the suture line will cause significant narrowing, a saphenous vein patch graft will be necessary. With an infected vena caval suture line, this can always be simply excised and closed. Absorbable sutures (4–0 catgut) have been used previously with success. Again, broad-spectrum antibiotic treatment and suction drainage are essential for a successful result.

VENOUS PROBLEMS

Tumor Involvement of the Vena Cava

Renal cell carcinoma will extend into the inferior vena cava in up to 10 percent of patients.[16] Previously thought to be incurable, involvement of the vena cava with tumor thrombus is now routinely managed with good prognosis. Half of these patients can be expected to have no clinical manifestations of caval obstruction. Complicating factors include tumor thrombus extension into hepatic veins or right atrium and direct tumor invasion of the vena caval wall.

A thoracoabdominal or transperitoneal approach can be utilized; however, we prefer the thoracoabdominal incision for infradiaphragmatic cases. Early ligation of the renal artery and isolation of the vena cava by isolating all lumbar veins are essential to this procedure. After mobilizing the inferior vena cava, a Rumel tourniquet is placed around it distally. The kidney is mobilized en bloc with renal hilar and periaortic lymph nodes. With a subhepatic thrombus, a Rumel tourniquet can be placed around the vena cava just below the liver. If the tumor extends into the hepatic portion of the vena cava, a Rumel tourniquet is placed around the suprahepatic inferior vena cava after the triangular and coronary ligaments of the liver have been taken down. The superior mesenteric artery, porta hepatis, and contralateral renal artery must be carefully controlled. All venous inflow must be controlled into the vena cava before making the cavotomy for removal of the thrombus.

If the tumor thrombus extends into the atrium or supradiaphragmatic vena cava, a midline anterior approach is indicated, using a generous midline abdominal incision carried upward as a median sternotomy. A thoracic team with bypass capability must be in attendance. Often tumors in the atrium can be extracted without bypass; however, if there is a "mushroom" extension of the tumor into the atrium, bypass is essential. Also, if the tumor is adherent to the caval wall, bypass is necessary to allow the operating surgeon to have a bloodless field for careful examination of the interior of the vena cava to enable all tumor fragments to be removed. A piecemeal removal of the tumor thrombus does not seem to compromise cure as long as the removal is complete. Cardiopulmonary bypass with hypothermia and exsanguination has been reported to decrease morbidity and mortality associated with major tumor thrombi that occur lower in the vena cava, but we question the need for its routine use in such cases.

All air must be removed from the vena cava by aspiration or by opening the distal clamp before the suture line is complete (with the proximal vena cava still controlled). Caval excision can be performed proximal to the first hepatic vein in patients with caval invasion. If it is a left-sided tumor, establishment of the right renal venous outflow is essential.

For left-sided tumors that invade the inferior diaphragmatic portion of the vena cava, a left or a right thoracoabdominal incision or an anterior incision can be utilized. If a left-sided renal tumor thrombus extends into the hepatic portion of the vena cava, a left thoracoabdominal incision should not be used. A right thoracoabdominal approach is preferable in such patients because it facilitates control of the suprahepatic subdiaphragmatic portion of the vena cava. A midline anterior incision can also be used.

Inferior Vena Caval Hemorrhage

Hemorrhage from the inferior vena cava is usually secondary to inadvertent laceration or avulsion of large fragile veins. A thorough knowledge of the vascular anatomy can help avoid these problems. Common areas of trouble include lumbar vessels during mobilization of the vena cava (particularly at the level of the renal vein) and injury to the right gonadal vein into the inferior vena cava as well as avulsion of the right adrenal vein.

Lumbar veins enter the posterolateral aspect of the vena cava and generally can be found to run with its corresponding artery at each vertebral level. Traction on the vena cava can easily avulse one of these fragile veins. The vena cava should be retracted gently with curved vein retractors and each lumbar vein doubly clamped and securely ligated using 3–0 or 4–0 silk. If these ligatures are tied too tightly, they can easily shear through the vessel. Particular care should be taken with the lumbar vessels when mobilizing the renal veins.

In the event of hemorrhage from the vena cava, immediate control often can be obtained by direct pressure on the bleeding site. Allis's clamps can be used to grasp the edges of the laceration, providing control and visualization for oversewing. If the bleeding is from a posterior lumbar vessel, the vena cava can be rolled medially with digital compression above and below the level of the involved area. A Satinsky clamp can be placed on the vena cava for larger lacerations.

Persistent bleeding from the proximal end of an avulsed lumbar vessel can be difficult to control if it retracts into the psoas muscle. Control often can be obtained by grasping the end of the vessel with a hemostat, twisting it, and finally placing a suture ligature. Alternatively, figure-of-8 sutures can be placed into the overlying psoas muscle, which may control the bleeding. If persistent bleeding occurs, retropsoas exploration may be necessary to find the origin of the lumbar vein.

Vena Caval Thrombosis

Vena caval thrombosis can be a complication with patients undergoing excision of a vena caval tumor thrombus or dissection of a retroperitoneal node for testis cancer, or in patients with large primary retroperitoneal tumors such as sarcomas. In cases in which the patient's vena cava has been invaded by intraluminal or extraluminal tumor, total or partial caval resection is necessary. If such a resection is performed, one must be careful not to leave a stump of vena cava below the resected margin, which has no inflow. In patients in whom infrarenal caval resection for retroperitoneal malignancy is performed, the cava should be resected flush with the right and left renal veins. A stump of vena cava left below this level may allow a thrombus to form, which could break loose and cause a pulmonary embolus.

If more extensive caval resection is necessary, as is occasionally the case in patients with renal cell carcinoma, retroperitoneal sarcoma, or stage B_3 testis tumors, the level of resection should be as proximal as possible (i.e., at the level of the hepatics), presuming that the renal vein insertion cannot be preserved. In such patients, the outflow of the right renal vein must be restored with anastomosis to the portal vein or by an autotransplant to the ipsilateral iliac fossa. It is possible to replace a segment of suprarenal vena cava that has to be excised with a segment of infrarenal cava.

Generally the vena cava can be narrowed considerably without complication; however, on occasion thrombosis has occurred. If the patient is symptomatic or if the outflow of the right renal vein is compromised, thrombectomy with anticoagulation therapy is necessary, with the possible placement of a vena caval clip. On occasion, recurrent thrombosis may cause venous hypertension or severe peripheral edema. Augmentation of the cava may be necessary. Pericardium has been used for this purpose when the problem has occurred at the time of tumor thrombus resection for renal cell carcinoma.[18] When augmentation of the vena cava is necessary on a delayed basis, Gore-Tex has been used successfully. Some surgeons advocate the creation of a distal arteriovenous fistula to increase blood flow in the inferior vena cava in such patients.

Renal Vein Thrombosis

Renal vein thrombosis can occur at any age, but it is most common in the neonatal period. Early diagnosis is dependent upon a high index of suspicion.

Renal vein thrombosis in infancy affects males and females, as well as left and right kidneys equally. More than half the cases occur in the first 2 weeks of life, usually in neonates with diarrhea and severe dehydration or in infants of diabetic mothers. Less commonly associated causes include sepsis, traumatic deliveries, congenital heart disease, and maternal ingestion of thiazide and the presence of cytomegalovirus infection.

Renal vein thrombosis in adults is rare and is usually associated with underlying renal disease such as glomerulopathies,nephrotic syndrome, or pyelonephritis. Other etiologies include infection, trauma, malignancies, amyloidosis, sickle cell disease, and estrogen ingestion. Any low flow state with hypoperfusion of the kidney can predispose to renal vein thrombosis.

Infants present with flank mass, hematuria, thrombocytopenia, and non-visualization of the involved kidney on intravenous urography (IVU). Adults have a more variable presentation but often seek medical attention because of pain and hematuria. Chronic renal vein thrombosis in adults may present with flank pain, hematuria, proteinuria, and flank mass. A left varicocele that does not collapse with recumbency should suggest left renal vein occlusion. The differential diagnosis of renal vein thrombosis includes ureteral stone, pyelonephritis, renal artery thrombosis, malignancy, perinephric abscess, and extrinsic compression of the renal vein ("nutcracker" syndrome).

The diagnosis is generally made by history, non-visualization on IVU, and a high index of suspicion. Intravenous urographic findings usually reveal a unilaterally enlarged kidney with poor or absent renal function. Exclusion of post-renal obstruction can be made by ultrasonography or retrograde pyelography. The definitive diagnosis is established by venography while evaluating for inferior vena caval involvement or bilateral renal vein involvement.

Once treated only with surgical intervention, unilateral renal vein thrombosis is now treated medically, at least initially. Correction of underlying disorders such as dehydration or sepsis is usually followed by systemic heparinization with subsequent oral anticoagulation with warfarin in adults. The use of anticoagulation therapy in infants is not universally accepted.

Indications for surgical intervention include bilateral renal vein thrombosis or thrombosis in a solitary kidney, inferior vena caval thrombosis, development of uncontrollable hypertension or sepsis, and renal vein thrombosis secondary to tumor. Surgery for primary renal vein thrombosis is often a very unsatisfying operative experience. Thrombus rarely involves only the main renal vein and usually extends far out into the smaller venous radicles, making them difficult to totally extract. Often venous bleeding is not optimal. This, however, coupled with anticoagulation, can be of benefit in selected patients.

If surgical intervention is deemed mandatory, a transperitoneal surgical approach allows for good control as well as for inspection of the inferior vena cava above and below in both renal veins prior to embolectomy. A vertical cavotomy is made, through which the thrombus is removed. The vena cava is closed with running 5–0 cardiovascular silk sutures. A nephrectomy may be indicated in certain patients.

Deep Venous Thrombosis

Venous thrombosis is a common problem among hospitalized patients as measured by ^{123}I fibrinogen leg scanning. Fortunately most of these thrombi are small and asymptomatic. Pulmonary embolism is the most common preventable cause of hospital and postoperative deaths, with a reported incidence of 0.1 to 0.8 percent of general surgical patients.[19] Most fatal emboli arise from more proximal vein thrombosis (i.e., popliteal, femoral, or iliac veins). Manifestations of venous thrombosis are a result of perivascular inflammation, obstruction to venous flow, and embolization into pulmonary circulation. Symptoms primarily occur in large occlusive thrombi that extend into the popliteal or more proximal veins. Risk factors for the development of thrombosis include tissue injury, venous stasis, vascular damage, and hypercoagulable states.

Complications of Deep Venous Thrombosis

Postphlebitic syndrome is caused by venous hypertension as a result of recanalization of organized thrombus with destruction of venous valves or by persistent obstruction of large proximal veins. Impaired venous circulation produces changes in the subcutaneous tissue and ultimately leads to venous ulceration. It is a complication primarily of proximal venous thrombosis, usually iliofemoral. Patients undergoing surgery who have a prevous history of venous thrombosis have a four-fold increased risk of developing recurrent venous thrombosis.

Pulmonary embolism (PE) is the most feared complication of venous thrombosis. More than 600,000 symptomatic cases occur each year in the United States, and about one third of these patients die, making pulmonary embolism the third most common cause of death. The rate of mortality is high because the majority of patients (60 to 90 percent) die within the first hour and are, therefore, never treated. Patients at the greatest risk of dying are those with massive PE obstructing more than 50 percent of the pulmonary circulation, accompanied by hypotension. The patients with venous thrombosis who are at greatest risk of developing complicating PE are those with involvement of the proximal leg veins, particularly the iliofemoral.

The clinical diagnosis of deep venous thrombosis (DVT) is highly unreliable and must therefore be confirmed by objective diagnostic tests before therapy can be initiated. However, the clinical evaluation of patients with suspected DVT is still important and is based on physical examination and a history of risk factors. Deep venous thrombosis rarely occurs in the absence of risk factors, and the frequency of its occurrence increases cumulatively with each additional risk factor that a patient demonstrates.[20] The occurrence of DVT in a patient without risk factors is unlikely.

Risk factors for DVT include: (1) prolonged venous stasis (e.g., bedrest, immobilization, or surgery); (2) advanced age (incidence progresses after age 40); (3) prior history of DVT; (4) malignancy; (5) obesity; (6) excessive estrogen levels (e.g., due to oral contraceptives or pregnancy).

Unilateral swelling is the most reliable physical finding of DVT. The mnaximal circumference of both calves should be compared, looking for unilateral pitting and prominent superficial veins. A palpable tender cord in the calf is highly suggestive. Only about 10 percent of patients will have a positive Homans's sign (pain in the calf on passive dorsiflexion of the foot). Venous obstruction may occasionally become so advanced as to cause marked swelling, cyanosis, and signs of tissue hypoxia. The majority of patients with DVT, however, are asymptomatic. More than half of patients with documented PE have no physical findings involving the leg.

Diagnostic Studies

Radioiodine-labeled fibrinogen uptake tests record the uptake and incorporation of labeled fibrinogen in new fibrin thrombi as monitored by external scintillation 24 hours after intravenous dose. This technique is very sensitive and reliable for detecting small calf thrombi. However, it is essentially useless for more proximal thrombi above the mid-thigh and in the groin or pelvis, and the 24-hour waiting period for results is a major drawback.

Duplex ultrasound scanning instruments allow both Doppler flow assessment and B mode imaging of the venous system. It is a non-invasive means of making an immediate evaluation. However, as with all ultrasonic techniques, it is highly operator-dependent, and accurate results require experienced hands.

Impedence plethysmography (IPG), the most widely used technique, measures changes in blood volume of the calf indirectly by changes in the electrical resistance of the leg. Venous occlusion plethysmography plots the initial venous filling of the calf after inflation of a thigh cuff against a 3-second venous outflow following deflation. Proximal venous occlusion of the popliteal, femoral, or iliac veins by thrombi will impair the 3-second venous runoff. This method has an overall sensitivity and specificity of 94 percent and a 100 percent sensitivity for identifying proximal thrombi. Its positive predictive value is >95 percent.

Venography continues to be regarded as the gold standard for assessment of the venous circulation because of its 90+ percent accuracy rate and because it provides a very reasssuring anatomic image.

In performing pelvic surgery, one must be particularly concerned about more proximal pelvic thrombi. These are not only more likely to occur after pelvic surgery but are also the most likely to lead to fatal pulmonary embolism. Impedence plethysmography is an excellent screening method for patients suspected of having proximal thrombi. The likelihood of subsequent DVT or PE following a negative IPG alone has been reported to be only 1 to 2 percent.[21] A positive IPG or an equivocal study in a patient with multiple risk factors or a highly suggestive physical examination should be followed by venography.

Treatment

The goals in treating patients with venous thrombosis are to prevent the morbidity and mortality from pulmonary embolism and to minimize postphlebitic syndrome. Thromboembolic therapy entails significant risk of complication and should not be undertaken without a definitive diagnosis confirmed by objective tests. Treatment options for venous thrombosis include anticoagulants, thrombolysis, vena caval interruption, and thromboembolectomy.

The anticoagulant drugs heparin and warfarin (Coumadin) are highly effective in preventing acute recurrent PE and reducing its consequences. Current guidelines support the initial treatment with continuous IV heparin or b.i.d. adjusted-dose subcutaneous heparin for 7 to 10 days in patients with documented proximal thrombosis or pulmonary embolus. Therapy should be monitored by keeping the activated partial thromboplastin time (APTT) between 1½ and 2 times the control value or by keeping the serum heparin levels between 0.3 and 0.5 U/ml by protamine titration assay. Patients who fail to lower their APTT with heparin doses greater than 50,000 units/day are considered to be heparin-resistant. Most cases of true heparin resistance are secondary to rapid heparin clearance in the early stages of pulmonary embolism or major venous thrombosis. However, be sure that it is not just an artifact (e.g., failure to administer heparin or laboratory error) by rechecking the APTT and checking the serum heparin level by protamine titration assay. If heparin levels are greater than 0.3 units/ml, the heparin dose should not be increased.

Oral therapy with Coumadin should be started 4 to 5 days after heparin therapy is begun and overlap for 4 to 5 days before stopping heparin. Oral therapy should be continued for at least 3 months and monitored by maintaining the prothrombin time at 1.3 to 1.4 times the control value. Patients suffering from recurrent episodes of DVT should be maintained on oral anticoagulation therapy for at least 1 year. Pregnant patients should be treated with an adjusted dose of subcutaneous heparin because oral therapy is contraindicated.

Untreated calf vein thrombosis will extend more proximally in only 20 percent of patients. Calf vein thrombosis can be monitored by periodic IPG for evidence of extension and treatment begun if extension is documented. However, if monitoring for extension cannot be done, anticoagulation therapy should be instituted.

The thrombolytic agents streptokinase and urokinase are primarily indicated for patients with massive PE and shock. Their value in treating routine venous thrombosis is unclear. In view of the significantly greater risk of hemorrhagic complications (approximately 3 times greater), their use should probably be limited to young patients experiencing extensive proximal DVT with no contraindications to therapy.

Placement of inferior vena caval clips or filters is effective in preventing acute or recurrent PE. This option is usually reserved for patients with major contraindications to anticoagulant or thrombolytic therapy.

Thombectomy is primarily reserved for patients with iliofemoral vein thrombosis and a painful, tensely swollen leg with evidence of arterial compromise (phlegmasia cerulea dolens) despite heparinization and leg elevation.[22] In instances of major proximal thrombosis, venous outflow obstruction will lead to progressively increased compartmental pressures and impeded arterial inflow. The technique of thrombectomy with adjunctive temporary AV fistula and postoperative anticoagulation therapy is warranted under these severe conditions. Embolectomy from the pulmonary artery is reserved for patients with acute, life-threatening PE when blood pressure cannot be maintained despite thrombolytic therapy and the administration of vasopressor agents.

Prophylaxis Against Deep Venous Thrombosis

Approximately 100,000 people die from massive PE in the United States each year, and over 90 percent of these deaths arise from DVT of the legs.[23] Although anticoagulant therapy is highly effective in preventing deaths, two thirds of these patients die within the first 30 minutes after the acute event, emphasizing the need for prophylaxis if we are going to improve this outcome. There is also significant morbidity from

Table 17–2. FACTORS THAT FAVOR PROPHYLAXIS IN UROLOGIC PATIENTS UNDERGOING EXTENSIVE PELVIC SURGERY FOR MALIGNANT DISEASE

1. These patients are in the highest risk group for developing venous thromboembolism (40 to 80% calf DVT, 10 to 20% proximal DVT, 1 to 5% fatal PE).
2. Proximal DVTs, particularly pelvic DVTs, are at greatest risk of causing fatal pulmonary embolism.
3. Almost all of these patients will have two or more risk factors for DVT (age >40, malignant disease, obesity, prolonged immobility, varicose veins, previous DVT, or CHF).

complications of venous thrombosis such as postphlebitic syndrome, which often cannot be prevented after the fact, despite anticoagulation therapy.

Patients undergoing extensive pelvic surgery for malignant disease have been shown to be in the highest risk group for developing postoperative thromboembolism.[24] Forty to 80 percent are at risk for developing calf vein thrombosis, 10 to 20 percent for developing proximal vein thrombosis, and 1 to 5 percent for developing fatal PE. Patients undergoing a transurethral resection of the prostate have a 7 to 10 percent risk for developing calf vein thrombosis, whereas a retropublic prostatectomy or equivalent operation has a 20 to 50 percent risk to patients (moderate risk group). In addition, many of these patients will have more than one of the known risk factors for DVT (i.e., age over 40, prolonged immobility, malignant disease, obesity, varicose veins, estrogen therapy, previous history of DVT, or congestive heart failure).

The factor of age alone, with surgery lasting more than 30 minutes, puts many in a moderate risk group (i.e., risk of calf thrombosis, 10 to 40 percent; proximal vein thrombosis, 2 to 10 percent; and fatal pulmonary embolism, 0.1 to 0.7 percent). These data strongly indicate the need for prophylaxis in all patients undergoing extensive pelvic surgery for malignant disease, and indeed this has been recommended by the NIH Consensus Conference on prevention of venous thrombosis and PE (Table 17–2).[25,26]

Primary prophylaxis using drugs such as low-dose subcutaneous heparin, IV dextran, and oral anticoagulants, or physical methods such as intermittent pneumatic compression of the legs and graduated compression stockings has proved to be more effective than secondary prevention by early detection and treatment of venous thrombosis after it occurs. Venous thrombosis develops by three principal mechanisms called Virchow's triad. They are venous stasis, activation of blood coagulation, and vascular endothelial damage resulting in activation of platelets. Prophylactic methods have, therefore, focused on three corresponding mechanisms, which are mechanical devices, anticoagulant drugs, and antiplatelet drugs.

Low-dose heparin has been shown to be highly effective in preventing venous thrombosis and pulmonary embolism in urologic patients. Several studies have demonstrated a 75 percent reduction in the incidence of postoperative DVT using low-dose, subcutaneous heparin.[26] Prophylaxis usually consists of 5000 units 2 hours preoperatively and every 8 to 12 hours postoperatively for 2 days.

Intermittent pneumatic leg compression works by enhancing blood flow to the deep veins in the legs and thus preventing venous stasis. It is an effective prophylaxis against DVT, especially in patients undergoing prostate surgery, and it is virtually free of clinically important side effects.[27,28]

Oral anticoagulation therapy is effective prophylaxis. However, its association with a high frequency of clinically important bleeding complications and with an increase in the incidence of lymphoceles in patients in whom pelvic lymph node dissection has been performed has severely limited its acceptence.

Low-molecular-weight, intravenous dextran 40 is effective prophylaxis for moderate-risk, general surgical patients. Its disadvantage is occasional hypersensitivity reactions and potential volume overload, particularly in patients with impaired cardiac function. Experience in the urologic setting is limited.

Aspirin's antiplatelet action is relatively ineffective as prophylaxis for venous thrombosis in randomized controlled trials.

Adjusted-dose, subcutaneous heparin, in which administration is determined by monitoring APTT, has been shown to be highly effective in high-risk patients undergoing hip replacement without associated increased frequency of bleeding complications. Data for urologic patients do not exist at present. The addition of a mild venous constrictor dihydroergotamine (DHE) to standard subcutaneous, low-dose heparin prophylaxis was suggested as a pharmacologic attack on venous stasis to complement the anticoagulant effect of heparin. The idea was an attempt to affect two limbs of Virchow's triad of venous thrombosis. A number of randomized trials have now confirmed that subcutaneous DHE (0.5 mg) plus heparin 5000 units b.i.d. results in a 50 percent reduced risk of developing DVT as compared with the risk when heparin is used alone.[29,30] In addition, no significant difference in bleeding complications was noted between treatment groups (DHE 0.5 mg/heparin 5000 units b.i.d.) and placebo control.[31]

General Guidelines for Prophylaxis

Patients undergoing transurethral resection (TUR) of the prostate do not require prophylaxis, based on the low risk of developing calf vein thrombosis (7 to 10 percent). Patients undergoing open prostatectomy or extensive pelvic surgery for malignancy are at moderate to high risk of developing venous thrombosis and should be considered for prophylaxis. Recommendations have supported either low-dose subcutaneous heparin (with or without DHE) or external pneumatic compression. Both of these modalities have been demonstrated effective, although most studies are based on low-dose heparin. Both modalities are cost-effective, according to studies in general surgical patients. Other workers favor the use of oral anticoagulants, extending the prothrombin time to 15 to 18 seconds (1.2 to 1.5 times the normal control value).

PULMONARY EMBOLISM

Pulmonary embolism remains the most serious complication of deep venous thrombosis. As with DVT, the clinical diagnosis of PE is highly non-specific. More than half of all patients with clinically suspected PE will have negative pulmonary angiograms.

The history and physical examination should be focused on determining if there are other causes for the patient's condition. The clinical diagnosis of PE is primarily one of exclusion. The clinical features of PE include dyspnea, hemoptysis, pleuritic chest pain, and acute right heart failure. None of these is specific, and other pulmonary and cardiac diseases must be ruled out. Chest x-ray, electrocardiogram, and arterial blood gases are all non-specific studies that are helpful in demonstrating other causes for the patient's condition.

Clinical suspicion of PE must be confirmed by objective testing.[32] Ventilation perfusion scans are obtained by making lung images after intravenous injection of ^{99}Tc-labeled albumin particles. Two thirds of patients with one or more segmental defects or larger defects in pulmonary blood flow will have a documented PE on angiography, whereas only 20 percent of subsegmental defects will be associated with PE.

The addition of a xenon ventilation study will improve sensitivity and specificity of the combined study for detecting PE. Washout images from normal ventilated segments of the lung will be cleared of tracer within 3 to 4 minutes, whereas poorly ventilated segments will take longer. The finding of a ventilation/perfusion mismatch (i.e., normal ventilation with defective perfusion) significantly increases the accuracy of diagnosing a PE. Poorly ventilated areas from other pulmonary diseases would be expected also to be underperfused. Ventilation/perfusion scan results are reported according to the probability that PE is present, i.e., normal, (0 percent); low probability, (less than 20 percent); intermediate, (35 to 50 percent); and high probability, (over 90 percent). Unfortunately the majority of studies—-about 75 percent—are reported as low, intermediate, or indeterminate possibility, with only 25 percent reading as definitive diagnosis of normal (10 percent) or high probability (15 percent). This often necessitates pulmonary angiography to make a definitive diagnosis.

Pulmonary angiography is the accepted gold standard for determining the presence or absence of PE. It allows direct visualization of intraluminal filling defects caused by thromboemboli. Significant complications, however, occur in 3 to 4 percent of patients who undergo pulmonary angiography, including tachyarrhythmias, endocardial or myocardial injury, cardiac perforation, cardiac arrest, and hypersensitivity reactions.

All patients suspected of having a PE after history and physical examination, chest x-ray, and electrocardiogram should undergo V/Q lung scanning. The normal V/Q scan excludes PE. A high probability scan is sufficient evidence to proceed with treatment. Again, up to 75 percent of the scans will be reported as indeterminate and the patient may require further tests. In view of data that report approximately 70 percent of patients with a documented PE will have an identifiable DVT, it is reasonable to proceeed with impedence plethysmography. A positive IPG would be a good indication for treatment and would, therefore, avoid pulmonary angiography in up to 70 percent of patients with indeterminate V/Q scans.

References

1. Stanley JC, et al: Fate of 100 aortorenal vein grafts: characteristics of late graft expansion, aneurysmal dilatation, and stenosis. Surgery 74:931, 1973.

2. Straffon RA, Siegel DF: Saphenous vein bypass graft in the treatment of renovascular hypertension. Urol Clin North Am 2:337, 1975.
3. Kaufman JJ: Renovascular hypertension: UCLA experience. J Urol 121:139, 1979.
4. Wichterman KA, Stansel HC: Simplified splanchnic artery revascularization using extra-anatomic bypass grafts. Arch Surg 114:1052, 1979.
5. Novick AC, Straffon RA, Stewart BH, et al: Surgical treatment of renovascular hypertension in the pediatric patient. J Urol 119:794, 1978.
6. Lye CR, String ST, Wylie EJ, et al: Aortorenal arterial autografts. Arch Surg 110:132, 1975.
7. Novick AC, Stewart BH, Straffon RA: Autogenous arterial grafts in the treatment of renal artery stenosis. J Urol 118:919, 1977.
8. Libertino JA, Zinman L, Breslin DJ, et al: Renal artery revascularization: restoration of renal function. JAMA 244:1340, 1980.
9. Brest AN, Bower R, Heider C: Renal functional recovery following anuria secondary to renal artery embolism. JAMA 187:540, 1964.
10. Perkins RP, Jacobsen, DS, Feeler FP, et al: Return of renal function after late embolectomy: report of a case. N Engl J Med 276:1194, 1967.
11. O'Brien DP, Parrott TS, Walton KN, et al: Renal arteriovenous fistulas. Surg Gynecol Obstet 139:739, 1974.
12. Muller WH, Goodwin WE: Renal arteriovenous fistula following nephrectomy. Ann Surg 144:240, 1956.
13. Chew QT, Madayag MA: Post-nephrectomy arteriovenous fistula. J Urol 109:546, 1973.
14. Kelly DG: Renal arteriovenous fistula: a review of four cases and review of the literature. Br J Urol 39:162, 1967.
15. Ekelund L, Lindholm T: Arteriovenous fistula following percutaneous renal biopsy. Acta Radiol 11:38, 1979.
16. Lieskovsky G, Pritchett R, Skinner DG: Surgical Management of Renal Cell Carcinoma. Monogr Urol 1984.
17. Shahalislamov F: Closure of defect of vena cava above renal vein by transposition of its lower segment. Kazan Med Zh 1:13, 1962.
18. Marshall FF, Reitz BA: Supradiapharagmatic renal cell carcinoma tumor thrombus: indication for vena caval reconstruction with pericardium. J Urol 133:266, 1985.
19. Dalen JE, Paraskos JA, Ockene IS, Alpert JS, Hirsh J: Venous thromboembolism: scope of the problem. Chest 84:370S, 1986.
20. Wheeler HB, Anderson FA: Diagnostic approaches for deep vein thrombosis. Chest 89:407S, 1986.
21. Hull RD, Hirsh J, Carter CJ, Jay RM, Ockerlford PA, Buller HR, et al: Diagnostic efficacy of impedance plethysmography for clinically suspected deep-vein thrombosis: a randomized trial. Ann Intern Med 102:21, 1985.
22. Rutherford RB: Role of surgery in iliofemoral venous thrombosis. Chest 89:434S, 1986.
23. Dalen JE, Alpert JS: Natural history of pulmonary embolism. Prog Cardiovasc Dis 17:259, 1975.
24. Salzman EW, Hirsh J: Prevention of venous thromboembolism. In Coleman RW, Hirsh J, Marder V, et al eds: Hemostasis and Thrombosis: Basic Principles and Clinical Practice. Philadelphia, JB Lippincott Co, pp 986–999.
25. NIH Consensus Conference: Prevention of venous thrombosis and pulmonary embolism. JAMA 256:744, 1986.
26. Hull RD, Raskob GE, Hirsch J: Prophylaxis of venous thromboembolism. Chest 89:374S, 1986.
27. Coe NP, Collins REC, Klein LA, Bettmann MA, Skillman JJ, Shapiro RM, et al: Prevention of deep-vein thrombosis in urological patients: a controlled, randomized trial of low-dose heparin and external pneumatic compression boots. Surgery 83:220, 1978.
28. Scurr JH, Ibrahim SZ, Faber RG, LeQuesne LP: The efficacy of graduated compression stockings in the prevention of deep-vein thrombosis. Br J Surg 64:371, 1977.
29. Gent M, Roberts RS: A meta-analysis of the studies of dihydroergotamine plus heparin in the prophylaxis of deep vein thrombosis. Chest 89:396S, 1986.
30. Multicenter Trial Committee: Dihydroergotamine–heparin prophylaxis of postoperative deep vein thrombosis: a multicenter trial. JAMA 251:2960, 1984.
31. Comerota AJ, White JV: The use of dihydroergotamine and heparin in the prophylaxis of deep venous thrombosis. Chest 89:389S, 1986.
32. Hull RD, Raskob GE, Hirsh J: The diagnosis of clinically suspected pulmonary embolism: practical approaches. Chest 89:417S, 1986.

COMPLICATIONS OF GENITOURINARY TRAUMA

18

George R. Fournier, Jr. • Jack W. McAninch

Genitourinary trauma occurs in 10 to 15 percent of all major abdominal injuries, either blunt or penetrating, and are therefore an important consideration in the initial evaluation. The best management of complications due to genitourinary trauma is prevention—that is, early recognition of the injury and its extent and appropriate treatment. Intravenous pyelography (IVP), retrograde cystourethrography, computed tomography (CT), and ultrasonography provide the genitourinary surgeon with extremely accurate and reliable information in most cases, and these procedures should be used to the fullest extent to augment the history and physical examination. Evaluation and management of genitourinary injuries in major multisystem trauma should take second place only to airway management, fluid resuscitation, control of hemorrhage, and recognition of central nervous system injury.

This chapter reviews both the complications that develop when genitourinary injuries go unrecognized or are treated inappropriately and the complications that arise despite appropriate initial management. We do not address in great detail specific reconstructive procedures, although the general approaches most appropriate to a specific set of circumstances are noted. The more speculative points regarding the "best" initial evaluation are not discussed; rather, the discussion stresses the more practical approach of maximizing the amount of information gathered in the shortest possible time, using the least number of studies to minimize interference with overall patient care and to maximize the benefit of any initial or subsequent intervention.

COMPLICATIONS OF RENAL TRAUMA

From a mechanistic point of view, renal trauma results from either blunt or penetrating injuries. In general, blunt injuries are by far the most common (80 to 90 percent); of these, 90 percent comprise parenchymal contusions or small lacerations that do not extend into the medulla or collecting system.[1] The collecting system can be injured as a result of deep parenchymal lacerations that extend into it or as a result of a pre-existing anatomic abnormality, such as congenital obstruction of the ureteropelvic junction (UPJ), which increases the risk of UPJ avulsion. Children are at greater risk of UPJ disruption than are adults, presumably because of the greater mobility of their kidneys.[2,3]

Renal pedicle injuries are rare (1 to 3 percent of all injuries) and are most frequently seen in conjunction with multisystem trauma.[4] The major site of renal injury is the parenchyma, and the immediate consequence is bleeding (subcapsular, perinephric, or intrarenal), with or without urinary extravasation (depending on whether or not the collecting system is disrupted). Contusion is a factor in all cases and accounts for the presence of some degree of hematuria in 90 percent of all renal injuries. In some cases contusions are so severe that the kidney is visualized poorly on IVP, even in the absence of severe lacerations.

Renal pedicle injuries lead to renal artery thrombosis and/or renal vein disruption. Disruption of the arterial intima, which is much less elastic than are the adventitia and media, creates an endothelial-intimal flap that obstructs the flow of blood and leads to distal thrombosis (Fig. 18–1). This injury is perhaps the most severe to the kidney because it leads to ischemic infarction of the parenchyma; it can be completely silent in its presentation (i.e., no hematuria) and can be easily overlooked in consideration of more immediately life-threatening injuries. Renal vein disruption is manifested as hypotension and, therefore, can be more readily diagnosed.

Failure to recognize and treat major renal lacerations and major collecting system lacerations or disruptions can lead to early complications (occurring within the first 4 weeks after injury) such as delayed bleeding, abscess formation, sepsis, urinary fistulas, hypertension, and urinoma formation. Delayed bleeding results from clot dissolution and from the release of whatever degree of tamponade the clot exerted on the injured vessel. Hypertension is probably renin-mediated and in most cases is transient.[5,6]

Late complications include hypertension, hydronephrosis, chronic pyelonephritis, and arteriovenous (AV) fistulas and calculus formation. The percentage of renal injuries in which hypertension develops is difficult to estimate, but a 1 to 5 percent prevalence has been reported.[7] The hypertension appears to be renin-mediated (as are cases of early hypertension) because of arterial stenosis, constricting perinephric hematoma, or segmental arterial thrombosis (Fig. 18–2).[5,6]

Early Complications

Delayed Renal Bleeding

Delayed renal bleeding is generally manifested 5 to 20 days after a major renal parenchymal laceration. Symptoms are gross hematuria (frequently massive and total) and flank pain (either from obstructing clots in the ureter or from the formation of large perinephric hematomas). Patients may have symptoms of orthostatic hypotension or may lapse into hypovolemic shock. They may also complain of urinary frequency or may present in clot retention. The bleeding may be spontaneous or may follow excessive activity, prolonged Valsalva maneuver, the lifting of heavy objects, or minor flank trauma. Physical findings can range from a normal presentation to anterior abdominal tenderness (with or without a palpable mass ipsilateral to the previous injury), pallor of mucous membranes and nail beds, tachycardia, hypotension, tachypnea, and altered mental status. It is important to remember that young patients have a greater capacity to compensate for a reduction in blood volume; thus the absence of hypotension that accompanies tachycardia and pallor in this patient population does not mean that blood loss is insignificant. The hematocrit level may be low initially, but in the acute situation it may be within normal limits and may decrease with fluid replacement (because of he-

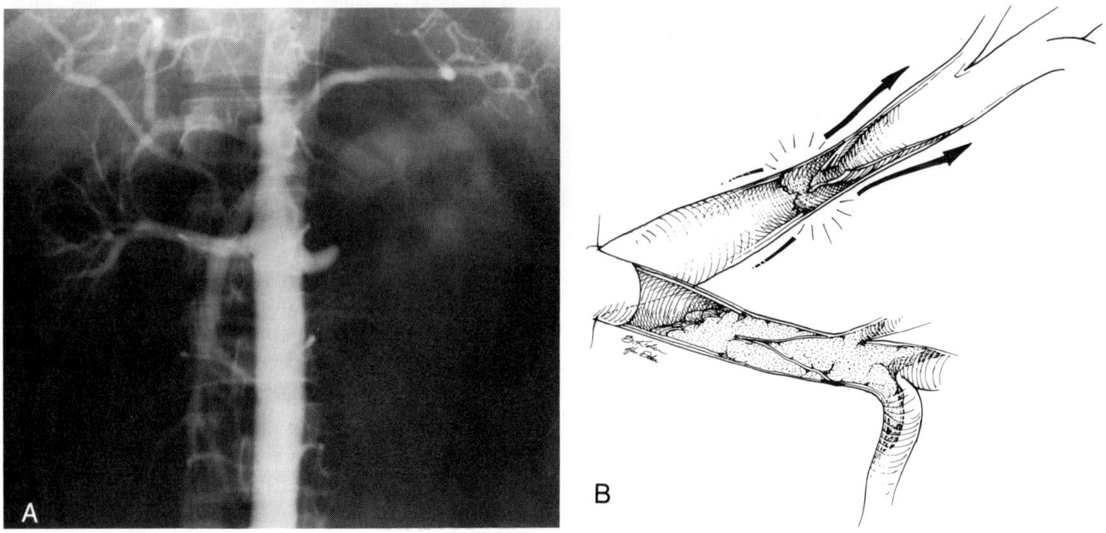

Figure 18–1. *A*, Abdominal aortogram showing classic finding of left renal artery thrombosis resulting from an intimal tear after blunt abdominal trauma. *B*, Mechanism of injury. Sudden forceful stretching of renal artery causes tearing of intima and endothelium. Rapidly flowing blood dissects under the intima, raising a flap that closes the lumen, which leads to stagnation of blood distally and proximally. Clotting factors released at the site of injury cause activation of the clotting cascade in the stagnant blood.

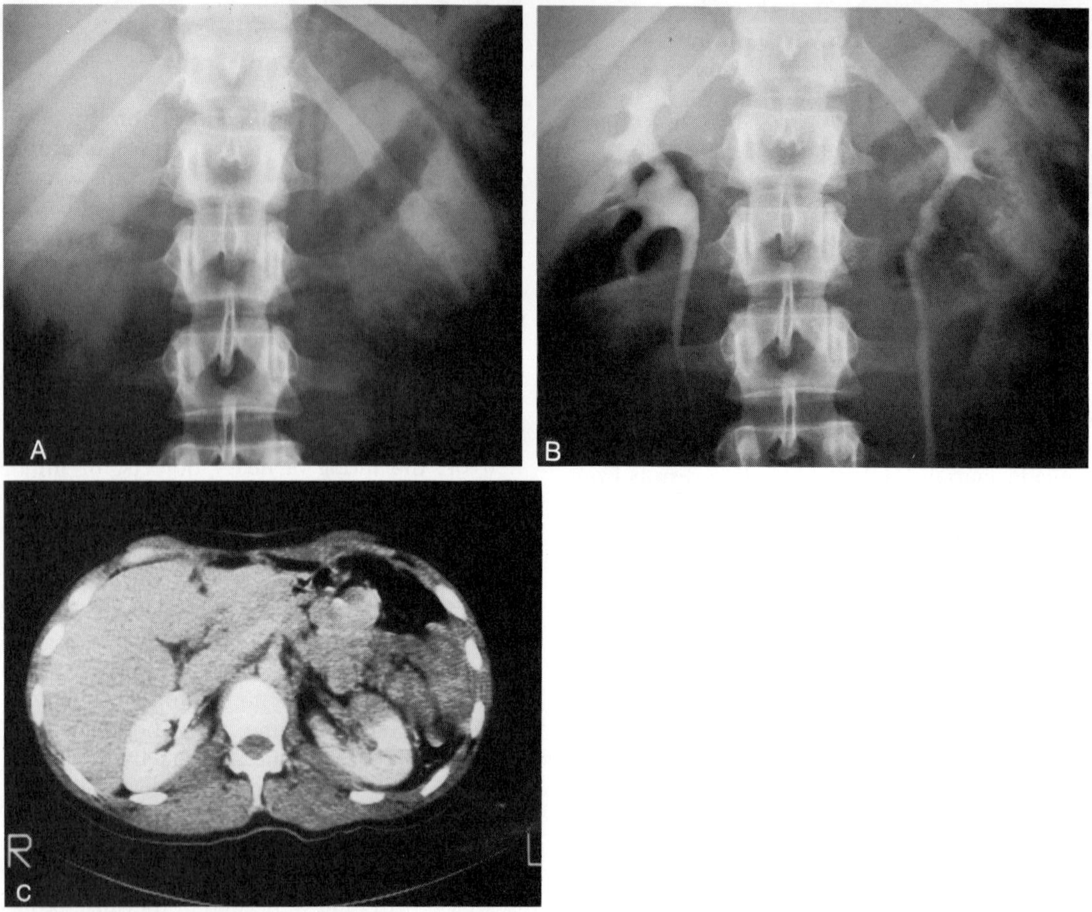

Figure 18–2. Lower-pole infarction after thrombosis of segmental renal artery. *A*, An intravenous pyelogram (IVP) in a 23-year-old man who presented with hypertension 8 months after blunt renal trauma. Note loss of function of lower pole of left kidney on nephrogram phase. *B*, Pyelogram phase shows loss of lower-pole calyces. *C*, CT confirms absence of any mass and shows nonfunctioning tissue that is sharply demarcated from functioning parenchyma.

modilution) if the red blood cell mass is not replaced.

In any case, some form of evaluation is necessary, and its mode is dictated by the acuteness of the situation and the availability of prior studies. For example, in the patient experiencing massive renal bleeding leading to hypovolemic shock that does not respond to fluid and blood replacement, immediate exploration is necessary *if* a prior study has documented the status of the contralateral kidney. Otherwise, a high-dose IVP should be performed immediately after the first 1000 to 1500 ml of fluid replacement to determine whether the contralateral kidney is present and functioning. The study can be done by infusing 1.5 to 2 ml/kg of intravenous contrast material as a bolus and using a portable x-ray source to obtain a KUB (kidney, ureter, and bladder profile) while the patient is on the gurney in the emergency room or after he or she has been positioned on the operating room table. This tactic is also extremely useful for initial evaluation and can be performed as rapidly as a plain abdominal film in the multiply injured, hypotensive, unconscious patient. For the patient who can be stabilized by fluid or blood replacement, a CT scan with intravenous contrast material is the procedure of choice: This yields the maximum amount of specific anatomic information (including size and extent of renal lacerations and retroperitoneal hematomas) and demonstrates the presence of non-viable renal parenchyma, urinary extravasation, and position and functional integrity of the contralateral kidney. If CT is not available, a reasonable alternative is an IVP with conventional tomography. In traumatized patients, ultrasonography is not an acceptable alternative to intravenous contrast studies because it cannot provide functional information about the contralateral kidney. In addition, results are subject to error of interpretation in direct proportion to the inexperience of the technician, radiologist, or urologist performing the procedure. Also, large retroperitoneal hematomas may not be detected in ultrasonographic studies because the echogenicity of the hematomas may not differ from that of normal perinephric tissue.

Delayed renal bleeding can occur after blunt or penetrating renal parenchymal injury (particularly from stab wounds) because of the formation of an AV fistula. This complication is not always preventable even when the kidney has been explored initially. The patient presents with gross hematuria.[1] The evaluative procedure of choice is selective renal arteriography, with digital subtraction angiography being the most preferable alternative. Management of small AV fistulas is within the purview of the angiographer experienced in embolization techniques. Larger AV fistulas may necessitate partial or total nephrectomy.[8]

The Surgical Approach to the Kidney. Gaining exposure of the renal vessels and controlling bleeding are of paramount importance and frequently mean the difference between renal salvage and nephrectomy (Fig. 18–3). A midline incision extending from the xiphoid process to the pubic symphysis provides the most rapid and extensive access to the abdominal cavity and permits examination of all intraperitoneal and extraperitoneal organs. The inferior mesenteric vein is localized, the mesentery incised medially and inferior to the vein over the aorta, and the incision extended superiorly to the ligament of Treitz. Frequently, the hematoma extends across the midline and into the root of the mesentery; this necessitates blunt dissection through the clot to identify the aorta. Once identified, the aorta is followed superiorly to the left renal vein; care should be taken to avoid the only major tributary, the inferior mesenteric artery.

Vascular loops are placed around all major renal vessels, and the artery to the injured kidney is occluded if the hematoma is expanding. (The surgeon should be alert to the possibility of multiple renal arteries.) Only at this point is Gerota's fascia entered. If bleeding is encountered as the kidney is mobilized, the artery should be occluded. Bleeding can often be controlled by simply squeezing the kidney and placing figure-

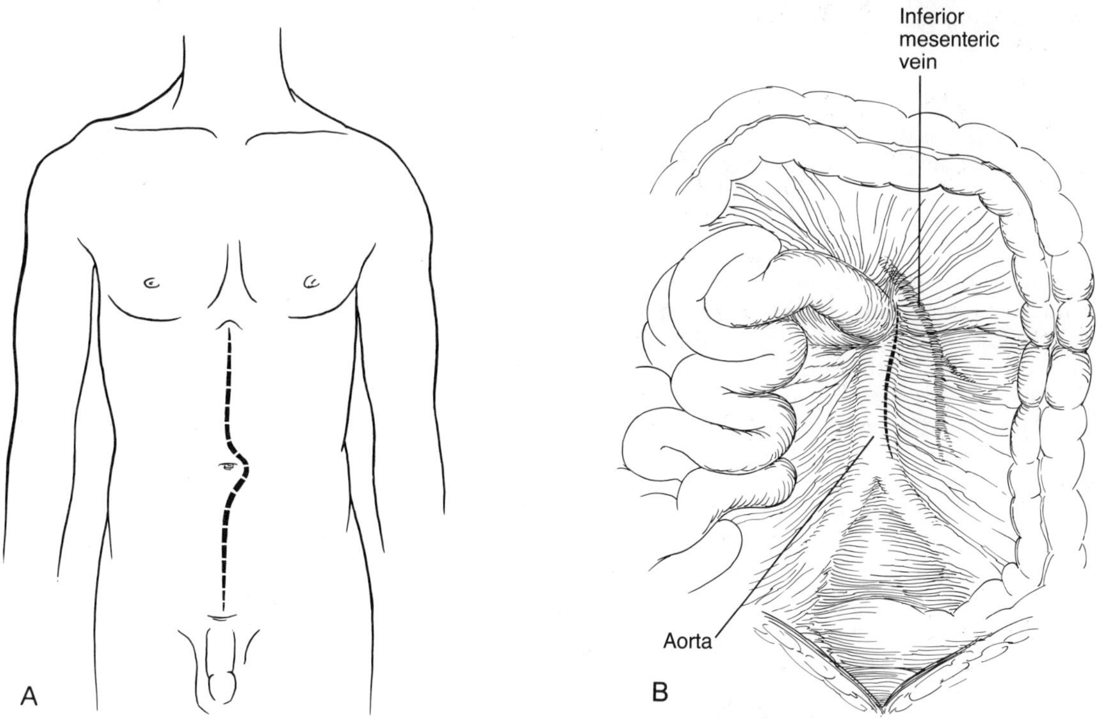

Figure 18–3. Transabdominal approach to renal vessels for control of renal blood flow before entering Gerota's fascia to explore perinephric hematomas. *A*, Midline laparotomy incision. *B*, Approach to renal vessels by incision of parietal peritoneum on the ventral surface of the aorta.

of-eight 3–0 or 4–0 absorbable sutures; an absorbable gelatin sponge (Gelfoam) or collagen hemostat (Avitene) can be used for added hemostasis. The purposes of the surgery are to debride devitalized tissue sharply, to ligate arterial and venous bleeding points, and to close collecting system lacerations (if needed). (Absorbable sutures should be used for the latter two procedures.)

In cases of blunt injuries, the integrity of the UPJ can be confirmed and the parenchymal laceration covered with renal capsule or omentum. A 1-inch Penrose drain should be placed through the flank if the collecting system is damaged, and as much of the hematoma as possible should be drained. The area is then irrigated with saline and the mesentery closed after removing all vascular loops.

In penetrating injuries (e.g., those resulting from stab or gunshot wounds) the ureter should be examined down to the pelvic brim. In most cases, methylene blue is given intravenously before the abdominal incision is made to color the urine and thereby facilitate detection of collecting system injury. The drain is removed 24 hours after placement if no drainage has occurred; otherwise, it is left in place until drainage stops.

Prolonged or Delayed Urinary Extravasation

Gunshot wounds pose a special risk of delayed urinary extravasation because blast injury to the ureter is not always evident at exploration (Fig. 18–4). A high index of suspicion of urinary leakage should be maintained when persistent fever, a great degree of abdominal distention, persistent ileus, or worsening of abdominal or flank tenderness is present. In this situation an IVP or retrograde pyelogram is indicated to rule out delayed ureteral fistula formation and to localize the site of extravasation. Another cause of delayed urinary extravasation is conservative treatment of major renal lacerations in the patient in whom urinary extravasation was not evident or recognized on initial evaluation. The extravasation can become evident up to several weeks after injury and may reach enormous proportions (Fig. 18–5). In patients with blunt trauma in whom extravasation is minor and there are no large parenchymal lacerations, exploration is not necessary. However, extravasation consequent to penetrating trauma probably should be explored.

Urinomas must be drained because they present a high risk of infection and abscess formation. In certain instances, percutaneous drainage can be achieved if there are only a few loculations. Separate drainage of each loculation is needed. Exploration and drainage through a flank incision are otherwise indicated, and care must be taken not to violate the peritoneal cavity. The collecting system injury must be localized and repaired, and further leakage should be minimized by augmenting drainage of the kidney with a nephrostomy tube.

Retroperitoneal Abscess Formation

Abscess formation is the result of infection of an undrained hematoma or urinoma that is seeded during the original exploration through a drain tract or by bowel content soilage resulting from concomitant bowel injury. Abscesses may be manifested within 5 to 7 days of the injury, or they may fester undetected for some weeks. Acute abscesses will betray their presence by causing persistent spiking fevers, flank tenderness, ileus, and, occasionally, flank erythema and "pointing" in the area of Petit's triangle. Chronic abscesses may cause lethargy, night sweats, weight loss, varying degrees of anorexia, and failure to thrive, especially in children. The urine may or may not be infected. The most expedient and definitive method of diagnosis is CT scanning. The abscess will be seen as a mass with a density of 10 to 60 Hounsfield units with or without loculations. Drainage should always be through a retroperitoneal approach. Recently, percutaneous drainage with CT scan or ultrasound guidance has been achieved, but this necessitates a persistent and experienced radiologist or endouroradiologist and demands that, as in the surgical approach, each and every loculation be drained.

Hypertension

Hypertension consequent to renal trauma is renin-mediated. Renin secretion by the acutely traumatized kidney can range from three to eight times that secreted by the normal kidney; as a result, peripheral plasma renin activity is elevated.[5,6,9] Appropriate management of acute traumatic injuries or nephrectomy lowers the plasma renin activity and relieves the hypertension.[5,6,9]

In a Cleveland Clinic study of renal trauma and associated hypertension, initially untreated renal arterial injuries accounted for 6 of 11 cases of hypertension detected 37 days to 12 years after the injury; subcapsular and perinephric he-

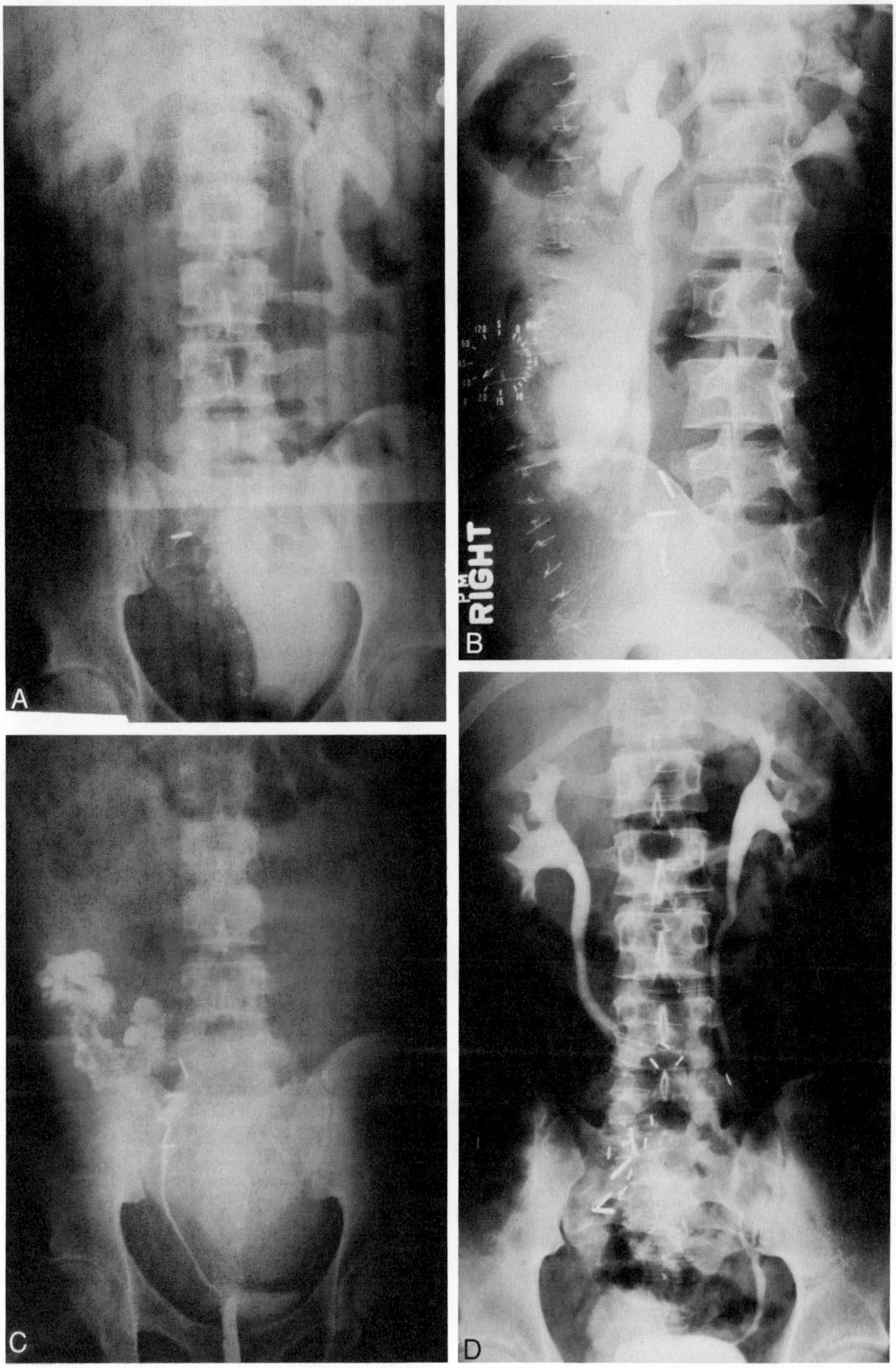

Figure 18–4. Delayed ureteral fistulization secondary to blast injury. *A*, An intravenous pyelogram (IVP) in an 18-year-old man who sustained a gunshot wound to the abdomen. The bullet lacerated the iliac vein and artery, but not the ureter. There was no evidence of ureteral injury at exploration; an intraoperative IVP demonstrated neither extravasation of urine nor obstruction of the right ureter. Note medial deviation of the ureter and compression of right bladder wall by large retroperitoneal hematoma. *B*, Oblique view of abdomen during IVP showing large amount of extravasation. *C*, Retrograde pyelogram 3 weeks after injury when sepsis and persistent ileus complicated the postoperative course. Note extravasation of urine into the abscess cavity. (Surgical clips are merely overlying the ureter.) *D*, An IVP 2 months after drainage of abscess and repair of the right ureteral injury by a right-to-left transureteroureterostomy and proximal drainage of right kidney through a nephrostomy tube (which was removed 2 weeks postoperatively).

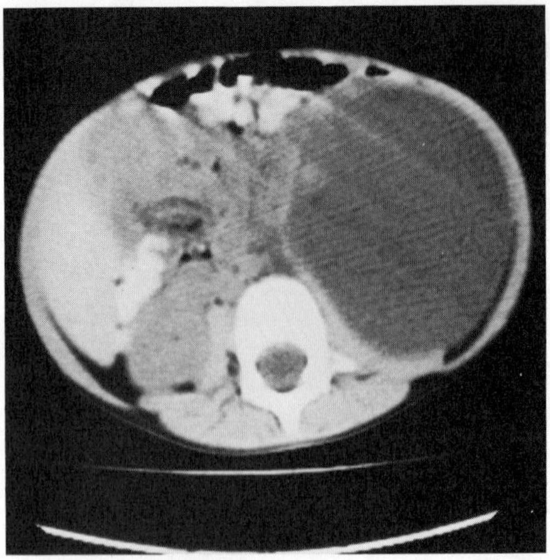

Figure 18–5. Urinoma. Abdominal CT scan in a 3-year-old child in whom an abdominal mass was noted 3 months after untreated blunt abdominal trauma. Note huge proportions of the urinoma, which fills the entire left abdomen and is confined by Gerota's fascia.

matomas accounted for four of the five remaining cases.[9] Nephrectomy relieved the hypertension in five of the six patients with renal artery injuries. When evaluating these studies, one is struck by the failure of early diagnosis and treatment of the renal injury as well as by the subsequent frequency of nephrectomy.

Late Complications

Late complications of renal trauma—those that occur 4 or more weeks after injury—include hydronephrosis, calculus formation, and chronic pyelonephritis. Any of these may result from an unrecognized injury of the collecting system, calcification of a retained blood clot, or fibrosis of a perirenal hematoma. In addition, hypertension and AV fistula formation may also be seen as late complications of renal trauma, although, as noted in the previous section, they may also be manifested as early complications. Indeed, they are often difficult to categorize as either early or late because some degree of overlap exists between cases that occur within the first 4 weeks of injury and those that develop later. For example, an AV fistula may form during the early post-injury stage, remain asymptomatic initially, and enlarge slowly over time, eventually becoming symptomatic. An extreme example of this was seen in a patient in whom an AV fistula formed subsequent to blunt renal trauma, enlarged over a 10-year period (Fig. 18–6), and became manifest as hypertension.

COMPLICATIONS OF VESICAL TRAUMA: ETIOLOGIC AND DIAGNOSTIC CONSIDERATIONS

Perforation and rupture are the most serious consequences of penetrating or blunt trauma to the urinary bladder and, unlike contusions, demand surgical attention in almost all cases. (Small iatrogenic bladder perforations resulting from endoscopic surgical procedures constitute a noted exception to this generality.) Failure to recognize and repair bladder perforation or rupture can lead to pelvic urinoma formation, urinary ascites, and abscess; in certain cases, incontinence and formation of vesicovaginal fistulas can result.

Blunt trauma is the most frequent cause of bladder rupture, accounting for 64 percent of cases of bladder rupture at our institution.[10] There is a high association between bladder rupture and pelvic fractures resulting from blunt trauma.[11,12] The site of rupture is most frequently the dome in blunt trauma and the lateral walls in penetrating trauma.[10] Cystography is the most expedient method of diagnosis, but its reliability is contingent upon proper technique.[11]

To avoid a misdiagnosis, the urologist should be able to recognize deficiencies in the study technique. A prerequisite is adequate filling of the bladder by gravity with sterile, water-soluble contrast material (350 ml or more in adults; to the point of urgency in children) through a retention catheter. Full abdominal anteroposterior (AP) and drainage films should always be taken. The objective of the procedure is to demonstrate extravasation of contrast material without inducing further injury. Inadequate filling is recognized by visualization of folds in the contrast outline on the AP view; extravasation may be seen only on the drainage film. Outlining of loops of bowel by the contrast medium signifies intraperitoneal rupture; a "starburst" or "feather-like" pattern implies extraperitoneal extravasation. Large ruptures can exist in the face of subtle findings on the cystogram, even when proper technique is followed; e.g., clots or overlying bowel can partially occlude large ruptures and significantly limit extravasation of contrast from them. If cystographic findings are equivocal in a patient who presents in clot retention with suprapubic tenderness, little or no flank pain, and a history of blunt abdominal

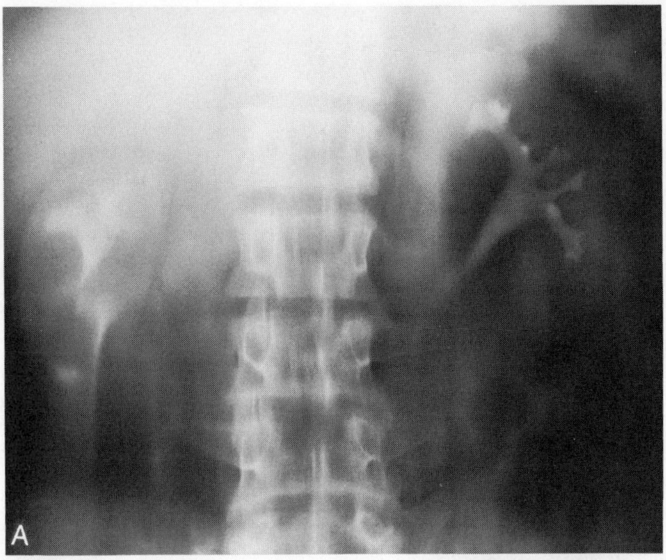

Figure 18–6. A 20-year-old man presented with gross hematuria 10 years after a blunt right renal injury. He was found to have hypertension. *A*, An IVP tomogram showing atrophic parenchyma of the right kidney with calyceal compression and calicectasis. The left kidney is normal. *B*, Abdominal aortogram showing the large right renal artery, which fills more rapidly than the left renal artery. *C*, Rapid venous filling immediately after contrast injection. Note huge tortuous arteriovenous malformation overlying the renal pelvis and early filling of renal vein (arrow) and vena cava. This lesion, much too large to be managed by embolization, was treated with nephrectomy.

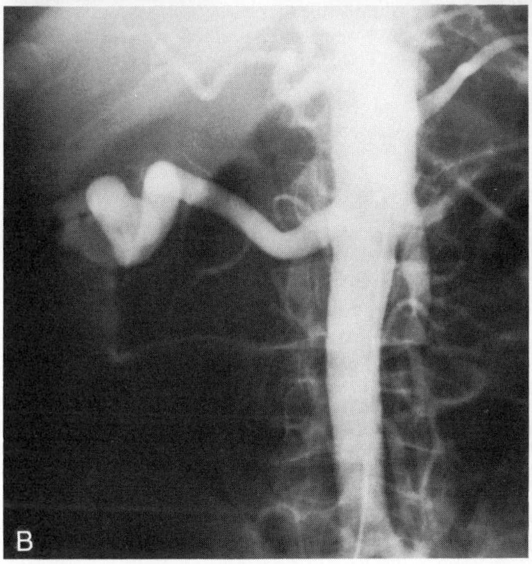

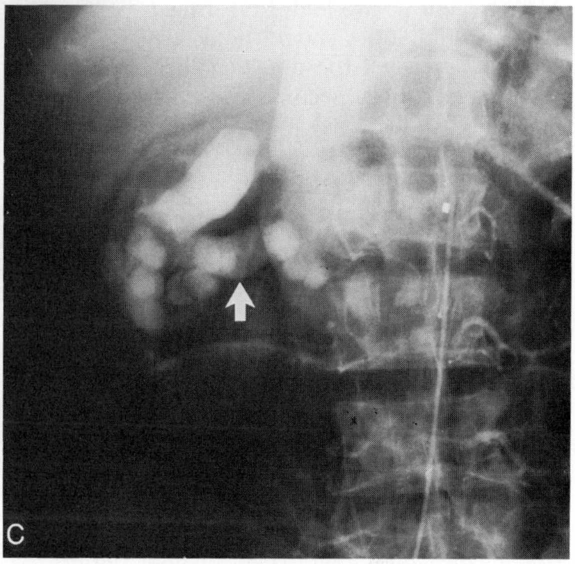

trauma, the index of suspicion of bladder rupture is high and a repeat cystogram, with instillation of a larger volume of contrast solution, is warranted. If findings of the second study are equivocal, exploration is justified.

Complications arising from bladder rupture include formation of pelvic abscesses, incontinence, and fistulas.

Pelvic Abscess Formation

A pelvic abscess can develop subsequent to conservative treatment of a bladder rupture because of either blunt or penetrating trauma. It can also result from infection of a pelvic hematoma after pelvic fracture. There are two crucial points of diagnosis and management that, if remembered, will lessen the risk of abscess formation. First, *the size of the bladder laceration does not correlate with the extent of extravasation.* Our own experience and that of others support this contention.[11,13] Second, *drains should not be placed into pelvic hematomas when bladder rupture is accompanied by pelvic fracture.* Proper closure of the bladder (by two to three layers of 3–0 absorbable suture) and either urethral or suprapubic catheter drainage for 7 to 14 days will prevent leakage of urine from the bladder.

It should be remembered that drains serve only to provide a passage for fluids to exit. Pelvic hematomas are basically large clots that liquefy over a prolonged period. Thus, the drain does not provide drainage of the clot but simply acts as a portal of entry for bacteria. Dissection of the pelvic hematoma(s) should be avoided, if possible, or at least limited to the extent necessary to expose the bladder dome or anterior wall. The bladder can be approached through a midline suprapubic incision, and entry into the bladder lumen can be gained by a cystotomy incision. Urine and clots should be completely evacuated, and repair of lacerations on the lateral and posterior walls can be accomplished from the bladder lumen.

If a pelvic hematoma develops into an abscess despite the avoidance of drains in the hematoma, the process will usually occur within the first 2 weeks of injury, and will be signaled by lower abdominal discomfort, night sweats, spiking fevers, and, in more severe cases, sepsis. Management is two-fold; first, broad-spectrum systemic antibiotics should be administered to prevent spread of the infection (in contrast to curing the abscess); second, *all* loculations must be accurately localized and drained. Computed tomography and ultrasonography are valuable techniques to facilitate localization of loculations. Drainage can be accomplished either percutaneously or surgically. Although percutaneous drainage as performed by a highly skilled and persistent interventional radiologist can be adequate to handle remarkably complex abscesses,[14] surgical drainage is indicated in most cases.

An abscess or chronic extravasation can develop subsequent to treatment of bladder rupture by catheter drainage alone (Fig. 18–7).[13] The only way to "stage" a bladder laceration accurately is to see it, and in the trauma setting this means exploration. Small bladder perforations resulting from endoscopic, prostatic, or bladder surgery seem to be the only instances of bladder rupture for which catheter drainage alone is sufficient management.

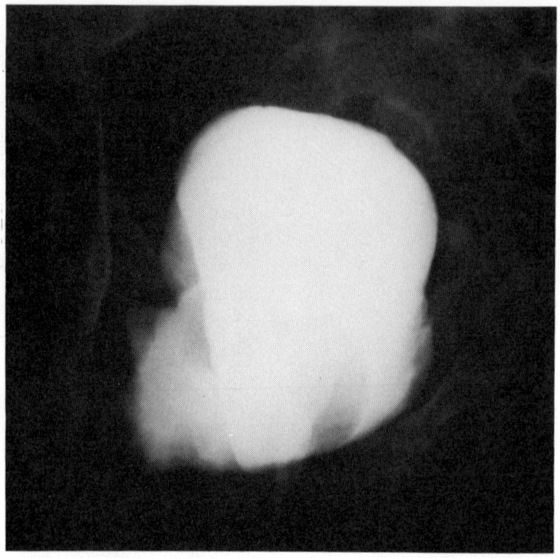

Figure 18–7. Chronic bladder extravasation. Cystogram in an adult woman 4 weeks after urethral catheter treatment of a bladder neck laceration that was not recognized (or repaired) at the time the patient sustained a pelvic fracture. The injury was subsequently repaired transvesically through a suprapubic cystotomy.

Incontinence

Incontinence is generally not a long-lasting complication of bladder rupture. During the period immediately following catheter removal, urgency incontinence may be seen but is usually transient. Stress incontinence is common in women and subsides within a few weeks. Injuries to the bladder neck (e.g., laceration of the trigone extending into the bladder neck) are those most likely to lead to total incontinence. This is especially true in women, in whom the bladder neck constitutes the major continence mechanism.

Incontinence can be avoided by meticulous anatomic reconstruction with interrupted 4–0 chromic sutures at the time of injury. Bladder neck lacerations are associated to a great degree with massive pelvic trauma (i.e., comminuted fractures [type 1] or fractures involving the anterior and posterior pelvic elements [type II]).[10,15] In such cases, bladder drainage by suprapubic, rather than urethral, catheters is preferred because the prolonged convalescent period attendant to massive pelvic injury may necessitate prolonged bladder drainage.

Fistulas

Vesicocutaneous and/or vesicovaginal fistulas are uncommon complications of bladder rupture. Vesicocutaneous fistula formation can result from failure of the suprapubic catheter tract to close after catheter removal. Risk factors include poor nutrition (leading to poor wound healing) and bladder outlet obstruction. Vesicovaginal fistula formation is often attendant to penetrating injuries of the vagina and bladder or to major ruptures resulting from massive blunt trauma to the bladder and vagina.

Management of a vesicocutaneous fistula includes simple urethral catheter drainage of the bladder, nutritional support, and elimination of any bladder outlet obstruction. As a last resort, excision of the fistulous tract with separate bladder and skin closures may be required. Management of a vesicovaginal fistula includes prevention of fistula formation by meticulous reconstitution of the laceration with multilayered, fine absorbable sutures (4–0 or 5–0 chromic or polyglycolic acid [Dexon]) at the time of injury and nutritional support (either enteral or parenteral). A soft silicone urethral catheter and suprapubic bladder drain should be placed for 10 to 14 days. Chronic vesicovaginal fistulas are best managed after sufficient time has elapsed to allow them to mature and contract (usually 4 to 6 months), thereby facilitating excision and repair. (For more detailed descriptions of fistula repair, consult the references.[16–19])

COMPLICATIONS OF URETHRAL TRAUMA

In women, the urethra is so short (2.0 to 2.5 cm) that it can simply be regarded as a single anatomic unit. In men, however, the urethra must be envisaged as two basic units: (1) the anterior urethra (consisting of the pendulous and bulbar portions) and (2) the posterior urethra (the prostatic and membranous portions). In essence, the urethra has one basic response to injury: stricture formation. Secondary complications include formation of urethrocutaneous fistulas (Fig. 18–8), urinary tract infection, and, in rare cases, necrotizing fasciitis (resulting from distal obstruction and fistula formation caused by the stricture in the presence of infected urine).

In men, injuries to the posterior urethra, such as prostatomembranous disruption, can result in the most severe and debilitating complications. Incontinence has been reported in 5 to 30 percent.[20,21] Impotence occurs initially in most patients but usually resolves after 1 year, although some patients may not regain potency for up to 3 years. Pelvic abscess formation can result from infection of the pelvic hematoma universally present acutely in posterior urethral injury.

To prevent or minimize the occurrence of these severe complications, two basic guidelines should be followed. First, blood at the urethral meatus at presentation should be interpreted as a clear signal to delay the insertion of any catheter until the urethra is evaluated by retrograde urethrography. (Injudicious placement of the catheter can serve two counterproductive functions: [1] the catheter can provide a portal for bacterial seeding of the pelvic hematoma, and [2] its placement may complete what may have been only a partial prostatomembranous disruption.) Second, primary repair may not always be the best course, although one report professes good results.[22] It should be noted that when acute repair is attempted, the disrupted urethra is fragmented and embedded in a large pelvic hematoma that must first be evacuated before adequate exposure can be achieved. Also, the nervi erigentes course by the prostatomembranous junction at about the 4 o'clock and 8 o'clock positions,[23,24] and the probability of iatrogenic injury to these nerves in such a bloody field is high.

We have found that examination of the bladder interior and placement of a catheter through a suprapubic cystotomy incision, with no attempt to enter and drain the pelvic hematoma, results in fewer complications. Any resultant stricture can be reconstructed 3 to 6 months later. In some cases of partial prostatomembranous urethral disruption, the stricture can be managed by endoscopic incision. However, most often, repair will require excision of the stricture and primary reanastomosis through either a perineal or a transpubic approach;[25,26] alternatively, a two-stage Johansen repair can be performed.[21,25]

Delayed reconstruction results in lower incontinence and impotence rates, as reported by Morehouse and MacKinnon.[20] Our personal experience substantiates their results. Virtually all patients in whom delayed reconstruction is the primary mode of treatment can expect to be continent, and only 10 to 15 percent will remain impotent.[26] Theoretically, the patients are at risk of incontinence after transurethral prostatic resection because of the potential for damage to the external sphincteric mechanism, from either the injury itself or from subsequent repair of the stricture. Persistent impotence can be due to irreparable damage to the nervi erigentes or the internal pudendal vessels along Alcock's canal in cases of associated pelvic fracture involving the posterior pubic rami.

Anterior urethral injuries are complicated most often by urethral strictures, and if these go untreated, urethrocutaneous fistulas may result. Additionally, a potentially fatal complication can occur if the urethral rupture extends through Colles' fascia. Because this fascial layer is continuous with Scarpa's fascia, blood and/or infected urine can move along the anterior abdominal wall and into the perineum. Straddle injuries classically involve rupture of Colles' fas-

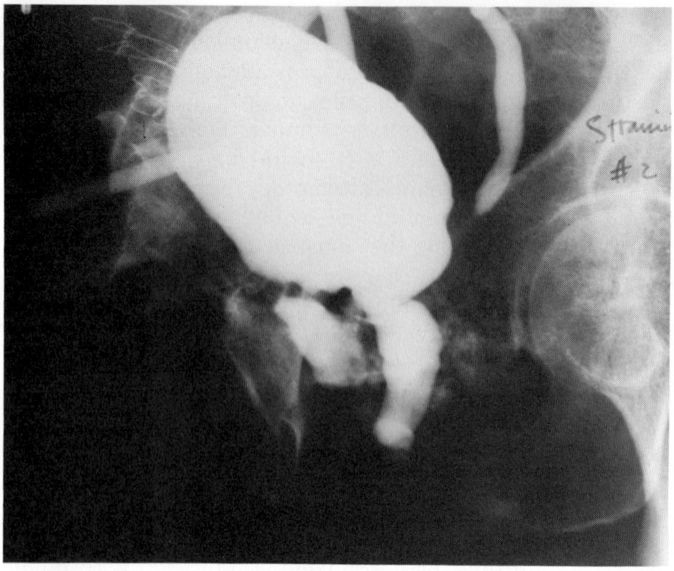

Figure 18–8. Prostatic urethral fistula 6 months after disruption of prostatomembranous urethra, a complication of a pelvic fracture. Oblique view of bladder filling during cystography. Contrast was introduced through a suprapubic cystostomy tube that was used to manage the original injury. Note bilateral ureteral reflux and extravasation of urine from fistula tract close to the bladder neck. Injury was successfully repaired through a transpubic approach to the urethroplasty.

cia, which clinically is signaled by a large perineal hematoma and ecchymosis. The diagnosis is confirmed by retrograde urethrography, and suprapubic diversion of the urine is then accomplished with the expectation that the patient will recover without incident, except for, perhaps, a bulbar stricture (which can be managed on an elective basis). A potentially lethal situation also arises in debilitated patients with chronic indwelling urethral catheters when the catheter is replaced incorrectly by inexperienced personnel and a false passage is created or the catheter balloon is inflated in the bulbar urethra. In the latter situation, the bladder is inadequately drained, overflow incontinence results, grossly infected urine extravasates into the perineum, and necrotizing fasciitis results. Management demands emergent wide debridement of necrotic tissue, suprapubic bladder drainage, administration of systemic antibiotics, and enteral or parenteral nutritional support. Debridement may need to be repeated, and meticulous and vigorous wound care invariably is required.

COMPLICATIONS OF URETERAL TRAUMA

Injuries to the ureter from non-iatrogenic trauma are rare and almost always result from penetrating injury. Early recognition and primary repair and drainage of the injury, with or without nephrostomy drainage, will prevent retroperitoneal abscess and/or urinoma and ureterocutaneous fistula formation. Hydronephrosis resulting from ureteral stricture may simply require ureterolysis, with or without an omental wrap, or excision and primary anastomosis. When dealing with ureteral injuries, especially iatrogenic injuries, which present the greatest challenge surgically, the urologic surgeon should have a repertoire of procedures for which the specific applications are clearly understood.

Ureteral injury is highly likely in the patient who has sustained a penetrating abdominal wound and presents with microscopic hematuria. This situation demands an IVP. If the entrance wound is in the lower abdomen, a cystogram should also be obtained. Retrograde ureteropyelography should be performed only as an adjunct to the IVP or in the patient with a history of contrast allergy. Simple transection of the ureter, if caused by gunshot wound, can be successfully managed by careful debridement and primary anastomosis over a 7 to 10 Fr. stent with 5–0 chromic sutures in a watertight interrupted closure. A Penrose drain is left in place and channeled through a separate flank stab incision. The stent can be internal or brought out through the bladder and removed in 10 days.

Special attention should be given to gunshot wounds. It is important to remember that a projectile creates damage in two ways: (1) by penetration of the tissues directly in its path and (2) by severe contusion of adjacent tissue. This latter type of damage, the so-called blast injury, results from a shock wave that precedes the bullet's tip and extends radially from its tract, creating a temporary cavity behind the bullet. The strength of the shock wave, and thus the size of the cavity, are a function of the bullet's velocity.

Delayed fistulization of the ureter can occur if the bullet passes sufficiently close despite the absence of gross anatomic disruption at the time of injury (Fig. 18–4). If the complication is not diagnosed and treated promptly, urinoma formation, persistent ileus, and sepsis will result. Management involves nephrostomy tube drainage of the urine, drainage of the urinoma, and either immediate or delayed ureteral repair.

Loss of ureteral tissue to a degree sufficient to preclude reanastomosis or vesicoureteral reimplantation is the greatest single challenge to the urologic surgeon treating extensive ureteral trauma. Such loss can occur after suction curettage abortions or shotgun or high-velocity rifle injuries. Five basic options are employed for immediate management of these injuries:

1. The kidney can be mobilized downward and the bladder moved upward by a psoas hitch.
2. The contralateral obliterated umbilical artery can be transected, increasing bladder mobility. (A Boari flap can be used in addition to the previous two maneuvers.)
3. The proximal and distal ureteral stumps can be tied off and tagged and a nephrostomy tube placed, with reconstruction done on an elective basis. This alternative is viable if the condition of the patient is sufficiently grave to preclude devoting time to an attempt at primary reconstruction.
4. A transureteroureterostomy can be performed, using fenestrated stents to drain both ureters separately.
5. Autotransplantation of the involved kidney may be possible, although this procedure is best done electively and by a surgeon experienced in renal transplantation.

Extensive loss of the ureter may necessitate the use of an ileal segment with a tapered implantation into the bladder, but this procedure should be done electively. Ultimately, nephrectomy is the final option for either immediate or elective management when the patient's general condition or the injuries dictate management associated with minimal complications.

Iatrogenic causes of ureteral injury are many (see Table 18–1), but in general they lead to obstruction, reflux, or fistula or urinoma formation. The pelvic ureter is the segment most frequently injured, and the risk arises in any major pelvic surgery, be it gynecologic, general, or urologic.

Transurethral resection of the ureteral orifice more frequently leads to reflux than to stenosis. The decision to correct depends more on the effect the reflux has on the kidney than on its mere presence. As long as the renal unit is not damaged by high-pressure reflux, as may occur with bladder-outlet obstruction or recurrent infection, the reflux can simply be followed periodically; otherwise, ureteral reimplantation is necessary.

Bilateral ureteral catheterization can lead to anuria because of mucosal edema, which causes obstruction within the intramural ureter. If bi-

Table 18–1. IATROGENIC CAUSES OF URETERAL INJURIES AND ATTENDANT COMPLICATIONS

	Common Complications			
Cause	***Reflux***	***Fistulas***	***Disruption***	***Obstruction***
Obstetric/Gynecologic Procedures				
Radical hysterectomy			x	x
Vaginal hysterectomy		x		x
Oophorectomy				x
Forceps delivery		x		x
Suction curettage			x	
Radiation		x		x
General Surgical Procedures				
Colonic resection			x	x
Correction of rectal prolapse				x
Abdominal perineal resection			x	x
Retrocecal appendectomy			x	x
Retroperitoneal tumor removal		x	x	x
Vascular Surgical Procedures				
Aortofemoral bypass graft				x
Lumbar sympathectomy			x	x
Vena caval ligation				x
Urologic Procedures				
Transurethral resection	x			x
Ureterorenoscopy	x		x	x
Vesical diverticulectomy	x		x	x

lateral stents are to be removed, it is prudent to stagger their removal by 24 to 48 hours to avoid azotemia.

Finally, the formation of ureterovaginal fistulas can be a complication of a difficult vaginal forceps delivery or vaginal hysterectomy. Ureteral catheterization and nephrostomy placement to aid spontaneous closure are viable initial approaches, but reimplantation of the ureter will most probably be needed because of a persistent fistula, sepsis, or ureteral stricture after fistula closure.

References

1. McAninch JW: Renal injuries. In McAninch JW, ed: Urogenital Trauma, Vol II. Blaisdell FW, Trunkey DD, series eds: Trauma Management, New York, Thieme-Stratton, Inc, 1985, pp. 27–49.
2. Cass AS: Blunt renal trauma in children. J Trauma 23:123–127, 1983.
3. Kuzmarov IW, Morehouse DD, Gibson S: Blunt renal trauma in the pediatric population: a retrospective study. J Urol 126:648–649, 1981.
4. Guerriero WG, Carlton CE Jr, Scott R Jr, Beall AC Jr: Renal pedicle injuries. J Trauma 11:53–62, 1971.
5. Spark RF, Berg S: Renal trauma and hypertension: the role of renin. Arch Intern Med 136:1097–1100, 1976.
6. Von Knorring J, Fyhrquist F, Ahonen J: Varying course of hypertension following renal trauma. J Urol 126:798–801, 1981.
7. Kossow AS: Hypertension complicating blunt renal trauma. Urology 16:84–86, 1980.
8. Cosgrove MD, Mendez R, Morrow JW: Traumatic renal arterio-venous fistulae: report of 12 cases. J Urol 110:627–631, 1973.
9. Grant RP, Gifford RW Jr, Pudvan WR, Meaney TF, Straffon RA, McCormack LJ: Renal trauma and hypertension. Am J Cardiol 27:173–176, 1971.
10. Carroll PR, McAninch JW: Major bladder trauma: mechanisms of injury and a unified method of diagnosis and repair. J Urol 132:254–257, 1984.
11. Carroll PR, McAninch JW: Major bladder trauma: the accuracy of cystography. J Urol 130:887–888, 1983.
12. Nowak A, Zielinski J: Difficulties in bladder rupture diagnostics. Eur Urol 3:351–354, 1977.
13. Cass AS, Johnson CF, Kahn AU, Matsuura JK, Godec CJ: Nonoperative management of bladder rupture from external trauma. Urology 22:27–29, 1983.
14. Jeffrey RB Jr: Percutaneous drainage of abdominal abscesses: the role of the radiologist. In Root RK, Trunkey DD, Sande MA, eds: New Surgical and Medical Approaches in Infectious Diseases, Vol 6. (Sande MA, Root RK, series eds: *Contemporary Issues in Infectious Diseases.*) New York, Churchill Livingstone; 1987, pp 133–150.
15. Trunkey DD, Chapman MW, Lim RC Jr, Dunphy JE: Management of pelvic fractures in blunt trauma injury. J Trauma 14:912–923, 1984.
16. Kiricuta I, Goldstein AMB: The repair of extensive vesicovaginal fistulas with pedicled omentum: a review of 27 cases. J Urol 108:724–727, 1972.
17. O'Connor VJ: Vesicovaginal fistulas. In Smith RB, Skinner DG, eds. Complications of Urologic Surgery: Prevention and Management. Philadelphia, WB Saunders Co, 1976.
18. Spence HM, Duckett JW Jr: Diverticulum of the female urethra: clinical aspects and presentation of a simple operative technique for cure. J Urol 104:432–437, 1970.
19. Turner-Warwick RT: The use of pedicle grafts in the repair of urinary tract fistulae. Br J Urol 44:644–656, 1972.
20. Morehouse DD, MacKinnon KJ: Management of prostatomembranous urethral disruption: 13-year experience. J Urol 123:173–174, 1980.
21. Gibson GR: Impotence following fractured pelvis and ruptured urethra. Br J Urol 42:86–88, 1970.
22. DeWeerd JH: Immediate realignment of posterior urethral injury. Urol Clin North Am 4:75–80, 1977.
23. Walsh PC, Donker PJ: Impotence following radical prostatectomy: insight into etiology and prevention. J Urol 128:492–497, 1982.
24. Lue TF, Zeineh SJ, Schmidt RA, Tanagho EA: Neuroanatomy of penile erection: its relevance to iatrogenic impotence. J Urol 131:273–280, 1984.
25. Johansen B: Reconstruction of the male urethra and strictures. Acta Chir Scand 176(Suppl):1–103, 1953.
26. McAninch JW: Traumatic injuries to the urethra. J Trauma 21:291–297, 1981.

19 COMPLICATIONS OF RENAL TRANSPLANTATION AND AUTOTRANSPLANTATION

J.T. Rosenthal

There have been dramatic decreases in morbidity and mortality rates associated with kidney transplantation in the past 10 years. The incidence of graft and patient survival of first cadaver grafts reported from a large multicenter study in 1981 were 1-year graft survival, 48 percent and 1-year patient mortality, 14 percent.[1] One-year cadaver graft survival now averages about 80 percent, although some centers report one-year cadaver graft survival of over 90 percent.[2–4] Average patient mortality has been reduced from above 15 percent to 3 to 4 percent. At the same time, the rate of complications and graft losses from complications have also declined dramatically. One important reason for these changes is the improvements in immunosuppression regimens, especially with the introduction of cyclosporine into routine clinical use in 1983. Every transplant center in the United States now uses cyclosporine as part of the immunosuppression regimen, usually in combination with steroids. However, the steroid doses are about one quarter of those administered before the use of cyclosporine. Whereas patients previously may have been maintained on 30 to 40 mg/day of prednisone, with cyclosporine immunosuppression, doses < 10 mg/day of prednisone are commonly given. Some centers are using no steroids at all in selected patients.[5] The effect of this is that steroid-related complications, such as cataracts, aseptic hip necrosis, and cushingoid appearance, are significantly reduced.

There are other factors that also play a role in the reduced complication rates. One is that patients are now healthier prior to transplantation because of improvements in dialysis therapy. Patients also undergo the procedure earlier in the course of treatment because of more widespread acceptance of transplantation as a therapy for end-stage renal disease. In addition, there has been an emphasis in clinical transplantation on developing networks for cadaver organ retrieval, which means that cadaver kidneys are unlikely to be injured during removal, reducing the risk for ureteral necrosis or stenosis. The development of new radiologic techniques has allowed prompt diagnosis and intervention, improving the rate of graft salvage when complications occur. The incidence of surgical complications such as wound infections is also reduced, and if complications do occur they are now much safer to treat. Despite these improvements, technical complications do occur and can result in disaster; every effort should be directed at prevention.

This chapter focuses on technical aspects of renal transplantation. (Such important nontechnical complications such as hypertension, infection, bowel problems, and rejection are important but are not discussed here.) The first part of the chapter presents some of the surgical principles that, if employed, should minimize the risk of serious complications. Meticulous technique and attention to detail are the hallmarks of success. The second part addresses diagnostic and therapeutic options for recognizing and treating the more common surgical complications.

LIVE DONOR MANAGEMENT

Screening

Live kidney donors should be carefully screened to be sure that two normal kidneys are present and that no conditions likely to progress after unilateral nephrectomy exist. Diabetes and renal cystic disease are two examples of progressive diseases that preclude live donation. Pyelography, renal arteriography, careful creatinine clearance measurements, and urinalysis are indicated. Attempts have been made to use digital subtraction angiography to screen potential live donors; however, these efforts have not been successful in detecting all renal arteries.[6] If there are single renal arteries on both sides, the left kidney is usually chosen for transplantation because of the longer renal vein on the left side. If the left side has multiple renal arteries, the right side can be used. If both kidneys have two renal arteries, it is still possible to use the kidney. This has been done many times in the UCLA series, using one of the many techniques available for managing two renal arteries. The only unacceptable technique in living donors is using a patch of aorta.

Hydration

Adequate hydration of the donor the night before surgery and supplementation with mannitol (25 to 50 gm) intraoperatively will minimize the risk of delayed graft function. Some surgeons use an anterotransabdominal approach in live donation procedures to ensure early exposure of the vessels. Our preference is an extrapleural, extraperitoneal 11th or 12th intercostal flank incision. Hilar fat should be left as undisturbed as possible to prevent damageto the ureteral blood supply from the main renal artery flowing down the ureter via the periadventitial arteries. If this blood supply is compromised, ureteral necrosis and slough can occur in the recipient. Because the hilar dissection tends to be more complete in live donor nephrectomy than in cadaver donor nephrectomy, there is greater risk of ureteral injury. The artery and vein should be securely suture ligated to prevent exsanguinating postoperative hemorrhage in the donor.

On completion of the nephrectomy, the kidney is immediately placed in an ice slush solution and infused with ice-cold intracellular type electrolyte solution to which heparin (5000 units) has been added. Systemic heparin administration of the donor is not necessary and may result in bleeding complications. Soft intracatheters or IV tubing can be used for infusion to avoid damage to the intima of the renal artery.

Serious morbidity and deaths have occurred in live kidney donation, making this a procedure not to be lightly undertaken. Bay reported on his own series and on the results from the literature of 2495 living related donors in which there were three deaths (0.1 percent mortality rate).[7] The deaths resulted from myocardial infarction and pulmonary embolism. Another report by Dunn and associates documented a 7 percent incidence of major complications from living related donor procedures, including wound infections, spleen or adrenal injuries, pulmonary embolism, and bowel obstruction.[8] If great care is taken in patient selection and surgical technique, such risks can be minimized. At UCLA, in over 400 live kidney donor procedures over a 20-year period, there have been no deaths and no serious morbidity. No long-term risk from hypertension or delayed renal insufficiency following unilateral nephrectomy in live kidney donors has been identified.[9]

CADAVER DONOR MANAGEMENT

Donor maintenance is also important in cadaver kidney donors. When brain death occurs, diabetes insipidus often ensues, resulting in a massive diuresis. Coupled with the therapy of reducing cerebral edema through dehydration prior to brain death, this may result in hypotension. Hypernatremia and prerenal azotemia may also develop. Massive rehydration is necessary as an initial step in restoring cardiovascular stability, and, usually, this is all that is necessary, although vasopressin injection (Pitressen) sometimes must be used to reduce the diuresis. Pressor agents may be necessary to maintain the blood pressure; however, every attempt should be made to maintain blood pressure and urine output with the lowest amount. Usually, dopamine can be used for weaning as rehydration proceeds. Thyroid hormone replacement has been shown to be an important adjunct in maintaining normal cellular functions in brain-dead donors.[10] Mannitol, steroids, and antibiotics are given perioperatively. Alpha blockers can be given just prior to aortic cross-clamping to reduce renal artery spasm.[11] Heparin (10,000 to 20,000 U) is given systemically at the same time.

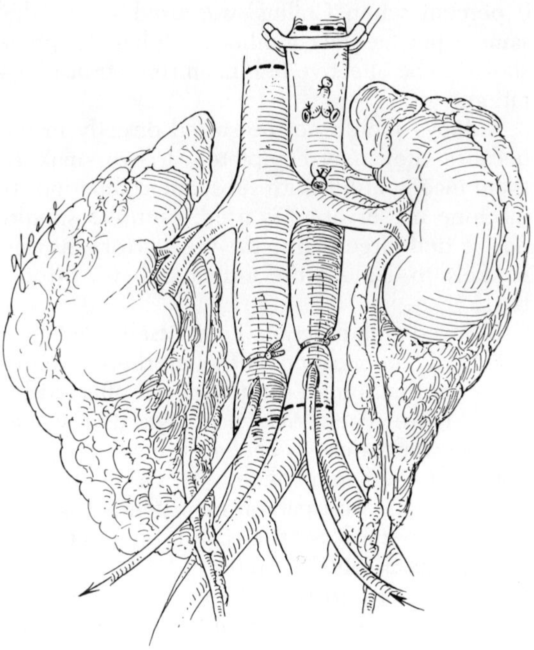

Figure 19–1. En bloc dissection for cadaver kidney donation with cannulas in place for in situ perfusion. Notice perihilar and periureteral fat are left in place.

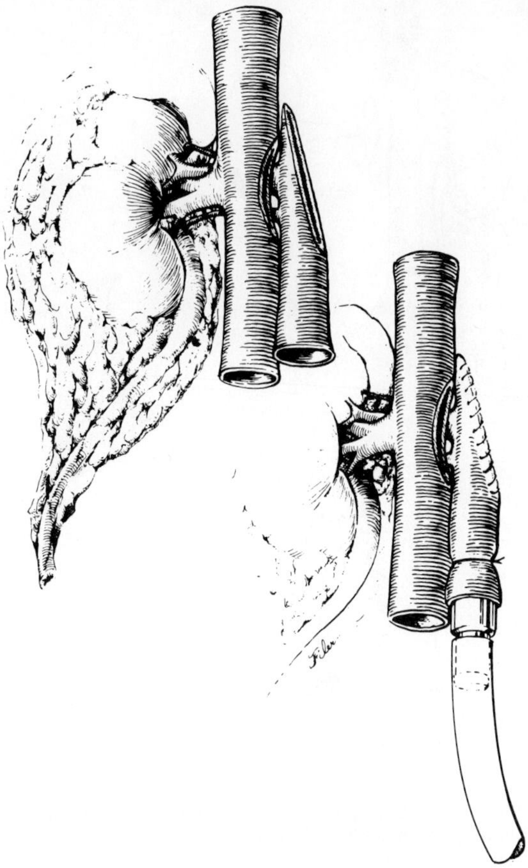

Figure 19–2. Right cadaver kidney after back-table separation. Notice cannula placed in the aorta for machine preservation and the entire vena cava left on the right side.

SURGICAL PROCEDURE

Wide exposure is obtained by a cruciate abdominal incision or a sternum-splitting midline incision. Since many donors now are multiple organ donors, the sternum-splitting incision has great versatility.[12,13] Whereas dissection of each individual kidney can be carried out as in the live donor nephrectomy, the en bloc technique is much safer and less likely to result in damage to hilar structures (Fig. 19–1).[14] In situ perfusion of the cold solution reduces warm ischemia time to zero and makes delayed graft function less likely. This is quick and easy to perform. Often, the main renal artery or upper-pole artery arises from the aorta at the level of the superior mesenteric artery (SMA). The aorta is not easy to expose and control between the superior mesenteric artery and the celiac artery; therefore, it is easiest to control the aorta above the celiac takeoff. This exposure can be easily obtained by mass ligation of the porta hepatis or by controlling the SMA and celiac artery with a vascular clamp, as described by Maley.[15,16]

If this is not possible, the aorta can be crossclamped in the left chest by elevating the left lung. Care must be taken not to put traction on either kidney, as an intimal dissection can occur in the renal artery, resulting in arterial thrombosis or stenosis in the recipient. This risk is minimized in the en bloc approach. In fact, some surgeons prefer to postpone any dissection on the renal hilum until cold infusion has been completed to minimize this risk and the risk of reflex vasospasm.

The kidneys are separated in the basin with cold slush (Fig. 19–2). The entire vena cava should be left with the right kidney to allow one of the right renal vein lengthening methods to be performed (Fig. 19–3).[17,18] All the renal arteries to each kidney should be left on a common patch of aorta for maximum flexibility in the recipient operation. Low-pole arteries that supply the ureter must be preserved; one artery that is easily damaged is a lower-pole artery to the right kidney, which crosses the vena cava at the level of the inferior mesenteric artery.

As noted in the foregoing discussion, hilar fat should be preserved. Belzer cautions that "no dissection should be performed on the left kidney in the triangle measured from the lower pole

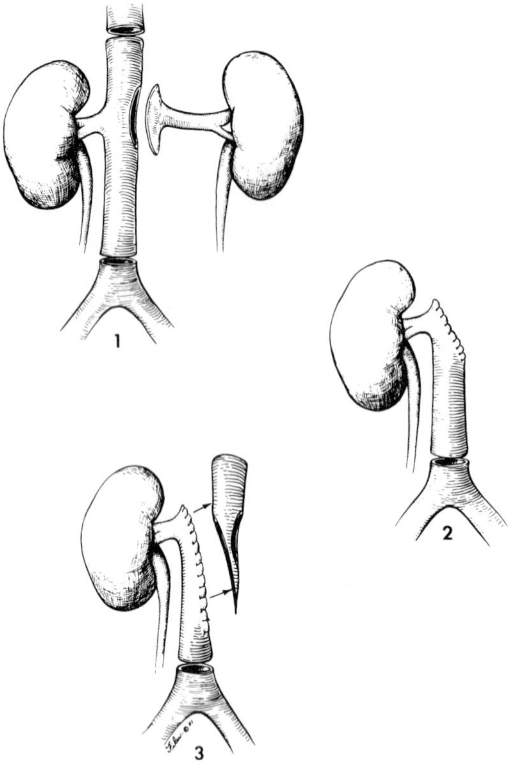

Figure 19–3. Separation of cadaver kidneys on the back table showing one technique for lengthening the right renal vein using vena cava.

to the insertion of the gonadal vessels into the renal vein, and on the right kidney from the lower pole to the inferior aspect of the junction of the right renal vein and vena cava."[19] Occasionally, there are capsular arteries that supply nickel-sized areas on the surface of the kidney. These are sometimes difficult to include in any of the vascular repairs and are the only arteries that should be considered for ligation.

Most preservation now is by simple cold storage after flushing with an intracellular-type electrolyte solution such as Collins' solution because of its simplicity compared with perfusion preservation. For periods of cold ischemia up to 48 hours, the results are similar to those of machine preservation.[20] Machine preservation does allow for longer cold ischemia times and is still used in some transplant centers. A new solution developed by Belzer and Southerd at the University of Wisconsin has been developed that may be a significant improvement over currently used solutions for flushing prior to cold storage preservation. In a study comparing it to Collins' solution in dogs, 100 percent graft survival was achieved at 72 hours cold ischemia time versus 0 percent when Collins' was used under the same experimental conditions.[21] It has also been shown to be effective in human renal transplantation.[22]

Kidneys should not be stored directly in ice because they may completely freeze, making them incompatible with subsequent function. If machine preservation is used, cannulas should not be tied directly into the renal artery, as this is likely to damage the intima and risk thrombosis.

Delayed graft function (DGF) itself is not considered a complication. Although there is some evidence that long-term graft is not affected by DGF, more recent evidence suggests a worse outcome for patients receiving kidneys that have not functioned immediately.[23,24] Certainly, initial post-transplant patient management is simpler, safer, and less expensive if the graft functions immediately. The rates of DGF vary from 5 to 85 percent and average about 25 percent.[22,25]

There are both donor and recipient factors that appear to affect the rate of delayed graft function.[26] The most important determinant of immediate function is cold ischemia time, a variable that may not always be possible to control. There are other factors that have been shown to reduce the incidence of DGF. Cardiovascular stability in the donor, delicate handling of tissues, minimization of warm ischemia and rewarm times, and volume expansion of the recipient are all beneficial.[27] Mannitol administered to both the donor and recipient before the vessels are unclamped seems to be particularly useful.[28] It may act directly by reducing cell swelling on reperfusion or simply as a volume expander. Touraine showed that with careful and controlled volume expansion in renal transplant recipients, DGF was reduced from 21 to 4.2 percent.[29] The only complications from the use of mannitol are fluid overload and myocardial depression, if given too rapidly. Calcium channel blockers, such as diltiazem and verapamil, free oxygen radical scavengers, and prostaglandins have been used experimentally and shown to improve immediate renal function.[30–32] None as yet is in routine clinical use.

Recipient Management

In an earlier edition of this chapter, it was noted that "surgical techniques have become standardized; however, meticulous attention to small detail will obviate potentially disastrous complications for both the allograft and the recipient."[33] This admonition is applicable today. On which side the kidney is placed makes little difference. Initially, it was placed in the contralateral iliac fossa. Others have routinely used the right side because of easier exposure of the external iliac vein, even placing the kidney upside down if necessary. I prefer the ipsilateral iliac fossa, if an end-to-side arterial anastomosis is used, and the contralateral iliac fossa, if an end-to-end arterial anastomosis is used. This allows the artery and vein to lie normally, without tension or kinking of the vessels. The only disadvantage of this approach is that the renal pelvis may lie posteriorly and make percutaneous access more difficult.

If the "correct" side has been used in a previous transplant or a peritoneal dialysis catheter is in the way, the opposite side can also be used. In women, the round ligament can be ligated to increase exposure without risk. In men, it had been routine to ligate the spermatic cord to improve exposure, but there are several good reasons not to do this. One is that since many patients now undergo second transplants, dividing the cord on both sides will produce infertility, which is unacceptable for many men.[34] Another reason is that testicular atrophy is likely to result. Finally, it is really not necessary to divide the cord to provide good exposure; the ureter should be brought under the cord when being put into the bladder.

In most patients, an extraperitoneal approach is possible. Any peritoneal holes made should be closed to prevent lodging of a loop of bowel producing intestinal obstruction. There are two situations in which an intra-abdominal approach may be necessary. One is in small children receiving a large adult kidney. A midline incision or an extended oblique incision to expose aorta and vena cava may be used instead. The other circumstance is in patients with multiple transplants, in which both sets of iliac vessels have already been used. Sometimes an extraperitoneal approach is still possible in this situation, but if scarring is great, a transabdominal approach is necessary. In these third, fourth, or fifth transplants it is sometimes possible to expose the external iliac arteries; however, more often, it is necessary to move higher into the common iliac artery. Whichever route is chosen, great care must be exercised in gaining proximal and distal vessel control, particularly avoiding venotomies before adequate control is obtained. Severe, difficult-to-control hemorrhage may be the result.

The external iliac artery or hypogastric artery

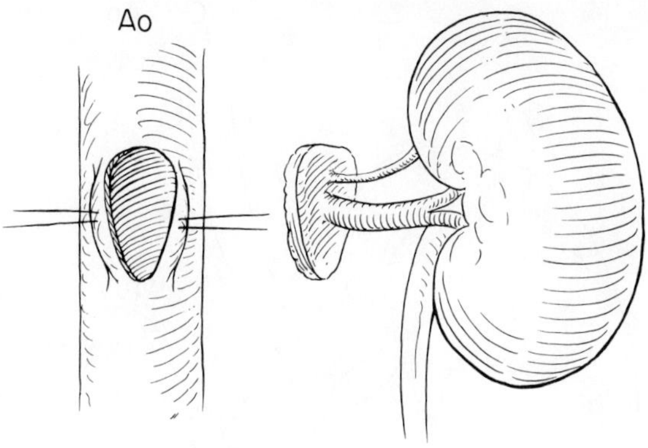

Figure 19–4. Diagrammatic view of Carrel patch. This method should be used in all cadaveric donor nephrectomies because it leaves all options open to the transplant surgeon performing the implantation.

is isolated. Many surgeons have switched to the external iliac artery, even for living related donor transplants, because it is usually easier than the end-to-end anastomosis. When the hypogastric artery was used in the first transplant, the hypogastric on the second side should not be used in a second transplant because impotence can result.[34] Dissection of the vessels should be the mimimum procedure used for control, and lymphatics should be clipped or tied. These measures will minimize the risk of lymphocele.[35]

In cadaver grafts, multiple renal arteries are easily handled by use of a Carrel patch of aorta (Fig. 19–4). If the arteries are far apart, two patches can be sewn together, allowing for a single end-to-side anastomosis. Occasionally, a small vessel exists without an aortic patch (Fig. 19–5). In these instances, there are several techniques that can be used. One is to use multiple branches from the hypogastric artery. Another is to sew the vessel into the side of the main renal artery. Still another is to create a patch from a piece of the iliac vein. The technique I prefer is to use the epigastric artery end-to-end, as is done for testicular or penile revascularization.[36] The variety of techniques to handle multiple renal arteries was well reviewed by Novick and included excellent illustrations.[37] Regardless of the technique chosen in arterial anastomosis, any intimal disruption must be tacked down to prevent dissection or thrombosis.

Multiple veins usually can be ligated, leaving one for anastomosis, except where there are two veins of equal size. It may be necessary to patch them together to provide adequate venous drainage of the kidney. A variety of techniques

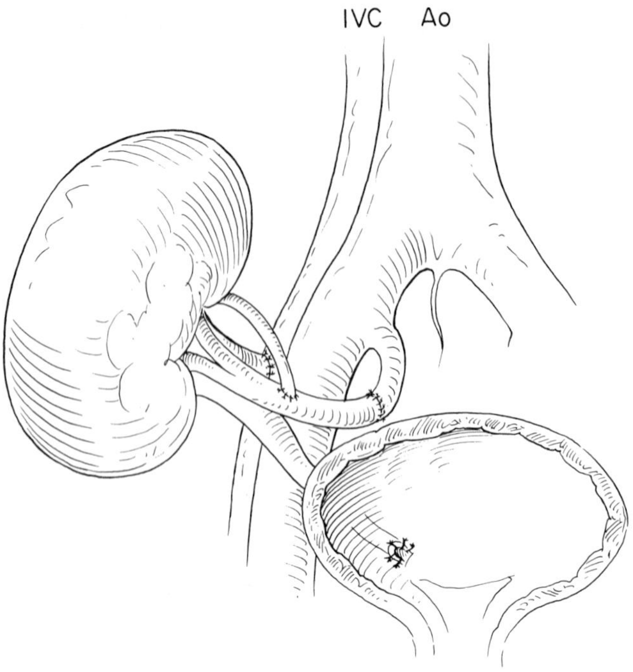

Figure 19–5. One method of vascularization of transected polar vessel. This can also be used in living related donors where there is a second small artery. Using the inferior epigastric artery end to end is another option.

exist for lengthening the right renal vein, which makes the use of the right kidney much simpler and safer. The kidney should be wrapped in ice during the vascular anastomosis, since prolonged rewarm times are associated with less successful outcomes.[38] Even though it is usually possible to complete the vascular repair in a short time, the use of ice obviates the need to hurry, and it protects the kidney. If ice is used, the kidney should be rewarmed with saline prior to release of the vascular clamps to prevent vasospasm from cold agglutinins.[39] If the kidney has been treated gently throughout the donor and recipient operations, it will become diffusely purple when the vein clamp is first released. It will then become diffusely pink and firm when the arterial clamp is released.

Some controversy exists about the use of small kidneys—those from donors less than 5 years of age. Both technical complications and losses from rejection have been reported as higher than when kidneys from older donors are used.[40–42] To obviate the thrombosis problem when kidneys from donors under age two are used, en bloc transplantation has been successfully employed. Taylor described a technique in which these kidneys can be used, even when liver removal has sacrificed the suprarenal aorta.[43] Although kidneys from anencephalic patients have been used, these kidneys have a higher incidence of abnormalities, and the use of these children as donors is now in question because they fail to meet the usual criteria for brain death.[44,45]

When large kidneys are used for children weighing less than 10 kg, it is critical to ensure adequate volume expansion intraoperatively to avoid hypotension that can result when the kidney compromises a large percentage of the child's cardiac output (Fig. 19–6). If this care is not taken, graft thrombosis is a frequent complication.[46]

Evaluation of the urinary tract is essential prior to transplantation to avoid unexpected problems. Voiding cystourethrography is a simple screening test to rule out significant abnormalities and ensure adequate bladder function required for ureteral reimplantation. In any adult with prior urinary tract abnormality and in children undergoing renal transplantation, of whom up to 20 percent have serious anomalies, more intensive evaluation of the lower urinary tract should be done.[47] A low pressure reservoir with adequate capacity and a means of emptying should be determined. The usual gamut of urologic modalities should be employed, including careful urodynamics. Most transplant surgeons feel that reconstruction should be done to fully rehabilitate the lower urinary tract prior to transplantation.[48]

The particular technique chosen to reaffix the ureter is less important than the ease and familiarity the surgeon has with a given technique. A nonrefluxing reimplant must be used unless

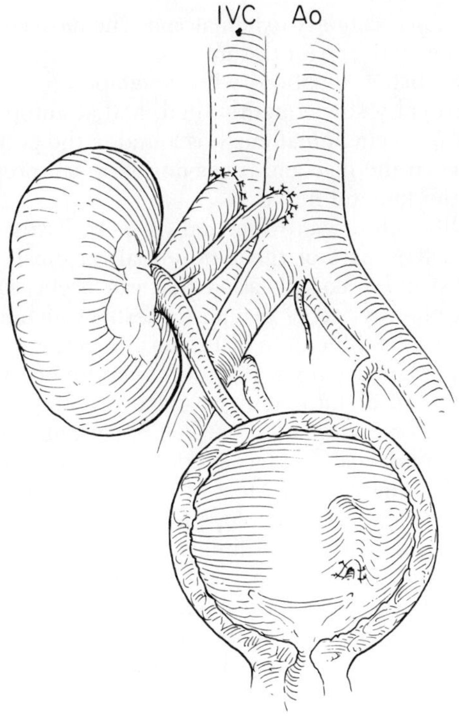

Figure 19–6. Standard technique of implantation of an adult kidney in a pediatric patient. The kidney may be placed extraperitoneally in children weighing between 15 and 20 kg and is more often placed intraperitoneally in children under 15 kg.

it is technically impossible. Higher rates of infection and pyelonephritis and lower rates of graft function have been demonstrated when reflux was present after transplantation than when a satisfactory antireflux mechanism was obtained.[49] Hanevold documented 22 cases in which grafts refluxed in children, and in five of these, one or more episodes of clinically significant pyelonephritis developed. There were no cases of pyelonephritis in nonrefluxing units. These are standard urologic principles.

Satisfactory results have been reported with a variety of reimplants, including the Leadbetter-Politano technique, extravesical reimplants, and pyeloureterostomy and ureteroureterostomy.[50–56] Our preference is to use an extravesical ureteroneocystostomy, similar to that described by Lich.[57] The advantages over intravesical reimplants are that it is easier and quicker to perform, requires less exposure, and does not necessitate a large bladder incision. In small disuse-type bladders, creating a submucosal tunnel intravesically can be difficult. In very thin-walled bladders, we often will still perform a more classic intravesical reimplant. Nonetheless, good results can be obtained with any technique if the ureter is handled gently and minimally, made short but without tension, and sewn with fine suture material. Nonabsorbable sutures have been used with the predictable development of sutureline stones.[56] Sutures of fine chromic catgut still are a reliable choice for ureter and bladder, as are the new synthetic absorbable sutures such as Maxon or PDS. Few transplant surgeons routinely use indwelling stents.

GENERAL COMPLICATIONS

Meticulous surgical technique is one of the most important determinants of a successful outcome. Hemostasis should be an obsession. Suturing techniques that do not strangulate tissue is another important tenet. Whether or not drains should be used is a matter of preference. Some surgeons do not use drains at all; others may use closed drainage systems for 24 to 48 hours. Penrose drains are less preferable because they are more likely to produce wound contamination.

In the early experience of renal transplantation, wound infections were a major cause of morbidity and mortality. These infections were sometimes superficial, but often they were deep infections, resulting in kidney exposure. Graft loss was not uncommon. High steroid doses, poorly functioning grafts, and poor general nutritional patient status were contributing factors. In the first report from the University of Minnesota hospitals in 1967, the wound infection rate in renal transplant patients was 30 percent.[58] A few years later, a series reported from San Francisco noted only a 1.7 percent wound infection rate in primary allografts but a 28.6 percent wound infection rate in any wound that was reopened (usually for allograft nephrectomy or drainage of hematoma).[59] The use of perioperative antibiotics has been demonstrated to be one way of reducing the rate of wound infections.[60,61] In the San Francisco series, the wound infection rate in the reoperation group was lowered to 5.3 percent by the combined use of parenteral and topical antibiotics.[62] Tilney and colleagues reported a wound infection rate of 2 percent when prophylactic antibiotics were added to their regimen.[63] Wound infection rates less than 1 percent are now frequently reported, and graft loss from wound sepsis is even rarer.[64]

Deep space infections and perinephric abscesses used to be common and often resulted in kidney exposure after open drainage of the abscess. Skin grafting techniques had been developed to manage this problem.[65] Now deep infections are rare, and when they do occur, they are usually easily diagnosed by ultrasonography.[66] Drainage and antibiotics make graft loss and mortality exceedingly rare. Percutaneous closed drainage is often possible.[66] If this is not successful, classic open drainage is necessary. Whereas a general principle in renal transplantation is to lower or stop immunosuppression in cases of infection, especially opportunistic infections, it is seldom necessary to stop immunosuppression for superficial wound infections. The development of generalized sepsis or a wound that does not respond to antibiotics and local treatment are two reasons to consider reducing immunosuppression.

Scrotal problems are uncommon. Catheter-related epididymitis can occur. It is minimized by early catheter removal after transplantation. Antibiotic treatment is usually also effective. It has been routine in some centers to leave the Foley catheter indwelling for up to 14 days after transplant. In most cases, we remove the catheter in 24 to 48 hours to reduce the risk of urinary tract infection. This practice has not resulted in any increased incidence of bladder leaks. Other authors have also shown a lower incidence of urinary tract infections when the catheter is removed early after transplantation.[67–69] Testicular atrophy seldom occurs if the cord is not ligated. Scrotal edema can occur, although the exact incidence is not known. It usually resolves spontaneously, although this may take several weeks. A lymphocele may drain spontaneously through the oblique fasciae into the scrotum and present as a scrotal mass. This can be distinguished from other causes of scrotal swelling by ultrasonography.

Many patients will have temporary superficial numbness from the cutting of cutaneous nerves around the incision or occasionally in the upper thigh area. The lateral femoral cutaneous nerve may be compressed by a self-retaining retraction.[70] A more severe femoral neuropathy has also been reported and may be more common than previously thought.[71] Several etiologies have been proposed. Yazbeck and coworkers recently reported two cases of presumed femoral nerve compression that resulted in significant quadricep weakness.[72] In both cases, the weakness resolved, but one case took 1 year to do so. They hypothesized that an ischemic injury to the nerve, secondary to a steal phenomena to the graft, caused the femoral nerve compression. The most likely etiology is from nerve compression secondary to hematoma. The most compelling evidence for this involves a case reported by Probst.[73] A patient who developed femoral nerve palsy subsequently died, and at autopsy, a $5 \times 5 \times 3$ cm hematoma was found in the gutter between the iliac and psoas muscles, compressing the femoral nerve.

Although organ rejection is not discussed here, it is part of the differential diagnosis of almost every complication that can occur. Despite the myriad of diagnostic tests available it still may be difficult to distinguish rejection with 100 percent accuracy. It requires experience and good clinical judgment to make correct decisions. For example, 50 percent of patients have small perirenal fluid collections demonstrated on ultrasonography. Most of these are insignificant. If a patient develops fever, graft tenderness, and rising creatinine indicative of acute rejection, it is not necessary to perform needle aspiration of every fluid collection prior to treatment of rejection to make sure that there is no abscess. It is necessary, however, to needle aspirate the abscess when it is present.

Lymphocele

Lymph leakage into the perirenal space results in formation of a lymphocele. This may present as early as 1 week after transplantation, although most often it occurs several weeks afterwards. The reported incidence is from less than 1 percent to as high as 8 to 10 percent.[35,74] A mass may be obvious in the area of the kidney; ipsilateral deep vein thrombosis or leg swelling may be present; or ureteral compression and rise in creatinine may be the only manifestation. Some lymphoceles cause no symptoms and are detected on ultrasonogram as an incidental finding (Fig. 19–7). Rarer presentations of lymphocele are incontinence secondary to bladder compression, scrotal mass secondary to spontaneous drainage into the scrotum, and vena cava or portal vein obstruction.[75] An unusual case of a lymphocele occurring years after kidney transplantation was reported by DeCamp.[76] Intractable ascites and pleural effusions developed. Multiple procedures were performed, including a Leveen peritoneal-venous shunt, before control was achieved.

In the past, pyelography, cystography, or lymphangiography would have been performed to detect a lymphocele. Now, ultrasonography is a standard test when there are significant alterations in renal function. The characteristic ul-

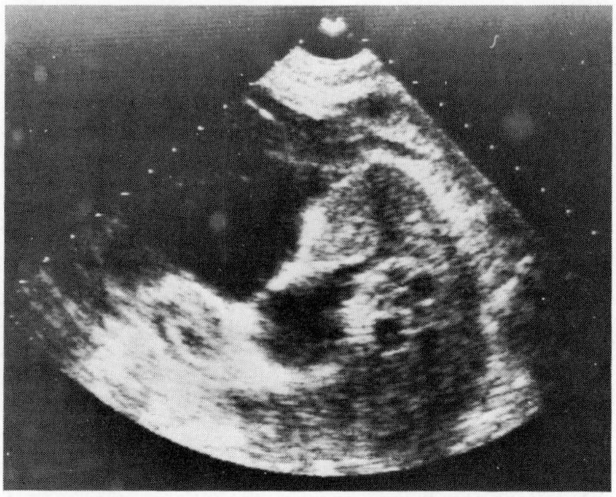

Figure 19–7. Ultrasonogram performed 1 month after transplant in an 18-year-old girl who had a gradual rise in serum creatinine over a 1 week period. Ultrasonogram shows moderate hydronephrosis and a large fluid collection, which proved to be a lymphocele producing ureteral obstruction. Marsupialization into the peritoneal cavity resolved the obstruction.

trasonogram of a lymphocele shows a roundish sonolucent, septated mass. Hydronephrosis may be present. More complex internal echos may signal an infected lymphocele, but this should occur only if a lymphocele has previously been needle aspirated and become contaminated.[77] These findings should distinguish the lymphocele from other perirenal fluid collections except a urinoma. Urinomas can be distinguished from lymphoceles by needle aspiration of the fluid using sterile technique, and comparing the creatinine in the fluid with the serum creatinine. Small, perirenal fluid collections that produce no symptoms should be left alone, because aspiration may result in infection.

It remains uncertain whether lymph leakages occur from the donor renal hilar lymphatics, the recipient periarterial lymphatics, or both.[78] Regardless, the best approach is prevention by careful thorough ligation of all lymphatics in both donor and recipient. Electrocoagulation does not seem to be sufficient to prevent lymph leakage. Minimizing the recipient arterial dissection to that required for vascular control has also been shown to be of value in preventing lymphocele formation. Carrying out all of these measures, Burleson reported 198 consecutive transplants without a lymphocele.[35]

There are several options for treatment; however, repeated simple aspiration is *not* one of them. If the lymphocele is large enough to warrant treatment, it will almost always reaccumulate within hours after simple aspiration. Sclerosing agents such as tetracycline and betadine have been instilled into drained lymphocele cavities with some reports of success, although more often this does not work.[79] Closed drainage is an option and may also be useful on occasion to determine if a lymphocele is responsible for a creatinine elevation by temporarily relieving the presumed obstruction.[66] If the creatinine falls, the obstruction probably was the cause. If the creatinine does not fall, another cause for graft dysfunction, such as rejection, must be sought.

External drainage has also been used. For this to work, the lymphocele cavity probably must become secondarily infected, causing fibrosis of the lymphatics. Certainly, the lymphocele that is already infected must be drained externally. The cleanest and potentially least morbid treatment is the transperitoneal window technique, which drains the lymphocele into the peritoneal cavity, where the fluid is resorbed.[80] The main risk of this procedure occurs when too small an opening is made, which can then seal over. Also, if the opening is small, there is a greater chance of a loop of bowel becoming entrapped, producing bowel obstruction or necrosis. Marsupializing the cavity by oversewing the peritoneal edges, making a large window and bringing omentum into the opening, will minimize this possibility.[80] One novel suggestion has been to make a prophylactic peritoneal window at the time of transplantation in children.[81] With the low incidence of lymphocele formation in most centers, the higher risk brought on by making the operation essentially an intra-abdominal one would not seem to justify this procedure routinely.

VASCULAR COMPLICATIONS

Arterial Thrombosis

The incidence of acute thrombosis of the renal artery has been reported to be as high as 3.5 percent.[82] More recent series have documented thromboses rates at less than 1 percent, and rates of less than 0.5 percent are achievable.[83] Although some thromboses may be secondary to hyperacute or accelerated rejection, most result from technical errors. Most often, the thrombosis will occur in the first or second posttransplant day. If the kidney is producing urine, then the thrombosis is manifested by acute anuria. Renal flow scan or Doppler ultrasonography will determine the other causes of acute anuria, such as acute rejection or urologic problems

(Fig. 19–8).[84,85] The flow scan will show an area of photopenia where the kidney should be (Fig. 19–9). Occasionally, the scan will show diffuse haze, either secondary to a poor bolus of isotope or to reduced flow secondary to acute rejection. In such cases, an arteriogram may be necessary to distinguish these, although the Doppler ultrasonography is proving to be excellent for detecting levels of flow within the kidney. If there is no urine output, the thrombosis may be silent and detectable only when no flow to the graft is seen on scan or on ultrasonogram. Graft salvage can occur if immediate surgical repair is carried out.[86] In one unusual case, graft function was restored after 51 hours of occlusion.[87] Most often, the graft is lost.

Segmental arteries may thrombose. This may produce hypertension from the underperfused renal mass or a mass effect from the infarct, and if a lower-pole artery thromboses, ureteral necrosis can result.[88]

Cyclosporine has been implicated by some surgeons in an increased incidence of graft thrombosis.[89] The evidence has been largely anecdotal or from series comparing cyclosporine-treated patients with historic controls. In a series from Houston, of 325 transplant procedures, six patients suffered acute renal artery thrombosis that occurred between 4 and 12 days after transplantation. In contrast, there were no thromboses in 297 azathioprine-treated patients.[90] These were not controlled cases, however. Studies have shown that cyclosporine does affect platelet function in vitro. Grace and associates showed that the addition of cyclosporine, at therapeutic concentrations to platelet-rich plasma from normal subjects in vitro, was found to increase platelet aggregration in response to adrenaline, collagen, and ADP.[91] Likewise, elevations of plasma fibrinogen and factor VIII levels have been found in cyclosporine-treated patients.[92] However, in a study in rats, the rate of thrombosis of a femoral artery anastomosis was no different between rats given cyclosporine and those not given the drug.[93]

In the Minnesota prospective, randomized trial of cyclosporine versus conventional immunosuppression, there was no difference in the rate of thrombotic events in either group.[94] It may be that since there is a demonstrable effect of cyclosporine on the clotting system, it can contribute to a propensity to thrombosis, if other factors exist to promote thrombosis. However, in a technically well-done anastomosis, cyclosporine does not seem to cause thrombosis.

Venous Thrombosis

Venous thrombosis is rarer and may result primarily from kinking of the vein or from a poorly constructed anastomosis. It may be secondary to rejection or glomerulonephritis. Renal vein thrombosis has been reported from progression of deep vein thrombosis of the leg, although most leg vein thromboses do not progress to include the kidney.[95] Oliguria, proteinuria, gross hematuria, and graft swelling are characteristic of graft vein thrombosis. If the

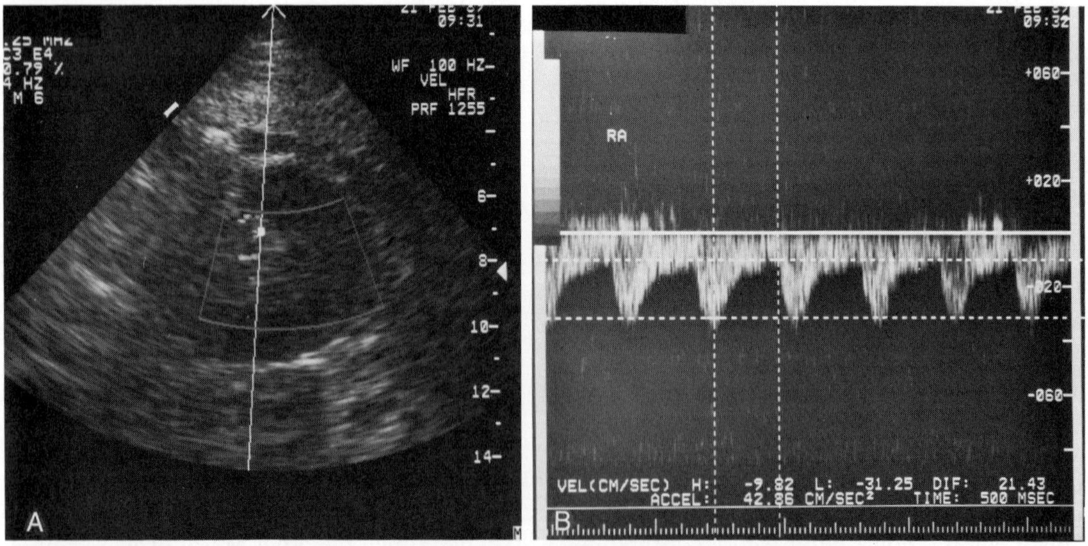

Figure 19–8. *A,B.* Post-transplant Doppler ultrasonogram showing normal arterial flow pattern.

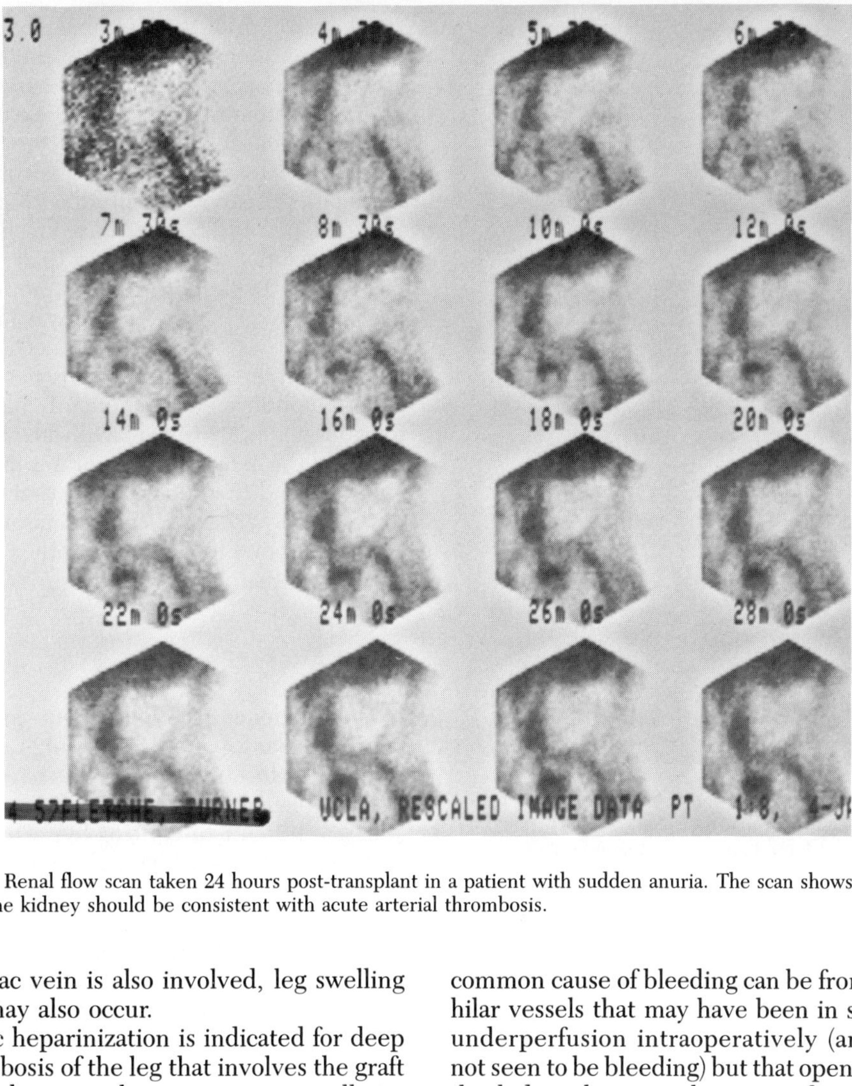

Figure 19–9. Renal flow scan taken 24 hours post-transplant in a patient with sudden anuria. The scan shows a photopenic area where the kidney should be consistent with acute arterial thrombosis.

external iliac vein is also involved, leg swelling and pain may also occur.

Systemic heparinization is indicated for deep vein thrombosis of the leg that involves the graft also. Thrombectomy, however, is not usually indicated. In cases of total graft occlusion, even if the thrombosis is secondary to rejection, the graft is usually lost. One case has been reported of late graft venous thrombosis occurring in association with deep vein thrombosis of the leg, which was successfully treated with intravenous streptokinase.[96]

Hemorrhage

Bleeding from the graft site can be profuse and, if not treated promptly, can result in patient death. There are several possible causes of post-traumatic hemorrhage. The most obvious cause of acute bleeding is due to an improperly performed vascular anastomosis. This is unusual, however, since anastomotic bleeding is usually easily recognized at the time of surgery. A more common cause of bleeding can be from small cut hilar vessels that may have been in spasm from underperfusion intraoperatively (and, hence, not seen to be bleeding) but that open later when the kidney becomes better perfused. Surgical exploration may be necessary if the bleeding is severe. Late hemorrhage (developing after 2 days) can result from graft rupture caused by rejection. Capsulotomy used to be routinely performed at the time of implantation to prevent graft rupture, but this is not done now, both because graft rupture is rare and because capsulotomy is unlikely to prevent graft rupture. Aggressive treatment of rejection and surgical repair may salvage the kidney, but most often, nephrectomy is required.[97]

Smith identified the following factors that would determine the management of graft rupture as the (1) length of time from implantation to rupture; (2) severity of the associated rejection episode; (3) number of prior rejection episodes; (4) source of the graft, i.e., living related or cadaver donor; (5) overall condition of the patient; (6) angiographic appearance of the graft, if avail-

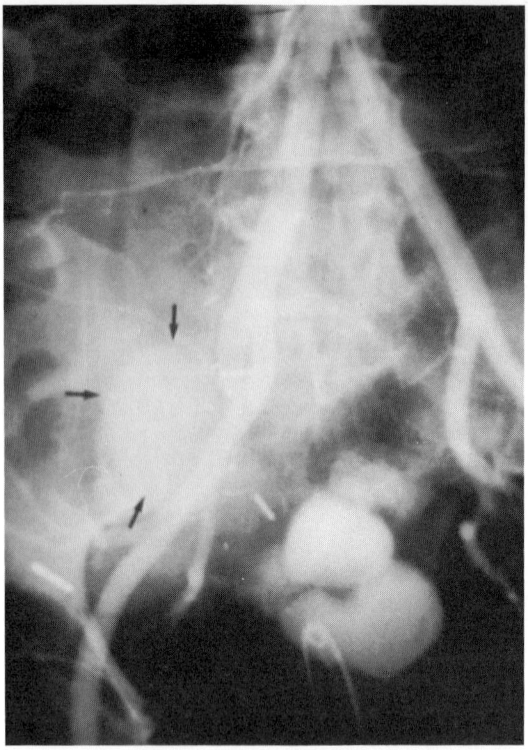

Figure 19–10. Mycotic aneurysm in a 45-year-old man 3 weeks after a cadaver renal transplant. Nephrectomy and femoral-femoral arterial bypass were carried out.

able; and (7) gross appearance at the time of exploration.[33] Three of seven cases of rupture at UCLA were repaired, one of which provided excellent long-term graft survival. These cases were all carried out under azathioprine/prednisone immunosuppression. In a more recent series of over 1200 cadaver transplants with cyclosporine immunosuppression, there were no cases of graft rupture.[98]

Another cause of late hemorrhage is leakage of a mycotic aneurysm (Fig. 19–10). Bleeding is often severe and life-threatening. Immediate surgical exploration is mandatory.[99] In fact, opening the incision while the patient is in bed and applying direct pressure may be necessary, even to make it to the operating room. I know of one patient who exsanguinated in bed from this and of another whose graft was salvaged in this situation. In the latter case, the artery was repaired, the wound was left open, and the patient was treated intensively with antibiotics and monitored by a bedside nurse. However, in most cases, nephrectomy is required in addition to arterial repair.

Placement of a balloon catheter via the femoral artery is useful for obtaining proximal arterial control prior to surgical exploration. If the arterial anastomosis is made to the hypogastric artery, ligation of the artery is curative. If the arterial anastomosis is made to the external iliac, several options for repair exist. One is to simply ligate the external iliac artery; surprisingly, on occasion, this does not produce leg ischemia. Blohm reported 35 cases of acute hemorrhage from infected arteriotomies of 1526 renal transplants.[100] In 13 patients, the common or external iliac artery was ligated. There was no mortality and no limb loss in these cases. Clearly, close observation for limb ischemia is necessary if ligation is performed. Anatomic bypass with autologous material prevent artificial material from entering the infected area, or suture-line excision with end-to-end anastomosis of the iliac artery can be performed. Extra-anatomic bypass, such as femoral-femoral, is another option and sometimes the only solution.

Renal Artery Stenosis

The incidence of hypertension in the stable post-transplant patient is as high as 50 percent.[101,102] Most of these patients have mild, easily controlled hypertension, but some develop severe, difficult-to-control hypertension, despite modern multidrug therapy. There are many causes of post-transplant hypertension, including cyclosporine and prednisone treatment, native kidney hyperreninemia, chronic allograft rejection, and graft renal artery stenosis (RAS). The incidence of RAS is reported as being from 1 to 12 percent.[83,103]

Which hypertensive patients to study with arteriography for the detection of RAS is not absolutely certain. The presence of a bruit has been felt to be one indicator. New onset hypertension and hypertension that is refractory to multidrug therapy probably are other indications for further evaluation (Fig. 19–11). A patient's response to the converting enzyme-inhibitor captopril may suggest significant RAS.[104] Eighteen patients with proven RAS had a significant, though reversible, fall in glomerular filtration rate (GFR) in response to captopril administration. Absence of this fall in GFR, however, may not rule out significant RAS. Detection sometimes occurs clinically when captopril is chosen for antihypertensive treatment and the serum creatinine acutely rises. Arteriography may also be indicated when a graft is failing in the absence of any apparent cause, and graft biopsy shows no evidence of chronic rejection.[105]

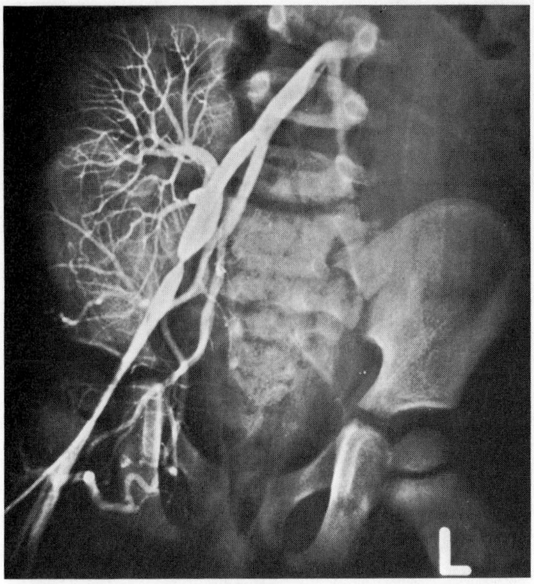

Figure 19–11. Arteriogram performed in 6-year-old boy 1 year after transplant for difficult-to-control hypertension. Arteriogram shows narrowing in the external iliac artery, secondary to intimal injury from vascular clamp.

There are several proposed etiologies for post-transplant RAS. One group is technical and therefore, presumably avoidable. In the series reported by Ricotta, the authors felt at least two thirds of their significant stenoses were secondary to identifiable technical factors.[106] These include inaccurate intimal approximation, harvesting injury to the intima, clamp injuries to donor or recipient vessels, kinking and fibrosis from a donor artery that is too long, and donor artery injury from perfusion cannulas. Whether or not RAS can result from rejection is uncertain; however, if it can, rejection is not the predominant cause of graft RAS.

There are two angiographic appearances of transplant RAS. One is a short anastomotic stenosis that almost always occurs following end-to-end anastomosis to the hypogastric artery.[107] The other is a longer postanastomotic stricture, which most often occurs after end-to-side anastomosis to the external iliac artery, and can occur even when a Carrel patch is used (Figs. 19–12 and 19–13).[108,109] Some have felt this to be largely a result of undetected intimal injury occurring either during harvesting or from cannulation injury to the intima.[110] Whether stenosis is more likely to occur following end-to-end anastomosis or end-to-side anastomosis is uncertain because no study has been done to directly compare them and so many other factors play a role in the development of RAS. It does seem that using a generous Carrel patch in an end-to-side fashion is technically less demanding than in an end-to-end anastomosis, and, if other factors are equal, a lower stenosis rate should result.

Surgical correction used to be the only treatment option available for RAS. When performed, the approach recommended is transperitoneal to the iliac and renal vessels. Repair can be achieved by resection and reanastomosis by bypass using autologous artery or vein, or by bypass with Gore-tex. Graft loss rates of 30 to 40 percent have been reported following surgical repair.[111,112]

Percutaneous transluminal angioplasty (PTA) has emerged as a reasonable alternative to surgical correction.[113] In a recent review of the literature, 76 of 90 patients after a 2-year follow-up were successfully treated by PTA.[114] Only one graft was lost as a result of the procedure. Results of PTA in pediatric grafts have been less impressive, with success rates of less than 50 percent being reported.[105] In most cases, if PTA is technically feasible, it can be tried first. If it fails to correct the stenosis, the more perilous surgical repair can still be undertaken.

Urologic Complications

Perhaps no area of transplantation has changed more dramatically in the past 10 years than the management of urologic complications. The incidence is lower now, and complications are easier to diagnose. Graft loss or patient death as a result of a urologic complication is much less likely. In the first decade that clinical transplantation was performed, the incidence of urinary fistula was 10 to 25 percent.[115,116] The mortality in those patients who sustained a fistula was 25 to 50 percent, leading Walsh to argue for pre-emptive allograft nephrectomy as the routine treatment for urinary fistula and Starzl to write in 1970, "With a urinary leak, the urgency of establishment of a water-tight urinary system has no parallel in standard urologic practice."[69,117,118] Now the usual rate of urologic complication is well under 5 percent.[67]

Loss of the graft from urologic complications is rare, and patient survival is seldom at issue as a direct result of such complications (see Table 19–1).[119,120] Several factors are credited with these changes. There is a greater degree of expertise in surgical techniques than ever before. Patients are healthier at the time of transplant now. Steroid doses are lower, allowing healing to occur much more readily. Ultrasonography

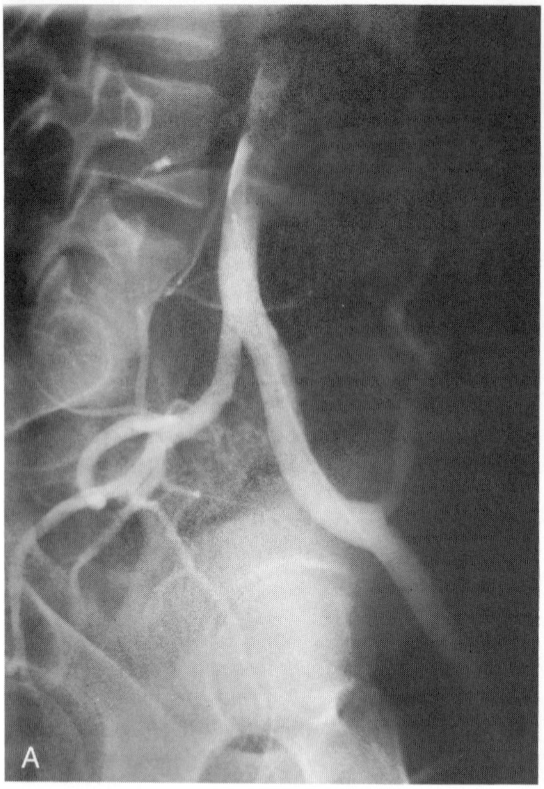

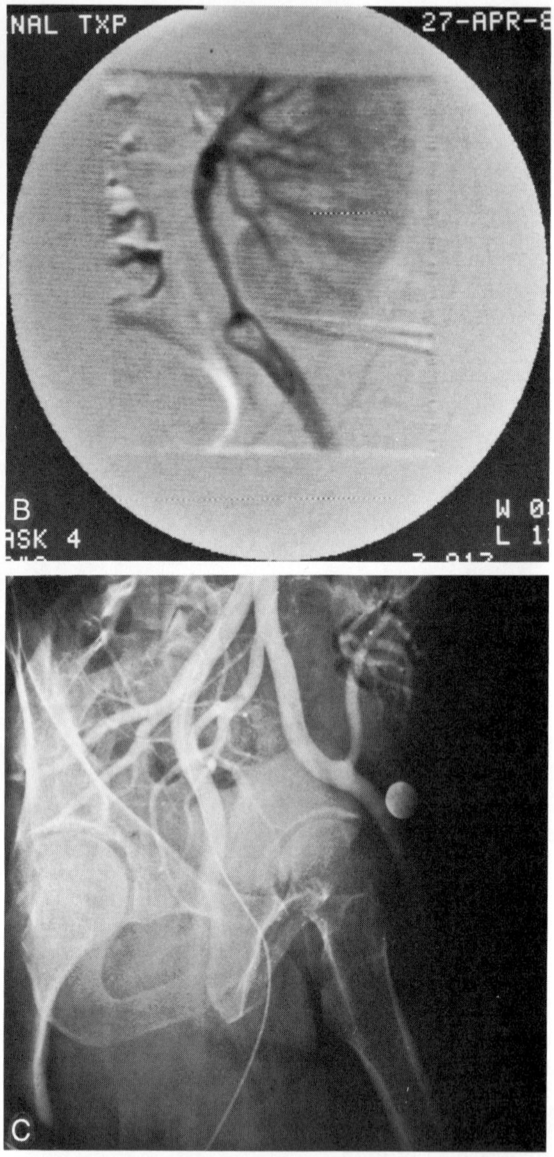

Figure 19–12. *A*, Renal arteriogram performed 14 months after cadaver transplant with end-to-side arterial anastomosis to the external iliac artery using a Carrel patch. Patient had difficult-to-control hypertension and a bruit over the graft. Seventy-five percent narrowing is present beyond the ostium, with 100 mm Hg gradient probably secondary to intimal injury at the time of donor nephrectomy. *B*, Dilatation with 8 mm balloon. *C*, The stenosis is resolved and blood pressure is normal. Follow-up is now 1 year, with no recurrence.

and percutaneous techniques give prompt and accurate diagnoses. The need for prompt treatment is well established.

In the early years of renal transplantation, urinary obstruction or fistulization was often difficult to diagnose because the clinical development of rising serum creatinine and falling urine output and, possibly, fever and graft tenderness were difficult to distinguish from symptoms of rejection. Intravenous pyelography may not have been possible, owing to poor renal function, and retrograde pyelography was often technically difficult. It was not uncommon for patients with urologic problems to be treated empirically with bolus steroids for presumed rejection. This was one of the factors that resulted in such high morbidity and mortality.

Now ultrasonography and renal scans are performed whenever there is any significant change in renal function, so that it is unusual for there to be a delay in the diagnosis of a urine leak or obstruction or any significant difficulty in distinguishing these from other cases of renal insufficiency. Retrograde pyelography has been replaced by percutaneous nephrostography as the first study to provide anatomic definition to ureteral problems in many centers.[121,122] Percutaneous techniques are helpful in two other ways in addition to helping to determine a diagnosis. One is that these techniques may indicate that repair is possible without the necessity of surgery. This was demonstrated in a recent case of a 35-year-old diabetic man who underwent ca-

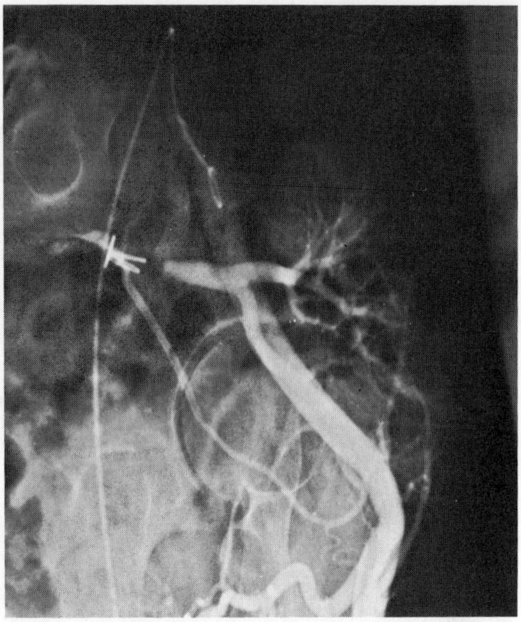

Figure 19–13. Anastomotic stenosis in an end-to-end hypogastric-to-renal artery anastomosis 2 years after transplantation. This was not amenable to balloon dilatation and required surgical repair.

Table 19–1. URETERAL COMPLICATIONS

Surgeon/Medical Facility	Date	Number of Leaks/Obstructions		Number of Grafts Lost
Jeffers Massachusetts General Hospital	1982	25/371	(7%)	8
Mundy Guys Hospital	1981	117/1000	(11.7%)	27
Cos Walter Reed Army Hospital	1985	11/184	(6%)	1
Loughlin Peter Bent Brigham Hospital	1984	88/718	(12%)	12
Jaskowski Oxford Infirmary	1987	44/600	(7%)	0
McDonald LSU	1987	12/204	(5%)	0
Sagalowski U. Texas, S.W.	1983	16/505	(3.1%)	2
Taylor U. Pittsburgh	1984	11/400	(2.7%)	0
Salvatierra UCSF	1977	29/860	(3.4%)	5
Starzl U. Colorado	1970	18/234	(7.7%)	5
Walzer Mayo Clinic	1980	14/500	(2.8%)	2

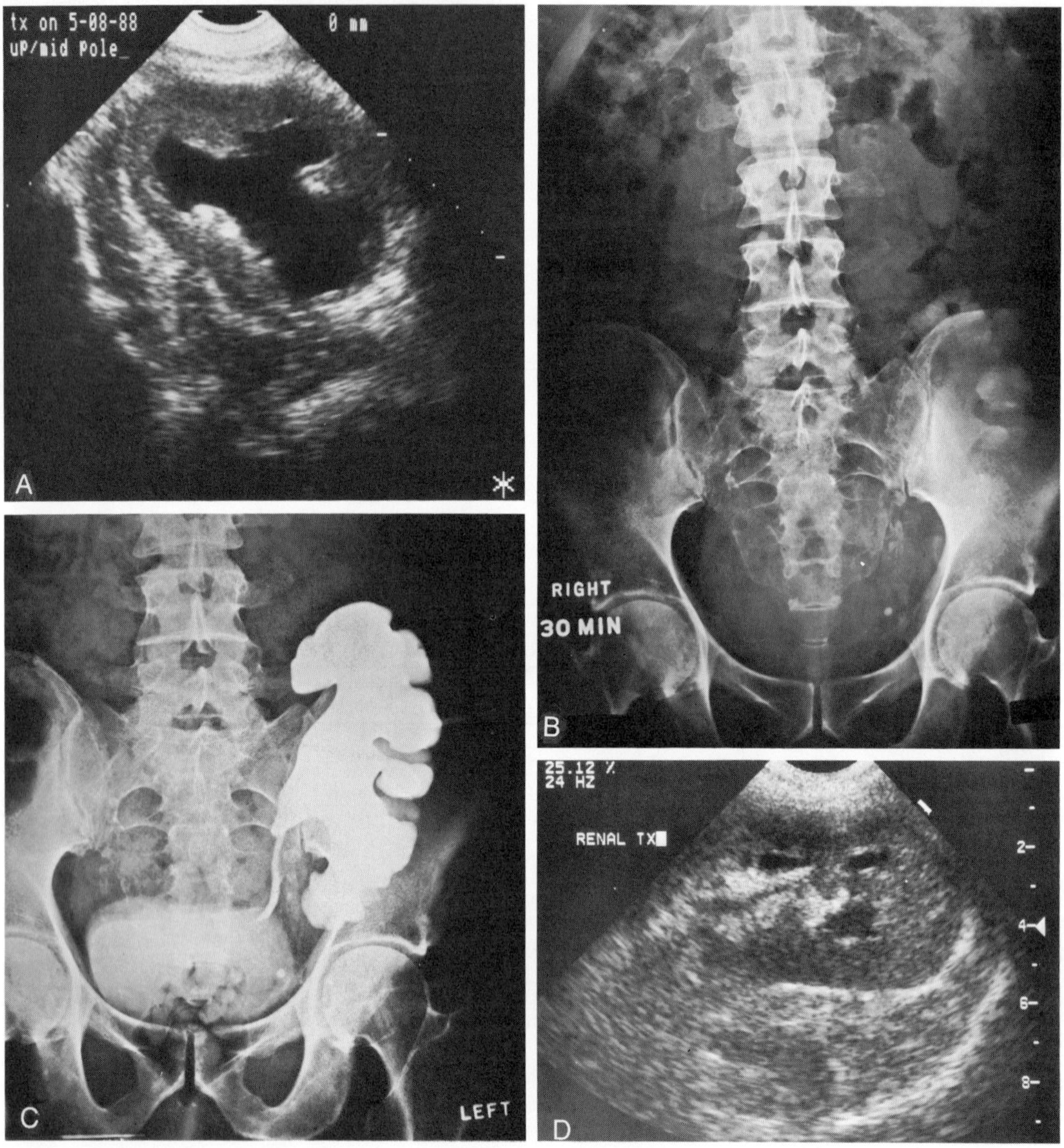

Figure 19–14. *A*, Ultrasonogram 3 weeks after a cadaver renal transplant in a 35-year-old diabetic man taken because of creatinine rise from 1.2 mg/cc to 2.5 mg/cc, showing 3+ hydronephrosis. *B*, Intravenous urogram taken the same day, consistent with obstruction. *C*, Percutaneous nephrostogram placed for relief of obstruction and showing ureteropelvic junction obstruction. *D*, Ultrasonogram performed 6 months after percutaneous balloon dilatation of ureteral stricture showing resolution of hydronephrosis. Serum creatinine stable at 1.2 mm/cc.

daver renal transplant (Fig. 19–14). Six weeks after surgery, his serum creatinine rose from a baseline of 1.0 to 2.5 mg/dl. An ultrasonogram of the allograft revealed severe hydronephrosis, and a percutaneous nephrostogram showed a ureteropelvic junction obstruction. This was balloon dilated, and a indwelling stent was left in place for 6 weeks. The creatinine returned to baseline levels. After removal of the stent, the renal function remained stable, and no further intervention was necessary.

The second way in which percutaneous techniques are helpful is that they are temporizing, allowing reconstructive surgery to be done under optimal conditions. An example is a case of a 30-year-old diabetic patient who underwent living related donor renal transplantation. Two weeks post-transplant, she developed fever and a rising creatinine. An ultrasonogram showed moderate hydronephrosis, and a percutaneous renal biopsy showed moderate rejection. A percutaneous nephrostogram showed severe mid-ureteral obstruction, apparently due to a kink in the ureter. The nephrostomy tube was left in place, the patient was treated for rejection, and, ultimately, renal function returned to normal. When the steroid doses were reduced to baseline, the ureter was repaired.

The first description of the use of percutaneous nephrostomy in transplant patients was in 1978 by Barbaric.[123] Since then, numerous series have been published by many centers documenting the use of endourologic techniques in transplant patients.[124–130]

The two major types of urologic problems after transplantation are leaks and obstructions. Although ureteral necrosis often presents as a urine leak, sometimes the initial manifestation of necrosis is obstruction. Obstruction that occurs early after transplantation may be confused with the other common causes of early graft dysfunction such as rejection. If the graft has been making urine, there will be sudden anuria. Hydronephrosis may not be present, although increasing hydronephrosis, if seen on ultrasonogram, is good evidence of obstruction.[131] Low-grade dilatation of the collecting system seen on early routine ultrasonogram usually results from edema and should not necessarily encourage further intervention.

The causes of acute obstruction are blood clots in the submucosal tunnel, technically poor reimplant, and, occasionally, ureteral slough. Usually, an acute postoperative obstruction will require surgical repair (Fig. 19–15). Late obstruction will usually present with decreasing graft function and progressive hydronephrosis on renal ultrasonogram. Extrinsic compression from abscess or lymphocele, kinking, subacute ischemia, stones, and, possibly, rejection are some of the causes of late obstruction. As with acute obstructions, percutaneous antegrade pyelography under fluoroscopy and pressure-flow measurements are the most useful procedures to confirm the diagnosis and identify the possible causes and site of late obstruction.

Leaks can occur at a number of levels in the post-transplant urinary tract including the blad-

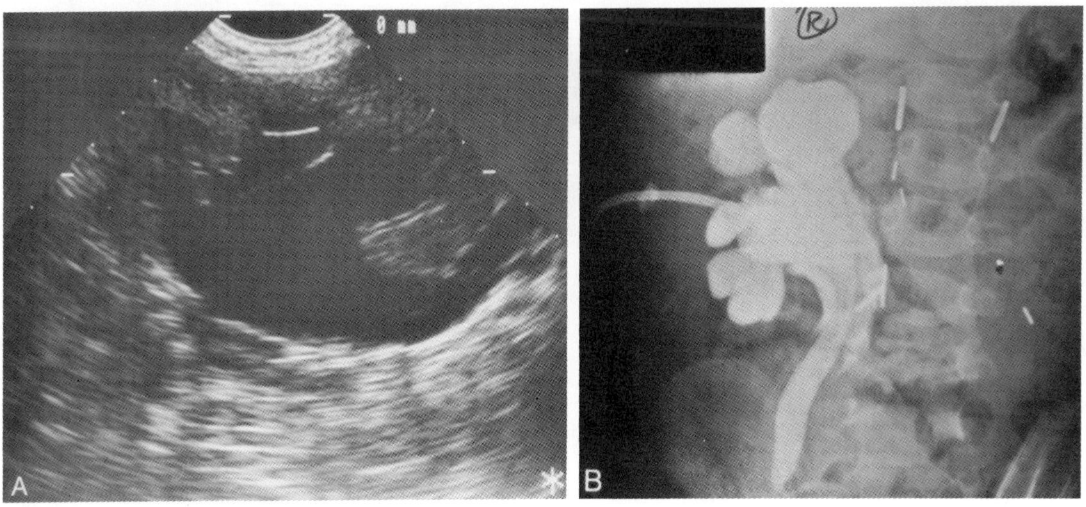

Figure 19–15. *A*, Ultrasonogram performed 6 months after transplant in six-year-old boy, following a creatinine rise from 0.4 mg/cc to 0.8 mg/cc showing grade 4 hydronephrosis. *B*, Antegrade nephrostogram demonstrates a kink in the distal ureter about 1 cm from the ureterovesical junction. This required surgical repair.

der, at the ureteroneocystostomy site, more proximally on the ureter or pelvis from a ureteral slough, at the calyceal level owing to a pressure-type blowout from an obstructed ureter, or from a segmental infarct of the kidney itself. If the wound is drained, the initial manifestation of a leak may be copious drainage of urine from the drain. If the wound is not drained, deteriorating renal function, pain, and a fluid mass on ultrasonogram may be the only signs. Occasionally, sepsis from the extravasation of infected urine may be the first sign.

A cystogram will document a bladder leak. A nuclear scan will sometimes reveal radioisotope outside of the urinary tract.[133] If the kidney is functioning well enough to provide large volumes of urine, measurement of the creatinine in the draining fluid is usually sufficient to distinguish urine leaks from lymph drainage, which also can be copious at times. Occasionally, intraveous methylene blue is helpful to indicate the leak.

The treatment of urinary leaks must be initiated at once. Delays in diagnosis and treatment have been associated with graft loss and mortality. If satisfactory drainage and control of the fistula are obtained by appropriate stenting and nephrostomy tube placement, some leaks may heal without operative intervention. These, however, are the exception. Most urinary leaks require surgical repair (Fig. 19–16). Percutaneous techniques may allow temporization. For example, a patient who develops a urinary leak and rejection simultaneously could have appro-

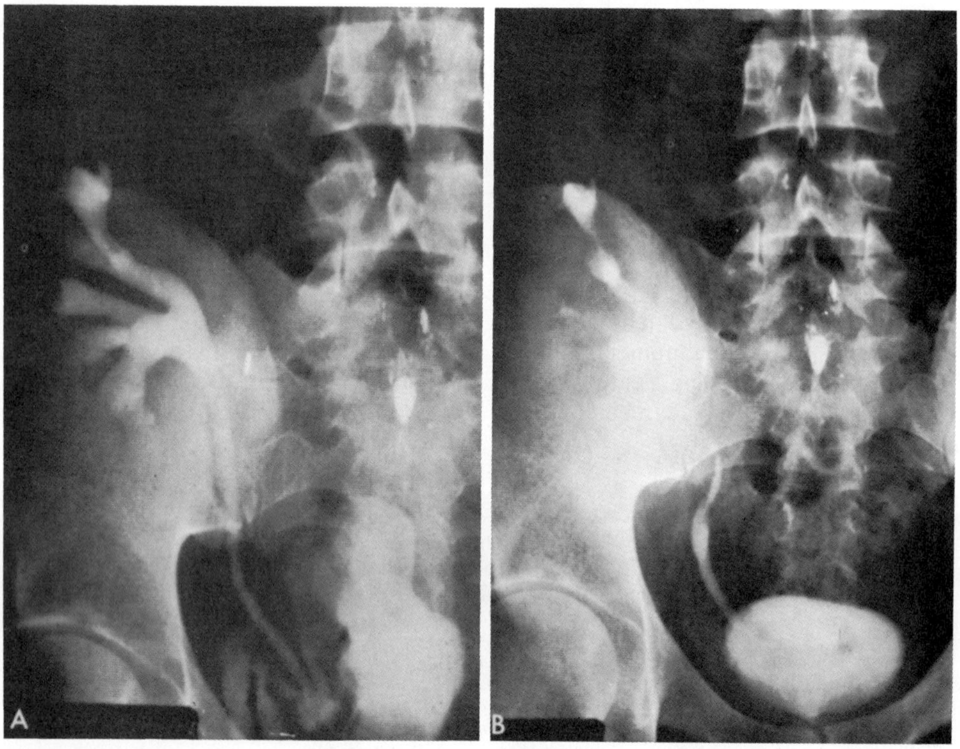

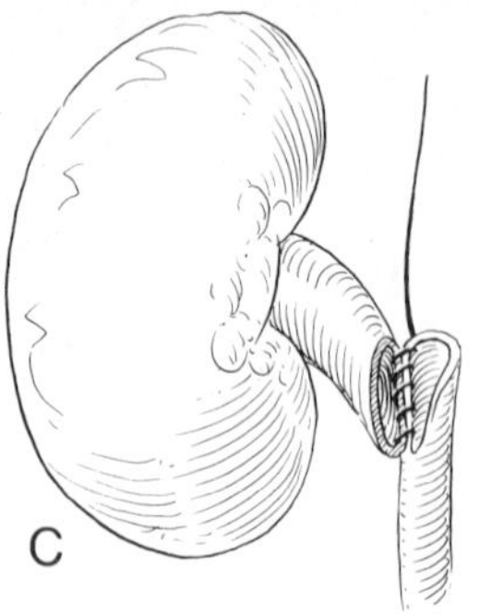

Figure 19–16. *A*, Ureteral fistula secondary to distal ureteral necrosis (7 days post-transplant). *B*, Repair with pyeloureteral anastomosis (recipient ureter to donor pelvis). *C*, Diagram of technique of pyeloureteral anastomosis.

priate percutaneous stents and drains placed, the rejection treated, and reconstruction performed when renal function is stabilized and steroid levels are reduced to baseline doses.

The type of surgical repair depends on the level of leak and viability of the tissues. Bladder fistulas should be closed primarily with three layers of suture. Some surgeons have advocated the use of nonabsorbable sutures here, but if the patient's nutritional status is good, absorbable sutures should be satisfactory. A calyceal leak resulting from obstruction is managed by treatment of the obstruction. A calyceal leak resulting from a segmental infarct is, fortunately, rare. When it has been reported, segmental nephrectomy and primary closure of the intrarenal collecting system have salvaged these grafts.[134]

Ureteral leaks can be the most troublesome, particularly if the entire ureter has sloughed. If it is a simple anastomotic leak, resection of the distal ureter and reimplantation are usually sufficient and the simplest solution. If more of the ureter is not viable, the entire gamut of urologic procedures is available for ureteral reconstruction. The only procedure that I have not seen reported is interposition of bowel, although it also is now feasible. Among the options that have been reported, one is a ureteropyelostomy using the native ureter. A native nephrectomy is not usually necessary. There is usually no morbidity resulting from ligation of the proximal native ureter if that native kidney is not making much urine. Despite the fact that an indwelling stent is not necessary at the time of transplant, most surgeons will place an indwelling double-J stent after secondary repair. Nephrostomy drainage is not essential, although if a prior percutaneous nephrostomy has been done, it is wise to leave it in place, since it can be used later to test the adequacy of the repair.

A variation of the ureteropyelostomy that can be performed even if the ipsilateral ureter is not viable is to use the contralateral ureter in the same fashion. Starzl first reported this in 1970, and I have seen this done in one other case.[69] Another option for repair of total ureteral loss is a cystopyelostomy, mobilizing the bladder widely and bringing it up to the renal pelvis to perform a psoas hitch. The advantage of the native ureter repair over the cystopyelostomy is that it is antirefluxing, which may result in less infection problems and stabilization of long-term renal function. However, Rajfer reported eight cases of cystopyelostomy with no long-term adverse effects.[135] When the native ureter cannot be used, this is an option. If the entire pelvis is sloughed along with the ureter, a ureterocalycostomy can be done, as reported by Flechner.[136] Togumi utilized a long Boari flap for ureteral reconstruction after a total slough.[137]

Complications of Percutaneous Biopsy

Although fine needle aspiration can now be done to diagnose rejection, it is not always sensitive or specific.[138] Needle biopsy is still performed in cases of acute graft dysfunction. The complication rate is less than 10 percent in our series. Most complications of percutaneous needle biopsy are minor, such as self-limiting hematuria. The most common complication is intragraft bleeding, causing hematuria. Usually, this will resolve spontaneously. If bladder clot retention occurs, catheter placement and irrigation may be required. Significant collecting system bleeding may result in clot obstruction of the kidney, causing anuria and azotemia. This may be mistaken for rejection, although an ultrasonogram will usually show the hydronephrosis and may also show the clot in the collecting system. Usually, the clots will lyse within a day so that no intervention is required.

Some clot obstructions can be prolonged. Kallash reported clot obstruction lasting 3 days which was treated with percutaneous nephrostomy.[139] We have had one case in which the obstruction lasted 2 weeks, which resolved with percutaneous nephrostomy drainage (Fig. 19–17). Intracollecting system streptokinase via percutaneous nephrostomy has been used, although there is the risk of inducing further hemorrhage with its use.[140]

There also have been serious complications resulting from needle biopsy, such as acute hemorrhage. This may be manifested by shock and a large mass seen on ultrasonogram. It is more likely to occur if the biopsy is done in a severely rejecting, necrotic graft or if a large vessel is inadvertently injured during the biopsy. Calne reported a case in which the biopsy needle lacerated the epigastric artery, resulting in exsanguinating hemorrhage.[141] Direct pressure and transfusion may stop severe bleeding, but the necessity for immediate surgical treatment is more likely.

Puncture of a lage intrarenal vessel may result in an AV fistula or pseudoaneurysm.[142,143] Moreau reported one such case, which was treated by angiographic embolization.[144] We have seen one case in over 300 biopsies performed in the

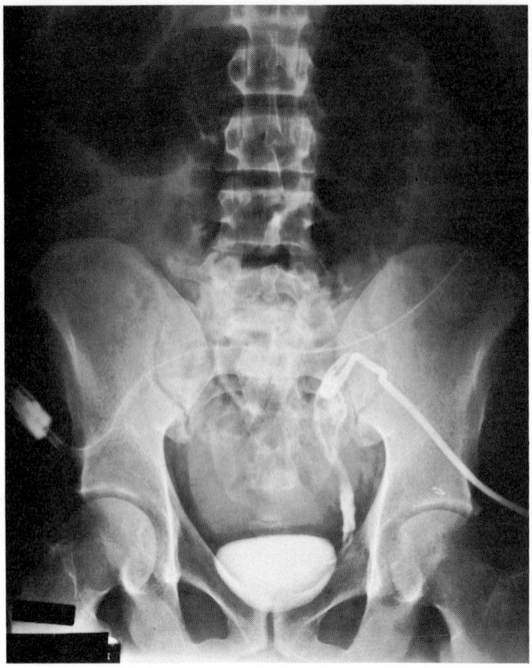

Figure 19–17. Percutaneous nephrostogram in a patient after a percutaneous renal biopsy and gross hematuria. The clot in the pelvis creates a negative filling defect. Clot lysis was complete after 3 weeks, and the nephrostomy tube was removed.

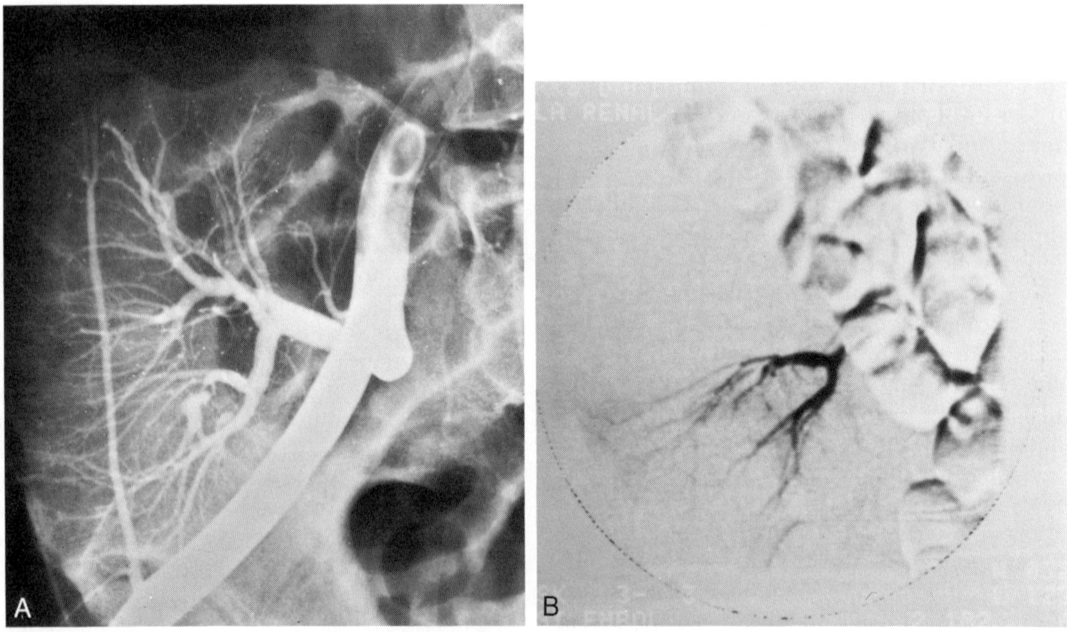

Figure 19–18. *A*, Twenty-nine-year-old man had undergone living related donor transplant 1 month previously and percutaneous allograft biopsy for rising creatinine. Persistent severe gross hematuria followed. The arteriogram shows a small arterial bleeding site. *B*, Angiographic control of arterial bleeding was carried out, with resolution of the hematuria and normal appearing arteriogram. (Courtesy T. Cochran)

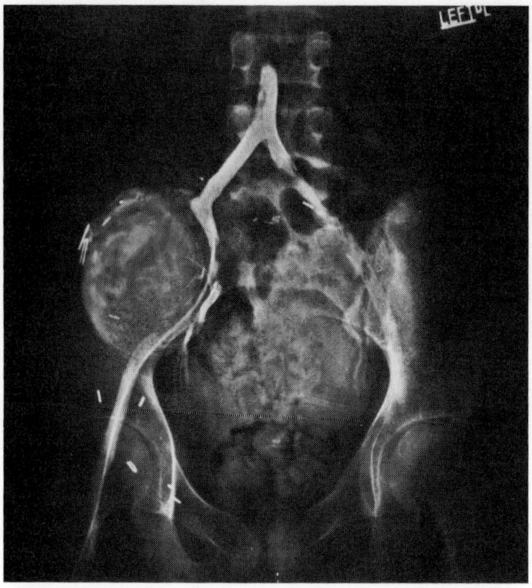

Figure 19–19. Arteriogram from a 19-year-old girl 11 years after allograft nephrectomy on the left side and 3 days after the sudden onset of a left groin mass. The arteriogram shows a large iliac artery pseudoaneurysm. This was surgically resected, and the defect in the iliac artery repaired with a Gore-tex patch.

last 5 years. It was detected by the development of a loud bruit several days after the biopsy and was successfully treated by transcatheter embolization without any effect on renal function (Fig. 19–18). Puncture of a large extrarenal vessel may result in a pseudoaneurysm; surgical repair is required in this situation. Rao reported a calyceal-cutaneous fistula resulting from a percutaneous needle biopsy.[145]

Complications of Allograft Nephrectomy

Every graft that fails does not require allograft nephrectomy. Most that fail early will require removal to avoid pain, fever, hematuria, and, possibly, graft rupture, which may occur if the graft is left in place as immunosuppression is withdrawn. Occasionally, severe hypertension may necessitate graft removal. The reported morbidity for allograft nephrectomy, however, is considerable. Morris reported 154 allograft nephrectomies performed over a 10-year period.[146] There was a 6 percent major intraoperative complication rate and a 14 percent major postoperative complication rate involving bleeding, infection, or lymph leaks. If the kidney is acutely rejected within a few weeks of transplantation, an extracapsular nephrectomy may be helpful. If the kidney is rejected later, especially if there is an element of chronic rejection, the kidney capsule is extremely adherent to the surrounding structures. If an extracapsular nephrectomy is attempted, damage to surrounding structures, e.g., bowel or iliac vessels, is likely. It is much safer to perform a subcapsular nephrectomy in this situation. It is not necessary to remove all the vessels; in fact, the closer to the hilum the dissection is carried out, the less likely damage to the iliac vessels will occur. Surprisingly, there are very few sequelae to leaving segments of the donor vessels in place. It may be thought that they would be prone to ongoing rejection and possibly result in severe acute hemorrhage (Fig. 19–19). I have yet to see delayed hemorrhage after allograft nephrectomy, although Starnes reported this complication in four patients of a group of 92 who underwent allograft nephrectomy.[147] Leaving a small amount of donor ureter in place can result in hematuria later, although this also is uncommon.[148] Removal of the bulk of the graft is sufficient to alleviate pain and fever, which are common indications for allograft nephrectomy after graft failure.

Stone Disease

Renal calculi occur infrequently after transplantation. Steroid use, hyperparathyroidism, renal tubular acidosis, and bacteriuria may be precipitating causes.[149,150] Also, stones may be transplanted with the kidney. Few transplant patients with stones will have colic. Decreased urine output, hematuria, rising creatinine, or infection may be the only presenting symptom. Ultrasonography is done routinely for any of these problems, especially before steroid pulsing is considered for rejection, so that most stones should be detected.

The same options for treatment of stones in native kidneys are available for treatment of stones in transplant kidneys, including surgery, endourologic techniques, and extracorporeal shockwave lithotripsy (ESWL), Fuchs reported ESWL treatment of five transplant patients (Fig. 19–20).[151] All patients developed stones more than 3 years after transplantation. One patient with a staghorn calculus also required nephrostomy tube placement. All patients were determined to be stone free. In two of these cases, it was necessary to perform the ESWL in the prone position.

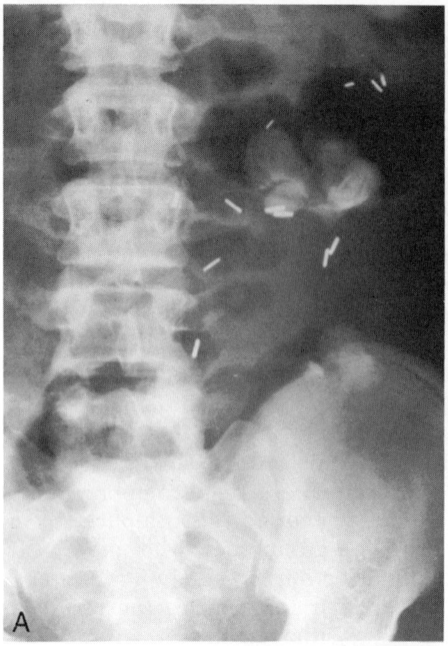

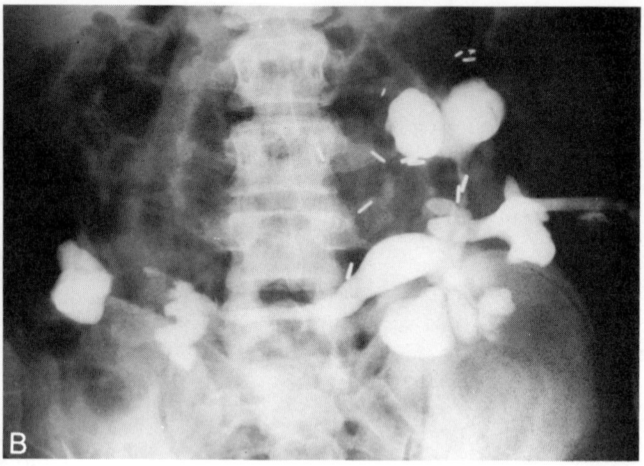

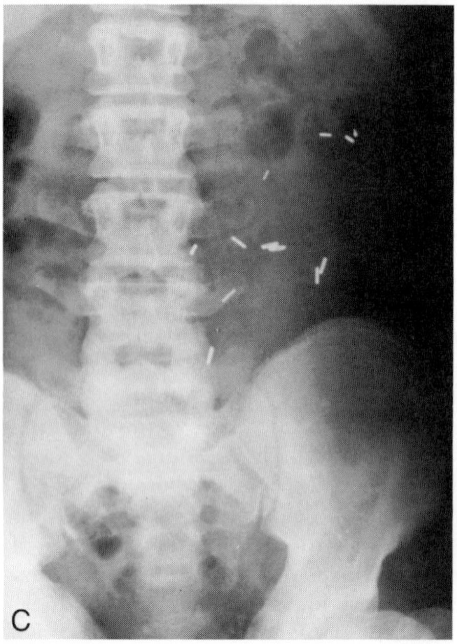

Figure 19–20. *A*, KUB done in a 20-year-old male who had a renal transplant 12 years previously. The ureter was placed into an ilial conduit. He had had two previous pyelolithotomies. Creatinine had risen to 3.5 mg/cc. *B*, Percutaneous nephrostogram. *C*, Combination percutaneous lithotripsy and ESWL resulted in complete stone dissolution and return of serum creatinine to 2.0 mg/cc. (Courtesy A. Fuchs)

REFERENCES

1. McDonald JC, Vaughn W, Filo RS, et al: Cadaver donor renal transplantation by centers of the Southeastern Organ Procurement Foundation. Ann Surg 193:1, 1981.
2. Tiwari J, Terasaki PI, Mickey MR: Factors influencing kidney graft survival in the cyclosporine era. Transplant Proc 19:1839, 1987.
3. Rosenthal JT, Hakala TR, Iwatsuki S, et al: Cadaveric renal transplantation under cyclosporine-steroid therapy. Surg Gynecol Obstet 157:309, 1983.
4. Simmons RL, Canafax DM, Fryd DS, et al: New immunosuppressive drug combinations for mismatched related and cadaver renal transplantation. Transplant Proc 18(Supp)1:76, 1986.
5. Calne RY, Rolles K, White DJG, et al: Cyclosporin A in clinical organ grafting. Transplant Proc 13:349, 1981.
6. Flechner SM, Rauschkolb EN, Cohen G, et al: Use of digital subtraction angiography for evaluation of the living related transplant donors. Transplantation 33:645, 1982.
7. Bay, WH, Hebert LA: The living donor in kidney transplantation. Ann Intern Med 106:877, 1987.
8. Dunn JF, Nylander WA Jr, Richie RE, et al: Living related kidney donors. Ann Surg 203:637, 1986.
9. Williams SL, Oler J, Jorkasky DK: Long-term renal function in kidney donors. Ann Intern Med 105:1, 1986.

10. Novitizky D, Cooper DKC, Reichard B: Hemodynamic and metabolic responses to hormonal therapy in brain-dead potential organ donors. Transplantation 43:852, 1987.
11. Belzer FO, Reed TW, Pryor MB, et al: Cause of renal injury in kidneys obtained from cadaver donors. Surg Gynecol Obstet 130:367, 1970.
12. Rosenthal JT: Kidney recovery from the multiple organ donor. Urol Clin North Am 12:571, 1985.
13. Rosenthal JT, Shaw BW, Hardesty RL, et al: Principles of multiple organ procurement from cadaver donors. Ann Surg 198:617, 1983.
14. Rosenthal JT, Denny D, Hakala TR: Results of a single kidney procurement center. J Urol 129:1111, 1983.
15. Rosenthal JT, Taylor RJ, Hakala TR: Sternotomy and portal triad division for cadaver donor nephrectomy. Urology 28:26, 1986.
16. Maley WR, Williams GM, Colombani P, et al.: Simple instrument occlusion of the anterior visceral branches of the aorta during en bloc renal allograft procurement. Surg Gynecol Obstet 167:442, 1988.
17. Taylor RT, Hakala TR, Rosenthal JT: Use of vena cava to extend right renal vein in cadaveric transplants. Surg Gynecol Obstet 160:279, 1985.
18. Barry JM, Fuchs EF: Right renal vein extension in cadaver kidney transplantation. Arch Surg 113:300, 1978.
19. Belzer FO, Glass N, Sollinger H: Technical complications after renal transplantation. In Morris PJ, ed: Renal Transplantation. Philadelphia, Grune & Stratton 1984, 407–426.
20. Rosenthal JT, Herman JB, Taylor RJ, et al.: Comparison of pulsatile machine perfusion with cold storage for cadaver kidney preservation. Transplantation 37:425, 1984.
21. Ploeg PJ, Goossens D, McAnulty JF, et al: Successful 72-hour cold storage of dog kidneys with UW solution. Transplantation 46:191, 1988.
22. Hoffman B, Sollinger H, Kalayoglu M, et al: Use of UW solution for kidney transplantation. Transplantation 46:338, 1988.
23. Mendez-Picon G, Posner MP, McGeorge MB, et al: Effects of delayed function on long term survival of renal allografts. Surg Gynecol Obstet 161:351, 1985.
24. Carpenter BJ, Rosenthal JT, Taylor RJ, et al: The impact of acute tubular necrosis on graft outcome in patients receiving cyclosporine. Transplant Proc 17:1282, 1985.
25. Barry JM, Fischer S, Lieberman C, et al: Successful human kidney preservation by intracellular electrolyte flush followed by cold storage for more than 48 hours. J Urol 129:473, 1983.
26. Taylor RJ, Zheng S, Ptachinski R, Rosenthal JT et al.: Cyclosporine therapy independent of graft diuresis in cadaveric renal transplants. Transplant Proc 18:5, 1986.
27. Rajagopalan PR, Kay NA, Fitts CT, et al: Prevention of acute tubular necrosis after transplantation: effect of pretransplantation volume expansion. South Med J 79:972, 1986.
28. van Valenberg PLJ, Hoitsma AJ, Tiggeler RGWL, et al: Mannitol as an indispensable constituent of an intraoperative hydration protocol for the prevention of acute renal failure after renal cadaveric transplantation. Transplantation 44:784, 1987.
29. Touraine JL, Garnier JL, Mercatello A, et al: Post-transplant acute renal failure. Adv Exp Med Biol 212:205, 1987.
30. Wagner K: Diltiazem in the prevention of delayed graft function in cadaveric renal transplantation. Lancet 1:1355, 1985.
31. Anaise D, Bachvaroff R, Sato K, et al: A membrane stabilization approach to long-term renal preservation. Transplant Proc 17:1457, 1985.
32. Tobimatsu M, Ueda Y, Katsumoto F, et al: A new prostacyclin analogue: its protective effect on ischemia-induced acute renal failure in dogs. Transplant Proc 17:1461, 1985.
33. Smith RB, Ehrlich RM: Complications of renal transplant surgery. In Smith RB, Ehrlich RM, eds: Complications of Urologic Surgery. Philadelphia, WB Saunders Co, 1976.
34. Gittes RF, Waters WB: Sexual impotence: the overlooked complication of a second renal transplant. J Urol 121:719, 1979.
35. Burleson RL, Marbarger PD: Prevention of lymphocele formation following renal allotransplantation. J Urol 127:18, 1982.
36. Merkel FK, Straus AK, Anderson O, et al.: Microvascular techniques for polar artery reconstruction in kidney transplants. Surgery 79:253, 1976.
37. Novick AC, Magnusson M, Braun WE: Multiple-artery renal transplantation: emphasis on extracorporeal methods of donor arterial reconstruction. J Urol 122:731, 1979.
38. The Canadian Transplant Study Group: Examination of parameters influencing the benefit : detriment ratio of cyclosporine in renal transplantation. Am J Kidney Dis 5:328, 1985.
39. Lobo PI, Strugill BC, Bolton WK: Cold-reactive alloantibodies and allograft malfunction occurring immediately post-transplant. Transplantation 37:76, 1984.
40. Churchill BM, Sheldon CA, McLorie GA, et al: Factors influencing patient and graft survival in 300 cadaveric pediatric renal transplants. J Urol 140:1129, 1988.
41. Wengerter K, Matas AJ, Tellis VA, et al: Transplantation of pediatric donor kidneys to adult recipients. Ann Surg 204:172, 1986.
42. Moel DI, Butt KMH: Renal transplantation in children less than 2 years of age. J Pediatr 99:535, 1981.
43. Taylor RJ, Rosenthal JT, Hakala TR: Combined cadaver hepatic and renal organ procurement in infants. Arch Surg 120:1084, 1985.
44. Iitaka K, Martin LW, Cox JA, et al: Transplantation of cadaver kidneys from anencephalic donors. J Pediatr 93:216, 1978.
45. Holzgreve W, Beller FK, Buchholz B, et al: Kidney transplantation from anencephalic donors. N Engl J Med 316:1069, 1987.
46. Churchill BM, Sheldon CA, McLorie GA, et al: Factors influencing patient and graft survival in 300 cadaveric pediatric renal transplants. J Urol 140:1129, 1988.
47. Najarian JS, So, SKS, Simmons RL, et al: The outcome of 304 primary renal transplants in children. Ann Surg 204:246, 1986.
48. Gonzalez R, Lapointe S, et al: Undiversion in children with renal failure. J Pediatr Surg 19:632, 1984.
49. Hanevold CD, Kaiser BA, Palmer JA et al: Vesicoureteral reflux and urinary tract infections in renal transplant recipients. Am J Dis Child 141:982, 1987.
50. Cos DLR, Light JA, Stutzman RE: External ureteroneocystostomy in renal transplantation. Urology 26:362, 1985.

51. Hefty TR: Experience with parallel incision extravesical ureteroneocystostomy in renal transplantation. J Urol 134:455, 1985.
52. Waltke EA, Adams MB, Kauffman HM, et al.: Prospective randomized comparison of urologic complications in end-to-side versus Politano-Leadbetter ureteroneocystostomy in 131 human cadaver renal transplants. J Urol 128:1170, 1982.
53. McDonald JC, Landreneau MD, Hargroder DE, et al: External ureteroneocystostomy and ureteroureterostomy in renal transplantation. Ann Surg 205:428, 1987.
54. Barry JM, Hatch DA: Parallel incision, unstented extravesical ureteroneocystostomy. J Urol 134:249, 1984.
55. Landau R, Botha JR, Myburgh JA: Pyeloureterostomy or ureteroneocystostomy in renal transplantation? Br J Urol 58:6, 1986.
56. Jeffers GJ, Cosimi AB, Delmonico FL, et al: Experience with pyeloureterostomy in renal transplantation. Ann Surg 196:588, 1982.
57. Lich R, Howerton LW, Davis LA: Recurrent urosepsis in children. J Urol 86:554, 1961.
58. Kelly WD, Lillehei RC, Aust, JB, et al: Kidney transplantation: experiences at the University of Minnesota hospitals. Surgery 62:704, 1967.
59. Schweizer RT, Kountz DS, Belzer FO: Wound complications in recipients of renal transplants. Ann Surg 177:58, 1973.
60. Tillegard A: Renal transplant wound infection: the value of prophylactic antibiotic treatment. Scand J Urol Nephrol 18:215, 1984.
61. Muakkassa WF, Goldman MH, Mendez-Picon G: Wound infections in renal transplant patients. J Urol 130:17, 1983.
62. Belzer FO, Salvatierra O, Schweizer RT, et al: Prevention of wound infections by topical antibiotics in high risk patients. Am J Surg 126:180, 1973.
63. Tilney NL, Strom TB, Vineyard GC, et al: Factors contributing to the declining mortality rate in renal transplantation. N Engl J Med 299:1321, 1978.
64. Koyle MA, Ward HJ, Twomey PA, et al: Declining incidence of wound infection in cadaveric renal transplant recipient. Urology 31:103, 1988.
65. Paley D, Spees EK, Zachary JB, et al: Skin autografts to cover exposed renal allografts. Surgery 90:910, 1981.
66. Cohan RH: Percutaneous drainage of pelvic lymphatic fluid collections in the renal transplant patient. Invest Radiol 22:864–867, 1987.
67. Sagalowsky AI, Ransler CW, Peters PC, et al: Urologic complications in 505 renal transplants with early catheter removal. J Urol 129:929, 1983.
68. Zaontz MR, Hatch DA, Firlit CF: Urological complications in pediatric renal transplantation: management and prevention. J Urol 140:1123, 1988.
69. Starzl TE, Groth CG, Putnam CW, et al: Urologic complications in 216 human recipients of renal transplants. Ann Surg 172:1, 1970.
70. Vaziri ND, Barnes, J, Mirahmadi Khosrow, et al: Compression neuropathy subsequent to renal transplantation. Urology 7:145, 1976.
71. Sisto D, Chiu WS, Geelhoed GW, et al: Femoral neuropathy after renal transplantation. South Med J 73:1464, 1980.
72. Yazbech S, Larbrisseau A, O'Regan S: Femoral neuropathy after renal transplantation. J Urol 134:720, 1985.
73. Probst A, Harder F, Hofer H, et al: Femoral nerve lesion subsequent to renal transplantation. Eur Urol 8:314, 1982.
74. Lerut T, Lerut J, Broos P, et al: Lymphatic complications in renal transplantation. Eur Urol 6:83, 1980.
75. Sollinger HW, Glass NR, Belzer FO: Post-transplant lymphocele causing obstruction of the inferior vena cava and portal vein. Transplant Proc 14:440, 1982.
76. DeCamp MM, Tilney NL: Late development of intractable lymphocele after renal transplantation. Transplant Proc 20:105, 1988.
77. Ridge JA, Manco-Johnson ML, Weil R: Ultrasonographic diagnosis of infected lymphocele after kidney transplantation. Eur Urol 13:31, 1987.
78. Pontes JE, McDonald FD, Midgal SD, et al: Lymphatic complications in renal allografts. Urology 17:26, 1981.
79. Teruel JL, Escobar EM, Quereda C, et al: A simple and safe method for management of lymphocele after renal transplantation. J Urol 130:1058, 1983.
80. Williams G, Howard N: Management of lymphatic leakage after renal transplantation. Transplantation 31:134, 1981.
81. Zaontz MR, Firlit CF: Pelvic lymphocele after pediatric renal transplantation. J Urol 139:557, 1988.
82. Jordan ML, Cook GT, Cardella CJ: Ten years of experience with vascular complications in renal transplantation. J Urol 128:689, 1982.
83. Palleschi J, Novick AC, Braun LWE, et al: Vascular complications of renal transplantation. Urology 16:61, 1980.
84. Lopatkin NA, Gleizer YY, Jarmolinskij JS, et al: Radioisotope studies in the diagnosis of acute complications in the post-transplantation stage. Int Urol Nephrol 12:169, 1980.
85. Needleman L, Kurtz AB: Doppler evaluation of the renal transplant. JCU 15:661, 1987.
86. Okiye SE, Zincke H: Renal allograft salvage after prolonged early post-transplant renal occlusion. J Urol 129:1216, 1983.
87. Gerard DF, Devin JB, Halasz NA, et al: Transplantation renal artery thrombosis. Revascularization after 51 hours of ischemia. Arch Surg 117:361, 1982.
88. Sussman SK, Baker ME, Saeed M, et al: Polar infarct in a transplanted kidney: cause of a pseudomass. Urol Radiol 9:42, 1987.
89. Samara EN, Voss BL, Pederson JA: Renal artery thrombosis associated with elevated cyclosporine levels. Transplant Proc 20:119, 1988.
90. Rigotti P, Flechner SM, VanBuren CT, et al: Increased incidence of renal allograft thrombosis under cyclosporine immunosuppression. Int Surg 71:38, 1986.
91. Grace AA, Barrados MA, Mikhailidis DP, et al: Cyclosporin A enhances platelet aggregation. Kidney Int 32:889, 1987.
92. Vanrenterghem Y, Roels L, Lerut T, et al: Thromboembolic complications and hemostatic changes in Cyclosporin A-treated cadaveric kidney allograft recipients. Lancet 4:1, 1985.
93. Colonna JO, Quinones-Baldrich W, Ray R, et al: Does Cyclosporin A increase arterial anastomotic thrombosis? Curr Surg 44:485, 1987.
94. Gruber SA, Pescovitz MD, Simmons RL, et al: Thromboembolic complications in renal allograft recipients. Transplantation 44:775, 1987.
95. Brunkwall J, Bergqvist D, Bergentz SE, et al: Postoperative deep venous thrombosis after renal transplantation. Effects of cyclosporine. Transplantation 43:647, 1987.
96. Robinson JM, Cockrell CH, Tisnado J, et al.: Selective low-dose streptokinase infusion in the treatment of acute transplant renal vein thrombosis. Cardiovasc Intervent Radiol 9:86, 1986.

97. Nghiem DD, Corry RJ: Long-term result of conservative surgical management of the ruptured renal transplant. Am Surg 49:392, 1983.
98. Markus BH, Hakala TR, Tzakis A, et al: Kidney transplantation in Pittsburgh. In Terasaki P, ed: Clinical Transplants 1987. Los Angeles UCLA Tissue Typing Laboratory, 1987, p 141.
99. Benoit G, Icard P, LeBaleur A, et al: Mycotic aneurysm and renal transplantation. Urology 31:63, 1988.
100. Blohm I, Brynger H: Emergency ligation of the external iliac artery. Ann Surg 201:505, 1985.
101. Luke RG: Hypertension in renal transplant recipients. Kidney Int 31:1024, 1987.
102. Curtis JJ: Hypertension and kidney transplantation. Am J Kidney Dis 7:181, 1986.
103. Rijksen JF, Koolen MI, Walaszewski JE, et al: Vascular complications in 400 consecutive renal allotransplants. J Cardiovasc Surg 23:91, 1982.
104. Dubovsky EV, Curtis JJ, Luke RG, et al: Captopril as a predictor of curable hypertension in renal transplant recipients. Contrib Nephrol 56:117, 1987.
105. Gedroyc WM, Reidy JF, Saxton HM: Arteriography of renal transplantation. Clin Radiol 38:239, 1987.
106. Ricotta JJ, Schaff HV, Williams GM, et al: Renal artery stenosis following transplantation. Surgery 84:595, 1978.
107. Chandrasoma P, Aberle AM: Anastomotic line renal artery stenosis after transplantation. J Urol 135:1159, 1986.
108. Sagalowsky AI, Peters PC: Renovascular hypertension following renal transplantation. Urol Clin North Am 11:491, 1984.
109. Stanley P, Malekzadeh M, Diament MJ: Post-transplant renal artery stenosis: angiographic study in 32 children. Am J Roentgenol 148:487, 1987.
110. Morris PJ, Yadav RVS, Kincaid-Smith DP, et al: Renal artery stenosis in renal transplantation. Med J Aust 1:1255, 1971.
111. Dickerman RM, Peters PC, Hull AR, et al: Surgical correction of post-transplant renovascular hypertension. Ann Surg 192:639, 1980.
112. Smith RB, Cosimi AB, London R, et al: Diagnosis and management of arterial stenosis causing hypertension after successful renal transplantation. J Urol 115:639, 1976.
113. Clements R, Evans C, Salaman JR: Percutaneous transluminal angioplasty of renal transplant artery stenosis. Clin Radiol 38:235, 1987.
114. Lohr DJW, MacDougall ML, Chonko AM, et al: Percutaneous transluminal angioplasty in transplant renal artery stenosis. Am J Kidney Dis 7:363, 1986.
115. O'Donoghue R, Chisholm GD, Shackman R: The urologic complications of transplantation. Proc Eur Dial Transplant Assoc 8:252, 1971.
116. Hamburger J, Crosnier J, Dormont J, et al: Urinary fistulas. In Renal Transplantation. Baltimore, Williams & Wilkins, 1972, p 205.
117. May J, Sands J, Lawrence JR, et al: Australasian renal transplant survey. Proc Eur Dial Transplant Assoc 8:223, 1971.
118. Walsh A: Technical considerations in renal transplantation. Transplant Proc 1:178, 1969.
119. Loughlin KR, Tilney NL, Richie JP: Urologic complications in 718 renal transplant patients. Surgery 95:297, 1984.
120. Mundy AR, Podesta ML, Bewick M, et al: The urologic complications of 1000 renal transplants. Br J Urol 53:397, 1981.
121. Mitchell A, Fellows GJ, Wright FW, et al: Hydronephrosis in a transplanted kidney: the use of pressure-flow studies to exclude ureteric obstruction. Transplantation 32:152, 1981.
122. Lieberman RP, Crummy AB, Glass NR, et al: Fine needle antegrade pyelography in the renal transplant. J Urol 126:155, 1981.
123. Barbaric ZL, Thompson KR: Percutaneous nephrostomy in the management of obstructed renal transplants. Radiology 126:639, 1978.
124. Glanz S, Rotter MR, Gordon DH, et al: Interventional radiologic procedure in the management of the renal transplant patient. Urol Radiol 7:97, 1985.
125. Curry NS, Cochran S, Barbaric ZL, et al: Interventional radiologic procedures in the renal transplant. Radiology 152:647, 1984.
126. Hunter DW, Castaneda-zuniga WR, Coleman CC, et al: Percutaneous techniques in the management of urological complications in renal transplant patients. Radiology 148:407, 1983.
127. Jarowenko MV, Flechner SM, Snadler CM, et al: Salvage of difficult transplant complications by percutaneous techniques. J Urol 133:840, 1985.
128. Bennett LN, Voegeli DR, Crummy AB, et al: Urologic complications following renal transplantation: role of interventional radiologic procedures. Radiology 160:531, 1986.
129. Ehrlichman RJ, Bettman M, Kirkman RL, et al: The use of percutaneous nephrostomy in patients with ureteric obstruction undergoing renal transplantation. Surg Gynecol Obstet 162:125, 1986.
130. Streem SB, Novick AC, Steinmuller DR, et al: Percutaneous techniques for the management of urological renal transplant complications. J Urol 135:456, 1986.
131. McWhinnie DL, Bradley JA, Briggs JD, et al: Early detection of obstructed ureter by ultrasound following renal transplantation. Proc Eur Dial Transplant Assoc 20:320, 1983.
132. Kinnaert P, Hall M, Janssen F, et al: Ureteral stenosis after kidney transplantation. J Urol 133:17, 1985.
133. Bushnell DL, Wilson DG, Lieberman LM: Scintigraphic assessment of perivesical urinary extravasation following renal transplantation. Clin Nucl Med 9:92, 1984.
134. Van Poppel H, Arango O, Gilovernet JM: Caliceal urinary fistula in renal allotransplantation. Eur Urol 11:277, 1985.
135. Rajfer J, Koyle MA, Ehrlich RM, et al: Pyelovesicostomy as a form of urinary reconstruction in renal transplantation. J Urol 136:372, 1986.
136. Jarowenko MV, Flechner SM: Recipient ureterocalycostomy in a renal allograft. J Urol 133:844, 1985.
137. Toguri AG, Emtage JB, Jarzylo SV: Management of total loss after kidney transplantation. Can J Surg 26:498, 1983.
138. Danovitch GM, Nast C, Rosenthal JT, et al: Evaluation of fine needle aspiration biopsy in the diagnosis of renal transplant dysfunction. Am J Kidney Dis (in press).
139. Kallash SS, Murakkassa WF, Campbell EW, et al: Persistent clot anuria complicating renal transplant biopsy. Urology 25:591, 1985.
140. Stegmayr B, Orsten PA: Lysis of obstructive renal pelvic clots with retrograde instillation of streptokinase. Scand J Urol 18:347, 1984.
141. Salaman JR, Calne RY, Pena J, et al: Surgical aspects of clinical renal transplantation. Br J Surg 56:413, 1969.
142. Pigott JP, Sharp WV: Arteriovenous fistula involving a transplant kidney. Transplantation 44:156, 1987.

143. Lehr HA, Waltzer WC, Anaise D, et al: Management of a postbiopsy arterial pseudoaneurysm in a transplanted kidney. Transplant Proc 18:976, 1986.
144. Moreau JF, Merland JJ, Descamps JM: Post-biopsy false arterial aneurysm of a transplanted kidney. J Urol 128:116, 1982.
145. Rao KV: Urological complications associated with a kidney transplant biopsy. J Urol 135:768, 1986.
146. Chiverton SG, Musie JA, Allen RD, et al: Renal transplant nephrectomy. Surg Gynecol Obstet 164:324, 1987.
147. Starnes HF, McWhinnie DL, Bradley JA, et al: Delayed major arterial hemorrhage after transplant nephrectomy. Transplant Proc 16:1320, 1984.
148. Dumler F: Gross hematuria caused by ureteral remnant hemorrhage in a renal transplant recipient. South Med J 74:81, 1981.
149. Van Gansbeke D, Zalcman M, Matos C, et al: Lithiasis complications of renal transplantation: the donor graft lithiasis concept. Urol Radiol 7:157, 1985.
150. Brien G, Scholz D, Oesterwitz H, et al: Urolithiasis after kidney transplantation. Urol Res 8:211, 1980.
151. Fuchs AM, Fuchs GJ, Stenzl A: Extracorporeal shock wave lithotripsy of urinary calculi in transplanted kidneys. J Urol (in press).
152. Taylor RJ, Rosenthal JT, Schwentker FN, et al: Factors in urologic complications in 400 cadaveric renal transplants. J Urol 131:336A, 1984.
153. Salvatierra O, Olcott C, Amend WJ, et al: Urologic complications of renal transplantation can be prevented or controlled. J Urol 117:421, 1977.
154. Walzer WC, Zincke H, Leary FJ, et al: Urinary tract reconstruction in renal transplantation. Urology 16:233, 1980.
155. Jaskowski A, Jones RM, Muri JA, et al: Urologic complications in 600 consecutive renal transplants. Br J Surg 74:922, 1987.

COMPLICATIONS OF URETERAL SURGERY

20

Alan M. Freedman • Richard M. Ehrlich • Richard David

Perhaps the most surprising aspect of ueteral injuries is that they do not occur more often. With the number of surgeries on the abdomen and pelvis, including hysterectomies, colon resections, aortoiliac procedures, and urologic operations done yearly in this country, it is rare that the urologist is called to treat an obstructed or transected ureter. Despite the number of accidents seen in our emergency rooms, there are remarkably few ureteral injuries resulting from abdominal trauma.

Ureteral injuries may be occult and may present on a delayed basis with vague abdominal symptoms or fevers. There is no question that whenever a ureteral injury does occur, it is a major problem for the patient, surgeon, and urologist and needs to be diagnosed and treated as expediently as possible. The trend over the last 10 years has been to treat the injury as soon as it is discovered. If given the opportunity, most urologists would prefer to evaluate and treat a ureteral complication in the operating room as soon as it occurs. Failing this, an aggressive approach as soon as the injury is discovered is needed. Careful preoperative and operative evaluations are necessary for optimal results. Radiographic studies of ureteral trauma are not complete until they demonstrate the entire ureter.[1,2] This may require combinations of intravenous, antegrade, and retrograde pyelograms. Even if one has a preoperative plan of how to repair the injured ureter, one must enter the operating room with complete flexibility to change plans in case the injury is different or more extensive than originally anticipated. One of the problems with our ability to assess a ureteral injury is that there is often a discrepancy between the radiographic and intraoperative findings. Although there are certain radiographic criteria for assessing viability of the ureter, including segmental narrowing, lack of peristalsis, hydronephrosis, and so forth, these often underestimate the actual amount of ureter that needs to be sacrificed to restore function.

In repairing the ureteral injury, basic tenets apply: debridement to leave only viable tissue even if this means removing or bypassing much more ureter than one would have expected; anastomosis with no tension; the use of indwelling ureteral stents; adequate periureteral drainage; and, at times, proximal diversion of urine, especially in emergency situations or when there has been recent infection in the vicinity of the ureteral repair.

SURGICAL ANATOMY

Most surgeons, gynecologists, and urologists are knowledgeable about ureteral anatomy. If all operations were performed through a generous midline incision, without adhesions or distortion of intraperitoneal or retroperitoneal structures, the ureters would be easy to identify and protect. The task becomes more difficult when pathology distorts the ureters. Also, with a different or limited surgical approach, the surgeon needs three-dimensional perception to relate the ureter to adjacent structures. For example, the Pfannenstiel incision, often used for gynecologic surgery, rarely allows the degree of mobilization needed above and below the ureter to aid in its identification and repair.

The upper two thirds of the ureter is adherent to overlying peritoneum. On flank and lateral surgical approaches, the ureter is always more anterior and medial than expected. On transperitoneal approaches, the upper two thirds is found most easily by medial reflection (kocherization) of the duodenum. The ureter's adherence to the peritoneum may lead to its inclusion during the process of peritonealization, often undetaken at the end of vascular and gynecologic procedures. On both sides, the ureter passes anteriorly over the psoas muscle posterior to the colonic mesentery. On the right side, it is crossed anteriorly by right colic, ileocolic, and superior mesenteric vessels; on the left side, it is crossed by left colic vessels at its entrance into the true pelvis (Fig. 20–1). The inferior mesenteric vein is medial and parallel to the left ureter but is slightly more anterior. However, its branches pass laterally in the sigmoid mesocolon directly over the ureter. Caution must be exercised during the course of a left hemicolectomy because this is a common site of ureteral injury.

The lower third of the ureter begins at the pelvic inlet, where the ureter crosses the bifurcation of the common iliac artery. The pelvic ureter is far more at risk than its abdominal counterpart. At the level of the bifurcation of the common iliac artery, the ureter descends posterolaterally and then anteriorly at the level of the ischial spine. At this point, it courses on top of the levator ani muscle to reach the trigone of the bladder. Below the iliac bifurcation, the ureter becomes more difficult to identify as it is eventually entangled in the small anterior branches of the hypogastric vessels, passing laterally to medially to reach the pelvic viscera.

In the female, the ureter lies behind the posterior peritoneum in the bed of the ovary (Fig. 20–2). This is at the level of the uterosacral ligaments. Just distal to this point, the ureter

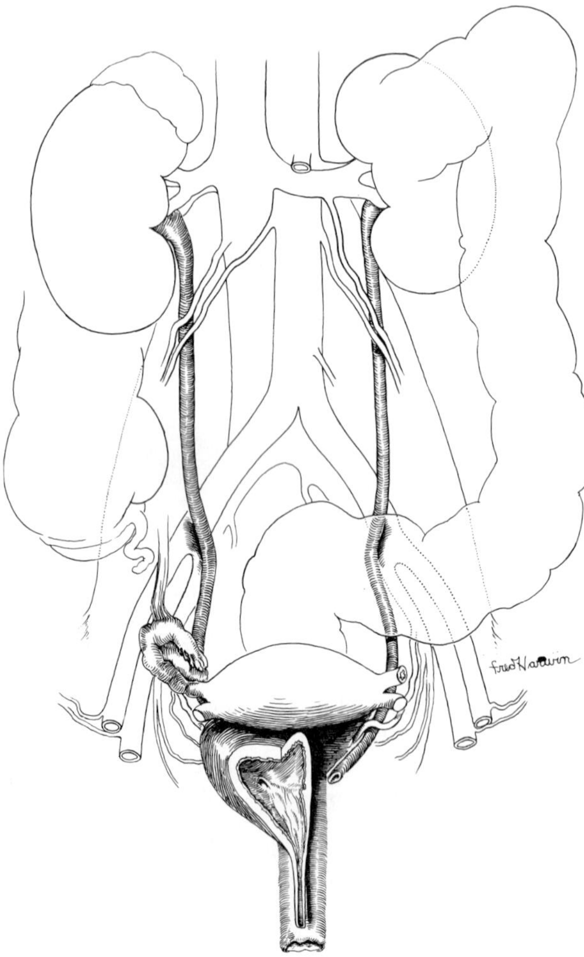

Figure 20–1. Anatomy of the ureter. (From Smith RB, Skinner DG, eds: Complications of Urologic Disorders. Philadelphia, WB Saunders Co, 1976, by permission.)

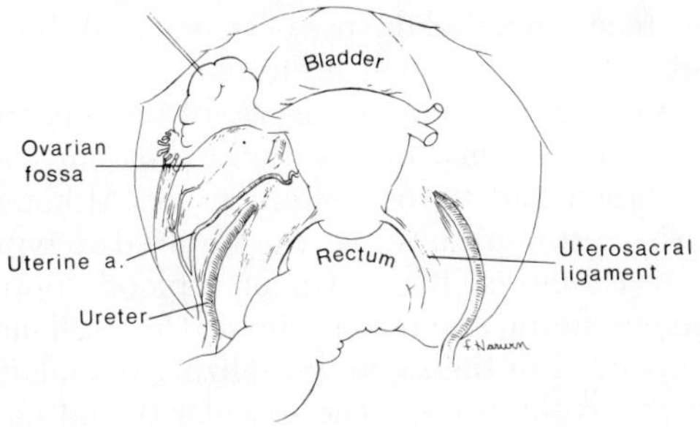

Figure 20–2. Anatomic relationships of the female pelvic ureter. (From Smith RB, Skinner DB, eds: Complications of Urologic Disorders. Philadelphia, WB Saunders Co, 1976, by permission.)

enters the base of the broad ligament. (Some authors refer to an anterior and posterior compartment of the broad ligament, placing the ureter in the posterior compartment.) At this point, the ureter first lies parallel to the proximal uterine arteries and is then crossed by them, 1 to 2 cm lateral to the uterocervical junction. The uterine vessels are most safely approached and ligated as close to their origin as possible, especially if the ureter has not been mobilized more inferiorly. Other sources on radical hysterectomy recommend ligating the uterine vessels medial to the ureter so as to preserve perforating branches of the uterine artery to the lateral aspect of the deep pelvic ureter.[3]

In the male, the ureter is seen coursing lateral to the anterior rectal wall, in the cul-de-sac between the rectum and bladder, behind the peritoneal reflection. The ureter is then crossed lateral to medial by the vas deferens, which arises from the internal ring inferiorly. When the posterior peritoneum is incised over the rectum for rectal resection, the incision should not be extended too far laterally since injury may occur to the vas deferens or the ureter at this point.

The ureter receives blood from almost all vessels near it (Fig. 20–3). Ureteral branches of the renal, gonadal, and internal iliac vessels reach the fibrous sheath of the ureter and form a freely anastomotic network within the adventitia. Because of this network, it is generally safe to sacrifice any one perforating blood vessel in order to mobilize the ureter. An attempt should be made, however, to mobilize the abdominal ureter laterally and the pelvic ureter medially. Also, the mid-ureter is the weak point in the adventitial blood supply. In this area, it is particularly important to avoid dissecting within the sheath of the ureter and, if at all possible, to avoid sacrificing the perforating perpendicular blood vessels.

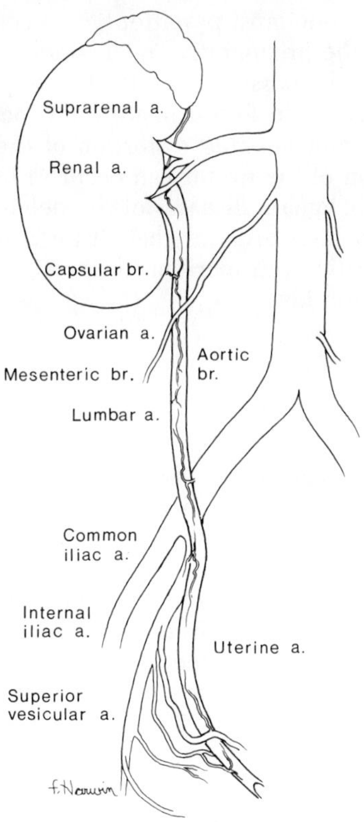

Figure 20–3. Blood supply of the ureter. (From Smith RB, Skinner DG, eds: Complications of Urologic Disorders. Philadelphia, WB Saunders Co, 1976, by permission.)

There are several important points in the anatomic identification of the ureter. It is very difficult to identify the ureteral course by trying to see through the posterior peritoneum. If there is any question about the ureter being involved by suture, scar tissue, and so on, it is preferable to incise the posterior peritoneum away from the suspect area and to dissect toward the area carefully, staying lateral to the abdominal ureter and medial to the pelvic ureter. In this manner, one can actually identify the ureter without entering its adventitial sheath.

The presence of peristalsis is a good sign; the usual test for this is to "pinch" the ureter and observe for vermiculation, or a worm-like peristaltic movement for approximately 10 seconds. However, if the ureter is involved in a pathologic process, one may have to identify what he thinks is the ureter without being able to induce peristalsis. If one is concerned about the integrity of the pelvic ureter, it is best to isolate the ureter overlying the common iliac vesels at the pelvic inlet and to carefully dissect the ureter inferiorly to identify its course in the posterior compartment of the broad ligament.

Finally, one must pay attention to certain nuances of the preoperative pyelographic studies, including the possibility of ureteral duplication, which occurs in approximately 0.6 percent of patients, and possible distortion of the ureter. Distortion of the ureter can occur in benign as well as malignant diseases of the pelvis. Examples of benign diseases that distort the ureter are idiopathic retroperitoneal fibrosis and large uterine fibroids.

VIABILITY

The fact that the ureteral tissue is present in any area of trauma cannot be taken as evidence of viability. Viability means not only that the tissue is alive and healthy at the time of surgery but also that the tissue can be expected to remain healthy after it is repaired. Devitalization of the ureter can be predicted by knowledge of the mechanism of injury and, sometimes, by preoperative radiography. The field of damage induced by radiotherapy, metastatic tumor, or blast trauma will always be greater than what is apparent radiographically or surgically. Turner-Warwick has described "gray zones" around urethral strictures; so, too, are there gray zones proximal and distal to a ureteral injury.[4]

Operative signs of devitalization include dense periureteral scarring, friability of tissues ("cheesy" ureter), lack of bleeding from cut edges, and inability to induce peristalsis by stroking the ureter. One technique found useful to determine viability is to inject intravenous fluorescein (1 ampule) and then inspect the injured ureter carefully with a Wood's lamp (ultraviolet light). We have found that this will often reveal an absence of fluorescence in an area that was deemed to be viable on gross examination.

Vigorous debridement is the key to avoiding postoperative complications. The best results of ureteral repair are undoubtedly achieved when all questionable tissue is removed and innovative techniques are used to bridge what sometimes may be lengthy ureteral gaps. Problems arise especially in ureteroureterostomies, which are often performed for abdominal ureteral injuries. During this procedure, the surgeon may fear that exuberant debridement may lead to tension on the anastomosis. Because of inadequate debridement, what often results is a tension-free anastomosis of tissue at risk for postoperative necrosis.

To improve the viability of the ureter, some have recommended the use of an omental sleeve graft.[5] It is known that ureteroureterostomies, for example, may not be successful if the ureter is allowed to lie in contact with the psoas muscle. Angulation and fibrosis often result. Although nearby retroperitoneal fat can be used to wrap the anastomosis, it has a poorer blood supply than omentum, and retroperitoneal fat itself may be involved in the same devitalizing pathologic process as the ureter. The vascularity and easy mobility of the omental pedicle, which is transferred from an atraumatic site to the traumatized area, is the key. The amount of omentum needed depends on the extent of the ureteral injury as well as its location. An omental graft of distal ureter may require total detachment of the omentum from left to right and from the greater curvature of the stomach and transverse colon. This, of course, necessitates an extensive abdominal exposure. Lesser injuries of the upper ureter may require only a small portion of the ipsilateral omentum to be mobilized through a peritoneal window to comfortably reach the ureteral anastomosis.

ETIOLOGY

There are several mechanisms of ureteral injury. By far the most common mechanisms are direct laceration, ligation, and devascularization during abdominal or pelvic surgery. Pathologic processes may involve the ureter secondarily. These processes include benign diseases, such as idiopathic retroperitoneal fibrosis and fibrosis secondary to prior pelvic surgery, and malignant processes, such as metastatic tumor in the aortoiliac lymph node chains. Abdominal aortic aneurysms often induce an intense fibroblastic reaction around them, thereby not only distorting the ureter, but also helping to devascularize it. Traumatic injuries need to be addressed separately since there are often adjacent organs injured at the same time, and the ureteral repair may depend on the kind of repair peformed on contiguous structures. Also, prior radiation therapy, which is being used increasingly, has deleterious effects on the ureter and implications in terms of the type of repair performed.

Trauma

Traumatic ureteral injuries may be blunt or penetrating. Blunt trauma is less likely to be associated with ureteral injury than penetrating trauma, and low-velocity penetrating trauma, such as stab wounds and low-velocity bullets, is implicated less than high-velocity penetrating trauma. The amount of ureteral trauma is determined by the amount of kinetic energy of the missile, which, in turn, is arithmetically related to the square of the velocity. Higher-velocity accidents result in wider zones of devitalized ureteral tissue.[6]

Unfortunately, several studies have demonstrated that neither hematuria nor an abnormal intravenous urogram can be used as a reliable indicator of traumatic ureteral injury.[7] In one series, nearly 20 percent of patients with surgically proven ureteral injuries had preoperative urograms that were interpreted as normal. There are several explanations for this. Intraveneous urography done prior to emergency laparotomy is often a hasty (one-shot) film that may demonstrate function of both kidneys but rarely demonstrates the entire course of the ureters. Because of shock and hypoperfusion of the kidneys, urine output may be low and, therefore, intraureteral pressure too low to demonstrate extravasation or dilation. Periureteral hematoma or urinoma can actually tamponade the partially transected ureter and allow contrast to remain intraluminally. Also, the ureter can be devitalized by periureteral interruption of blood supply, without the acute-phase urogram showing either hydronephrosis or extravasation. Only a repeat urogram, when symptoms arise, may reveal a missed injury.

Seldom is a patient with blunt abdominal trauma explored only for a suspected ureteral injury. If the urogram suggests a partial ureteral disruption, and the patient is not going to undergo laparotomy for other reasons, a retrograde pyelogram with placement of a ureteral stent monitored fluoroscopically is a reasonable approach. If laparotomy is otherwise necessary, there is usually inadequate time to perform retrograde pyelography, and the ureter will need to be carefully explored after incising the posterior peritoneum.

When laparotomy is needed for blunt or penetrating trauma, ureteral exploration should be done if the associated injuries indicate a likelihood of ureteral trauma. Ureteral exploration must consist of more than palpation of the ureter through the posterior peritoneum. If, after carefully mobilizing the ureter outside of its adventitial sheath, suspicion of injury persists, a ureteral catheter should be passed intraluminally through a remote ureterotomy. If the ureter is intact but may be devitalized, the minimal requirement is stenting the ureter and placing a drain next to the traumatized area. In this case, one may also consider wrapping the intact but traumatized area of ureter in an omental sleeve. When ureter and adjacent bowel are lacerated, requiring suturing of both, it is essential that the suture lines not lie in apposition to each other. If spatial separation cannot be guaranteed, the urine should be diverted by a nephrostomy tube, and a pad of omentum or retroperitoneal fat must be interposed between the two suture lines. Failure to do this may lead to a ureteroenteric fistula (in the case of a bowel injury) or a ureteroiliac fistula (in the case of an iliac artery injury).

The association between ureteral and duodenal injury from penetrating trauma is illustrated in the following case report. In this case, paradoxically, the ureteral injury was apparent, but the duodenal injury was not.

Case Report. A 28-year-old male was involved in an altercation during which he allegedly stabbed another male, who thereupon stabbed the patient in the right flank area. The patient was conscious, had normal vital signs and presented with an expanding mass in the right flank, which was tender. Serial examinations revealed no evidence of peritonitis, but tenderness in the flank. A computed axial tomography (CAT) scan was performed (Fig. 20–4), which revealed obvious extravasation of intravenously administered contrast material from the region of the upper ureter. No bowel or pancreatic injury was apparent on the CAT scan. There was no extravasation of orally administered meglumine diatrizoate (Gastrografin). A retrograde pyelogram (Fig. 20–5) revealed extravasation of contrast material from the upper ureter, below the ureteropelvic junction, but continuity of the ureter above this point. The patient was then explored through a midline transperitoneal incision.

A transverse 3-mm laceration was noted on the anterior surface of the upper ureter, which was sutured, stented, and drained. However, upon further examination of the kocherized duodenum, a 3-mm full thickness laceration was noted in the duodenum with leakage of duodenal contents. This was closed in two layers, inverting the mucosa, and was spatially separated from the ureteral closure using a locally mobilized piece of omentum. The postoperative clinical and radiographic results were excellent.

The literature does not report a vast experience in dealing with blunt injuries to the ureter. Over the last 10 years, there have been sporadic reports of interesting injuries resulting from blunt traumas, often to a large extrarenal pelvis. These are often deceleration injuries, in which there is a clean disruption of the renal pelvis from the upper ureter.[8]

On the other hand, there is an extensive ex-

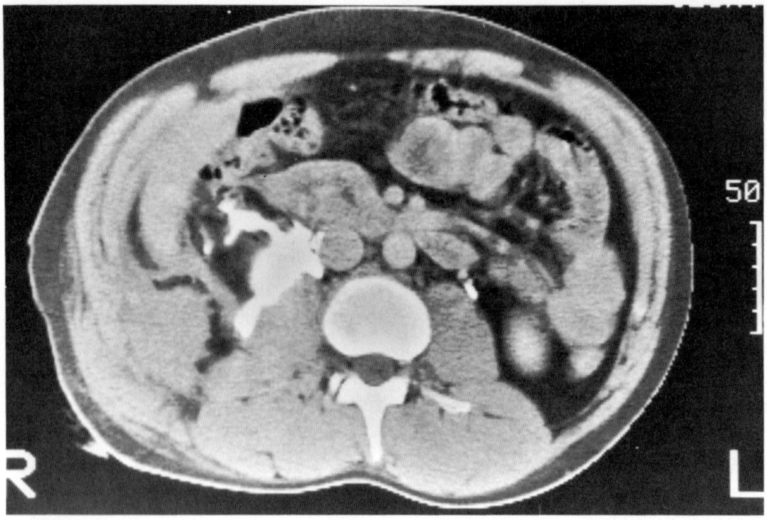

Figure 20–4. CT scan with intravenous contrast showing free extravasation of urine from upper ureter.

perience with penetrating trauma to the ureter, much of which was obtained during the Vietnam War.[6] The Vietnam experience taught surgeons that in patients with extensive injury with necrosis, proximal urinary diversion with a nephrostomy tube is extremely important. Many of the problems resulting from attempts at primary repair were related to breakdown of the anastomosis, with extravasation of urine, formation of fistulas, and sepsis. It is quite possible that in these patients, proximal diversion would not have totally obviated the need for further surgery of the ureter but might have reduced postoperative morbidity and allowed for a less scarred field in which to operate. The literature points out that stents alone are not adequate to divert the urine in patients with high-velocity ballistic injuries. Obviously, if the anastomosis is of adequate caliber, there is going to be leakage of urine around the catheter, out through the poorly healing suture line.

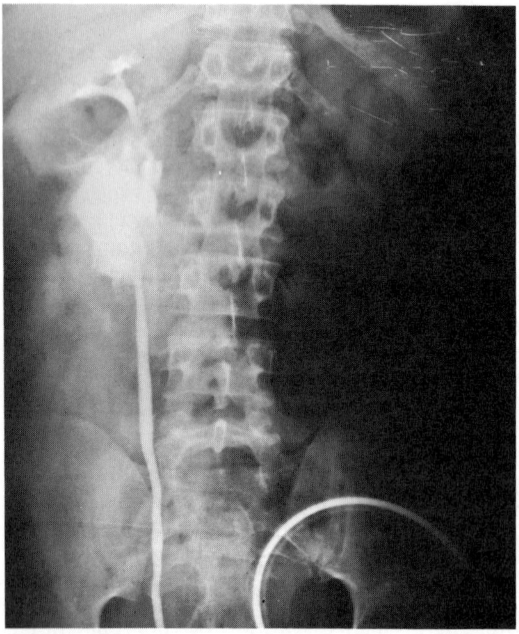

Figure 20–5. Operative retrograde pyelogram shows ureteral continuity despite gross urinary extravasation.

Delay in diagnosis of ureteral injury resulting from trauma carries with it significant morbidity. This is especially tragic when an opportunity to assess the ureter at the time of the initial laparotomy is not utilized by the surgeon. Rohrer reports on three cases of war-related bullet wounds to the abdomen; in two cases, intravenous indigo carmine was given and was not seen extravasating from the ureter.[9] In all three cases, the path of the bullet was unquestionably near the ureter, and in all three, a delayed fistula resulted. Besides the blast effect with high focal kinetic energy and thrombosis of periureteral vessels, a heat effect was also postulated which, along with bacterial contamination, was thought to produce delayed breakdown of tissue and fistula.

Post-irradiation Ureteral Injuries

Radiation-induced ureteral injuries, generally obstructions, occur approximately 22 to 30 months after primary therapy, with an incidence of 0.4 to 8 percent.[10] The variabilty in incidence may relate to techniques employed; interestingly, some of the newer series of radiation injuries to the ureter actually report higher incidences of obstruction than reported in the older series. This may be due to better detection or more aggressive follow-up of ureteral injuries in more recent series.

Although the average elapsed time between radiation therapy and ureteral injury is 2 years, the range can be anywhere from 6 months to 10 or more years. The etiology of ureteral obstruction following radiation includes reduced vascular supply secondary to endarteritis obliterans and proliferation of connective tissue, with contraction of the periureteral fibrous tissue. The end result is either a localized stricture or sometime, a long, thread-like stenosis, usually in the pelvic ureter.

Progressive ureteral obstruction demonstrated within 1 year of radiotherapy for pelvic malignancy generally results from recurrent tumor and not from radiation effect. Computed tomography (CT) scan or magnetic resonance imaging (MRI) may be beneficial in distinguishing these etiologies. In the irradiated pelvis, the parametric and paravesical tissues are often fibrotic, and mobilization of the bladder is not possible. Surgeries to repair post-irradiation ureteral structures may, therefore, be more difficult than repairs in the non-radiation setting. Transureteroureterostomy (TUU) may be helpful here. The benefit of TUU is that it bypasses irradiated bladder and paravesical tissues that may make the creation of either a bladder flap or a psoas hitch too difficult. The problem with TUU is that if the contralateral pelvic ureter develops a delayed stricture, the patient will have bilateral ureteral obstruction secondary to the obstructed common distal ureter. The best solution for the irradiated structure may, indeed, be one of the more aggressive approaches. Use of an ileal ureter will allow for ipsilateral drainage and bypass of the stenotic segment, without placing the contralateral renal unit at risk. The ileal ureteroneocystostomy is less likely to obstruct because of its wide orifice (see discussion below).

Gynecologic Ureteral Injuries

There are several mechanisms for pelvic ureteral injury during gynecologic surgery. Although readily apparent in most cases, these injuries may be confirmed by intravenous injection of indigo carmine with observation of leakage of stained urine. Ligation without laceration could easily go unrecognized. Stripping of the ureter by entering the sheath, or ligation of the periureteral tissues may be the most common mechanism leading to fistulas. As always, fistulas result from two opposing viscera, each with loss of integrity. The sutured vaginal stump is indeed in apposition to the injured pelvic ureter, and the usual postoperative inflammatory reaction enhances the adhesiveness between these two structures.

An attempt to control sudden bleeding from the uterine arteries may lead to placement of a clamp or suture material too far posteriorly, thus including periureteral tissue or the ureter itself. If possible, the bleeding area should be tamponaded with a sponge stick, and a precise bleeder identified. Fine absorbable hemostatic suture material should be used in the vicinity of the ureter. Failing this, one can find the plane between the uterine vessels and the ureter, while continuing to compress the hemorrhagic vessels. If the clamp or suture has already been placed, integrity of the ureter should be aggressively established. This may require a cystotomy or distant ureterotomy, with passage of a ureteral catheter through the suspect area.

Traditionally, radical hysterectomy has been associated with a high percentage of gynecologic ureteral injuries.[3,10,11] The stage of the uterine or cervical malignancy, prior radiation, and technique employed are interactive in leading to injuries. Several modifications have been recommended to diminish ureteral injury and fistula. Most of these pertain to the management of the ureter after the uterus has been removed. Buschbaum reported no fistulas in 23 patients with reperitonealization and drainage of the retroperitoneal space with suction catheters brought out through the abdominal wound.[3] This technique was previously advocated by Symmonds and Pratt in 1961.[12] Drainage of serous fluid seems to favor adherence of the ureter to the lateral pelvic sidewall, thus spatially separating it from the vaginal stump. Other techniques, including suspending the ureteral adventitia from the superior vesical artery and placing the ureter in the envelope of peritoneum, have their advocates but are seldom used in this country.[13,14] Besides radical hysterectomy, there are other gynecologic surgeries that have an undue association with ureteral injuries. Operations for endometriosis are often difficult because of the diffuse nature of the disease, secondary involvement of the ureter and/or bladder wall, and inflammatory reaction and adhesions induced by the endometrial ectopic tissues. Uterine fibroids are an example of a benign disease that can result in significant distortion of the ureter. In some cases, the ureter may actually lie quite medial to the fibroid extensions of the uterine fundus.

During vaginal hysterectomy, the anatomy may be difficult for those surgeons more familiar with the abdominal approach to the uterus and retroperitoneum. Vaginal hysterectomy requires an anterior and posterior colpotomy, through which the peritoneal cavity anterior and posterior to the uterus is entered. Following the anterior colpotomy, a retractor is placed under the bladder to elevate it anteriorly. This leaves a thick fold of tissue on either side of the midline, which gynecologists refer to as "bladder pillars." Cruikshank uses a technique in which the ureters are not only palpated in the bladder pillars but are actually mobilized after incision of the peritoneum on either bladder pillar.[15] He advises entering the retroperitoneal space lateral to the peritoneum over the bladder pillar and sweeping the ureter anteromedially to displace it from the underlying hypogastric artery. With sufficient lateral retraction of the vagina the ureter can actually be visualized and is seen to be clear of the branches of the hypogastric artery. Following this, the uterine vessels are ligated at the point of their origin, and the specimen is removed.

If recognized intraoperatively, most gynecologic ureteral injuries can be repaired with a very high success rate. Most of the techniques involve direct reimplantation of the ureter into the bladder, sometimes with the aid of a psoas hitch. More problematic, however, is the delayed injury.[16] This is compounded by the fact that ureteral obstructions that occur during the course of gynecologic surgery may be asymptomatic, thus leading to silent hydronephrosis and loss of renal function. Follow-up intravenous urograms or ultrasonograms are advocated by many but may be misleading in that it is not uncommon to find mild to moderate hydronephrosis for several months postoperatively. Certainly, after 2 to 3 months postoperatively, hydronephrosis due to simple ureteral atony should have subsided. Therefore, by this time, an aggressive approach to diagnosis and treatment is indicated, even if there is not yet evidence of any renal atrophy. A urogram or nuclear renogram, with Lasix washout, is highly recommended to differentiate obstructive hydronephrosis from nonobstructive hydronephrosis following gynecologic surgery.

General Surgical Ureteral Injuries

There is a scant number of reports in the literature of general surgical injuries to the ureter.[17] The ureter is in intimate contact with many of the abdominal and pelvic viscera treated by the general surgeon. In particular, the left colon and the colorectal area are at risk as well as the area of the aortoiliac bifurcation. Diseases that induce an inflammatory and fibrous reaction, such as abdominal aortic aneurysm and diverticulitis of the colon, are more likely not only to involve the ureter, but also to draw the ureter toward the area of inflammation. Thus, the ureter is at especially high risk during procedures for extirpation of these diseases, although less so with mass lesions, such as tumors, which tend to compress the ureter or to deviate it laterally.

Although, in general, the preoperative placement of ureteral stents has not been shown to diminish the risk of ureteral injury, in some patients, its benefit is more clear. During procedures such as left hemicolectomy for diverticulitis, in which the ureter is likely to be involved in the inflammatory reaction, a preoperative stent will be helpful in identification and will make it easier to repair the ureter if it is lacerated during the procedure.

One problematic area is that of ureteral injury incurred during the course of a prosthetic vascular graft operation.[18] In patients undergoing this procedure, not only is there a risk of having opposing suture lines of ureter and the vascular anastomosis, but there is also the problem of potential infection of the prosthetic material. If an injury to the ureter is discovered intraoperatively, a meticulous repair should be performed and spatial separation made using omentum between the ureteral repair and the vascular anastomosis. Urinary diversion using a nephrostomy tube for at least 10 days to 2 weeks postoperatively is important.

If the injury is noted postoperatively, a decision must be made as to whether the involved renal unit needs to be salvaged. In an elderly patient or a patient who may not withstand another abdominal exploration, a simple ipsilateral nephrectomy, using a flank approach, must be strongly considered. In some cases of ureteral obstruction, it is discovered that a vascular graft has been placed anterior to the ureter. In these patients, it may be beneficial to revise the vascular graft by dividing it and placing it posterior to the ureter.

When a decision is made to re-explore a vascular graft patient with ureteral obstruction alone, extreme care must be taken to avoid injuring the ureter; in these patients, a fistula is far worse than the obstruction. In the case of a delayed fistula, it is an extremely difficult task to reconstruct the ureter anywhere near the area of the fistula. Because these fistulas tend to be higher in the abdomen than gynecologic fistulas, procedures such as reimplantation with a psoas hitch or Boari flap are not possible. Transureteroureterostomy may be considered, but this, too, may be limited by the pathologic process in and around the aorta, which may prevent mobilizing the ipsilateral ureter across the midline. Therefore, even in the younger, healthier patient, the best decision may be to sacrifice the ipsilateral kidney. If the patient presents with septicemia and a ureteral obstruction or fistula, a percutaneous nephrostomy is placed, and after resolution of the acute infection, a nephrectomy is performed.

Urologic Injuries to the Ureter

An increasing percentage of ureteral injuries occur during the course of urologic surgeries. A number of these are being seen following ureteroscopy. The literature on ureteroscopic injury alludes to several technical points, including the placement of a guidewire, adequate dilation of the ureter, the use of the C-arm fluoroscopy (if available), and careful advancement of the ureteroscope under direct vision.

Most of the ureteral injuries during ureteral endoscopy are minor and consist of small perforations. If these are in the pelvic ureter, they have no significance, as long as the ureter is either stented or the urine is proximally diverted with a nephrostomy tube. The more significant injuries during ureteral endoscopy are avulsions. These may occur with forceful placement of the ureterscope but more often occur during the course of ureteral stone extraction, in which care must be taken to be sure that the stone is completely free of the surrounding ureteral mucosa. As opposed to perforation injuries, which are focal and small and generally heal primarily, avulsion injuries may leave a large gap of ureter. These gaps cannot heal primarily and often require delayed open surgery, despite what seems to be adequate stenting or proximal diversion.

During the course of surgery on the upper ureter or ureteropelvic junction, the ureter will occasionally be avulsed from the renal pelvis. Attempts to directly reanastomose these structures may involve anastomotic tension. Therefore, one must be familiar with other techniques (discussed below) to bridge the gap in the ureter at this level. The lower ureter is vulnerable to several kinds of open urologic procedures. During the course of vesical diverticulectomy or radical prostatectomy, the distal or intramural ureter may be injured. Injuries to this portion of the ureter are usually managed easily but may require remobilization of the uninjured ureter outside the bladder and a combined extravesical and intravesical reimplantation. During radical prostatectomy, the ureter may be injured during ligation of the proximal branches of the inferior vesical artery or during retrovesical dissection of the seminal vesicle, the tip of which is in close proximity to the ureter as it enters the trigone. The intramural ureter may also be injured during transection of the posterior bladder neck if the dissection progresses cephalad within the layers of the detrusor, instead of in a straight anteroposterior direction.

In general, ureteral injuries sustained during urologic surgeries are often not reported because they tend to be readily noted at the time of the surgery and correctly repaired. Furthermore the urologist's knowledge of internal urinary diversion probably accounts for the relatively low complication rate after ureteral injuries sustained during urologic surgery.

PATIENT PREPARATION AND TIMING OF PROCEDURES

An important guideline in repairing ureteral injuries is to have several creative options available to handle any particular situation. Some techniques demand transperitoneal exposure. These include use of an ileal ureter and TUU. Other techniques, such as the psoas hitch and ureteroureterostomy, can be done extraperitoneally; however, because of extensive retroperitoneal scarring in the area of the injury, even these techniques are sometime more easily performed transperitoneally. One must not be overly concerned with avoiding entry into the peritoneal cavity unless there is suspicion of gross bacterial infection in the area. In patients with overt contamination, especially abscess, the preliminary procedure should probably be extraperitoneal drainage and percutaneous nephrostomy. This should precede any attempt to repair the injury. In difficult elective repairs, it is always wise to perform a complete bowel preparation. This will permit use of an ileal ureter as an option, and will also decrease postoperative morbidity should the bowel be inadvertently entered during an transperitoneal approach.

Concepts of when to repair a ureteral injury

have changed greatly with the advent of percutaneous techniques. The former practice was to repair the injury immediately (i.e., within a few days of discovering it) or to wait several months. It is very rare now that a nonoperative approach for several months is undertaken. If it is considered unwise to proceed immediately with surgery, temporization of the patient's symptoms can often be achieved by endourologic techniques. Although it is possible to actually cure some patients with endourologic techniques, it is the extent of the ureteral damage, rather than the means by which it is treated endourologically, that will determine the eventual outcome. For example, an extensive avulsion of the ureter (larger than 2 cm) may be temporized by percutaneous nephrostomy and even antegrade placement of a ureteral stent over a guidewire, but it is likely that the patient will require operative intervention later because the injured area would probably obstruct completely after removal of the stent.

Most of the recent literature has taught us that an aggressive approach, as early as when the ureteral injury is discovered, is preferred.[11,19,20] There is definitely a higher failure rate when either the injuries are not recognized early or they are intentionally treated on a delayed basis. There are conditions, however, for which the definitive procedure should be delayed. These are well known, including severe sepsis, fluid and electrolyte abnormalities, and severe inanition. Also, patients with limited life expectancy, including those with incurable cancer, should be considered for palliation with endourologic techniques alone.

The urologist should recall that, in general, a ureteral stricture is easier to palliate than a ureteral fistula. Although a percutaneous nephrostomy can be performed to treat a fistula, it may fail to completely stop leakage of urine through the fistula and may be technically difficult because hydronephrosis may be absent. In patients with a ureteral fistula, it is probably a better practice to attempt antegrade passage of a guidewire through the narrrowed area and to place a double pigtail stent over the guidewire. These techniques are exemplified in the following case report.

Case Report. A 37-year-old woman underwent a difficult removal of a benign soft tissue tumor of the deep pelvis that had caused marked deviation of the left ureter and left bladder sidewall, with attendant mild hydronephrosis. Preoperative retrograde ureteral stenting was impossible. The operative procedure went well, with minimal blood loss, and there was no evidence of urinary leakage prior to closure.

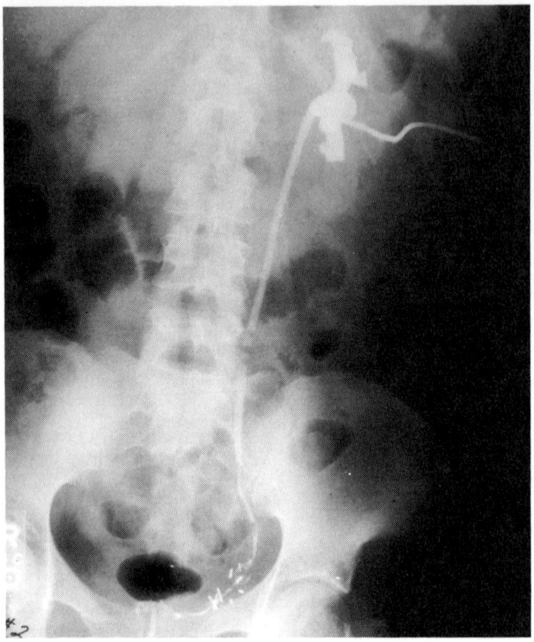

Figure 20–6. Left antegrade pyelogram demonstrates abnormal strictured area of pelvic ureter, previous site of uretero-cutaneous fistula.

However, on the third postoperative day, increasing amounts of urinary leakage were seen through the abdominal drains. X-rays revealed leakage of urine, from both the bladder and the left ureter. Hydronephrosis was absent. The patient was left on prolonged Foley catheter drainage, and the pelvic drain was advanced out. The urinary leakage stopped and the patient was released with bladder catheter drainage for several weeks. Following this, she developed acute pyelonephritis on the left side and was found to have hydronephrosis. A percutaneous nephrostomy was placed, and after the patient's sepsis resolved, an antegrade study demonstrated a stricture at the site of the prior ureterocutaneous fistula, with continuity for the ureter distal to the fistula (Fig. 20–6). An antegrade double pigtail stent was successfully placed, which temporized the patient until several months later, when she chose to have an elective ureteral reimplantation.

SPECIFIC PROCEDURES

The ureter is quite sensitive to trauma. Sometimes, even placement of a solitary absorbable suture around the ureter will result in a focal necrosis and stricture or fistula. Experimental studies on dogs have shown that simple deligation may yield satisfactory results if the interval of ligation is less than 1 week.[21] If, however, the interval is longer, the results are less impressive, although there may be some recovery of function over time. Sometimes, if ureteral ligation by an absorbable suture is suspected by the presence of postoperative hydronephrosis, it is reasonable to place a percutaneous nephrostomy and to observe the lower ureter for evidence of recanalization. If, however, within the time one would expect suture resorption (i.e., a few weeks) there is no change radiographically, one can assume that there has been some degree of irreversible injury to that ureteral segment.

Ureteroureterostomy

Ureteroureterostomy is the most commonly performed procedure for repairing an injury in the proximal two thirds of the ureter. Although some use this procedure for pelvic ureteral injuries, it is generally less preferable than direct reanastomosis of ureter to bladder. In patients with pelvic ureteral injuries, there is often significant devascularization of the distal ureteral stump, which would result in anastomotic failure.

The two most important principles in ureteroureterostomy, as in other reparative surgeries, are adequate debridement and ensuring lack of tension. If these are accomplished, the results will be excellent, whether or not the ureter is stented. The trend recently, however, has been to place an indwelling double pigtail catheter in most patients. It may also be wise to choose a double pigtail catheter without holes throughout the length of the catheter ("fistula" stent) to avoid leakage of urine from the inside to the outside of the stent, where the urine may get through the suture line.

After proper debridement, the ureter should be mobilized without compromising its blood supply. This requires sparing the larger perpendicular blood vessels in the mid-ureter, which is more tenuous in its blood supply than the proximal or distal ureter. The ureter should be handled atraumatically with a fine nontoothed forceps. Downward mobilization of the kidney is a useful adjunct to the ureteroureterostomy because it may yield several extra centimeters of ureter proximally, without tension. The anastomosis itself should always be oblique to allow for the greatest luminal diameter, which will always shrink a bit postoperatively (Fig. 20–7). Sutures should be absorbable, and we have found chromic to be ideal. The anastomosis should be watertight, and interrupted sutures avoid the problem of purse-string suturing of the oblique anastomosis. The sutures should be very fine and should be placed at appropriate intervals to ensure that no leakage occurs between them. Although some feel that placement of too many sutures may compromise the blood supply to the anastomotic region, we have found that this is not a problem with the use of fine suture material. Wrapping the anastomosis with healthy surrounding tissue, retroperitoneal fat at the minimum, or better, pedicled omentum, will prevent angulation and fixation of the anastomosis to the psoas muscle, with resulting cicatrix formation.

The duration of placement of intraureteral stenting is variable, but if one is going to use a stent, it is generally advisable that it be left in for a minimum of 2 weeks. A urogram, retrograde pyelogram or both can be performed prior to removing the stent to visualize contrast around the double J stent and to verify absence of periureteral leakage.

Some investigators have shown interest in microsurgical ureteroureterostomy.[22] Further experience will be needed to determine if this technique offers an advantage over standard ureteral anastomosis.

Transureteroureterostomy

Transureteroureterostomy (TUU) has a somewhat negative reputation. To be sure, it should not be among the first few procedures of choice for repairing a ureteral injury. It is, however, an important technique for patients in whom the pelvis must be avoided. Transureteroureterostomy would be ideal in patients with a pelvic abscess or in those who have suffered extensive "blast" injury to one side of the bladder and the ipsilateral ureter. In such patients, it may be impossible to reimplant the ureter ipsilaterally or even to mobilize the ipsilateral bladder to create a psoas hitch or Boari flap. Transureteroureterostomy can also be used in the management of a failured psoas hitch or Boari flap. Its use in urinary undiversion has been well documented by Hendren and others.[23] Well-known contraindications to TUU remain. In patients with recurrent urolithiasis or ureteral transitional cell carcinomas, we would prefer use of an ileal ureter over TUU.

The operation is done through a generous midline incision, with initial mobilization of the lateral aspect of the donor ureter through the peritoneal reflection lateral to the colon. The donor ureter is divided above the level of the injury, with adequate assessment of the viability

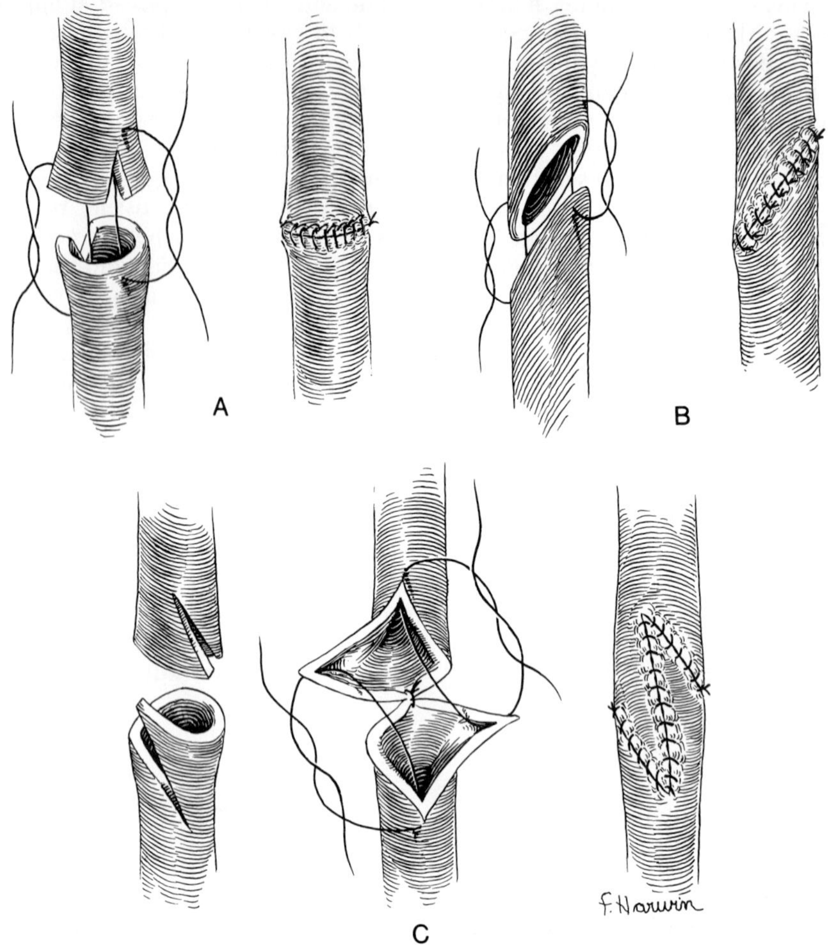

Figure 20–7. Ureteroureterostomy. *A*, spatulation of ureteral margins and placement of running locked sutures. Preferred technique. *B*, oblique anastomosis. (From Smith RB, Skinner DG, eds: Complications of Urologic Disorders. Philadelphia, WB Saunders Co, 1976, by permission.)

of the cut edge. The medial attachments of the donor ureter should be preserved. This may include an en bloc transfer of the ipsilateral gonadal vessels with their ureteral branches along with the donor ureter (Fig. 20–8). The peritoneum over the recipient ureter is then incised.

The donor ureter is transferred in a tunnel created below the posterior peritoneum. The ureteral course is anterior to the great vessels on a gentle curve, in much the same way as mobilization of the left ureter across the midline to reach an ileal conduit. (Some advocate that the donor ureter cross above the level of the inferior mesenteric artery to diminish anastomotic tension.[5]) The donor ureter is then spatulated over a 2 cm area. Although the anastomosis is end-to-side, the donor ureter should approach the recipient ureter at a 45-degree angle to allow for good drainage. If the available length of donor ureter is inadequate for an oblique anastomosis to the contralateral side, the TUU is less advisable. The available donor ureteral length is best assessed preoperatively by intravenous urography and retrograde pyelography, if necessary.

Interrupted suture material of fine chromic (5–0) or other suitable material such as Vicryl or Dexon is used to obtain a watertight anastomosis. In the case of TUU, it is especially important to avoid even a minimally leaky anastomosis. Although the traditional literature advises an unstented anastomosis, we would strongly consider passing two narrow stents up the common ureter with one of each continuing proximally up the donor and recipient ureters, respectively. The delicate No. 4.8 Fr. double

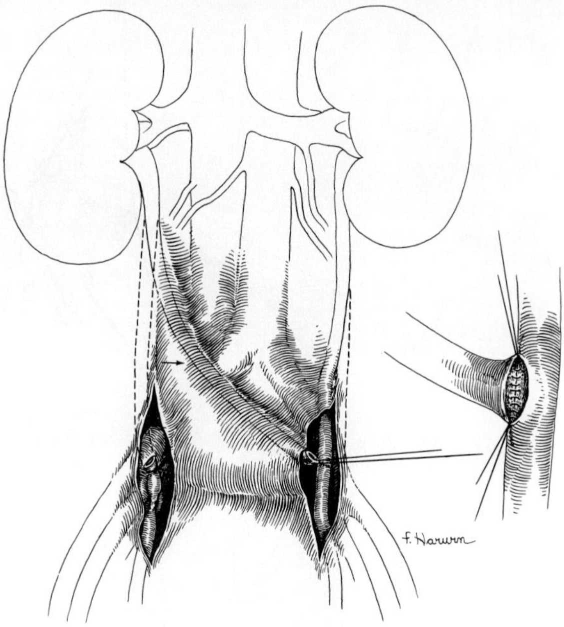

Figure 20–8. Transureteroureterostomy. Right-to-left transureteroureterostomy showing retroperitoneal tunnel anterior to great vessels. Careful mobilization prevents acute ureteral angulation and permits an anastomosis without tension. (From Smith RB, Skinner DG, eds: Complications of Urologic Disorders. Philadelphia, WB Saunders Co, 1976, by permission.)

pigtail stents currently available for use through the rigid ureteroscope would not cause undue internal pressure on the anastomosis. A large drain is placed lateral to the recipient ureter, next to, but not directly on top of, the anastomosis.

The broad exposure needed for TUU permits access to both kidneys. This lends itself to placement of a nephrostomy tube, which should be seriously considered when there has been significant infection, ischemia, or a concurrent visceral injury along the path of the donor ureter.

Although there have been reports of less than successful outcomes with TUU, there has been an equal number of successful series.[24] It should be noted that in the case of some of the negative reports on TUU, the procedure was carried out "in the middle of the night" as a salvage-type procedure, in days prior to the employment of modern endourologic techniques. It is quite likely that future reports of TUU in well-selected patients will be more sanguine.

Ureteral Reimplantation with Psoas Hitch

In patients with pelvic ureteral injuries, which are most commonly seen after hysterectomy, it is seldom possible to obtain a good tunneled reanastomosis of ureter to bladder without placing the ureter on tension. The psoas hitch is one of the best procedures for treating these kinds of injuries because it permits movement of healthier tissue (bladder) above the area of injury.

The bladder is extremely well vascularized and is surprisingly mobile. Unlike the ureter, its vascular integrity is seldom disturbed by radical gynecologic surgery. Its mobility may be increased by taking down the contralateral and, sometimes, the ipsilateral superior vesical pedicle. A horizontal cystotomy seems to allow greater upward displacement of the bladder. The ipsilateral posterior wall is then pushed cranially over the psoas minor tendon or the psoas muscle itself, above and lateral to the site of the ureteral injury (Fig. 20–9). In this position, the seromuscular bladder wall is sutured with two or three sutures of heavy Vicryl or Dexon to the psoas muscle. The previously mobilized ureter is then transected above the injured segment, taking into account the possibility of a "gray zone" of poorly vascularized ureter. Several techniques are available for a nonrefluxing anastomosis of ureter to bladder. The most commonly used has been the Leadbetter-Politano reimplantation.

Sometimes, after the bladder has been hitched and the ureter transected, the ureter barely reaches the "horn" of the bladder. To avoid tension on the reimplantation and to permit tunneling of the intravesical ureter, the psoas hitch should be taken down and recreated, using a more medial portion of the posterior bladder wall. In this procedure, the contralateral superior vesical pedicle should be divided, if it

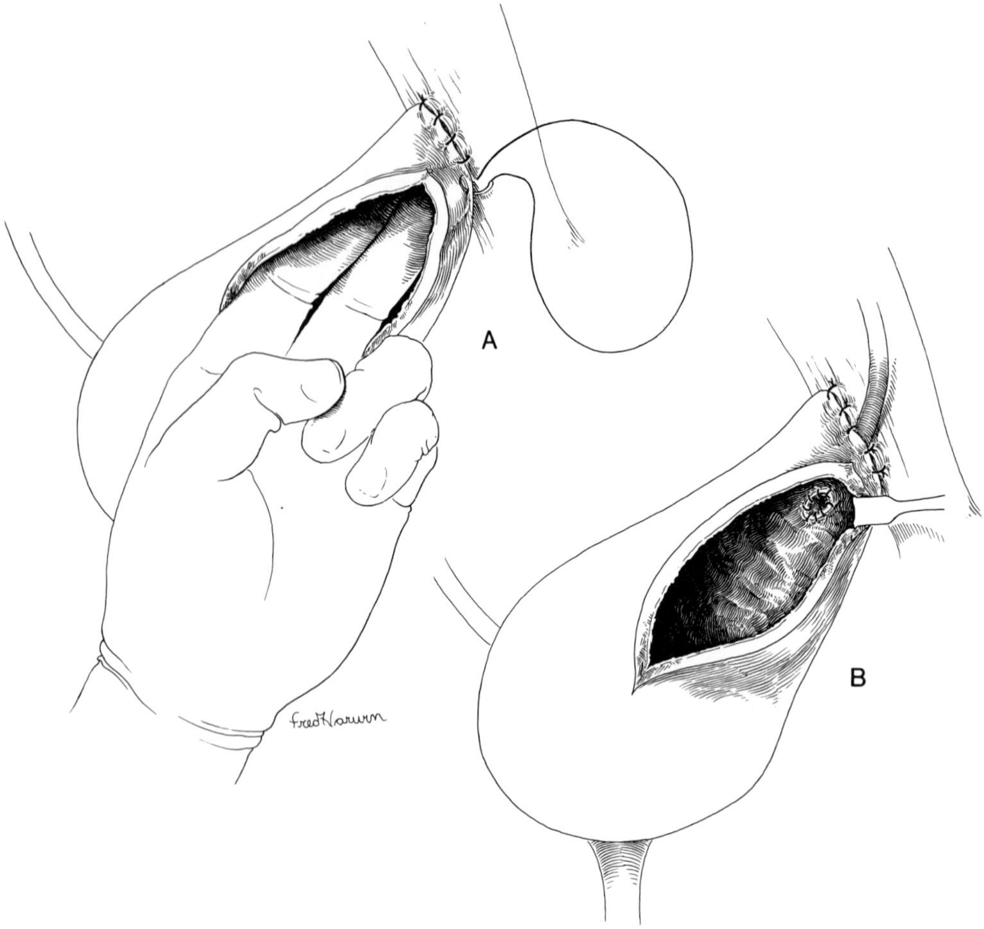

Figure 20–9. Psoas bladder hitch. *A*, previously mobilized bladder being anchored to psoas muscle, *B*, ureteral implantation. (From Smith RB, Skinner DG, eds: Complications of Urologic Disorders. Philadelphia, WB Saunders Co, 1976, by permission.)

has not already been done. If tension still exists on the anastomosis, we have found it preferable to create a Boari flap rather than to attempt to mobilize the ureter further (Fig. 20–10). In these cases, the viability of the healthy midureter could be jeopardized by overmobilization. There have been reports of combining a Boari flap and a psoas hitch to replace two thirds or more of the ureter.

The psoas hitch operation is remarkably free of complications. Stenting of the ureter is practical but not absolutely necessary. A double pigtail catheter may be left indwelling for 2 to 3 weeks. Despite the cystotomy, it is seldom necessary to leave a Foley catheter in place for more than 3 to 5 days unless there is some other complicating factor such as pelvic radiation therapy or steroid use. Adequate drainage should be used, including one extravesical drain anterior to the bladder and another lateral to the bladder horn created by the psoas hitch.

With an adequate tunneled reimplantation technique, the chance of reflux is minimal. However, in the experience of most, even when reflux is present, it usually does not harm the patient. This is consistent with the general notion that reflux in the adult kidney is not likely to result in permanent scarring or loss of parenchyma.

Boari Flap

The Boari flap has stood the test of time since its inception by Boari in 1894. Over the years, it has become popularized by several other investigators.[25,26] It is second to the psoas hitch as the method of choice for bridging a lower ure-

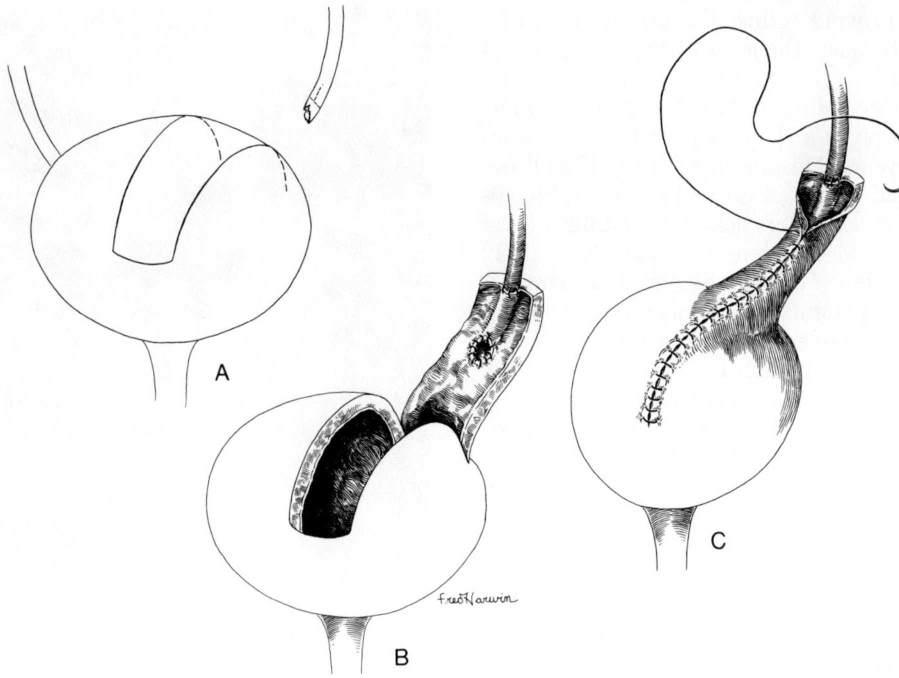

Figure 20–10. Bladder flap procedure. *A*, creation of tapered bladder flap, based posteriorly. *B*, submucosal ureteral reimplantation. *C*, closure of bladder flap. (From Smith RB, Skinner DG, eds: Complications of Urologic Disorders. Philadelphia, WB Saunders Co, 1976, by permission.)

teral defect. Because it is a pedicled flap, it has greater inherent risks than the psoas hitch. Physiologically, the Boari flap never totally fulfills the function of the ureter, although normal ureter above the flap allows for proper peristalsis and emptying of urine into the bladder. When the rectangular or oblong flap is rolled into a tube, the wall of the tube is quite thick, leaving the luminal diameter small. The most tenuous part of the flap is at its apex, where the ureteroneocystostomy is placed. Most authors advise a flap at least 4 cm wide at the base and generously spiraled from the ipsilateral posterior bladder wall to the contralateral anterior wall. The base of the flap should not be at the dome of the bladder, but neither should it be placed too close to the trigone, to prevent both ureteral injury and injury to branches to the inferior and middle vesical arteries, which provide important blood flow to the base of the flap. It is not readily appreciated that the amount of bladder necessary for the Boari flap does diminish bladder capacity. Furthermore, closure of the wide bladder defect created by the cephalad repositioning of the flap leads to narrowing of the junction between the bladder and the bladder tube.

The Boari flap can easily be used to bridge a defect of 12 to 14 cm, and, if the bladder is normal, a tube can be constructed that reaches well above the pelvic inlet. Certain technical considerations are important. The longer the length of the tube, the wider the base should be. In widening the base, one should recognize that bladder capacity can be reduced. The base of the flap should be in a posterolateral position; free bleeding should be demonstrated from the apex of the flap. The entire flap should be fixed to the psoas muscle lateral to the iliac vessels before actually tubularizing it. Two layers of interrupted absorbable sutures are used to tubularize the flap, using larger bites of the seromuscular layer than of the mucosa. Too large a bite of the mucosa will result in an inadequate lumen. If one wishes, one may use a continuous suture technique, beginning with the inner layer of the bladder defect closure and continuing cranially to tubularize the flap. The second layer, also in continuity, would begin with the seromuscular layer of the bladder defect and end with the seromuscular layer of the Boari tube.

As with the psoas hitch, it is controversial as to whether an antireflux procedure is necessary. If one chooses to avoid an antireflux procedure, the ureter can be directly anastomosed to the open tubularized flap, using an oblique or spatulated anastomotic technique. However, if one wishes to prevent reflux, the ureter should be tunneled through the wall of the flap prior to tubularizing the flap. One series reported on the effects of free reflux in 23 patients who underwent creation of a Boari flap, with a follow-up of 5 to 14 years. Despite free reflux, 17 of these patients had return of normal pyelographic appearance, and 5 others achieved stabilization of hydroureter on intravenous pyelography (IVP) with no evidence of progressive renal damage. Twenty-one patients experienced improvement or stabilization of creatinine clearance. No negative effect could be ascribed to reflux.[27] It may be that reflux in these adult patients simply is not injurious to the kidneys or that there is an actual buffering effect against increased intrarenal pressure provided by the base of the flap, which contains thick but compliant bladder muscle.

Complications are more frequently seen with the Boari flap than with the psoas hitch. The apex (cranial aspect) of the flap may necrose, leading to hydronephrosis or fistula. In fact, stenosis of the apical region of the tubularized flap is far more common than anastomotic stricture between the ureter and bladder. When postoperative leakage of urine occurs, it is often at the point where the base of the flap meets the remainder of the bladder. To prevent this complication, the tenuous area between the bladder and the flap must be reinforced by extra suture material at the time of closure. Leakage may occur early postoperatively if there is inadequate Foley catheter drainage. It is far more important to leave the patient on a longer period of catheter drainage for the Boari flap than for the psoas hitch. A complication is illustrated in the following case report.

Case Report. A 36-year-old female underwent a somewhat difficult Boari flap procedure for a distal ureteral stricture. On the seventh postoperative day, the Foley catheter was inadvertently clamped for over 45 minutes during the course of a urography examination. The delayed films revealed evidence of extravasation (Fig. 20–11). Following this—and despite being kept on catheter drainage—the patient developed signs of progressive pelvic pain and psoas irritation with low-grade fever. A pelvic CAT scan revealed an extensive fluid collection that, on percutaneous aspiration, proved to be non-infected urine. Percutaneous drainage was contemplated, although the catheter would have to traverse the peritoneal cavity. Therefore, the patient's urinoma was incised and drained surgically. Recovery was uneventful.

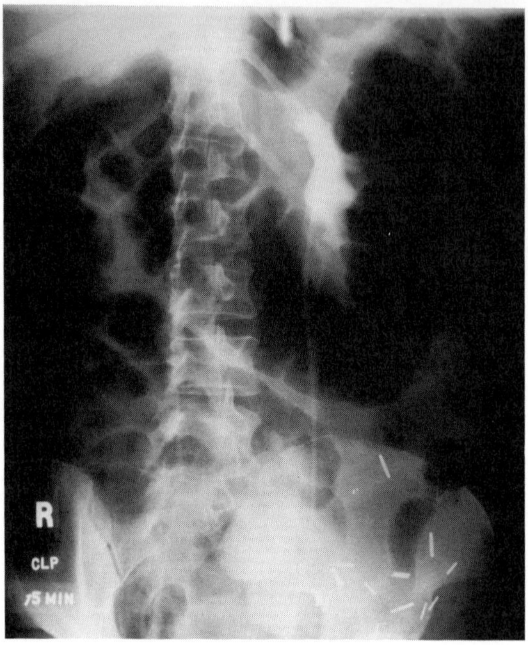

Figure 20–11. Oblique pyelogram shows urinary extravasation from Boari flap. This resulted in a pelvic urinoma.

Another complication associated with the Boari flap reported by Gregoir is the delayed development of pelvic abscess.[28] In the four cases in his report, the Boari tube was completely destroyed by an intense periureteritis, whether or not the abscess was drained. He does not state whether the abscess in itself may have resulted primarily from necrosis of the Boari tube.

Mention should be made of one other technique similar to the Boari tube with which we have not had experience. This is referred to as a reverse Boari flap, and, as opposed to the Boari flap, it is based anteriorly. The apex of the flap includes the ipsilateral ureteral orifice, with a circumscribing incision made around the orifice. This procedure may be of some use to patients with injuries to the middle part of the ureter, where the vascularity to the distal and intramural ureter is unquestioned. The reverse Boari flap can easily bridge a defect of 10 cm.[29]

ILEAL URETER

The ileal ureter is an excellent technique for replacing substantial ureteral losses. It is certainly within the technical grasp of any urologist who performs ileal conduits. Of all substitutes for the ureter, the ileum comes closest to retaining the native peristaltic behavior of the ureter. However, the ileum is different from the ureter in that it maintains segmentation contractions when filled with urine just as it previously did when filled with enteric material. Although segmentation is adaptive for enteric function to allow better contact between the digested food and the surface area of absorptive villi, it permits stasis of urine with resorption of urea and electrolytes. Because of this physiology, the ileal ureter should be used only in patients with overall good renal function and a functioning ipsilateral renal unit. Any patient with a serum creatinine greater than 2.0 should be excluded. Also, the length of the ileal segment should be kept as short as possible to diminish the surface area available for direct contact with urine. Therefore, if the entire lower two thirds of the ureter needs to be replaced, the proximal ureter can be implanted into the ileal segment, which can be anastomosed directly into the bladder. A psoas hitch or Boari flap can help minimize the length of ileal segment.

Although the ileal ureter has been used extensively in treating patients with multiple ureteral strictures, tuberculosis, schistosomiasis, and transitional cell carcinoma, it is gaining wider acceptance in the treatment of refractory operative injuries, especially when the patient has already had one failed repair.

Ileal ureter should certainly be one of the main options in a patient undergoing a second ureteral repair. The bowel is prepared in the same manner as for ileal conduit. On entering the abdomen, an estimate is made of the length of the ureteral defect, and a piece of ileum is then chosen. One should choose a piece of ileum in close proximity to the injury; prior to taking down the mesentery of the ileal segment, the prospective piece of ileum should be measured against the actual defect. In this manner, one will be certain that the proximal and distal anastomoses are not under undue tension.

After the segment is excluded from the remainder of the ileum, it will sometimes appear that the segment seems to have shrunk. This, however, is transitory, and after the ileum relaxes more, it will comfortably fill the defect, as originally anticipated. The segment should be oriented in an isoperistaltic fashion (Fig. 20–12). The proximal anastomosis, if performed to the renal pelvis directly, may be difficult because of prior surgery in the area. However, in a majority of these patients, the most scarred portion of the renal pelvis is posterior, in the area of prior pyelolithotomy or pyeloplasty. Indeed, the anterior or modified flank-torque exposure needed for the ileal substitution may avoid some of the problems more posteriorly.

In mobilizing the renal pelvis for the pyeloileal anastomosis, one must protect the basilar renal artery, which often courses just anterior to the renal pelvis. If either the proximal or the distal anastomosis is directly to the ureter, the same techniques are employed as with ureteroileostomy for conduit surgery.

The ileovesical anastomosis is usually done from inside the bladder, removing a sufficiently large portion of bladder wall on or near the trigone. The contralateral ureteral orifice should be protected. Some authors advocate tapering of the distal ileal segment.[30] Not only does this diminish the total absorptive capacity of ileum and reduce contact with urine, it also may make reimplantation of the ileal segment in a nonrefluxing manner more possible. Another way to prevent reflux is to create a nipple of ileum by turning redundant ileum back on itself inside the bladder. The ileovesical anastomosis is created with 3–0 chromic or other appropriate absorbable suture material.

Despite these techniques, it is not clear that prevention of reflux is necessary. The ileal segment is very compliant and probably buffers the ipsilateral kidney against the pressure of refluxing urine. Furthermore, the status of the bladder is probably more important than the nature of the reimplantation in that a low-pressure bladder will result in low-pressure reflux, which is unlikely to harm the kidney.[31]

The ileal ureter should be kept in an extraperitoneal position as much as possible to reduce the risk of postoperative adhesions and obstruction. This is easier on the right side, where the entire ileal ureter can be passed through the right colonic mesentery and allowed to lie completely lateral to the ascending colon. On the left side, the ileal ureter can also be taken laterally through a colonic mesentery window and kept retro-colic, entering the bladder below the peritoneal reflection.

Mucus formation will continue in the ileal segment when it is substituted for ureter. This is generally not a problem if the patient has competent bladder function and a patent bladder outlet. The presence of significant bladder outlet or uretheral obstruction is a contraindication to the use of an ileal ureter.

COMPLICATIONS OF RENAL AUTOTRANSPLANTATION

Since it was first described by Hardy in 1963, renal autotransplantation has become an impor-

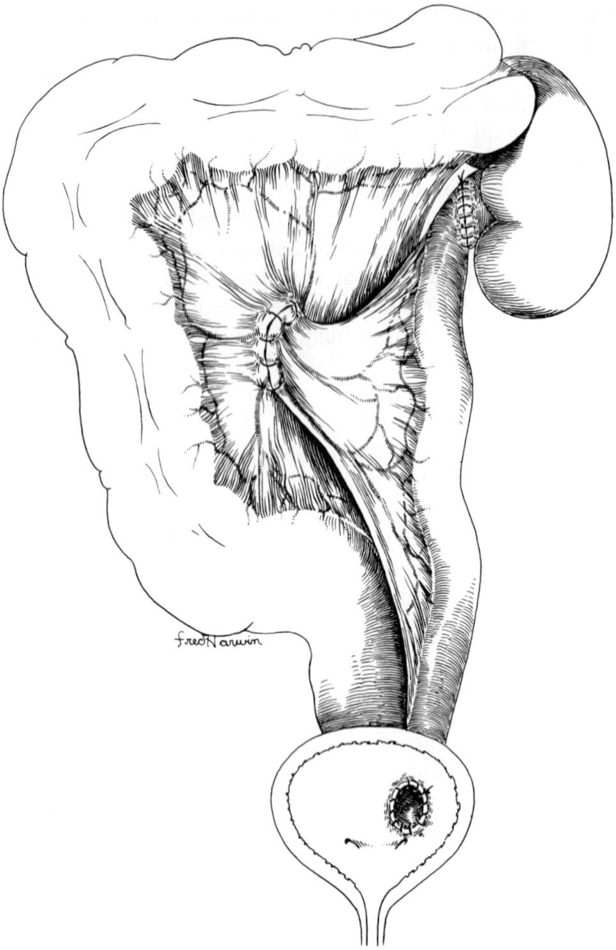

Figure 20–12. Ureteral replacement by ileum. Left colon retracted medially. Ileum brought through a hiatus in the colonic mesentery. Ileal ureter is in retroperitoneal position. (From Smith RB, Skinner DG, eds: Complications of Urologic Disorders. Philadelphia, WB Saunders Co, 1976, by permission.)

tant part of the urologic armamentarium.[32] Surgical experience with renal transplantation both technically and with respect to methods of renal preservation has improved greatly. The facility and familiarity with the procedure at major centers have led to wider indications and excellent results.

Renal autotransplantation has become the procedure of choice for some patients with especially difficult urologic problems. The procedure was initially described as a treatment for extensive ureteral loss. However, today, the most common indication for autotransplantation is for the surgical treatment of renal arterial lesions, both occlusive and aneurysmal. Other common indications include ureteral loss (from trauma, tumor, or extensive stricture disease), renal pelvic and hilar tumors, and complex stone disease. Most patients who require replacement of a segment of ureter can be managed by conservative means, reimplantation, psoas hitch, Boari flap, or TUU. In some patients, the entire ureter can be replaced with the combination of psoas hitch and Boari flap, but this requires a large and mobile bladder. In patients for whom the aforementioned techniques are not possible, creation of an ileal ureter and renal autotransplantation are the only two remaining options to preserve the affected renal unit.[33]

Ex vivo surgery with autotransplantation is a specialized technique with specific indications. Most commonly, this is performed for renal arterial disease extending into branches of the renal artery. Bench surgery also provides improved access to the renal hilum, and combined with microvascular techniques, it can facilitate the treatment of renal pelvic tumors with preservation of the ureteral blood supply.

Reviews of the literature show autotransplantation to be a safe technique. Complications directly related to the procedure are rare.[34,35] Autotransplantation has the added benefit of not requiring immunosuppression. Similarly, prosthetic materials are not used, reducing the incidence of infectious complications.

Urine leakage with fistula formation is the most common complication occurring with renal transplantation. This is usually associated with ureteral devascularization. It has been shown that with autotransplantation, ureteral transection and reimplantation should be avoided whenever possible to avoid this problem. This reduces operative time, preserves the collateral ureteral blood flow, and safely permits more extensive hilar dissection. The intact, long, redundant ureter does not lead to alterations in urine flow.[36,37]

The other major class of complications associated with autotransplantation relates to renal nonfunction. Vascular problems related to renal nonfunction can present early or late. Early complications include postoperative bleeding and artrial thrombosis. Bleeding has occurred up to 12 days after autotransplantation.[33] Immediate arterial thrombosis is a technical complication that, fortunately, is rare and normally requires immediate re-exploration. This can usually be detected and differentiated by a diethylenetriamine pentaacetic acid (DTPA) renal flow scan or arteriography.

Acute tubular necrosis can also be a cause of renal nonfunction after autotransplantation. The reversible cases usually relate to either prolonged warm ischemia time or inadequate flushing of the kidney. The kidney is very susceptible to damage from warm ischemia owing to its dependence on aerobic metabolism. Human renal tolerance to warm ischemia approximates that seen in canine kidneys, in which the maximal arterial occlusion time tolerated before irreversible damage ensues is generally 30 minutes.[38]

Surface hypothermia can be achieved by simply applying ice slush to the surface of the kidney. This is effective but has the disadvantage of nonhomogeneous cooling, with slower cooling occurring at the core of the kidney. Inducing perfusion hypothermia is also simple and effective and avoids these problems. With short ischemic intervals, the perfusion solution's composition is probably not important. As the ischemic interval increases (2 to 3 hours), perfusion with an intracellular solution high in potassium (i.e., Collins solution) is superior in preserving renal function because of its ability to maintain intracellular concentrations and to prevent cellular swelling.[39]

Adjunctive measures to minimize tubular necrosis include generous preoperative and intraoperative hydration, avoidance of intraoperative hypotension during anesthesia, and administration of mannitol. Mannitol given 5 to 15 minutes before arterial occlusion increases renal plasma flow, minimizes intracellular edema, and promotes an osmotic diuresis when renal circulation is restored.[40] Finally, autotransplantation of kidneys with severe renal parenchymal disease should be avoided since such kidneys generally flush poorly. This can lead to irreversible damage and renal nonfunction postoperatively.

References

1. Barbaric ZL, Wolfe DE, Segal AJ: Intraoperative ureteral trauma: a radiologic approach. J Assoc Can Radiol 29:40, 1978.
2. Demos TC, Churchill R, Flisak ME, Poor CT: The radiologic diagnosis of complications following gynecologic surgery: radiography, computed tomography, sonography, and scintigraphy. CRC Crit Rev Diagn Imaging 22(1):43, 1984.
3. Buchsbaum, HJ: The urinary tract and radical hysterectomy. In Buchsbaum HJ, Schmidt J, eds: Gynecologic and Obstetric Urology, 2nd ed. Philadelphia, WB Saunders Co., 1982.
4. Turner-Warwick RT: Urethral stricture surgery. In Glenn JF ed: Urologic Surgery, 3rd ed, Philadelphia, JB Lippincott Co, 1983, p 710.
5. Zinman LM, Libertino JA, Roth RA: Management of operative ureteral injury. Urology 12(3):290, 1978.
6. Stutzman RE: Ballistics and the management of ureteral injuries from high velocity missiles. J Urol 118:947, 1977.
7. Bright TC: Emergency management of the injured ureter. Urol Clin North Am 9(2):285, 1982.
8. Hopkins TB, Klein LA: Disruption of the renal pelvis by blunt trauma. J Trauma 15:250, 1975.
9. Rohrer TJ Jr: Delayed ureteral fistula from high velocity missiles. J Urol 105:63, 1971.
10. Kontturi M, Kauppila A: Ureteric complications following treatment of gynaecological cancer. Ann Chir Gynaecol 71:232, 1982.
11. Beland G: Early treatment of ureteral injuries found after gynecological surgery. J Urol (1):25, 1977.
12. Symmonds RE, Pratt JH: Prevention of fistulas and lymphocysts in radical hysterectomy. Obstet Gynecol 17:57, 1961.
13. Green TH Jr: Ureteral suspension for prevention of ureteral complications following radical Wertheim hysterectomy. Obstet Gynecol 28:1, 1966.
14. Okhawa K: Ureteral management in radical pelvic surgery with special reference to the peritoneal flap. New York, Sixth World Congress of Gynecology and Obstetrics, April, 1970.
15. Cruikshank SH. Avoiding ureteral injury during total vaginal hysterectomy. South Med J (12):1447, 1985.
16. Mendez R, McGinty DM: The management of delayed recognized ureteral injuries. J Urol (2):199, 1978.
17. Jordan WP Jr, Scaljon W: Anatomic complications of abdominal surgery with special reference to the ureter. Am Surg (9):565, 1979.
18. Schapira HE, Li R, Gribetz M, Wulfjohn MA, Brendler H: Ureteral injuries during vascular surgery. J Urol (3):293, 1981.
19. Flynn JT, Tiptaft RC, Woodhouse CRJ, Paris AMI,

Blandy JP: The early and aggressive repair of iatrogenic ureteric injuries. Br J Urol 51:454, 1979.
20. Witters S, Cornelissen M, Vereecker R: Iatrogenic ureteral injury: aggressive or conservative treatment. Am J Obstet Gynecol 155:582, 1986.
21. Raney AM: Ureteral trauma: effects of ureteral ligation with and without deligation—experimental studies and case reports. J Urol 119(3):326, 1978.
22. Ponig BF: Microsurgical ureteroureterostomy in ureteral injuries. J Urol 128:594,1982.
23. Hendren WH, Hensle TW: Transureteroureterostomy: experience with 75 cases. J Urol 123:826, 1980.
24. Ehrlich RM, Skinner DG: Complications of transureteroureterostomy. J Urol 113:467, 1975.
25. Spies JW, Johnson CE, Wilson CS: Reconstruction of the ureter by means of bladder flaps. Proc Soc Exp Biol Med 230:425, 1933.
26. Ockerblad NF: Reimplantation of the ureter into the bladder by the flap method. J Urol 57:845, 1947.
27. Thompson IM, Ross G Jr: Long-term results of bladder-flap repair of ureteral injuries. J Urol 3:483, 1974.
28. Gregoir WL: Commentary: bladder flap: indications and technique. In Whitehead ED, Leiter E, eds: Current Operative Urology. 2nd ed. New York, Harper & Row, 1984.
29. Ehrlich RM, Freedman A: Surgical treatment of long ureteral defects. AUA Update Series, Vol IV, Washington, DC, AUA Office of Education, 1985.
30. Middleton AW Jr: Tapered ileum as ureter substitution in severe renal damage. Urology 9:509, 1977.
31. Boxer RJ, Johnson SF, Ehrlich RM: Ureteral substitution. Urology 12:3, 1978.
32. Hardy JD: High ureteral injuries: management by autotransplantation of the kidney. JAMA 184:97, 1963.
33. Bodie B, Novick AC, Rose M: Long term results with renal autotransplantation for ureteral replacement. J Urol 136(6):1187, 1986.
34. Lawson RK: Extracorporeal Surgery. J Urol 123:301, 1980.
35. Salvatierra O, Olcott C, Stoney RJ: Ex vivo renal artery reconstruction using perfusion preservation. J Urol 119:16, 1978.
36. Whitsell JC, Goldsmith EI, Nakamura H: Renal autotransplantation without ureteral division: an experimental study and case report. J Urol 103:577, 1970.
37. Milsten R, Neifield J, Koontz WW Jr: Extracorporeal renal surgery. J Urol 112:425, 1974.
38. Novick AC: Renal hypothermia: in vivo and ex vivo. Urol Clin North Am 10(4):637, 1983.
39. Collins GM, Green RD, et al: Protection of kidneys from warm ischemic injury: dosage and timing of mannitol administration. Transplantation 29:83, 1980.
40. Novick AC: Extracorporeal renal surgery and autotransplantation for complicated stone disease. Cleve Clin Q 52(1):21, 1985.

COMPLICATIONS OF URETEROSCOPY

21

Jerry J. Weinberg • Arthur D. Smith

Ureteroscopy has become vital for today's urologist as an investigative tool as well as a method for diagnosing and treating ureteral and renal pelvic disease. Its success in the treatment of lower ureteral stones is even greater than that achieved with percutaneous extraction of upper ureteral stones,[1] and it is complementary to extracorporeal shock wave lithotripsy (ESWL). Recently, ureteroscopy has proved to be more accurate than a standard diagnostic protocol in the diagnosis of upper-tract filling defects.[2]

Originally thought of as an art exclusively for the experienced endourologist, ureteroscopy is now being undertaken routinely by nearly all urologists. With the advent of flexible ureteroscopes, flexible grasping forceps, new stone baskets, and various types of lithotripsy, the indications for and ways to use ureteroscopy have gradually expanded. With the ever-growing demand for cost-effective, minimally invasive procedures, ureteroscopy seems certain to become even more popular.

OVERVIEW OF URETEROSCOPY

Indications and Contraindications

The indications for ureteroscopy are similar to those for cystourethroscopy, and therefore the new technique has been adopted, slowly, on an intuitive basis for both diagnosis and therapy (Table 21–1).[3–5] Its present diagnostic uses include investigation of filling defects or unilateral hematuria in the ureter or renal pelvis that cannot be discerned by radiographic means; biopsy of lesions; and follow-up after chemotherapy or resection of tumors. Its therapeutic uses include extraction of stones with baskets or graspers or by electrohydraulic, ultrasonic, or laser lithotripsy; removal of foreign bodies, such as displaced stents; dilating or incising strictures; manipulation beyond a fistula; and resection of tumors. The indications for stone removal are similar to those for percutaneous extraction, viz, upper-tract obstruction and dilatation, declining renal function, recurrent infection, and recurrent colic.

Table 21–1. INDICATIONS FOR URETEROSCOPY

Diagnostic
Filling defects in the ureter or renal pelvis
Unilateral hematuria
Examination and biopsy of ureteral or renal pelvic lesions
Follow-up of previously treated lesions
Therapeutic
Stone extraction (intact or with lithotripsy)
Removal of foreign bodies
Examination/dilatation of ureteral strictures
Manipulation beyond a fistula
Resection of ureteral or pelvic tumors

Relative contraindications to ureteroscopy are previous pelvic surgery, radiation, or trauma, which may leave the ureter fibrosed, tortuous, or kinked, making it particularly vulnerable to injury. Under these circumstances, ureteroscopy is associated with a significant failure rate. Urethral stricture and prostatic obstruction are relative contraindications: if the obstruction can be relieved, ureteroscopy is often possible.

Table 21–2. INDICATIONS AND OUTCOME OF URETEROSCOPY AT LONG ISLAND JEWISH MEDICAL CENTER

Indication	No. (Males/Females)	Age (Years)	Success (Percent)
Diagnostic	20 (15/5)	19–58	20 (100%)
Mid-ureteral stone	8 (6/2)	37–62	5 (62%)
Distal ureteral stone	119 (94/25)	19–89	99 (83%)

Results in Authors' Series

At Long Island Jewish Medical Center, we performed ureteroscopy in 147 patients from 1982 through the middle of 1985 (Table 21–2). Of these procedures, 20 were for diagnostic purposes (to rule out stone disease in 15 patients and ureteral tumor in five) and 127 were for stone removal from the mid-ureter (eight patients) or distal ureter (119 patients). The overall success rate was 84 percent (124/147), including all of the procedures done for diagnosis. The causes and outcome of the failures of stone removal are shown in Table 21–3.

The 15 complications in the series consisted of one ureteral avulsion, which was managed successfully by ureteral reimplantation; two ureteral perforations with displacement of the stone into the retroperitoneum and an uneventful postoperative course; 11 cases of postoperative fever (101° F), for which intravenous antibiotics were given; and one case of bleeding, necessitating transfusion. Thus, the complication rate was 10 percent, and the rate of ureteral injury was 2 percent (Table 21–4).

Comment

The increasing success and low morbidity of ureteroscopic removal of distal and mid-ureteral stones are particularly encouraging in view of the drawbacks of other approaches. For example, approaching these stones via a percutaneous nephrostomy tract is associated with higher morbidity.[6] In fact, unless the ureteral stone can be pushed, flushed, or blown up into the renal pelvis, an approach via a percutaneous nephrostomy tract is not warranted.[7] Also, ESWL is not appropriate for many stones in the distal or mid-ureter, as they are shielded from the stone-destroying shock waves by bone. The extracorporeal method also is ill suited for removing impacted stones (because successful lithotripsy necessitates expansion of the stone) or for stones trapped above an obstruction.[8,9] Cystoscopic use of baskets is problematic in many patients, such as those with multiple or impacted stones or distal ureteral obstruction. Most of these cases are suitable for management by ureteroscopy.

Therefore, we believe that the effort needed to master ureteroscopy is amply repaid. The success rates are gratifying, and the incidence of complications is low. Moreover, if the procedure fails, none of the alternatives has been precluded; indeed, prior ureteroscopy may facilitate them, e.g., by moving a stone into a more convenient position for extraction. As a further aid, a percutaneous nephrostomy tract can be created by retrograde puncture of an appropriate calyx while the instrument in the ureter prevents the stone from escaping back into the ureter.[10]

Table 21–3. CAUSES AND OUTCOME OF FAILURES OF URETEROSCOPIC STONE REMOVAL IN 127 PATIENTS

	Stone Location		
	Distal Ureter (N=119)	*Mid-Ureter (N=8)*	Total (Percent)
Stone migration; percutaneous extraction required	2	1	3 (2%)
Spontaneous passage postoperatively	5	0	5 (4%)
Migration into calyx; no further treatment needed	4	0	4 (3%)
Displacement into retroperitoneum (no treatment needed)	2	0	2 (2%)
Open ureterolithotomy	7	2	9 (7%)
	20	3	23 (18%)

Table 21–4. COMPLICATIONS OF URETEROSCOPY IN 147 PATIENTS AT LONG ISLAND JEWISH MEDICAL CENTER

	Indication		
	Distal Stone	*Mid-ureteral Stone*	Total (Percent)
Ureteral avulsion	1	0	1 (0.7%)
Ureteral perforation	1	1	2 (1%)
Fever	7	4	11 (7%)
Blood loss necessitating transfusion	1	0	1 (0.7%)
	10	5	15 (10%)

COMPLICATIONS AND THEIR PREVENTION

Several of the more common complications of ureteroscopy result from difficulties in introducing or advancing the instrument. Short-term complications that result include ureteral perforation and avulsion; long-term complications are stricture and stenosis. A rule of successful ureteroscopy is that resistance to instrument passage must always be overcome by deft manipulation, never by force. Even after the ureteroscope has been advanced, the procedure—especially stone extraction—may fail: the operator may not find the stone, or it may be displaced into the collecting system or the retroperitoneum. The ureter can be damaged by grasping forceps, baskets, or lithotripsy probes if these are not used with sufficient caution. Postoperative complications include colic, fever, infection, and sepsis (Table 21–5). In the remainder of this chapter, we review these complications according to the point in the procedure at which they arise and offer advice on minimizing their frequency.

Preoperative Evaluation

Some ureteroscopy procedures fail or cause complications because of inadequate planning. During the initial interview, the patient must be asked about voiding symptoms and signs. A urethral stricture precludes introduction of the ureteroscope, whereas prostatic hyperplasia may make it difficult to introduce the instrument into the ureteral orifice as well as to manipulate it up the ureter. It also is important to know whether the patient has had previous pelvic surgery, radiation, or trauma, as these alter the anatomy in the pelvis and often lead to strictures, kinks, or tortuosity of the ureter.

During the physical examination, the size of the prostate must be determined. Signs of enlargement and symptoms of prostatism may be a signal that trouble lies ahead if the problem is not corrected before ureteroscopy.

A plain radiograph of the abdomen taken within 24 hours prior to ureteroscopy is essential. One of the leading causes of failure to find a stone is that it is, in fact, not there; a small calculus can easily pass unnoticed or can migrate and be bypassed with the ureteroscope. Either occurrence will leave the unprepared endourologist searching the ureter fruitlessly.

Failure of Ureteral Dilatation

Before ureteroscopy, a ureteral catheter and guide wire should be advanced up to the renal pelvis to serve as a guide for the ureteroscope. As a bonus, this stent may straighten out any redundancy in the ureter. Failure to advance

Table 21–5. COMPLICATIONS OF URETEROSCOPY*

Mechanical Problems
Difficulty dilating ureteral orifice
Inability to advance ureteroscope
Difficulty seeing calculus
Inability to basket calculus
Displacement of calculus
Ureteral Injury
Extravasation†
Perforation of ureter or ureterovesical junction
Avulsion
Late stenosis†
Late stricture†
Postoperative Problems
Ureteral colic
Fever
Infection, sepsis
Instrument Breakage
Late Problems
Vesicoureteral reflux
Infection
Retroperitoneal fibrosis

*Information from references 11 to 38 listed at the end of this chapter.

†May be result of abrasions by instruments or damage to ureteral mucosa by ultrasonic or electrohydraulic lithotripsy probe.

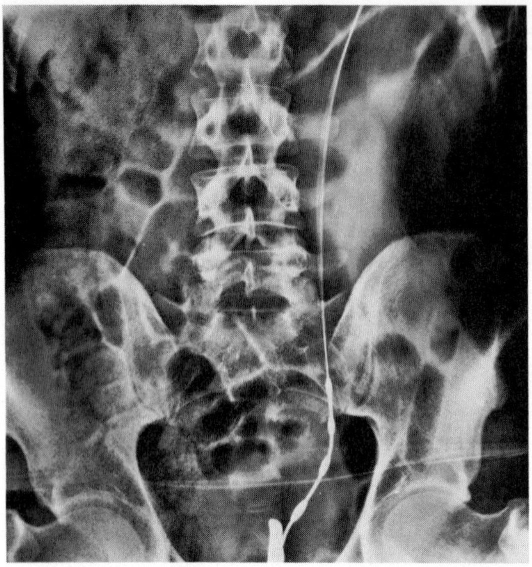

Figure 21–1. The Smith rapid-sequence ureteral dilators. The ureterovesical junction can be dilated rapidly over a guide wire.

this wire or catheter beyond the orifice can have several causes. Prostatic hyperplasia can cause "J-ing" of the ureters, making advancement of a catheter impossible. With suitable preoperative assessment, this problem would be discovered and eliminated. Difficulty in locating the orifice may lead the operator to stab the area surrounding it repeatedly, causing edema and hemorrhage that may prevent catheter passage. To avoid this problem, no attempt should be made to stent the ureter unless the orifice is clearly visible, perhaps with the aid of intravenous indigo carmine.

The next step is a retrograde ureteropyelogram, not only to confirm the site of obstruction, either stone or tumor, but also to forewarn of the troublesome spots that lie ahead, e.g., strictures, kinks, or redundancy. The contrast medium also reveals whether the guide wire is in the ureteral lumen or a submucosal tunnel.

The ureterovesical junction is the narrowest portion of the ureter, and ureteroscope passage across it without dilatation can lead to disruption, avulsion, bleeding that reduces visibility, and, in the long term, stricture formation. Dilatation should be carried out over a metal guide wire. The most useful devices are the Smith rapid-sequence ureteral dilator[23] (Fig. 21–1) and balloon catheters. The former provides rapid dilatation, which decreases intraoperative time, and can be reused. The devices are passed under fluoroscopic guidance. After the guide wire has been advanced through the cystoscope up to the renal pelvis, removing the inner workings of the cystoscope and leaving its sheath pointed at the ureteral orifice often make advancement of the dilators easier. When the rapid-sequence dilators cannot be advanced, individual acorn dilators can be used.

For balloon dilatation, two types of catheters can be used. To dilate just the orifice, a high-pressure 4-cm balloon is available. Part of the balloon will be in the submucosal tunnel, the remaining portion outside the ureter; this arrangement guarantees dilatation of the orifice itself. A balloon, 5 to 6 mm in diameter, enlarges the orifice to 15 to 18 French (Fr.). The other option, a 20-cm balloon, will dilate the entire ureter, which may facilitate passage of the stone as well as advancement of the ureteroscope.[24,25] With either type of balloon, a pressure gauge should be attached to the injecting syringe. Even though the balloons have an indicator of the volume that can be injected, it is still possible to rupture them, which can cause rupture of the ureter as well as hemorrhage.

The ureterovesical tunnel always has petechiae after dilatation regardless of the type of dilator used. It is not clear whether the procedure has any permanent effects. There are scattered reports of vesicoureteral reflux as a result of such dilatation, but other authors deny that reflux occurs.[26] Because sterile reflux in the adult does not damage the kidney, the question is probably of minor importance anyway.[27]

Failure to Introduce and Advance the Ureteroscope

Introduction and advancement of the ureteroscope can be difficult or hazardous even with adequate dilatation. With ureteroscopes having a high-angle beak, inverting the sheath 180° may make negotiation of the orifice easier. If introduction is still difficult and the stone is near the ureterovesical junction, a ureteral meatotomy can be performed: a small incision at the 12 o'clock position opens the orifice and enables the stone to be delivered without the ureteroscope being passed. This operation does not appear to create long-term problems. Of the 14 patients in whom we have performed it, only two have experienced postoperative reflux.

In patients with complete duplication (Fig. 21–2), one may perform ureteroscopy in the unobstructed ureter and not visualize the stone. This can be easily prevented with an adequate retrograde pyelogram prior to insertion of the ureteroscope.

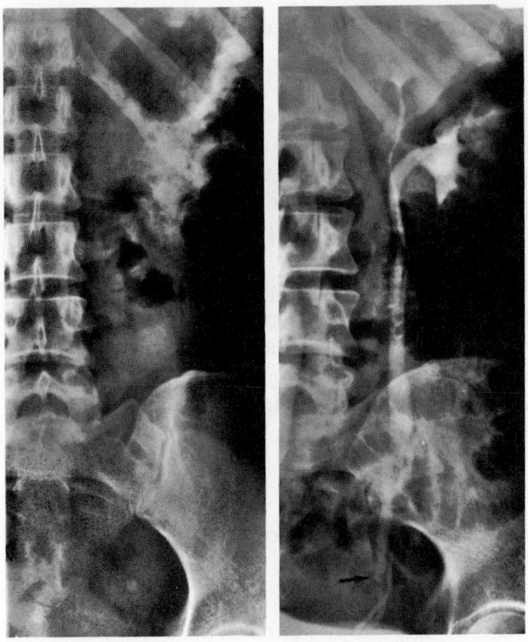

Figure 21–2. Left distal ureteral stone. Intravenous urogram prior to ureteroscopy demonstrates the calculus to be in the lower-pole ureter of a duplicated system.

When introduction of the ureteroscope beyond the ureterovesical junction is difficult, a false passage may be the problem. Placing the ureteroscope at the orifice, identifying the false passage visually, passing a guide wire beyond the area under vision, and redilating may facilitate ureteroscope passage. Once the ureterovesical junction and intramural ureter have been bypassed, advancement of the instrument is easier.

If areas of tortuosity are met further up the ureter, a 4 Fr. ureteral catheter or stone basket advanced through the sheath ahead of the ureteroscope often straightens the ureter. Strictures can be dilated with a 4 Fr. balloon catheter.[28]

One of the most difficult segments to traverse with the ureteroscope is where the iliac vessels cross the ureter. Here, the lumen of the ureter tends to narrow, and often the path of the ureter dips, making forward observation impossible. To keep the problems at this point to a minimum, two steps can be taken. First, if the patient is placed in the dorsal lithotomy position with the contralateral hip maximally abducted and the other leg in a more central position, the angle between the ureter and the iliac vessels tends to be minimized, affording the ureteroscope a straighter path. Second, the table should permit C-arm fluoroscopy so that the entire urinary tract can be examined from several angles, permitting visualization of the path to be taken by the ureteroscope.

Instrument Breakage

Rarely, the ureteroscope or the baskets or probes that operate through its working sheath crack or break. Pieces may then become lodged in the ureter. The type of ureteroscope affects the likelihood of this problem: the more versatile the instrument, the less likely it is to be damaged. At present, ureteroscopes with 12 Fr. or 13 Fr. working sheaths can be used with a variety of graspers, baskets, and lithotripsy probes. The smaller ureteroscopes can be used for diagnostic procedures. If a piece of instrument does become detached, the best course is to remove it carefully inside the working sheath. This measure reduces the risk of mucosal damage.

Stone Extraction

For stone removal, the patient should be placed in the reverse Trendelenburg position to enhance the stone's downward migration.[22] If a stone is identified, it can be grasped, basketed, or fragmented, but all procedures must be done under direct vision. Grasping should be attempted only if the stone fits easily into the jaws of the forceps. Basketing is appropriate only if the ureter is dilated sufficiently to permit the basket to be advanced alongside and beyond the stone and then withdrawn after the stone has been captured without disrupting the ureteral mucosa. Forceps or basket removal of stones is much more likely to fail when not done under direct vision.[30]

The complications of basket extraction include eversion of the ureter, entrapment of the basket, and mucosal damage.[29] Disruption of the mucosa can cause bleeding and interference with visibility. Also possible is disruption or avulsion of the ureter. Infringement of the ureteral blood supply may lead to fibrosis or stenosis. If the stone and basket become entrapped in the mucosa, the stone probably is too large to be removed in one piece. No further attempt should be made to do so; rather, lithotripsy should be undertaken.

Once a stone of suitable size has been seized, the basket or forceps should be withdrawn under direct vision with the stone held close to the tip of the ureteroscope. This maneuver decreases the likelihood of ureteral injury.

Lithotripsy

When the stone cannot be extracted easily, it is best to initiate ultrasonic or electrohydraulic lithotripsy.[31–34] For ultrasonic lithotripsy, it is best to trap the stone in a basket. Constant irrigation must be supplied to prevent thermal injury to the ureteral mucosa.[35] Operating the probe in small, short bursts is also helpful. Other complications of ultrasound use are residual microfragments of calculus, hemorrhage, and breakage of the instrument.[34,36,37]

For electrohydraulic lithotripsy, the stone should not be held in position. Rather, the probe is kept several millimeters beyond the end of the ureteroscope and observed constantly to be certain that it does not make contact with the ureteral mucosa. Once the stone has broken up, the fragments must be removed with forceps or a basket. Another precaution is to work only on stones that are not impacted. Complications of early electrohydraulic ureteral lithotripsy are now attributed to direct contact of the probe with the mucosa as a result of attempting the procedure under fluoroscopy. Trials by Green and Lytton[33] and by Raney[38] demonstrated no complications at all when electrohydraulic lithotripsy is performed under direct vision.[33]

Displacement of Stones

Attempts to remove or fragment a stone can result in its displacement either further up the ureter or into the retroperitoneum. The former is the more common problem.

Proximal displacement of the stone can occur at several points in the procedure. Introduction of the guide wire can be sufficient to displace a small calculus. During advancement of the ureteroscope, the pressure of the continuously flowing irrigant may do likewise. Finally, continued manipulation of the stone with a basket or forceps may displace it. In our series, there were seven cases of displacement of the stone into the renal pelvis or calyces; the stone was removed percutaneously in three.

Several precautions can be taken to avoid displacing the stone. First, placing the patient in the reverse Trendelenburg position not only facilitates stone capture but also eliminates gravity as a cause of stone migration. Second, once the stone is visible, the flow of irrigant should be reduced or halted (except during lithotripsy). Finally, baskets or forceps should not be used carelessly but only when the stone has been located visually and is seen to be readily accessible.

Displacement of a stone into the retroperitoneum follows ureteral perforation. Although such loss of a stone is not an ideal outcome for either the urologist or the patient, it is usually not necessary to pursue the stone. Stenting the ureter until the perforation has healed is usually sufficient, as it was in our two cases. However, if the stone is infected and adheres to the ureter at the site of the perforation, there is a considerable risk of fibrosis and stricture formation as a result of tissue reaction. In such cases, surgical exploration, stone retrieval, and ureteral stenting may be a necessity.

Ureteral Perforation or Avulsion

Mechanical perforation of the ureter can take place at any point in the procedure beginning with dilatation of the ureterovesical junction.[11–13] Small perforations are rather common, as extravasation occurs in 10 to 15 percent of patients immediately after the procedure. Usually, 48 hours of drainage with the original catheter used for the retrograde pyelogram is sufficient if subsequent films show no extravasation. If extensive trauma is suspected, a pigtail stent can be inserted for 6 weeks, at which stage the intravenous urogram usually shows healing; however, the films must be repeated without the stent a few weeks later to exclude a delayed stricture (Fig. 21–3*A*). If stent insertion is not possible or if the disruption is more extensive, a percutaneous nephrostomy tube will divert the urine until edema subsides. Without stenting or other form of urinary diversion, urine leakage may produce retroperitoneal fibrosis,[14] abscess, stricture, or obstruction that presents as abdominal pain and renal colic (Figs. 21–3*B* and *C*).[15]

Complete disruption of the ureter is caused by forceful advancement of the ureteroscope beyond a narrowed area or pulling on a basket or forceps that have grasped mucosa. Obviously, avulsion requires open surgical repair; the question is when. If avulsion occurs early in the procedure, before much manipulation has taken place, immediate repair with the patient under the original anesthesia is appropriate. However, if avulsion occurs after considerable manipulation has taken place, the tissues will be friable and reimplantation is likely to fail. In these cases, a percutaneous nephrostomy tube should be inserted and the repair delayed until the edema has subsided.

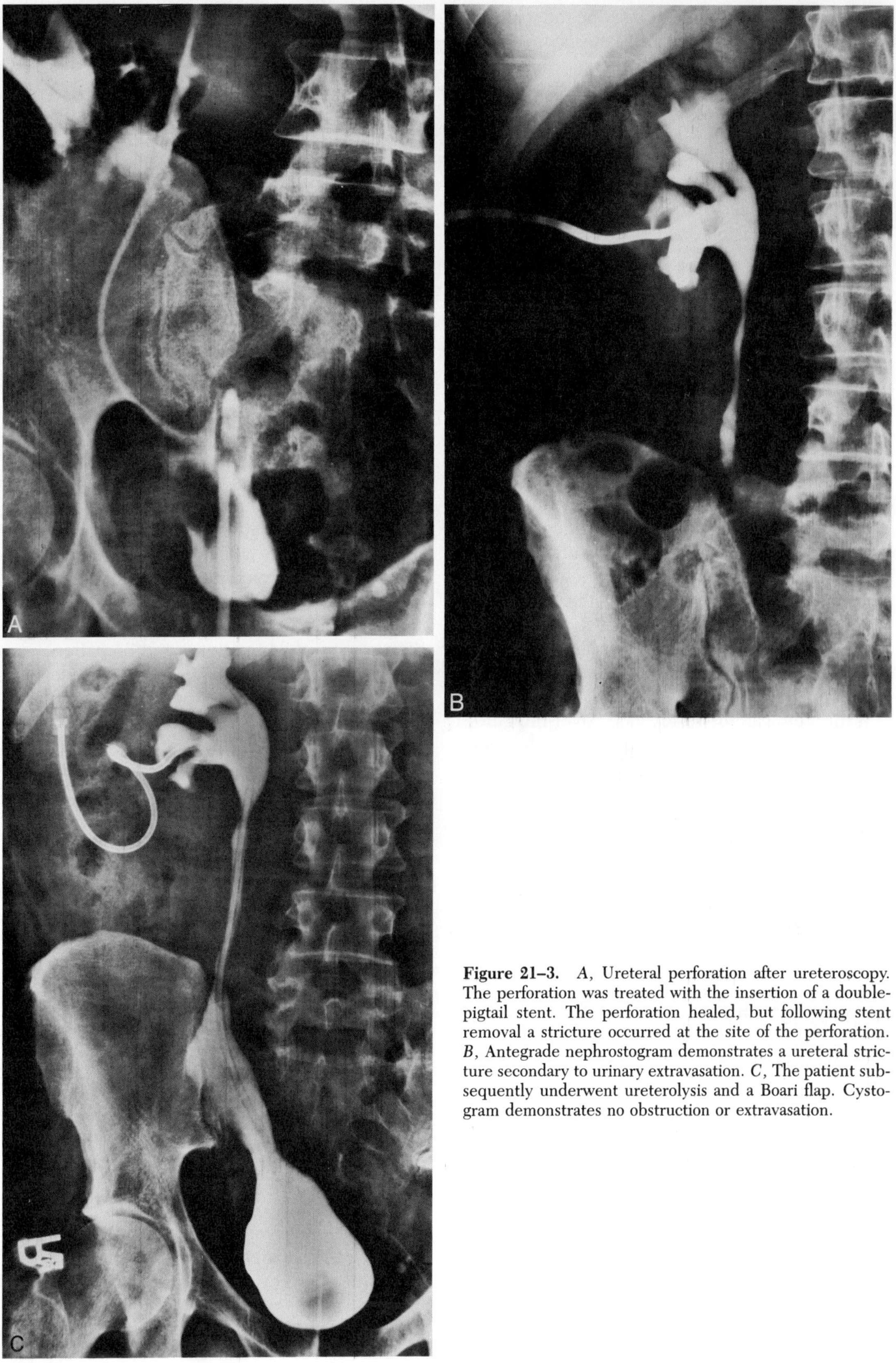

Figure 21–3. *A*, Ureteral perforation after ureteroscopy. The perforation was treated with the insertion of a double-pigtail stent. The perforation healed, but following stent removal a stricture occurred at the site of the perforation. *B*, Antegrade nephrostogram demonstrates a ureteral stricture secondary to urinary extravasation. *C*, The patient subsequently underwent ureterolysis and a Boari flap. Cystogram demonstrates no obstruction or extravasation.

To avoid these complications, one must always handle the ureteroscope gently. Resistance to its advancement signals a turn or kink in the ureter or a stenotic segment. It may be possible to straighten the area or dilate it with a catheter or balloon passed ahead of the ureteroscope. If this is not possible, ureteroscopy should be abandoned. Moreover, the ureteroscope should never be advanced unless the guide wire and the ureter are visible.

Postoperative Stenting

Only if a stone has been removed with minimal trauma is a stent forgone. In most cases, therefore, a stent is inserted. Generally, this can be done easily over the guide wire used for the procedure. Some endourologists prefer to use a double-pigtail stent with a monofilament thread at its distal end that hangs out through the urethra, permitting removal in the office without cystoscopy. However, some operators prefer to perform a retrograde pyelogram before removing the stent to confirm the absence of perforation, extravasation, or residual stone fragments; therefore, an externally draining ureteral catheter is placed and removed approximately 48 hours later.

If the stent cannot be advanced over the guide wire, a retrograde pyelogram should be performed to locate the point of obstruction. Often, a flexible guide wire can be negotiated across the obstruction, over which the stent will usually pass. If this, too, fails, a percutaneous nephrostomy can be performed for antegrade insertion of a guide wire and stent. If antegrade insertion likewise fails, nephrostomy drainage will suffice during further investigation of the problem.

Hemorrhage and Infection

Ureteroscopy is just as likely to cause bleeding and infection as are other types of instrumentation. Prophylactic antibiotics are needed in all cases. In a patient with a known urinary infection, it is advisable simply to pass a ureteral catheter beyond the obstruction in the first session and delay ureteroscopy until the infection has been eradicated.

Hemorrhage is rarely of major significance, and in only one of our patients was a transfusion required. Occasionally, a blod clot causes postoperative obstruction of the ureteral stent, resulting in colic. Gentle irrigation with a syringe will flush out the clot, restoring catheter patency.

Delayed Complications

Ureteral stenosis and stricture formation have been reported after ureteroscopy[16] but are not necessarily caused by the procedure. An impacted stone disrupts the ureteral mucosa and may cause scarring no matter how it is removed. Similarly, pressure by the stent may result in tissue ischemia and fibrosis, which also leads to stricture formation.[14,17,18] A few cases of periureteral fibrosis are attributable to urinary extravasation through a perforation.

The few reports of long-term results of ureteroscopy are most encouraging. Stackl and Marberger found no ureteral stenosis or renal scarring in 38 of 42 patients studied by intravenous urography 19 to 20 months after ureteroscopy, and none of the patients had symptoms of obstruction.[17] There was no increase in the incidence of urinary tract infection or hypertension. Lyon and associates[4] and Ford and Wickham[19] had no significant long-term complications in their review of 242 patients and 31 patients, respectively. Furthermore, ureteroscopy clearly is associated with a lower incidence of both immediate and delayed complications than are ureterolithotomy and transureteral stone manipulation. Bucchiere and Furlow, who reviewed the effects of those more traditional procedures performed in 1061 patients between 1950 and 1966, found morbidity rates of 10 to 25 percent, depending on the procedure[20]; and Amar and associates found a 4 to 5 percent incidence of ureteral stricture after open operation.[21]

Several options are available to manage ureteral strictures. We recommend that balloon dilatation, either retrograde or antegrade (via a percutaneous nephrostomy) with at least 6 weeks of ureteral stenting, be the initial approach. If this fails, open operation is appropriate, with the procedure depending on the location and length of the stricture.

CONCLUSION

The incidence of complications of ureteroscopy is low, provided that the operator is careful and patient. Even in the presence of ureteral tortuosity or stenosis, ureteroscopy may be possible. Certainly, it is more prudent to perform intraureteral manipulations under direct vision than blindly or under fluoroscopy alone. If the procedure fails or complications occur, other options have not been precluded. If ureteroscopy succeeds, both patient and urologist are gratified.

References

1. White EC, Smith AD: Percutaneous stone extraction from 200 patients. J Urol 132:437, 1984.
2. Streem SB, Pontes JE, Novick AC, Montie JE: Ureteropyeloscopy in the evaluation of upper tract filling defects. J Urol 136:383, 1986.
3. Ford TF, Watson GM, Wickham JEA: Transurethral ureteroscopic retrieval of ureteric stones. Br J Urol 55:626, 1983.
4. Lyon ES, Huffman JL, Bagley DH: Ureteroscopy and ureteropyeloscopy. Urology 23 (Suppl 5):29, 1984.
5. Khuri FJ, Peartree RJ, Ruotolo RA, Valvo JR: Rigid ureteropyeloscopy: diagnostic and therapeutic indications. NY State J Med 85:205, 1985.
6. Clayman RV, Surya, V, Miller RP, Costaneda-Zuniga WR, Smith AD, Hunter DH, Amplatz K, Lange PH: Percutaneous nephrolithotomy: extraction of renal and ureteral calculi from 100 patients. J Urol 131:868, 1984.
7. Coleman CC, Kimura Y, Castaneda-Zuniga WR, Hunter DW, Castaneda F, Young A, Amplatz K: Interventional techniques in the ureter. Semin Intervent Radiol 1:24, 1984.
8. Lupu AN, Fuch GJ, Chaussy CG: A new approach to ureteral stone manipulation for ESWL. Endourol Newslett 1(1):13, 1986.
9. Chaussy CG, Fuchs GJ: World experience with extracorporeal shock-wave lithotripsy (ESWL) for the treatment of urinary stones: an assessment of its role after 5 years of clinical use. Endourol Newslett 1(1):7, 1986.
10. Hawkins IF, Jr: Retrograde nephrostomy tract creation. Semin Intervent Radiol 1:9, 1984.
11. Huffman JL, Bagley DH, Lyon ES: Extending cystoscopic techniques into the ureter and renal pelvis. JAMA 250:2002, 1983.
12. Huffman JL: Transurethral endoscopy of the upper urinary tract. NY State J Med 85:194, 1985.
13. Kaufman JJ: Ureteral injury from ureteroscopic stone manipulation. Urology 23:267, 1984.
14. Mitchinson MJ, Bird DR: Urinary leakage and retroperitoneal fibrosis. J Urol 105:56, 1971.
15. Bagley DH: Ureteropyeloscopy. NY State J Med 85:193, 1985.
16. Biester R, Gillenwater JY: Complications following ureteroscopy. J Urol 136:380, 1986.
17. Stackl W, Marberger M: Late sequelae of the management of ureteral calculi with the ureterorenoscope. J Urol 136:386, 1986.
18. Davis DM: The process of ureteral repair: a recapitulation of the splinting question. J Urol 79:215, 1958.
19. Ford TF, Wickham JEA: Transurethral ureteroscopic stone extraction. Br J Surg 71:777, 1984.
20. Bucchiere JJ, Furlow WL: The surgical fate of ureteral calculi: review of Mayo Clinic experience. J Urol 116:559, 1976.
21. Amar AD, Das S, Bulusu NV: Ureteral strictures following ureterolithotomy. J Urol 125:416, 1981.
22. Huffman JL, Bagley DH, Lyon ES: Treatment of distal ureteral calculi using rigid ureteroscope. Urology 20:574, 1982.
23. Smith AD: Rapid dilatation of ureteral orifice for ureteroscopy. Urology 26:407, 1985.
24. Daughtry JD, Bean WJ, Rodan BA, Mullin DM: Balloon dilatation of the ureter: a means to facilitate passage of ureteral and renal calculi. J Urol 136:1063, 1986.
25. Rutner AB: Balloon dilatation of lower ureter to facilitate cystoscopic extraction of large ureteral calculi. Urology 21:226, 1983.
26. Maddocks RA, Leadbetter GW: Absence of vesicoureteral reflux after stone basket manipulation. Urology 7:272, 1976.
27. Ransle PG, Risdon RA: Reflux and renal scarring. Br J Radiol 14(Suppl):1, 1978.
28. Banner MP, Pollack HM: Dilatation of ureteral stenosis: techniques and experience in 44 patients. Am J Roentgenol 143:789, 1984.
29. Alterbarmakian VK, Caldamone AA, Davis RS, Peartree RJ: Stricture of ureter caused by stone basket manipulation. Urology 19:13, 1982.
30. Drach GW: Stone manipulation. Urology 12:286, 1978.
31. Howard SS, Merrill E, Harris S, Cohen J: Ultrasonic lithotripsy: laboratory evaluation. Invest Urol 1:273, 1974.
32. Miller RA: Endoscopic application of shock wave technology for the destruction of renal calculi. World J Urol 3:36, 1985.
33. Green DF, Lytton B: Early experience with direct vision electrohydraulic lithotripsy of ureteral calculi. J Urol 133:767, 1985.
34. Huffman JL, Bagley DH, Schoenberg HW, Lyon ES: Transurethral removal of large ureteral and renal pelvic calculi using ureteroscopic ultrasonic lithotripsy. J Urol 130:31, 1983.
35. Marberger M, Stackl W, Hruby W, Wurster H, Schendl W: Ultrasonic lithotripsy and soft tissue. World J Urol 3:27, 1985.
36. Marberger M, Stackl W, Hruby W, Kroiss A: Late sequelae of ultrasonic lithotripsy of renal calculi. J Urol 133:170, 1985.
37. Marberger M: Disintegration of renal and ureteral calculi with ultrasound. Urol Clin North Am 10:729, 1983.
38. Raney AM: Electrohydraulic ureterolithotripsy: preliminary report. Urology 12:284, 1978.

COMPLICATIONS OF RETROPERITONEAL LYMPHADENECTOMY

22

Steven M. Weiner • E. David Crawford

Retroperitoneal lymphadenectomy (RPLND) is a well-established modality for the accurate staging and treatment of nonseminomatous germ cell testis tumors (NSGCTT). With the development of extremely effective multidrug chemotherapy regimens, patients with tumors previously judged unresectable may now be candidates for curative surgery.

HISTORICAL PERSPECTIVES

The first RPLND for testis cancer was performed in 1902 by Roberts and demonstrated that the operation was technically feasible, although the patient died of complications.[65,70] In 1910, Chevassu reported on performing the procedure using an incision extending from the tenth rib to the internal ring on the involved side.[65] Hinman[26] described a two-stage procedure consisting of an initial inguinal-scrotal orchiectomy and, upon pathologic confirmation of tumor, an RPLND via extension of the incision to the costal margin in the mid-axillary line. Enthusiam for this procedure waned until rekindled by Kimbrough and Lewis at the Walter Reed Hospital in the post–World War II era.[70] Here, Lewis reported on 169 consecutive RPLNDs without an operative fatality. Cooper[10] demonstrated the usefulness and superb exposure afforded by the thoracoabdominal approach to the retroperitoneum and suprahilar area in 1950. Patton and Mallis[49] emphasized the transabdominal approach in 1959 and noted the ease with which bilateral dissections could be performed. Modified node dissections have been advocated since then by many authors[17,21,36] as a way of preserving ejaculatory competence in the absence of gross retroperitoneal disease at the time of lymphadenectomy.

FACTORS CONTRIBUTING TO PERIOPERATIVE COMPLICATIONS

Young adult males who are otherwise healthy have very little difficulty tolerating a routine RPLND. The overall operative mortality is less than 1 percent, and the overall morbidity, excluding ejaculatory impotence, varies from between 6 and 30 percent, with the majority of authors reporting complications in the 8 to 15 percent range.[2,17,29,38,51,54–56,60,63,66–68,70,71]

It is clear from the literature that, in addition to the recognized surgical risk factors, various other conditions unique to patients with this tumor increase the susceptibility to developing operative-related complications. These factors include preoperative chemotherapy, bulky retroperitoneal disease, extent of dissection, and, possibly, the surgical approach.

Preoperative *cis*-platinum-based chemotherapy regimens have revolutionized the treatment of metastatic NSGCTT, with survival rates approaching those achieved for stage A disease. The potentially adverse effects of *cis*-platinum on renal function and the temporary myelosuppression associated with vinblastine may increase the potential for postoperative morbidity in the patient with metastatic NSGCTT.

The reduction in tumor burden afforded by the chemotherapy can facilitate the removal of bulky disease while decreasing the operating time and reducing blood loss. Unfortunately, the tissue reaction to multiple courses of chemotherapy also can obscure natural cleavage planes, which may make the dissection particularly hazardous around major vascular structures.[17] For example, it is quite easy to strip the adventitia off the aorta, resulting in a weakened vessel wall that is prone to rupture. Should this occur, it may be necessary to bolster or replace the aorta with a woven or knitted Dacron graft.

As a corollary of the foregoing discussion, it would appear that the more advanced the disease, the greater the likelihood of a postoperative complication. Sago[54] reported no difference in operative morbidity for stages I(A1), IIA(B_1), and IIB(B_2) disease. Donohue[16] reported a complication incidence of 15.8 percent for stage I(A), 13.2 percent for stage II(B_1, B_2, B_3), and 26.0 percent for stage III(C) patients. McLorie[42] encountered no significant complications in patients operated on for stage II(B_1, B_2, B_3) disease but reported nine complications in 20 patients operated on for stage III(C) disease, including one death. Finally, Skinner[56] reported a major complication incidence of only 3.1 percent for stages I(A), IIA(B_1), IIB(B_2) disease in contrast to 17.3 percent for stages IIC(B_3) and III(C) disease.

Similarly, the more extensive the RPLND, the greater the morbidity. As the scope of infrahilar dissection is expanded, the likelihood of postoperative ejaculatory incompetence increases. This is especially true if the area around the aortic bifurcation is extensively resected. Modified bilateral dissections can minimize this complication but are suggested only in patients with stages I(A) and IIA(B_1) disease.[21,35]

The need for suprahilar dissection depends on the extent of disease below the renal vessels. Donohue[16] routinely performed suprahilar dissection for all stages of NSGCTT prior to 1982, and he noted an increase in operating time of at least 1.5 hours as well as an increased risk to major vessels. Sago[54] suggested that pancreatic complications increased if suprahilar dissection was performed, but others have noted that these can be minimized if proper attention is paid to packing and retraction in this area.[16] Donohue[16] reviewed the distribution of nodal metastases in his first 235 retroperitoneal lymphadenectomy procedures and noted that the incidence of suprahilar metastases in the absence of gross infrahilar disease was less than 1 percent. In the presence of advanced stage IIB(B_2) disease (≥ 5 grossly involved nodes or nodes ≥ 2 cm), there was nearly a 30 percent incidence of suprahilar metastases. It is now generally recommended that suprahilar dissection be reserved for those patients with advanced infrahilar disease.

Finally, the relationship between the approach to the retroperitoneum and subsequent postoperative complications is unknown because no prospective randomized trials comparing any two approaches have ever been done. However, when all series are compared, the complication rates appear to be similar regardless of the route chosen. The incidence of postoperative small bowel obstruction tends to be lower if a pure extraperitoneal approach is utilized; however, the ability to perform contralateral dissections is often compromised.

MORTALITY

The overall mortality of RPLND is approximately 1 percent.[2,8,16,18,21,27,29,38,42,51,54,56,60,66,67,70,71] In Hinman's 1919 review of 51 patients who underwent retroperitoneal lymph node dissections,[27] five deaths were reported. Since then, however, operative-related mortality has become a rare occurrence, although surgery following preoperative chemotherapy is associated with an increased mortality, especially in patients with advanced disease.[70]

MORBIDITY

Wound Complications

Wound infection incidence after RPLND ranges from 0 to 17 percent and varies from superficial infection to frank and life-threatening wound dehiscence.[2,17,19,26,29,38,54,56,60,63,69] Although not specifically addressed in the literature, it can generally be assumed that patients who are nutritionally depleted or who have received preoperative chemotherapy are at greater risk for developing wound complications. Likewise, routine preoperative mechanical bowel preparation and perioperative antibiotics have not been extensively discussed in the literature, but they probably are not needed for the routine stage I(A) or IIA(B_1) lymphadenectomy.

There is no evidence that routine perioperative antibiotics decrease the incidence of wound infections. Consideration should be given to their use, however, in high-risk patients such as those with bulky disease or those who have had previous chemotherapy. Some authors recommend the routine use of external retention sutures in high-risk patients.[9,60,73]

The percentage of patients undergoing RPLND with incidental appendectomy is unknown. Sago[54] reported that of 24 retroperitoneal lymphadenectomies performed with incidental appendectomies, six (25 percent) developed wound infections, compared with only two infections in 23 patients who did not have incidental appendectomies. He recommended that incidental appendectomy be discouraged in the setting of RPLND and that it be avoided in patients who have not undergone preoperative mechanical bowel preparation. We do not recommend a routine appendectomy in these patients.

Pulmonary Complications

The adult respiratory distress syndrome (ARDS) associated with bleomycin-induced pulmonary fibrosis is clearly a devastating sequela of RPLND. Goldiner and colleagues[23,24] correctly identified the hazards associated with anesthesia and surgery in patients treated with bleomycin. Bleomycin is well known to produce chronic fibrotic changes in the lung that lead to restrictive pulmonary disease and impaired carbon monoxide diffusion capacity (Fig. 22–1). These changes are quite subtle and may require pulmonary-function testing to be appreciated. Overhydration during surgery in the face of fixed pulmonary-artery resistance may lead to interstitial edema, thereby enhancing the diffusion-deficit caused by the bleomycin. Raising inspired FI_{O_2} concentrations to maintain adequate arterial saturations may then lead to the destruction of type I and type II pneumocytes, producing the classic clinical picture of the ARDS. This theory assumes that the pneumocytes have become sensitized to relatively low FI_{O_2} concentrations because these levels are not toxic to normal respiratory epithelium. Using this theory as a guideline, Goldiner recommended maintaining a relatively hypovolemic status as measured by Swan-Ganz catheterization monitoring of central and pulmonary pressure, judicious use of crystalloids and preferential use of colloid in fluid replacement, and avoiding FI_{O_2} percentages greater than 25. Following these guidelines, no further ARDS has been reported in their series of over 200 patients.[23]

Other reported pulmonary complications following RPLND include atelectasis, pneumonia, pleural effusion, hemothorax and/or pneumothorax, empyema, lung abrasion secondary to a cut rib edge, and pulmonary embolism.[16,17,21,42,43,51,54,67,69]

Atelectasis is a common complication in the early postoperative period and is more likely to occur in patients who have had a large abdominal or chest incision and prolonged general anesthesia. Clinically, it is manifested by fever, tachycardia, rales, and poor air movement. Early, aggressive respiratory physiotherapy, including incentive spirometry, intermittent positive airway pressure breathing, the use of nebulized bronchodilators and mucolytics, and early ambulation, are all needed to prevent the development of consolidation or pneumonia. Preoperative instruction to the patient on the techniques of deep breathing and coughing can facilitate early postoperative recovery of pulmonary function. Also, the judicious use of parenteral narcotics can help minimize the respiratory depressant effects associated with these medications. We have reported on the beneficial effects of perioperative intercostal nerve-blocking agents in reducing both atelectasis and analgesic requirements following the thoracoabdominal approach for retroperitoneal lymph node dissection.[12]

Hemopneumothorax is a rare complication associated with the thoracoabdominal approach to the retroperitoneum, now that closed-tube thoracostomy is routinely used in the postoperative period. Skinner[57] reported that of 20 patients who had no intraoperative chest tubes placed, seven (35 percent) developed hemopneumothorax and required postoperative chest tube placement. Of 38 patients who had had an intraoperative chest tube placed, only one required another chest tube for hemopneumothorax.

Pleural effusions in the postoperative period are not uncommon and are nearly always transudative in patients who have undergone thoracoabdominal incision. Ileus with subsequent third spacing of fluid, fluid overload, and transient depletion of oncotically active proteins all contribute to the development of pleural effusions. Persistent or loculated effusions, fever, and/or leukocytosis well into the postoperative period suggest possible empyema, and consideration should be given to diagnostic thoracentesis.

Pulmonary embolism is a rare but life-threatening complication following RPLND. Clinical thrombophlebitis, which is often associated with

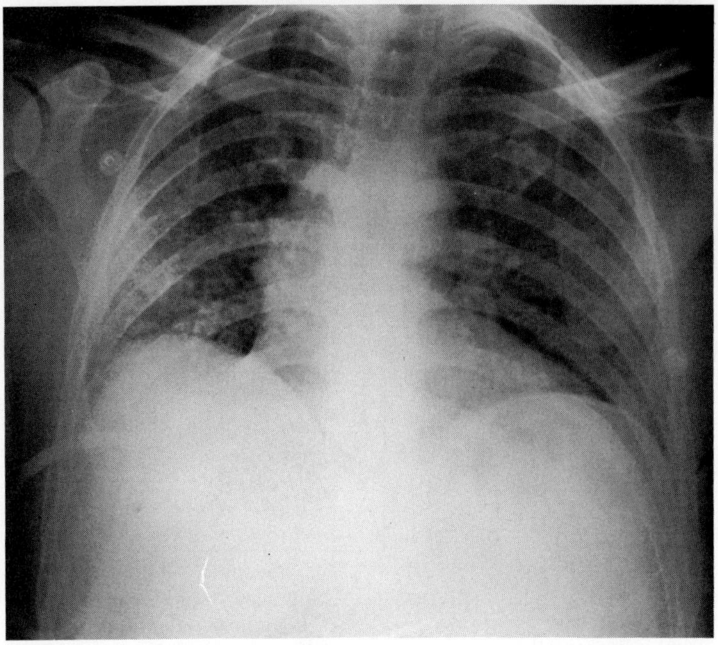

Figure 22–1. Posterior/anterior (PA) chest radiograph of 32-year-old man with bleomycin pulmonary toxicity. Note patchy bilateral pulmonary infiltrates and elevated fixed hemidiaphragms. (Courtesy of John N. Wettlaufer, M.D.)

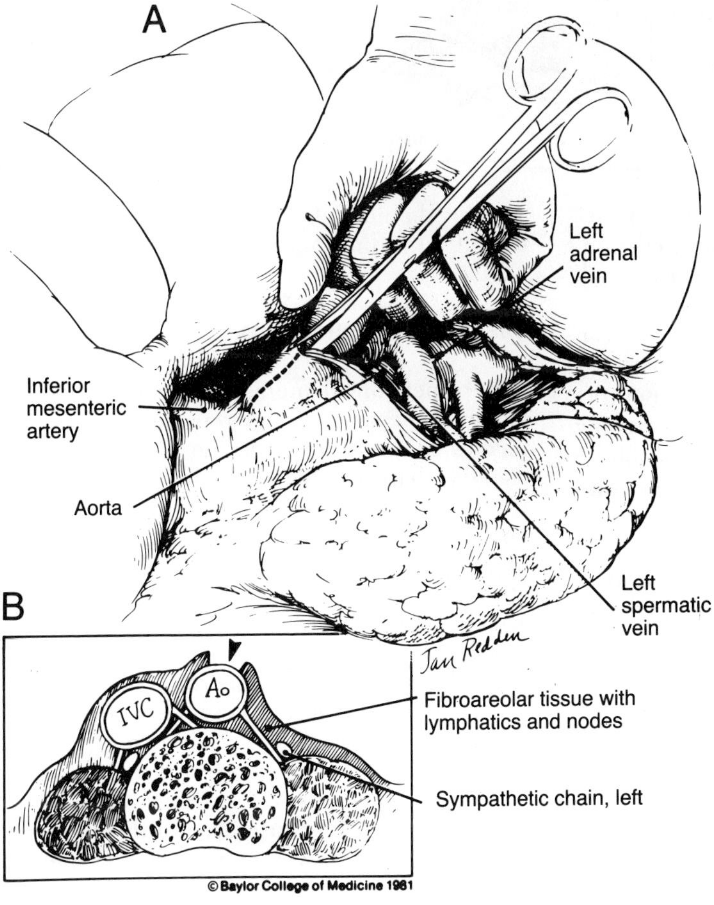

Figure 22–2. Split-and-roll technique. *A*, The left renal vein is mobilized by dividing the adrenal and spermatic veins. The plane between the aorta and the retroperitoneal tissue to be dissected can be established bluntly as illustrated. *B*, The dissection is viewed in cross section to illustrate the tissue to be dissected from the great vessels. (From Scardino PT: Thoracoabdominal retroperitoneal lymphadenectomy for testicular cancer. In Crawford ED and Borden TA eds: Genitourinary Cancer Surgery. Philadelphia, Lea & Febiger, 1982, with permission.)

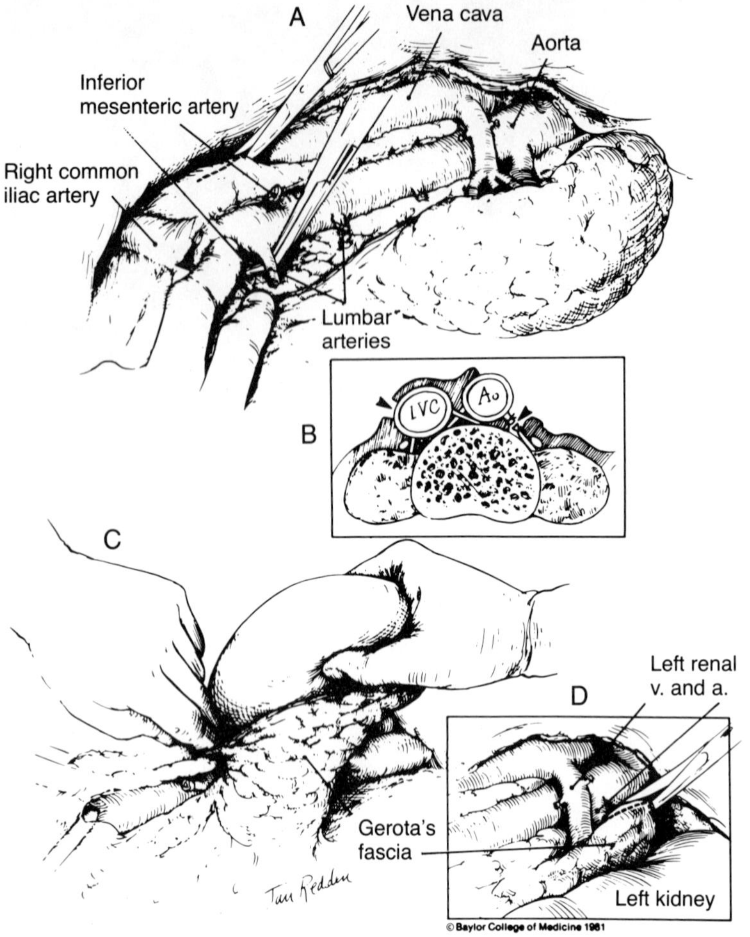

Figure 22–3. Split-and-roll technique (continued). *A*, The lateral border of the dissection is the lateral aspect of the inferior vena cava. Hemoclips must be applied along this margin. The lumbar arteries are identified, ligated, and divided. *B*, Cross-sectional view. *C*, Gerota's fascia is divided over the lateral border of the kidney and split into an anterior and posterior bundle. *D*, The ring of perirenal fat is divided at the renal hilum while the renal vessels are directly visible. (From Scardino PT: Thoracoabdominal retroperitoneal lymphadenectomy for testicular cancer. In Crawford ED and Borden TA eds: Genitourinary Cancer Surgery. Philadelphia, Lea & Febiger, 1982, with permission.)

the subsequent development of pulmonary embolism, is not always present in affected individuals. Factors that deter venous stasis, such as intermittent calf compression, early ambulation, and low-dose anticoagulation therapy, can help minimize the risk to patients undergoing prolonged and extensive operations. Routine use of mini-dose heparin in patients undergoing RPLND has not been advocated because of the small but definite increase in hemorrhagic complications associated with heparin therapy as well as its questionable efficacy in patients having this extensive dissection. Leyvraz and associates[37] have reported on adjusting mini-dose heparin levels to the activated partial thromboplastin times. This approach appears ideally suited for high-risk patients undergoing lymphadenectomy because tissue thromboplastin levels frequently override the effect of mini-dose heparin. Should pulmonary embolism occur, the patient should be hemodynamically stabilized and treated with full-dose heparin IV therapy for a time sufficient to allow fibrinolysis to occur, and this should be followed by oral sodium warfarin (Coumadin) therapy for 3 to 6 months.

Vascular Complications

Retroperitoneal metastases from NSGCTT follow the course of the retroperitoneal lymphatics and, as such, become intimately associated with the vascular structures traversing the retroperitoneum. In the course of retroperitoneal dissection, many of these vessels can be inadvertently traumatized. Review of the literature reveals that injury has occurred to renal arteries and renal veins, aorta, vena cava, iliac arteries and veins, and the ileocolic artery. No reports have appeared concerning injury to the celiac axis or superior mesenteric artery, although this undoubtedly has occurred.

The inferior mesenteric artery is routinely sacrificed by many urologic surgeons to facilitate exposure, and it has caused very little morbidity (e.g., diarrhea) in young patients. However, complications may occur in older patients. Di-

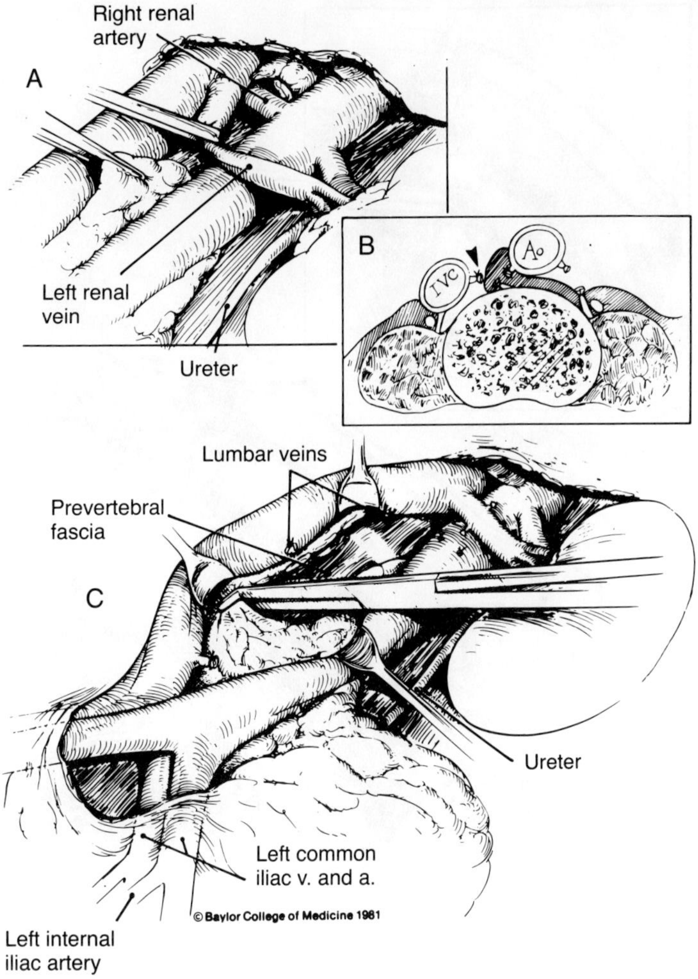

Figure 22–4. Split-and-roll technique (continued). With the left renal vein and right renal artery retracted inferiorly, the interaortocaval tissue above the right renal artery can be mobilized as a packet, clipped, and divided. This is the right "suprahilar" tissue. *B*, All of the tissue anterior, medial, and posterior to the inferior vena cava is dissected; the left lumbar veins are ligated and divided to expose the prevertebral fascia so that all interaortocaval tissue is removed. *C*, The dissection is facilitated if the vena cava is retracted laterally and hemoclips are applied just adjacent to the right lumbar veins. The dissection continues inferiorly to a level several centimeters below the aortic bifurcation. The right lumbar arteries are divided, and the aorta is lifted anteriorly and laterally, allowing the node-bearing tissue to be passed beneath. (From Scardino PT: Thoracoabdominal retroperitoneal lymphadenectomy for testicular cancer. In Crawford ED and Borden TA eds: Genitourinary Cancer Surgery. Philadelphia, Lea & Febiger, 1982, with permission.)

vision of the inferior mesenteric artery is contraindicated in patients who have had prior left colon surgery. Blood loss and vascular injury can be minimized by complete vascular dissection and mobilization of the aorta and vena cava with planned ligation of the lumbar vessels using the split-and-roll technique (Figs. 22–2 through 22–5).[17] Dissecting Gerota's fascia off the kidney and identifying the vessels at the hilum serve to reduce both vascular injury (Fig. 22–4) and polar vessel injury.

We routinely administer 12.5 gm of mannitol IV prior to manipulation of the renal vessels. Segmental and polar renal artery ligation has been reported.[17,67] Skinner[56] reported one patient who developed postoperative hypertension after a lower-pole renal artery ligation. The renovascular nature of the hypertension was confirmed by angiography and by differential renal vein renins. Others, however,[17,67] have reported no adverse effects from such an injury. Clearly, it is always best to anticipate the presence of aberrant vessels and to preserve them if at all possible (Figs. 22–6 and 22–7).

A comprehensive review of the literature has revealed only 11 reported cases of injury to the main renal artery during RPLND.[4,17,18,57,60,63,73] Seven injuries led to loss of the involved renal unit, and four of these injuries were primarly repaired. No postoperative problems have been noted in the patients who had primary repair of the artery. Young[73] reported nine postoperative nephrectomies following 67 lymphadenectomies in patients in the Walter Reed series but did not discuss the factors leading to nephrectomy. Beck[4] described a dramatic case in which the left renal artery was inadvertently clipped during a RPLND and remained undetected until after the patient was noted to have developed malignant hypertension when he sustained a grand mal seizure and developed papilledema and decerebrate posturing on the 17th postop-

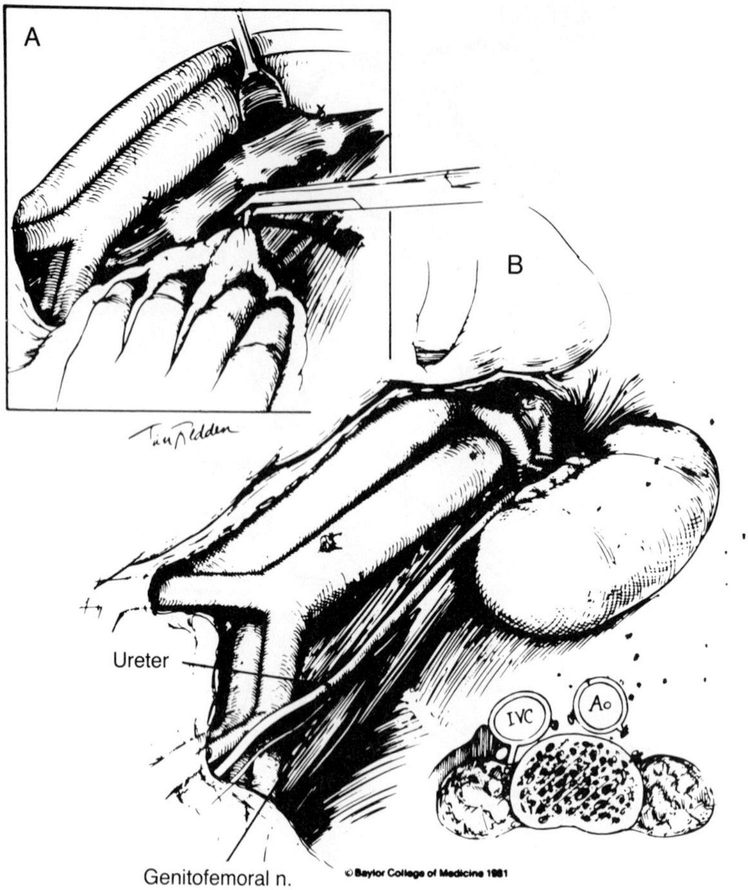

Figure 22–5. Split-and-roll technique (continued). *A*, Clips are applied to the vessels along the left aortic groove in the area of the sympathetic chain. *B*, The completed dissection is illustrated both as an overview and as a cross-section. The left common iliac artery and vein are dissected to a point just beyond their bifurcation. (From Scardino PT: Retroperitoneal lymphadenectomy for testicular cancer. In Crawford ED and Borden TA eds: Genitourinary Cancer Surgery. Philadelphia, Lea & Febiger, 1982, with permission.)

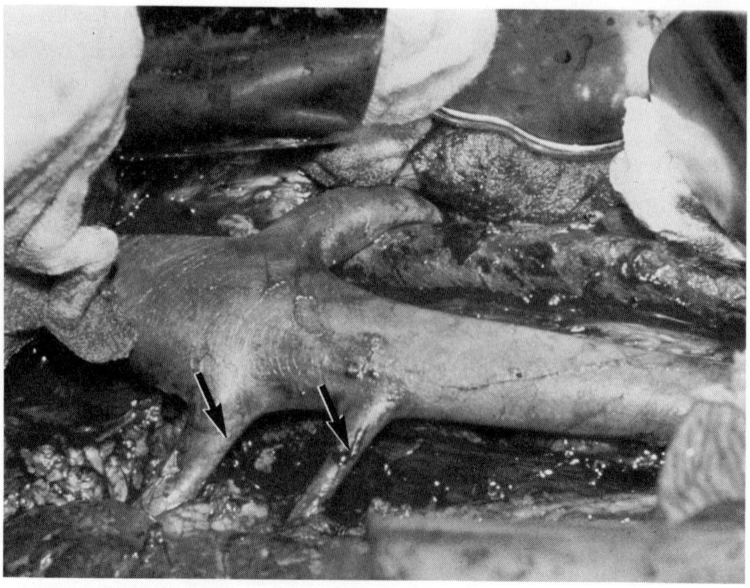

Figure 22–6. Intraoperative photograph demonstrating a double right renal vein (arrows).

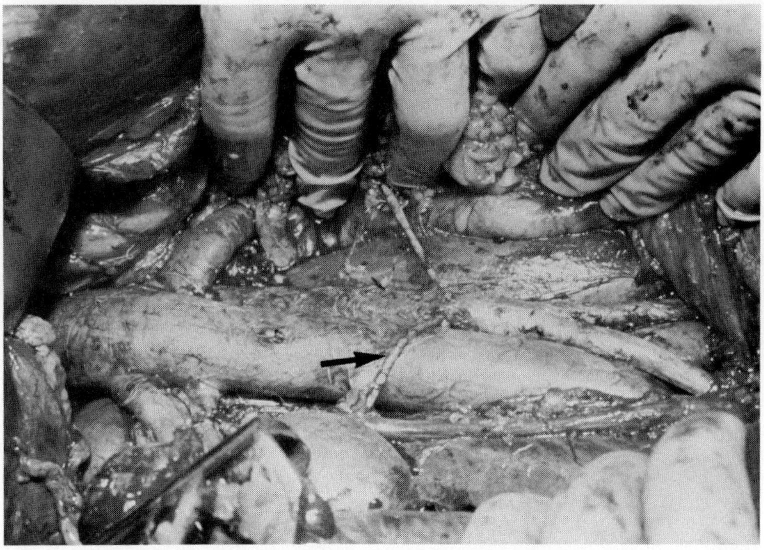

Figure 22–7. Intraoperative photograph demonstrating bilateral lower polar renal vessels originating quite distally on the aorta (arrows).

erative day. Tests revealed the occluded left renal artery, and he underwent a left nephrectomy after blood pressure stabilization. In the immediate postoperative period, he was noted to be paralyzed in the lower extremities and completely blind. Computed tomography scan revealed an infarct in the region of the calcarine cortex.

If inadvertent renal artery injury is recognized at the time of lymphadenectomy, an effort should be made to repair it. It is best not to close lacerations primarily because stenosis and subsequent hypertension may result. Saphenous vein or hypogastric artery patches have been used successfully in renal artery repair. Dacron and Gore-Tex can also be used but are less desirable.

Injuries to the renal vein, on the other hand, nearly always can be repaired primarily and should rarely necessitate nephrectomy. Renal vein thrombosis has been reported following RPLND.[17,38,73] Dissection of the left renal hilum is more tedious because of the multiple branches involved, including the lumbar and adrenal branches (Figs. 22–8 and 22–9). Failure to be cognizant of these vessels can lead to significant intraoperative blood loss.

Special consideration should be given to the dissection of bulky retroperitoneal metastases, which may be intimately associated with the great vessels. Sharp dissection using a surgical knife is frequently necessary. Unfortunately, the most readily developed plane of dissection along the aorta is often subadventitial. Should aortic injury occur during such a dissection, repair is nearly impossible because the ability of the aortic wall to hold sutures is based largely on its dense adventitia. Additionally, these injuries tend to occur during the dissection of bulky tumor, making closure difficult. Extreme measures, such as placing a Foley catheter inside the aorta, may be necessary to control large rents while proximal and distal control is attained. Donohue[17] reported on five patients who needed aortic and/or iliac artery replacement with knitted or woven Dacron grafts because the adventitia had been stripped away and the vessel so compromised that it was deemed unsafe. Indeed, one postoperative aortic rupture occurred and necessitated emergency aortic graft replacement.

Many authors have reported on the success of the en bloc resection of the infrarenal inferior vena cava when it is obstructed, thrombosed, or invaded by large retroperitoneal tumors.[17,40,42,43,56] Mathisen and Javadpour[40] reported on six patients who underwent debulking surgery prior to chemotherapy in which the inferior vena cava and aorta were completely encased by tumor. They noted that, by removing the infrarenal vena cava en bloc with the tumor, they were able to facilitate the dissection of the tumor from the aorta, improve access to the interaortocaval nodes, and eliminate the vena cava as a source of hemorrhage. Postoperatively, they noted no mortality and only minor morbidity (temporary leg edema). One patient developed an iliofemoral thrombosis that was successfully treated with anticoagulants.

Other authors have addressed the morbidity associated with interruption of the inferior vena cava, mostly in reference to the treatment and prevention of pulmonary embolism.[11,25,50,55] These authors report a rather high morbidity

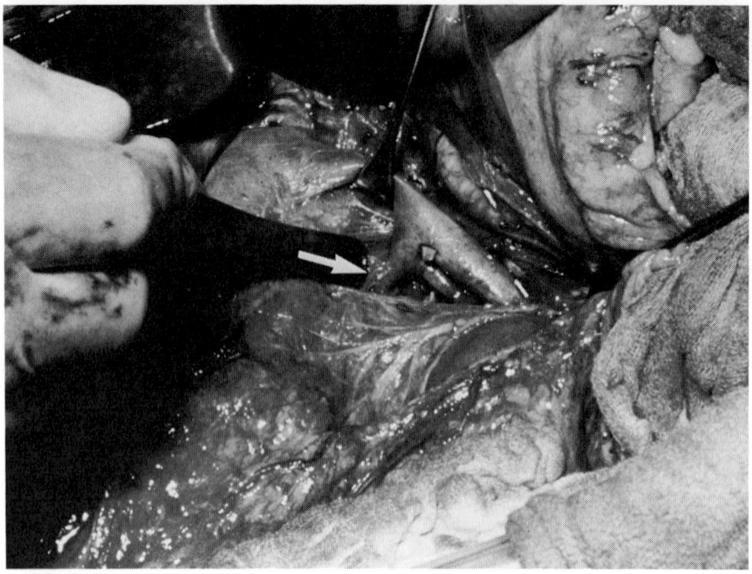

Figure 22–8. Intraoperative photograph demonstrating a lumbar vein joining the left renal vein (arrow).

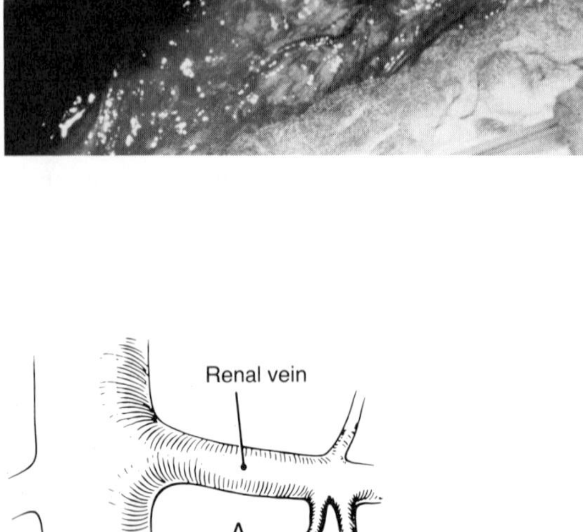

Figure 22–9. Variation in location of the lumbar vein. (From Wise HA II and Crooks KK: Anterior transabdominal approach for radical retroperitoneal lymphadenectomy. In Crawford ED and Borden TA eds: Genitourinary Cancer Surgery. Philadelphia, Lea & Febiger, 1982, with permission.)

rate, including refractory lower extremity edema and chronic venous stasis disease. Whether these patients can be compared with patients with testis tumor who have an obstructed vena cava and previously developed collateral circulation is not known.

One final point should be made regarding vena cava resection. Often, the tumor is so extensive that the right renal pedicle is hopelessly involved, necessitating a right nephrectomy. Although the left renal vein has been ligated successfully without postoperative renal failure during the course of a right nephrectomy,[41] every attempt should be made to preserve it. Skinner[59] reported on five patients who underwent RPLND in whom the left renal vein had been ligated during the course of a right nephrectomy. He noted that acute renal failure ensued, requiring hemodialysis for periods of up to 6 weeks in over half the patients. Although results are encouraging, the enthusiasm for aggressive dissections such as these is not shared universally. Whitmore[70] feels that, with the exception of inferior vena cava thrombosis by tumor, deliberate attempts to perform major vascular replacements are of little therapeutic value compared with the risks and that it is preferable to leave tumor capsule behind and control the tumor with adjuvant chemotherapy.

It is our opinion that every effort should be made to remove all of the retroperitoneal node tissue. We have reported that survival rates in patients who have not received a thorough radical retroperitoneal lymph node dissection are markedly compromised (Table 22–1). Retroperitoneal lymph node dissection after cytoreduc-

Table 22–1. SURVIVAL RELATION TO HISTOLOGY AND SURGICAL REJECTION

	Incomplete Resection (n=16)		Complete Resection (n=38)	
	No. of Patients	*Percent*	*No. of Patients*	*Percent*
Histology				
Cancer	11	(69)*	6	(16)†
Fibrosis	1	(7)*	22	(58)§
Teratoma	4	(25)‡	10	(27)‖
Thoracotomy	6	(35)	12	(31)
Serum Markers				
Positive prechemotherapy	12	(75)	29	(76)
Positive postchemotherapy	7	(43)	2	(5)
Platinum Dose				
High	7	(43)	22	(57)
Low	9	(56)	16	(43)
Survival	5	(31)	37	(97)

*one survivor
†five survivors
‡three survivors
§twenty-two survivors
‖ten survivors
Crawford ED: The Southwest Oncology Group Study for Advanced Testicular Cancer. Semin Urol 2(4):244–253, 1984. Reprinted with permission.

tive chemotherapy is a formidable task and should be undertaken only by a urologic surgeon well trained in retroperitoneal surgery who treats enough patients with this disease to maintain his surgical expertise. These operations are tedious and may require 10 to 14 hours of operating time to complete.

Intestinal Complications

The most common bowel complication reported in the literature following RPLND is bowel obstruction.[2,4,20,38,51,56,67,69] Mechanical obstruction occurs in 1 to 5 percent of patients and often requires re-exploration. It occurs almost exclusively in patients whose peritoneal cavity has been violated. Careful attention to techniques designed to minimize serosal trauma, e.g., using a bowel bag, avoiding laparotomy pads and rigid retractors, minimizing operating time, and carefully reapproximating the posterior peritoneum to close the retroperitoneal space, will all help to reduce the incidence of this complication. The use of a thoracoabdominal incision with an extraperitoneal approach reduces the chance of bowel complications; however, this extraperitoneal approach is suitable only for patients with low-stage disease.

Other complications include bowel ischemia and necrosis,[4] massive gastrointestinal bleeding,[60] and isolated cases of both small bowel and large bowel fistulas.[13,17,20,63] If the fistulas are uncomplicated, i.e., not associated with intra-abdominal sepsis, they can often be treated non-operatively with hyperalimentation or low-residue diets.

Lymphatic Complications

Lymphoceles

A lymphocele or lymphocyst is an abnormal, well-encapsulated collection of lymphatic fluid that occasionally forms after transection of efferent lymphatic channels during lymphadenectomy. The vast majority of lymphoceles have occurred in the pelvis following radical gynecologic procedures and renal transplantation.[45] In the mid-1970s, lymphoceles became a recognized complication of RPLND, and numerous reports have appeared since.[2,22,29,31,39,56,63]

The genesis of lymphoceles has been well established.[31,45] After transection (without ligation) of a lymphatic channel, there is an outpouring of lymph. The proximal ends of the cut lymphatic channel remain open for up to 48 hours and act as a siphon to carry the fluid away from the area of injury before the proximal ends become occluded by fibrin clots. If collateral channels are undisturbed and if the injured segment is short enough to regenerate, a lymphocele will not develop. If, however, collateral channels are disrupted and long segments are injured or removed, a lymphocele is likely to occur (Fig. 22–10).

The symptoms of lymphoceles are nonspecific or absent, and these fluid collections are often noted on follow-up CT scans or ultrasonography examinations. A palpable abdominal mass or feeling of fullness may be noted on physical examination. Lymphoceles have a propensity to cause varying degrees of ureteral obstruction, and, therefore, flank pain may be the presenting symptom. Wettlaufer[72] correctly points out that a lymphocele is not always easily differentiated from a cystic teratoma on radiographic analysis alone. He notes that, although lymphoceles usually have a thin wall, they may indeed be thick-walled. Therefore, it is incumbent upon the urologist to explore the capsules of these cystic masses and to perform biopsy to make a definitive diagnosis. The capsule of a lymphocele will not have an epithelial lining as is found in cystic teratomas.

The management of lymphoceles is varied, with no single treatment modality universally applicable. Small, asymptomatic lymphoceles may require no therapy at all and may resolve spontaneously.[31] In general, simple aspiration is unsuccessful because lymphoceles tend to recur rapidly. Repeated aspirations invariably lead to infection and sepsis. The use of external drainage via a Penrose or Jackson-Pratt drain is a widely advocated method and is usually successful.[39,45] A radiologically placed percutaneous drain using an indwelling pigtail catheter is another method of external drainage. We prefer the creation of a peritoneal window by marsupialization of the cyst wall to the peritoneum. This is usually quite successful—although at times technically demanding—and obviates the need for drains to be left in place for prolonged periods, which is usually the case with methods of external drainage.

Chylous Ascites

Chylous ascites and chylothorax are the other major lymphatic complications occurring after RPLND. Their occurrence can be devastating in terms of morbidity and prolonged hospital stay. Fortunately, they are quite rare, with fewer than 15 cases being reported in the English literature.[1,5,14,28,44,51,63] Chylous ascites results most commonly from parasitic, neoplastic, or inflammatory diseases involving the lymphatic system.[5,14] Following RPLND, it is caused by a rent in the cisterna chyli, thoracic duct, or major intestinal lymphatic tributaries in association with distal lymphatic obstruction.

The cisterna is a dilated ampullary portion of the thoracic duct located medial to the aorta at the level of the L_1 and L_2 vertebral bodies. Up to 50 percent of patients have no specific cisternae, but a coalescence of intestinal lymphatics at this level where they join the thoracic duct.

Patients with chylous ascites and chylothorax most often present with increasing abdominal distention and shortness of breath, usually within the first few weeks postoperatively. Diagnosis is confirmed by paracentesis and/or thoracentesis that demonstrates a milky-appearing fluid with a content high in cholesterol, calcium, lactate dehydrogenase (LDH), alkaline phosphatase, albumin, and total protein in contrast

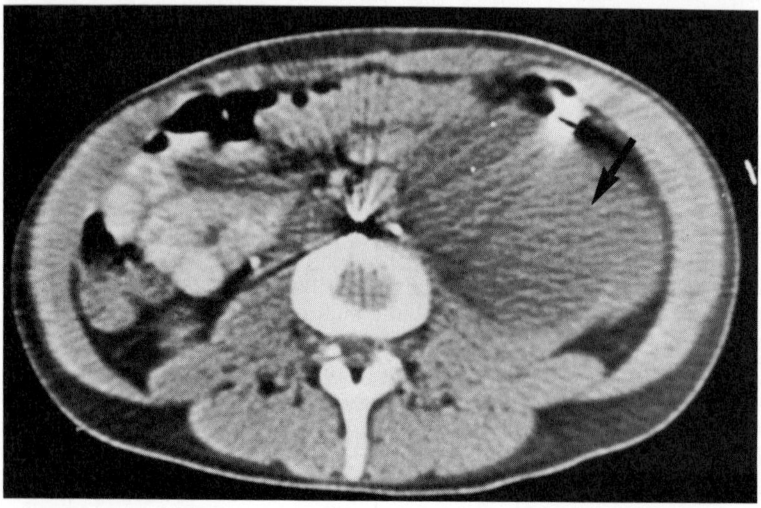

Figure 22–10. Computerized abdominal tomogram demonstrating a large left retroperitoneal lymphocele (arrow).

to urine containing higher concentrations of urea, creatinine, and potassium.

Initial treatment of this condition should be conservative and aimed at decreasing the amount of long-chain fatty acids in the diet. A diet of medium-chain triglycerides rich in protein and otherwise fat free should first be tried. Medium-chain triglycerides are transported directly to the portal circulation, thus bypassing the intestinal lymphatics. Long-chain fatty acids, however, must first be transported through the intestinal lymphatics. If this diet is not tolerated or fails to resolve the ascites within a few weeks, a trial of total parenteral nutrition should be employed to put the bowel totally to rest. These methods will succeed in most patients. Repeat paracentesis or thoracentesis should be avoided except to relieve the discomfort of abdominal distension or shortness of breath.

If conservative measures fail to relieve the ascites, surgical intervention may be necessary. It is unlikely that the point of lymphatic leakage can be identified and oversewn directly. The LeVeen peritoneovenous shunt has been used successfully in a number of patients to control refractory chylous ascites.[44]

Ureteral Injury

Ureteral injury is an uncommon complication associated with RPLND and, when it occurs, results in substantial morbidity.[2,17,38,51,60,63,65] The most common site of ureteral injury is at the point where the gonadal vessel crosses anteriorly to the ureter. Here, tenting up the tissues around the gonadal vein can angulate the ureter if it has not been previously isolated. This can lead to inadvertent ureterotomy or ureteral transection. Small defects may be closed primarily with appropriate stenting. A complete transection of the ureter may not be reparable by ureteroneocystostomy because of the already compromised blood supply caused by the node dissection. This is especially true if the injury has occurred in the upper and middle thirds of the ureter. A transection in the lower third of the ureter often can be managed by a ureter reimplantation or ureteroneocystotomy in conjunction with a psoas hitch. A proximal ureteral injury may necessitate nephrectomy if the contralateral kidney is normal. Transureteroureterostomy may be employed in distal or midureteral transections. Autotransplantation should be considered only in rare instances in which patients have solitary kidney function with a proximal ureteral injury.[58] Vahlensieck[63] noted that of nine patients with ureteral injuries, six required nephrectomy, two required stenting and suffered subsequent stricture formation, and one died from complications after the repair failed.

Infertility

Fertility following RPLND has been discussed extensively in the urologic literature and focuses primarily on two issues. The first is that the affected population is young men in their reproductive years. The second issue is that research into the anatomy and physiology of seminal emission and into the distribution of nodal metastases from testis tumors has made the problem of seminal emission, and possibly infertility, preventable in a large number of patients.

Ejaculatory control is the result of the following three distinct phenomena that are all dependent on intact reflex neural processes: seminal emission, antegrade ejaculation, and closure of the bladder neck.[32] Afferent sensory stimuli are transmitted from the genitalia via the pudendal nerves to the cerebral cortex where efferent fibers send the impulse through the anterolateral columns of the spinal cord to the thoracolumbar sympathetic outflow tract. The sympathetic outflow tract of T_{12}–L_3 then sends signals via the paravertebral ganglion, the aortomesenteric plexus, and the ureteral plexus to the hypogastric plexus, which causes smooth muscle contraction of the vas, ampulla, prostate, and seminal vesicles as well as causes partial closure of the bladder neck. This leads to seminal emission into the posterior urethra. Parasympathetic sacral outflow causes clonic contraction of the striated bulbocavernosus and ischiocavernosus muscles, complete closure of the bladder neck, and relaxation of the external sphincter, which lead to rhythmic, projectile ejaculation through the urethra.[32,35]

There is no doubt that extensive bilateral RPLND leads to permanent ejaculatory incompetence in a vast majority of patients.[6,10,16,21,29,33,35,46,48,56,66,67,69] This fact alone has been the main impetus in the development of techniques of modified or unilateral node dissections to spare the contralateral sympathetic chain and hypogastric plexus as it decussates about the aortic bifurcation.[21,35,63] For these modifications to be practical, the "cancer-curing" tenets that RPLND is based upon cannot be compromised.

The majority of authors who advocate limited node dissection are careful to point out that these operations should be used only in low-stage (stages I(A) and IIA(B_1)) disease and that a more thorough bilateral dissection should be performed if obvious metastatic involvement is present. Others[29] extend these limitations to clinical stage I(A) left-sided tumors only because right-sided tumors have a high incidence of metastatic crossover.[19,53] When these principles are applied, the cure rates for unilateral or modified dissections appear comparable with more extensive bilateral dissections, and retroperitoneal failures are uncommon.[21,35,63]

Lange[35] reported a 51 percent spontaneous return of ejaculation following his modified bilateral node dissection for patients with pathologic stages I(A) and IIA(B_1) disease. In addition, eight of 14 other patients treated with alpha-adrenergic medication had return of ejaculation, and there were 14 pregnancies associated with patients in his series. Fossa[21] reported normal ejaculation in 28 of 36 patients following unilateral RPLND, whereas only three of 16 patients experienced normal ejaculation following standard bilateral lymphadenectomy. Interestingly, in a series of 18 patients, all who underwent unilateral right-sided dissections had a better chance at maintaining normal ejaculation compared with 10 of 18 patients who underwent unilateral left-sided dissections. The authors attributed at least part of the difference to more extensive dissection at the aortic bifurcation for patients with left-sided tumors.

It would appear, therefore, that ejaculatory competence, if not fertility, can be preserved in a large percentage of carefully selected patients. Some authors have questioned the importance of maintaining ejaculatory competence at the expense of a less thorough node dissection.[2,6,16,29,56] They cite data regarding the fertility status of men with testis tumors after orchiectomy but prior to other therapy as well as the patient's desire to father children. In a retrospective study, Bracken and Johnson[6] noted that only 12 of 37 cured married men responding to a questionnaire desired to father children and that of these 12 men, seven eventually impregnated their wives. Other studies have shown that up to 80 percent of men with testis tumors have sperm concentrations less than 20 million per ml immediately before or after orchiectomy.[7,19,56,62] The reason for this is not entirely clear.

Men who develop testis tumors do not appear to be subfertile.[6] Lange[36] noted an average sperm concentration of 90 million per ml in men with spontaneous return of ejaculation following RPLND. Unfortunately, preoperative semen analyses were not routinely performed. These data suggest the presence of one or more reversible factors that may be responsible for the poor semen quality in the periorchiectomy period. These factors may include tumor products such as beta human chorionic gonadotropin (BHCG) or the psychological stress that accompanies a diagnosis of cancer. Lange[36] has estimated that of all patients with testis tumors, perhaps 40 percent will be fertile at the time of diagnosis and that of the remaining 60 percent, 35 percent will have temporary subfertility, and 25 percent will be permanently sterile.

The use of alpha-adrenergic drugs in treating postlymphadenectomy fertility disorders has received much attention in the urologic literature.[32,33,46,47,52,61] Many agents have been shown to be effective, including brompheniramine maleate, phenylephrine HCl, pseudoephedrine HCl, ephedrine, and imipramine. Their effectiveness, however, appears to be limited almost exclusively to patients who suffer from retrograde ejaculation. Unfortunately, this occurs in the minority of men with ejaculatory disorders following RPLND. An occasional patient with absent seminal emission will respond to sympathomimetic therapy,[52] but this is clearly the exception rather than the rule.

Finally, what effect does chemotherapy have on fertility? The deleterious effects of the alkylating agents and vinblastine on semen quality are well known.[19,62] The effects of *cis*-platinum and bleomycin have been examined in regard to spermatogenesis.[19,36] It appears that up to 60 percent of patients treated by chemotherapy alone have sperm counts greater than 20 million per ml within 24 months of treatment.

CONCLUSION

Retroperitoneal lymphadenectomy is a well-established procedure for the staging and treatment of NSGCTT and is easily performed with minimal morbidity and mortality. Meticulous attention to detail combined with a well-thought-out and an orderly approach to the dissection will help minimize the morbidity. Modified dissections for low-stage disease do not appear to contradict the principles of cancer surgery and may prevent postoperative ejaculatory incompetence in a large number of patients.

References

1. Allen W, Parrott TS, Saripkin L, Allan C: Chylous ascites following retroperitoneal lymphadenectomy for granulosa cell tumor of the testis. J Urol 135:797–798, 1986.
2. Babaian RJ, Backen RB, Johnson DE: Complications of transabdominal retroperitoneal lymphadenectomy. Urology 27:126–128, 1981.
3. Barakos JA, Jeffrey RV Jr, McAninch JW, Bottles K: Computerized tomography diagnosis of diffuse intraperitoneal metastases after retroperitoneal lymphadenectomy for testicular carcinoma. J Urol 136:680–681, 1986.
4. Beck PH, Stutzman RE: Complications of retroperitoneal lymphadenectomy for nonseminomatous tumors of testis. Urology 13:244–247, 1979.
5. Bigley HA Jr, Chenault OW Jr: Chylous ascites following retroperitoneal lymphadenectomy. J Urol 114:948–950, 1975.
6. Bracken RB, Johnson DE: Sexual function and fecundity after treatment for testicular tumors. Urology 7:35–38, 1976.
7. Bracken RB, Smith KD: Is semen cryopreservation helpful in testicular cancer? Urology 25:581–583, 1980.
8. Brenner J, Vugrin D, Whitmore WF: Cytoreductive surgery for advanced nonseminomatous germ cell tumors of testis. Urology 19:571–575, 1982.
9. Catalona WJ, Rubenstein MA: An incision for extended suprahilar retroperitoneal lymphadenectomy. J Urol 119:316–319, 1978.
10. Cooper JF, Leadbetter WF, Chute R: The thoracoabdominal approach for retroperitoneal gland dissection: its application to testis tumors. Surg Gynecol Obstet 90:486–496, 1950.
11. Couch NP, Baldwin SS, Crane C: Mortality and morbidity rates after inferior vena cava clipping. Surgery 77:106–112, 1975.
12. Crawford ED, Skinner DG, Capparel DB: Intercostal nerve block with thoracoabdominal incision. J Urol 121:290–291, 1979.
13. Crosse JEW, Soderdahl DW, Schamber DT: Colocutaneous fistula: an unusual complication of retroperitoneal lymphadenectomy. J Urol 115:614–615, 1976.
14. Dharman K, Temes SP, Wetherell FE, Kendrick MJ: Chyloperitoneum and chylothorax: a combined rare occurrence after retroperitoneal lymphadenectomy and radiotherapy for testis tumor. J Urol 131:346–347, 1984.
15. Donohue JP, Einhorn LH, Perez JM: Improved management of nonseminomatous testis tumors. Cancer 42:2903–2908, 1978.
16. Donohue JP, Rowland RG: Complications of retroperitoneal lymph node dissection. J Urol 125:338–340, 1981.
17. Donohue JP: Complications of lymph node dissection. In Marshall FF, ed: Urologic Complications. Chicago, Year Book Medical Publishers, 1986.
18. Dowd JB, Chute R, Weinert SD: Retroperitoneal lymph node dissection for testicular cancer. J Urol 81:448–456, 1959.
19. Drasga RE, Einhorn LH, Williams SD: Fertility after chemotherapy for testicular cancer. J Clin Oncol 1:179–183, 1983.
20. Dykhuizen RF, George FW III, Kurohara S, Rotner M, Sargent CR, Varney JK: The use of cobalt 60 teleculietherapy or x-ray therapy with and without lymphadenectomy in the treatment of testis germinal tumors: a 20-year comparative study. J Urol 10:321–328, 1968.
21. Fossa SD, Klepp O, Ous S, Lien HH, Stenwig AE, Abyholm T, Kaalhus O: Unilateral retroperitoneal lymph node dissection in patients with non-seminomatous testicular tumor in clinical stage I. Eur Urol 10:17–23, 1984.
22. Fried AM, Williams CB, Litvak AS: High retroperitoneal lymphocele: an unusual clinical presentation and diagnosis by ultrasonography. J Urol 123:583–584, 1980.
23. Goldiner PL, Schweizer O: The hazards of anesthesia and surgery in bleomycin-treated patients. Semin Oncol 6:121–124, 1979.
24. Goldiner PL, Carlon GC, Cvitkovic E, Schweizer O, Howland WS: Factors influencing postoperative morbidity and mortality in patients treated with bleomycin. Br Med J 1:1664–1667, 1978.
25. Haimov M, Kirschner P, Kark AE: Fatal complications following inferior vena cava interruption. Vasc Surg 5:228–233,1971.
26. Hinman F: The radical operation for teratoma testis. Surg Gynecol Obstet 28:495–508, 1919.
27. Hinman F, Gibson TE, Kutzmann AA: The radical operation for teratoma testis. Surg Gynecol Obstet 37:429–451, 1923.
28. Jansen TTH, Debruyne FMJ, Delaere KPJ, De Vries JDM: Chylous ascites after retroperitoneal lymph node dissection. Urology 23:565–567, 1984.
29. Johnson DE: Retroperitoneal lymphadenectomy: indications, complications and expectations. Recent Results Cancer Res 60:221–230, 1977.
30. Johnson DE, Bracken RB, Blight EM: Prognosis or pathologic stage I non-seminomatous germ cell tumors of the testis managed by retroperitoneal lymphadenectomy. J Urol 116:63–65, 1976.
31. Jonsson K, Wallace S, Jing B, Johnson DE, Dodd GD: Changes in the lymphatic dynamics after retroperitoneal lymph node dissection. J Urol 118:814–818, 1977.
32. Kedia K, Markland C: The effect of pharmacological agents on ejaculation. J Urol 114:569–573, 1975.
33. Kedia KR, Markland C, Fraley EE: Sexual function after high retroperitoneal lymphadenectomy. Urol Clin North Am 4:523–528, 1977.
34. Klimberg I, Wajsman Z: Duplicated inferior vena cava simulating retroperitoneal lymphadenopathy in the patient with embryonal cell carcinoma of the testicle. J Urol 136:678–679, 1986.
35. Lange PH, Narayan P, Fraley EE: Fertility issues following therapy for testicular cancer. Semin Urol 2:264–274, 1984.
36. Lange PH, Narayan P, Vogelzang NJ: Return of fertility after treatment for nonseminomatous testicular cancer: changing concepts. J Urol 129:1131–1135, 1983.
37. Leyvraz PF, Richard J, Bachmann F, et al: Adjusted versus fixed dose subcutaneous heparin in the prevention of deep venous thrombosis after total hip replacement. N Engl J Med 309:954, 1983.
38. Lindsey CM, Glenn JF: Germinal malignancies of the testis: experience, management and prognosis. J Urol 116:59–62, 1976.
39. Livingston WD, Confer DJ, Smith RB: Large lymphoceles resulting from retroperitoneal lymphadenectomy. J Urol 124:543–546, 1980.
40. Mathisen DJ, Javadpour N: En bloc resection of inferior vena cava in cytoreductive surgery for bulky retroperitoneal metastatic testicular cancer. Urology 16:51–54, 1980.
41. McCullough DL, Gittes RF: Ligation of the renal vein in the solitary kidney: effects on renal function. J Urol 113:295–298, 1975.
42. McLorie GA, Skinner DG: Metastatic non-seminoma-

tous testis tumors: morbidity of treatment. J Urol 124:479–481, 1980.
43. Merrin CE, Takita MH: Cancer reductive surgery: report on the simultaneous excision of abdominal and thoracic metastases from widespread testicular tumors. Cancer 42:495–501, 1978.
44. Miedema EB, Bissada NK, Finkbeiner AE, Casali RE: Chylous ascites complicating retroperitoneal lymphadenectomy for testis tumors: management with peritoneovenous shunting. J Urol 120:377–378, 1978.
45. Mott C, Shreiber MH: Lymphoceles following renal transplantation. Am J Roentgenol 122:821–827, 1974.
46. Narayan P, Lange PH, Fraley EE: Ejaculation and fertility after extended retroperitoneal lymph node dissection for testicular cancer. J Urol 127:685–688, 1982.
47. Nijman JM, Jager S, Boer PW, Kremer J, Oldhoff J, Koops HS: The treatment of ejaculation disorders after retroperitoneal lymph node dissection. Cancer 50:2967–2971, 1982.
48. Orecklin JR, Kaufman JJ, Thompson RW: Fertility in patients treated for malignant testicular tumors. J Urol 109:293–295, 1973.
49. Patton JF, Mallis N: Tumors of the testis. J Urol 81: 457–461, 1959.
50. Piccone VA, Vidal E, Yarnoz M, Glass P, LeVeen HH: The late results of caval ligation. Surgery 68:980–998, 1970.
51. Pizzocaro G, Durand JC, Fuchs WA, Merrin CE, Musumeci R, Schmucki O, Vahlensieck W, Whitmore WF, Zvara VL: Staging and surgery in testicular cancer. Eur Urol 7:1–10, 1981.
52. Proctor KG, Howards SS: The effect of sympathomimetic drugs on post-lymphadenectomy aspermia. J Urol 129:837–838, 1983.
53. Ray B, Hajdu SI, Whitmore WF: Distribution of retroperitoneal lymph node metastases in testicular germinal tumors. Cancer 33:340–348, 1974.
54. Sago AL, Ball TP, Novicki DE: Complications of retroperitoneal lymphadenectomy. Urology 13:241–243, 1979.
55. Shea PC Jr, Robertson RL: Late sequelae of inferior vena cava ligation. Surg Gynecol Obstet 93:153–158, 1951.
56. Skinner DG, Melamud A, Lieskosky G: Complications of thoracoabdominal lymph node dissection. J Urol 127:1107–1110, 1982.
57. Skinner DG, Leadbetter WF: The surgical management of testis tumors. J Urol 106:84–93, 1971.
58. Skinner DG: Complications of lymph node dissection. In Smith, RB, Skinner DG, eds: Complications of Urologic Surgery, Philadelphia, WB Saunders Co, 1976.
59. Skinner DG: Surgical management of advanced nonseminomatous tumors of the testis. Urol Clin North Am 4:465, 1977.
60. Staubitz WJ, Early KS, Magoss IV, Murphy GP: Surgical treatment of non-seminomatous germinal testes tumors. Cancer 32:1206–1211, 1973.
61. Stockamp K, Schreiter F, Altwein JE: Alpha-adrenergic drugs in retrograde ejaculation. Fertil Steril 25:817–820, 1974.
62. Thachil JV, Jewett MAS, Rider WD: The effects of cancer and cancer therapy on male fertility. J Urol 126:141–145, 1981.
63. Vahlensieck W, Jaeger N: Diagnostics and therapy of germinal testicular tumors. Urol Int 40:48–59, 1985.
64. Vahlensieck W, Weissbach L: The combined surgical and chemotherapeutic approach to non-seminomatous cancer of the testicle. Recent Results Cancer Res 22:231–237, 1977.
65. Van Buskirk KE, Young JG: The evolution of the bilateral antegrade retroperitoneal lymph node dissection in the treatment of testicular tumors. Milit Med 133:575–577, 1968.
66. Walsh PC, Kaufman JJ, Coulson WF, Goodwin WE: Retroperitoneal lymphadenectomy for testicular tumors. JAMA 217:309–312, 1971.
67. Waters WB, Richie JP: Complications of retroperitoneal lymphadenectomy in the management of non-seminomatous tumors of the testis. Surg Gynecol Obstet 154:501–504, 1982.
68. Weissbach L, Boedefeld EA, Oberdorster W, Vahlensieck W: Therapy in stage I non-seminomatous testicular tumor. Eur Urol 10:1–9, 1984.
69. Whitmore WF: Surgical treatment of adult germinal testis tumors. Semin Oncol 6:55–68, 1979.
70. Whitmore WF Jr, Morse MJ: Surgery of testicular neoplasms. In Walsh PC, Gittes RF, Perlmutter AD, Stamey TA, eds: Campbell's Urology, Vol 3, 5th ed. Philadelphia, WB Saunders Co, 1986.
71. Weisler M, Thurston OG, McCarten AB: Bilateral transabdominal retroperitoneal node dissection in embryonal carcinoma and teratocarcinoma of the testis. Can J Surg 15:256–259, 1972.
72. Wettlaufer JN: Personal communication.
73. Young J: Complications of simultaneous radical retroperitoneal lymphadenectomy. Proc Kimbrough Urol Sem 1:56–57, 1967.

COMPLICATIONS OF URINARY CONDUIT DIVERSION

23

Kevin R. Loughlin • Jerome P. Richie

Perhaps no area of urologic surgery has undergone greater change in the past decade than the techniques involving urinary diversion. Because of the pioneering effort of Kock[1,2] toward the development of a continent ileal reservoir and the further work by Skinner[3,4] to popularize and apply the technique to urinary diversion, continent urinary diversion is now a viable option in the hands of many urologists. Alternative techniques of continent diversion have been described by Rowland,[5] Camey,[6] Thuroff,[7] Light,[8] and others. The principles used to avoid complications in standard urinary diversion, however, become even more paramount when employing the complex techniques of any type of continent urinary diversion. This chapter reviews the principles involved in all forms of urinary diversion with special emphasis on avoiding and managing complications associated with this complex surgical procedure.

HISTORY OF URINARY CONDUIT DIVERSION

The incorporation of the intestinal tract for urinary diversion dates back to at least 1888, when Tizzoni and Pozzi performed experimental transplantation of ureters into isolated ileal segments.[9] The numerous techniques and variations since adopted, ranging from the use of intact sigmoid to isolated ileal segments to antirefluxing conduits to continent urinary diversion, represent four eras of evolutionary progress in the maturation of diversionary procedures in conjunction with the bowel.

Ureterosigmoidostomy Era

Diversion of the urinary stream into the intact gastrointestinal tract led to the development of such techniques as the direct buried anastomosis of Mayo and Coffee,[10] elliptic mucosal anastomosis,[11] the many methods of antirefluxing tunneled anastomosis, and finally, the combined techniques of Leadbetter and Clark.[12] The classic paper by Ferris and Odel[13] on electrolyte imbalance in ureterosigmoidostomy focused attention on many of the problems inherent in the reservoir system of urinary-intestinal diversion and provided much of the impetus toward the "ileal conduit era."

Ileal Conduit Era

Bricker[14] popularized the concept of the ileal conduit. When first introduced, the conduit system, which seemed to eliminate most of the disadvantages of electrolyte imbalance, pyelonephritis, calculus formation, and renal deterioration, rapidly emerged as a more effective procedure for urinary diversion in patients with malignant disease. As long-term results of ileal cutaneous diversion became available, progressive renal deterioration was noted in a significant percentage of patients. The role of reflux, with or without infection, was inculpated for much of this deterioration, and numerous techniques were developed to prevent reflux in ileal conduits or to use colonic or ileocecal conduits with nonrefluxing anastomoses.

Nonrefluxing Conduit Era

Owing to the potential damage of the upper urinary tract by reflux,[15] particularly in children, efforts were made to develop a reliable nonrefluxing conduit. Mogg[16] contributed much of the early work on the use of the sigmoid conduit, and Zinman and Libertino[17] popularized the use of the ileocecal segment as a nonrefluxing conduit. With the establishment of such techniques that ensured nonrefluxing anastomoses, the next logical progression was to the development of continent urinary diversion techniques.

Continent Diversion Era

The concept of continent urinary diversion is attractive to both surgeon and patient. Gilchrist and associates[18] performed some of the very important early experimental and clinical work that became the foundation for the next generation of surgeons who popularized these techniques. Kock and Skinner did much of the modern work that established continent urinary diversion as the procedure of choice in many patients requiring urinary tract diversion.

URINARY DIVERSION

Any form of urinary diversion is a major surgical undertaking. Significant morbidity and mortality can occur if proper preoperative planning, meticulous surgical technique, attention to detail, and thorough postoperative care are not performed.

Basic Preparation

The following principles of diversion are essential to urinary diversion surgical procedures:

1. Achievement of the shortest possible intestinal segment should be the final objective. A longer segment may be chosen initially and subsequently shortened at the stomal site. The segment must reach the surface and form a stomal "bud" without tension.
2. The segment acts as a conduit and rapidly causes peristalsis of the urine into an external collecting device, eliminating any reservoir of urine in contact with bowel mucosa.
3. The segment is discontinuous with the fecal stream, eliminating any possible cross-contamination.
4. The segment maintains a low resting pressure in the absence of obstruction.

A short intestinal segment used as a conduit virtually eliminates problems of electrolyte imbalance and hyperchloremic acidosis so prevalent when the intact bowel is used as a reservoir.

Patient Preparation

In order to ensure good bowel preparation, a clear liquid diet is initiated 24 hours preoperatively. A castor oil preparation (Neoloid, 120 ml, or castor oil, 60 ml) is given 24 hours prior to surgery for mechanical cleansing, and oral neomycin (1.0 gm every hour for 4 doses, followed by 1.0 gm every 4 hours) and erythromycin base (1.0 gm every 6 hours) are given beginning at 10 A.M. the morning before operation. Erythromycin is added to neomycin to inhibit the growth of colonic anaerobes more effectively, particularly of *Bacteroides fragilis*.[19] Neomycin retention enemas are used when a colonic segment is to be incorporated.

Adequate preoperative hydration is imperative, and intravenous volume expanders are begun the night before surgery. When diversion is to be an adjunct to a radical extirpative procedure, a central venous catheter is placed and checked for position.

Placement of the Stoma

From the patient's point of view, the stoma will be the single most important part of the surgical procedure. The success of the patient's adaptation to a new lifestyle will be governed by his ability to wear an external appliance and his relief from the worries of urinary leakage. Therefore, it is incumbent upon the surgeon to exercise sound judgment in the placement and construction of a stoma that will function in a physiologic manner. In order to accommodate a collecting appliance, the stomal site should not impinge on any adjacent bony structure such as the anterosuperior iliac spine or the costal margin, nor should it be near any abdominal deformity, such as the umbilicus or a previous surgical scar (Fig. 23–1). The abdominal incision is chosen relative to the stoma site, care being taken to keep the incision, retention sutures, and drains well away from the stoma. The site should be a relatively flat surface of the abdomen, at least an inch and a half in diameter, and its location determined after the abdomen is vis-

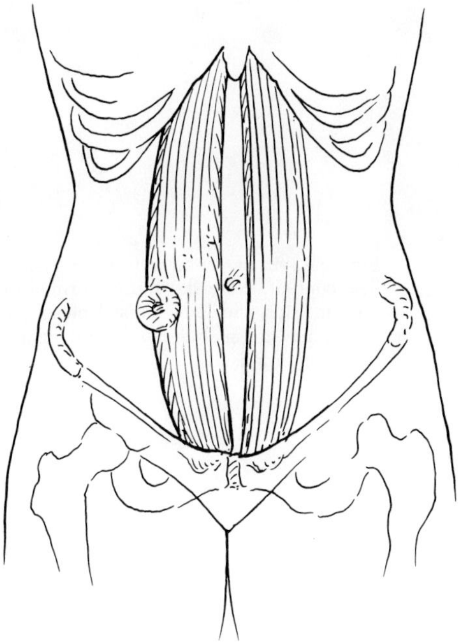

Figure 23–1. Stomal placement. Ample margins from adjacent protuberances and deformities are imperative.

ualized with the patient in the sitting, standing, and supine positions. The ideal site is usually just below the center of a line connecting the umbilicus with the anterosuperior iliac spine. In an obese patient or in one whose status is questionable, fitting with an appliance for several days preoperatively will ensure the best placement. An additional consideration in obese individuals is placement of the stoma at a slightly higher level than usual because visualization is an important aspect in the proper positioning of the appliance. Preoperative scratching of the site selected for the stoma will prevent accidental erasure of ink marking during the preoperative shaving and preparation for surgery.

URETEROILEAL CUTANEOUS DIVERSION

Incision and Mobilization of Ureters

A paramedian incision (above the umbilicus) converted to a lower mid-line incision is employed, depending on the proposed location of the stoma. To facilitate node dissection in conjunction with a radical cystectomy, the ascending colon and terminal ileum are mobilized up to the second portion of the duodenum. The descending and sigmoid colon are then mobilized to the same level. Obstructing bands between the sigmoid colon and sacral promontory must be divided to allow for eventual free passage of the left ureter. The ureters identified during the colonic mobilization are divided at a convenient level, usually several centimeters distal to the iliac vessels. In patients with carcinoma of the bladder, frozen sections of the ureters are essential to ascertain lack of intraureteral or periureteral involvement with tumor prior to implantation into the bowel segment.

Ligation of the distal end of the proximal ureteral segment with a large hemoclip will allow dilation and subsequent ease of implantation; the area that has been ligated is discarded at the time of implantation. The left ureter is passed underneath the sigmoid mesentery to lie adjacent to the right ureter. Because this is the most common site of ureteral obstruction, great care must be taken to ensure free passage without kinking or obstruction by vascular bands to the sacral promontory. With both ureters prepared for implantation, attention is turned to the creation of the intestinal segment.

Preparation of the Segment and Closure of the Base of the Loop

Prior to isolation of the ileal segment, routine appendectomy is performed. The ideal segment of bowel to be isolated is usually found 15 to 20 cm from the ileocecal valve (Fig. 23–2). However, anatomic variations in the vascular arcades as well as the thickness of the abdominal panniculus will dictate the best choice of segment. Care should be taken not to include heavily irradiated intestine. Irradiation changes usually are identified by a thickened or edematous muscularis with ischemic appearance of the serosa. Sufficient length of the segment must be utilized so that the skin can be reached and an everting bud formed without tension.

Preservation of blood supply to the segment and to the areas of ileum to be reconnected is of paramount importance in isolation of the ileal segment. Mesenteric incisions need be only 2 to 4 cm deep for the proximal segment, which will be anchored near the root of the mesentery. The distal segment, in order to reach the skin level, will require a longer mesenteric incision (see Fig. 23–2). By utilization of the short proximal incision, the blood supply to the segment is virtually assured without the necessity of visual identification of the vascular arcade. In obese patients, a satisfactory alternative technique described by Ehrlich[20] involves isolation of an en-

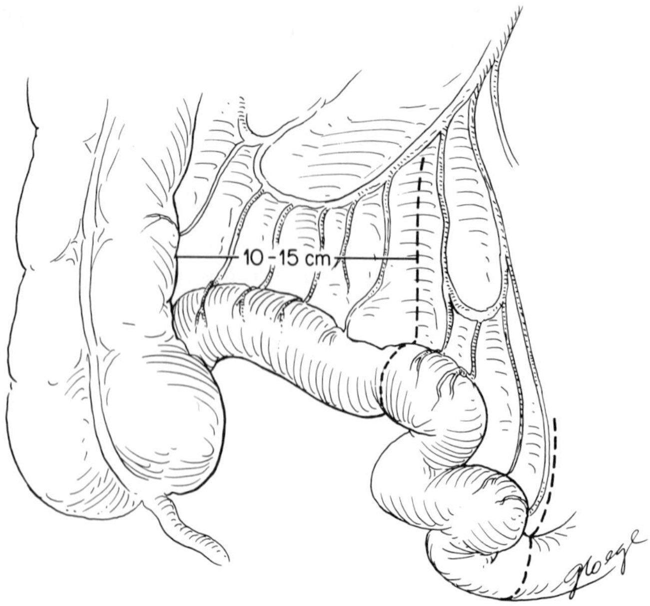

Figure 23–2. Selection of isolated segment for ileal conduit. Note the short proximal mesenteric incision and longer distal mesenteric incision, allowing mobility without danger of vascular compromise.

tire loop of bowel and disposal of the distal half of the loop (Fig. 23–3). As soon as the proximal segment is severed from the intact bowel, the end is closed with an inverting Parker-Kerr suture of 3–0 chromic catgut in two layers, reinforced by interrupted 4–0 silk Lembert sutures. This early closure of the proximal end of the bowel segment ensures an isoperistaltic segment. The distal segment of the isolated loop remains closed in a non-crushing bowel clamp until delivered to the site of the external stoma. Prior to reconstruction of the bowel, the lumen is enlarged by an incision in the antimesenteric border (Fig. 23–4) to guarantee an adequate lumen. The bowel anastomosis is performed according to the surgeon's preferred technique.

Ureteroileal Anastomosis

It is our preference to anchor the base of the ileal conduit to the sacral promontory, the psoas muscle, or the fibrous connective tissue at the aortic bifurcation. The ureter is then spatulated along its medial surface and anastomosed end-to-side into the ileal segment with closely spaced, mucosal-to-mucosal, interrupted 4–0 polyglycolic acid (Dexon) sutures. Placement of the sutures in the ileum should incorporate the edge of the mucosa with a generous (1 cm) cuff of serosa (Fig. 23–5*A*). Incorporation of the large cuff of serosa prevents tension on the mucosal anastomosis. Trauma to the ureter by forceps should be avoided. Introduction and spreading of fine forceps into the ureteral lumen allow visualization to determine the exact apposition of ureter to bowel without luminal compromise (Fig. 23–5*B*).

Ileostomy

Creation of Stomal Site. At the predetermined stomal site, a circular piece of skin—approximately the size of a quarter—is excised, and a core of subcutaneous fat is removed down to the anterior rectus fascia. Tension on the Kocher forceps, placed on the fascia on the side of the stoma, properly aligns the fascia with the skin incision. A cruciate incision is made in the anterior rectus fascia, and straight clamps are applied at each corner. The rectus muscles are split with lateral perineal retractors to expose the posterior fascia, which is opened in cruciate fashion. Curved clamps are applied at each corner. The openings in the skin and fascia should be in alignment and should permit two fingers to be inserted snugly. A non-crushing bowel clamp delivers the distal end of the segment. Care must be taken not to twist or otherwise compromise the mesentery and its vascular supply to the loop.

Fixation of the Stoma. Approximately 1 inch of ileum should protrude above the skin level without tension to create an adequate stoma. The anterior and posterior fasciae are then sewn to the ileum with approximately eight circumferentially placed 3–0 chromic catgut sutures to prevent peristomal herniation. Care must be

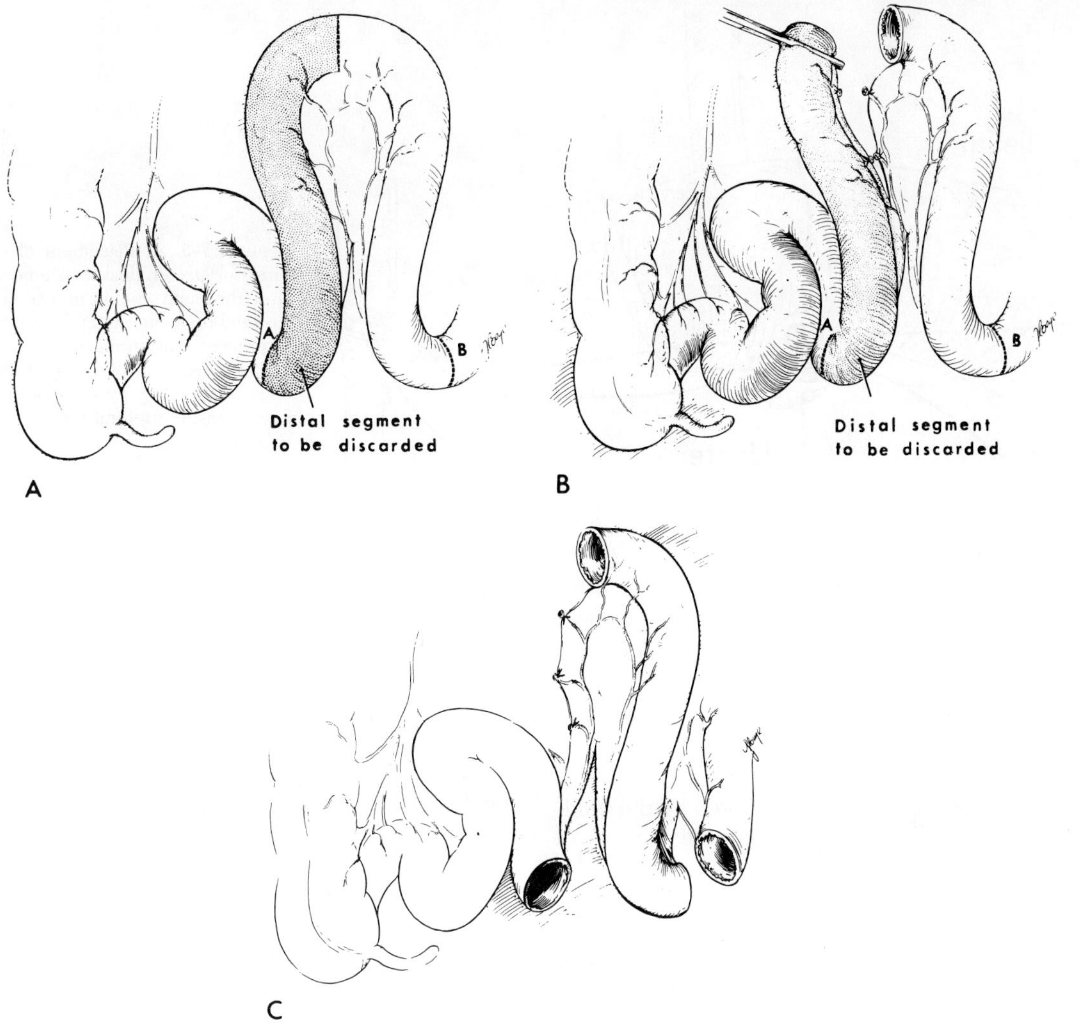

Figure 23–3. Daniel's technique of discarding the distal half of the loop in creating an isolated segment. (From Ehrlich R: Ileal conduit. J Urol 109:994, 1973.)

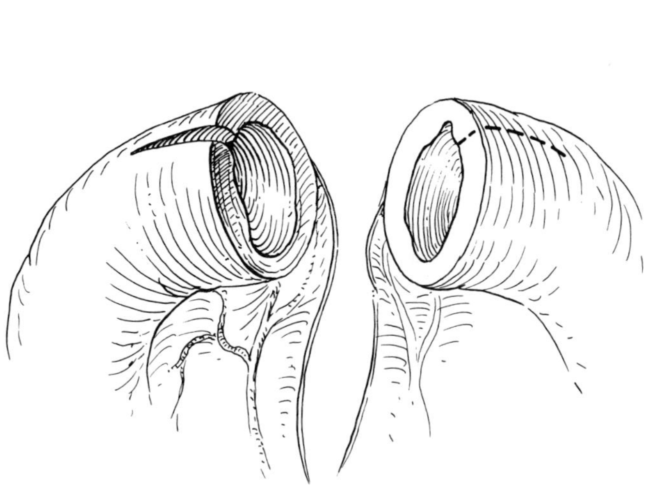

Figure 23–4. Antimesenteric incisions to enlarge ileal lumen prior to enteroenterostomy.

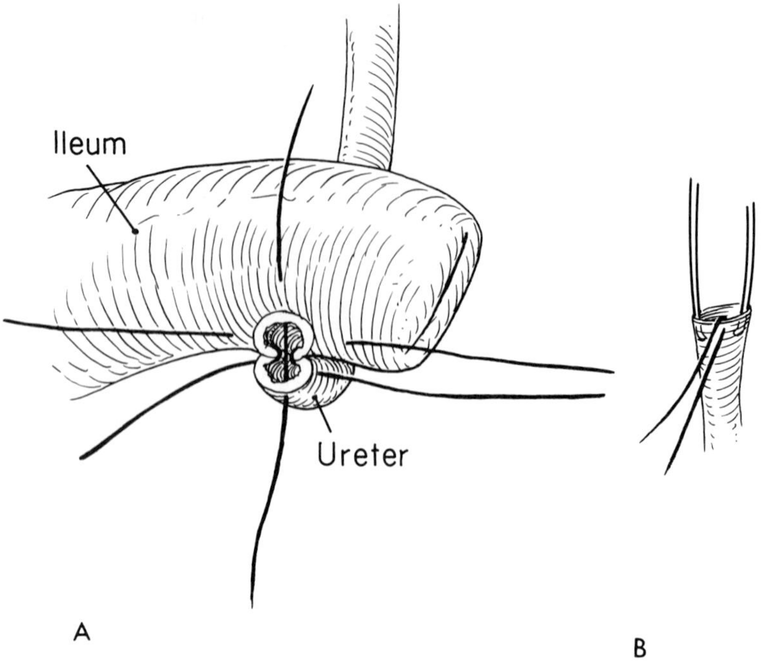

Figure 23–5. *A*, Placement of sutures for ureteroileal anastomosis. Note the small amount of ileal mucosa and the generous cuff of serosa to prevent tension on the mucosal anastomosis. *B*, Prevention of ureteral crush injury by placement of forceps inside ureteral lumen.

taken in the placement of sutures in the mesentery.

Eversion of the Stoma. Eversion of the stoma with creation of a "bud" is achieved by the modified Brooke technique.[21] Quadrant sutures of 3–0 Dexon are placed through the subcuticular tissue at the cutaneous skin edge, through the seromuscular layer of the ileum (just above the fixation of the fascia), and through the full thickness of the bowel at its distal edge (Fig. 23–6). This will create a bud of 1 to 2 cm and will allow diversion of efflux into an external collecting device and prevent ileostomy dysfunction.

According to Artz and Hardy, 90 percent of patients will have absolutely no problem should the stoma protrude ½ inch above the skin level.[22] The question of the efficacy of ligating the distal mesentery to prevent stomal bowing remains unresolved. Although Turnbull[23] has stated that the distal 5 cm may be ligated with impunity, a well-controlled study by McEwan and Clarke[24] clearly demonstrated a substantially increased residual urine, a decrease in renal function, and an increased complication rate when the mesentery has been divided.

EARLY COMPLICATIONS

Urinary Leakage

Urinary leakage is the most dreaded and lethal of all the complications associated with urinary diversion. In our series of 141 patients under-

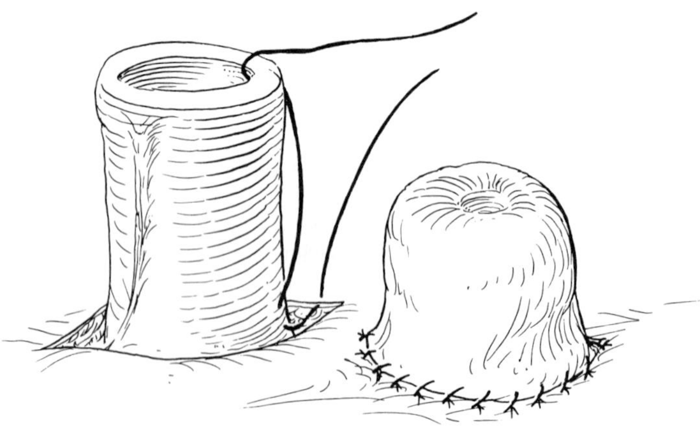

Figure 23–6. Creation of an ileostomy stoma. Sutures are placed through subcuticular tissue, emerging ileum, and everting ileum.

going this procedure, urinary leakage was present in eleven. Five of the eleven patients died; the remaining six were hospitalized an average of 42 days.[25]

The role of stents in the postoperative management of urinary diversion remains controversial. Regan and Barrett[19] reported a very positive experience in which no urinary leakage occurred in 126 patients in whom a stent was used after urinary diversion.[26] Walther, however, presented a more sobering experience with ureteral stents that became obstructed after urinary diversion, resulting in urosepsis and death.[27] The modification of silicone ureteral diversion without side holes to prevent obstruction by intestinal mucus appears to be a real improvement.[28,29] Nonetheless, there is no consensus among urologists about whether stents should be used routinely during urinary diversion. In the absence of a diseased bowel, leakage rarely occurs at sites other than that of the ureteroileal anastomosis, although it may occur at the site of closure of the proximal margin of the ileal loop. Meticulous closure and attention to detail are essential in reducing the frequency of this complication.

When leakage and fistula occur, various methods of treatment may be instituted depending on the severity of the leakage and the patient's general condition. In a stable and non-septic patient, conservative therapy with catheter drainage and low intermittent sump suction may be tried initially for both ease of institution and noninvasiveness.

In patients who experience failure with other management techniques, exploration and formal revision are necessary. These procedures are always extremely difficult, secondary to the reaction from the urinary extravasation. In older patients with a normal contralateral kidney, nephrectomy should be given reasonable consideration as the most expeditious procedure. Simple closure of the leakage site is theoretically sound but seldom achieved in practice. Most often, the ureteroileal anastomosis that caused the leak will have to be resected, reanastomosed at a different site, stented, and drained. A catheter placed in the conduit aids in the identification of the conduit during dissection. Occasionally, methylene blue may be necessary to identify the loop or the leak, but this technique should be reserved because of increased difficulty with determination of the viability of the base of the loop, a common cause of leakage.

Acute Intestinal Obstruction

Resolution of edema at the site of enteroenterostomy and return of peristaltic activity of the bowel ordinarily occur within 3 to 5 days postoperatively. The presence of bowel sounds and the passage of flatus are reliable indicators to discontinue gastric decompression and to reinstitute alimentation.

In the presence of large retroperitoneal hematoma or excessive manipulation of the bowel, prolonged ileus may result and must be distinguished from acute small bowel obstruction. Making this differentiation may be a formidable task, and one must utilize radiographic studies, laboratory data, and serial abdominal examinations coupled with expertise and clinical judgment to determine the most likely diagnosis.

Paralytic ileus, characterized radiographically by a stepladder appearance, can be adequately treated by nasogastric decompression and "tincture of time."

Mechanical bowel obstruction, due to either internal herniation or failure to create a patent anastomosis, often reveals multiple air-fluid levels on radiographs and may have a sentinel (solitary) loop of dilated bowel. Although decompression with a long Miller-Abbott or Cantor tube may relieve the problem, the inherent danger of ischemia and perforation must always be considered, and judicious early re-exploration is often the therapy of choice.

Intestinal Leak

Leakage from the enteric anastomosis rarely occurs regardless of the type of anastomosis utilized. Should it occur, the most likely site is the mesenteric border of the enteroenterostomy. Overzealous and extended denuding of the mesentery prior to division of the bowel predisposes to ischemia at the anastomotic site.

Intestinal fistulas usually respond to drainage, decompression with the long Miller-Abbott tube, and intravenous hyperalimentation. Occasionally, re-exploration is necessary.

Thrombosis of Ileal Segment

Excessive tension on the mesentery to the ileal loop, hematoma in the mesentery, or inadvertent ligation of the major blood supply to the loop may result in ischemia and thrombosis of the stoma or, on rare occasions, of the entire ileal segment. When this occurs, the stoma, which may normally appear dusky at the end of the procedure, fails to regain its healthy appearance over the ensuing hours or days. Endoscopy of the segment can be used to ascertain the extent of involvement. Although rarely resulting in urinary leakage in the first 7 to 10 days, this complication should be recognized and corrected on a semiemergent basis, preferably at the time of the initial surgery. Re-exploration and either attachment of an additional isolated ileal segment (ileoileostomy to the ileal loop) or reconstruction of an entire new segment are the treatments of choice, depending on the extent of thrombosis.

Wound Infection

The incidence of wound infection after ileal diversion when combined with radical cystectomy is high, occurring in 25 percent of 141 patients studied at the UCLA Hospital.[25] The addition of high-dose preoperative radiotherapy (5000 rad) substantially increases the incidence of complications. We therefore routinely employ anterior fascial retention sutures, placed approximately ½ inch apart, in all patients undergoing cystectomy and Bricker's diversion. Those retention sutures that would emerge near the stoma are placed parallel to the incision and tied on the contralateral side to prevent interference with placement of the postoperative collection bag. Should dehiscence occur, emergency secondary fascial closure with number 28 wire is recommended.

LATE COMPLICATIONS

Stomal Complications

Difficulties involving the stoma continue to be the most common complication associated with urinary diversion. A review of pediatric patients at the UCLA Hospital disclosed that stomal stenosis developed in 25 percent of those who had undergone urinary diversion. Each patient required at least one revision.[30] This finding parallels the experience reported in the literature. The overall incidence of stomal complications ranges from 15 to 43 percent.[31] Some of these complications are the consequence of errors in construction of the stoma, and correction may require reconstruction or repositioning of the stoma. Others result from a lack of education or understanding of postoperative care by the patient and his family and can be corrected by proper instruction. Conservative measures should be employed in the management of some stoma problem such as dermatitis, incrustation, and even stenosis before surgical intervention is attempted.

Since many stomal problems originate during surgery, attention to stomal management must begin in the operating suite. Application of the postoperative collective device should not be relegated to the least experienced (junior) member of the team. A watertight seal is of the utmost importance; frequent changes and reapplication of collecting devices rapidly lead to maceration and stomatitis. The temporary collection device ideally stays in place for 4 to 5 days and then is changed electively, not because of leakage. The skin margin between the stoma and the base plate should be less than ⅛ of an inch, preferably less than $\frac{1}{16}$ of an inch. Since shrinkage will occur with healing, recalibration should be performed at 3- to 6-week intervals for the first 6 months[32] and corrections to the base plate made by cementing an appropriately sized foam pad to the inner circumference. The enterostomal therapist is an extremely valuable adjunct in this part of the patient's overall management as well as in efforts to correct complications.

Faulty Placement of the Stoma

As previously mentioned, the site of placement must be decided preoperatively and must take into account the flange of the appliance as well as the patient's bony protuberances, scars, and skin depressions. The most common error is placing the stoma too low on the abdomen, causing the face plate to ride up on the stoma with hip flexion. This problem is manifested by ulceration of the lower portion of the stoma and urinary leakage.

In dealing with the incorrectly placed stoma, attempts may be made to use an appliance with a different flange or to use a different type of adhesive. These methods are not often successful, and the best long-term solution is complete reconstruction of the ileostomy at a new site, bearing in mind the additional deformity from the old stomal site.

After first marking the proposed site, the surgeon can mobilize the old ileostomy by making a circumferential incision just outside the mucosal margin, carefully freeing the bowel wall down to the fascial level. Great care must be exercised in handling the mesentery, and its early identification is helpful. If stomas are created with the ileal mesentery in a standard position such as in the upper medial quadrant, later revision will be simplified by prior knowledge of its position.

Faulty Length

Controversy has existed for many years concerning the efficacy of flat versus everted stomas. Indeed, Schmidt and coworkers maintained that both work well.[33] A detailed comparison by McEwan and Clarke clearly demonstrated the advantages of the everted stoma, showing a significant decrease in residual urine, basic pressures, deterioration in renal function, and incidence of stomal complications.[24]

The ideal stomal bud should protrude 1 to 2 cm above the skin in order to direct urinary efflux into the collecting apparatus, prevent leakage, and allow easy adaptation to appliances.[34] A longer stoma is more prone to damage and may not be readily drained by the collecting device.

In stomas that are excessively long, circumferential incision and freeing of the everted ileum from the emerging ileum can be accomplished, with resuturing performed after trimming the redundant ileum.

Short or flush stomas create more difficulty in management. Prior to corrective operation, evaluation with retrograde conduitogram will ascertain the length of the ileal segment and the presence of any intraperitoneal redundancy. If redundancy exists, this extra portion of the ileal segment can be drawn out through the stomal site and the mesentery partially divided. Otherwise, the addition of a second ileal segment (ileoileostomy) or construction of an entirely new ileal segment and reanastomosis of the ureters are required.

Prolapse and Recession of the Stoma

This complication is invariably related to inadequate internal fixation of the segment to the fascia, or it is associated with a peristomal hernia. The treatment in both cases requires fixation at multiple points of the anterior and posterior fascia to the seromuscular layer of the bowel.

Cutaneous Problems

Peristomal dermatitis, stomal bleeding, plaque, and incrustation are among the most frequent complications associated with ileal conduit urinary diversion. Although proper construction and placement of the stoma aid in reducing the frequency of these complications, other factors, such as careful and adequate management of the stomal appliances and maintenance of urinary acidification, play a key role.

Education of the patient and his family must be initiated prior to surgery. A thorough knowledge of and familiarity with all of the requirements of stomal management will virtually eliminate complications resulting from neglect, poor hygiene, or misunderstanding. This education must be continued through the postoperative and convalescent periods until the patient is thoroughly versed in the management of his appliance. Ideally, the collecting device should not require changes more frequently than every 5 to 7 days.[32]

Peristomal dermatitis, characterized by an excoriated, red, weeping lesion, is usually caused by improper fitting of the collecting device, prolonged urinary contact with the peristomal skin, or reaction to the adhesive used to fix the bag in place. The opening of the appliance should be checked, and no more than $\frac{1}{16}$ to $\frac{1}{8}$ of an inch in excess of the stoma diameter should protrude.[34]

Conservative therapy, as outlined by Jeter and Lattimer,[32] consists of removal of the appliance and treatment with cool air from a hair dryer for 30 minutes twice a day. Application of heat from a gooseneck lamp with a 60-watt bulb placed 12 inches from the skin will aid in preventing further skin maceration by rapidly drying the affected areas. Anti-inflammatory sprays that contain cortisone are useful for severe cases. A temporary appliance may be used between treatments.

Bathing of the unprotected skin in alkaline urine may result in formation of granulation tissue. In patients with sterile urine (pH greater than 6.5), urinary acidification should be initiated with ascorbic acid (1 gm orally 4 times daily). In addition, cutaneous soaks with a 0.25 percent acetic acid solution (vinegar diluted 1:3 with water) should be applied twice daily, followed by cool air, gooseneck lamp heat, and a new temporary appliance. The collecting device should be treated with acetic acid solution or other agents to rid it of contamination by resident colonies of urea splitters.

Stomal bleeding, incrustation, and plaque are problems that are almost always secondary to alkaline urine and poor hygiene associated with the collecting device. Acidification should be instituted immediately, and the permanent appliance may have to be replaced. Use of a bedside collecting device to prevent bathing of the stoma in alkaline urine at night is also an integral part of the therapy.

Stomal Stenosis

Stenosis may be secondary to the technique of construction of the stoma such as the flush stoma with subsequent skin retraction, but in patients with a bud stoma, this phenomenon is often the result of inflammation at the ileal segment. This inflammation results from bathing of the stoma in alkaline urine and can be treated with oral and topical acidification preparations. Keratinization around the stoma is believed to be the first sign of impending stomal stenosis, and if the process cannot be reversed by conservative therapy, the stoma should be reconstructed.

The surgical approach to correction of stomal stenosis varies with the patient's anatomy. Richardson and associates described a rotated lateral skin flap with excision of the scarred area.[35] In most patients, however, stomal stenosis is associated with loop redundancy and is best corrected by excision of the stenotic area and delivery of an additional bowel segment from the peritoneal cavity.[36] In severe or recalcitrant cases, reposition of the stoma at a site completely away from the scan may be necessary.

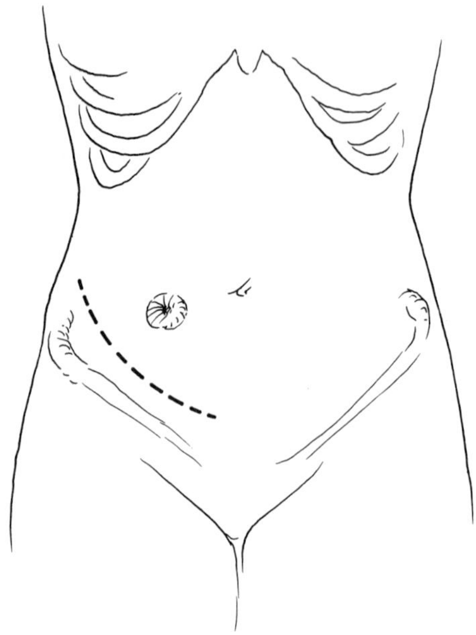

Figure 23–7. Modified Gibson incision for repair of ureteroileal stenosis allows complete extraperitoneal approach.

Peristomal Herniation

This complication is the result of inadequate fixation at the fascial level. There usually is obvious evidence of herniation, and the patient has difficulty maintaining an appliance. Treatment requires open reduction and proper fixation at the fascial level. Careful suturing of the bowel serosa to both fascial layers and all quadrants will effectively prevent this complication.

Ureterointestinal Obstruction

Because of its asymptomatic nature, obstruction can be the most ominous complication. If undetected, it leads to progressive renal deterioration. Careful follow-up with routine 6- to 12-month radiographic studies is the best way to recognize this problem early.

Obstruction may occur at various levels, most commonly at the ureteroileal anastomosis or where the ureter crosses under the sigmoid mesentery and less commonly, at the fascial level. Although some hydronephrotic changes are routinely noted in the early postoperative period, persistence of more than minimal changes beyond 3 to 6 months is cause for alarm.

Ureteroileal Stenosis

Stenosis of the ureteroileal anastomosis may be caused by technical failure at the original anastomosis, ischemia to the distal ureter with subsequent fibrosis and stricture, recurrent tumor in the ureter, or abscess formation with reaction and scarring. One additional cause of apparent stenosis may be the lodging of a calculus at the ureteroileal junction. Efforts to evaluate this problem should include an excretory urogram, a retrograde conduitogram, and when indicated, an antegrade pyelogram.

Therapy may be instituted via endoscopic (percutaneous) or open procedures.[37] In patients who require surgical exploration, a retroperitoneal approach through a modified Gibson incision is preferred (Fig. 23–7). This route avoids tedious dissection in the previously dissected peritoneal cavity and allows direct access to the area in question. Care must be taken not to interfere with the stomal area when these incisions are made. The exposure of the left ureter may be complicated by the overlying sigmoid mesocolon. The rent in the mesentery through which the ureter passes may be enlarged to expose the base of the loop.

Heineke-Mikulicz pyloroplasty may be utilized for patients in whom the exposure has been relatively uncomplicated. With the ureter left attached at the ureteroileal anastomosis, ureterotomy is made proximally, and the ureter and bowel wall are incised parallel to the ureter. These incisions are then closed perpendicular to the original incision, shortening and widening the ureteroileal anastomosis (Fig. 23–8).

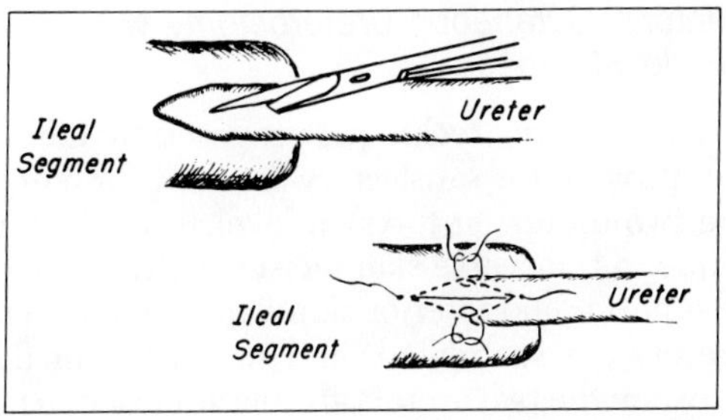

Figure 23–8. Repair of ureteroileal stenosis. (From Bowles WT, et al: Uretero-ileal stenosis. J Urol 92:630, 1964. By permission.)

An elliptic ureteral incision may be made just proximal to the site of stricture and a similar incision made in the ileum just lateral to the ureteral incision. The ureter can then be rolled over onto the ileal incision, and a side-to-side anastomosis bypassing the stricture can be performed with 4–0 Dexon sutures.

When the ureteroileal anastomosis is difficult to identify, which is often the case, an incision may be made near the base of the loop on its antimesenteric border and carried down to the ureteroileal anastomosis, which can then be repaired by one of the methods described. An advantage of these methods is that they do not dismember the ureter from the ileum and thereby provide additional strength and support.

In difficult cases, the ureter can be detached and reimplanted end-to-side into the ileal loop. This is probably the most common technique of revision for ureteroileal obstruction. If exposure of the loop itself is difficult, the ureter may be brought to the contralateral ureter as a transureteroureterostomy, while exercising great caution not to place any tension on either ureter.

Fascial Stenosis

This complication is often the result of either an inadequate incision of the fascia or a shuttering effect created by improper alignment of the anterior and posterior fasciae. A helpful preventive technique is to grasp the abdominal fascia with clamps and pull toward the midline, approximating final closure before making the cruciate fascial incision. Revision requires circumferential incision and opening of the fascial area in question.

Pyelonephritis

In a review of collected series of ileal diversion procedures performed for benign disease, pyelonephritis occurred in 29 of 500 patients (5.8 percent).[38] This complication occurs more frequently in patients in whom the upper urinary tracts have been damaged. Although the incidence of positive urinary cultures from the ileal segment is reportedly much greater, the correlation with clinical symptoms of pyelonephritis is notoriously poor. Colonization occurs at the distal 2 to 3 cm of ileal mucosa; therefore, to detect true evidence of loop infection, a double-lumen sterile catheter to bypass the distal segment is required. In this series, the number of positive cultures decreased by 50 percent and more closely correlated with clinical pyelonephritis.

Treatment includes the administration of fluids and appropriate antibiotics. Evaluation to rule out obstruction or other contributing anatomic factors should be undertaken after the acute process subsides. Recurrent bouts of pyelonephritis indicate the need for long-term antibiotic therapy or conversion of the conduit to a nonrefluxing system.

Calculi

Renal calculi formation occurred in 5 percent of patients undergoing diversions for benign disease.[15] However, the average follow-up period was only 3 to 5 years. Koehler and coworkers reported that calculi occurred most commonly more than five years postdiversion and almost never formed in upper urinary tracts that were normal prior to diversion.[38] Dretler's postulation of the pathogenesis of renal calculi in patients with ileal conduits related it to obstruction, increased chloride-bicarbonate exchange, acidosis, buffering by calcium absorption from bone, and precipitation of calcium in the acid urine.[39]

The mainstay of therapy is directed toward prophylaxis: adequate fluid intake, vigorous treatment of infection, and close surveillance for early detection and correction of any urinary obstruction. Large calculi require surgical intervention.

Ureterostomy

The seemingly ideal form of cutaneous diversion is cutaneous ureterostomy with no interposed bowel to cause electrolyte imbalance, bowel obstruction, or anastomotic stenosis or leakage. Major difficulties are encountered when two separate stomas must be created or

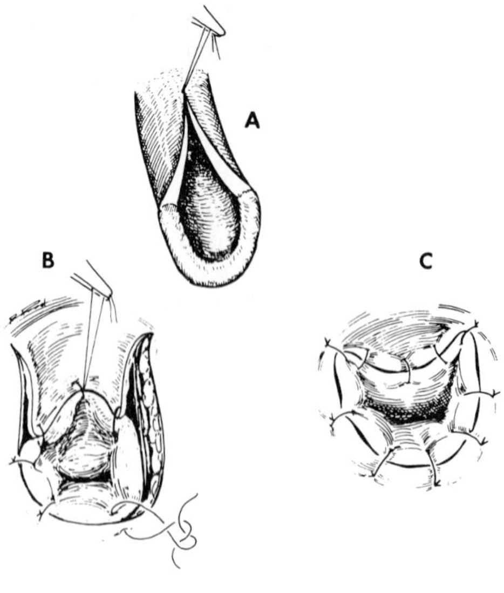

Figure 23–9. Unilateral cutaneous ureterostomy with cutaneous skin flap to prevent stenosis. (From Straffon RA: Cutaneous ureterostomy. J Urol 103:140, 1970. By permission.)

when the two ureters are joined by a procedure such as transureteroureterostomy. Most important, a patent stoma must be maintained. In the normal caliber (unobstructed) ureter, the blood supply to the distal end is extremely poor, predisposing to stenosis and failure.[40] In the obstructed dilated ureter, the blood supply is markedly increased because of a vast plexus of arteries and veins throughout the ureter, allowing for a viable stoma without imminent danger of ischemia.[41] If the ureter is too dilated, however, peristalsis will be virtually ineffective; thus, the aperistaltic "floppy" ureter is a contraindication to cutaneous ureterostomy.

Several techniques may be utilized to construct the cutaneous ureterostomy. The stoma requires the same exacting considerations as does the ileal conduit stoma.

Unilateral Cutaneous Ureterostomy

In patients with a solitary kidney and hydronephrosis, the technique described by Straffon and associates is utilized.[42] A U-shaped flap is created, with the base of the flap superior. The ureter is spatulated on its ventral surface so that the cutaneous skin can be approximated to the most proximal margin of the spatulation. The skin flap acts as a retardant to prevent stenosis of the orifice (Fig. 23–9). This technique is also applicable to a dual system with one dilated ureter in which the second ureter is joined to the first by transureteroureterostomy.

Bilateral Cutaneous Ureterostomy with Single Stoma

The butterfly technique proposed by Lapides has provided a satisfactory method for joining the two ureters at the skin level.[43] In this technique, a transverse skin incision with formation of superior and inferior skin flaps is made, both ureters are spatulated, and the two skin flaps between the two ureters are anastomosed to prevent stricture (Fig. 23–10).

A modification of this technique consists of creation of a Z-plasty at the skin level and subsequent excision of a core of subcutaneous fat, anterior rectus sheath, transversalis fascia, and anterior peritoneum.[42] Longitudinal incisions are made at the opposite ends of each ureter, and the skin flaps are sutured deeply into each ureter (Fig. 23–11).

Results

Complications have been minimal in properly selected patients. In Straffon's series of 51 patients, five died and four suffered progressive renal failure; however, the renal status was tenuous when diversion was performed in all nine of these patients.[42] The majority of the other patients in the series demonstrated improved renal function and decreased hydronephrosis on the excretory urogram. Stomal problems included bleeding (three patients), ischemic ureter with obstruction (one patient), difficulty with appliance fitting (two patients), and phosphate precipitation on the stoma (one patient). Kendall and Karafin reported no stomal stenosis in 28 patients who underwent cutaneous ureterostomy.[34] Although these statistics are encouraging, one must be aware that these patients were carefully selected and that many problems become evident only after long-term follow-up.

Although it is sometimes possible to revise the cutaneous ureterostomy stoma by using one of the aforementioned methods, the most prudent course in many cases may be to incorporate a segment of bowel. In patients with adynamic dilated segments, the bowel should be placed high in the ureter, even high enough to function as a pyeloileal diversion, completely bypassing the poorly functioning segments.

SIGMOID CONDUITS

The ever-increasing number of ureteroileocutaneous diversions attests to the ascendancy

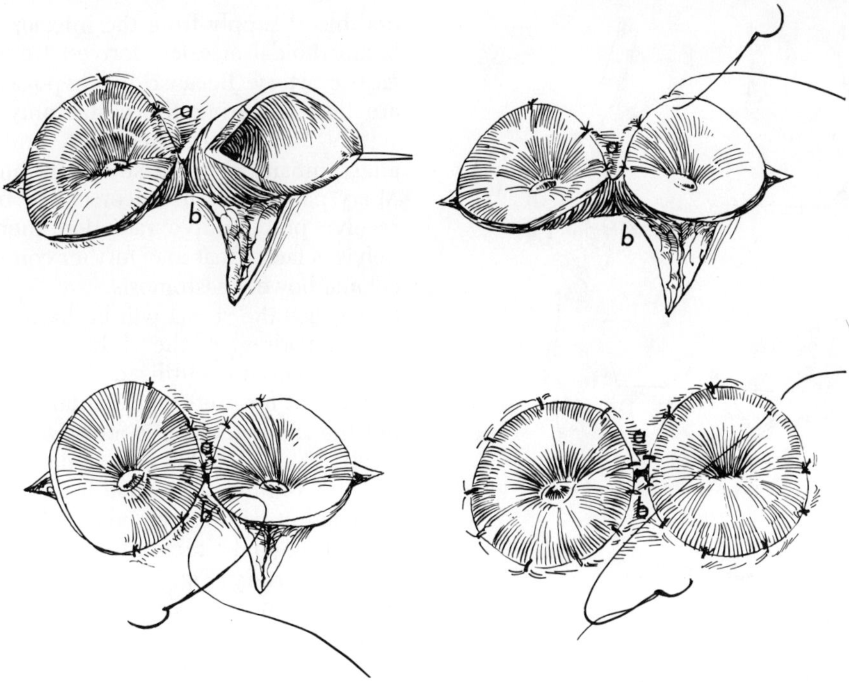

Figure 23–10. Technique for bilateral cutaneous ureterostomy. Transverse skin flaps are anastomosed between spatulated ureters. (From Lapides J: Butterfly ureterostomy. J Urol 88:736, 1962. By permission.)

of Bricker's operation as the procedure of choice for urinary diversion. The life span of the patient who undergoes urinary diversion for malignant disease is usually determined by the aggressive potential of the malignancy itself rather than by the efficacy of the diversional procedure. In the patient undergoing diversion for benign disease, however, the life span will be limited by the renal reserve, which is directly attributable to the ability of the diversion to protect the remaining renal parenchyma. Furthermore, because many of these diversions for benign disease are performed in children with neurogenic bladders, the diversionary procedure must continue to function for many decades.

These factors place rigid demands on any long-term form of urinary diversion, demands that are not entirely satisfied by the current cutaneous ureteroileostomy. A review of several large series of patients undergoing urinary diversion for benign disease disclosed that 10 percent of children with normal upper urinary tracts prior to diversion will show radiographic evidence of renal deterioration in the first 3 to 5 years postoperatively.[15] Long-term follow-up data revealed that an even more striking number will show deterioration 10 years postoperatively. Although obstruction at the stoma, fascia, or ureteroileal anastomoses accounts for some of this deterioration, for much of it, the etiologic factors are unknown.

Reflux of infected urine produces chronic pyelonephritis in patients with an intact urinary system and in those who have undergone diversion by ureterosigmoidostomy into the intact colon. It seems probable that ileoureteral reflux also will cause pyelonephritis and renal deterioration.

Attention has thus focused on the development of more effective conduit systems, and Mogg has turned to the use of sigmoid colon as a conduit rather than a reservoir.[16] Prevention of reflux has clearly shown to be feasible by the previous work of Leadbetter and Clarke in ureterosigmoidostomies.[12] Adapting this principle to colonic conduits, we and others have been able to prevent reflux in colonic conduits, both in the experimental laboratory and in clinical patients.

Indications

The colon offers major theoretical advantages over the ileum as an isolated segment for long-term urinary diversion. The colon absorbs far less per unit surface area than does the ileum. We have demonstrated conclusively that the co-

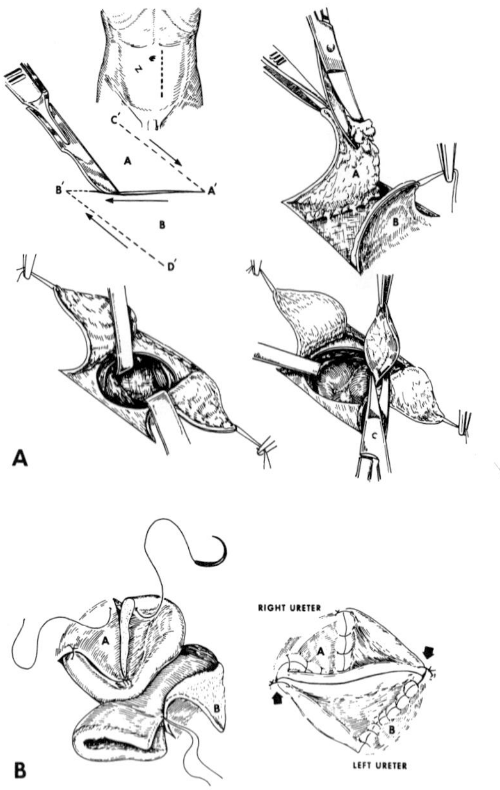

Figure 23–11. Alternative technique to reduce the incidence of stomal stenosis in bilateral cutaneous ureterostomy. *A*, Z-plasty creation of skin flaps and excision of core of subcutaneous tissue and fascia. *B*, Spatulation of ureters and sutering of skin flaps into cleft in each ureter. (From Straffon RA: Cutaneous ureterostomy. J Urol 103:140, 1970. By permission.)

lon maintains a lower resting pressure and adapts more readily to acute occlusion. The functional emptying of both conduits is identical, and stomal problems are encountered less frequently with colonic stomas. The bowel anastomosis in the left lower quadrant allows for complete retroperitonealization with a marked decrease in internal herniation and obstruction. Most significantly, animal experiments have clearly shown the increased incidence of histologic pyelonephritis in freely refluxing ileal conduits when compared with nonrefluxing colonic conduits (83 percent and 7 percent, respectively).[30]

We believe, however, that the colonic conduit is inadvisable for diversion in conjunction with radical cystectomy for malignant disease. The creation of antirefluxing anastomoses adds about 45 minutes to an already lengthy surgical procedure. More importantly, healing of the colonic anastomosis (colocolostomy) depends on collateral blood supply from the inferior and middle hemorrhoidal arteries derived from the hypogastric artery. Because the hypogastric vessels are ligated during the cystectomy, the blood supply to the distal segment, and hence the anastomosis, may be severely embarrassed. Many patients with cancer of the bladder also receive preoperative radiation therapy to the pelvis, a factor that may further compromise the colonic bowel anastomosis.

Because the stoma will be located in the left lower quadrant of the abdomen, a right paramedian incision is utilized. Mobilization is similar to that for ureteroileal cutaneous diversion, but the sigmoid colon is mobilized more extensively. The sigmoid is almost always redundant, and this redundant portion is incorporated into the conduit with the blood supply derived from the last sigmoid artery or from the superior hemorrhoidal artery (Fig. 23–12). The colocolostomy is performed using a two-layer silk anastomosis medial to the conduit.

The key to this operation is creation of the submucosal tunnels, and we advocate the method described by Leadbetter and Clarke.[12] The surgical technique has been recorded on film and is available through the American College of Surgeons Film Library and the Eaton Medical Film Library.[44]

Complications

Between 1971 and 1974, colonic conduits were performed in twelve of our patients, with a follow-up period of 6 to 42 months. There have been no instances of electrolyte imbalance, stomal stenosis, or ureteral leakage or obstruction. One patient suffered a single episode of pyelonephritis, which resolved promptly on antibiotic therapy. Excretory urograms have demonstrated no evidence of renal deterioration.

A series by Altwein and Hohenfeller of 42 colonic conduits revealed a low mortality rate (1 of 42) and a "small" number of complications encountered from 6 months to 6 years postdiversion.[45] They have employed the sigmoid conduit as a salvage procedure for failed ureterosigmoidostomy or ureteroileal diversion with success. Although extensive follow-up is necessary, these preliminary data support solid laboratory evidence of the major advantages of colonic conduits for long-term urinary diversions.

CONTINENT URINARY DIVERSION

The fundamental surgical principles of traditional methods of urinary diversion have direct

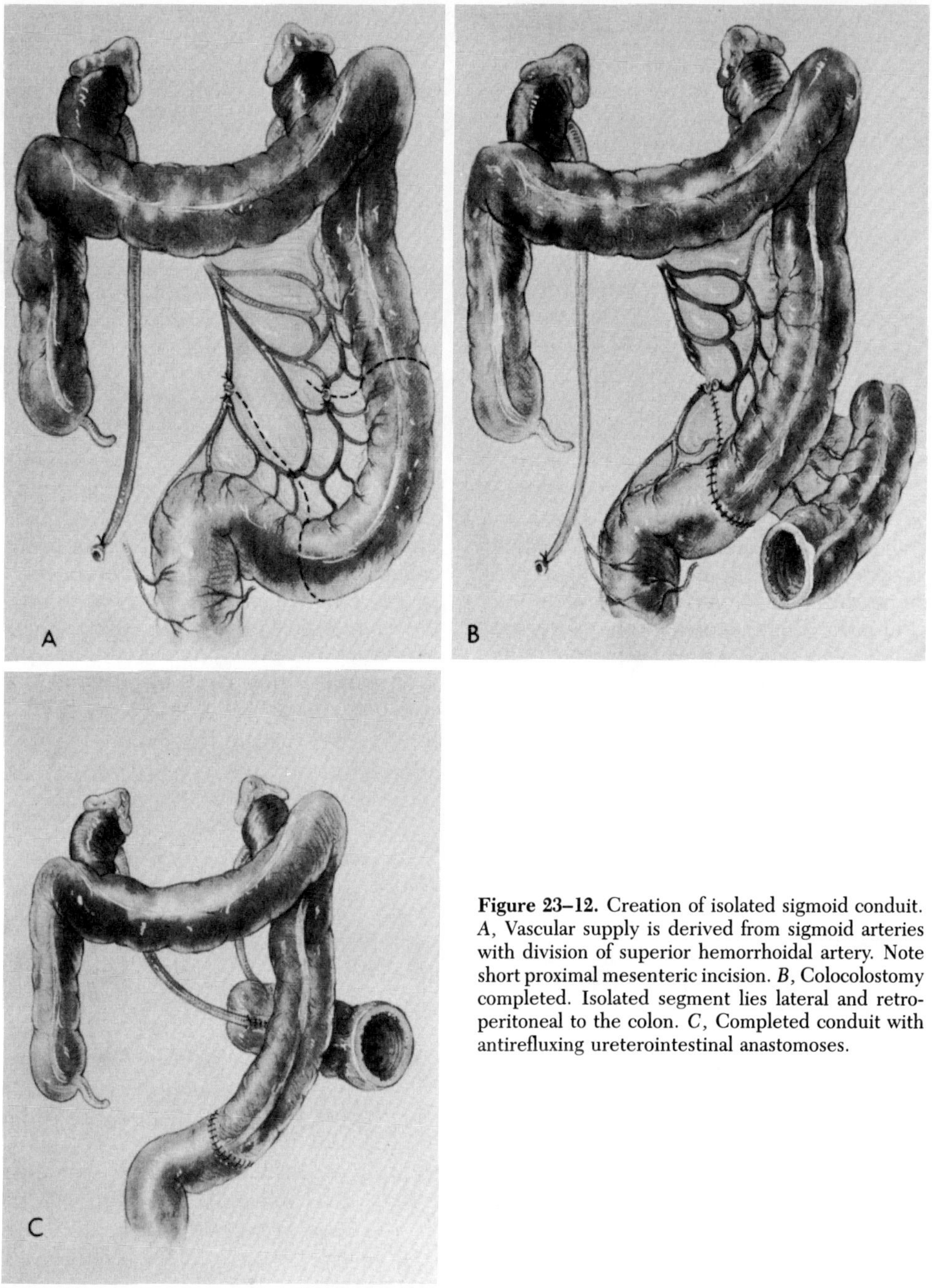

Figure 23–12. Creation of isolated sigmoid conduit. *A*, Vascular supply is derived from sigmoid arteries with division of superior hemorrhoidal artery. Note short proximal mesenteric incision. *B*, Colocolostomy completed. Isolated segment lies lateral and retroperitoneal to the colon. *C*, Completed conduit with antirefluxing ureterointestinal anastomoses.

application to continent urinary diversion. Any method of continent urinary diversion is a major undertaking, and meticulous technique and attention to detail are even more critical than with standard diversion techniques. Many of the complications such as urinary leakage, anastomotic stricture, and bowel obstruction are common to both traditional and continent forms of diversion. However, certain complications are unique to continent diversion techniques.

Integrity of Nipple Valve

All methods of continent diversion are dependent on some type of nipple valve. The Kock pouch utilizes intussuscepted ileum, and the Indiana pouch makes use of intussusception of the ileocecal valve. Whichever type of bowel segment is chosen, formation of a reliable nipple valve is crucial to the maintenance of a continent stoma. Skinner[3] made important modifications

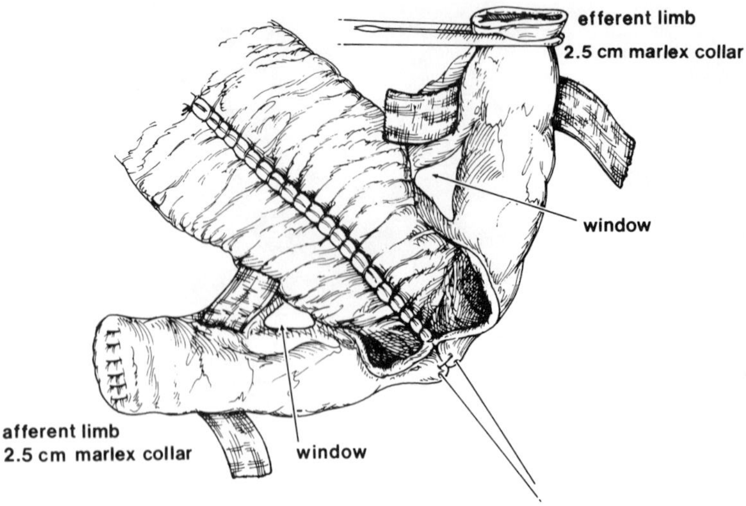

Figure 23–13. The mesentery is divided adjacent to the serosa of the afferent-efferent limb for a distance of nearly 8 cm. One usually leaves an arcade and places a 2 cm-wide strip of Marlex that will serve as a collar to fix the afferent-efferent limb to the pouch once the intussusception technique has been accomplished. (From Skinner DG, Lieskovsky G, and Boyd SD: Technique of creation of a continent internal ileal reservoir (Kock pouch) for urinary diversion. Urol Clin North Am 11:744, 1984.)

that provided a more reliable, durable nipple valve. Approximately 7 to 8 cm of mesentery is stripped off the ileum from the afferent and efferent limbs for the creation of antireflux and continence valve mechanisms. This technique was originally described by Hendren[46] and was applied by Skinner for use in the Kock pouch. Skinner[4] has also advocated the use of a Marlex (now polyglactin 910 [Vicryl]) strip to serve as a collar to fix the afferent or efferent limb to the pouch once the intussusception technique has been accomplished (Figs. 23–13 and 23–14A,B). The intussuscepted nipple is created by utilizing four longitudinal rows of automatic staples, which are placed with the TA–55 automatic stapling device.

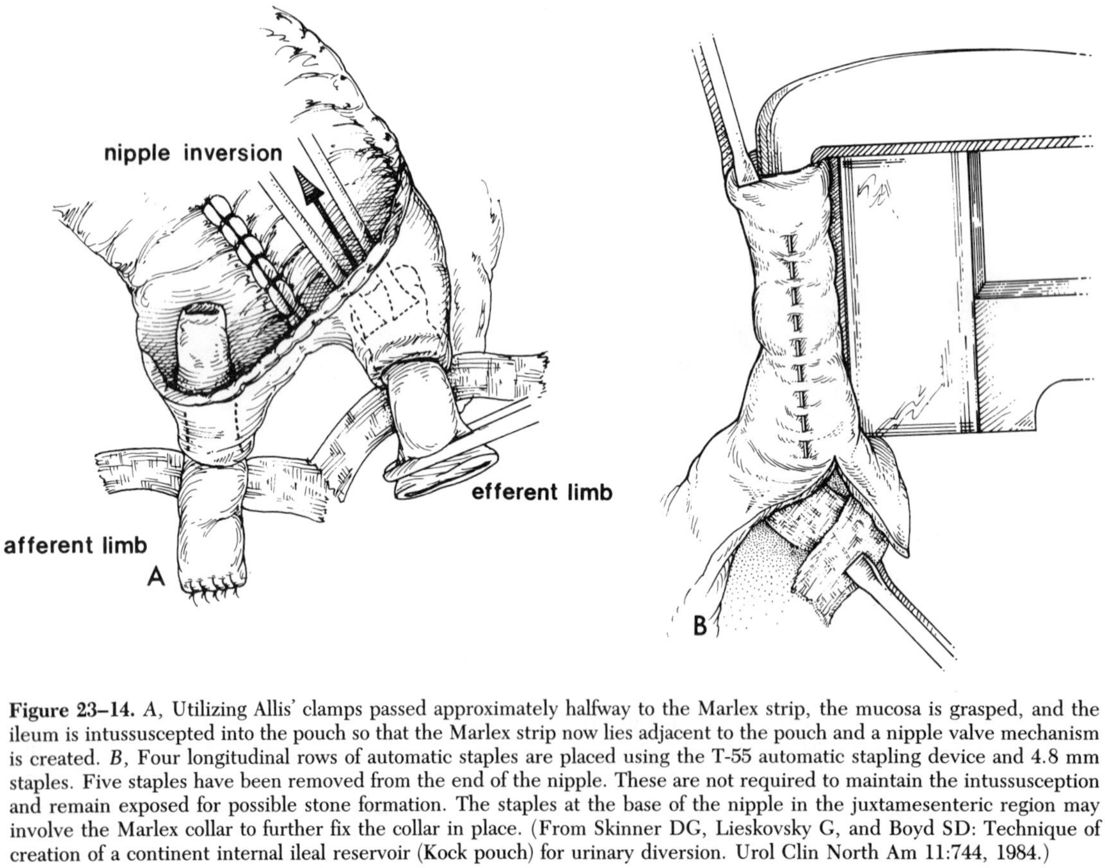

Figure 23–14. *A*, Utilizing Allis' clamps passed approximately halfway to the Marlex strip, the mucosa is grasped, and the ileum is intussuscepted into the pouch so that the Marlex strip now lies adjacent to the pouch and a nipple valve mechanism is created. *B*, Four longitudinal rows of automatic staples are placed using the T-55 automatic stapling device and 4.8 mm staples. Five staples have been removed from the end of the nipple. These are not required to maintain the intussusception and remain exposed for possible stone formation. The staples at the base of the nipple in the juxtamesenteric region may involve the Marlex collar to further fix the collar in place. (From Skinner DG, Lieskovsky G, and Boyd SD: Technique of creation of a continent internal ileal reservoir (Kock pouch) for urinary diversion. Urol Clin North Am 11:744, 1984.)

POUCH LEAK

Any form of continent urinary diversion requires the creation of a bowel reservoir. Postoperative leaks usually occur secondary to technical problems with closure of suture line or with inadvertent overdistention of the reservoir. The former problem is best avoided by careful intraoperative closure and by testing the integrity of the closure intraoperatively by distending the reservoir with saline. The latter problem is best alleviated by providing adequate postoperative drainage of the pouch with a #30 Medena catheter or some other large-diameter catheter. Regular irrigation of the catheter to prevent mucus obstruction of the tube and therefore overdistention of the reservoir is important. Skinner[3] also reports migration of the Penrose drain into the reservoir and therefore advocates anchoring the drain to the psoas muscle with a 3–0 chromic suture several centimeters away from the pouch.

STONE FORMATION

With the reliance of staples to construct the nipples of most continent reservoirs, some degree of stone formation is inevitable. Fortunately, most of the staples erode beneath the mucosa and in effect become submucosal. When stone formation does occur, it can usually be managed endoscopically.

Ultrasonic or electrohydraulic shock-wave therapy can be employed by using standard cystoscopic instruments placed directly into the pouch. The stones can therefore be distintegrated under direct vision. In addition, removal of the distal five to ten rows of staples in the TA-55 stapler will also decrease the number of staples exposed to urine without compromising the integrity of the nipple.

STOMA PROBLEMS

If the patient cannot perform catheterization of his stoma postoperatively, the operation has failed. The surgeon must be satisfied at the conclusion of surgery that the stoma can be easily catheterized. Certain principles are important to achieve a satisfactory continent stoma. The efferent limb of the reservoir should not be too long or redundant. If a Marlex collar is used, it should be sutured directly to the abdominal wall fascia. The surgeon should be satisfied that the efferent limb provides a straight path from the skin to the bowel reservoir for ease of catheterization. If these fundamental principles are followed, the success of the continent diversion will be rewarding to both the patient and the surgeon.

References

1. Kock NG: Intra-abdominal 'reservoir' in patients with permanent ileostomy: preliminary observations on a procedure resulting in fecal 'continence' in five ileostomy patients. Arch Surg 99:223, 1969.
2. Kock NG, Nilson AE, Nilsson LO, et al: Urinary diversion via a continent ileal reservoir: clinical results in 12 patients. J Urol 128:469, 1982.
3. Skinner DG, Boyd SD, Lieskovsky G: Clinical experience with the Koch continent ileal reservoir for urinary diversion. J Urol 132:1101, 1984.
4. Skinner DG, Lieskovsky G, Boyd SD: Technique of creation of a continent internal ileal reservoir (Koch pouch) for urinary diversion. Urol Clin North Am 11:741, 1984.
5. Rowland RG, Mitchell ME, Bihrle R, et al: Indiana continent urinary reservoir. J Urol 137:1136, 1987.
6. Camey M, LeDuc A: L'enterocystoplastie apres cystoprostatectomie totale poor cancer de la vessie. Ann Urol 13:114, 1979.
7. Thuroff JW, Alken P, Hohenfellner R: The Mainz pouch for bladder augmentation and continent diversion. In King LR, Stone AR, Webster GD, eds: Bladder Reconstruction and Continent Urinary Diversion. Chicago, Year Book Medical Publishers Inc, 1987, pp 252–268.
8. Light JK, Scardino PT: Radical cystectomy with presentation of sexual and urinary function: use of the ileocolonic pouch ("Le bag"). Urol Clin North Am 13:261, 1986.
9. Tizzoni G, Poggi A: Die wiederherstellung der harnblase: Experimentelle untersuchungen. Zentralbl Chir 15:921, 1888.
10. Coffee RC: Transplantation of the ureters into the large intestine. Surg Gynecol Obstet 47:593, 1928.
11. Nesbit RM: Ureterosigmoid anastomosis by direct elliptical connection: a preliminary report. J Urol 61:728, 1949.
12. Leadbetter WF, Clarke BG: Five years' experience with uretero-enterostomy by the 'combined' technique. J Urol 73:67, 1954.
13. Ferris DO, Odel HM: Electrolyte pattern of the blood after bilateral ureterosigmoidostomy. JAMA 142:634, 1950.
14. Bricker EM: Bladder substitution after pelvic evisceration. Surg Clin North Am 30:1511, 1950.
15. Richie JP: Intestinal loop urinary diversion in children. J Urol 111:687, 1974.
16. Mogg RA: The treatment of neurogenic urinary incontinence using the colonic conduit. Br J Urol 37:681, 1965.
17. Zinman LM, Libertino JA: Ileocecal bladder for temporary and permanent urinary diversion. J Urol 113:317, 1975.
18. Gilchrist RK, Merricks JW, Hamlin, HH, et al: Construction of a substitute bladder and urethra. Surg Gynecol Obstet 90:752, 1950.
19. Nichols RL, Broido P, Condon RE, Gorbach SL, Nyhus LM: Effect of preoperative neomycin-erythromycin intestinal preparation on the incidence of infectious com-

plications following colon surgery. Ann Surg 178:453, 1973.
20. Ehrlich RM: An improved method of creating an ileac conduit: the importance of a better vascular supply. J Urol 109:993, 1973.
21. Brooke BN: Management of ileostomy including its complications. Lancet 2:102, 1952.
22. Artz CP, Hardy JD: Management of surgical complications, 3rd ed. Philadelphia, WB Saunders Co, 1975.
23. Turnbull RB, Jr: Management of ileostomy. Am J Surg 86:617, 1953.
24. McEwan AB, Clarke P: The stoma of the ileal conduit. Br J Urol 45:600, 1973.
25. Richie JP, Skinner DG, Kaufman J: Radical cystectomy for carcinoma of the bladder: 16 years of experience. J Urol 113:186, 1975.
26. Regan JB, Barrett DM: Stented versus non-stented ureteroileal anastomoses: is there a difference with regard to leak and stricture? J Urol 134:1101, 1985.
27. Walther PJ, Robertson CN, Paulson DF: Lethal complications of standard self-retaining ureteral stents in patients with ileal conduit urinary diversion. J Urol 133:851, 1985.
28. Walther PJ: The management of the Koch continent ileal reservoir urinary diversion with single pigtail self-retaining ileal conduit stents. J Urol 134:1104, 1985.
29. Gittes RF: To stent or not to stent. J Urol 134:1179, 1985.
30. Richie JP, Skinner DG, Waisman J: The effect of reflux in the development of pyelonephritis in urinary diversion: an experimental study. J Surg Res 16:256, 1974.
31. Pekarovic E, Robinson A, Lister J, Zachary RB: Pressure variations in intestinal loops used for urinary diversion. Dev Med Child Neurol (Suppl) 16:87, 1968.
32. Jeter KF, Lattimer JK: Common stomal problems following ileal conduit urinary diversion. Urology 3:399, 1974.
33. Schmidt JD, Hawtrey CE, Flocks RH, Culp DA: Complications, results and problems of ileal conduit diversions. J Urol 109:210, 1973.
34. Kendall AR, Karafin, L: Urinary diversion in children. J Urol 109:717, 1973.
35. Richardson JR, Jr, Linton PC, Leadbetter GW, Jr: A new concept in treatment of stomal stenosis. J Urol 108:159, 1972.
36. Derrick WA, Jr, Hodges CV: Ileal conduit stasis: treatment and prevention. J Urol 107:747, 1972.
37. Kramolowsky EV, Clayman RV, Weyman PJ: Management of ureterointestinal anastomotic stricture: Comparison of open surgical and endourological repair. J Urol 139:1195, 1988.
38. Koehler PR, Bowles WT, McAlister WH: Roentgenographic evaluation of late results of ileal loop urinary diversion in infants and children. Am J Roentgenol Radium Ther Nucl Med 100:177, 1967.
39. Dretler SP: Urinary tract calculi and ileal conduit diversion. Am J Surg 123:480, 1972.
40. Mingledorff WE, Rinker JR, Owen G: Experimental study of the blood supply of the distal ureter with reference to cutaneous ureterostomy. J Urol 92:424, 1964.
41. Rinker JR, Blanchard TW: Improvement of the circulation of the ureter prior to cutaneous ureterostomy: a clinical study. J Urol 96:44, 1966.
42. Straffon RA, Kyle K, Corvalan J: Technique of cutaneous ureterostomy and results in 51 patients. J Urol 103:138, 1970.
43. Lapides J: Bufferfly cutaneous ureterostomy. J Urol 88:735, 1962.
44. Skinner DG, Richie JP: Urinary diversion: the isolated sigmoid segment. Film; available from American College of Surgeons Film Library and Eaton Medical Film Library, 1973.
45. Altwein JE, Hohenfeller R: Use of the colon as a conduit for urinary diversion. Surg Gynecol Obstet 140:33, 1975.
46. Hendren WH: Reoperative ureteral reimplantation: management of the difficult case. J Pediatr Surg 15:1980.

COMPLICATIONS OF URINARY STOMAS

24

David A. Bloom • Edward J. McGuire

The stoma is the weak link of external urinary diversion. Stomal complications with Bricker's ileal conduit exceeded 50 percent in some series, and reoperation on an ileal conduit was most likely for stomal dysfunction, typically stomal stenosis.[1] Other problems, such as bleeding, ulceration, peristomal dermatitis, malposition, and appliance leakage, add to the burden of a draining stoma. Judicious site selection, improvements in surgical technique, enterostomal expertise, and improved appliance technology have minimized but have not eliminated stomal woes.[2] New types of urinary diversions, including dry stomas, have added to the spectrum of stomal complications.

ILEAL AND JEJUNAL STOMAS

Free-draining ileal conduits are constructed with flush, bud, or loop stomas, each of which has its own advantages and drawbacks. Ileal conduit stomas should be examined periodically with and without their appliances in place to ensure proper fit of the device, underlying skin condition, and stomal health. A catheter is passed to assess stomal caliber and residual urine volume. We no longer routinely evaluate stomas with digital examination. A residual urine volume of less than 10 ml, free passage of a 12-French (Fr) catheter, and normal upper tracts generally attest to a satisfactory stoma.

Observation of stomal drainage is useful: intermittent prolonged squirting suggests stenosis. A contrast study of the conduit not only offers evidence of stomal stenosis in terms of conduit elongation and distention but also localizes the site of stenosis. Conduit leak pressure can be measured with a simple manometer, although a triple-lumen catheter, fluoroscopic guidance, and continuously recording equipment provide a more complete picture of conduit urodynamics. Significant stomal stenosis causing upper tract deterioration may exist without suggestive residual urine volumes, and urodynamics may provide the best means of diagnosis.[3] Leak pressures should be less than 10 cm of water in a freely draining ileal conduit, and resting pressures are normally less than 5 cm of water.[4] To culture urine from a conduit, the stoma is prepared and catheterization is performed with a double-catheter technique (Fig. 24–1).[5] Bacterial colonization of a urinary stoma is common, and antimicrobial treatment is not usually required in the absence of clinical manifestations. Colonization of the inner conduit, on the other hand, is unusual, perhaps, as Mansson and colleagues postulated, because of secretory IgA produced by intestinal mucosa.[6]

Peristomal skin complications are usually related to appliance care. Allergic reactions to appliance materials, contact dermatitis, cellulitis, or irritation from prolonged contact with urine are managed by local skin care and substitution of appliance materials. Peristomal dermatitis occurs when a poorly fitting appliance allows urine to pool in contact with skin. Alkaline urine is particularly irritative, and chronic irritation produces hyperkeratosis, cicatrix formation, and stomal stenosis. A tight-fitting appliance may cause a pressure sore. Stomal excoriations are secondary to local trauma and repair themselves

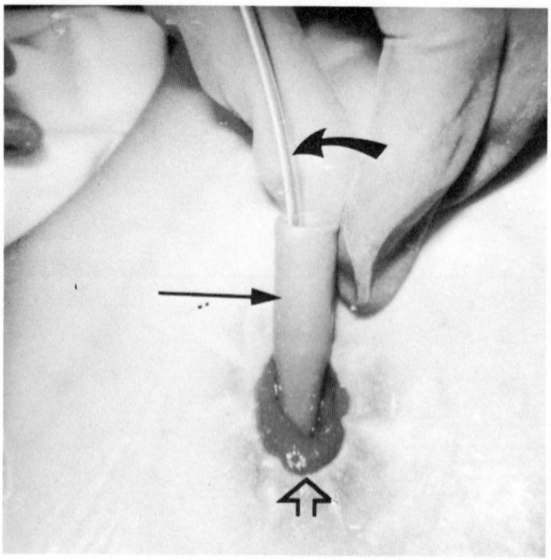

Figure 24–1. Double-catheter intubation of stoma. A cut-off 14 French Robinson catheter containing a No. 5 pediatric feeding tube is passed into the stoma. The conduit is aspirated with a syringe through the feeding tube. Open arrow: stoma; narrow arrow: Robinson catheter; curved arrow: feeding tube.

quickly after the traumatic factor is removed. Encrustations are also related to stomal care and usually dissolve with 2.5 percent acetic acid soaks. Local care usually suffices for most peristomal skin problems, although stomal revision is occasionally necessary. Temporary catheter diversion of urine provides peristomal skin additional respite to heal. Richardson and associates reported resolution of severe hyperkeratosis with radiation.[7] Flush stomas are more susceptible to skin complications, although Filmer and Honesty found that some flush stomas do surprisingly well.[8]

Appliance leakage is due to faulty appliance care or stomal malposition. A satisfactory location at one point in time may become unsatisfactory later in life because of growth, postural changes, interim abdominal/spinal surgery, or alteration in weight. When leakage interferes with lifestyle, relocation of the stoma is necessary. A new location is selected and marked preoperatively, but it may be modified by intraoperative restrictions, such as conduit mobility. Given a choice at the time of stomal revision, some patients prefer conversion to a dry diversion.

Stomal odor occurs with leakage, infection, or infrequent appliance emptying. Alkaline urine is particularly foul, and addition of two aspirin tablets to the bag just after emptying may minimize this embarrassment. Filmer and Honesty preferred oral acidification with 1 gm ascorbic acid daily, believing that topical aspirin caused stomal bleeding and ulceration.[8]

Stomal bleeding is related to minor trauma, and although it is generally self-limited, the stoma, appliance, and urine must be examined to be certain that there is no other source of bleeding. When there is suspicion that the source of bleeding is proximal to the stoma, the upper tracts are studied urographically and the conduit is examined endoscopically. Gross parastomal hemorrhage is occasionally related to portal hypertension by virtue of peristomal and stomal varices. Digital compression and varix ligation generally solve the immediate bleed, but ultimately correction of the portal hypertension or stomal revision may be required.[9] Stomal lesions are usually inflammatory, but persisting or unusual ones must be excised and biopsy must be done. Stomal malignancy can masquerade as necrosis and granulation tissue.[10]

Stomal stenosis is the most serious complication of the ileal conduit stoma. The conduit initially bears the brunt of stomal obstruction, but in the long run upper tracts will be damaged. Stomal stenosis occurs in as many as a third of patients with flush or bud stomas, and children are particularly at risk.[1] The Turnbull loop stoma is unlikely to develop distal stenosis.[11] Stomal stenosis develops at any of several levels in the distal conduit but should be distinguished radiologically from midloop stenosis or pan conduit fibrosis (old loop syndrome).

Fascial stenosis is generally the result of an inadequate anterior rectus fascial aperture or an angulated passage through the fascia causing a shuttering effect on the distal conduit. The angulation may occur over a period of years because differential growth displaces the visceral portion of the conduit from its stomal site. Whether the initial fasciotomy was a simple longitudinal or a cruciate incision matters less than the caliber of the aperture, which should be at least 2 fingerbreadths in diameter. Depending upon the factors that contribute to the problem, correction of fascial stenosis requires fasciotomy, conduit mobilization, or construction of a new end stoma. When the fascial opening is enlarged, it must be approximated to the conduit to prevent subsequent parastomal herniation.

Muscular stenosis is a peculiar form of distal obstruction that occurs in occasional paraplegics because of a shuttering effect from spastic anterior abdominal muscle. Angulation through the abdominal aperture may exacerbate this problem, but antispasmodic medications are usually effective in solving this complication.

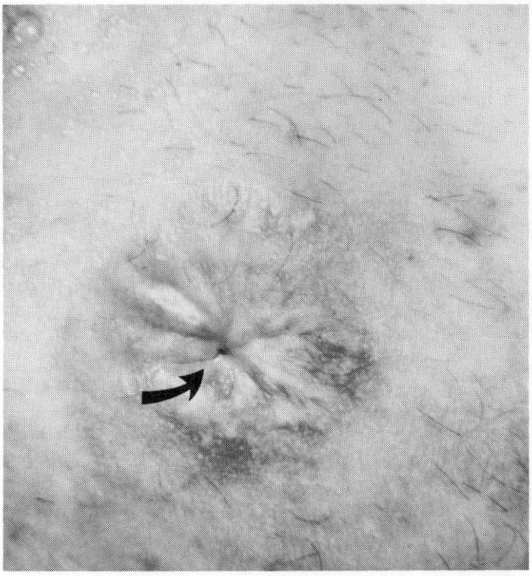

Figure 24–2. Terminal stomal stenosis.

Distal stomal stenosis is the result of skin cicatrix, which is related to peristomal dermatitis, although terminal conduit ischemia is an occasional factor, especially when stenosis occurs soon after stomal construction. Terminal stomal stenosis can reduce the opening to a pinpoint caliber (Fig. 24–2). The consequent elongation of the conduit facilitates stomal revision by permitting sacrifice of the stenotic terminal portion. Stomas are locally refashioned or resited with distal amputation and reconstruction (Fig. 24–3). A circumferential incision permits mobilization of the terminal conduit from subcutaneous tissue, muscle, and peritoneum. Coincidental parastomal herniation is identified and corrected. Further intraperitoneal mobilization is usually not necessary, and stenotic stoma is excised. The operative field is irrigated with saline throughout the procedure, and perioperative antibiotics are administered. Peritoneal defects are corrected, terminal conduit is fixed to fascia, and refashioning is completed at the skin with a flush, bud, or loop stoma. The split-cuff and skin flap inlays described by Notley and Thomson are helpful (Fig. 24–4).[12] Synthetic absorbable suture materials are preferred. Relocation of a stoma, because of peristomal scarring or poor siting, usually necessitates laparotomy. Stomal dilation, with rigid devices or balloon catheters, is an easy alternative to stomal reconstruction and is often worth a try in moderate instances of stenosis.

Parastomal hernia is an incisional hernia along the circumference of the distal conduit as it passes through abdominal wall; the likely point for the defect is at the mesenteric border. These are common complications in alimentary diversions and are particularly apt to occur when a stoma is brought out lateral to the rectus muscle rather than through it.[13] Marshall and co-workers reported a 4.5 percent incidence of parastomal hernia in patients with bud-type ileal conduits.[14] The main complication of the Turnbull loop stoma has been parastomal hernia, although this can be minimized by careful surgical technique.[11] Most parastomal hernias are small and cause little difficulty, but large hernias interfere with appliance security, thereby producing leakage and peristomal dermatitis. Pain,

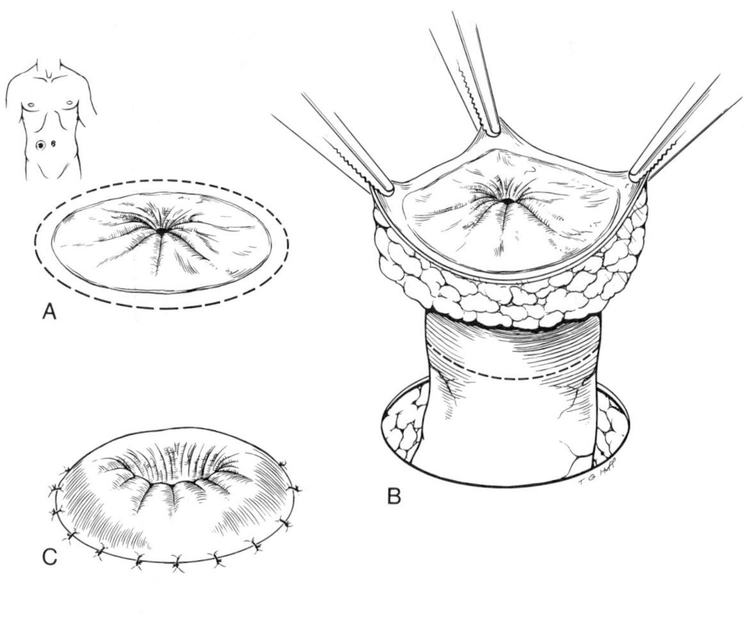

Figure 24–3. Reconstruction with distal amputation. *A*, Circumferential incision is made around stoma. *B*, Mobilization of stoma and distal conduit and amputation of distal segment are performed. *C*, New stoma is fashioned.

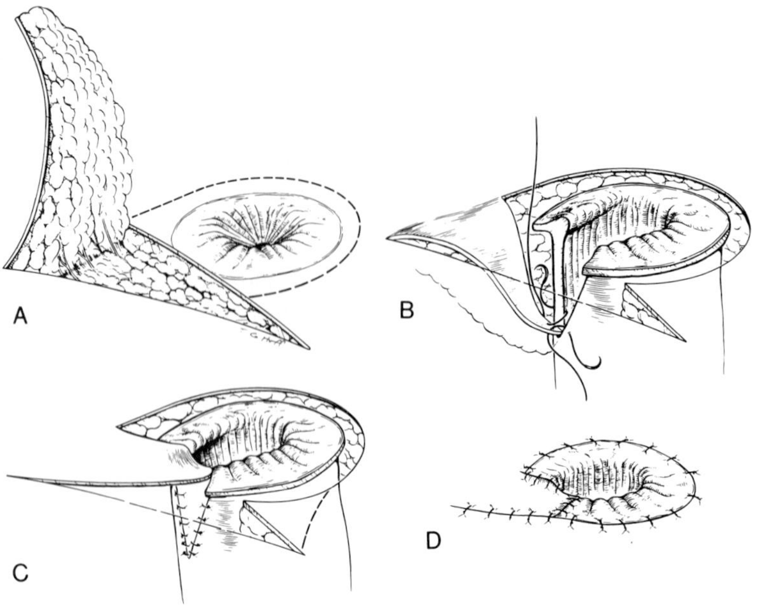

Figure 24–4. Skin inlay reconstruction. *A*, Old stoma and skin flap are mobilized. *B*, Stoma is spatulated. *C*, Skin flap is inlayed. *D*, Skin edges are reapproximated.

bowel incarceration, conduit-enteric fistula, and conduit obstruction are rare complications of parastomal hernias.[16,17] Small hernias are corrected by closure of the defect. Large defects are difficult to localize and necessitate excision of herniated peritoneal sac, complete stomal revision, and relocation to a portion of abdominal wall with less attenuated musculature. Kaufman described a technique of stomal relocation without laparotomy.[18] Mesh is sometimes necessary to repair the defect.[19] Leslie's principles of parastomal hernia repair are particularly well conceived and apply nicely to urinary tract parastomal hernias.[13] Parastomal herniorrhaphy is attended by recurrence in as many as one third of patients.[11]

Stomal retraction makes it difficult to maintain a watertight appliance. Early postoperative retraction is related to inadequate intraoperative conduit mobility and excessive abdominal wall thickness. Late retraction occurs in patients who become very obese or who undergo major postural changes. Stomal revision is necessary for severe retraction (Fig. 24–5).

Stomal prolapse occurs to minor degrees in many ileal conduits, occasionally progressing to the point that revision is needed. Prolapse is a consequence of inadequate fascial attachment, although one must always consider the possibility of increased abdominal pressure as a contributory factor. Prolapse of the blind end of a Turnbull stoma leaves a fascial defect and is a prelude to parastomal hernia. Stomal fistula is a rare complication, which is not a problem unless it interferes with appliance security.[1]

Jejunum is used much less frequently than ileum for urinary conduits and experience with jejunal stomas is limited, one reason for this being the characteristic electrolyte complications of hyponatremia, hypochloremic acidosis, and hyperkalemia. This syndrome occurs in as many as 36 percent of patients, particularly those with limited renal function, and is correctable with sodium chloride supplementation.[20] The shortest possible length of jejunum should be used for this conduit. Stomal problems in these systems parallel those of ileal conduits.[21]

COLONIC STOMAS

Although the ileum gained greatest initial favor for urinary diversion, Moog and Syme reported satisfactory experience with large bowel.[22] Their review of 40 patients in 1969 described stomal stenosis in at least nine patients (22 percent) and stomal bleeding requiring hospitalization in four patients. They advised colonic stoma construction with skin flaps and a modified Z-plasty.[46] Hendren substituted nonrefluxing colon conduits for refluxing ileal conduits and found no stomal complications in 21 patients.[23] A later report amplified the relative immunity of the colon stoma to stenosis with two instances of stomal stenosis and two of parastomal hernia in 70 patients.[24]

Most other authors have shared this experience; however, Elder and associates[25] traced 26 of the pediatric patients with colon conduits (58 percent had reflux at the ureterocolic anasto-

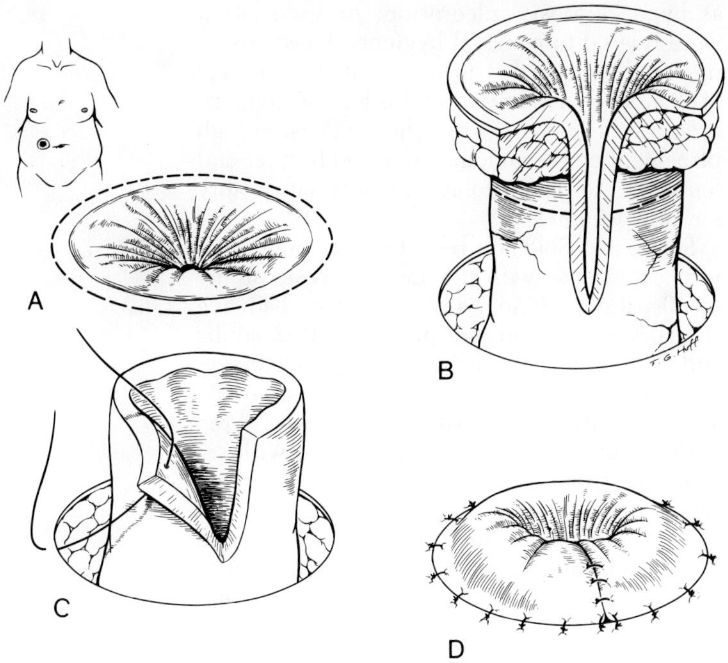

Figure 24–5. Reconstruction of retracted stoma. *A*, Skin incision is made. *B*, Distal segment is amputated. *C*, Spatulation for split cuff stoma is made. *D*, Final stoma.

mosis) in the Moog and Syme study and demonstrated stomal stenosis in 16 patients and significant stomal prolapse in four patients 9 to 20 years postoperatively (average 13.2 years). This 61.5 percent incidence of stomal stenosis remains unmatched, as yet, in the colonic stomal literature. Whereas three patients were managed by dilations, 13 required one to five stomal revisions.

In contrast, Loening and co-authors described no instances of stenosis in 62 colon conduits, although 8 percent had parastomal hernia or prolapse.[26] In a study by Altwein and colleagues, 64 children with colon conduits for neuropathic bladders had a 4.2 percent rate of stomal stenosis, with the authors commenting on the satisfactory appearance of flush colon stomas.[27] Libertino and Zinman encountered three stomal prolapses and one parastomal hernia but no stenoses among 100 colon stomas in ileocecal diversions.[28]

As with small bowel, the likely stomal complications with colon are peristomal dermatitis, parastomal hernia, bleeding, prolapse, and stenosis. Prolapse and parastomal hernia are the usual reasons for reconstruction and the principles of stomal revision generally parallel those of small bowel stomas. Stomal stenosis seems unusual with colon conduits, apart from the experience of the Cardiff group reported by Elder.[15] The optimal colon stoma has a small bud or may be flush. When colon is used for a continent stoma and no appliance is to be worn, the stoma should be flush. Turnbull stomas using large bowel do not provide any advantage and are excessively bulky.

BLADDER STOMAS

Drainage Vesicostomy

In 1957 Blocksom[29] was an early proponent of urinary diversion via vesicostomy and reported a successful experience in a 75-year-old man with urethral cancer and a troublesome indwelling suprapubic tube. Blocksom additionally proposed temporary vesicostomy in infants with obstructive uropathy.

Taking up this suggestion, Carlson[15] in 1960 described tubeless cystostomy in ten children, observing that an adequate stoma on follow-up examinations contained little or no residual urine and freely admitted a 32 Fr sound. Two patients required revision of stomal prolapse, which he ascribed to excessive stomal aperture.

Lapides and associates[30] advocated vesicostomy for permanent drainage in children and adults, adding an inlaid skin flap to prevent prolapse and stomal stenosis. After their experience exceeded 200 vesicostomies, the Lapides group updated their report with a long-term follow-up on 45 patients, of whom only one had stomal stenosis needing revision. Skin problems such as hyperkeratosis, ulceration, or excoriation were related to personal hygiene. These investigators believed that urine residuals in excess of 30 ml were not detrimental as long as drainage occurred at low pressure. They suggested high placement on the abdomen to avoid fissures and found their own ileostomy appliance satisfactory for vesicostomies.[31]

Sonda and Solomon reported a favorable 20-year experience with the Lapides vesicostomy in 30 patients.[32] Ross and colleagues had five stomal stenoses and one prolapse in 22 adults and two children in whom permanent diversion was accomplished by vesicostomy.[33] Laskowski and Scott studied 45 patients including three with stenoses, one with prolapse, two with serious peristomal skin inflammations, and two with chronic appliance leakages.[34] Hair encrustations were simply wiped away, but the authors advised placing stomas high on abdominal wall to avoid hairy areas. Findings by Paquin and others[35]—two prolapses among five Lapides vesicostomies—led to a modification of the procedure adding posterior rectus support, which apparently saved the next eight vesicostomies from prolapse. Ireland and Geist described difficulties with vesicostomy in 15 children with myelomeningocele and ultimately preferred ileal conduit for long-term diversion.[36] Three revisions were required, but the main problems seemed to relate to appliance security. In spite of the favorable experiences of the Lapides group, permanent vesicostomy has generally been avoided because of difficulty with appliances in hair-bearing areas.

Temporary Vesicostomy

Temporary vesicostomies, unlike cutaneous vesicostomies, which have their main value in infants, are associated with a good outcome (Fig. 24–6). Ross and colleagues performed diversions in 12 children with temporary vesicostomy, resulting in seven instances of stomal stenosis.[33] Lytton and Weiss also used a flap technique for temporary diversion in 13 infants and encountered four prolapses (one of which persisted), and three instances of dermatitis.[37] Duckett adapted the Blocksom vesicostomy in children.[38] Diaper drainage is satisfactory in infants, although in larger older children the abdominal stoma is susceptible to leakage over the top of the diaper. Bruce and Gonzales reported 24 vesicostomies in children with four instances of stenosis, requiring one revision, and no prolapse

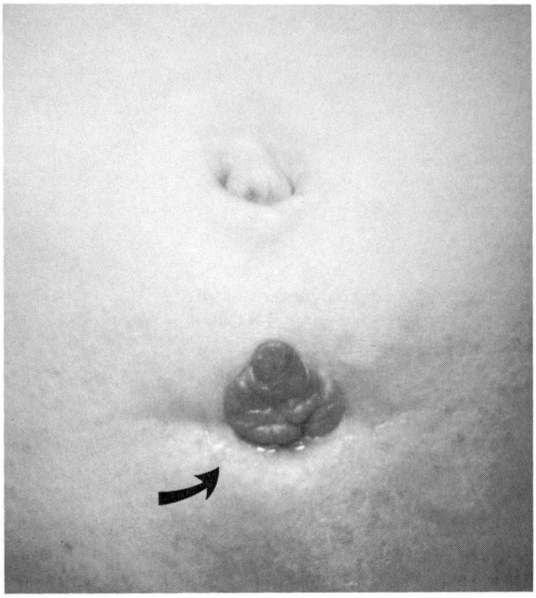

Figure 24–6. Normal vesicostomy in infant.

or dermatitis.[39] Allen noted four prolapses (only one required revision), one stenosis, and three skin rashes in 13 Lapides vesicostomies, whereas three simple vesicostomies resulted in one stomal stenosis.[40]

Stomal stenosis in vesicostomies is usually managed by dilation. Once stenosis is evident, a program of daily catheterization may keep the stoma open, but revision is sometimes necessary and inlay skin flaps help prevent recurrence. Intubation is a suboptimal solution except as a temporizing measure. Stomal prolapse results from poor initial stomal location, such as a caudal position on the abdominal wall, use of the anterior detrusor wall instead of dome, excessive fascial aperture, failure to anchor outgoing bladder to anterior abdominal fascia, or increased abdominal pressure. Prolapsed bladder becomes irritated and bleeds readily. Mild degrees of prolapse may be left until the time of anticipated vesicostomy closure, but severe prolapse necessitates revision or advancement of the closure timetable (Fig. 24–7). Peristomal skin inflammation is managed by local wound care with zinc oxide or antibiotic ointments. Frequent changes of highly absorbent diapers help minimize contact with urine, but temporary catheter diversion is occasionally required. Peristomal fungal infections occur in some children, particularly neonates on broad-spectrum antibiotics.

Vesicostomy closure is accomplished with a transverse incision that includes the stoma in a central ellipse. If a skin tube is present, it is

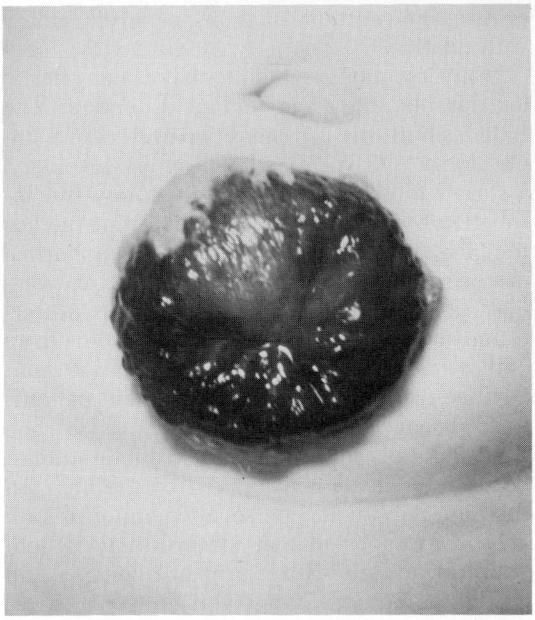

Figure 24–7. Vesicostomy prolapse.

preserved. The bladder is freed from subcutaneous tissue, fascia, and muscle. Stoma and adjacent skin are excised and bladder is closed in two layers with synthetic absorbable suture and dropped beneath muscle and fascia. The wound is closed in layers with the same material after vigorous irrigation of the operative field.

Continent Vesicostomy

Continent vesicostomy was described by Lapides in 1966.[41] Schneider and associates were other early enthusiasts of continent vesicostomy and reported on their technique and its modifications in 18 patients.[42] The stomas were flush, and no problems were described. Naude's hidden vesicostomy was continent in 19 of 20 patients.[43] McGuire[43a] has had favorable long-term experience with a continent vesicostomy in selected adults. Koff updated the Lapides abdominal neourethra and reported successful clinical experience with continence in six children.[44] The stomas were flush and catheterized intermittently or self-voiding. Patients for continent vesicostomy must have high-volume and low-pressure bladders. The most serious complication of this form of vesicostomy is inability to catheterize the stoma. Failure of the continence mechanism may be due to technical failure or to bladder hyperreflexia, and the management of these two problems is substantially different. We have had favorable experience with continent vesicostomy stomas. In one patient, simultaneous peristomal abscess and deep stomal stenosis developed a little more than 1 year after construction of the device. We postulated that the abscess was secondary to traumatic catheterization after access to the reservoir became difficult because of the stenosis. The abscess was incised and drained, and the stoma was dilated with a balloon catheter.

Mitrofanoff reported a continent abdominal stoma in 1980 made from appendix interspersed between bladder and skin. Duckett and Snyder expanded this concept to include ureter or bowel channels for catheterization without many stomal complications.[45]

OTHER STOMAS

Cutaneous Pyelostomy

Cutaneous pyelostomy is primarily useful for temporary high diversion in infants with severe obstructive uropathy after lower diversion has failed or when extreme upper-tract tortuosity suggests that more distal diversion would be unsuccessful. In infants, drainage is managed by diapering, which becomes inadequate as the children outgrow their diapers. Immergut and co-workers[46] found no stomal stenosis in seven long-term patients and cautioned that the ureteropelvic junction may be intimately involved in a cutaneous pyelostomy. We had encountered this phenomenon, which requires pyeloplasty at the time of stomal closure. A subsequent experience by Schmidt and others with this technique in 41 patients noted eight problematic skin irritations, three stomal stenoses, and one prolapse.[47] Because this is a temporary diversion, when late complications occur, the time may be right for undiversion.

Loop Ureterostomy

Temporary diversion with loop ureterostomy in infants with obstructive uropathy is surprisingly free of complications. These systems rarely obstruct unless they are kinked at the time of operation. Success with these diversions is largely related to the dilation of the systems, although, as with the Turnbull loop, the nature of the stoma largely precludes stenosis. Loop ureterostomy was advocated by Johnston in 1963,[48] and Perlmutter and Patil demonstrated

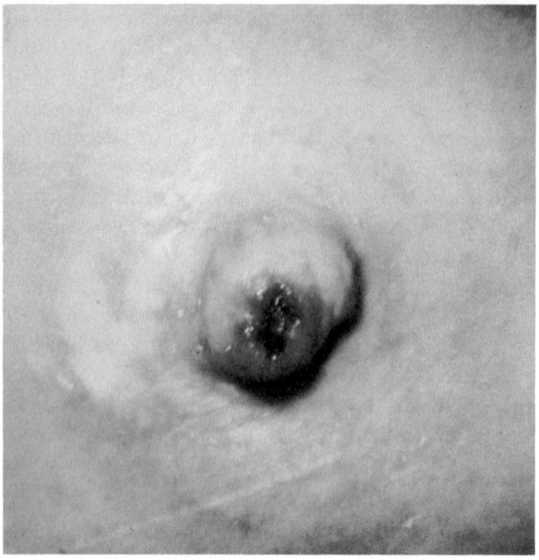

Figure 24–8. Cutaneous ureterostomy at 12-year follow-up.

its value in 32 patients but noted no stomal problems.[49]

End Ureterostomy

End ureterostomy is usually successful in a dilated ureter, particularly when the ureter is larger than 8 mm in diameter (Fig. 24–8).[50] When a normal ureter must be diverted, stomal stenosis becomes a high probability. An intestinal conduit would usually provide satisfactory diversion, but this adds another order of magnitude of effort and complication to the operation.

Straffon and associates[51] described favorable experience with cutaneous ureterostomy in 51 patients, most of whom had dilated ureters. A skin flap technique was used. Three patients had occasional bleeding; two had appliance difficulty; and one each had encrustation, yeast infection, and stomal stenosis.

Shafik found 17 instances of stenosis among 110 patients with end ureterostomy for bladder cancer.[52] He suggested that the causes for stenosis were avascularity of distal ureter, tension, improper anastomosis to skin, malignant infiltration, and bilharzial stricture. Incidence of stricture depended on technique, 55 percent with stenosis after free nipple to skin anastomosis, 10 percent with direct anastomosis, and no stomal stenosis with an everted nipple-cuff technique. Management options consisted of amputation with reimplantation of stenotic distal ureter, intermittent dilation, or urethrotomy with dilation.[52]

Many ingenious techniques have been offered for durable stomas in undilated ureters. The Lapides butterfly combines two ureters in a single stoma.[53] Ariyoshi and colleagues developed a staged method of end ureterostomy, but intubation was often necessary.[54] In canine models they created satisfactory stomas from normal ureters using vaginal mucosa autografts and vaginal cuffs.[55] A terminal loop cutaneous ureterostomy adds the advantage of a loop stoma to an end stoma in a normal ureter and has occasionally been successful in renal transplant patients with damaged lower tracts.[56] The biocarbon stoma has led the way among prosthetic stomas, but success remains hampered by the high fistula rate (Grossman, personal communication). Hendren suggested that ureterostomy is generally an unsatisfactory form of diversion and described methods of undiversion.[23]

Intubated Stoma

Intubated stomas are occasionally of use and produce few complications when used for short durations, although problems ensue during longer periods of use. Granulation tissue may creep up along the tube requiring cauterization with silver nitrate and occasionally excision. Stiff tubes cause erosion at the stomal site as well as internally. Asymptomatic bacterial colonization is expected, but for frank suppuration, replacement of the tube or revision of the stomal site may be required.

Continent Stoma

Continent stomas are made with large bowel, small bowel, appendix, bladder, ureter, or urethra. Ideally, no appliance or cover is needed (Fig. 24–9). Because appliance seal is not a problem and protrusion of an unprotected dry stoma offers more opportunity for trauma or irritation, flush construction is preferred, as there is no need for a bud or loop. Intermittent catheterization usually obviates stomal stenosis. Continent stomas are susceptible to the usual range of stomal complications in addition to the problem of catheter impassability. This is related to terminal conduit fibrosis, distortion by a parastomal hernia, bowel angulation, or edema from overzealous attempts at intubation.

When revision is necessary, the refashioned

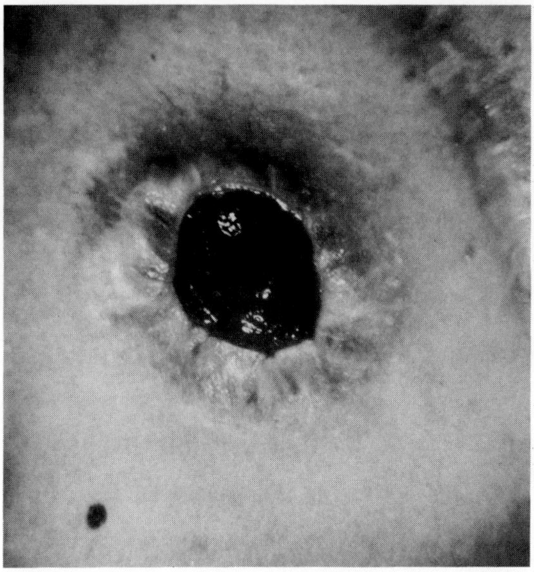

Figure 24–9. Continent ileocecal conduit stoma without problems.

distal limb and stoma must provide a straight shot for intermittent catheterization into the reservoir. This angle must be tailored to the patient's upper extremity capabilities. Incontinence is not a stomal problem per se; it is related to valve failure or to high-reservoir pressures.

References

Cited References

1. Bloom DA, Grossman HB, Konnak JW: Stomal construction and reconstruction. Urol Clin North Am 13:275–283, 1986.
2. Jeter KF, Lattimer JK: Common stomal problems following ileal conduit urinary diversion. Urology 3:399–403, 1974.
3. Knapp PM Jr, Konnak JW, McGuire EJ, Savastano JA: Urodynamic evaluation of ileal conduit function. J Urol 137:929–932, 1987.
4. Mayo ME, Chapman WH: Stomal obstruction of ileal conduits in children: a urodynamic study. J Urol 121:68–70, 1979.
5. Smith ED: Follow-up studies on 150 ileal conduits in children. J Pediatr Surg 7:1–10, 1972.
6. Mansson W, Colleen S, Low K, Mardh P-A, Lunblad A: Immunoglobulins in urine from patients with ileal and colonic conduits and reservoirs. J Urol 133:713–716, 1985.
7. Richardson JR Jr, Linton PC, Leadbetter GW Jr: A new concept in the treatment of stomal stenosis. J Urol 108:159–161, 1972.
8. Filmer RB, Honesty H: Problems with urinary conduit stomas in children. Urol Clin North Am 1:531–547, 1974.
9. Eckhauser FE, Sonda LP, Strodel WE, Edgecomb LP, Turcotte JG: Parastomal ileal conduit hemorrhage and portal hypertension. Ann Surg 192:620–624, 1980.
10. Grabstald H: Carcinoma of ileal bladder stoma. J Urol 112:332–334, 1974.
11. Bloom DA, Lieskovsky G, Rainwater G, Skinner DG: The Turnbull loop stoma. J Urol 129:715–718, 1983.
12. Notley RG, Thomson AAG: Split cuff ileal stoma. J Urol 120:159–161, 1978.
13. Leslie D: The parastomal hernia. Surg Clin North Am 64:407–415, 1984.
14. Marshall FF, Leadbetter WF, Dretler SP: Ileal conduit parastomal hernias. J Urol 114:40–42, 1975.
15. Carlson HE: Tubeless cystostomy in childhood. J Urol 83:669–671, 1960.
16. Hampel N, Zabbo A: Parastomal ileal conduit–enteric fistula. J Urol 134:956–957, 1985.
17. Lynne CM, Politano VA, Cohen RL: Parastomal hernia causing anuria. Urology 4:603–604, 1974.
18. Kaufman JJ: Repair of parastomal hernia by translocation of the stoma without laparotomy. J Urol 129:278–279, 1983.
19. Hopkins TB, Trento A.: Parastomal ileal loop hernia repair with Marlex mesh. J Urol 128:811–812, 1982.
20. Golimbu M, Morales P: Electrolyte disturbances in jejunal urinary diversion. Urology 1:432–438, 1973.
21. Klein EA, Montie JE, Montague DK, Kay R, Straffon RA: Jejunal conduit urinary diversion. J Urol 135:244–246, 1986.
22. Moog RA, Syme RRA: The results of urinary diversion using the colon conduit. Br J Urol 41:434–447, 1969.
23. Hendren WH: Nonrefluxing colon conduit for temporary or permanent urinary diversion in children. J Pediatr Surg 10:381–398, 1975.
24. Althausen AF, Hagen-Cook K, Hendren WH III: Nonrefluxing colon conduit: experience with 70 cases. J Urol 120:35–38, 1978.
25. Elder DD, Moisey CU, Rees RWM: A long-term follow-up of the colonic conduit operation in children. Br J Urol 51:462–465, 1979.
26. Loening SA, Navarre RJ, Narayana AS, Culp DA: Transverse colon conduit urinary diversion. J Urol 127:37–39, 1982.
27. Altwein J, Jonas U, Hohenfellner R: Long-term follow-up of children with colon conduit urinary diversion and ureterosigmoidostomy. J Urol 118:832–835, 1977.
28. Libertino JA, Zinman L: Ileocecal antirefluxing conduit. Surg Clin North Am 62:999–1008, 1982.
29. Blocksom BH Jr: Bladder pouch for prolonged tubeless cystostomy. J Urol 78:398–401, 1957.
30. Lapides J, Ajemian EP, Lichtwardt JR: Cutaneous vesicostomy. J Urol 84:609–614, 1960.
31. Lapides J, Bourne RB, Lanning RJ: Present status of cutaneous vesicostomy. J Urol 93:192–201, 1965.
32. Sonda LP, Solomon MH: Twenty-year outcome of cutaneous vesicostomy. J Urol 124:326–328, 1980.
33. Ross G Jr, Michener FR, Brady C Jr, Thompson IM: Cutaneous vesicostomy as means of urinary diversion. J Urol 94:549–555, 1965.
34. Laskowski TZ, Scott FB: Cutaneous vesicostomy as means of urinary diversion. J Urol 94:549–555, 1965.
35. Paquin AJ Jr, Howard RS, Gillenwater JY: Cutaneous vesicostomy: a modification of technique. J Urol 99:270–273, 1968.
36. Ireland GW, Geist RW: Difficulties with vesicostomies in 15 children with myelomeningocele. J Urol 103:341–342, 1970.
37. Lytton B, Weiss RM: Cutaneous vesicostomy for temporary diversion in infants. J Urol 105:888–891, 1971.
38. Duckett JW Jr: Cutaneous vesicostomy in childhood. The Blocksom technique. Urol Clin North Am 1:485–495, 1974.

39. Bruce RR, Gonzales ET Jr: Cutaneous vesicostomy: a useful form of temporary diversion in children. J Urol 123:927–928, 1980.
40. Allen TD: Vesicostomy for the temporary diversion of urine in small children. J Urol 123:929–931, 1980.
41. Lapides J: Follow-up of abdominal neourethra. J Urol 119:219–222, 1978.
42. Schneider KM, Reid RE, Fruchtman B, Ewing RS, Levitt SB: Continent vesicostomy, surgical technique. Urology 6:741–744, 1975.
43. Naude JH: The hidden vesicostomy. Br J Urol 54:686–688, 1982.
43a. McGuire EJ: Personal data, Ann Arbor, Michigan, 1985.
44. Koff SA: The abdominal neourethra in children: technique and long-term results. J Urol 133:244–247, 1985.
45. Duckett JW, Synder HM III: The Mitrofanoff principle in continent urinary reservoirs. Semin Urol 5:55–62, 1987.
46. Immergut MA, Jacobson JJ, Culp DA, Flocks RH: Cutaneous pyelostomy. J Urol 101:276–279, 1969.
47. Schmidt JD, Hawtrey CE, Culp DA, Flocks RH: Experience with cutaneous pyelostomy diversion. J Urol 109:990–992, 1973.
48. Johnston JH: Temporary cutaneous ureterostomy in the management of advanced congenital urinary obstruction. Arch Dis Child 38:161–166, 1963.
49. Perlmutter AP, Patil J: Loop cutaneous ureterostomy. J Urol 107:655–659, 1972.
50. Feminella JG Jr, Lattimer JK: A retrospective analysis of 70 cases of cutaneous ureterostomy. J Urol 106:538–540, 1971.
51. Straffon RA, Kyle K, Corvalan J: Techniques of cutaneous ureterostomy and results in 51 patients. J Urol 103:138–146, 1970.
52. Shafik A: Stomal stenosis after cutaneous ureterostomy; etiology and management. J Urol 105:65–70, 1971.
53. Kendall AR, Karafin L: Urinary diversion in children. J Urol 109:717–722, 1973.
54. Ariyoshi A, Fujisawa Y, Oshima K, Hiratsuka Y, Sakamoto K: Catheterless cutaneous ureterostomy. J Urol 114:533–535, 1975.
55. Ariyoshi A, Hiratsuka Y: Vaginal cuff cutaneous ureterostomy as a model for split renal function study in dog. Urol Int 38:346–350, 1983.
56. Amin M, Clark R, Howerton LW, Lich R Jr: Terminal loop cutaneous ureterostomy: an experimental study and its clinical application. J Urol 118:383–385, 1977.

Uncited References

Hendren WH: Complications of ureterostomy. J Urol 120:269–281, 1978.

THE KOCK POUCH

25

Clinical Experience in the Management of Late Complications

Donald G. Skinner • Gary Lieskovsky • Stuart D. Boyd

OVERVIEW

Continent urinary diversion has become increasingly popular and today represents an attractive alternative to the ileal conduit or ureterosigmoidostomy for those patients requiring diversion for any reason. It is estimated that over one thousand Kock pouch forms of continent diversion were constructed over the initial 5-year period following its introduction by Kock in 1982. Future demand will continue to escalate.

The majority of patients are those with invasive bladder cancer for which optimal therapy requires radical cystectomy and some form of cutaneous urinary diversion. Annually, it is estimated that nearly 10,000 patients within the United States are diagnosed as having high-grade invasive bladder cancer and as such become potential candidates for Kock pouch construction. In addition, many patients with neurogenic bladder or congenital anomalies of the lower urinary tract, as well as those having undergone previous diversion by other methods, seek conversion to the continent form of internal diversion. The future impact of this operation on urologic surgery cannot be underestimated both in terms of its construction and the management of late complications.

From July 1982 through December 1986, we performed 395 Kock pouch procedures. This chapter reviews our experience in terms of the management of late complications and discusses changes in surgical technique designed to reduce the complication rate and the need for reoperation.

POUCH CONSTRUCTION

Original Technique

The technique for pouch construction has been described in detail both in print and on video.[1–5] It has been shown that the early complication rate is not significantly different from that associated with single-stage radical cystectomy and ileal loop cutaneous urinary diversion.[6] In the original report by Kock and associates,[7] it was noted that more than half of their 12 patients required one or more reoperations to achieve continence, and to date there have been only two articles addressing the management of late complications.[8,9]

The goal of a suitable internal reservoir for urinary bladder replacement is to construct a reservoir to hold 500 to 1000 ml, with maintenance of low pressure on filling and elimination of pressure spikes. The ileal reservoir, as developed by Kock, is so far the only internal bladder substitute that fulfills this basic requirement, with follow-up in excess of 10 years.[10]

Although the principle and technique of reservoir construction have remained constant, modifications have developed in the technique of valve construction in order to achieve true continence with ease of emptying and elimination of reflux.[11] In Kock's original report,[7] seven of the 12 patients needed one or more reoperations to achieve continence. Experience in our first 245 patients revealed that 58 (24 percent) had to undergo revisional surgery to resolve problems with continence (44 patients), difficult catheterization without leakage (eight patients), or the development of a parastomal hernia without leakage (six patients).[9]

Modifications

In order to reduce the need for reoperation and lessen the late complication rate, we have made a series of modifications from Kock's original surgical description.[11] These are now described.

1. A slightly longer segment of ileum is used than described originally by Kock and associates. The afferent and efferent limbs are 17 cm long, and the pouch is constructed from two 22-cm segments. In addition, a 4- to 6-cm segment of bowel proximal to the measured segment is discarded with its mesentery divided adjacent to the serosa (Fig. 25–1). This is done to ensure a broad mesenteric blood supply to the pouch, to increase the mobility of the afferent limb, and to move the small bowel anastomosis from proximity to the suture lines.

2. Approximately 8 cm of mesentery are stripped off the serosa of the ileum from the afferent and efferent limbs adjacent to the pouch, according to the method originally described by Hendren.[12] At least one or two vascular arcades are left intact and then a strip of polyglycolic acid (PGA) mesh, 2 cm wide, soaked with a tetracycline solution is passed through the next window of Deaver (Fig. 25–2). Stripping of the mesentery in this way allows ileal intussusception without incorporation of the mesentery. The thickness and bulk of the mesentery can promote subsequent slippage or late loss of this critical valve construction. During the intussusception process, the PGA mesh moves to become adjacent to the pouch wall, where it will be fixed with 2–0 chromic catgut sutures. By fixation of the PGA mesh to the pouch wall, the intact vascular arcades remain between the mesh and the stripped mesenteric portion of the intussusception to further fix the valve mechanism and prevent slippage. The PGA mesh serves the same function and has replaced the Marlex collar described in our earlier publications.

3. Three rows of the 4.8-mm stainless steel staples, which are nonhemostatic and do not crush the bowel, are applied to the intussuscepted segment. The PGA mesh should not be incorporated into the staple because its thickness may prevent proper closure of the staple. It is important to use the pin of the stapler to avoid malaligned staples, but the pinhole must be closed with 3–0 PGA suture to prevent urine leakage from bypassing the intussuscepted nipple. Initially, two rows of staples are evenly placed around the anterior 180° of the intussusception. We use the PI-55 automatic stapler with custom cartridges provided by the manufacturer (3M Company) in which six staples from the proximal portion of the cartridge are removed at the factory. Since staples at the end of the nipple do not contribute to maintenance of the intussusception, may remain exposed, and form a nidus for subsequent stone formation, these staples are removed from the stapling cartridge. The third row of staples fixes the intussuscepted nipple to the back wall of the pouch. There are two methods to accomplish this:

(a) the anvil of the stapling device can be passed into the inside of the nipple from outside the pouch, initiating the procedure at the region of the mesentery at the base of the nipple. This technique fixes two layers of bowel: the back wall of the pouch to one layer of the nipple valve. A full cartridge with all staples should be used because important staples are those at the nipple base (Fig. 25–3). The pinhole must again be closed.

(b) A small hole may be made in the pouch wall just beyond the point where the intussuscepted nipple will lie. The anvil of the stapler can then be brought through this hole from outside the pouch, the intussuscepted nipple advanced over the anvil, which slips up the ileum beyond the intussusception and then stapled full thickness to the back wall (Fig. 25–3). This staples three thicknesses of ileum: the back wall and two layers of the intussusception. A custom cartridge is used with this technique. In addition, the ends of both nipples are sutured to the pouch wall with 3–0 PGA sutures. The hole in the pouch wall must also be closed.

4. A number 30 Medina tube is then passed through the nipple, and the PGA mesh is sewn around the ileal segment with 2–0 chromic catgut interrupted sutures to fix the mesh to the

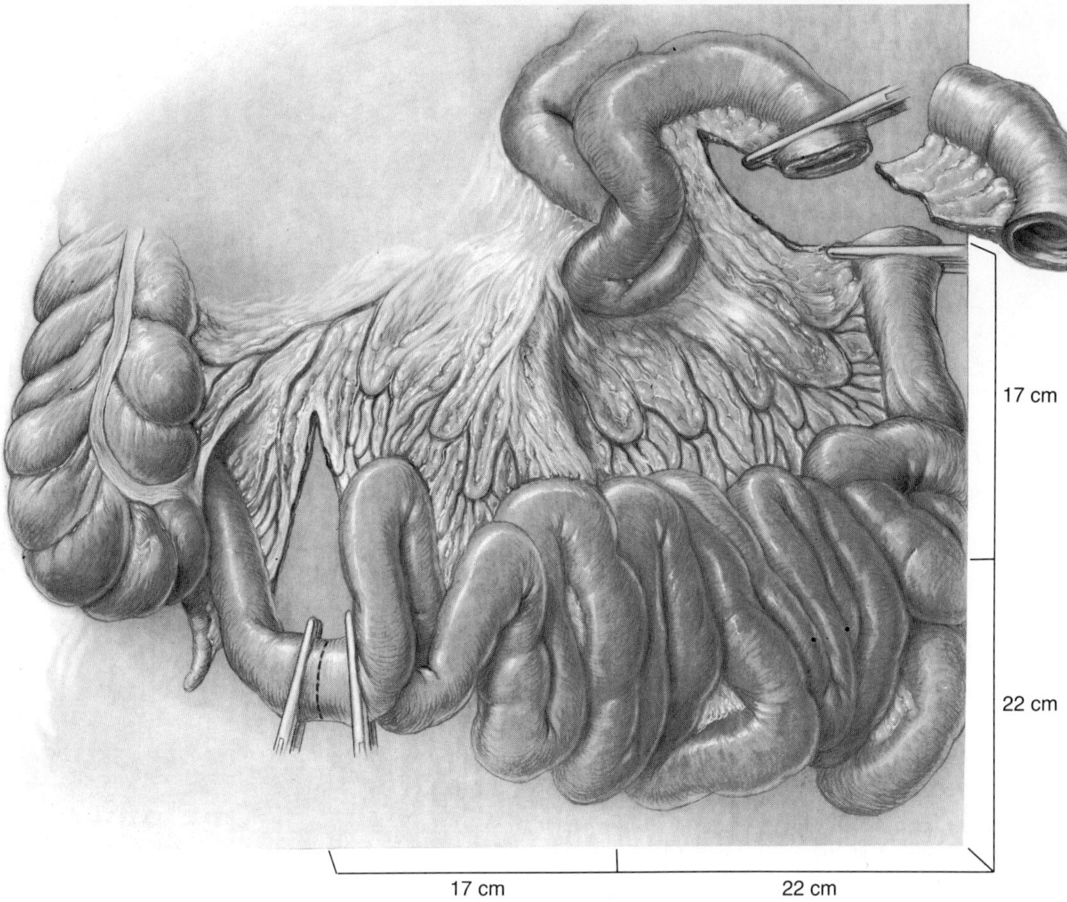

Figure 25–1. Various segments of terminal ileum chosen for creation of the Kock pouch. Note that the distal mesentery division is usually between the ileal colic artery and the terminal ileal branches of the superior mesenteric artery and that it extends deep into the avascular plane of the mesentery. The proximal mesenteric division is quite short to ensure a broad vascular supply to the pouch. Usually a small window of mesentery and an additional 3 to 5 cm of small bowel are discarded proximal to the overall segment in order to ensure good mobility to the pouch and the small bowel anastomosis. The pouch itself is created from two central 22-cm segments, with each limb extending to or away from it; the pouch is approximately 17 cm in length. If there is an existing ileal conduit, the afferent limb is created from only 13 to 15 cm of small bowel. (From Skinner DG, Boyd SD, Lieskovsky G: Creation of the continent Kock ileal reservoir as an alternative to cutaneous urinary diversion. In Skinner DG, Lieskovsky G, eds: Philadelphia, WB Saunders Co, Diagnosis and Management of Genitourinary Cancer, 1988, p 658. By permission.)

pouch and ileal segment. The pouch is then closed and the ureters implanted as originally described.

5. This last important modification was added in July 1985. A strip of Marlex, 2 cm wide, is fixed with a No. 1 nylon suture to the peritoneum and abdominal wall fascia, lateral and slightly cephalad to the foramen in the abdominal wall through which the efferent limb of ileum will exit. The Marlex strip is then brought through the window of Deaver of the ileal mesentery at the base of the efferent intussusception adjacent to the PGA mesh collar. Two No. 1 PGA sutures are then placed as horizontal mattress sutures entering through the abdominal wall fascia, through the PGA mesh, and back out through the abdominal wall fascia, one lateral to the pouch and one medial (Fig. 25–4). The efferent limb is then brought out through the abdominal wall, and the redundant ileum is excised. The horizontal mattress sutures then fix the bowel and the continent valve mechanism to the abdominal wall fascia. The Marlex strip is then fixed to the peritoneum and posterior rectus fascia medial to the pouch. This Marlex strip, located away from the catheterization process, does not cause erosion but is important to prevent parastomal herniation at the region of the mesentery and further fixes the continent valve mechanism to facilitate catheterization and prevent valve slippage.

We find that these modifications have solved

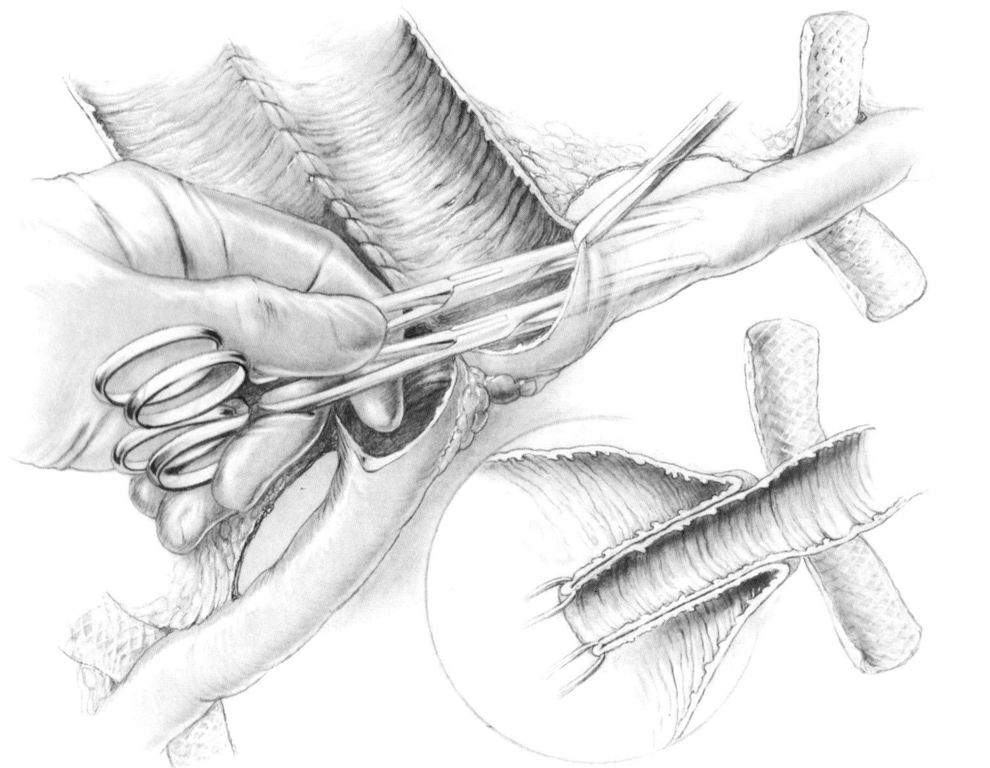

Figure 25–2. Technique of intussusception of valve construction. Note that the mesentery has been denuded for approximately 8 cm along each limb. A Dexon mesh is then passed through a distant window of Deaver, leaving several vascular arcades in between. In this way, the intussusception does not incorporate the mesentery, and the Dexon mesh, when secured to the pouch, further locks in the intact remaining vascular arcade. (From Skinner DG, Boyd SD, Lieskovsky G: Urinary diversion: evolution of the continent ileal reservoir; surgical technique and clinical results. In Skinner DG and Lieskovsky G, eds: Diagnosis and Management of Genitourinary Cancer, Philadelphia, WB Saunders Co, 1988, p 662. By permission.)

most of the problems associated with catheterization, leakage, and development of parastomal hernias. Other aspects of the operation and postoperative management remain as previously described.

CLINICAL RESULTS

From August 1982 through December 1986, construction of the Kock continent ileal reservoir for cutaneous urinary diversion has been performed in 395 patients. Two hundred-sixty were men ranging in age from 15 to 87 years, and 135 were women between 13 and 87 years.

Single-stage radical cystectomy and Kock pouch construction constituted the primary treatment used for bladder malignancy in 278 patients. An additional 37 patients underwent simultaneous cystectomy and Kock pouch construction to relieve symptoms and/or complications of neurogenic bladder (21), end-stage interstitial cystitis (eight), or traumatic bladder injury not amenable to primary repair (eight). Eighty additional patients underwent Kock pouch conversion from an existing form of urinary diversion, 68 from an ileal conduit, and 12 from uterosigmoidostomy. Of the 395 patients, 72 had received varying degrees of radiation therapy prior to Kock pouch construction (four, 1000 to 2000 rads; 25, 4000 to 5000 rads; and 43, greater than 6000 rads with or without brachytherapy implants).

The average operating time to construct a Kock pouch is approximately 1 to 1½ hours longer than that for the construction of a standard ileal conduit. The operating time remains approximately the same, whether the pouch is done in conjunction with cystectomy or is a conversion of an existing ileal conduit. Patients with fat mesenteries present the greatest challenge because closure of the pouch is tedious and may be difficult. Other than the patient with the fat mesentery, the operation is not technically difficult; however, it is tedious, and attention to

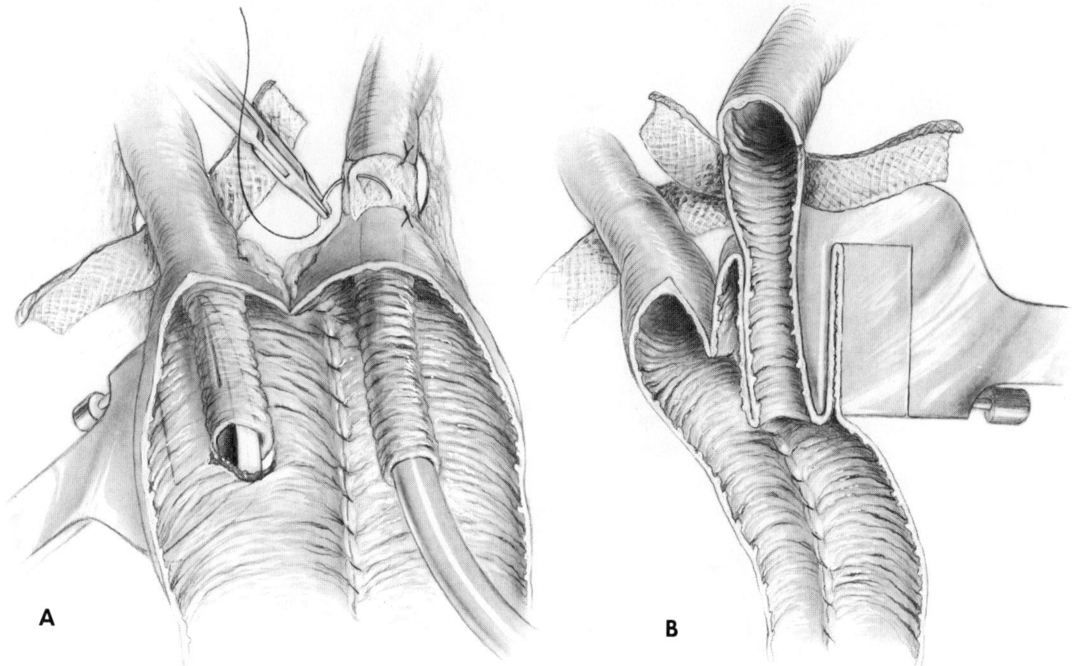

Figure 25–3. Two methods to fix the nipple valve to the back wall of the pouch. *A,* A small hole has been made in the posterior wall of the pouch several centimeters distal from the nipple. The anvil of the stapling device can be inserted through this hole, with the anvil arm of the staple device passed through the nipple. This allows the intussuscepted nipple to be fixed to the back wall of the pouch as further protection against slippage or extussusception. A custom cartridge with six staples removed should be used with this method. *B,* The anvil of the stapler is inserted between the two walls of the nipple at the region of the mesentery from outside the pouch. This will fix the nipple wall to the back wall of the pouch without any staples exposed within the urinary pouch. A standard cartridge with all staples in place should be used with this technique. This figure also depicts fixation of the polyglycolic acid (PGA) mesh at the base of the nipple. A No. 30 Medina tube has been inserted through the nipple and on through the PGA mesh so that the mesh can then be positioned around the afferent and efferent limbs. The catheter is used to ensure that the PGA collar is not too tight to avoid the possibility of erosion. The mesh is secured both to the pouch and to the respective ileum with interrupted 2–0 chromic sutures. (From Skinner DG, Boyd SD, Lieskovsky G: Creation of the continent Kock ileal reservoir as an alternative to cutaneous urinary diversion. In Skinner DG, Lieskovsky G, eds: Diagnosis and management of genitourinary cancer. Philadelphia, WB Saunders Co, 1988, p 664. By permission.)

every detail is essential to its ultimate success. Follow-up ranges to 53 months.

Sixty-eight patients (17 percent) suffered one or more early complications, resulting in an operative mortality rate of 2.3 percent (9/395). As reported previously,[3] our continuing experience reveals that those undergoing simultaneous cystectomy and Kock pouch construction had a higher complication rate than those undergoing conversion: 19 percent (53/278) compared with 12.8 percent (15/117). Once the importance of adequate pelvic drainage was recognized and achieved, the overall early complication rate has remained stable throughout our experience and does not significantly differ from that we have reported among patients undergoing single-stage radical cystectomy and ileal conduit cutaneous urinary diversion.[6]

Follow-up of the 386 patients surviving the operation ranges from the minimum of 6 months to a maximum of 53 months. Late complications are often difficult to assess in a population of patients for whom the operation is part of the treatment of malignancy and whose age makes them prey to other serious medical conditions. We have analyzed our data in terms of late complications directly resulting from the operation or as a direct result of this form of urinary diversion. In this context, 119 of the 386 patients surviving the operation have suffered one or more late complications. The late complications and the number of episodes are listed according to sequential groups of patients in Table 25–1. Some patients suffered more than one complication and those additional complications were usually corrected at the time of initial reoperation. For example, only eight patients presented with a late complication directly related to Mar-

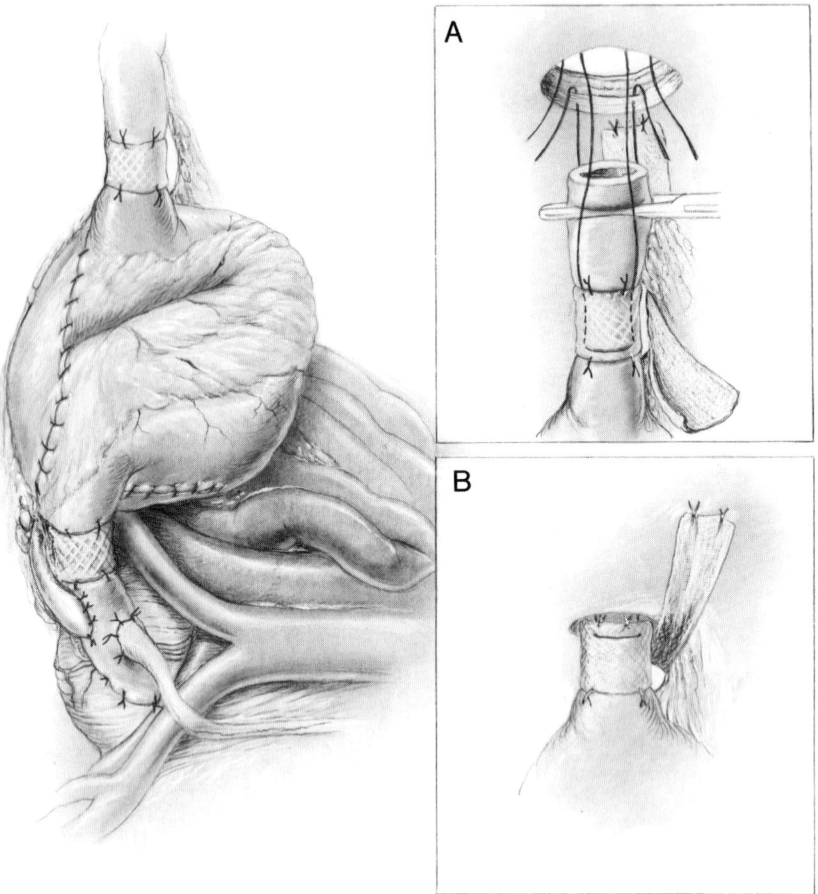

Figure 25–4. Final location of the pouch with completed ureteroileal anastomosis. Horizontal mattress sutures of No. 1 polyglycolic acid (PGA) sutures are passed through the anterior rectus fascia and collar of the efferent limb of the Kock pouch and back out through the anterior rectus fascia. One suture is placed lateral and one medial to the pouch, and the efferent limb is drawn through the abdominal wall. The suture is then secured so that the PGA mesh is fixed to the anterior rectus fascia, thus providing a very short segment from the PGA mesh collar to the skin. The redundant efferent ileum is excised providing a flesh stoma. Note the use of a narrow Marlex strip fixed to the posterior abdominal wall both lateral and medial to the pouch (insets). This strip is passed through the window of Deaver, through which the PGA mesh was placed. This strip is important in preventing a parastomal hernia and helps fix the continence valve mechanism to the abdominal wall. (From Skinner DG, Boyd SD, Lieskovsky G: Creation of the continent Kock ileal reservoir as an alternative to cutaneous urinary diversion. In Skinner DG, Lieskovsky G, eds: Diagnosis and management of genitourinary cancer. Philadelphia, WB Saunders Co, 1988, p 667. By permission.)

Table 25–1. LATE COMPLICATIONS AND NUMBER OF EPISODES ACCORDING TO SEQUENTIAL GROUPS OF PATIENTS UNDERGOING KOCK POUCH CONSTRUCTION (AUGUST 1982–DECEMBER 1986)

Sequential Groups of Patients (No.)	No. of Patients With Late Complications	Percent	No. of Complications
50	24	48	41
52	22	42	31
51	15	29	25
41	15	36	23
50	16	32	19
46	15	32	15
50	07	14	07
45	05	11	05
386	119	31%	166

lex erosion, but 15 additional patients were found to have Marlex erosion while undergoing reoperation for another problem, such as difficult catheterization or urinary leakage. The late complications have involved problems mainly with continence or ease of catheterization. Most of the problems were detected within the first 6 months of surgery. The following sections discuss the specific problems and their solutions.

Leakage of Urine

The most common complaint was excessive urine leakage at the stoma noted in 66 patients (17.8 percent). This leakage was often seen in conjunction with difficulty in catheterization and could be categorized into three groups of patients:

1. Those with leakage from the very beginning who were never dry. Chronic leakage was noted in 35 patients (9 percent) and was the result of a shortened fibrotic nipple valve, a split nipple, or a fistulous false pass at the base of the nipple, perhaps the residual of a pinhole caused by the pin at the end of the stapling device used to secure the intussusception. We believe that, other than those patients with the pinholes, this problem is most likely related to an ischemic intussuscepted nipple.
2. In 25 patients, the onset of leakage was sudden and due to acute prolapse of the efferent valve; in all these patients, continence had been perfect prior to the event. We believe that the described modification in surgical technique that staples the intussuscepted nipple to the pouch wall can eliminate this problem.
3. The other six patients had parastomal hernias that were responsible for, or associated with, leakage.

Overall, 63 of the 66 patients with leakage have undergone a total of 84 revisional operations to achieve continence. Three have yet to undergo revision; they wear an appliance and intermittently catheterize themselves two to three times during a 24-hour period. We have found that once significant leakage occurs, or if a patient is having difficulty with catheterization, revision should be done promptly because continence and ease of catheterization can be achieved and should be the goal in all cases.

To repair leakage or efferent limb redundancy, we routinely dissect out the efferent limb from the abdominal wall, continuing that part of the dissection through the rectus fascia as far as possible before incising the old midline abdominal incision. Care must be taken not to damage the blood supply to the efferent limb, particularly in the region of its mesentery, which will be found cephalad. The abdomen is then opened and the pouch dissected off the anterior abdominal wall. Once the efferent limb and pouch have been mobilized, the pouch is opened several centimeters away from the nipple and away from the mesentery of the pouch, allowing the cause of the failure to be determined. If the nipple looks healthy and the cause of leakage was prolapse or hypermobility, the nipple is stapled to the wall of the pouch and further fixed with No. 3–0 PGA sutures securing the muscularis of the nipple to the muscularis of the pouch wall. Because we have started to do this routinely at the time of the initial surgery, this problem is now rarely seen.

Occasionally, a fistula may be found at the base of the nipple as a result of forced catheter false pass or the pinhole from the stapling device; or a split nipple may be found as the cause of leakage. These valves can often be further intussuscepted into the pouch, repaired, restapled, and again fixed to the wall of the pouch over the Medina tube. If, however, the nipple length was found to be inadequate or fibrotic, suggestive of vascular insufficiency or slough of the original nipple, a new efferent limb and nipple need to be created from an adjacent 15-cm segment of small bowel.

Once it has been determined that the efferent continent valve mechanism cannot be salvaged or is inadequate, a new efferent limb should be constructed. This requires lysis of additional intra-abdominal adhesions in order to identify the ileal small bowel anastomosis, usually found medially adjacent to the pouch, and to free up sufficient proximal small bowel for mobility. The old anastomotic site is divided, and approximately 15 cm of small bowel is freed proximal to the anastomosis (Fig. 25–5*A*). Again, a small wedge of mesentery and approximately 3 to 5 cm of proximal bowel are discarded to enhance mobility of the segment and to facilitate the small bowel reanastomosis. The segment can then be rotated between 90 and 180° so that it reaches toward the skin in an antiperistaltic manner. That is, the proximal or afferent limb of this segment becomes the stoma and the distal end is sewn to the existing pouch. Beginning approximately 5 cm from the end to be anastomosed to the pouch, the mesentery should be stripped with the cautery for 8 cm similar to the method described in our original Kock pouch technique.[1–3] A strip of PGA 2 cm wide is then

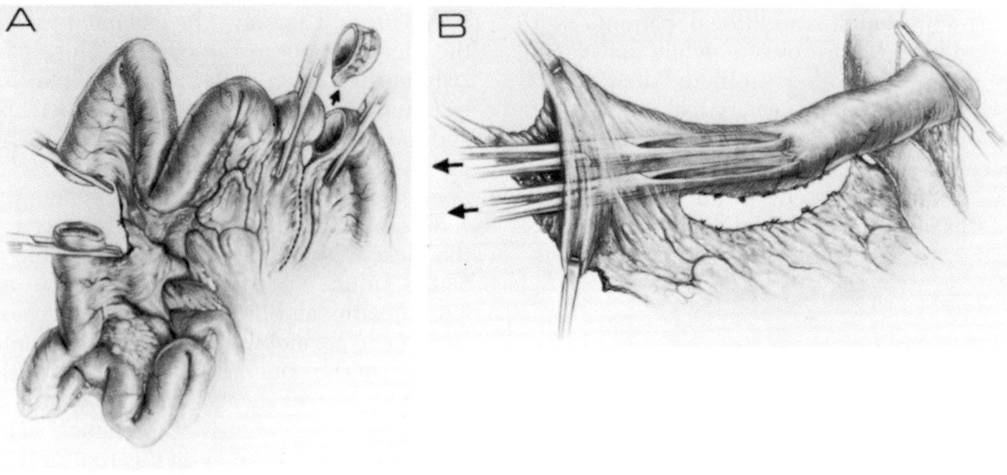

Figure 25–5. *A*, Excision of previous enteroenterostomy and isolation of a suitable segment of ileum for construction of a new efferent limb. *B*, The mesentery is divided immediately adjacent to the serosa of the new efferent limb for a distance of approximately 8 cm. At least one, and preferably two, vascular arcades are preserved, and a 2.5-cm-wide strip of polyglycolic acid (PGA) mesh can then be placed through the window of Deaver distal to the arcade(s). Utilizing Allis' clamps passed about two thirds the way to the PGA mesh, the intraluminal mucosa is grasped in preparation for intussusception. (From Lieskovsky G, Boyd SD, Skinner DG: Management of late complications of the Kock pouch form of urinary diversion. J Urol 137:1147, 1987. By permission.)

passed through a distal window of Deaver, leaving an intact vascular arcade (Fig. 25–5*B*). Next, the ileum to be sewn to the pouch is opened along its antimesenteric border with the cautery. The ileum is then intussuscepted into this opening with Allis forcep clamps, similar to the technique described previously (Fig. 25–6*A*).[1,2] Two rows of staples are applied along the anterior 180° and a third row fixes the nipple to the opened ileal wall as described on page 330.[3] The PGA mesh is then fixed to the ileal "patch" or efferent limb over a No. 30 Medina tube with 2–0 chromic sutures. This ileal "patch" with intussuscepted nipple is then sewn to the opened pouch after the original efferent limb has been excised (Fig. 25–6*B*,*C*). The new segment of ileum thus serves as a "patch graft" onto the pouch, which is then secured to the abdominal wall with the horizontal mattress sutures of No. 1 PGA and the Marlex strip as previously described.

In patients needing revision who previously had Marlex used as a collar, we routinely dissect out the foreign material and replace it with PGA mesh. In addition, the afferent antireflux nipple should be checked for evidence of Marlex erosion, seen in two of our patients. When this is noted, the Marlex has been dissected out from inside the pouch but no replacement mesh has been used on the afferent nipple.

The leakage resulting from a parastomal hernia or diastasis in the obese patient is the most difficult to resolve. Fifteen reoperations have been required to solve this problem, which occurred in six patients. Use of the Marlex strip, as denoted in Fig. 25–4, may prevent this problem or help resolve the complication. However, most of these patients required at least one additional surgical procedure to relocate the stoma in order to achieve a satisfactory result. From experience, we would recommend against using a sheet of Marlex mesh as a flange around the efferent limb, because of the difficulties encountered at reoperation as well as the ongoing risk of infection. It is of interest that most of the hernia problems occurred after we substituted the PGA mesh for Marlex as a collar around the efferent limb and observed that the region of the mesentery was the usual site for development of a parastomal hernia. Our additional experience in more than 200 patients since adopting the Marlex strip concept (see Fig. 25–4) indicates that the parastomal hernia problem has been largely eliminated.

All 63 patients who have undergone revisional surgery for leakage are currently "dry," although additional surgery was required in several. The remaining three patients with chronic leakage are either awaiting surgery or tolerating their condition.

An additional nine patients returned with a bothersome parastomal hernia not associated with leakage. The hernias were usually cephalad

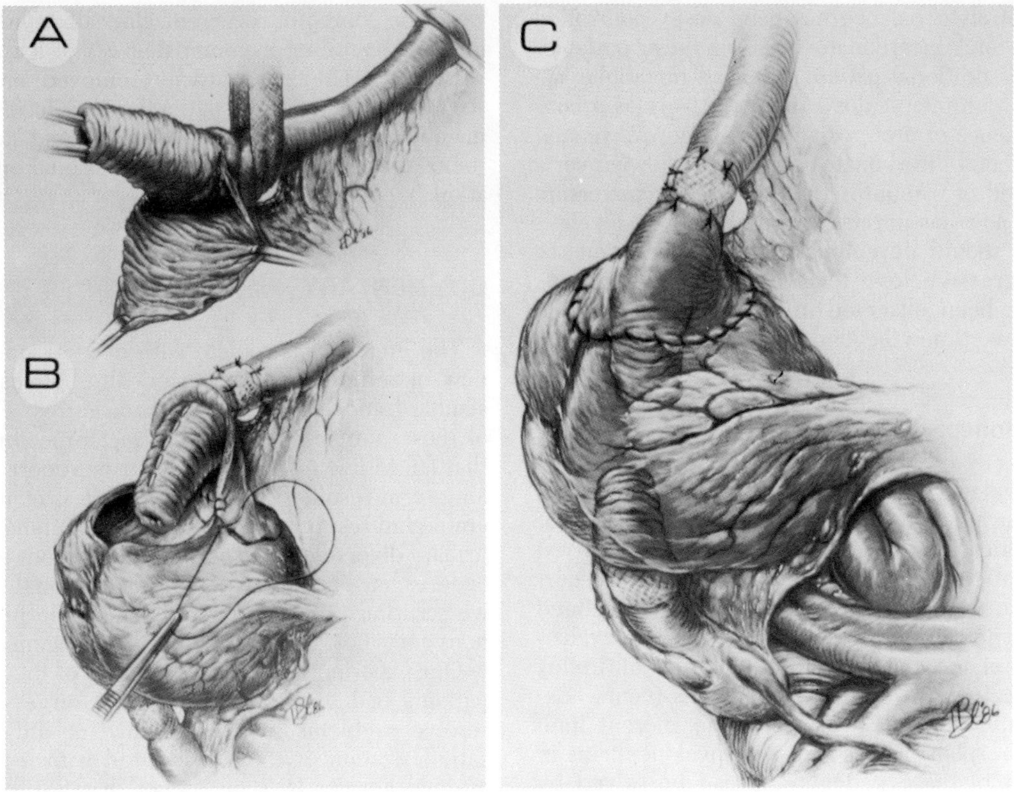

Figure 25–6. The ileum is now intussuscepted so that the polyglycolic acid (PGA) mesh lies adjacent to the base of the efferent limb and a nipple valve mechanism is created (*A*). Two longitudinal rows of staples are placed using the PI-55 automatic stapler and 4.8-mm staples. Note the absence of staples from the end of the nipple to prevent possible stone formation. The staples at the base of the nipple should not extend beyond the end of the mucosa so as to leave a sufficient lip of ileum to be sewn to the pouch away from the mesh collar. The two staple lines should be positioned over approximately 180° so that a third staple row can be placed, fixing the nipple to the open ileal wall of the efferent limb, and not interfering with the two previously placed staple lines. The PGA mesh strip is formed into a collar and the edges secured to the adjacent serosa with No. 2–0 interrupted sutures (*B*). The base of the new efferent limb is then sewn to the open end of the original pouch with two layers of continuous No. 3–0 running PGA sutures to provide meticulous and watertight closure (*C*). (From Lieskovsky G, Boyd SD, Skinner DG: Management of late complications of the Kock pouch form of urinary diversion. J Urol 137:1148, 1987. By permission.)

in the region of the mesentery and occurred primarily during the hiatus between use of the Marlex collar and reinstitution of the Marlex strip. Twelve reoperations were required to solve this problem and the use of the Marlex strip; in some cases, additional Marlex to reinforce the abdominal wall cephalad to the pouch proved successful without the need for stomal relocation.

Difficult Catheterization

Difficulty in catheterizing without associated leakage was noted in ten patients. This problem was corrected by removing the redundancy and angulation of the efferent limb and usually reanchoring the fixation collar to the anterior rectus fascia, especially on the mesenteric side. An infected Marlex collar secondary to erosion was observed in several patients and corrected by removal of the Marlex collar and substitution with PGA mesh, which is now routinely used. Again, the Marlex strip should be used in the reoperation to eliminate the tendency for redundancy and creation of false pass in the region of the mesentery, a common tendency in obese patients with a fat mesentery.

Electrolyte Abnormality

Hyperchloremic metabolic acidosis has been noted to a minor degree in three patients, two of whom required brief periods of rehospitalization for hydration and electrolyte correction.

Electrolyte balance has been easily controlled with oral bicarbonate in all of these patients. One additional patient who had metabolic hyperchloremic acidosis preoperatively as a consequence of ureterosigmoidostomy was weaned from oral bicarbonate supplement slowly over a period of 6 months following Kock conversion and now has normal serum electrolyte levels.

It should be emphasized that no serious or progressive long-term electrolyte problems have been observed in any patient, with the follow-up now beyond 3 years.

Pyelonephritis

Pyelonephritis has been noted in ten patients requiring rehospitalization for intravenous antibiotics. Eight of these episodes have occurred in patients with reflux, and one solitary occurrence was noted in a diabetic who remained asymptomatic for over 2 years. Careful evaluation of the function of the afferent antireflux valve is required if pyelonephritis recurs. Extussusception or prolapse of the afferent limb was responsible for recurrent pyelonephritis in eight of these patients and can be solved by securing the afferent nipple to the wall of the pouch; we now do this routinely.

Hydronephrosis

Hydronephrosis was noted on follow-up intravenous pyelogram (IVP) secondary to ureteroileal anastomotic stenosis in nine patients; six of these patients have undergone revision. The other three remain stable and are asymptomatic. Hydronephrosis as a result of afferent nipple stenosis was seen only early in our experience associated with Marlex collar erosion and subsequent stone formation.

Stone Formation

Stone formation in the pouch has been found in 22 of the early patients. The stones tended to form on staples near the end of the nipples, on eroded Marlex collars, or on the heavy No. 0 PGA sutures we originally utilized that were not absorbed. Because staples are no longer employed on the exposed end of the nipple valves and the Marlex collar has been replaced by PGA mesh, the anticipated stone problem has not materialized. In seven of the 22 patients, stones were the source of recurrent clinically evident infection resulting in minor degrees of leakage *"Kockitis"*. They were easily removed endoscopically. The other 15 patients either have remained asymptomatic or have undergone stone removal at the time of another revisional operation.

COMMENTARY

The literature is replete with descriptions of new operations and suggested alternatives to standard and tested urologic procedures. Few of these authors, however, retract procedures that fail to live up to early claims or report the long-term results. Inasmuch as there is considerable interest in new alternatives to cutaneous urinary diversion and a number of different procedures have been advocated, it is essential that we scrutinize our results and report the problems and, most importantly, their management.

Our experience has shown that 66 of the 386 patients had to undergo revisional surgery to resolve problems with continence or difficult catheterization or those associated with a parastomal hernia. It is our belief that fastidious attention to details with ongoing surgical modifications will further reduce the burden of additional surgery required to achieve our ultimate goal. For example, we are looking for a better alternative to the PGA mesh currently employed as a collar around the base of the efferent limb to fix the pouch to the abdominal wall and to facilitate catheterization. The replacement of Marlex by PGA mesh was a step forward by preventing erosion, but its lack of reaction and early resorption led to late slippage and an increased incidence of parastomal hernia development. Search for a better alternative, perhaps a collagen-derived product, continues, but so far no better absorbable alternative has emerged.

SUMMARY

We have analyzed our experience in terms of late complications resulting directly from the operation or from this form of urinary diversion. In this context, 119 of the 386 patients surviving the operation have suffered one or more late complications. Most of the complications have involved problems with continence or ease of catheterization and were detected within the first 6 months of surgery. We believe that these problems can be resolved successfully, leading to overwhelming patient acceptance of the operation. It is hoped that further refinements and modifications in surgical technique will continue to reduce the incidence of late complications. The basic surgical premise as conceived by Kock remains: a low-pressure, high-capacity reservoir with continent and non-refluxing valves that can be constructed from ileum. It is a sound concept that currently offers the best alternative to the patient who reqires cutaneous urinary diversion.

References

1. Skinner DG, Boyd SD, Lieskovsky G: Clinical experience with the Kock continent ileal reservoir for urinary diversion. J Urol 132:1101, 1984.
2. Skinner DG, Lieskovsky G, Boyd SD: Technique of creation of a continent internal ileal reservoir (Kock pouch) for urinary diversion. Urol Clin North Am 11:741, 1984.
3. Skinner DG, Lieskovsky G, Boyd SD: Continuing experience with the continent ileal reservoir (Kock pouch) as an alternative to cutaneous urinary diversion: an update after 250 cases. J Urol 137:1140, 1987.
4. Skinner DG, Boyd SD, Lieskovsky G, Hardy BE: Construction of a continent ileal reservoir (Kock pouch) for urinary diversion: an update after the first 250. Video presented before the annual meeting of the American Urological Association, New York, 1986. (Available AUA Film Library and American V. Mueller Video Library.)
5. Skinner DG, Lieskovsky G: Creation of the continent Kock ileal reservoir as an alternative to cutaneous urinary diversion. In Skinner DG, Lieskovsky G, eds: Diagnosis and Management of Genitourinary Cancer. Philadelphia, WB Saunders Co, 1988.
6. Skinner DG, Lieskovsky G: Contemporary cystectomy with pelvic node dissection compared to preoperative radiation therapy plus cystectomy in management of invasive bladder cancer. J Urol 131:1069, 1984.
7. Kock NG, Nilson AE, Nilsson LO, Norlen LJ, Philipson BM: Urinary diversion via a continent ileal reservoir: clinical results in 12 patients. J Urol 128:469, 1982.
8. Kock NG, Norlen L, Philipson BM: Management of complications after construction of a continent ileal reservoir for urinary diversion. World J Urol 3:152, 1985.
9. Lieskovsky G, Boyd SD, Skinner DG: Management of late complications of the Kock pouch form of urinary diversion. J Urol 137:1146, 1987.
10. Kock N: Material presented at the 1985 Postgraduate Course in Urologic Oncology. Los Angeles, University of Southern California School of Medicine, January 1985.
11. Skinner DG, Boyd SD, Lieskovsky G: An update on the Kock pouch for continent urinary diversion. Urol Clin North Am 14:789, 1987.
12. Hendren WH: Reoperative ureteral reimplantation: management of the difficult case. J Pediatr Surg 15:770, 1980.

COMPLICATIONS OF BLADDER SUBSTITUTION AND CONTINENT URINARY DIVERSION

26

Jacob Golomb • Carl G. Klutke • Shlomo Raz

INTRODUCTION

During the past several years, there has been a remarkable surge in the use of bowel segments for replacement of the native bladder, either as bladder substitutes that empty through the intact urethra or as continent urinary reservoirs that must be drained by clean intermittent catheterization via a cutaneous stoma. As the various forms of continent urinary reservoirs have evolved, three basic requirements have been addressed. First is the need to preserve upper urinary tract function by avoiding reflux and obstruction. Second is that the reservoir needs to have a high capacity while maintaining low pressures. Finally, there should be a mechanism to allow reasonable continence yet ease of emptying. Surgical creativity and ingenuity have led to the development of a large variety of ureteric reimplantation techniques and to the construction of various continent valve mechanisms and pouches using different configurations of bowel segments.

The creation of a urinary reservoir may be indicated in cases of bladder ablation secondary to malignant diseases, or as a last resort, in benign processes such as neurogenic bladder, exstrophy, and trauma. However, in the adult, the ileal conduit should be the gold standard with which the risks and benefits of continent reservoir and bladder substitution procedures are compared. Patient selection for these procedures is extremely important since intelligence, strong motivation, psychosocial stability, and manual dexterity are important factors for a successful ultimate result.

The four basic factors that govern the function of bowel as a reservoir are geometric capacity, accommodation, compliance, and contractility.[1] *Geometric capacity* refers to the fact that the volume of a tubular segment (cylinder) increases by the square of the radius and by only the first power of length. This means that simple detubularization or reconfiguration of a bowel segment may double its capacity.

Accommodation and *compliance* relate to Laplace's law, which states that with increasing radius of a spherical reservoir, mural tension increases while intraluminal pressure remains approximately constant up to the limits of the viscoelastic elements in the wall of the reservoir. A reservoir with a larger radius will not only accommodate a larger volume at the same pressure of a smaller reservoir, but also produce a higher wall tension. This will promote successive enlargement of the reservoir by stretching the wall without increasing pressure. Therefore, the compliance (changes in volume per increments of pressure) will be higher in reservoirs with larger diameters.

The fourth important factor to determine reservoir characteristics is bowel *contractility.* Three patterns of contractions are found in the bowel: phasic contractions (a start, a peak, and a return to baseline) and tonal contractions (volume related, ascending loop) or a combination of both. These contraction patterns can be either segmental or diffuse mass contractions. The basic electrical rhythm in the ileum and colon lies in the longitudinal muscle layer and spreads quickly into the circular layer, thus inducing a contraction ring that increases the intraluminal pressure. After detubularization, the contraction is limited to half of the circumference at most. Therefore, the basic contractile rhythm arising from the longitudinal coat is not sequentially propagated but becomes disorganized and discontinuous, and the pressure wave is blunted and dampened.

The resting pressure of a continent reservoir is a function of compliance of the bowel wall and tonic contractile activity of the muscularis. The resting pressures of intact or reconfigurated bowel are usually less than 15 to 20 cm water, and variability is directly related to reservoir volume. The magnitude and frequency of contraction pressures are a function of reservoir volume as well as the technique of construction. An intact bowel segment, like a cecal reservoir, can generate pressures as high as 60 to 90 cm water at high volumes, whereas in reconfigurated segments, the pressures rarely exceed 40 cm water at high volumes.[2]

Reservoir distention is usually accompanied by vague abdominal fullness or cramping. At 3 to 6 months after surgery, those reservoirs that require catheterization for emptying need to be catheterized at intervals of 4 to 8 hours during the day. Catheterization at night may not be required. The reservoirs tend to become more capacious over time, and large capacities are usually observed in patients who catheterize infrequently.[2]

The continence mechanism, other than that of the native urethra or the anal sphincter, is based either on ileal intussusception or on plication, incorporating the ileocecal valve in some patients. Ileal intussusception or plication provides resistance to urinary flow that exceeds the intraluminal pressures of the reservoir, which are a summation of intra-abdominal and intrareservoir pressures. Phasic contractions of the intussusception may contribute in part to this resistance. Contraction of the cecal or Kock reservoir is accompanied by simultaneous increase in the pressures within the intussusception. These changes are volume- and pressure-related. Coordinated contractions of the ileal intussusception through the ileocecal valve with the cecal segment are expected because in the intact gastrointestinal tract, distention of the cecum normally results in increased pressures within the ileum as well as contraction of the ileocecal valve.[2,3]

Undoubtedly, malfunction of the continence mechanism and difficulties in catheterization are the most frequent problems with continent reservoirs. Malfunction of an intussuscepted nipple usually results from nipple instability and is manifested by valve slippage (disintussusception) or prolapse without slippage (eversion or devagination), subsequently causing difficulties in catheterization and incontinence. Valve slippage results from the detachment of opposing walls of the intussuscepted ileum. The reservoirs particularly vulnerable to this complication are those with free intraluminal nipple because the intussuscepted segment is a direct extension of the reservoir, and overdistention of the pouch tends to pull apart the walls of the intussusception.

Fixation of the nipple to the side wall of the reservoir can prevent this complication. Valve prolapse may follow dilatation of the reservoir outlet, which can result from parastomal herniation or oversized abdominal wall defect and high intraluminal pressures. Angulation of the reservoir outlet at the abdominal wall or dilatation of the outlet can also cause difficulties in catheterization. Modifications aimed at stabilizing the ileal intussusception include strengthening the reservoir outlet with a collar of synthetic material or autologous fascia, mesenteric exclusion, the use of staples for fixation of the intussusception, and attachment of the nipple to the reservoir wall.[2]

In colonic reservoirs, ureteric reimplantation is usually based on traditional methods of tunneled non-refluxing anastomosis. When small bowel is involved, different techniques are used because of the friability of the small bowel mucosa and the absence of thick muscularis. These include antireflux tunneled anastomosis, antireflux non-tunneled ureteroileal implantation technique (Le Duc), and creation of an afferent intussuscepted ileal nipple to which the ureters are anastomosed end-to-side.

The various procedures that are in practice for bladder substitution and continent diversion can be classified according to the patient's sex, the part of the bowel that is utilized, use of an intact or a detubularized bowel segment, outlet continence mechanism, and type of ureteric reimplant.[5–10,12–45] Each of the procedures differs in bowel configuration, continence mechanism, and antireflux measures, and thus some of the possible complications are inherent to the surgical technique, whereas others are related to usage of bowel per se for urinary tract reconstruction. We, therefore, elect to review the specific complications related to each type of the most common operative techniques, followed by general clinical considerations. These bladder substitution and continent urinary diversion techniques are classified as follows:

1. Continent diversion with neither the urethra nor a cutaneous stoma:
   A. Ureterosigmoidostomy
2. Bladder substitution:
   A. Intact ileal bladder (Camey procedure)
   B. Intact colonic and ileocolonic bladder substitutes
   C. Bladder substitutes of reconfigurated bowel:
      a. Bladder substitutes based on an intact urethral sphincter (Le Bag, Mainz pouch, UCLA pouch in males, urethral Kock pouch, and others).
      b. Bladder substitutes with reinforced outlet sphincteric mechanism (Indiana pouch, UCLA pouch in females, and others).
3. Continent cutaneous diversion:
   A. Intact cecal reservoir (Gilchrist et al., Mansson et al., and others).
   B. Reconfigurated ileocolonic reservoirs with plicated terminal ileal segment (Indiana pouch, Lockhart, Bejany and Politano)
   C. Open ileal reservoir (Kock pouch)
   D. Reconfigurated ileocolonic reservoir with intussuscepted continence mechanism:
      a. Mainz pouch
      b. UCLA right colonic pouch

URETEROSIGMOIDOSTOMY

Ureterosigmoidostomy is one of the oldest forms of urinary diversion and provides continent diversion in appropriate candidates. Early experiences with this procedure were associated with prohibitive mortality because of the absence of effective antimicrobial agents and reliable operative techniques. Peritonitis, renal infection, anastomotic obstruction, and fistulas were common causes of death. Evolution of techniques for ureterocolonic anastomosis from the non-refluxing but frequently obstructive submucosal method of Coffey to the submucosal tunnel with direct mucosa-to-mucosa anastomosis described by Leadbetter and Goodwin and associates reduced the incidence of anastomotic complications.[4–6] However, even though the general infectious problems inherent to bowel surgery are more easily avoided and controlled since the development of better antibiotics, only about a third of all patients undergoing ureterosigmoidostomy avoid major complications. Clinical bouts of acute pyelonephritis occurred in 20 to 57 percent of the patients; abnormal upper urinary tract findings were reported in 17 percent of the patients with preoperatively normal excretory urograms; deterioration of preoperatively abnormal excretory urograms was diagnosed in 12.5 to 32 percent of the patients; and electrolyte disturbances, mainly hyperchloremic metabolic acidosis, were recorded in the vast majority of patients.[7,8]

As for continence, Marberger and Straub have found that 19 percent of the children who were believed to have anal continence preoperatively experienced occasional diurnal or nocturnal soiling, associated particularly with liquid stools.[9] Adults also may suffer frequency during the day and night, which may compromise their quality of life.

There is also growing evidence of an increased rate of colonic neoplasms associated with ureterosigmoidostomy. A review of several series of patients with ureterosigmoidostomy reveals that the incidence of polyps or colonic adenocarcinoma occurring at the anastomotic site is as high as 5 to 40 percent, a 500- to 7000-fold increased incidence compared with its incidence in the general population in selected decades of life. The incubation period observed between the procedure and the finding of a tumor varies between 7 and 49 years, with an average period of 20 years.[10]

Carcinogenesis clearly depends on the presence of urine, feces, urothelium, and colonic epithelium in close apposition at a healing anastomotic suture line. This theory is supported by findings in animal models.[10] This is a major shortcoming of ureterosigmoidostomy, especially in children and young adults with benign diseases who have a long life expectancy.

BLADDER SUBSTITUTION

Bladder substitutes are structures that collect and store urine and empty per urethram either by spontaneous micturition or by intermittent catheterization. The methods for construction of the storage component and creation of the antireflux ureteric mechanism are similar to those for the continent reservoirs; however, the normal bladder outlet and urethral sphincter serve as the continence mechanism, with or without reinforcement of the reservoir outlet, especially in female patients. Spontaneous voiding is accomplished by coordinated relaxation of the pelvic floor and abdominal straining when pelvic fullness or cramps are sensed. Pre-existing sphincteric incompetence can be managed by bowel intussusception, plication procedures, or an artificial sphincter.

A distressing complication of all bladder substitutes is enuresis, which reportedly affects up to 91 percent of the patients, mainly following the Camey procedure. The causes of nocturnal incontinence after bladder substitution are not entirely clear. Apparently, the sensation of reservoir fullness is not sufficient to awaken the patient, and the reservoir pressures are capable of overcoming the resistance of perineal musculature, which is relaxed during sleep.[11] However, although perineal muscle tone clearly decreases when one assumes the horizontal position, there is a difference in nocturnal continence between bladder substitution and radical prostatectomy, even though the urethral stump and the external sphincter are the same in both procedures. It seems that after radical prostatectomy, by preserving the normal bladder innervation and local reflexes, patients are better able to maintain continence than following cystectomy (with urethral denervation, which leads to decreased urethral resistance during bladder filling). An intact reservoir, as opposed to a detubularized segment, has a higher risk of leakage by generating high pressures that may overcome the outlet resistance.

A major technical factor in creating a bladder substitute is the mobility of the intestinal segment that needs to reach the urethra. A short mesentery may in some cases compel the surgeon to resort to an alternative form of reconstruction or to an ileal conduit diversion.

Intact Ileal Bladder (Camey Procedure)

In 1959, Camey first performed this procedure utilizing a 40 cm, U-shaped isolated segment of ileum as a bladder substitute following radical cystoprostatectomy in men. Since 1977, antireflux implantation of the ureters has been added to the technique.

The clinical experience with this techique was reported by several authors. In Camey's series of 185 patients who underwent the procedure between 1958 and 1986, the incidence of major complications was as follows: Gastrointestinal (colic or ileal fistula, small bowel obstruction, prolonged paralytic ileus, peptic disorders)—14 percent. Urologic (ileourethral fistula, ureteroileal fistula, ileal stump fistula, ileosigmoid fistula, ureteroileal obstruction, transient acidosis)—15 percent. Infectious (wound infection, septicemia and septic shock, pelvic abscess, persistent fever, persistent urinary infection, pulmonary infection)—25 percent.

The incidence of early and late complications at the urethral anastomosis was greater among patients treated with radiation therapy before or after surgery. He further reported that 95 percent of the patients in his series since 1977 achieved daytime continence; nighttime incontinence, however, has been a problem in approximately 50 percent of the patients. He noted that patients can overcome this problem by a combination of awakening to void 2 or 3 times per night and by limiting nocturnal fluid intake. Reflux has been prevented in 85 percent of the patients, and 70 percent of patients maintained sterile urine.[12]

Allen and associates published their experience in 11 patients with a short-term follow-up. Three patients experienced mucous plugging of the urethral catheter, causing obstruction until recognized. Metabolic acidosis occurred in two patients but was easily controlled, and one patient developed an enteric fistula. Reflux persisted in 29 percent of the patients. As for continence, only 45 percent of the patients had complete daytime continence, and 91 percent were enuretic.[13]

Roehrborn and coworkers studied 14 men who underwent the Camey ileal bladder procedure, with a mean follow-up period of 15 months. Eleven patients had diurnal continence and only two had nighttime continence. Reflux was prevented successfully in 86 percent of the renal units. Metabolic acidosis was seen in 43 percent of the patients.[14]

Goldwasser and colleagues reviewed their experience with the Camey procedure at the Mayo Clinic. From ten patients with a follow-up of 3 to 18 months, two had diurnal and nocturnal continence, one was totally incontinent, and six were incontinent to various degrees that necessitated the use of pads or diapers. In the eight incontinent patients, a spurting type of incontinence was present that was related to high pressure contractions of the ileal bladder. The patients tended to leak from their "bladder" when the intrareservoir pressures exceeded 40 to 50 cm water. The only two patients who were totally continent had no contractions on cystometry. Reflux occurred in three of 20 renal units.[15]

A urodynamic evaluation of the ileal bladder by several authors revealed an average capacity of 300 ml and intraluminal pressures of 40 to 80 cm water recorded at maximum volumes. The average urinary flow rate was 9 to 19 ml per second. Residual urine volumes averaged 60 ml.[12,14,15]

Intact Colonic and Ileocolonic Bladder Substitutes

The sigmoid and ileocecal segments have been used successfully for bladder replacement by several authors. Bladder substitutes from intact sigmoid are generally constructed in a manner identical to the Camey procedure. Hradec reported a series of 79 patients with sigmoid bladder substitutes and concluded that, in his hands, the capacities of the sigmoid bladder (200 to 400 ml) were greater than those of the ileal bladder and that the urinary flow and the ability to empty were superior. Even though the pressures ranged from 20 to 40 cm water, enuresis was less common. Because in many patients, the distal prostate and even the entire trigone were preserved, incontinence was infrequent. When comparing the use of different bowel segments for bladder replacement in 114 patients, he concluded that the use of ileocolonic segment or sigmoid colon was superior to small bowel.[16]

Gil-Vernet popularized the use of ileocolonic segment for bladder substitution, and favorable experiences with this segment have been reported by Turner-Warwick and Ashken, Khafagy and associates, Zinman and Libertino, and others.[17–19] Recently McDougal published his results in five patients in whom he used the entire ascending colon and distal 12 cm of ileum to create an intact reservoir. The antireflux mechanism was based on creating an ileocecal intussusception and anastomosing the ureters to the ileum in a conjoined fashion (Wallace technique). In four males, the distal end of the colon segment was anastomosed end-to-end to the prostatic urethra, and in one woman, 0.5 cm of bladder was left attached to the circumference of the urethra. In all cancer patients, frozen biopsies confirmed the absence of malignant changes at the resection line.

The follow-up ranged from 9 to 16 months. All five patients voided spontaneously and had diurnal continence, whereas one required intermittent catheterization twice daily and one had significant enuresis. The average capacity was 315 ml, and the average peak flow was 24 ml per second. In two patients, the reservoir pressures ranged between 20 and 40 cm water at low volumes. Two patients developed metabolic acidosis that required treatment. One patient, a boy with compromised renal function, developed recurrent episodes of septicemia that required hospitalization.[20]

Bladder Substitutes of Reconfigurated Bowel

The creation of reservoirs from detubularized and reconfigurated bowel segments was carried out by several authors, utilizing ileum, ileocecum, and right colon for this purpose. These bladder substitutes differ mainly in the continence mechanism and are therefore easily classifed according to the continence mechanism as follows: (1) sphincteric mechanism of the native urethra, (2) intussuscepted ileum (with or without using the ileocecal valve), and (3) imbricated bowel.

Bladder Substitutes Based on an Intact Urethral Sphincter

Light and Engelmann described a method of bladder substitution using a reconfigured ileocolonic segment and anastomosing the intact ileum to the urethra after a 180-degree rotation. The ureters are reimplanted to the colonic segment with conventional tunneling technique (Le Bag pouch). Ten patients have undergone the procedure, with a follow-up of 4 to 15 months. The results were reported for four patients. Three patients were continent, two with an artificial sphincter and one with an intact sphincteric mechanism. The remaining patient with a neuropathic sphincter is incontinent and awaits implantation of an artificial sphincter. Mild reflux was documented in only one case.[21]

Thuroff and associates reported their experience with 100 patients with the Mainz pouch, 15 of whom underwent complete bladder substitution. In these patients, a buttonhole incision was created in the lowest part of the detubularized cecum and anastomosed to the urethra. The ureters were reimplanted to the cecum in an antireflux tunneling technique. In this group, one patient had grade I stress urinary incontinence and the remainder had good diurnal continence. However, at night four patients were incontinent. The mean capacity of the bladder was 510 ml, and the pressures ranged from 33 cm water (50 percent capacity) to 41 cm water (100 percent capacity). Most patients initially needed alkalizing drugs to balance a compensated hyperchloremic acidosis. After a follow-up of 6 months, about 50 percent of the patients stabilized without any alkalizing drugs, and no patient with a follow-up longer than 12 months required therapy.[22]

Goldwasser and associates recently reported their technique with detubularized right colonic segment and direct urethrocecal anastomosis. With a mean follow-up period of 5.1 months, six of seven patients had diurnal and nocturnal continence. The average "bladder" capacity was 641 ml, and the recorded contractions ranged from 24 to 42 cm water.[23,24] In another paper, these authors compared the cystometric properties of the detubularized right colon with those of tubular right colon, tubular ileum, and detubularized ileum. They found that the compliance curves were normal in nearly all patients except those who underwent tubular cystoplasty. As for capacity and magnitude of contractions, detubularized right colon had more favorable results compared with tubular right colon and tubular ileum but did worse compared with detubularized ileum.[25]

Lockhart reported a method in which he has used a remodeled right colon based on the cecum, ascending colon, and the right third of the transverse colon. The continence mechanism depended on partial or total preservation of the sphincteric mechanism, and the lower end of the reconfigured bowel was sutured to the trigone. He reported that of three patients, all of whom were continent, one is voiding spontaneously, whereas the other two are on self-catheterization. The average capacity was 450 ml and the maximum reservoir pressure ranged between 18 and 30 cm water.[26]

Ghoneim and associates reported their experience with bladder substitution using the Kock reservoir.[27] They eliminated the efferent nipple and anastomosed the reservoir directly to the urethra. They reviewed 37 patients, with a follow-up ranging from 3 to 18 months. Six patients were dropped from evaluation because of tumor recurrence or metastatic disease. All of the remaining 31 patients were continent during the day, urinating 3 to 5 times daily, and 28 were dry at night, with nocturia of 0 to 3. Four of these patients had occasional enuresis that improved upon treatment with imipramine. Three patients out of 31 had nocturnal incontinence. The mean reservoir capacity was 579 ml, and the pressure at maximum capacity was 56 cm water. Urography revealed slight dilatation in 11 renal units, and reflux was corrected surgically in nine patients. Eversion of the antireflux valve was noted in 13 cases.

Continent lower urinary tract reconstruction with Kock pouch urethrostomy is also utilized by Skinner and associates in highly selected male patients following cystectomy, but no follow-up results have been reported yet.[28]

At UCLA, we have performed 12 bladder substitution procedures in male patients between 1986 and 1988, utilizing 50 to 60 cm of detubularized ileum to create the reservoir. The continence mechanism was based on intact urethral sphincter without reinforcement, to which the distal part of the ileum was anastomosed. Emptying was accomplished by spontaneous voiding. The ureters were reimplanted with a submucosal tunnel.

The follow-up ranged from 2 to 30 months with an average of 13.2 months. Only ten patients were considered for follow-up because two patients were dropped from the survey; one patient suffered a urethral recurrence and underwent urethrectomy and conversion to a continent pouch, and the second patient had difficulties in voiding and catheterization owing to kinking and adhesions of the distal ileal segment. Following revision he became incontinent and underwent placement of an artificial urinary sphincter around the bulbar urethra. The remaining ten patients void spontaneously with residual volumes of less than 100 ml, and all have diurnal continence. Seven out of ten are fully continent at night, one has mild nocturnal incontinence, and two have moderate nocturnal incontinence. One patient developed a spontaneous urinoma 5 months after surgery that had to be drained surgically, without any apparent leakage. One patient developed recurrent carcinoma and a fistula between the terminal ileum and the urinary reservoir that necessitated surgical repair.

Reddy and Lange compared their results with ileal versus sigmoid segments in the construction of a detubularized bladder substitute anastomosed to the urethra following cystoprostatectomy.[29] In six men, ileum was used, whereas sigmoid was utilized in 14 patients. Follow-up ranged from 3 to 15 months. All patients had excellent daytime continence; however, 80 percent of patients with sigmoid bladder achieved nocturnal continence compared with only 50 percent of patients with ileal bladder, and nocturnal continence was regained quicker in sigmoid substitutes. At 3 months, sigmoid reservoirs appeared superior to ileal reservoirs by urodynamic studies.

Bladder Substitutes With Reinforced Outlet Sphincteric Mechanism

When the urethral sphincteric mechanism is weakened or cannot be depended on, the outlet of the bladder substitute can be reinforced by one of the following means: bowel intussusception, bowel plication, or placement of an artificial sphincter around the urethra or bowel segment.

Rowland and associates have designed a modification of the Gilchrist procedure, which is based on a reconfigured cecal segment to which the ureters are reimplanted in an antireflux tunneled technique.[30] The continent outlet is created by plicating the terminal ileum in its entire length over a 12 Fr. catheter, using Lembert sutures, and anastomosing it end-to-end to the urethra (the Indiana valve). Continence is thus based to some extent on the reinforced ileocecal valve along with the tapering of the terminal ileum. This technique was used in five patients with exstrophy as the primary diagnosis; in three males, the tapered ileal segment was anastomosed to the reconstructed uretha, and two women had a stoma created on the anterior vaginal wall. All patients emptied the reservoir by intermittent catheterization. Two patients required reoperation and placement of an artificial sphincter around the ileal segment for continence. The average frequency of catheterization was every 3.7 hours, and the average maximal volume was 508 ml.

At UCLA, we have performed bladder substitution with a reinforced outlet in seven female patients between 1986 and 1988. The reservoir was created from a reconfigurated ileocecal segment. Continence was based on an intussuscepted ileal segment through the ileocecal valve, stabilized by three rows of SGIA staples (which also secured the nipple to the side wall of the reservoir) and by a Dexon mesh. The proximal ileum was anastomosed to the anterior vaginal wall at the urethral meatus. The ureters were reimplanted to the colonic segment in a tunneled technique. Emptying of the reservoir was accomplished by intermittent self-catheterization. The follow-up ranged from 9 to 17 months, with an average of 12 months.

Only five patients were considered for follow-up because two patients were dropped from the survey; one patient with interstitial cystitis suffered recurrent episodes of infection and "bladder" pain and underwent conversion to an ileal conduit, and the second patient experienced malfunction of the nipple with difficulties in catheterization that necessitated revision and, finally, conversion to a continent stoma. Four of the five patients evaluated have diurnal and nocturnal continence on self-catheterization every 4 to 6 hours, whereas one patient has moderate leakage, mainly when the urine is infected. Two patients have protracted diarrhea, which is controlled by medication. Two patients formed calculi around staples that migrated into the reservoir and were removed through cystoscopy.

CONTINENT CUTANEOUS DIVERSION

Continent urinary reservoirs are structures that collect and store urine and are emptied by catheterization through a cutaneous stoma. Because the different reservoirs vary mainly in the storage component and continence mechanism, the classification will be done accordingly.

Intact Cecal Reservoir

Construction of an intact continent cecal reservoir was first described by Gilchrist and associates in 1950.[31] They used the isolated ileocecal segment, with the cecum functioning as a urinary reservoir and the ileum forming the outflow tract and the cutaneous stoma. Continence depended on the antiperistaltic function of the terminal ileum and the action of the ileocecal valve and the small ileal skin stoma. They reported complete continence in 37 patients (94 percent).[32] However, the authors acknowledged that continence improved with time and that stomal contracture was a significant factor in providing continence.

Mansson and colleagues have reported extensively on the cecal reservoir. Initially, they created the continence-providing intussuscepted ileal nipple proximal to the ileocecal valve to protect it from high-pressure cecal contractions. Angulation of ileal segment when the reservoir was full made catheterization difficult. Therefore, the technique was modified with distal mesenteric exclusion, intussusception of the terminal ileum into the cecal lumen, and reinforcement with fascial sling. With this technique, all eight patients in the series had good functional results, and revision of the reservoir outlet was indicated in one of the eight patients.[33]

Hedlund and coworkers studied the dynamics of intact cecal reservoirs and found low basal pressures in the reservoir even at high-volume fillings. However, they recorded intermittent pressure waves in the reservoir at a frequency of every 2 to 3 minutes. These waves increased in frequency, duration, and amplitude with increasing volume.

In patients with continence, the basal pressure at the outlet always was higher than that in the reservoir, and the pressure waves peaked simultaneously in the reservoir and the outlet. In two incontinent patients, relatively long delays occurred in the peaking of the outlet pressure. The amplitude of the pressure waves in the reservoir diminished with time, whereas no such change occurred in the frequency or duration of the waves.[34]

Reconfigurated Ileocolonic Reservoirs With Plicated Terminal Ileal Segment

Rowland and associates have reported on their results with a modified Gilchrist reservoir, namely, reconfigurated cecal segment with either ileal or sigmoid patch or reconfiguration of the ascending colon in a Heineke-Mikulicz type of closure and tapering of the terminal ileum to provide continence (Indiana pouch).[30] They stress that patient selection is critical to the ultimate success and patient satisfaction. It is imperative for them to verify that the patient is willing to take the added responsibility of a continent reservoir and is able to perform clean intermittent catheterization and irrigation of the reservoir. Impaired renal function, limited life expectancy (less than 1 year), serious intercurrent illness, psychological instability, primary disease of the colon, and prior high-dose irradiation to the pelvis are contraindications for the procedure. These apply to both bladder substitution and continent diversion.[35]

Rowland and associates report their experience in 29 patients (including five patients with bladder substitution) between 1982 and 1986. In the initial ten patients, no attempt was made to disrupt the tubular configuration of the cecum. Poor compliance and mass contractions produced poor continence in five of these ten patients, who subsequently underwent a procedure to disrupt the tubular nature of the bowel. The remaining 19 patients underwent cecal reconfiguration at the time of reservoir construction. The *continence* mechanism was created by plicating the terminal ileum over a 12 Fr. Robinson catheter in two layers. The first layer was composed of series of Lembert sutures beginning at the ileocecal valve and extending to the end of the ileal segment, with a second reinforcing suture layer. The terminal ileum was brought out to the lower abdominal wall as a cutaneous stoma. The ureters were reimplanted in the tenia line in a tunneled technique.

Twenty-seven of the 29 patients (93 percent) had acceptable daytime continence. The remaining two patients had significant diurnal and nocturnal leakage, requiring a cutaneous bag between catheterizations. However, cystometrograms did not demonstrate bolus contractions. Of 22 patients who were dry at night, 15 underwent catheterization once at night and seven were able to sleep all night without catheterization. The remaining seven who experienced nocturnal incontinence wore a cutaneous drainage bag at night. The average volume removed by catheterization was approximately 300 ml during the day and 500 ml at night.

Cystograms showed asymptomatic grade I reflux in one patient and a higher grade reflux in a second patient that required a secondary reimplantation. The postoperative complications included one patient who had urinary leakage with sepsis and peritonitis, which required reoperation and a lengthy hospital stay; two patients with pouch leaks, which were treated by conservative measures and by percutaneous drainage, respectively; one patient with small bowel obstruction, treated conservatively; one patient with myocardial infarction; and one patient with parastomal hernia.[30,35]

Lockhart has published his results with remodeled right colon and continence mechanism, which was based on infolded imbricated terminal ileum around a 12 Fr. Robinson catheter, anastomosed to the abdominal wall. Ureterocolonic reimplantation was done via two techniques: the transcolonic Goodwin technique and the nontunneled modified Le Duc technique. Lockhart's technique was applied in eight patients. Six patients were completely dry between catheterizations performed every 4 to 6 hours, one male patient required more frequent catheterizations, and one female patient refused self-catheterization and wears an external appliance.

Vesicoureteral reflux has not been demonstrated. One patient suffered mild ureterectasis and required percutaneous dilatation. Mild hyperchloremia without acidosis was present in four patients. All but one patient had creatinine levels of 1.5 mg/100 ml or less. Reservoir capacities ranged from 400 to 1200 ml, with maximal reservoir pressures at capacity ranging from 18 to 55 cm water. No patient had diarrhea.[26]

Bejany and Politano have created a reconfigurated reservoir from distal ileum, cecum, and ascending and transverse colon in ten patients. Continence was achieved by tapering of the distal ileum; the distal ileum was intubated with a 14 Fr. catheter, Allis's clamps were placed on the antimesenteric border to provide traction, and GIA staples (five patients) or bowel clamp (five patients) were applied snugly to reduce the size to 14 Fr., the excess tissue was excised, and the edges were oversewn. Three pursestring sutures were placed, one at the ileocecal junction and two—1 cm apart—distally and tied snugly over the catheter. The distal ileum was brought to the abdominal wall and a flush stoma was created. The ureters were reimplanted in a nontunneled ureterocolonic anastomosis.

In a follow-up of a 3 to 24 months, all ten patients were continent, employing catheterization every 4 to 6 hours. Mucus production initially was abdundant and decreased progressively to become minimal at 4 to 5 months. The maximum capacity of the pouch ranged from 750 to 800 ml, and the pressure fluctuated between 10 and 20 cm water. Hydronephrosis was noted in one ureter and was successfully treated percutaneously; the same patient developed also a subphrenic abscess, which was drained percutaneously.[36] No acid-base imbalance was seen.

Open Ileal Reservoir (Kock Pouch)

The Kock pouch, developed initially as a continent ileostomy, was later applied for the urinary tract, with Kock and associates reporting their initial experience with 12 patients in 1982. They constructed an ileal pouch in which continence and the prevention of reflux were maintained by an intussusception technique. Their first clinical application resulted in a high reoperation rate, although the feasibility of the technique was proved.[37]

Subsequently, the use of open ileal reservoirs for continent urinary diversion was popularized by several authors, with the largest series reported by Skinner and associates.[38–41] They reviewed their experience in 395 patients who underwent the procedure between 1982 and 1987, and have made a series of modifications in the surgical technique designed to reduce the need for reoperation. These modifications included discarding a short bowel segment proximal to the measured segment to ensure broad mesenteric blood supply to the pouch; stripping the mesentery as described by Hendren; stapling the nipple with four rows of staples, including the back wall of the pouch, and removing the staples from the tip of the nipple (to prevent stone formation); and fixating Dexon mesh around the ileal segment and a Marlex strip around the mesentery of the efferent loop to prevent herniation.

In their series, 17 percent of the patients suffered at least one early complication, resulting in an operative mortality rate of 2.3 percent. As reported in the foregoing discussion, those undergoing simultaneous cystectomy and Kock pouch construction had a higher complication rate than those undergoing conversion; 18 percent compared with 13 percent. However, once the importance of adequate pelvic drainage was recognized and achieved, the overall early complication rate remained stable and did not differ significantly from the reported rate among patients undergoing one-stage radical cystectomy and ileal conduit construction.

Late complications were primarily associated with failure of the *continence* valve mechanism, characterized by leakage, difficult catheterization, or associated parastomal hernia. In their first 250 patients, late complications occurred in 77 of the 245 patients who survived the operation (31 percent), requiring 85 reoperations. Forty-four patients (18 percent) had leakage of urine at the stoma, often in conjunction with difficulty in catheterization, and 41 of the 44 patients have undergone a total of 55 revisions to achieve continence. Eight patients experienced difficulty in catheterization without associated leakage corrected by surgery. Three patients developed hyperchloremic metabolic acidosis, which in two resulted in hospitalization for hydration and electrolyte correction. Pyelonephritis was noted in five patients, requiring hospitalization for antibiotic treatment. Hydronephrosis secondary to stenosis of the uretero-ileal anastomosis occurred in five patients, and stone formation in the pouch was noted in seven patients.[39] Skinner and associates contend that although the aforementioned modifications have greatly reduced the risk of stomal prolapse, parastomal hernia, and stone formation, they expect that 8 to 10 percent of future patients will still require reoperation for late complications.[38]

In their series, the mean capacity of the reservoir was 800 to 1000 ml at 6 months (range 600 to 1400 ml). After 2 to 3 months, most patients performed self-catheterization every 4 to 6 hours during the day and at 8-hour intervals during the night, depending on fluid intake. Asymptomatic bacteriuria was noted in most patients, with a flora similar to that in the ileal conduit. However, since these patients had no reflux, asymptomatic bacteriuria has not been treated.[40]

In an effort to define the psychological effect of continent urinary diversion, Boyd and associates carried out an intensive psychosocial survey comparing the impact on patients who underwent Kock pouch construction with the impact on a matched control group of patients who had ileal conduits. Their study revealed a remarkable improvement in the quality of life and patient perception of self-image favoring the Kock pouch.[41]

Waters and coworkers reported their experience with 15 patients who underwent construction of the Kock pouch between 1984 and 1986.[42] There was no operative mortality. There were three (20 percent) early complications; a urinary leakage from the pouch in two patients that required re-exploration and an enteric Kock pouch fistula in one patient that required surgical repair. A late complication in three patients (20 percent) was incontinence of the efferent nipple valve with difficulty in catheterization, necessitating revision in two. The remaining 12 patients are continent and dry and have no metabolic abnormalities.

DeKernion and associates reviewed their results in 22 patients with Kock pouch construction between 1983 and 1984.[43] Late complications included one patient who required reoperation 2 months later for distal ureteral obstruction, which resulted in postoperative death from pulmonary embolus. One patient developed bilateral hydronephrosis secondary to fibrosis and underwent conversion to ileal conduit. Four patients (18 percent) required subsequent revision of the efferent valve for difficulties in catheterization. One patient underwent reoperation for small bowel obstruction, and the remaining patients experienced occasional minor difficulties with catheterization but overall had good results.

The authors comment on their results and conclude that complications related to the efferent nipple are due to two major factors: improper construction and fixation of the distal efferent segment in the abdominal wall and disintussusception of the nipple This can result in inability to catheterize the pouch, which may constitute a surgical emergency. They stress that since the major advantage of the Kock pouch over the ileal conduit is the absence of an external urinary appliance, in consideration of modern enterostomal therapy with excellent fitting of the external appliances, the patient trades the need for an external device with the need to carry a catheter and to catheterize the pouch at regular intervals. The patient must also accept the increased risk of difficulties in catheterizatoin and must usually wear a small pad over the stoma for minor leakage. Presented with the options in this manner, only about 50 percent of their patients preferred an internal reservoir over an ileal conduit, and only one in 40 patients with an existing ileal conduit wished to be converted to a Kock pouch.

In an editorial article summarizing the results of several authors, McDougal concludes that the cost of the Kock pouch in the first 2 years following surgery is that one in 50 patients will die of the procedure, 50 percent will have serious complications, one third will require at least one operation to create a functional stoma, a few will suffer early nutritional or metabolic problems, and a few will have early deterioration of the upper tracts. The benefit in the right patient is an improved lifestyle and body image.[44]

Reconfigurated Ileocolonic Reservoirs with Intussuscepted Continence Mechanism

Mainz Pouch

Thuroff and associates have published their experience in 51 patients who underwent construction of a Mainz pouch continent diversion.[22] The reservoir consisted of detubularized ileum, cecum, and ascending colon. The continence mechanism was based on an intussuscepted ileal segment through the ileocecal valve and stabilized with two rows of staples. Two additional rows of staples were used to fix the nipple to the back wall of the ileocecal valve and pouch. In addition, the tip of the intussusception was sutured circumferentially to the cecal opening of the ileocecal valve. In 30 patients, the stoma was placed in the region of the pubic hair; however, for 21 wheelchair-bound or obese patients, the stoma was located at the umbilicus with a shortened efferent loop. The ureters were reimplanted using a ureterocolonic tunneled technique.

At follow-up, all but two patients were completely dry on self-catheterization, mean capacity was 622 ml, and pressures ranged from 23 cm water (50 percent capacity) to 31 cm water (100 percent capacity). Contraction waves, recorded in the early postoperative phase only, began at about 50 percent capacity, with a mean maximal amplitude of 12 cm water. The majority of late complications were related to malfunction of the intussusception valve. Of eight patients in the initial series, in which the ileoileal intussusception had been sutured only, seven required reoperation because of prolapse of the valve. Another four patients with staple stabilization of the intussusception valve but no fixation of the ileocecal valve required surgical revision because of incontinence without prolapse (two patients) or because of difficulties in catheterization (two patients). All patients have remained completely dry since the revision. The umbilical stoma gave excellent cosmetic results and ease of catheterization in obese patients.

UCLA Right Colonic Pouch

At UCLA, early experience with construction of a right colonic pouch in two patients was noted for complications such as leakage and recurrent urinary infections due to staple extrusion. Therefore, technical modifications were applied in the subsequent 11 patients between 1986 and 1988. The bowel segment consisted of the distal 15 cm of the ileum, cecum, and ascending colon. The colonic segment was detubularized in its length along the tenia. The continent nipple was created by an ileoileal intussusception through the ileocecal valve, secured with SGIA staples (outside the lumen of the pouch), and fixed to the back wall of the reservoir with nonabsorbable sutures. A Dexon mesh was placed at the base of the nipple for stabilization and for fixation to the abdominal wall fascia. The ureters were reimplanted to the colonic segment in a submucosal tunneled technique.

The follow-up period ranged from 2 to 20 months (average 7.2 months). Ten of the 11 patients have total continence and perform self-catheterization every 4 to 6 hours during the day and at 8-hour intervals during the night, depending on fluid intake. One patient needs self-catheterization every 2 to 3 hours to prevent leakage. The later complications included a pelvic lymphocele drained percutaneously in one patient; unilateral hydronephrosis in two patients; and reoperation and reimplantation in one patient. The other is still followed expectantly. One patient died of metastatic bladder cancer. None of the patients devleoped stones or extrusion of staples into the pouch, and none had difficulties with catheterization.

These initial results are encouraging, but further experience will be necessary to determine the long-term results of this procedure.

GENERAL CLINICAL CONSIDERATIONS

Electrolyte Imbalance

The physiology of fluid and electrolyte absorption and secretion by intestinal segments exposed continuously to urine has been studied extensively. The nature of these events depends on the inherent function of the specific bowel segment. The impact on normal fluid and electrolyte balance is related to the surface area of the bowel exposed to the urine, the rapidity of urine drainage, renal function, and, possibly, the time since surgery.

The colon normally absorbs sodium and chloride by active transport from the fecal stream. Bicarbonate is excreted if chloride absorption exceeds sodium absorption. Water absorption or excretion and potassium excretion is passive. After ureterosigmoidostomy, hyperchloremic acidosis occurs to varying degrees in all patients because urinary chloride is absorbed in slight excess of sodium. Total body potassium depletion also occurs. Hyperchloremic acidosis occurs among patients with normal renal function but is amplified by renal insufficiency. Prevention of electrolyte imbalance is usually achieved by oral administration of sodium-potassium bicarbonate solution. The absorptive and secretory properties of the ileum parallel those of the colon.[11]

According to McDougal, all patients with intestine interposed in the urinary tract will absorb excess chloride and hydrogen ion and, if studied carefully, will demonstrate some degree of hyperchloremic metabolic acidosis, the degree depending upon the amount of intestinal surface exposed, length of exposure time, and the intrinsic renal function.[20] The primary cause of this acidosis is active chloride transport, and this transport can be limited by oral administration of chlorpromazine or nicotinic acid. However, in large series of patients with bladder substitution or continent diversion, the reported percentage of patients with electrolyte imbalance is variable.

Of interest is the report of Thuroff and associates on 100 patients with Mainz pouch. Most patients initially needed alkalizing drugs to balance a hyperchloremic acidosis, but at follow-up of 6 months, about 50 percent of the patients stabilized without any alkalizing drugs, and with follow-up over 12 months, no patient required therapy.

Despite these divergent observations, electrolyte imbalance among patients with continent reservoirs and bladder substitution is clearly less common compared with imbalance among patients who underwent ureterosigmoidostomy. This probably results from the small surface area of intestine exposed to urine, since after ureterosigmoidostomy, urine refluxes freely throughout the entire colon. It is also known that the histologic appearance of the epithelium of transposed intestinal segments changes over time. The normal density of villi and crypts is reduced and a somewhat flat epithelium evolves. This reduces the surface area of bowel exposed to urine and may inhibit both active and passive fluid and electrolyte absorption and secretion.[11] This can also explain the aforementioned findings by Thuroff and associates.[22]

Most workers do not consider mild renal insufficiency a contraindication to continent diversion or bladder substitution procedures; however, intermittent monitoring of serum electrolytes is prudent, and therapeutic intervention is advisable if minor degrees of hyperchloremic acidosis are detected.[11]

Malabsorption

Defects in the intestinal absorption of vitamin B_{12}, fat, water, and electrolytes may occur after excision of extended parts of small intestine. Vitamin B_{12} is absorbed exclusively in the lower ileum; however, vitamin B_{12} deficiency appears to be uncommon after any continent diversion or bladder substitution.

Fat and fluid malabsorption may be manifested by diarrhea, caused by unabsorbed soaps and fatty acids that are irritating to the colonic mucosa, or liquid stool. However, in most of the large series of continent diversion and bladder substitution, the incidence of diarrhea was small. Diarrhea and vitamin B_{12} deficiency have been reported in patients with continent cecal reservoirs when additional small bowel resection was needed for the treatment of postoperative complications.[45]

Renal Function, Bacteriuria, and Renal Infection

The impact of continent reservoirs and bladder substitutes on renal function will require decades of observation for proper assessment. Nonetheless, among 31 patients with Kock pouch and a mean follow-up of approximately 5 years, changes in the serum creatinine levels have not been observed.[11] Mansson found that the glomerular filtration rate, as measured by isotope studies, did not deteriorate in 10 patients followed for over 2 years after cecal reservoir construction, despite the finding of delayed ureteral drainage during reservoir contraction.[45] Lockhart has also demonstrated preservation of renal function in 10 of 11 patients with remodeled right colonic reservoir in a short-term follow-up.[26]

Over the long term, chronic bacteriuria may be an important factor in determining renal function. Renal deterioration caused in part by chronic bacterial colonization of the renal pelvis is observed in patients with ileal conduits and freely refluxing urine. Bacteriuria caused by one or more organisms is an inevitable consequence of urinary diversion to a cutaneous stoma. Experience with the ileal conduit indicates that acute renal infection is not common in the absence of obstruction or underlying systemic risk factors (diabetes mellitus, immunosuppression). The risk of acute infection is further reduced with the antireflux ureteral reimplantation techniques used in continent reservoirs and bladder substitutes. Colonization of the urine per se does not have an unfavorable impact on the function of continent reservoirs or bladder substitutes. Furthermore, it was demonstrated that the secretion of antibodies (IgA) by the intestinal mucosa, directed against enteric bacteria, appears to persist after transposition to the urinary tract, although the physiologic importance of this phenomenon is yet unknown.

Based on these considerations, it can be expected that the urine of continent reservoirs will be colonized but that acute infections will be rare. The urine of most patients with bladder substitutions that drain spontaneously is usually sterile.[11]

Urinary Calculi

In up to 30 percent of patients with ileal conduits, renal calculi develop during prolonged observation periods. Most are infection stones (struvite) and result from colonization of the urine by urea-splitting organisms. Urinary stasis caused by impaired drainage probably predisposes to formation of infection stones. As for continent reservoirs and bladder substitutes, the follow-up is too short to reach meaningful conclusions. From a conceptual standpoint, however, the development of infection stones should be less likely among patients with bladder substitutes because the urine is often sterile. Among patients with continent diversion, who usually drain by intermittent catheterization, chronic suppressive antimicrobial therapy or intermittent treatment when urea-splitting organisms are isolated may possibly reduce the incidence of infection stone formation.[11]

Encrustation and stone formation on staples used for the fixation of intussusceptions appear to be uncommon if the staples are well seated and buried in the mucosa during application. Staples applied in this fashion are usually covered by the healing mucosa. Skinner's observation that staples applied to the tip of the intussusception are more resistant to mucosal overgrowth led to his suggestion that staples be excluded from the tip of the intussusception. In his series of 250 patients, stone formation in the pouch was found in seven of the early patients and five have undergone successful endoscopic removal. The stones tended to form on staples near the end of the nipple, on eroded Marlex collars, or on a heavy polyglycolic suture that was not absorbed. After changes in the technique, the anticipated stone problem has not materialized.[39]

Carcinogenesis in Transposed Bowel

The development of polyps and adenocarcinomas of the sigmoid is now well recognized as an important long-term risk of ureterosigmoidostomy. Review of the literature also reveals ten reports of neoplasm formation following augmentation cystoplasty, with a latent period of 5 to 24 years (average 18 years).[46–52] The etiology of these malignant changes in augmentation cystoplasty is unclear. Most of the patients had concomitant risk factors (history of tuberculosis with chronic inflammatory changes, radiation therapy, multiple surgeries, poor drainage of the bladder, and recurrent infections).

Moorcraft and associates have studied the histologic changes in the mucosa of colon conduits and have demonstrated chronic inflammation with a dense infiltration of plasma cells and eosinophils, changes that were progressive and correlated with the duration of urinary diversion.[53] They assume that these persistent inflammatory changes may act as a precursor of malignancy. Mansson and Willen studied the mucosal morphology of cecal reservoirs and demonstrated interstitial inflammatory cell proliferation with a slight increase in collagen fibers.[54] No tumors arising in continent reservoirs or bladder substitutes have been reported to date, but long-term follow-up is necessary to verify this issue.

Increased Reservoir Pressures and Urinary Leakage

Intermittent pressure elevations can occur in continent reservoirs or bladder substitutes, mainly those constructed from intact bowel, and may cause urinary leakage and even predispose the pouch to prolapse or sliding of intussusception and to ureteral reflux. Mansson has found that the contraction pressures of cecal reservoirs decrease substantially with time.[45] Nonetheless, reduction of reservoir pressures may be beneficial to incontinent patients. This can be achieved either by secondary enteroplasty or by medical therapy with anticholinergic medications (oxybutynin, Pro-Banthine).

Fowler and associates have assessed the impact of instillations of diphenoxylate hydrochloride and atropine sulfate (Lomotil) directly into the reservoir in six patients with urinary leakage.[55] The treatments reduced the frequency of spontaneous reservoir contractions as well as the basal and contraction pressures of the reservoirs. All patients reported a decrease of cramping with reservoir distention and a decrease in the frequency of catheterization. Full continence was regained in two patients. No systemic side effects were observed.

Goldwasser and colleagues stress that whenever high intrareservoir pressures resulting from poor compliance or high-pressure contractions cause leakage by overcoming the outlet resistance, increasing outlet resistance by means of implanting an artificial sphincter around the bowel or urethra will only circumvent the problem and may result in upper tract deterioration over the years.[24]

SUMMARY

Procedures to create continent reservoirs and bladder substitutes are a major undertaking for both the patient and the surgeon. Even in the hands of experienced surgeons, 10 to 20 percent of patients will suffer major late complications requiring reoperation, which in some cases may involve complicated surgical techniques. Some of the delayed effects of reservoir construction from bowel are yet unknown, and decades of observation are required before final conclusions can be drawn. In the adult, the ileal conduit should be the standard against which the risks and benefits of continent reservoir and bladder substitution procedures must be measured. Because the sole benefit of a properly functioning continent reservoir is the avoidance of a urinary drainage appliance, with resulting better satisfaction and improved self-esteem, the patient is basically trading an external appliance for a catheter, which he needs to carry with him, and which may present difficulties in catheterization that can constitute a medical emergency. In patients with bladder substitutes, the most distressing complication is enuresis, which is not acceptable as a satisfactory result.

Patient selection is a key issue for a successful result. It is imperative that the patient have the desire and willingness to take on the added responsibility of a continent reservoir and the intelligence required to deal with it, mainly to empty it at regular intervals. The patient must also have sufficient manual dexterity to perform clean intermittent catheterization and irrigation of the reservoir. Some patients are incapable of handling the frustrations of reservoir malfunction or are unwilling to perform the perineal exercises that may be critical to the prevention of enuresis after bladder substitution procedures. These requirements underline the importance of maturity, intelligence, and psychosocial stability as factors in proper patient selection, which will enhance the chances of an ultimate success.

References

1. Hinman F Jr: Selection of intestinal segments for bladder substitution: physical and physiological characteristics. J Urol 139:519, 1988.
2. Fowler JE Jr: Continent urinary reservoirs and bladder substitutes in the adult: Part I. In Stamey TA, ed: 1987 Monographs in Urology, Vol 8, No 2. Princeton, Custom Publishing Services, Inc, 1987.
3. Cohen S, Harris LD, Levitan R: Manometric characteristics of the human ileocecal junctional zone. Gastroenterology 54:72,1968.
4. Coffey RC: Physiologic implantation of the severed ureter or common bile-duct into the intestine. JAMA 56:397, 1911.
5. Leadbetter WF: Consideration of problems incident to performance of uretero-enterostomy: report of a technique. J Urol 65:818, 1951.
6. Goodwin WE, Harris AP, Kaufman JJ, Beal JM: Open transcolonic ureterointestinal anastomosis: a new approach. Surg Gynecol Obstet 97:295, 1953.
7. Zincke H, Segura JW: Ureterosigmoidostomy: critical review of 173 cases. J Urol 113:324, 1975.
8. Wear JB Jr, and Barquin OP: Ureterosigmoidostomy: long-term results. Urology 1:192, 1973.
9. Marberger M, Straub E: Ureterosigmoidostomy in children. In Ashken MH, ed: Urinary Diversion. Springer-Verlag, 1982, p 59.
10. Gittes RF: Carcinogenesis in ureterosigmoidostomy. Urol Clin North Am 13(2):201, 1986.
11. Fowler JE Jr: Continent urinary reservoirs and bladder substitutes in the adult: Part II. In Stamey TA, ed: 1987 Monographs in Urology, Vol 8, No 3. Princeton, Custom Publishing Services, Inc, 1987.
12. Camey M: Bladder replacement by ileocystoplasty following radical cystectomy. Semin Urol 5(1):8, 1987.
13. Allen TD, Peters PC, Sagalowsky AI, Roehrborn C: The Camey procedure: preliminary results in 11 patients. World J Urol 3:167, 1985.
14. Roehrborn CG, Teigland CM, Sagalowsky AI: Functional characteristics of the Camey ileal bladder. J Urol 138:739, 1987.
15. Goldwasser B, Rife CC, Benson RC Jr, Furlow WL, Barrett DM: Urodynamic evaluation of patients after the Camey operation. J Urol 138:832, 1987.
16. Hradec EA: Bladder substitution: indications and results in 114 operations. J Urol 94:406, 1965.
17. Turner-Warwick RT, Ashken MH: The functional results of partial, subtotal and total cystoplasty with special reference to ureterocaecocystoplasty, selective sphincterotomy and cystocystoplasty. Br J Urol 39:3, 1967.
18. Khafagy M, El-Bolkainy MN, Barsoum RS, El-Tatawy S: The ileocecal bladder: a new method for urinary diversion after radical cystectomy (a preliminary report). J Urol 113:314, 1965.
19. Zinman L, Libertino JA: Right colocystoplasty for bladder replacement. Urol Clin North Am 13(2):321, 1986.
20. McDougal WS: Bladder reconstruction following cystectomy by uretero-ileo-colourethrostomy. J Urol 135:698, 1986.
21. Light JK, Englemann UH: Le Bag: total replacement of the bladder using an ileocolonic pouch. J Urol 136:27, 1986.
22. Thuroff JW, Alken P, Riedmiller H, Jacobi GH, Hohenfellner R: 100 cases of Mainz pouch: continuing experience and evolution. J Urol 140:283, 1988.
23. Goldwasser B, Barrett DM, Benson RC Jr: Bladder replacement with use of a detubularized right colonic segment: preliminary report of a new technique. Mayo Clin Proc 61:615, 1986.
24. Goldwasser B, Madgar I, Hanani Y: Urodynamic aspects of continent urinary diversion. Scand J Urol Nephrol 21:245, 1987.
25. Goldwasser B, Barrett DM, Webster GD, Kramer SA: Cystometric properties of ileum and right colon after bladder augmentation, substitution or replacement. J Urol 138:1007, 1987.
26. Lockhart JL: Remodeled right colon: an alternative urinary reservoir. J Urol 138:730, 1987.
27. Ghoneim MA, Mahran MR, Kock NG: The urethral Kock reservoir as a bladder substitute. J Urol 139:507A, 1988.
28. Skinner DG, Boyd S, Lieskovsky G: Technique of continent lower urinary tract reconstruction with Kock

pouch urethrostomy following cystectomy. J Urol 139:159A, 1988.
29. Reddy PK, Lange PH: A comparison of ileal versus sigmoid bowel segments in the construction of a new detubularized reservoir for total bladder replacement following cystoprostatectomy. J Urol 139:243A, 1988.
30. Rowland RG, Mitchell ME, Bihrle R, Kahnoski RJ, Piser JE: Indiana continent urinary reservoir. J Urol 137:1136, 1987.
31. Gilchrist RK, Merricks JW, Hamlin H, Rieger IT: Construction of a substitute bladder and urethra. Surg Gynecol Obstet 90:752, 1950.
32. Sullivan H, Gilchrist RK, Merricks JW: Ileocecal substitute bladder: long-term followup. J Urol 109:43, 1973.
33. Mansson W, Colleen S, Sundin T: The continent cecal reservoir for urinary diversion. World J Urol 3:173, 1985.
34. Hedlund H, Lindstrom K, Mansson W: Dynamics of a continent caecal reservoir for urinary diversion. Br J Urol 56:366, 1984.
35. Rowland RG, Mitchell ME, Bihrle R: Alternative techniques for a continent urinary reservoir. Urol. Clin. North Am 14(4):797, 1987.
36. Bejany DE, Politano VA: Stapled and nonstapled tapered distal ileum for construction of a continent colonic urinary reservoir. J Urol 140:491, 1988.
37. Kock NG, Nilson AE, Nilsson LO, Norlen LJ, Philipson BM: Urinary diversion via a continent ileal reservoir: clinical results in 12 patients. J Urol 128:469, 1982.
38. Skinner DG, Boyd SD, Lieskovsky L: An update on the Kock pouch for continent urinary diversion. Urol Clin North Am 14(4):789, 1987.
39. Lieskovsky G, Boyd SD, Skinner DG: Management of late complications of the Kock pouch form of urinary diversion. J Urol 137:1146, 1987.
40. Skinner DG, Lieskovsky G, Boyd SD: Continuing experience with the continent ileal reservoir (Kock pouch) as an alternative to cutaneous urinary diversion: an update after 250 cases. J Urol 137:1140, 1987.
41. Boyd SD, Feinberg SM, Skinner DG, Lieskovsky G, Baron D, Richardson J: Quality of life survey of urinary diversion patients: comparison of ileal conduits versus continent Kock ileal reservoirs. J Urol 138:1386, 1987.
42. Waters WB, Vaughan DJ, Harris RG, Brady SM: The Kock pouch: initial experience and complications. J Urol 137:1151, 1987.
43. deKernion JB, DenBesten L, Kaufman JJ, Ehrlich R: The Kock pouch as a urinary reservoir: pitfalls and perspectives. Am J Surg 150:83, 1985.
44. McDougal WS: The continent urinary diversion. Editorial. J Urol 137:1214, 1987.
45. Mansson W: The continent caecal reservoir for urine. Scand J Urol Nephrol 85:8, 1984.
46. Stone AR, Davies N, Stephenson TP: Carcinoma associated with augmentation cystoplasty. Br J Urol 60:236, 1987.
47. Smith P, Hardy GJ: Carcinoma occurring as a late complication of ileocystoplasty. Br J Urol 43:576, 1971.
48. Leedham PW, England HR: Adenocarcinoma developing in an ileocystoplasty. Brit J Surg 60:158, 1973.
49. Kirby RS, Lloyd-Davies RW: Adenocarcinoma occurring within a caecocystoplasty. Br J Urol 57:357, 1985.
50. Egbert BM, Kraft JK, Perkash I: Undifferentiated sarcoma arising in an augmented ileocystoplasty patch. J Urol 123:272, 1980.
51. Takasaki E, Murahashi I, Toyoda M, Honda M, Waku S: Signet ring adenocarcinoma of ileal segment following ileocystoplasty. J Urol 130:562, 1983.
52. Golomb J, Klutke CG, Lewin KJ, Goodwin WG, deKernion JB, Raz S: Bladder neoplasms associated with augmentation cystoplasty: report of two cases and literature review. J Urol, 142:377, 1989.
53. Moorcraft J, DuBoulay CEH, Isaacson P, Atwell JD: Changes in the mucosa of colon conduits with particular reference to the risk of malignant change. Br J Urol 55:185, 1983.
54. Mansson W, Willen R: Mucosal morphology and histochemistry of the continent cecal reservoir for urine. J Urol 139:1199,1988.
55. Fowler JE Jr, Clayton M, Mouli K, Reagan G: Effect of liquid diphenoxylate hydrochloride and atropine sulfate (Lomotil) instillation on dynamics and function of continent cecal urinary reservoirs. J Urol 138:735, 1987.

COMPLICATIONS OF TRANSURETHRAL SURGERY

27

Robert B. Smith

The technical aspects of transurethral surgery are perhaps the most difficult operative techniques for the neophyte surgeon to master. Limitations imposed by endoscopic teaching attachments involving light transmission, object clarity, up-and-down orientation, and instrument maneuverability have hampered the training of young endoscopic surgeons. The advent of the Hopkins lens system and the fiberoptic core has helped to circumvent these physical limitations. Advances in television technology have also greatly aided in the teaching of transurethral surgery. Many compact, lightweight cameras now exist which when placed on resectoscopes, limit maneuverability little more than the standard teaching attachments. Nevertheless, the teaching of transurethral surgery remains a challenge.

It is my conviction that a resident physician should have extensive endoscopic experience before performing a transurethral procedure of any type. Typically, the incidence of complications of transurethral surgery is inversely proportional to the experience of the surgeon. It is the purpose of this chapter not only to help the urologist handle such complications should they arise but, more importantly, to help obviate unnecessary complications by stressing basic techniques that should be utilized in everyday surgical endoscopic practice. Too often, complications occur when these basic concepts are circumvented in order to conserve that all-important commodity, time.

GENERAL CONSIDERATIONS

Surgical Instrumentation

When the surgeon begins an endoscopic procedure, it is essential that an appropriate array of instruments be immediately available to him. Certainly, many complications encountered in transurethral surgery are attributable to shortcuts employed because the surgeon did not have the appropriate instruments on hand.

The instrumentation for standard adult endoscopic procedures should include a full set of Van Buren sounds up to No. 30 Fr. All sizes should be available since overly rapid dilation of a stricture is a major cause of false passages. Likewise, a filiform of woven silk followers or LeForte sounds and a urethrotome should be included.

A full selection of insulated resectoscope sheaths in calibers to accommodate all loop sizes is mandatory, although it is rare that the largest sheath is utilized. Sheaths with short beaks are preferable because they are less likely to cause injury to the urethra or trigone than long-beaked sheaths. For similar reasons, the beaks should be inspected for smoothness. Appropriate obturators are necessary for each sheath. It is sometimes helpful to have on hand an obturator with a screw tip that can accommodate a filiform thread. Copious amounts of water-soluble jelly and 1 percent hydrocortisone ointment for proper lubrication of sounds and sheaths are required for any endoscopic procedure.

Lenses with 30- and 70-degree viewing angles are essential; the addition of a 0-degree (direct-vision) lens, although not mandatory, is often helpful. A fiberoptic light source should be part of a modern endoscopic surgical suite. Extra bulbs or an alternative light source should also be available.

Two resectoscopes should be available, the design of which may be the choice of the individual surgeon. A one-handed instrument of the Iglesias design that frees the opposite hand for rectal or suprapubic manipulation is a personal preference, but other endoscopic surgeons are equally at ease with two-handed instruments.

A full selection of appropriate resectoscope loops should be available in regard to both loop size and wire caliber. The thinner the wire, the better the cutting capability and the poorer the coagulating capacity of the loop. Several loops of each size should be available in the event of breakage.

When a one-handed instrument is employed, an O'Conor rectal shield should be used to enable the physician to perform periodic rectal manipulation without causing contamination. The rectal portion of the shield should be well lubricated to prevent irritation and possible rectal injury.

A lithotrite or electrohydraulic lithotriptor of the surgeon's choice should be available to handle unsuspected vesical or urethral calculi. Similarly, flexible and rigid grasping forceps are useful in the event that material cannot be removed from the bladder by manipulation of the resectoscope loop. Often, frequent levering of the resectoscope sheath successfully evacuates fragments of tissue from the bladder. The Toomey syringe or Ellik evacuator is helpful for rapid evacuation of vesical debris. To facilitate filling of the Ellik evacuator, a deep bowl of sterile irrigating solution should be prepared. The Ellik evacuator should be checked for bulb strength and signs of leakage. The connecting hose should be of large caliber, rigid, and short, with an airtight seal between the glass flange and the nozzle that adapts to the resectoscope sheath.

Generous stores of suitable irrigating fluid are imperative. Distilled water is safe for brief procedures such as bladder tumor resection, cystolithalapaxy, and resection of fibrous bladder necks. Because of the possible risk of hemolysis, use of distilled water should be discouraged in standard transurethral prostatic surgery, despite its advantage of low cost and superior optical properties. The advantage of superior optical properties is certainly not as important as it was before fiberoptics and the Hopkins telescope system were available. Despite a growing body of evidence indicating that the danger of hemolysis has been overstated, it is nevertheless unwise to use distilled water because of the current tendency of the patient population to litigate.

The ideal irrigating solution should be nonelectrolytic and isosmotic; those composed of 3.3 percent sorbitol, 5 percent mannitol, and 1.5 percent glycine readily satisfy these criteria. With improved optical and illumination systems, good visualization is not a problem with any solution. Glycine should not be used in patients with hepatic dysfunction because ammonia is a metabolic by-product in the breakdown of glycine, and hyperammonemia may result. Hyperglycemia can result with the use of sorbitol, which is metabolized to glucose. This may be a threat to high-risk diabetic patients who are poorly controlled when there are large amounts of fluid absorption or extravasation. In addition, lactic acidosis occurs. Mannitol has the advantage of being an osmotic diuretic, potentially helping to unload the patient from increased volume expansion. However, mannitol is not evenly distributed throughout the total body space. Hypervolemic changes may be temporarily compounded and further contribute to manifestations of transurethral resection (TUR) syndrome.

Surgical instruments for performing vasectomy, meatotomy, and perineal urethrotomy should be available. A minimal set should include two towel clips, four straight hemostats, one Adson thumb forceps, a scalpel, and a needle holder. The type of suture material depends on the preference of the surgeon.

Two electrosurgical units should be available in case of malfunction of the primary unit. The type is, again, the surgeon's choice. Desirable features include a weighted foot pedal that will remain relatively stationary during the procedure and a sound mechanism, with which cutting and coagulation currents can be differentiated by ear to help prevent the wrong pedal from being pressed inadvertently. A warning light or buzzer is imperative for detecting short circuits or improper patient grounding. (Thermal burns caused by inadequate grounding have become relatively rare.) In addition, there should be no contact between the patient and the metallic part of the operating table.

The operating table should be freely adjustable by the surgeon. The tray should be large enough to facilitate collection of irrigating fluid and resected tissue. The ideal table should have radiologic capabilities in case emergencies arise in which cystography or urethrography is necessary. Semi- or completely adjustable chairs are an added luxury for the endoscopic surgeon. Operating time may be decreased by minutes if the surgeon can easily adjust the patient's or his own relative position.

Patient Preparation and Evaluation

The identification and preoperative correction of potential medical problems are of primary importance in decreasing morbidity and mortality associated with transurethral surgery. It is incumbent upon the urologist to ensure that each urologic patient has undergone a thorough medical evaluation. The patient's cardiac status is especially important as he may be challenged by massive shifts in fluid volume and serum electrolyte composition, especially during transurethral resection of the prostate. Cardiac disease may account for as much as 50 percent of mortality associated with prostatectomy. In addition to proper preoperative evaluation, adequate intraoperative monitoring is essential. In high-risk patients, intraoperative monitoring with oxygen electrodes and Swan-Ganz catheters to measure central venous pressure and pulmonary wedge pressure has greatly reduced this mortality. Patients who have coronary artery disease or who have undergone status coronary angioplasty, or bypass and who are on aspirin or dipyridamole (Persantin) present an added dilemma to the transurethral surgeon. Discontinuing this medication increases the likelihood of a thrombotic cardiac event; remaining on the medication increases the probability of significant postoperative hemorrhage. The decision of whether to stop medication before surgery should be made in conjunction with the cardiologist, cardiothoracic surgeon, and urologist. It is my practice to continue anticoagulation therapy for most patients and to handle postoperative hemorrhage, should it occur. Meticulous hemostasis usually circumvents a major problem. Postoperative traction on the Foley catheter for longer periods of time will reduce the incidence of significant venous sinus bleeding. The Foley catheter balloon should be positioned just inside the bladder neck and not in the prostatic fossa.

It is important to know the renal reserve of the patient to determine his capability to handle the extra fluid volume. Serum creatinine and creatinine clearance tests are adequate for this purpose. If compromised renal reserve is detected, an attempt should be made to identify the cause and to correct it prior to surgery (e.g., catheter drainage for long-standing obstructive nephropathy). Bladder drainage should be instituted in patients with upper urinary tract obstruction and the creatinine level allowed to stabilize prior to transurethral resection.

Patients with compromised renal function have deficient clotting mechanisms due to abnormal platelet function. There is some evidence that uremic patients have a compromised resistance to infection, presumably secondary to decreased immunologic response. Most large transurethral series indicate a significantly higher mortality rate among patients undergoing transurethral surgery with compromised renal function. Patients who are uremic secondary to upper urinary tract obstruction and prostatism must be watched carefully for a post-obstructive diuresis after a catheter has been passed. This diuresis is caused by the inability of the obstructed kidney to concentrate urine, the abnormal handling of sodium by the obstructed kidney, and the hyperosmolar effect of the elevated urea. In addition, most of these patients start out in a fluid overloaded situation.

Daily weights should be monitored and urine output replaced on a ml per ml basis with 5 percent dextrose in ½ normal saline until the osmotic load of the urea has been stabilized. Potassium is replaced as it is excreted; frequent urine and serum electrolyte measurement is essential to properly manage these patients. In addition, adequate serum levels of calcium and magnesium are important because these minerals can be excreted as well. The substances should be replaced as necessary. When the blood urea nitrogen has stabilized, one can begin to reduce fluid replacement so as to not perpetuate this diuresis. Rarely should fluid replacement be less than 1500 ml of the total urine output per 24-hour period. When urine output is less than 250 ml per hour, fluid replacement less 50 ml of the urine output per hour is given. For ouptuts greater than 250 ml, generally 100 ml per hour is subtracted from the replacement until the diuresis slows down.

Urine culture and sensitivity determinations are mandatory in preparation for transurethral procedures, especially for patients with an indwelling catheter. Patients with significant urinary bacterial growth should be given appropriate parenteral antibiotic agents preoperatively, intraoperatively, and postoperatively to decrease the risk of bacteremia. Bacteremia has been noted in as many as 80 percent of patients undergoing transurethral surgery.[1] Prophylactic coverage with antibiotics in patients with sterile urine preoperatively is optional. Patients with valvular heart disease or prosthetic devices must receive full-spectrum prophylactic antibacterial coverage. It is our procedure to administer gentamicin (1.5 mg/kg) and ampicillin (1 gm) 1 hour prior to the transurethral procedure. Antibiotics should be continued for 36 hours postoperatively.

It is my feeling that "prophylactic" antibacterial therapy begun 1 hour prior to the procedure for patients with an indwelling catheter or active urinary tract infection is inadequate. Such patients are generally admitted to the hospital the night before surgery for antibacterial treatment beginning at least 12 hours prior to the proposed operation. This treatment is then continued with specific antibacterial therapy for 24 hours after the patient is catheter-free. Follow-up with oral antibacterial agents after the catheter has been removed is optional.

Since hemostasis in transurethral surgery is sometimes a problem, a coagulation profile should be obtained prior to any major procedure and specific deficiencies corrected (see Chapter 4). This profile should include a prothrombin time, partial thromboplastin time, platelet count, and bleeding time for patients with suspected platelet dysfunction. As mentioned previously, the decision to continue administering anticoagulant agents (e.g., aspirin, Persantin) is made by the surgeon and medical consultant. Patients on warfarin (Coumadin) who require the maintenance of anticoagulation devices (e.g., artificial mechanical heart valves) should be treated with heparin preoperatively for finer control of the coagulation system. Coumadin can be resumed in the postoperative period after the major risk of postoperative hemorrhage has passed. The length of the postoperative period depends on the size of the prostate. If severe coagulopathy exists, and it is refractory or unreasonably costly to correct, alternative surgical plans may be necessary. Under these circumstances, my preference is to perform total prostatectomy rather than transurethral prostatectomy, especially in patients with hemophilia. With the current nerve-sparing technique of Walsh available as well as with the decrease in morbidity and side effects associated with the procedure, total prostatectomy may be especially indicated.

Diabetic patients should be under the tightest control possible to help minimize their risk of developing a hyperosmolar syndrome. Patients with a high serum glucose level have increased serum osmolarity, which can cause increased water shift from the intracellular and extracellular spaces. Thus, extravasated fluid from TUR may move to the intravascular space at an accelerated rate, causing exacerbation of the hyponatremia associated with the TUR syndrome. Control of serum glucose levels will help to alleviate this problem. Patients in whom this is not possible may be treated with the early use of a loop diuretic.

Patients with other medical conditions, such as an obstructive pulmonary or a peptic ulcer disease should undergo appropriate preoperative management. Vigorous pulmonary toilet will prevent many of the pulmonary complications associated with transurethral resection. The use of histamine antagonists preoperatively will reduce the incidence of stress gastrointestinal (GI) bleeding in the postoperative period.

It is our practice to obtain preoperative intravenous pyelograms on most patients undergoing major transurethral surgery to serve as a baseline as well as to detect any pathologic process that could influence the operative approach. If vesical diverticula are found, cystograms with post-void films should be obtained to determine whether they are emptying. Uroflometric and cystometric determinations are helpful in differentiating confusing neurologic and obstructive lesions. In questionable cases, a complete urodynamic evaluation is essential.

Anesthesia

The choice of anesthetic agents may be determined by the anesthesiologist and patient. Spinal anesthesia is my preference, as opposed to general anesthesia, because in the immediate postoperative period, the patient is not as restless and coughs less, thus reducing the risks of increased Valsalva pressure and postoperative hemorrhage. Spinal anesthesia allows the patient to respond to pain in the event of complications such as intraperitoneal extravasation. It also permits better assessment of the central nervous status in case of TUR syndrome. The spinal anesthesia should be of sufficient duration to allow for unplanned occurrences. It should be given to a level of at least T_9 to prevent discomfort from vesical distention during the procedure.

Blood loss should be monitored by both the surgeon and the anesthetist, although estimation can be inadequate. In large resections, the volume and hemoglobin content of the irrigation should be measured, if possible. The anesthetist must watch for the signs and symptoms of water intoxication syndrome and be prepared to treat it. If the venous sinuses are opened early in the procedure, the anesthesiologist should be notified to be alert to the water intoxication syndrome. The serum sodium should be determined in the recovery room in such patients, and if the operating time is prolonged, intraoperative determinations should be made as well. Should the sodium be decreasing, IV replacement should not contain any free water, and furosemide (Lasix) should be administered intravenously. Intravascular sodium-sensitive electrodes are now available and can be used to determine plasma sodium concentration during transurethral resection. If these electrodes are available, it may be wise to utilize them in patients undergoing resection of large glands.

When hemostasis is being secured at the end of a procedure, the anesthetist should ensure that the patient's blood pressure is in the preoperative range. Hypotension occurring at the end of a procedure may mask significant arterial bleeding, which may be the source of troublesome hemorrhage in the postoperative period. Ephedrine or similar drugs should be administered to normalize the blood pressure at the end of the procedure, should hypotension exist.

When positioning the patient for an endoscopic procedure, the legs should be well padded at the knee brace to protect against peroneal nerve injury. For more extensive procedures, the legs should be wrapped to guard against venous stasis and possible subsequent embolic events. Up to 10 percent of patients undergoing transurethral resection develop deep venous thrombosis, which is related to the duration of resection and to positioning of the patient. Resections should be kept under 1 hour. For patients with a history of venous disease or with disease entities that predispose to a hypercoagulable state, pulsatile stockings should be employed.

INTRAOPERATIVE COMPLICATIONS

Mechanical Difficulties

It is beyond the scope of this chapter to describe all possible mechanical malfunctions that can occur during transurethral surgery. The best way to prevent problems is to require that the technicians who maintain the instruments routinely check all equipment after each use. If the surgeon closely inspects his instruments while assembling them, he may also discover potential soruces of difficulty.

Problems of Instrument Introduction

Phimosis may be severe enough to cause difficulty in passing instruments. In such cases, a circumcision should be performed to facilitate instrument introduction and to allow better antiseptic preparation. It should be possible to determine whether phimosis is likely to occur and to obtain proper preoperative patient consent. In the absence of consent for a circumcision, a limited dorsal slit will suffice to allow instrument introduction.

In the postoperative period, phimosis may trap secretions and cause periurethral drainage around the catheter, possibly leading to a severe urethritis and subsequent stricture formation. Endoscopic surgical instruments for vasectomy or meatotomy should include those needed for circumcision.

Meatal stenosis of congenital, inflammatory, traumatic, or iatrogenic origin may be present. Not only can this prevent passage of a resectoscope, but it may also cause instrument drag, which hampers the sheath's maneuverability and interferes with the tactile sensation of the surgeon. A meatal stenosis in the postoperative period is also a cause of purulent urethral drainage with all its potential sequelae. Meatotomy should be adequate. Incomplete incision will fail to prevent subsequent damage and possibly lead to a postoperative meatal stenosis, which is often more symptomatic than the original condition. Urethral calibration of the area may determine the proximal extent of the stenosis. If the stenotic area is long, it may be wise to perform an internal urethrostomy with a straight urethrotome or with the direct-vision Winter-Ivy instrument. Severe long strictures may be bypassed with this use of a perineal urethrostomy.

It is controversial whether the meatotomy incision should be made dorsally or ventrally. A dorsal meatotomy incision causes less subsequent splaying of the urinary stream but limits the extent of the incision; hemorrhage is often a consequent problem. The ventral meatotomy is usually satisfactory. If it becomes necessary to perform a radical meatotomy to ensure proper instrument mobility, reconstruction of the meatus, utilizing a frenular flap, may be performed at a later time.

Urethral strictures or the formation of false passages often present problems for the surgeon. Mild strictures may be dilated with Van Buren sounds. False passage formation is a common hazard when dilating anesthetized patients with these instruments. Sounds should never be forcibly introduced; the curve of the instrument should allow smooth passage using only pressure of the fingers to direct the sound. It is often helpful to place a free hand in the rectum to guide the sound, thus helping to prevent the formation of a false passage.

Should a false passage be encountered, a filiform may be passed through the urethra, utilizing a urethroscope with a 0- or 30-degree lens. Dilation with woven silk followers is then performed. Timberlake obturators with a screw tip to accommodate the filiform threads are useful in ensuring proper passage of the resectoscope sheath. If one cannot satisfactorily negotiate the true urethral passage, the procedure is best terminated and attempted at a later date.

Ninety percent of male patients can accept a No. 26 Fr. resectoscope without difficulty. If the resectoscope does not move freely in and out of the urethra after apparent satisfactory dilation and lubrication, an internal urethrotomy or perineal urethrostomy should be considered. It is *never* necessary to use a No. 28 Fr. sheath.

When an internal urethrotomy is performed for individual strictures, it is my preference to use the Winter-Ivy instrument, cutting the stricture under direct vision. If the urethra is too tight in general to allow the resectoscope to move freely, I prefer to perform the internal urethrotomy with an Otis urethrotome. The urethrotome need only be set at No. 36 Fr. and one cut made in the 12 o'clock position. If the penis is held perpendicular to the pubis during internal urethrotomy, injury to the membranous urethra is avoided (Fig. 27–1). Catheterization following this procedure is necessary for only 48 to 72 hours postoperatively.

Some surgeons routinely perform internal urethrotomy prior to transurethral resection of the prostate. I do not agree with this approach because associated complications including sepsis, hemorrhage, subsequent stricture formation, and severe chordee formation can develop (0.9 percent of patients).

Many urologists advocate perineal urethrostomy to bypass distal urethral strictures. In patients with a short suspensory ligament of the penis or a long phallus, it is also invaluable in facilitating maneuverability of the resectoscope. Some urologists routinely perform the procedure in transurethral prostatic resection when resectable tissue is expected to exceed 40 gm in weight. Also, should a patient develop an erection at the beginning of a procedure, it is one way to proceed with the operation, obviating potential urethral injury while maintaining the ability to maneuver the resectoscope with ease. Perineal urethrostomy, however, is considered by many surgeons to be a cumbersome, difficult, and often time-consuming procedure. Brisk

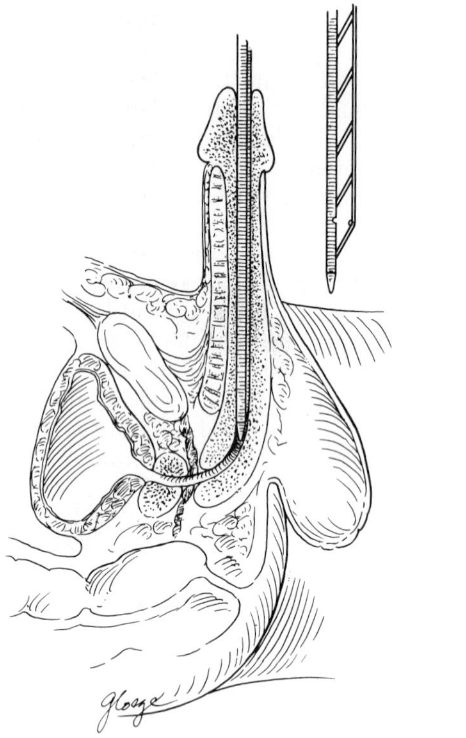

Figure 27–1. Technique for internal urethrotomy. Note that straight urethrotome is the preferred instrument. Penis is held perpendicular to the pubis to avoid injury to the membranous urethra.

hemorrhage can result if the incision is not kept in the midline.

A simple and successful method of performing perineal urethrostomy employs resectoscope sheaths of different sizes. With this technique, the distal urethra must be dilated to a sufficient caliber to accommodate a No. 24 Fr. resectoscope sheath. The sheath is passed into the bulbous urethra to the point at which the urethra turns upward toward the urogenital diaphragm. The fenestra of the resectoscope beak is then readily palpable in the perineum (Fig. 27–2*A*). After ensuring that the fenestra is in the midline, the surgeon makes an incision just large enough to allow the smaller sheath to be passed through the urethral wall and to exit via the perineum (Fig. 27–2*B*). Then, using a No. 26 Fr. sheath with the No. 24 Fr. Timberlake obturator fitted snugly into the proximal end of the No. 24 Fr. sheath, the larger sheath is passed into the distal urethra as the smaller sheath is withdrawn from the meatus (Fig. 27–2*C*). The No. 24 Fr. obturator is replaced in the larger sheath by its appropriate obturator. The surgeon then passes a larger sheath into the proximal urethra and bladder, taking care to hug the anterior wall of

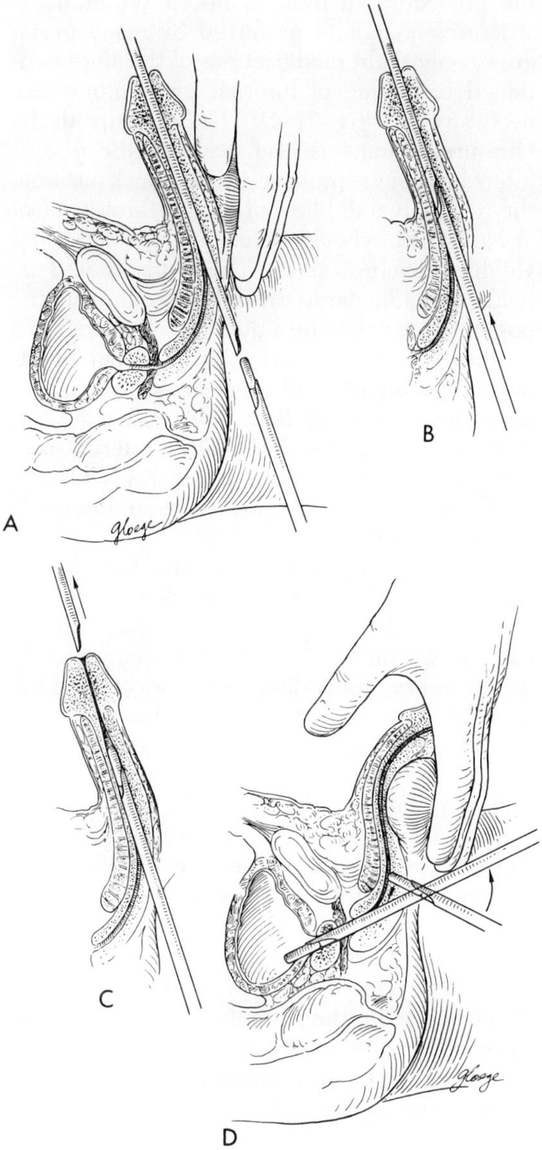

Figure 27–2. Technique for perineal urethrostomy. *A*, Fenestra of No. 24 Fr. resectoscope sheath palpated in perineum. *B*, Small incision over the No. 24 Fr. resectoscope beak has been made in perineal urethra. No. 28 Fr. sheath with No. 24 Fr. obturator has been inserted into fenestra of the No. 24 Fr. sheath. *C*, Both sheaths are advanced into urethra distal to perineal urethrostomy. No. 24 Fr. sheath has been withdrawn. No. 28 Fr. obturator is now placed in appropriate sheath. *D*, No. 28 Fr. sheath now advanced into bladder, taking care to "hug" the anterior wall of the bulbous urethra during introduction.

the bulbous urethrea when negotiating the turn toward the urogenital diaphragm (Fig. 27–2*D*). This is the crucial part of the procedure. If the surgeon is not successful in accomplishing this maneuver, the No. 24 Fr. sheath is reinserted into the distal urethra and advanced through the existing skin incision in the perineum and the entire procedure repeated until it is successful.

Sutures are not necessary with this technique; the larger sheath tamponades the perineal urethrostomy site during the procedure. Hemorrhage is rarely a problem. If the resectoscope is inadvertently extracted from the perineal urethrostomy site during the course of the procedure, the entire maneuver is repeated. *One should never attempt to simply push the sheath back through the perineal urethrostomy, as severe urethral injury and hemorrhage may result.*

During the postoperative period, the catheter should not exit via the perineal urethrostomy site; delayed wound healing and prolonged urinary leakage will occur from this site. A catheter guide is helpful in passing the catheter from the meatus and distal urethra into the bladder to avoid the urethrostomy site. If a Foley catheter is left indwelling for 72 hours after the transurethral resection, coursing the entire urethra, it is unusual for perineal leakage to occur when the catheter is removed. Urethral strictures at the site of the perineal urethrostomy have not been seen.

Erection during transurethral surgery is another possible cause of difficulty. It may occur with any mode of anesthesia and often persists stubbornly despite all therapeutic attempts. A trial of hypotensive anesthesia is of occasional benefit. When a patient is under spinal anesthesia, judicious administration of amyl nitrate may be helpful. Temporary cessation of manipulation may allow the phallus to detumesce. Under no circumstances should the procedure simply continue. Forcing the instruments through an erect penis may result in meatal and urethral injury. If erection persists, perineal urethrostomy can bypass the problem, but troublesome hemorrhage may occur if the incision veers from the midline. On occasion, a procedure must be terminated because of an erection.

TRANSURETHRAL SURGERY OF THE URETHRA

Urethral Strictures

In addition to the aforementioned incidence of urethral strictures that impede the passage of instruments for other transurethral procedures, strictures may also result from transurethral surgery. These are usually asymptomatic and are an incidental finding. As noted, most symptomatic urethral strictures may be managed by periodic dilatation, using either Van Buren sounds or filiforms and followers. A more aggressive approach in treating symptomatic urethral strictures depends on the ease and frequency of dilatation, the degree of patient discomfort, and the incidence of septic complications following the use of each instrument. If infected urine is present, the patient should be given an appropriate antibiotic agent 24 to 48 hours prior to dilatation. If a stricture is easily dilated with little chance of causing a false passage, and if dilation is not required more frequently than at 3-month intervals, conservative therapy is indicated. If dilations are technically difficult, must be performed at more frequent intervals, require general anesthesia to be accomplished, or are accompanied by frequent episodes of sepsis, consideration of a more aggressive approach is warranted (see Chapter 34).

Injection of local steroids such as dexamethasone into the area of the stricture at the time of dilation may retard its re-formation. This injection may be introduced percutaneously, using direct-vision urethroscopy to observe its accuracy. Malleable needles (No. 6 Fr. in caliber) are also available for transurethral instillation under direct vision. Injection of a solution of 6 parts of dexamethazone and 4 parts of lidocaine (Xylocaine) (1 percent) may decrease patient discomfort; 2 ml or less of this solution is usually sufficient. Reports regarding the efficacy of such treatment, however, show conflicting results.

If this approach is not successful, the surgeon should consider therapy with internal urethrotomy or open surgical urethroplasty. The indications and techniques of urethroplasty are beyond the purview of this chapter; however, it is my firm conviction that internal urethrotomy should be tried before open urethroplasty, because an unsuccessful internal urethrotomy rarely compromises subsequent open surgical repair.

The direct-vision urethrotome has become the most popular instrument employed for internal urethrotomy. Under direct vision, the stricture is incised deeply at the 12 o'clock position in the fibrous intercavernous septum. If this does not allow the stricture to spring open, cuts can be made at other points around the circumference of the stricture until the desired urethral caliber is reached. The injection of dexamethazone with internal urethrotomy may benefit the patient and certainly will not cause the patient harm.

When a straight Otis urethrotome is used for the procedure to treat stubborn symptomatic strictures (as is still preferred by many urologists), only slight modifications of the aforementioned technique of internal urethrotomy are necessary (see Fig. 27–1). The incision with the Otis urethrotome is also made in the fibrous intercavernous septum at the 12 o'clock position; the relatively dull blade of the urethrotome (set at No. 38 Fr.) should sever only the rigid, unyielding stricture areas. The penis should be held perpendicular to the pubis to eliminate the possibility of sphincter injury. Employment of a urethrotome with a screw tip that can be attached to a filiform will guard against the extension of a false passage. Because it is often difficult to pass a urethral catheter after internal urethrotomy, the subsequent use of this filiform in combination with a Councill catheter and guide is often helpful.

There is controversy regarding how long a catheter should be left in place after therapeutic internal urethrotomy. It is my feeling that the catheter should be left in place for approximately 4 to 6 weeks, depending on the severity of the stricture. Use of Silastic catheters has decreased the frequency of urethral reactions and improved the success rate of urethrotomy. Small fenestrae cut into the urethral portion of the catheter allow drainage of purulent material into the catheter, further decreasing the likelihood of urethritis and stricture formation. This, however, can lead to urinary leakage out of the fenestra, and drainage of urine around the catheter can be a nuisance to the patient. The main disadvantage for the patient who has undergone internal urethrotomy is the inconvenience of long-term catheter drainage. If a restricture should result, internal urethrotomy does not seem to compromise the success rate of subsequent urethroplasty.

Some endoscopic surgeons prefer to use a Colling's knife to incise strictures of short length electrically. Often, however, incision of these strictures may lead to dense scar tissue, resulting in a tighter or longer stricture than that originally treated. This may be partially circumvented if a low cutting current is used without coagulation. However, for dense, short strictures, open excision with primary reanastomosis may be preferable to endoscopic techniques. Recent experience with laser energy in the treatment of urethral strictures is interesting (see Chapter 43).

Urethral Polyps and Condylomas

These lesions, although rare, may be difficult to manage. Poorly planned attempts at transurethral resection may lead to widespread dissemination to areas of denuded, traumatized mucosa. Use of a flexible cup biopsy forceps to remove the bulk of the lesion, followed by chemcial or electrical fulguration of the base, is often successful. Resection with an electrosurgical loop is rarely indicated because of the high incidence of subsequent hemorrhage and stricture formation. Only localized lesions should be treated transurethrally.

Multiple lesions are best treated chemically with topical urethral instillation of 5 percent 5-fluorouracil cream or 0.5 percent colchicine; both medications have proved effective.[2,3] If these measures are not successful, open marsupialization of the involved segment of the urethra with an open incision of the lesions may be necessary. After a minimun 6-month period of observation for recurrences, the urethra may be closed with standard second-stage urethroplasty techniques.

Transurethral Sphincterotomy

Occasionally patients with neurogenic dysfunction of the detrusor muscle retain substantial residual urine despite all attemps to correct out fluid obstruction and to increase the tone of the detrusor by either medical or surgical means. External urinary sphincter spasm often causes such imbalance in micturition and may be suspected if the patient describes a hesitant, interrupted urine stream. Diagnosis may be determined by a urodynamic profile measuring the urethral resistance and the EMG activity of the sphincter during voiding. This can be confirmed with a pudendal block with 1 percent Xylocaine. External sphincter spasticity may also be caused by an increased tonus from lack of superspinal inhibition of gamma loop activity, and an adrenalitic agent such as Dibenzyline or methyl dopa (Aldomet) or prazosin hydrochloride (Minipress) may be beneficial in restoring balanced voiding.

If such pharmacologic measures fail, staged transurethral sphincterotomy can be successful in correcting this problem. However, whether the therapeutic result will lead to a successful outcome, continued retention, or incontinence is difficult to predict. If residual urine is still present, it is better to perform the procedure at a later date, than to risk incontinence, although often the latter is preferable in male patients with large amounts of residual urine and partially decompensated upper urinary tracts. Patients with retention, however, can be managed by intermittent self-catheterization. Candidates for sphincterotomy must be selected carefully indeed. For patients unable to perform self-catheterization, an external, condom type drainage device on the penis may be preferable to a stomal appliance. Sphincterotomy obviously presents less operative risk than the alternative of ileal loop diversion. If penile complications develop from the use of external collecting devices, supravesical diversion may be performed subsequently.

Transurethral sphincterotomy is performed with an Otis urethrotome, using direct-vision urethrotomy, or by electroresection of a sphincter with a Colling's knife. We favor the latter procedure. Pure cutting current is used in incising the sphincter area at the 12 o'clock position. An incision, 3 to 4 cm in length, should extend into the corpus spongiosum. Brisk bleeding is an expected sequela, and although bothersome, it rarely presents a signficant complication. Coagulation of bleeding points should not be performed, since stricture formation may occur. Significant hemorrhage can be managed with catheter traction and an Ace elastic compression dressing on the penis. If significant residual urine still remains, additional incisions are made judiciously at a later time. Incisions made laterally can result in impotence; all patients undergoing sphincterotomy should be advised that impotence may occur.

TRANSURETHRAL RESECTION OF THE BLADDER NECK

General Considerations

Bladder neck contractures may be primary or secondary. Great care should be exercised in making the diagnosis of *primary* bladder neck contracture, especially in the female patient, in whom this condition rarely, if ever, exists. In the male, primary bladder neck contracture is usually the result of adenomatous hypertrophy of the posterior commissure lobe rather than to a true fibrous median bar. The former is part of a more generalized process involving other prostatic lobes. Although primary bladder neck contracture due to median bar does exist, its incidence is much lower than previously cited.

Secondary bladder neck contractures are most commonly of iatrogenic origin but may occur as the sequelae to generalized detrusor hypertrophy, as in incidences of distal obstruction (e.g., posterior valves) and hypertonic neurogenic vesical dysfunction. Such secondary bladder neck contractures may cause significant continued obstruction after the primary etiologic factor has been corrected. Many feel that this lesion is often better treated by open Y-V plasty than by transurethral resection.

Iatrogenic fibrous contractures of the bladder neck most frequently result from transurethral open prostatectomy or prior bladder neck resection. Circumferential resection of the bladder neck with indiscriminate fulguration may lead to this complication. Occasionally, it is a sequel to radical prostatectomy. This type of contracture frequently causes high-grade obstructive lesions.

Neurogenic dysfunction of the bladder neck is another major cause of bladder neck obstruction. This purely functional obstruction should be distinguished from true anatomic obstruction often seen with generalized detrusor hypertrophy secondary to a spastic neurogenic dysfunction. A complete urodynamic evaluation, paying special attention to the electromyography of the bladder neck and sphincter area, should differentiate these entities. Use of beta blockers in such cases may obviate the need for surgical resection. The adrenalytic effect of these agents will relax the dysfunctional bladder neck as well as facilitate vesical contracture.

Transurethral Bladder Neck Resection in the Female

As noted, bladder neck resection in the female is rarely indicated. (It has been years since I have performed this procedure.) If the procedure is to be done, scrupulous attention to detail and technique is imperative. The distal extent of the resection must be carefully monitored. As the resection is carried distally, the urethra may appear to be obstructed and may lead the resectionist to cut too far distally, which can result in incontinence. Resection should be limited to the proximal one third of the urethra. It is helpful to mark the distal extent of the proposed resection with light fulguration prior to performing the resection.

Whenever possible, a resection should preserve the muscle fibers in the anterior and posterior portions of the bladder neck, since these fibers aid in vesical neck opening during micturition. A deep incision with the Colling's blade at the 5 and 7 o'clock positions is the preferred method; circumferential resection with loop invites subsequent fibrous contracture. Use of a pure, unblending cutting current with precise and minimal fulguration of bleeding points will further decrease the likelihood of this development. Vaginal palpation is helpful in determining the completeness of the resection. A catheter should be left indwelling for a minimum of 48 hours postoperatively.

Hemorrhage, recurrent bladder neck contracture, incontinence, perforation, and fistula formation are complications encountered in bladder neck resection in the female. Careful attention to technical detail will guard against incontinence. Postoperative hemorrhage rarely requires repeat fulguration. Perforation into the vagina will, in most instances, heal spontaneously with prolonged catheter drainage, although open surgical repair is occasionally necessary. Delayed fistula formation usually results from tissue necrosis. Open surgical repair in this instance is usually necessary but should be deferred for a minimum of 3 months.

Transurethral Bladder Neck Resection in the Male

Resection of only the apparent obstruction of the bladder neck rarely suffices when primary bladder neck contracture occurs in the male. It is usually necessary to resect adenomatous tissue involving other prostatic lobes. In patients with neurogenic dysfunction, a full resection of the prostatic fossa should be performed, with all adenomatous tissue resected to encourage a successful result. The prostatic fossa and bladder neck are converted into a conical funnel.

Fibrous contractures of the bladder neck in the male are best treated with the Colling's knife. An initial incision at the 6 o'clock position is usually adequate and should extend to transect all circular fibers. If this does not cause the bladder neck to spring open, incisions in additional quadrants (10 and 2 o'clock) may be made until the desired effect is obtained. Minimal use of a fulguration current is essential to prevent subsequent contracture. Cystoscope loops may also be used for this purpose. Concomitant circumferential local injection with triamcinolone transurethrally may decrease the incidence of subsequent contractures.[4] Patients who have fibrous contractures of the bladder neck following transurethral resection are at a very high risk of a recurrence after initial resection. Recurrence rates as high as 50 percent for the first recurrence have been noted, and after a second resection of the bladder neck contracture, recurrences as high as 75 percent have been reported. It is my recommendation that after two subsequent unsuccessful transurethral resections of bladder neck contracture following the original transurethral resection of the prostate, open Y-V plasty of the bladder neck be performed to give a reasonable expectation of correcting the problem.

Retrograde ejaculation is a common sequel to any surgical procedure involving the bladder neck. The patient should be informed of this possibility.

TRANSURETHRAL RESECTION OF THE PROSTATE

General Considerations

The decision to perform transurethral prostatic resection instead of open prostatectomy is largely one of individual preference. Prostate size is an important consideration; however, there is no absolute size limit for transurethral prostatectomy. Rather, a time limit of 1 hour for resection should be the surgeon's guide. Transurethral resections requiring over 1 hour to complete are associated with a higher incidence of complications such as water intoxication syndrome, urethral strictures, sepsis, and excessive blood loss. If a greater duration is anticipated, open prostatectomy should be selected.

It is important that an accurate preoperative assessment of the prostatic size be performed by digital rectal examination and cystoscopy if there is any question. Prostatic size may be misjudged if a rectal digital examination is performed when large amounts of residual urine are present, as the base of the distended bladder may be palpated, obscuring the prostate. Possibly, this can be mistaken for the prostate. I prefer to resect in two stages when the gland is too large to manage in a single 1-hour period. Although this is appropriate when the prostate is found to be larger than anticipated during resection, it is questionable, in my opinion, whether a *planned* two-stage resection is ever justified. The necessary second anesthesia and possible septic sequelae in such cases favor a one-stage open prostatectomy. On the other hand, in poor-risk or very old patients, it is possible to resect one lateral lobe or the middle lobe and one lateral lobe only and still obtain an excellent functional result. This is preferable to an incomplete resection of all lobes because the incidence of postoperative slough, hemorrhage, and obstruction is increased in the latter procedure.

Small, fibrotic glands should almost invariably be removed by the transurethral route. Transurethral incision of the prostate at the 4 and 8 o'clock positions may work well to relieve obstructive symptoms in such patients. Resection may not be necessary. Carcinoma of the prostate causing lower urinary tract obstructions should also be managed transurethrally, as cleavage planes often are not present during enucleation, and capsular tears, perforations, and even rectal injury can result.

Associated lesions, such as vesicoureteral reflux, vesical calculi, diverticula, vesical neoplasms, and stones, may alter the decision with regard to the route of prostatectomy.

Vasectomy

There is still controversy regarding the efficacy of prophylactic vasectomy to prevent epididymitis in patients undergoing transurethral resection of the prostate. Evidence exists both for and against vasectomy. In a well-controlled study by Rinker and associates of 1029 patients in whom unilateral vasectomy was performed, the incidence of epididymitis in the non-vasectomized side was 4.2 percent compared with 0.39 percent in the vasectomized patients.[5] Schmidt and Hinman noted a three-fold difference in the incidence in patients in the vasectomized and non-vasectomized groups.[6] Lynn and Nesbit and Haralambidis and Spinelli, however, noted no significant difference.[7,8] In 1963, Kendall reported a 30 percent incidence of bacterial growth when excised vas segments were cultured from patients who had had an indwelling catheter placed for more than 3 days.[9] Since then, it has been considered that vasectomy in this group would be hazardous because of the risk of trapping bacteria within the epididymis. A later study by Brooks and associates, however, demonstrated a reduction in the incidence of epididymitis after vasectomy in patients with prior catheter drainage (20.5 percent versus 0 percent).[10] Although the series is small, it does show that in certain instances, vasectomy may be beneficial in these groups. These diverse conclusions, all from seemingly well-conceived studies, most likely are the result of individual surgical variation. It is my practice not to routinely perform vasectomies in patients undergoing transurethral resection because in my experience, the incidence of epididymitis is low, and there is reasonable morbidity associated with vasectomy.

When vasectomy is to be performed, the percutaneous method or the standard exposure, excision, and ligation method is superior to the simple "vas crush."

Technique for Benign Adenomatous Hypertrophy

It is mandatory that thorough cystoscopic evaluation be performed before resection of obstructive adenomatous prostatic tissue. The bladder should be the first area examined because cystoscopic manipulation of the prostatic urethra may cause troublesome and obscuring hemorrhage. The 0- or 30-degree lens is employed for the resection, but the 70-degree lens allows more complete inspection of the bladder wall. The presence of co-existent bladder tumors, diverticula, or vesical calculi must be excluded. If found, they should be dealt with prior to the prostatic resection. Bladder diverticula of small capacity with an open neck need no therapy when the preoperative cystogram reveals complete emptying of the diverticulum. By contrast, if the neck is small and residual urine is present in the diverticulum, transurethral incision of the diverticulum is advisable. Vesical calculi, when present, should be handled by litholapaxy or electrohydraulic lithotripsy prior to resection. If the stone is too large for treatment by either of these techniques, perhaps open cystolithotomy and open prostatectomy should be considered.

After concomitant vesical disease has been excluded or properly treated, careful evaluation of the obstructing adenoma should be made in regard to its anatomic relationship to the trigone, bladder neck, verumontanum, and external urinary sphincter. These relationships must be indelibly fixed in the surgeon's mind before resection is performed.

The distance from the adenoma to the trigone is an important determination. As the trigone hypertrophies and the length of the prostatic fossa increases, this distance decreases, making trigonal injury more likely. The bladder neck and trigone should be inspected to determine the amount of middle lobe tissue present; the appropriate resection is then planned. The length of the prostatic urethra proximal to the verumontanum should be measured with respect to the length of the loop excursion. When the fossa is shorter than the loop excursion, care must be taken during the resection to avoid encroaching upon the trigone and ureteral orifices.

The amount of prostatic tissue distal to the verumontanum should also be determined to help protect against injury to the external sphincter. The bulk of the adenoma should be judged by palpating the cystoscope with the rectal finger. It is especially important to gauge the thickness of the adenoma at the posterior vesical neck, one of the common potential sites of perforation. The external sphincter should then be visualized in relation to the verumontanum at the apex of the prostate during resection; it is imperative that the surgeon be able to differentiate between the cut surface of adenoma and that of muscle tissue, as the spatial relationships of the external sphincter, verumontanum, and adenoma are constantly changing.

A No. 24 Fr. sheath will suffice for most resections and should be used in preference to larger sheaths, except when large adenomas exist. A No. 28 Fr. loop can be accommodated in a No. 26 Fr. sheath. Thus, it is never necessary to use a No. 28 Fr. sheath. In using a Stortz Iglesias resectoscope in large glands, a No. 27 Fr. sheath is necessary, as a smaller loop will not fit within this sheath. If, after satisfactory dilation and lubrication, the sheath is noted to "drag," an internal urethrotomy or perineal urethrostomy is indicated. If instrument drag occurs in mid-procedure, the smaller sheath should be substituted whenever possible. When a No. 24 Fr. sheath is already in use, an internal urethrotomy or a perineal urethrostomy in the middle of the procedure may be wise.

A detailed anatomic discussion of all techniques of transurethral prostatic resection is beyond the scope of this chapter. The order in which lobes are resected is largely one of personal preference. Ideally, the neophyte resectionist should employ various methods during the initial phases of his training so that he may determine which method best suits his talents. Variant adenomatous configuration may require that the surgeon deviate from his routine pattern, but a uniform method should be followed whenever possible.

By initially resecting the posterior bladder neck area and middle lobes, one improves the flow of irrigating fluid from the prostatic fossa into the bladder. Resected chips of adenomatous tissue may then flow more readily into the bladder and not hamper the resectionist. Another advantage of beginning in this area is that resection of the middle lobe and posterior bladder neck can be completed early in the procedure when the surgeon is fresh and when visualization is optimal. It reduces the risk of trigonal injury or perforation of the posterior bladder neck.

When circular muscle fibers of the posterior bladder neck are seen, resection in this area should be terminated. One should be especially careful not to use widespread coagulation in the area of the bladder neck; otherwise, a bladder neck contracture may develop. Only "pinpoint" fulguration of arterial bleeders should be employed. The posterior bladder neck is a very common site of perforation. Careful attention to detail without resecting through the circular muscles of the bladder neck will help obviate this complication. Also, when one is evacuating chips with the resectoscope, the beak of the resectoscope should be placed underneath the bladder neck because leverage on the resectoscope sheath emptying the bladder can cause a perforation.

The adenoma is thinnest in the anterior portion of the prostatic fossa, and care must be taken to avoid perforation. Multiple venous sinuses may be encountered in this area. Early entrance into venous sinuses may lead to water intoxication syndrome. During resection, the resectoscope beak should be positioned so that the verumontanum is often in view, thus protecting the external sphincter from injury. Whenever possible, full use of the loop's sweep should be made, and the entire length of the prostatic adenoma resected with each excursion.

Patients with small prostates in which a loop excursion may exceed the length of the prostatic fossa must be handled so as not to encroach upon the trigone. When the prostatic fossa is markedly elongated, two loop excursions may be necessary, or the sheath should be moved to the apex while the loop is still extended. The latter method is quicker and facilitates a smooth resection. If the lateral lobes appear so bulky that three loop widths will not complete the resection laterally into the area of the surgical capsule, it is preferable to employ an encirclement technique rather than the side-to-side, stepdown technique.

With large prostates, resection time may be greatly reduced if suprapubic punch cystostomy is performed prior to the procedure, making it unnecessary to stop resection periodically to empty the bladder. A suprapubic cystostomy tube allows continual run-off of irrigating fluid. Continuous flow resectoscopes are preferred by some resectionists.

In the final stage of the procedure, the apical adenomatous tissue lying distal to the verumontanum is resected. The external urinary sphincter should be visualized to guard against injuries, and the beak of the resectoscope should be placed just proximal to the sphincter. Any apical tissue that protrudes into the lumen of the prostatic fossa, as viewed from the area of the membranous urethra, should be resected. In patients who have considerable adenomatous tissue distal to the verumontanum, pushing the loop forward to resect in a proximal direction may help decrease the chance of sphincter damage.

After resection, the bladder is freed of prostatic chips with an Ellik evacuator or Toomey syringe, and final hemostasis is achieved. If open venous sinuses cause excessive bleeding, catheter traction should be employed in the initial postoperative period. It is rare, in my experience, not to enter venous sinuses in the terminal phase of a prostatic resection. The surgeon should ensure that the blood pressure level at the final stage of the procedure is nearly normal prior to removing the resectoscope. Hypertension at the end of the procedure may mask significant arterial bleeders that may open up when the blood pressure is restored to more normal levels in the recovery room, causing postoperative hemorrhage. If necessary, ephedrine should be administered by the anesthesiologist to normalize the blood pressure to guard against this occurrence.

A No. 22 or 24 Fr. Foley catheter is then inserted and connected to straight drainage. If clots form and obstruct the catheter lumen, intermittent hand irrigation usually suffices to remove them. It was my practice to use a standard catheter rather than a three-way Foley catheter because in many instances, I have seen bleeding exacerbated when a three-way catheter became occluded with a clot and the continuous irrigation persisted, thus overdistending the bladder and prostatic fossa. With careful observation, and good nursing care, this has not occurred as often as in the past, and I currently favor the use of the three-way Foley catheter with continuous irrigation using normal saline.

Catheter traction is employed, and at least 30 ml of fluid should be placed in the balloon to ensure that the catheter balloon remains outside the prostatic fossa. A balloon distending the prostatic fossa prevents contraction of the prostatic capsule, which is a major hemostatic mechanism. To prevent this, a correspondingly larger volume should be placed in balloons when larger adenomas are resected. Up to 90 ml may be placed in the "30 ml" balloon chamber. Traction necessary to control venous sinus bleeding can be applied initially with meatal pressure by tying a moist sponge around the catheter or by weighted traction (less than 1 pound over the end of bed). Traction utilizing meatal pressure should never be employed longer than a few minutes because necrosis of the meatus can result. Weighted traction over the end of the bed can be left on for longer periods of time as necessary. If bleeding persists, traction should be intermittently released to prevent pressure necrosis of the bladder neck. However, this has never occurred in my experience and may be more of a theoretic concern than a truly realistic problem.

Technique for Carcinoma of the Prostate

The same indications for operative intervention for hyperplasia apply to carcinoma of the prostate. When massive neoplastic involvement of the prostate occurs, causing obstruction, many urologists favor perineal needle biopsy to confirm the diagnosis of carcinoma, followed by orchiectomy or estrogen therapy, or both. Controversy exists as to whether hormone therapy is, in fact, justified for obstructive disease, or whether its use should be withheld until the patient becomes symptomatic for metastatic disease. We do not tend to advocate one approach over the other; however, when benign adenomatous hyperplasia exists in conjunction with carcinoma and is the prime lesion responsible for outlet obstruction, transurethral prostatectomy should be performed in preference to hormone manipulation.

Cystoscopic evalation is helpful in distinguishing between obstruction caused by adenomatous hyperplasia and that caused by massive infiltrative carcinoma. There is controversy regarding the traditional role of TURP in the management of such patients in urine retention with associated stage C carcinoma of the prostate. Many patients with complete or near-complete retention may be well managed by catheter drainage and radiation therapy, with or without adjunctive hormone treatment. It is essential, however, that patients experiencing retention should not undergo irradiation with a urethral Foley catheter in place. Such patients should be drained by a suprapubic tube during the course of radiation therapy. Severe urethral stricture can result if radiation therapy is given with a Foley catheter in the urethra. Seven weeks, however, are often required for sufficient shrinkage of the prostate and a decrease in the radiation reaction to occur before the catheter can be removed and the patient is allowed to void.

Although it is thus possible to obtain significant shrinkage of neoplastic glands with radiation therapy, we prefer transurethral resection for this group of patients. It is our feeling that transurethral resection of the prostate obviates the need for long-term suprapubic catheter drainage during the period of radiation therapy and also reduces the possibility that the procedure may be necessary following radiation therapy. In our experience, patients who undergo transurethral resection after definitive radiation therapy for stage C lesions often have a higher incidence of incontinence, bleeding, and infection because of compromise of the sphincter by fibrosis secondary to the therapy and inability of the prostatic fossa to heal following irradiation. The onset of incontinence may be delayed, as progressive fibrosis of the sphincter does occur following radiation therapy (administered by way of external beam only or combined with interstitial seeds).

When transurethral resection of a prostatic carcinoma has been performed and subsequent radiation therapy is contemplated, it is best to delay radiation therapy for 8 weeks to allow reepithelialization of the prostatic fossa. Fewer irritative symptoms result. If the patient has already received the full course of radiation therapy and later develops lower urinary tract obstruction, transurethral resection should be performed, but there is a greater risk of delayed healing in the prostatic fossa, bleeding, urinary incontinence, and urethral stricture formation, and the patient should be informed accordingly.

Special care must be taken when performing resection in cases of carcinoma of the prostate, since the incidence of postoperative bleeding is higher in these patients than in those who have benign disease. A prothrombin time, platelet count, and examination of the urine for fibrinolysis should be part of the preoperative evaluation. If troublesome postoperative hemorrhage ensues, primary fibrinolysis and primary intravascular coagulation must be considered as potential causes. Fibrinolysis may occur in conjunction with disseminated intravascular coagulation.[11] Fibrinolysis secondary to urokinase is easily detected by incubating the blood clot in a urine sample. If clot lysis occurs, intravenous epsilon-aminocaproic acid (EACA) should be administered immediately, and the patient later converted to oral therapy. Five gm are given at once, followed by 1 gm per hour until the bleeding stops.

The administration of EACA to patients who have both fibrinolysis and disseminated intravascular coagulation, however, is hazardous, and intravascular coagulation must be ruled out prior to its use. The diagnosis of disseminated intravascular coagulation is made when the patient is found to be thrombocytopenic and hypofibrinogenemic, with an associated increase in the prothrombin time (secondary to a decrease in the concentration of accelerator globulin). Decreased levels of prothrombin in factor VIII (anti-hemophilic factor) further substantiate the diagnosis.

Disseminated intravascular coagulation is managed with intravenous heparin in a dose of 140 to 400 mg per 24-hour period. Continuous intravenous infusion is preferable to the intermittent intravenous or subcutaneous method. If associated urokinase activity is present, EACA may be added to heparin after the clotting factors (platelet count, fibrinogen, and prothrombin) have begun to return to normal. Transfusion with appropriate blood components, such as platelet packs, fresh frozen plasma, and so on, is an important adjuvant in stubborn cases (see Chapter 4). The use of EACA routinely in transurethral resection for benign disease is not warranted.[12]

When carcinoma exists in conjunction with hyperplasia, the surgical technique remains essentially the same as with benign adenomatous obstruction. If the prostate is extensively involved with carcinoma, however, some modification in the technique may be necessary. Often there is anatomic distortion; the bladder neck and membranous urethra may be the only remaining landmarks. With extensive carcinoma, the urethra is often rigid so that maneuverability of the sheath is limited. In such cases, a perineal urethrostomy may allow improved maneuverability of the sheath, facilitating the resection. In patients with prostatic obstruction secondary to scirrhous carcinoma, a "channel cut" often suffices for relief of obstruction because tissue will not fall into the fossa as with adenomatous tissue. Exceptional care must be taken in the region of the apex in patients with carcinoma, especially those who have been irradiated. If the carcinoma appears to be infiltrating the prostatic apex, incontinence is a common sequela of resection, no matter how careful the surgical technique. The patient with such apical extension should be apprised preoperatively of this potentiality.

It is my approach to do a limited resection of the apex of such patients, giving consideration to postoperative hormone manipulation to cause enough softening and regression of the local lesion to allow satisfactory voiding. One can always resect persistent apical tissue at a later date should continued obstruction remain. It is difficult to put apical tissue back in a patient whom you have made incontinent.

Technique for Prostatic Abscess

Modern antibiotic treatment has made prostatic abscess a rare lesion. During the course of transurethral resection, however, it is not uncommon to encounter small pockets of purulent material that persist following acute or chronic episodes of infection. These pockets, however, usually are sterile.

Occasionally, a patient will present with acute obstructive symptoms secondary to a prostatic abscess. The abscess areas are often fluctuant but occasionally may be so firm as to resemble carcinoma. Prior to the use of modern antibacterial chemotherapy, incision and drainage by perineal exposure was the procedure of choice. Today, appropriate parenteral or broad-spectrum antibiotics alone will often suffice. If the patient presents with acute retention, however, a small urethral catheter or punch suprapubic cystostomy may be necessary until the appropriate antibiotic therapy has been administered and has had a chance to resolve the problem. Transurethral resection may be necessary and can be performed subsequently if continued obstruction is present. Also, transurethral resection may be necessary in patients who fail to defervesce following appropriate antibacterial therapy.

The abscess is often seen bulging into the lumen of the prostatic urethra. Simple unroofing of the most prominent portion of the bulge is usually all that is necessary. If significant hyperplasia is also present, it can be resected at this time or at a later date, depending upon the general status of the patient.

Technique for Prostatitis

Transurethral resection should be employed only rarely in patients with prostatitis, and patients should be properly forewarned that their symptoms may persist. Irritative symptoms must not be confused with obstructive symptoms; the former are often worsened by an ill-advised resection. When prostatitis is associated with adenomatous obstruction or prostatic calculi and if the patient has severe, debilitating symptoms, a properly performed resection may be of benefit. The radical transurethral resection offers the best chance for symptomatic relief in these patients. All tissue surrounding the prostatic calculi should be resected. Should prostatic calculi exist between the adenoma and the surgical capsule, resection should extend well into the surgical capsule in an attempt to remove most of the inflamed tissue. In patients with inflamed prostates, coagulation should be used sparingly to decrease the subsequent fibrosis in the prostatic fossa. When severe symptoms persist, total prostatectomy may be the only means of benefiting such patients.

COMPLICATIONS OF TRANSURETHRAL RESECTION OF THE PROSTATE

As noted, preoperative evaluation of the patient's coagulation profile is an essential prophylactic measure in preventing excess hemorrhage. Careful electrofulguration of arterial bleeders will decrease the chance of delayed hemorrhage resulting from sloughing of chronic tissue secondary to massive fulguration of the prostatic fossa. Blood pressure levels must be normal at the termination of the procedure to ensure that significant bleeding points are not masked by hypotension. When venous sinuses are opened during the procedure, it is not necessary to terminate the resection. The level of irrigating fluid should be lowered and Lasix administered. Free water should not be given.

Bleeding venous sinuses will respond to catheter traction; indiscriminate fulguration will not control this type of bleeding and may even cause an additional hemorrhage. Unroofing of venous sinus bleeders is a common occurrence if a truly complete resection is performed. Generally, a continuous three-way irrigation catheter is used, which lessens the chance of a blood clot occluding the catheter. One must be careful, however, because should the catheter occlude, continuous inflow of fluid may cause overdistention of the bladder and dilation of the prostatic urethra, causing further bleeding. Attentive nursing care is necessary if continuous irrigation is utilized. It is my feeling that a closed continuous irrigation system with intermittent hand irrigation as necessary is preferable to a standard two-way catheter.

If it is necessary to reoperate to control hemorrhage, thorough evacuation of clots from the bladder and prostatic fossa should be performed. Systematic examination of the entire prostatic fossa for bleeding sites should be conducted, using the irrigating fluid under low pressure. Appropriate fulguration may then be accomplished. It may be necessary to remove clots that adhere to the prostatic fossa with a resectoscope loop in order to visualize sites of hemorrhage. In my experience, a common area in which undetected postoperative hemorrhage occurs is the anterior bladder neck where, often, pieces of prostate tissue can be pulled in during resection only to "flip up" and reside just inside the bladder neck. Careful observation of this area is essential if an obvious bleeding site is not found on re-exploration elsewhere in the prostatic fossa. Occasionally, open surgical exploration may be necessary, with direct fulguration or suture ligation of bleeding sites. The circumferential bladder neck suture may be of benefit in stubborn cases; only rarely should it be necessary to leave a pack in the prostatic fossa.

In a randomized double-blind control study using EACA in patients undergoing transurethral resection for benign disease, we were unable to find any benefit in the EACA-treated group compared with the placebo-treated group.[12] It is my feeling that EACA is appropriate only if fibrinolysins are detected, and only after disseminated intravascular coagulation has been excluded. In cases of stubborn hemorrhage, some surgeons advocate the use of a Foley catheter balloon within the prostatic fossa. A No. 24 Fr. Foley catheter with a 30-ml balloon is inserted into the bladder and the balloon inflated to 15 ml. The catheter is withdrawn until resistance is felt. The balloon then resides in the prostatic fossa. An additional 15 ml of fluid is put in and the amount increased in 10 to 15 ml increments until hemostasis is achieved. While numerous surgeons favor this approach for stubborn bleeders, I have rarely used this technique and favor compression of the prostatic urethra with the balloon inflated within the bladder.[13] It is my feeling that compression of the prostatic fossa to allow the capsule to contract better accomplishes hemostasis.

Undermining the trigone with associated ureteral injury is the result of careless technique. Should this occur, a cystogram should be performed to exclude the possibility of intraperitoneal perforation. If there is no perforation, nothing further needs to be done. A catheter guide is often helpful in placing the catheter in these patients to prevent further undermining the trigone. Fulguration near the injured ureteral orifice should be avoided as this will increase the risk of subsequent obstruction. An intravenous pyelogram should be performed in these patients postoperatively (at two months) to exclude the possibility of subsequent obstruction.

The water intoxication syndrome may develop when venous sinus or capsular perforation occurs early in the course of resection or when the resection time is prolonged. Hypertension and mental confusion are the predominant symptoms. Hypotension, bradycardia, or restlessness secondary to hyponatremia may follow. When general anesthesia has been employed, restlessness, disorientation, and nausea may not be present. The only manifestations of delusional hyponatremia in such patients may be increasing hypertension and an increase in pulse or venous pressure. For this reason, spinal anesthesia is the preferred method of anesthesia. In patients with large prostates that require resection under general anesthesia, it is wise to use the intravascular sodium-sensitive electrodes to detect variations in plasma sodium concentrations during the procedure. If these are not available, frequent electrolyte determinations made during and after the procedure are essential.

If perforation occurs or if venous sinuses are open during the resection, the administration of a loop diuretic (Lasix, 40 to 120 mg) should be administered. In addition, intravenous fluids should be changed so that no free water is given. With severe hyponatremia, the judicious administration of hypertonic saline (3 percent) may be necessary. The use of 5 percent mannitol solution as an irrigating medium in such patients helps to obviate this complication because of its osmotic diuretic effect. Because of its hyperosmolar nature, however, mannitol may cause a more rapid intravascular volume expansion, allowing the extravasated fluid to be absorbed more easily, thus perhaps increasing the amount of hyponatremia. In patients who have had perforation with large amounts of extravasation, the intraoperative sodium value may be misleading, because significant absorption may occur in the first few postoperative hours. Frequent electrolyte determinations are necessary during this time, with the continued restriction of free water and the liberal use of loop diuretics.

During the procedure, if perforations have occurred, it is essential to reduce the height of the irrigating fluid to less than 60 cm to minimize the amount of fluid extravasated. Rarely, in my experience, has percutaneous drainage of this extravasated fluid been indicated.

Urethral strictures occur in approximately 5 percent of patients following transurethral resection of the prostate. The membranous urethra, penoscrotal junction, and fossa navicularis are the common sites for such strictures. Gentle technique, including proper preliminary urethral dilation and instrument lubrication, is an important prophylactic measure. By using the smallest available instrument and limiting the resection time to less than 1 hour, the incidence of stricture formation can be decreased further. If a pre-existing stricture is found or if the urethra is simply too small to accept the smallest resectoscope sheath comfortably, an internal urethrotomy or perineal urethrostomy should be performed. Assessment of the entire urethra by panendoscopy before attempting to insert the resectoscope blindly will lessen the incidence of false passage formation and permit a more accurate assessment of the urethral channel. Use of a small caliber Silastic catheter in the postoperative period also reduces the incidence of stricture formation. However, the caliber of the catheter should be sufficient to allow easy irrigation of clots. Rarely should a catheter smaller than No. 22 Fr. be used.

If catheter traction is necessary in the postoperative period, this should be removed as soon as possible to lessen the likelihood of trauma to the penoscrotal junction and possible subsequent stricture formation. The passage of a No. 22 Fr. sound 8 weeks postoperatively will allow a stricture to be detected before it becomes severe enough to cause a management problem. Periodic dilation usually prevents the development of this complication.

Symptomatic perforation of the bladder neck and prostatic capsule should occur only rarely. It is not uncommon, however, in performing complete transurethral resection to have small, insignificant perforations. If a major perforation occurs early during the resection, large amounts of fluid may extravasate into the retroperitoneal space causing significant discomfort or delayed resorption and an exacerbation of the water intoxication syndrome. Spinal anesthesia allows the symptomatic extravasation to be discovered while the patient is still in the cystoscopic room, where appropriate therapeutic measures may be immediately initiated. General anesthesia often delays the diagnosis, requiring the patient to be returned to the operating suite for possible treatment. General anesthesia further complicates the situation by masking many of the early symptoms of water intoxication syndrome.

Another sign indicating that significant perforation extravasation has occurred is a distortion of the prostatic urethra where the lumen is narrowed and the length of the prostatic urethra is elongated. The bladder neck and trigone may appear distant. Perforations posteriorly in the prostatic capsule usually occur at the bladder neck area. If the perforation is in this position or if there is severe distortion of the prostatic urethra, a cystogram should be performed. A cystogram is also indicated if abdominal distention is noted and if the patient complains of abdominal discomfort. In the event that an intraperitoneal perforation has occurred, the patient should be explored and the site of the perforation closed through a cystotomy incision. A careful search to rule out injury to a hollow viscus should be performed.

Rarely are lateral or anterior perforations associated with intraperitoneal extravasation. Expectant therapy with catheter drainage and diuretics may suffice for small and moderate perforations and even large perforations in the lateral and anterior area. Close observation of the patient is imperative. Careful monitoring of serum electrolytes for the initial 12 hours following surgery is mandatory to decrease the risk of undiagnosed water intoxication syndrome.

Retroperitoneal perforations are routinely managed with catheter drainage. These perforations occur quite commonly and usually remain undiagnosed; however, large retroperitoneal perforations are associated with severe discomfort. A small suprapubic incision should be made in such patients and a Penrose drain placed in the retropubic space. It is my feeling that this should be done only if the patient is symptomatic. If the patient is infected preoperatively and if parenteral antibiotic coverage has not already been administered, a Penrose drain should be placed at once. Prophylactic antibacterial coverage is not mandatory in patients with sterile urine preoperatively.

Incontinence is a feared complication of any form of prostatectomy, and the patient must be forewarned of this possibility. The incidence of permanent urinary incontinence after transurethral resection of the prostate should be less than 0.5 percent. Temporary incontinence is more common but usually resolves in a few days or weeks. The irritative symptoms such as urgency and urgency incontinence are generally due to irritability from the resected prostatic fossa. In addition, it is not uncommon to have detrusor instability in patients with prostatic obstruction, which can be a cause of postoperative incontinence of the urgency type. If this occurs, treatment with an anticholinergic agent is usually effective. Some degree of incontinence can be seen up to 1 year postoperatively. Rarely is an incontinence procedure indicated without observing the patient for signs of improvement during a minimum of several months to 1 year. Patients with continued incontinence of the urgency variety should undergo a urodynamic evaluation, especially if they are not responsive to anticholinergic agents. On occasion, augmentation enterocystoplasty is necessary for these patients.

Infected urine in the postoperative period is common and is difficult to remedy completely until the prostatic fossa has re-epithelialized. In such patients, appropriate antibacterial coverage should be given, followed by antibacterial suppression for 8 to 12 weeks postoperatively. During the healing phase, the presence of pyuria is expected and does not necessarily indicate infection. A culture should be taken to justify the administration of antibiotic agents. Even then, antimicrobial therapy may only lead to drug resistance or superinfection.

POSTOPERATIVE MANAGEMENT OF TRANSURETHRAL PROSTATECTOMY

It is imperative that the catheter drainage be employed well into the postoperative period. An obstructed catheter will cause distention of the prostatic capsule with resultant hemorrhage. A three-way catheter with continuous irrigation lessens the likelihood of clot formation. It must be carefully monitored, however. Should a clot occlude the lumen, bleeding could be worsened by the continuous infusion of irrigating fluid, which will further distend the bladder and prostatic capsule, perhaps opening venous sinuses. The use of postoperative prophylactic antibiotics is, of course, up to the surgeon. Bladder spasms may indicate an obstructed catheter. If clots in the bladder are ruled out as a cause of the spasms, appropriate anticholinergic agents may be administered. If a large amount of solution is left in the balloon at the time the catheter is placed in traction, reduction in the size of the balloon to 30 ml will lessen bladder spasms, when traction is discontinued.

Patients should be kept at bedrest in the initial 24-hour period following prostatectomy. Full ambulation is allowed during the first postoperative day, but the patient should be discouraged from sitting for prolonged periods. Bowel movements should be kept soft to prevent excessive strain during this period. If an enema is necessary, it should be given with extreme caution to avoid possible rectal perforation or manipulation of the prostate, which may result in bleeding. Heavy lifting should be avoided during the first 4 to 6 weeks postoperatively.

Delayed Complications of Transurethral Prostatectomy

In patients who have a less than optimal stream following prostatectomy, urethral stricture, bladder neck contracture, inadequate tissue resection, and atonic bladder all need to be considered in the differential diagnosis. Usually patients with an atonic bladder or inadequate resection will never have a good stream following surgery, whereas patients who develop urethral strictures or bladder neck contractures will initially have an excellent stream, only to experience a diminution in the caliber and force of their steam in the first few weeks following surgery. In such patients, a cystoscopic evaluation is essential. If no obstruction is noted, urodynamic evaluation of the bladder should be performed. Also, the urine flow rate should be documented and urethral resistance calculated. These can easily determine if there is truly an obstructive lesion.

The treatment of urethral strictures has been described in the foregoing discussion. Bladder neck contractures following transurethral resection can be a very troublesome problem. Contractures occur in up to 5 percent of patients following the procedure and seem to occur more commonly in patients with small, fibrotic prostates. The cause is unknown. However, indiscriminate fulguration of the bladder neck and excessive catheter traction of the bladder neck have been implicated as possible causes. When bladder neck contracture occurs, it may present a troublesome problem in the future. Initially, patients with a circumferential contracture of the bladder neck should be treated transurethrally with incision. If this does not allow the bladder neck to spring open, circumferential resection should be performed. Patients who demonstrate the tendency for bladder neck contracture have a very high risk of recurrent bladder neck contracture once the initial contracture has been surgically corrected. Forty to 50 percent of patients who develop a postoperative bladder neck contracture will experience some degree of recurrence after resection. Those patients who have had two resections of bladder neck contractures have an up to 75 percent chance of developing a third contracture. It is my feeling that if a patient has a third bladder neck contracture, consideration to open surgical repair with a Y-V plasty is warranted.

Continued obstructive symptoms secondary to inadequate tissue resection should be a relatively rare event. If a patient has a great deal of apical tissue distal to the verumontanum, extreme caution should be used in resecting this tissue. This is clearly the focus of most obstruction when inadequate tissue has been resected. In my opinion, this is not a terrible complication following surgery. It is far better to re-resect the patient for minor apical obstruction than to make the patient incontinent with an excessive resection at the first procedure.

A problem area of inadequate resection is the anterior prostatic tissue. Often during the course of the resection, if the resectionist does not recheck the anterior area at the termination of the procedure, anterior tissue will fall into the prostatic lumen after the supporting lateral lobe tissue has been removed. Paying attention to this possible cause of inadequate resection at the terminal phases of the procedure will lessen the likelihood of this occurrence. Also, one must carefully check for flaps of prostatic tissue that may act as a ball-valve in the postoperative period.

Most patients with poor bladder tone who void inadequately following an adequate transurethral resection will have to be managed with intermittent self-catheterization. This generally occurs in patients with long-standing chronic obstruction and perhaps with associated diabetes mellitus. It is my opinion that even if a relatively atonic bladder and a mild increased voiding resistance are diagnosed preoperatively, it is worth a transurethral resection. Many times, patients with poor detrusor tone can be placed in reasonable balance by lowering the voiding resistance by transurethral prostatectomy.

Retrograde ejaculation is an expected sequela of transurethral prostatic resection. Patients should be made aware that this will occur in the postoperative period. When patients have normal antegrade ejaculation following transurethral resection, the occurrence of a bladder neck contracture should be suspected. If the patient desires children following prostatectomy, he should be referred to a fertility specialist. Sperm can be collected by catheterization, pooled, and artificially inseminated if desired. A solution of sodium bicarbonate should be instilled in the bladder before ejaculation. It is my feeling that preserving the bladder neck during transurethral resection to preserve antegrade ejaculation is rarely indicated. Continued obstruction is the most likely sequela of this maneuver. Transurethral resection should rarely affect potency. Many patients, however, need something to "blame" their impotence on. Other patients who truly are impotent following the procedure and who had good erections before the transurethral resections may have potency problems on a psychological basis. Nocturnal tumescence studies are indicated.

TRANSURETHRAL BLADDER SURGERY

It is not the purpose of this section to discuss the indications for transurethral resection of malignant vesical neoplasms. Most low-grade, non-invasive bladder tumors may be managed satisfactorily by the transuretheral route. The extent to which higher-grade invasive carcinomas should be managed transurethrally depends on the patient in question and the skill of the endoscopic surgeon. Carcinoma in situ should be treated primarily with intravesical chemotherapy after the diagnosis has been established with cold cup biopsies. On occasion, in poor-risk patients with carcinoma in situ, persistence of this lesion despite intravesical chemotherapy can be managed with a roller electrode, cauterizing all areas of carcinoma in situ. Very close follow-up needs to be made in these patients, as it is often difficult to determine exactly where carcinoma in situ exists with the cystoscope.

SURGICAL TECHNIQUE OF THERAPEUTIC RESECTION

After the surgeon has determined that resection of the bladder tumor is indicated and feasible, the resection should proceed from the top of the lesion to the bottom. Tumors and the areas of likely perforation should be reserved for last. Thus resection of tumors in the dome area of the bladder or those near the the obturator nerve, where the obturator reflex may cause perforation, should be deferred until the end of the procedure. Distilled water is the preferred irrigating medium because of its superior optical properties and its potential cytotoxic osmotic effect on free-floating tumor cells. The bladder should be filled with sufficient fluid to carry the normal bladder away from the lesion but not overdistended. An overdistended bladder is thinner than one that is partially filled, making perforation more likely. One should attempt to secure hemostasis during the course of the resection to allow optimal visualization. However, this is often difficult to accomplish until one gets to the pedicle of the papillary lesion with a narrow stalk. When the lesion has been completely resected, further tissue below the obvious lesion should be resected and submitted as a separate pathologic specimen. Tissue around the entire circumference of the lesion should also be resected to ensure total removal of the tumor and submitted separately for pathologic examination as well. The border of the lesion should be fulgurated. If resection is complete, it is unnecessary for the base of the lesion to be widely fulgurated because this merely delays wound healing, causing necrosis and possible delayed hemorrhage.

In the later stages of resection, the bladder should not be overly distended, as perforations of thin areas may result. Lesions near ureteral orifices should be resected as if they were in any other area of the bladder. The fulguration in and around the ureteral orifice should be limited to prevent subsequent ureteral obstruction.

Stimulation of the obturator nerve is a major cause of vesical perforation. To avoid this problem, bladder resection should be performed in the area of the obturator nerve with the bladder only partially filled. If this problem does occur, it can be circumvented by administration of muscle relaxants when the patient is under general anesthesia; instillation of local anesthesia around the obturator nerve can be of benefit.[14] Whenever an obturator reflex occurs, the surgeon must immediately release the foot pedal to prevent serious injury. Perforation may lead to premature termination of the procedure and necessitate a second anesthesia at a later time.

With resection of a lesion less than 1 cm in size, it is rarely necessary to employ postoperative catheter drainage. Larger lesions require catheter drainage from 1 to 5 days, depending both on the size of the tumor and on the depth of resection.

Complications

Hemorrhage following endoscopic resection of bladder tumors can be exceedingly troublesome. It is imperative to keep the catheter free of clots, as overdistension of the bladder may lead to delayed perforation. Should repeated clot retention occur, it is best to return the patient immediately to the cystoscopy suite for clot evacuation and fulguration. In patients who have undergone large tumor resections, the use of a three-way catheter with constant irrigation may help prevent clot retention.

Extraperitoneal perforation is not a serious complication unless extensive extravasation has occurred. In these patients, suprapubic drainage as well as catheter drainage should be instituted for 5 to 7 days. Smaller extraperitoneal perforations require only catheter drainage for 4 to 5 days.

Intraperitoneal perforation requires immediate exploration to repair the perforation and to drain the extravasated fluid. Catheter drainage should be employed for 5 to 7 days postoperatively.

Transurethral Resection of Vesical Diverticula

Controversy exists regarding the indication for transurethral resection of diverticular orifices. Small diverticula without residual urine need no treatment, whereas larger ones should be managed by open surgical excision. Many urologists doubt that incision into the neck of a small diverticulum can improve drainage without producing concomitant vesical perforation and subsequent urine extravasation. In selected patients, however, careful incision into the muscular rim around the diverticular orifice can be successfully accomplished by using a Colling's knife. Improved drainage of the diverticulum is often noted subsequently. This is generally reserved for patients who represent a poor risk for surgery.

Perforations are managed as with any clinical situation. If open cystotomy is necessary for closure of an intraperitoneal perforation, it may be prudent to proceed with transvesical diverticulectomy at the same time.

TRANSURETHRAL RESECTION OF URETEROCELES

Indications

Transurethral resection has only limited application in intravesical management of ureteroceles. Obstruction caused by ureteroceles frequently will be replaced by vesical ureteral reflux if simple resection is performed. Therefore, large ureteroceles with high-grade obstruction should be excised by open surgery so that the involved renal segment can be managed concomitantly. In these patients, the base of the ureterocele must also be reinforced, as a hernia-like defect, which is often present behind the ureterocele will interfere with subsequent bladder emptying. Fragments of retained ureterocele tissue may act as the nidus for persistent urinary tract infection.

Small ureteroceles may be associated with significant obstruction or stones and may benefit from a transurethral unroofing. Careful follow-up for reflux is mandatory, since it can cause progressive upper urinary tract changes and recurrent infection. Should symptomatic reflux occur, an open antireflux procedure may be necessary.

Large ureteroceles with associated high-grade obstruction and pyonephrosis may be handled on an emergency basis with transurethral resection to effect a rapid decompression of an obstructed, infected system in this acute situation. When the condition of the patient stabilizes, open repair should then be accomplished on an elective basis.

Technique

A variety of instruments may be employed to perform transurethral resection of a ureterocele. Meatotomy scissors are useful if they can penetrate the wall of the ureterocele. If not, a Colling's knife or loop electrode may be used. The inferior portion of the ureterocele should be incised transversely, creating a flap valve mechanism that may prevent subsequent reflux. These patients must be followed closely in the postoperative period, using intravenous pyelograms and cystograms to monitor the status of the upper urinary tract.

TRANSURETHRAL URETERAL MEATOTOMY

Indications

Transurethral ureteral meatotomy should be performed in a very few patients because vesicoureteral reflux is a common sequel of this procedure. Meatotomy is occasionally indicated for ureteral reimplantation if obstruction appears to result in an excessively long submucosal tunnel. A carefully performed meatotomy may benefit these patients, relieving the obstruction without causing reflux. Meatotomy is also occasionally justified when a ureteral calculus is lodged in an intramural ureter. I find that the use of a ureteroscope and basket often facilitates stone passage in such patients. Flexible cystoscopic scissors offer precise control. Incision at the 6 o'clock position in the orifice will result in a lower incidence of reflux, as compared with an incision at the 12 o'clock position. Fulguration should not be performed after meatotomy.

A ureteral catheter with a stylet protruding from the end may also be used to perform transurethral meatotomy. An electrosurgical unit is connected to the stylet and a pure cutting current applied for meatotomy. This method facilitates a ventral 6 o'clock incision, which is often technically difficult to perform with meatotomy scissors.

References

1. Smith RB: Unpublished data, 1978.
2. Dretler SP, Klein LA: The eradication of intraurethral condyloma acuminata with five percent 5-fluorouracil cream. J Urol 113:195, 1975.
3. Gigax JH, Robinson JR: The successful treatment of intraurethral condyloma acuminata with colchicine. J Urol 105:809, 1971.
4. Damico CF, Mebust WK, Valk WL, Foret JD: Triamcinolone: adjuvant therapy for vesical neck contractures. J Urol 110:203, 1973.
5. Rinker JR, Hancock CV, Henderson WD: A statistical study of unilateral prophylactic vasectomy in the prevention of epididymitis: 1029 cases. J Urol 104:303, 1970.
6. Schmidt S, Hinman F: The effect of vasectomy upon the incidence of epididymitis after prostatectomy: an analysis of 810 operations. J Urol 63:872, 1950.
7. Lynn JM, Nesbit RM: The influence of vasectomy upon the incidence of epididymitis following transurethral prostatectomy. J Urol 59:72, 1948.
8. Haralambidis G, Spinelli AN: Vasectomy: an evaluation. J Urol 89:591, 1963.
9. Kendall AR: Rationale prophylactic vasectomy. J Urol 89:712, 1963.
10. Brooks MB, Lytton B, Weiss SA: Vasectomy in the control of epididymitis after prostatectomy following urethral catheter drainage. J Urol 105:694, 1971.
11. Brooks MB: Heparin in the treatment of hemorrhagic diathesis associated with prostatic carcinoma. J Urol 102:240, 1969.
12. Smith RB, Riach P, Kaufman JJ: Epsilon aminocaproic acid and control of post-prostatectomy bleeding: prospective double blind study. J Urol 131:1093, 1984.
13. Greene LF: Transurethral surgery. In Walsh PC, Perlmutter, AD, Gittes RF, Stamey TA, eds: Campbell's Urology, 5th Ed. WB Saunders Co, Philadelphia, 1986, p 2832.
14. Augspurger RR, Donohue RE: Prevention of obturator nerve stimulation during transurethral surgery. J Urol 123:170, 1980.

COMPLICATIONS OF TRANSABDOMINAL PROSTATECTOMY

28

Prevention and Management

Philippe E. Zimmern • Andrei N. Lupu

In one nationwide survey, prostatectomy accounted for more than 20 percent of all urologic operations and was ranked as the most common urologic procedure.[1] This chapter focuses on the recognition and management of intraoperative as well as short-term postoperative complications of transvesical, simple retropubic, and radical retropubic prostatectomies.

MODIFIED CYSTOSTOMY

Because adequate suprapubic drainage of the bladder is an essential part of suprapubic surgery, we would like to describe briefly, at this point, a modified technique of suprapubic cystostomy based on the creation of a U-shaped cutaneous aponeurotic flap over the rectus abdominis muscles.

A U-shaped suprapubic incision is made over the rectus abdominis muscles with the tip of the U one finger breadth above the symphysis pubis (Fig. 28–1). The anterior rectus sheath is divided in the same U-shaped fashion, and a cutaneous aponeurotic flap is raised. The rectus muscles are divided in the midline and retracted laterally.

After identification of the bladder, a small anterior cystotomy is made. With one finger introduced through the cystostomy, the dome of the bladder is brought anteriorly and a 2–0 chromic catgut purse-string suture is placed encompassing the pericystis and detrusor (Fig. 28–1).

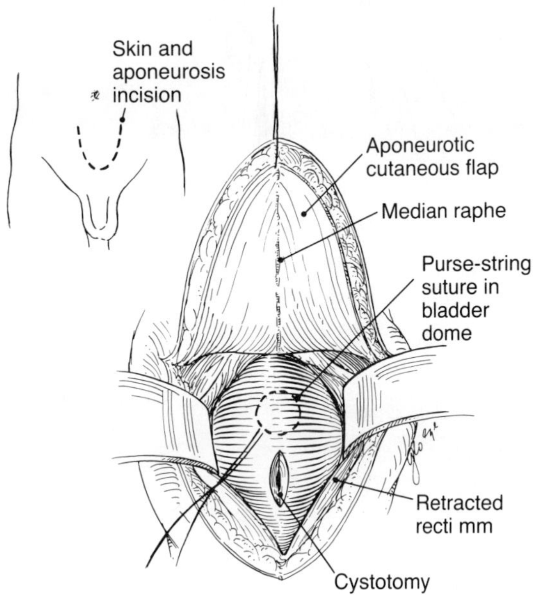

Figure 28–1. Line of incision. Identification of the bladder after reflection of the peritoneum upward. Cystotomy and purse-string placement.

If necessary, and prior to the placement of the purse-string suture, the peritoneal reflection can be bluntly freed. A tonsil forceps is passed through the cystostomy and brought out through the middle of the purse string (Fig. 28–2*A*). The cutaneous aponeurotic flap is lowered to its initial position, and the tonsil forceps is advanced through a stab wound placed toward the base of

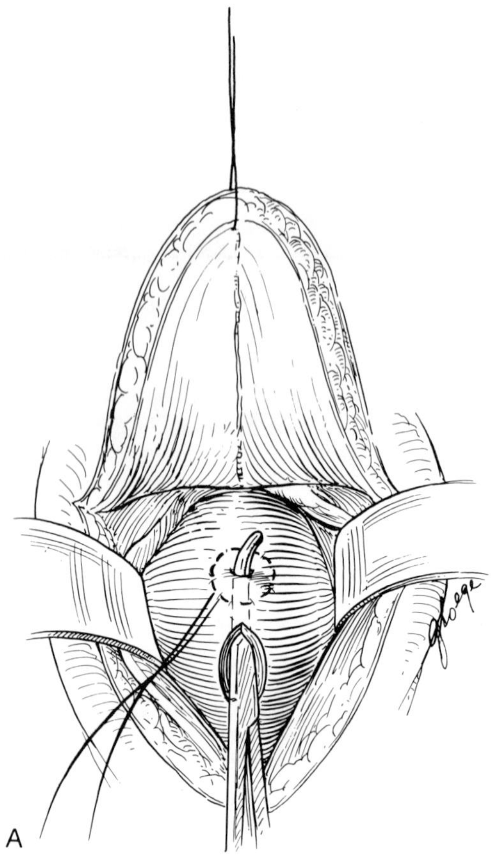

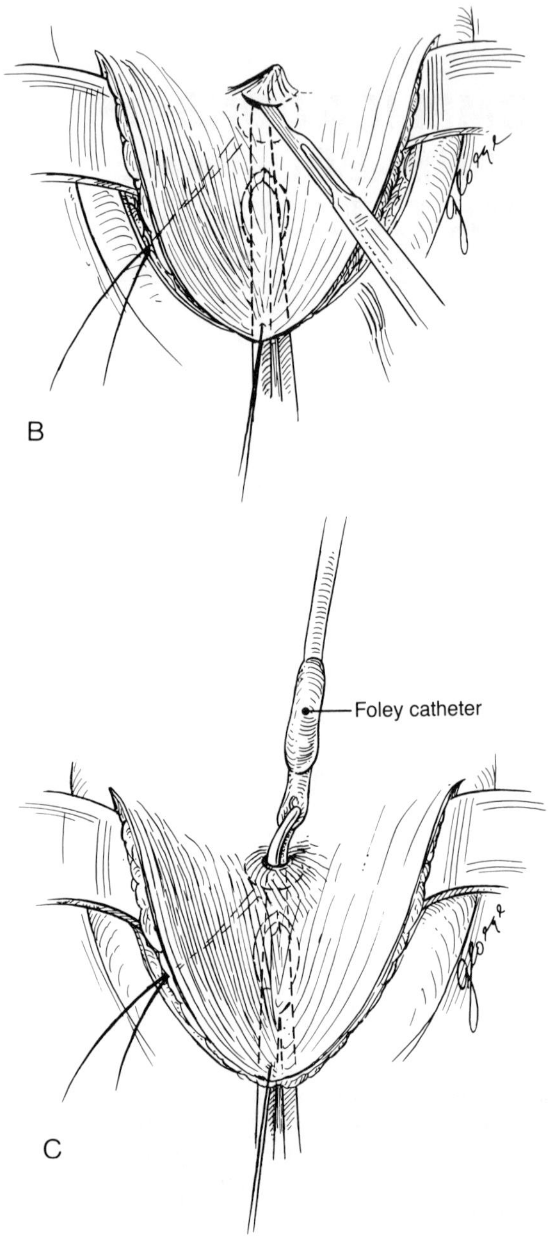

Figure 28–2. *A–C*, Placement of a large catheter in the dome of the bladder through separate abdominal and vesical incisions.

the flap and overlying the purse string (Fig. 28–2*B*). A large Foley or Malecot catheter is then grasped with the forceps and brought into the bladder (Fig. 28–2*C*).

The purse string suture is tied around the catheter, and the cystostomy is closed in two layers. A second purse string is placed and tied about the catheter and secured to the aponeurosis. A small *Penrose drain* is used, and the incision is closed in layers. The catheter is secured to the skin with two nonabsorbable sutures (Fig. 28–3).

The advantages of this simple technique reside in the short distance between bladder and skin, allowing for uncomplicated catheter change postoperatively, as well as in the placement of the catheter in the middle of the flap far removed from the incision line.

INTRAOPERATIVE COMPLICATIONS

Incision of the Abdominal Wall

With the patient under general or spinal anesthesia in a *supine* position with shoulder

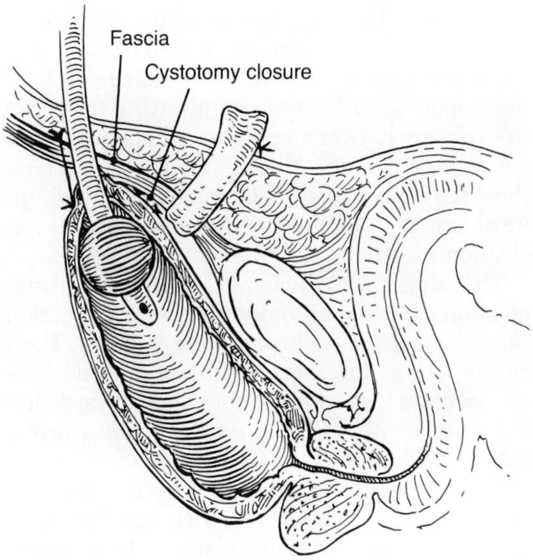

Figure 28–3. Final result after closure of the cystotomy with drainage of the retropubic space.

braces, the table can be flexed in the midline and tilted slightly in the Trendelenburg position, although some operators argue that the resulting tension on the abdominal muscles later prevents full extension of the retractors.[2] After adequate prepping and draping, the right-handed surgeon comes to stand on the left side of the patient and passes a 20 French (Fr.) catheter in the bladder.

A vertical *midline suprapubic incision*, extending from the pubis to the left border of the umbilicus, is made through the skin, subcutaneous tissue, and linea alba. The rectus abdomini muscles are separated in the midline. By incising the medial edge of their tendinous insertion on the symphysis pubis, one can often improve the *exposure* of the space of Retzius.

Medially, the prevesical and retropubic spaces are developed carefully in order to avoid injury to the *Santorini's venous plexus* coursing on the prostatic capsule and anterior bladder wall. Laterally, with the help of an Israel retractor lifting up the rectus muscle, the hand gently sweeps the peritoneum off the external iliac vessels and can easily expose the psoas muscle and the ureter if needed.

During this maneuver, however, the *epigastric vessels* can be torn and, in this case, should be ligated and divided. Also, if a small *peritoneotomy* occurs during the dissection of the dome of the bladder, especially in multioperated patients, it should be closed with a running absorbable suture.

Suprapubic Prostatectomy

In opposition to the incision described above, some authors recommend a transverse Pfannenstiel incision made two finger breadths above the symphysis.[3] After bladder distention (200 to 300 ml), two Allis clamps (or stay sutures) are placed on the anterior surface of the bladder 2 to 4 cm above the bladder neck. With these clamps elevated, a vertical or transverse *cystostomy* is performed and extended bluntly or sharply.

Long stay sutures are then placed on the edges of the cystostomy to facilitate bladder exposure, placement of a self-retaining retractor, and finger introduction later during the procedure. The bladder is inspected for stone, bladder diverticulum, and location of *the ureteric orifices*. Visualization of the orifices may necessitate intravenous injection of indigo carmine, lateral traction on the bladder neck area with narrow Deaver retractors, or flattening of the trigone by elevation of the prostatic lobes grasped with tenaculum forceps. Rarely is there a need for ureteral catheterization (proximity to the neck of a diverticulum to be resected).

The bladder mucosa covering the prostate is incised circumferentially with the long handle of a Bovie cautery to prevent mucosal tearings during the enucleation. The bladder retractor and sponges are removed. The index finger is inserted into the prostatic urethra and breaks the thin anterior prostatic adenoma against the symphysis pubis medially.

Next, the enucleation plane is developed laterally and posteriorly. At this point, some authors recommend freeing the apical attachments to prevent damage to the *external sphincteric mechanism* during the extraction of the adenoma later on.[3] Others complete the digital enucleation and, after retracting the adenoma superiorly, transect the prostatic urethra with blunt Satinsky scissors.

The prostate is withdrawn and inspected to determine whether all the adenoma has been removed, whereas the prostatic fossa is *packed* with sponges or head roll. Presence of seminal vesicles in the specimen signifies rupture of the posterior capsule. It must be repaired and reanastomosed to the bladder neck after careful examination of the rectal wall for tears.

The retractors are repositioned and the *bleeding points at the bladder neck* are controlled with figure-of-eight 2–0 chromic catgut sutures (routinely at 5 and 7 o'clock). The prostatic fossa is slowly unpacked after at least 5 minutes, and the remaining bleeding points are suture-ligated or coagulated.

Trigonization of the prostatic fossa by approximation of the mucosa to the posterior capsule is performed with the hope of reducing the incidence of bladder neck contracture. When excessive bleeding persists, a purse-string suture around the bladder neck, as described by Malament,[5] should be considered. It is tightly pulled over a large Foley catheter and brought out to the skin, where it is tied over a button. After 1 or 2 days, it is simply removed by cutting and pulling one end.

When hemostasis is achieved, a 22 Fr. Foley catheter is inserted in the bladder while a 26 Fr. Malecot suprapubic catheter is positioned in the dome of the bladder and brought out through a stab wound incision. However, since the use of the Malament encircling suture, we have found that a suprapubic cystostomy is seldom necessary.

The cystostomy is closed in two layers of running 2–0 chromic catgut. *Irrigation* is then performed and any vesical leak repaired. A prevesical Penrose drain is brought out through a lateral stab wound incision and secured to the skin.

The wound is irrigated and closed in layers. The dressing is applied with Montgomery straps and changed frequently over the subsequent postoperative days. Slow continuous saline irrigation as well as slight traction on the Foley catheter can be utilized when oozing persists in the immediate postoperative period.

Simple Retropubic Prostatectomy

For the first part of the procedure, the patient's position and the exposure to the prostate and retropubic space are the same as described under "Incision of the Abdominal Wall." The *preprostatic fat* is gently freed upward and laterally to expose the anterior surface of the prostatic capsule. Superficial veins should be ligated or coagulated to prevent retraction and troublesome bleeding under the pubic arch.

Before the prostatic capsule is incised, it is recommended that deep interrupted sutures be placed in the prostatic capsule around the future line of incision.[6] First, it helps to localize the midline of the capsular closure. Second, it offers good control of the blood vessels underrunning the capsule. The most lateral sutures that control the prostatic branches also prevent tearing of the capsule during enucleation of a large adenoma. With the long handle of the bovie cautery, the *prostatic capsule is incised transversely* down to the prostate. A *plane of cleavage* is then developed on either side by inserting the tip of the scissors between capsule and adenoma and spreading them gently. An Allis clamp placed on the edge of the capsular incision and pulled upward may help in entering the appropriate enucleation plane.

The adenoma is then enucleated using Metzenbaum scissors or blunt fingertip dissection starting medially and continuing laterally. Each lateral lobe of the prostate is then grasped with a tenaculum to retract the adenoma upward, and the attachments to the *prostatic urethra proximal to the veru montanum* are transected under vision or finger guidance using curved-tip Satinsky scissors.[7] The adenoma is elevated through the capsulotomy. An Allis clamp is now placed on the superior edge of the capsular incision and pulled upward to allow dissection toward the bladder neck.

The bladder neck mucosa is entered anteriorly and circumferentially incised on top of the adenoma in order to complete the enucleation. The anterior lip of the bladder neck can be retracted with a narrow Deaver to expose the trigone and *the ureteric orifices*. In case of a large median lobe, their exact location must be determined (indigo carmine intravenously, ureteral catheters) before incising the bladder neck mucosa. Despite a large capsulotomy, some large prostates can be extracted at the rate of only one lobe at a time.

The prostatic fossa is packed, and *absorbable hemostatic sutures* are placed in the bladder neck at 5 o'clock and 7 o'clock. After 5 minutes, the prostatic pack is irrigated with warm saline and slowly removed. Prostatic fossa bleeders are coagulated or suture-ligated. To prevent bladder neck contracture, trigonization of the prostatic fossa is performed by suturing the inferior edge of the trigone down inside of the posterior prostatic capsule. A 22 Fr. Foley catheter is inserted in the bladder, and the balloon is inflated. The capsulotomy is closed with interrupted 2–0 chromic catgut, and the Foley catheter is irrigated at the end of the closure to ensure its *watertightness*. The wound is then closed in layers and drained with a Penrose tube as described under "Suprapubic Prostatectomy."

Radical Retropubic Prostatectomy

The patient's position and the exposure to the prostate and bladder are the same as described under "Incision of the Abdominal Wall." Bilaterally, the *vas deferens* is isolated, freed up to the spermatic vessels, and followed cranially to the peritoneal reflection, from which it is bluntly freed by separation off the spermatic fascia. Its liberation is continued alongside the bladder wall and away from the peritoneum as deep as possible in the pelvis, where it is finally divided and ligated or clipped.

For better exposure of the iliac vessels and easy bladder mobilization, the peritoneum is bluntly and gently freed from the spermatic vessels. This maneuver allows cranial retraction of the peritoneum and ultimately facilitates the bladder descent at the time of vesicourethral anastomosis. At this point, the operator can position either a self-retaining Balfour retractor or a ring (Wilkinson retractor). Both permit the use of a malleable center blade to retract the peritoneum superiorly; however, the latter retractor allows the placement of an additional lateral malleable blade on the bladder to widen the exposure for pelvic lymphadenectomy.

The dissection for a limited staging lymphadenectomy proceeds medial to the external iliac artery and encompasses the lymphatics from the node of Cloquet up to the angle between the external iliac and hypogastric arteries. Care is taken to avoid injury to the *obturator nerve* and to the *obturator vessels*.[8] Careful clipping or tying of lymphatic vessels is of utmost importance in preventing postoperative *lymphocele*.

At this point, Walsh and colleagues recommend[9] placing bulldog clamps on the hypogastric arteries to reduce blood loss throughout the remainder of the procedure. In our experience, however, this was not necessary. In rare instances when access to the membranous urethra is difficult, we perform a *partial pubic symphysiectomy*. A triangle-shaped piece of bone is removed using the Gigli saw, and the opening is enlarged by further bone chipping. Bone wax is applied to the raw bony surfaces. We have not experienced any morbidity related to partial symphysiectomy.

The next step is the incision of the *endopelvic fascia* without entering the lateral venous plexuses. The safest place to enter the endopelvic fascia is at its reflection over the pelvic sidewall, just above the levator ani. After completing this incision bilaterally, the surgeon can palpate the apex of the prostate. By dividing the *puboprostatic ligaments* at this pubic attachment, the dorsal venous complex becomes easily accessible. Separate dissection and ligation of the superficial branch of the dorsal vein to facilitate the exposure of the *dorsal venous complex* at the prostatourethral junction is recommended by Catalona.[10]

Control of the dorsal venous complex is essential to minimize bleeding loss during the rest of the procedure.[11] After identification of the urethra by palpation of the Foley catheter, a right-angle clamp is passed through the avascular plane located anterior to the urethra and posterior to the dorsal venous complex. A heavy ligature—silk or polyglycolic acid for those concerned by leaving nonabsorbable material in close proximity to the urinary tract—is passed around the dorsal venous complex and tied. The right-angle clamp is passed again and can be gently opened to better define the plane between urethra and dorsal venous complex. Then using the closed right-angle clamp to protect the underlying urethra, the dorsal venous complex is transected on the bladder side of the ligature. Significant backflow, which is rare, must be controlled with running or interrupted figure-of-eight absorbable sutures on the anterior surface of the prostate. Additional suture ligation of the cut section of the dorsal venous complex can be performed to achieve hemostasis. *Fascial bands*, posterolateral to the urethra and containing the innervation of the corpora cavernosa, are sharply dissected off the urethra. With the help of an umbilical tape passed around the urethra, the *anterior urethra* is incised at its junction to the apex of the prostate.

Through the urethral opening, the Foley catheter is grasped with a curved heavy clamp and divided. Lifting the catheter exposes the posterior urethral wall, which is sharply divided. Excessive pulling on the Foley catheter may tear the membranous urethra. For fear of loosing the urethral stump, placement of sutures for later use during the vesicourethral anastomosis is suggested by Catalona.[10] However, others argue that the anatomic relationship between the ligated dorsal venous complex and the urethra prevents retraction of the urethral stump and that inadvertent pulling of the sutures during subsequent maneuvers is not uncommon.[2,9] We favor placing the anastomotic sutures after removal of the prostate and completion of the bladder neck reconstruction.

To free the apex of the prostate from the underlying rectum requires blunt or sharp incision of the *rectourethralis muscle* on the midline. Its division gives access to the plane between rectum and prostate *(Denonvillier's fascia)*, which can be defined by finger dissection on the midline. Although rare, a *rectotomy* can occur, especially in scarred tissues after either prior transurethral resection of the prostate or radiation. Depending on its extent and assuming an adequate preoperative colorectal cleansing, immediate two-layer closure of the rectum, placement of a nasogastric tube, prolonged alimentary restriction, and broad-spectrum antibiotics will prevent postoperative urethrorectal fistula. Diverting colostomy, however, should always be considered in face of fecal contamination, poorly vascularized tissues after radiation, and extended rectotomy.

Starting from the apex of the prostate and advancing cranially, the lateral surface of the prostate is progressively freed bilaterally from the *lateral pelvic fascia,* anteriorly enough on the lateral surface of the prostate to preserve the neurovascular bundle. If involved by tumor, the ipsilateral bundle is sacrificed. At this point of the procedure, the *seminal vesicles* can be identified posteriorly with their tips coming, laterally, close to the neurovascular bundle.

Next, the bladder neck is transected and the bladder entered on the midline. The balloon of the Foley is deflated, and its tip is grasped in a curved clamp to provide traction on the prostate. The bladder mucosa is incised circumferentially on top of the prostate, after localizing the *ureteric orifices* (indigo carmine IV). The prostatic pedicles are clamped and ligated laterally. Complete incision of the bladder neck is achieved, and the rectovesical space is entered by blunt dissection. Using further blunt dissection and gentle traction on the Foley catheter, the prostate is elevated. This exposes the *ampullae of the vasa deferentia* and the seminal vesicles.

The final step consists of freeing the vasa deferentia and mobilizing the seminal vesicles after careful ligation of their pedicles, which are near the neurovascular bundles. The specimen is removed and examined.

Narrowing of the bladder neck is then undertaken to fit in size with the remaining urethra. Rather than a horizontal closure, we recommend a vertical closure, which offers less chance of injuring the ureteric orifices and transposes the bladder neck anteriorly in a more mobile position than the fixed trigone, allowing a tension-free *vesicourethral anastomosis* later on. The *reconstituted bladder neck* should accept one finger breadth. Its mucosal lining is *everted* to provide better apposition with the urethral stump.[10]

At this point, the pelvis should be irrigated with antibiotic solution and the hemostasis completed carefully. Four to six absorbable ligatures are passed from the urethra to the bladder neck with special care not to injure the neurovascular bundle adjacent to the urethra and not to cross the sutures over. A two-way or three-way catheter is advanced in the bladder, and its balloon is inflated. If used, the kidney rest should be taken down before tying the vesicourethral sutures. The posterior sutures at 5 o'clock and 7 o'clock are tied first, so that if one breaks during tying, it can still be fairly easily replaced. Dropping the bladder down in the pelvis releases the tension during tying. To prevent inadvertent loss of the Foley catheter secondary to balloon deflation in the postoperative period, a nonabsorbable suture anchored at the tip of the catheter is transferred with a Keith needle to the outside through the bladder and abdominal walls and is secured over a button.[10] The danger, however, is to tilt up the tip of the catheter on the anterior bladder wall, thereby preventing adequate dependent drainage of the bladder.

Using a Toomey syringe, the bladder is filled slowly to assess the watertightness of the vesicourethral anastomosis. Slight traction on the Foley catheter can be applied and continuous bladder irrigation started if necessary. *Drainage of the retropubic space* is mandatory before wound closure.

Hemorrhage

There is little doubt that the most feared intraoperative complication of abdominal prostatic surgery is profuse beeding. During *suprapubic prostatectomy,* excessive bleeding may occur from the prostatic fossa after enucleation as well as from the incised bladder neck mucosa. In our experience, placement of a Malament suture has always resulted in satisfactory hemostasis (see above).

During *retropubic prostatectomy,* bleeding from the capsulotomy can be prevented by carefully "boxing" the incision line. Excessive bleeding from the prostatic fossa is usually due to a faulty plane of cleavage. If bleeding occurs at the start of the dissection, every effort should be made to find the adequate cleavage plane. When bleed occurs late in the dissection, the adenoma is removed and suture ligatures are placed. If control of bleeding is still inadequate, the capsulotomy is closed and the bladder is opened to place a Malament encircling suture.

During *radical retropubic prostatectomy,* the two most common points of bleeding result from

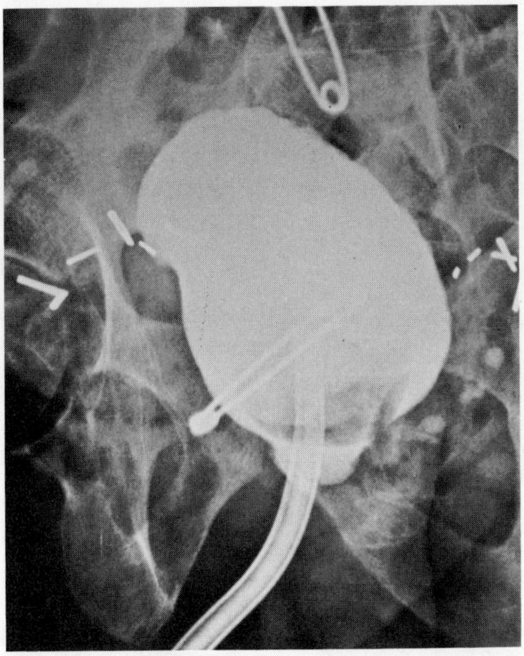

Figure 28–4. Two weeks after placement of Vest sutures, a cystogram demonstrates no extravasation.

injury to the obturator vessels during the lymph node dissection or from inadequate hemostatic control of the dorsal venous complex. In the first instance, the bleeding vessels can usually be identified, cross-clamped, and ligated. Great care should be taken not to injure the obturator nerve. In the presence of profuse bleeding from the plexus of Santorini, cross-clamping is mostly fruitless. A tourniquet is placed at the base of the penis,[12] and after transection of the membranous urethra, a 22 Fr. Foley catheter with a 30-ml balloon is advanced in the urethra. The balloon is inflated to 50 ml, and traction is applied. This maneuver reduces the bleeding to a minimum, allowing the surgeon to proceed with the rest of the procedure. If at the time of vesicourethral anastomosis and after balloon deflation bleeding recurs, placement of anastomotic sutures is forsaken. The catheter is advanced into the bladder, the balloon inflated to 50 ml, and the bladder is brought in contact to the membranous urethra and pubic arch by traction on the Foley catheter. This provides satisfactory tamponade to the retropubic bleeding vessels. Placement of Vest sutures is also useful to ensure a close vesicourethral contact,[13] and to maximize the likelihood of postoperative urinary continence (Figs. 28–4, 28–5). The tourniquet at the base of the penis is removed and additional urinary drainage is obtained by a suprapubic cystostomy. The Foley catheter is kept under light traction for 5 to 7 days. After the second day, a strong rubber band is attached to the catheter and placed under leg traction to permit ambulation without undue discomfort.

IMMEDIATE POSTOPERATIVE COMPLICATIONS

Catheter and Drain

Following *suprapubic prostatectomy,* the urethral catheter is removed early (in 5 to 7 days) as soon as the urine clears up. The suprapubic tube is removed at the seventh postoperative day if the patient can urinate adequately with the tube clamped and if the postvoid residual is less than 50 ml, determined twice. The Penrose drain is usually removed the next day if there is no urinary leakage.

Following *retropubic prostatectomy,* the urethral catheter is removed within 5 to 7 days postoperatively when the urine is clear. The drain is advanced and removed the following day if no urinary leakage occurs.

Following *radical retropubic prostatectomy,* the urethral catheter is left indwelling for 14 to 21 days and the drain is removed either as soon as it becomes dry or only after the urethral catheter has been discontinued. We recommend a voiding cystourethrogram before removing the urethral catheter to rule out vesicourethral extravasation.

Early inadvertent withdrawal of the catheter can be prevented with the button technique (see "Radical Retropubic Prostatectomy"). Otherwise, the options to reposition the urethral catheter in the bladder vary according to the time elapsed since the surgery. Immediately postoperatively, one simple catheterizing attempt can be done prior to open surgical repositioning. Careful cystoscopy can be attempted to guide a ureteral stent in the bladder, over which a Foley catheter can be advanced after removal of the cystoscope. After a few days, it is usually easy to recatheterize the patient with or without the help of cystoscopy.

Urinary Leakage

Leakage always stops after additional catheter drainage. Most authors advocate removal of the

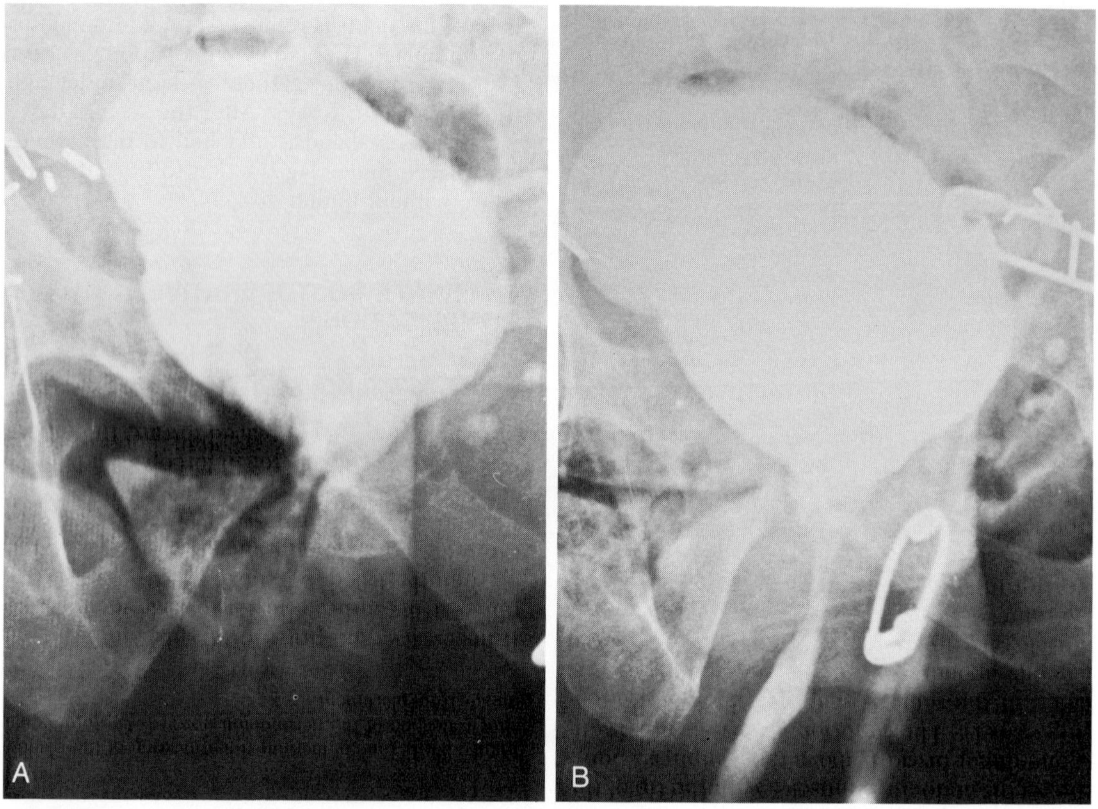

Figure 28–5. *A,B,* Two months later, a good level of continence is achieved with no evidence of bladder neck contracture on the voiding film.

retropubic drain 1 day after the catheter has been discontinued in case leakage should occur after removal of the catheter.

Additional Complications

Fever and Wound Infection. Infection of the retropubic space from undrained urinoma is no longer seen with the accepted practice of drainage.

Epididymitis. Epididymitis has become a rare complication. Prophylactic bilateral vasectomy, previously used, is seldom employed nowadays.

Atelectasis and Pneumonia. Both are preventable with incentive spirometry.

Deep Venous Thrombosis. This is a rare but feared complication. Heparin therapy started prior to the procedure is apparently the best preventive modality.[14] Elastic stockings and early mobilization may or may not be helpful.

References

1. Rutkow IM: Urological operations in United States. J Urol 135:1206, 1986.
2. Paulson DF: Management of prostatic malignancy. In DeKernion JB, Paulson DF, eds: Genitourinary Cancer Management. Philadelphia, Lea & Febiger, 1987.
3. O'Connor VJ, Jr: Suprapubic and retropubic prostatectomy. In Harrison JH, Gittes RF, Perlmutter AD, Stamey TA, Walsh AC, eds: Campbell's Urology. Philadelphia: WB Saunders Co, 1979, pp 2299–2313.
4. Hodges CV, Barry JM: Suprapubic and retropubic prostatectomy for prostatic hyperplasia. Urol Clin North Am 2:49, 1975.
5. Malament M: Maximal hemostasis in suprapubic prostatectomy. Surg Gynecol Obstet 120:1307, 1965.
6. Millin T: Retropubic prostatectomy: new extravesical technique. Report on 20 cases. Lancet 2:693, 1945.
7. Nanninga JB: Suprapubic and retropubic prostatectomy. American Urological Association, Update Series, Vol 3, Lesson 8. Houston, 1984.
8. Donohue JP: Lymphadenectomy in urologic cancers. Part II. American Urological Association, Update Series. Vol 3, Lesson 39. Houston, 1984.
9. Walsh PC, Lepor H, Eggleston JC: Radical prostatectomy with preservation of sexual function: anatomical and pathological considerations. Prostate 4:473, 1983.
10. Catalona WJ: Nerve-sparing radical retropubic prostatectomy. Urol Clin North Am 12:187, 1985.

11. Reiner WG, Walsh PC: An anatomical approach to the surgical management of the dorsal vein and Santorini's plexus during radical retropubic surgery. J Urol 121:198, 1979.
12. Kaufman JJ, Katske FA: Simple technique to control venous bleeding during radical retropubic prostatectomy and cystectomy. Urology 20:309, 1982.
13. Vest SA: Radical perineal prostatectomy: modification of closure. Surg Gynecol Obstet 70:935, 1940.
14. Roberts HR, Adel S, Bernstein EF, et al: Thrombosis and embolism: consensus conference. JAMA 256:744, 1986.

COMPLICATIONS OF RADICAL RETROPUBIC PROSTATECTOMY

29

Robert R. Bahnson • William J. Catalona

Recent modifications in operative technique have made conceptualization and performance of radical retropubic prostatectomy less difficult than previously. This operation offers the patient the greatest chance for cure without major functional sacrifices. In this chapter, the indications for operation, preoperative evaluation, intraoperative management, and postoperative care of the patient with clinically localized carcinoma of the prostate are presented, with emphasis on factors that minimize the morbidity of radical retropubic prostatectomy. In addition, the recognition and management of specific intraoperative, perioperative, and late postoperative complications are discussed.

INDICATIONS FOR RADICAL RETROPUBIC PROSTATECTOMY

A prerequisite for the surgical cure of prostatic cancer is complete excision of the tumor. Therefore, ideal candidates for radical prostatectomy are those patients with tumor confined to the prostate who have no evidence of regional or distant metastases (stages A and B). The available evidence suggests that young patients with stage A1 carcinoma are not free of risk of disease progression, and careful consideration should be given to radical prostatectomy.[1,2] Because more than one third of patients with stage A2 tumors can be expected to experience progressive cancer and approximately 20 percent of untreated patients will die of the disease, definite treatment should be recommended.[3] It is our opinion that radical prostatectomy usually is not more difficult to perform in patients who have undergone a prior transurethral resection of the prostate (TURP). We do not believe that the interval between TURP and radical prostatectomy is of critical importance in most instances, the exceptions being patients having capsular perforation. Operation should be delayed 2 to 3 months in these patients. We have not observed an increased incontinence rate among patients who have undergone prior TURP.

No form of treatment has been shown superior to the 15-year tumor-free survival achieved with radical prostatectomy in patients with disease limited to the prostate (stage B). In a series of 57 patients at the Johns Hopkins Hospital with stage B1 lesions undergoing radical prostatectomy from 1951 to 1963, there was a 51 percent, 15-year disease-free survival equal to the survival of an aged matched control population.[4] Therefore, patients having clinical stage B1 prostate cancer are considered to be ideal candidates for radical prostatectomy if they are acceptable surgical risks and have a life expectancy of at least 10 years.

Patients with clinical stage B2 prostate cancer traditionally have not been considered ideal candidates for radical prostatectomy because one half to two thirds of them may have seminal vesicle involvement compared with only about 17 percent of patients with clinical stage B1 lesions. However, the survival of patients with stage B2 tumors that were histologically confined to the prostate was comparable to that ob-

Dr. Bahnson is a recipient of the American Cancer Society Clinical Oncology Career Development Award 86–48.

served in patients with clinical stage B1 lesions.[5] If patients with B2 tumors are staged with pelvic lymphadenectomy and nodal metastases are not found, 63 to 85 percent can be expected to have tumors that are confined within the prostatic capsule and less than 10 percent will have seminal vesicle involvement.[6,7] Thus, radical prostatectomy is a legitimate option in patients having clinical stage B2 tumors in whom there is no evidence of lymph node metastases. Radical prostatectomy should probably not be recommended for patients who have unequivocal, palpable evidence of extracapsular tumor spread or persistent gross evidence of seminal vesicle involvement on radiologic imaging studies such as transrectal ultrasound, computed tomographic (CT) scanning, or magnetic resonance imaging (MRI).

There are insufficient data on the efficacy of radical prostatectomy combined with pelvic lymphadenectomy to control stage D1 disease. Kramer and associates[8] reported that the median time to treatment failure in patients with stage D1 tumors was similar among patients treated with delayed endocrine therapy, radical prostatectomy, or extended field radiation therapy. Further evidence limiting the applicability of radical prostatectomy to patients with stage D1 tumors is the fact that the vast majority of these patients also have extraprostatic tumor extension. Catalona and Stein reported that only 31 percent of patients with lymph node metastases had primary tumors that were histologically confined within the prostatic capsule.[9] Although long-term survival has been reported in a few patients with minimal nodal disease,[10] the great majority of patients with stage D1 disease experience progression irrespective of treatment. Therefore, it seems unjustified to categorically recommend that all patients with stage D1 prostate cancer undergo radical prostatectomy in an attempt to salvage the small proportion of patients having tumors that theoretically are curable.

PREOPERATIVE EVALUATION

Our preoperative staging evaluation consists of bone scan, transrectal ultrasound, serum acid phosphatase (enzymatic method), and serum prostate–specific antigen (Hybritech). A bone scan is the most sensitive means of detecting osseous metastases.[11] However, it is relatively nonspecific and suspected areas should be viewed along with roentgenograms or CT scans with bone windows. An area of increased radionuclide uptake that is not visualized on skeletal radiographs or CT scan should be subject to biopsy. Definitive localization of the appropriate site for bone biopsy using preoperative scintigraphic imaging can be performed.[12] An elevated prostatic acid phosphatase (PAP) level is generally indicative of metastatic disease. Interpretation is difficult because elevations of PAP can occur when the cancer is limited to the prostate or, conversely, because some patients with disseminated cancer may have normal PAP values. Because transrectal and transurethral manipulation of the prostate may produce transient elevation of PAP,[13] these determinations are best performed before or 48 hours after manipulation. Since it is well established that elevation of acid phosphatase in patients with clinically localized carcinoma of the prostate is an unfavorable prognostic sign,[14] these patients should probably not be subjected to radical prostatectomy. We do not find that routine CT scanning is necessary because it has been found to be relatively insensitive to extracapsular tumor spread and is generally inaccurate in predicting seminal vesicle invasion. CT scanning does not allow discrimination between tumor tissue and normal prostatic tissue. At the Washington University Medical Center, CT scanning has been found to have a sensitivity of 20 percent in detecting seminal vesicle invasion and a sensitivity of 14 percent in detecting tumor extension into the periprostatic fat.[15] However, CT scanning may show gross involvement of seminal vesicles or pelvic nodes.

Although early reports suggest that MRI may be more accurate for local staging of prostate cancer than CT scanning, we have not found this to be true. In the Washington University series, the sensitivity of MRI for detecting extracapsular extension of prostatic cancer was 29 percent using periprostatic fat extension as a criterion, 57 percent using disturbance of the periprostatic venous plexus as a criterion, and 50 percent using alterations of the seminal vesicles as a criterion. The overall sensitivity of using all three criteria was 87 percent with a specificity of 90 percent and accuracy of 89 percent, but in some instances extracapsular extension was read on the MRI scan for the wrong reasons.[16]

We have adopted transrectal ultrasonography of the prostate in an attempt to accurately stage the local extent of tumor in prostatic cancer patients. Scardino[28] reported that transrectal ultrasonography is more sensitive and accurate than digital rectal examination. Staging by digital rectal examination was accurate in only 52 percent of 81 cases, and when digital rectal examination indicated that the tumor was confined to the prostate, the tumor proved to be confined in only 46% of patients (positive predictive value). By contrast, transrectal ultrasound accurately staged 75 percent of the patients. The positive predictive power of transrectal ultrasound for indicating a tumor confined to the prostate was 70 percent. Both digital rectal examination and transrectal ultrasound showed high predictive power for tumors that were not confined (78 to 79 percent).[17]

It is recommended that patients with clinical stage A or B prostatic cancer and a life expectancy of 10 years or more be treated with radical prostatectomy. A careful history is taken with a thorough review of systems. It is particularly important to assess the relative health of the cardiovascular, pulmonary, and renal systems. Notation of previous ischemic heart disease, congestive failure, valvular heart disease, arrhythmias, and hypertension should be made. With patients who have suffered recent myocardial infarction, surgery should be delayed because perioperative reinfarction is frequent and the mortality from reinfarction is approximately 69 percent.[18] Patients with signs and symptoms of ischemic heart disease should be evaluated with a treadmill or thallium stress test. Hypertension should be brought under medical control. A preoperative pulmonary evaluation should include an estimate of the patient's exercise tolerance. If there is any suspicion of diminished pulmonary reserve, pulmonary function tests and room air blood gas determinations should be performed. Patients at high risk, i.e., forced expiratory volume (FEV_1) less than 15 ml/kg, vital capacity (VC) less than 1.5 liters, or maximal voluntary ventilation (MVV) less than 50 percent of predicted normal, should be evaluated further.[19] If there is any history of renal dysfunction, a creatinine clearance should be obtained, since it is the best measure of renal impairment and a better predictor of mortality than other measurements of renal function.[20]

Although it is uncommon in patients with low-stage prostatic cancer, a history of recent weight loss should signal the need for nutritional assessment. Skeletal muscle protein and fat stores can be adequately measured by mid-arm muscle circumference and the triceps skin-fold method, respectively. Visceral protein stores can be assessed by measurements of serum albumin, total lymphocyte count, and reactivity to recall skin-test antigens. An albumin of less than 3.5 gm/dl, a lymphocyte count of less than 15,000/ml, and anergy to skin test antigens such as mumps, *Candida*, and streptokinase-streptodornase are indicators of protein-calorie malnutrition. Such patients should receive preoperative nutritional support for 2 to 3 weeks to restore these deficits because an increased incidence of surgical complications and mortality accompanies individuals with protein-calorie malnutrition.[21]

Finally, historical questions that relate to hemostatic function and thromboembolic disease are especially important. If the patient has had previous surgery or tooth extraction complicated by excessive bleeding, a diligent laboratory search is needed to uncover minor bleeding tendencies. All patients are screened with a platelet count, bleeding time, prothrombin time (PT), and partial thromboplastin time (aPTT). Patients are asked to discontinue aspirin, aspirin-containing compounds, and nonsteroidal anti-inflammatory drugs for 2 weeks prior to surgery to minimize platelet dysfunction. A previous venous thromboembolism places the patient at high risk for subsequent deep venous thrombosis and mandates that prophylactic measures be instituted.

We now routinely recommend that patients donate blood preoperatively for autologous transfusion during radical prostatectomy. This reduces the incidence of complication from transfusions, the most serious of which is the transmission of infection.[22] Despite screening for hepatitis B surface antigen and the exclusive use of volunteer blood donors, the attack rate for post-transfusion hepatitis is still approximately 7 to 10 percent or about three to six cases per 1000 units transfused.[22a] Of more immediate concern to patients is the risk of transfusion-transmitted acquired immunodeficiency syndrome (AIDS). Although the risk is small and has been reduced by the introduction of anti-HIV-antibody screening, public awareness of this potential significantly frightens many surgical patients.

Several units (450 ml) of autologous blood may be collected in a relatively short period of time. We begin supplemental iron (325 mg $FeSO_4$ three times daily) at least 1 week prior to the first phlebotomy. Donations are usually performed once a week (but can be done every 3 days) up to 72 hours before surgery. Phlebotomies are not performed on individuals in whom hemoglobin/hematocrit values fall below 11 gm/dl/34 percent. The blood has a shelf life of 35 days in citrate phosphate-dextrose-adenine-1 (CPD-A1) anticoagulant. The safety of transfusing autologous blood is reassuring for the patient because the risks of antigenic sensitization and transmission of disease are eliminated.

OPERATIVE MANAGEMENT

The evening before surgery the patient is given a cleansing enema and intravenous fluids for overnight hydration. Thigh-high anti-embolism stockings are fitted, and 1 gm of a first-generation cephalosporin is given intramuscularly on call to the operating room. We do not use minidose heparin because it is associated with an increased incidence of prolonged lymphatic drainage and lymphocele formation.[23] The patient is positioned supine on the operating table and shaved. Sequential compression stockings are placed on the lower extremities. Unless contraindicated, an epidural or spinal anesthetic is administered because it is safe and has been shown to result in decreased operative blood loss.[24] A nerve-sparing technique is then utilized for radical retropubic prostatectomy, which was originally developed by Dr. Patrick C. Walsh.[25] The design of the operation was aided by a detailed dissection in stillborn male infants of the neurovascular bundles that innervate the corpora cavernosa.[26] A complete description of the technique that we use to perform potency-sparing surgery for localized prostate cancer has been published.[27] We begin the procedure by performing a limited bilateral pelvic lymphadenectomy with frozen section diagnosis. At the conclusion of the procedure, we place two suction drains deep in the pelvis and a Foley catheter is left to dependent drainage.

POSTOPERATIVE MANAGEMENT

The patient takes nothing by mouth until he passes flatus. The diet is then slowly advanced as tolerated. When a solid diet is tolerated, colace is given in order to avoid constipation. Antibiotics are administered for only two doses following surgery. Intermittent, sequential compression stockings are left on until the patient is fully ambulatory. The closed suction drains are removed no earlier than postoperative day 5 or until the drainage is less than 30 ml per day. If there is persistent drainage, the suction is discontinued. This usually results in diminished drainage. The Foley catheter is kept at dependent drainage, and the patient is usually discharged between the seventh and tenth postoperative days. The patient returns to the surgeon's office 2 weeks following the operation, and the Foley catheter is removed at that time.

COMPLICATIONS SPECIFIC TO RADICAL RETROPUBIC PROSTATECTOMY

Although generally well tolerated, radical retropubic prostatectomy has been previously reported to involve considerable morbidity. In early series, morbidity rates as high as 52 percent[28] were reported; in contemporary series, complications have diminished to 32[29] and 20 percent.[30] Mortality has been as high as 2.5 percent,[31] but more recent series have reported surgical deaths in only 0[29,32] to 1.5 percent of patients.[30] Morbidity can be grouped into *operative, early postoperative,* and *late postoperative* complications.

Operative Complications

Hemorrhage

The most common operative complication is severe hemorrhage. It has been reported that the use of regional anesthesia and bulldog clamps on the hypogastric arteries are associated with reduced blood loss.[33] Careful management of the dorsal venous complex is crucial to limit excessive blood loss. The puboprostatic ligaments must be sharply divided under direct vision to mobilize the prostate and facilitate separation of the dorsal venous complex from the urethra. In patients who have undergone previous transurethral resection of the prostate, the dorsal venous complex can be densely adherent to the anterior surface of the prostate. In this situation, a right-angle clamp must be passed further caudad beyond the area of scarring from the previous transurethral resection (Fig. 29–1). In our experience, back bleeding from the transected dorsal venous complex can be severe, and we routinely use a running, chromic suture ligature on the anterolateral surface of the prostate for control. During division of the lateral pelvic fascia, any small arteriolar or venous branches encountered should be individually tied using *fine sutures* as opposed to *cautery* or *mass ligatures,* which could produce injury to the neurovascular bundle. Troublesome, persistent bleeding can occasionally occur from the depths of the obturator fossa. This can almost always be managed by temporary packing with a laparot-

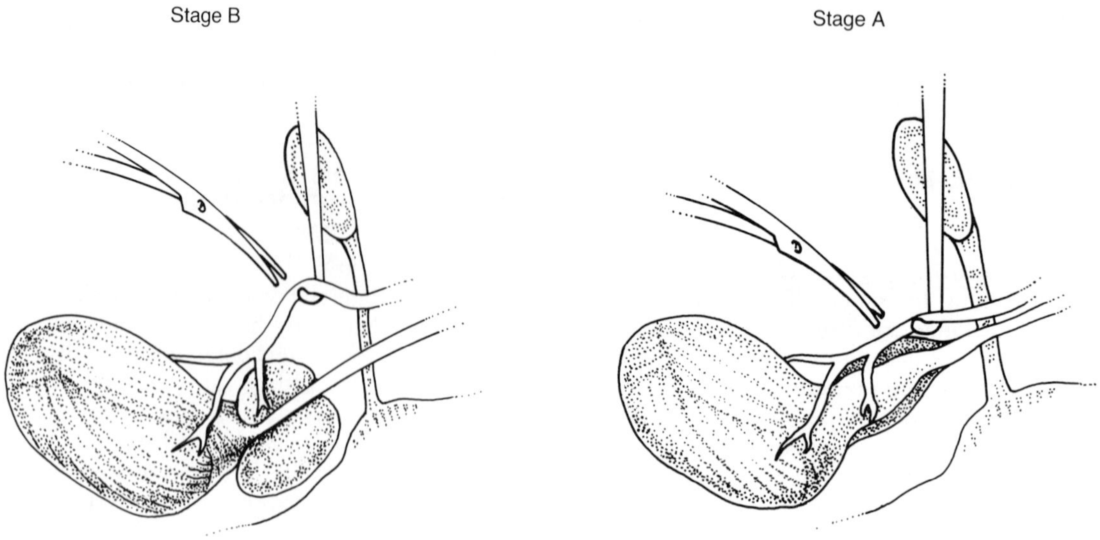

Figure 29–1. The dorsal venous complex is adherent to the anterior surface of the prostate following a transurethral resection (stage A). Ligation and division of the complex should be performed distally, where it can be more easily mobilized from the surface of the prostate.

omy sponge while surgical efforts are directed elsewhere.

Rectal Injury

Injury to the rectum has been reported to occur in 0 to 7 percent of radical retropubic prostatectomies. In patients with stage C or D1 carcinoma of the prostate, the reported incidence (17 percent) of rectal wall injury is considerably higher.[34] If a rectal laceration occurs, the safest, most prudent plan is to close the rectum in two layers, defunctionalize the anal sphincter by wide digital dilatation, and perform a diverting colostomy. In one series of 11 patients who underwent closure primarily without a colostomy, fistula developed in four; of the four patients who had undergone colostomy, fistula developed in none.[35]

Ureteral Injury

Although injury to the ureter is uncommon, it can occur during lymphadenectomy or when dissecting the bladder neck and trigone from the area of the seminal vesicles. This should be treated by ureteral reimplantation.

Obturator Nerve Injury

Accidental injury of the obturator nerve is an infrequent (1.3 percent) complication usually associated with pelvic lymph node dissection.[36] If complete transection occurs, primary reanastomosis with fine, permanent sutures should be performed.

Early Postoperative Complications

Deep Venous Thrombosis and Wound Infection

The most frequent early complications are deep venous thrombosis and wound infection. Deep venous thrombosis is reported to occur in 3 to 12 percent of patients.[37] It should be noted, however, that the incidence of deep venous thrombosis varies, depending on the physician's index of suspicion and on the sensitivity and specificity of the diagnostic test chosen for confirmation. Although some authors have recommended routine postoperative anticoagulation, we do not employ this approach. Intermittent, sequential compression stockings are utilized intraoperatively and are not removed until the patient is fully ambulatory. The patients are ambulated as soon as feasible after surgery, preferably on the first postoperative day.

Clinically documented pulmonary embolism has been reported in up to 4.6 percent of patients.[30] Patients with suspected pulmonary emboli undergo immediate ventilation perfusion scanning in the Nuclear Medicine department. Those with a high probability of pulmonary embolism are treated immediately with systemic anticoagulation utilizing a continuous heparin infusion sufficient to prolong the PTT to 1.5 to two times control. This is continued for 7 to 10 days with at least a 5-day overlap with oral anticoagulants. Anticoagulation is continued for 3 months using oral anticoagulants to prolong the prothrombin time to 1.2 to 1.5 times control. Patients with intermediate probability of pulmonary embolism on scanning undergo pulmonary angiography and are treated if findings are positive. Patients with a low probability of pulmonary embolism are followed expectantly with observation.

Wound infection has been reported in 0 to 16 percent of patients.[37] The incidence can be reduced by the use of perioperative antibiotics, shaving of the patient in the operating room immediately prior to surgery, and copious irrigation of subcutaneous tissues prior to wound closure.

Excessive Drainage

Prolonged drainage from the suction drains can be due to either a urine leak from the vesicourethral anastomosis or from excessive lymphatic fluid. During lymphadenectomy, we favor meticulous use of cautery and small hemoclips to reduce the incidence of postoperative lymphatic drainage. In cases of excessive drainage, a specimen of the drainage should be sent for blood urea nitrogen (BUN)/creatinine determination. If the drainage results parallel the serum values, the drains are taken off suction and the patient is observed. If a urine leak is confirmed by a high BUN and creatinine value, the drains are similarly taken off suction and the Foley catheter is left indwelling until the anastomotic leak seals. Lymphoceles are managed expectantly unless they have significant clinical manifestations. If treatment is required, we now favor percutaneous drainage with slow advancement of the drainage tube.

Loss of Catheter

Occasionally, loss of the urethral catheter owing to a defective retention balloon can occur. Testing of the catheter balloon should be performed prior to its insertion during bladder neck reconstruction. In this situation, if the catheter does not pass easily on the first gentle attempt, the patient is taken to the cystoscopy suite and a 0.035-inch, floppy tipped Bentson guide wire is passed into the bladder under direct vision using the cystoscope. A well-lubricated 20 French (Fr.) Council-tipped Foley catheter is then passed over the guide wire into the bladder utilizing fluoroscopic guidance. This ensures an atraumatic catheter passage and minimizes the chance of a vesicourethral anastomotic disruption.

Late Postoperative Complications

The most frequent late complications of radical retropubic prostatectomy are impotence, incontinence, and bladder neck contracture. Orchialgia may also occur.

Impotence

Until the introduction of the nerve-sparing modification, loss of sexual potency was nearly a universal consequence of radical retropubic prostatectomy. In 1982, Walsh and Donker suggested that impotence following radical prostatectomy was produced by injury to the pelvic nerve plexus, which provides the autonomic innervation to the corpora cavernosa.[26] A nerve-sparing procedure was designed aided by a detailed dissection in stillborn male infants of the neurovascular bundles that innervate the corpora cavernosa. Based upon these dissections, it was proposed that the nerves mediating erectile function were injured at the time of incision of the endopelvic fascia over the prostate, during the mobilization of the urethra, and during ligation of the lateral pedicle of the prostate. A review of the results of the nerve-sparing procedure at Johns Hopkins Hospital has been reported.[38] Sexual function was evaluated in 60 of the patients who were potent preoperatively and who had been followed for a minimum of 1 year. Of these men, 70 percent were potent postoperatively. A very definite correlation was observed between pathologic stage and postoperative potency. Surgical margins were not compromised owing to the nerve-sparing modification. In this series, the surgical margins of resection were positive in only seven patients. The adequacy of the operation has been confirmed in our series in which positive surgical margins were noted in seven (23 percent) and 24 (47 percent) of patients with clinical stage A/B1 and clinical stage B2, respectively. The data compare well to information obtained on 25 patients treated with standard radical retropubic prostatectomy in which a positive margin in two (18 percent) and seven (50 percent) of the clinical A/B1 and clinical stage B2 patients was demonstrated, respectively. Although slight differences in the incidences of positive surgical margins in the two groups were seen, these differences were not statistically significant.[27] Although the histopathologic observations suggest that the nerve-sparing modification achieved resected margins similar to those of the standard radical retropubic prostatectomy, conclusions based on histopathologic findings alone must remain tentative. Final judgment will only be known when the long-term survival free of disease in patients not treated with adjunctive endocrine or radiation therapy is known.

Most patients who exhibit onset of return of erectile activity within 3 months of surgery can be expected to have full return of erectile function but may not regain full function for up to 15 months. Most patients who regain erectile function do so within 6 months postoperatively. Patients with onset of return of erectile function delayed beyond 6 months postoperatively are unlikely to regain full function.

Patients who are impotent 12 months or more following nerve-sparing radical retropubic prostatectomy undergo papaverine testing. Early experience suggests that in many of these patients erectile dysfunction following surgery is predominantly vasculogenic in origin. Thus, factors other than injury to the neurovascular bundles may be responsible for postsurgical impotence. Patients whose erectile impotence persists beyond 15 months are offered papaverine injections or insertion of a penile prosthesis.

Incontinence

Significant incontinence persisting for more than 6 months has been reported in 0 to 57 percent of cases. Continence can be preserved after radical retropubic prostatectomy by avoiding injury to the pelvic floor musculature and the performance of an accurate mucosa-to-mucosa vesicourethral anastomosis. It has been speculated that the nerve-sparing procedure may enhance postoperative continence. It is not uncommon for patients to have stress urinary incontinence in the immediate postoperative period. These patients should be followed expectantly for a period of up to 6 months. Patients who have persistent stress urinary incontinence beyond 6 months can be treated pharmacologically with alpha-adrenergic agonists, anticholinergics, or imipramine, which mediates bladder neck tightening and detrusor relaxation. Patients with total urinary incontinence can be managed with a Cunningham clamp or a condom catheter. They can also be treated with periurethral injections of polytef (Teflon) paste or insertion of an artificial urinary sphincter around the bulbous urethra.

Bladder Neck Contracture

Stricture of the vesicourethral anastomosis (bladder neck contracture) has been reported in 2.6 to 23 percent of cases. Bladder neck contracture is usually caused by failure to achieve an accurate mucosa-to-mucosa apposition of bladder neck and urethra. Intraoperatively, the bladder neck is narrowed down to the size of an 18 Fr. Foley catheter and a technique described by Walsh is used to reconstruct the bladder neck.[39] In this technique, the mucosa of the bladder is advanced over the raw muscular edges of the bladder neck and sutured to the perivesical fascia with 4.0 chromic catgut sutures. This provides a stoma of mucosa that can be brought down to coapt accurately with the urethral mucosa using four interrupted 2–0 chromic catgut sutures placed at 2, 5, 7, and 10 o'clock. Patients with bladder neck contracture usually complain of a markedly diminished urinary stream. In these patients, a urethral sound is gently passed in the office. In many cases, an office dilation suffices in eliminating this problem. If passive dilation is not successful, patients should be returned to the operating room, where a cold knife incision of the bladder neck contracture should be made followed by transurethral injection of triamcinolone acetonide, 200 mg, to prevent further stricture formation.

Orchialgia

Another late complication is orchialgia. We believe that this is related to the ligation of the vasa deferentia at the time of the staging pelvic lymphadenectomy. In all cases, this problem has resolved spontaneously.

NERVE-SPARING RADICAL PROSTATECTOMY

At Washington University, we reviewed the complications, including continence and potency rates, in a series of 132 patients with clinically localized carcinoma of the prostate. The perioperative and postoperative complications are presented in Table 29–1. A total of 76 patients, or 58 percent of the entire population, suffered no complications related to the surgery. There were no operative mortalities. Although the initial incidence of stricture of the vesicoure-

Table 29–1. COMPLICATIONS RELATED TO NERVE-SPARING RADICAL PROSTATECTOMY IN 132 PATIENTS

	No. of Patients	Percent
Stricture	27	20.0
requiring transurethral incision	10	8.0
(stoma technique)	4/63	6.0
Pulmonary embolism	5	4.0
Retention	5	4.0
Wound infection	3	2.0
Deep vein thrombosis	2	1.5
Cholecystitis	2	1.5
Lymphocele	2	1.5
Lymph leak	1	0.8
Lymphedema	1	0.8
Epididymitis	1	0.8
Wound seroma	1	0.8
Pneumonitis	1	0.8

thral anastomosis was high, since October of 1985 (when the stoma technique was introduced for the vesicourethral anastomosis), the incidence of postoperative bladder neck contracture has been reduced to 6 percent; of those four patients, only one required transurethral incision of the bladder neck. The remaining three patients responded nicely to a single dilation with a male sound in the office.

Continence rates were computed from a total of 105 patients who were followed up for at least 6 months (Table 29–2). The majority (96 percent) had complete urinary control. Many patients for the first few weeks to months following surgery have stress-related urinary incontinence, but in the majority of these patients this totally resolves within a short period of follow-up.

Potency rates were assessed in 87 patients who were eligible for 12-month follow-up (Table 29–3). Of the 62 evaluable patients, erections sufficient for penetration were present in the majority (68 percent). The return to full erections usually occurs within the first 12 months following surgery, but an occasional patient in our series has required as much as 24 months postoperatively to achieve full erectile function.

Table 29–2. CONTINENCE (SIX-MONTH FOLLOW-UP IN 105 PATIENTS)

Condition	No. Patients (Percent)
Consistently wet	2* (2)
Precautionary pad for occasional drop	2 (2)
Continent (no pads)	101 (96)

*Postoperative radiation therapy (one patient).

Table 29–3. POTENCY (12-MONTH FOLLOW-UP IN 87 PATIENTS)

	No. of Patients (Percent)
Exclusions	
preoperative sexual dysfunction	23
endocrine therapy	1
Insufficient follow-up	2
Evaluable	62
Erections sufficient for penetration	42 (68)
Insufficient erections	20 (32)

SUMMARY

Radical retropubic prostatectomy is the best proven form of therapy for patients with a life expectancy of 10 years or more and clinically localized prostatic carcinoma. This operation can be performed safely with limited morbidity and mortality with preservation of continence and potency in the majority of patients. Although complications can and do occur, in most instances they can be prevented or easily managed. Therefore, in skilled hands, a nerve-sparing radical retropubic prostatectomy should be the treatment of choice for patients with potentially curable prostatic carcinoma.

References

1. Blute ML, Zincke H, Farrow GM: Longterm followup of young patients with stage A adenocarcinoma of the prostate. J Urol 136:849, 1986.
2. Epstein JI, Paull G, Eggleston JC, Walsh PC: Prognosis of untreated stage A1 prostatic carcinoma: a study of 94 cases with extended followup. J Urol 136:837, 1986.
3. Catalona WJ, Kelley DR: Indications for total prostatectomy. American Urological Association, Update Series, Vol 3, Lesson 2. Houston, 1983.
4. Walsh PC, Jewett HJ: Radical surgery for prostate cancer. Cancer 45:1906, 1980.
5. Elder JS, Jewett HJ, Walsh PC: Radical perineal prostatectomy for clinical stage B2 carcinoma of the prostate. J Urol 127:704, 1982.
6. Catalona WJ, Fleischmann JD, Menon M: Pelvic lymph node status as predictor of extracapsular tumor extension in clinical stage B prostatic cancer. J Urol 129:327, 1983.
7. Middleton RG, Smith JA, Jr: Radical prostatectomy for stage B2 prostatic cancer. J Urol 127:702, 1982.
8. Kramer SA, Cline WA, Jr, Farnham R, Carson CC, Cox EB, Hinshaw W, Paulson DF: Prognosis of patients with stage D1 prostatic adenocarcinoma. J Urol 125:817, 1981.
9. Catalona WJ, Stein AJ: Staging errors in clinically localized prostatic cancer. J Urol 127:452, 1982.
10. Zincke H, Utz DC, Myers RP, Farrow GM, Patterson DE, Furlow WL: Bilateral pelvic lymphadenectomy and radical retropubic prostatectomy for adenocarcinoma of the prostate with regional lymph node involvement. Urology 19:238, 1982.

11. Schaeffer DL, Pendergrass HP: Comparison of enzyme, clinical, radiographic and radionuclide methods of detecting bone metastases from carcinoma of the prostate. Radiology 121:431, 1976.
12. Durzinsky DS, Messing EM, Myerowitz PD, Pellett JR, Wilson MA: Method for assuring accuracy of bone biopsy using technetium 99 bone scan. Cancer 59:723, 1987.
13. Pearson JC, Dombrovskis S, Dreyer J, Williams RD: Radioimmunoassay of serum acid phosphatase after prostatic massage. Urology 21:37, 1983.
14. Whitesel JA, Donohue RE, Mani JH, Mohr J, Scanaveino EJ, Augsburger RR, Biber RJ, Fauver HE, Wettlaufer JN, Pfister RR: Acid phosphatase: its influence on the management of carcinoma of the prostate. J Urol 131:70, 1984.
15. Catalona WJ: Unpublished data, cited in reference 16.
16. Biondetti PR, Lee JKT, Ling D, Catalona WJ: Clinical stage B prostate carcinoma: staging with MR imaging. Radiology 162:325, 1987.
17. Scardino PT: UTZ suggested for staging prostate cancer. Urology Times 14:2, 1987.
18. Steen PA, Tinker JH, Tarhan S: Myocardial reinfarction after anesthesia and surgery. JAMA 239:2566, 1978.
19. Hodgkin JE: Preoperative evaluation of pulmonary function. Am J Surg 138:355, 1979.
20. Wilson RF, Soullier G, Antonenko D: Creatinine clearance in critically ill surgical patients. Arch Surg 114:461, 1979.
21. Mullen JL: Consequences of malnutrition in the surgical patient. Surg Clin North Am 61:465, 1981.
22. Conrad M: Diseases transmissible by blood transfusion: viral hepatitis and other infectious disorders. Semin Hematol 18:122, 1981.
22a. Aach RD, Khan RA: Post-transfusion hepatitis: current perspectives. Ann Intern Med 92:539, 1980.
23. Catalona WJ, Kadmon D, Crane DB: Effect of minidose heparin on lymphocele formation following extraperitoneal pelvic lymphadenectomy. J Urol 123:890, 1980.
24. Ryan DW: Anaesthesia for cystectomy: a comparison of two anaesthetic techniques. Anaesthesia 37:554, 1982.
25. Walsh PC, Lepor H, Eggleston JC: Radical prostatectomy with preservation of sexual function: anatomical and pathological considerations. Prostate 4:473, 1983.
26. Walsh PC, Donker PJ: Impotence following radical prostatectomy: insight into etiology and prevention. J Urol 128:492, 1982.
27. Bahnson RR, Catalona WJ: Potency-sparing surgery for localized prostate cancer. Urol Ann 1:41, 1987.
28. Boxer RJ, Kaufman JJ, Goodwin WE: Radical prostatectomy for carcinoma of the prostate: 1951 through 1976. A review of 329 patients. J Urol 117:208, 1977.
29. Crawford ED, Kiker JD: Radical retropubic prostatectomy. J Urol 129:1145, 1983.
30. Lieskovsky G, Skinner DG: Technique of radical retropubic prostatectomy with limited pelvic node dissection. Urol Clin North Am 10:187, 1983.
31. Veenema RJ, Gursel EO, Lattimer JK: Radical retropubic prostatectomy for cancer: a 20 year experience. J Urol 117:330, 1977.
32. Middleton AW, Jr: Pelvic lymphadenectomy with modified radical retropubic prostatectomy as a single operation: technique used and results in 50 consecutive cases. J Urol 125:353, 1981.
33. Peters CA, Walsh PC: Blood transfusion and anesthetic practices in radical retropubic prostatectomy. J Urol 134:81, 1985.
34. Patterson DE, Zincke H: Perioperative complications of pelvic lymphadenectomy and radical retropubic prostatectomy for stages C and D1 prostate cancer. Urology 23:243, 1984.
35. Smith AM, Veenema RJ: Management of rectal injury and rectourethral fistulas following radical retropubic prostatectomy. J Urol 108:778, 1972.
36. Paul DP, Loening SA, Narayana AS, Culp DA: Morbidity from pelvic lymphadenectomy in staging carcinoma of the prostate. J Urol 129:1141, 1983.
37. Walsh PC: Radical retropubic prostatectomy. In Walsh PC, Gittes RF, Perlmutter AD, Stamey TA, eds: Campbell's Urology, Philadelphia, WB Saunders Co, 1986, pp 2754–2775.
38. Eggleston JC, Walsh PC: Radical prostatectomy with preservation of sexual function: pathological findings in the first 100 cases. J Urol 134:1146, 1985.
39. Walsh PC: Radical prostatectomy with preservation of sexual function: evolution of a surgical procedure. American Urological Association, Update Series, Vol 5, Lesson 5. Houston, 1986.

COMPLICATIONS OF PERINEAL PROSTATECTOMY

30

David F. Paulson

This chapter examines specifically the complications of a perineal approach to the apex of the prostate and the prostate itself, as well as the complications of the radical perineal prostatectomy. Today, a discussion of the complications of a simple prostatectomy is deemed inappropriate because as an operative procedure, simple prostatectomy has been largely abandoned in favor of transurethral resection or suprapubic transcapsular or transvesical prostatectomy. The discussion that follows is, therefore, divided into three sections: (1) the positioning and surgical approach to the apex of the prostate and the prostate itself, (2) the surgical technique for radical prostatectomy, and (3) the complications attendant to surgical approach to the apex of the prostate and the prostate itself and the complications attendant to radical prostatectomy.

TECHNIQUE FOR SURGICAL APPROACH TO THE PROSTATIC APEX AND PROSTATE

Positioning the patient is important to ensure easy access to the anatomic area of interest. The exaggerated lithotomy position is optimal and should be encouraged. To establish the exaggerated lithotomy position, the patient's sacrum is brought to the edge of the table with the buttocks extending several inches over the end of the table (Fig. 30–1). The patient is stabilized with padded shoulder braces to produce counterpressure and to hold the patient in position. These shoulder braces are placed laterally against the acromial processes in such a way as to prevent stress or pressure injury to the brachial plexus. The sacrum may be further elevated on sandbags or folded towels to aid in positioning. However, this is often not necessary. The legs should be well padded to prevent damage to both the nerves and the vascular structures. The legs are rotated superiorly and fixed in place by wrapping them to the braces. Correct positioning places the perineum parallel to the floor and provides optimum exposure. Failure to elevate the patient adequately reduces exposure and forces the surgeon to operate while looking up into the operative field rather than horizontally or downward.

When the patient is placed in the exaggerated lithotomy position, a Lowsley prostatic tractor is placed through the urethra into the bladder, and the blades are opened (Fig. 30–2). If the Lowsley tractor cannot be passed into the bladder because of stricture formation, a sound or a Foley catheter may be used. Alternatively, a urethral catheter, secured to the end of the Lowsley tractor with interrupted silk sutures, can be used to bypass false passages or strictures. The ureteral catheter will then guide the Lowsley tractor into the bladder, and the operation can be conducted in a standard manner.

The skin incision is established approximately 1.5 cm anterior to the anus and is curved posterolaterally on either side within the medial borders of the ischial tuberosities. The skin incision should be extended to the posterior anal margin on both sides; failure to do so will limit exposure. The superficial perineal fascia may then be incised and the ischiorectal fossa de-

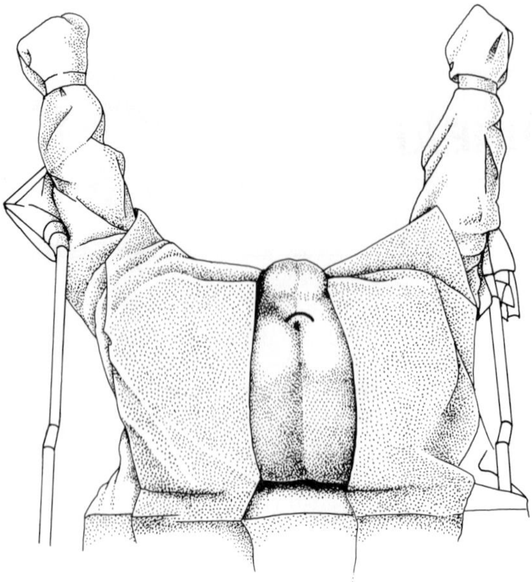

Figure 30–1. The patient is in the exaggerated lithotomy position, with the line of incision indicated anterior to the rectum.

veloped by placing an index finger slightly forward and down along either side of the rectum. The superficial perineal fascia must be incised; otherwise, access to the ischiorectal fossa cannot be secured. Use of the cutting cautery allows incision with hemostasis.

Following completion of this incision on either side of the rectum, the central tendon becomes prominent in the mid-portion of the operative field. The central tendon extends from the trans-

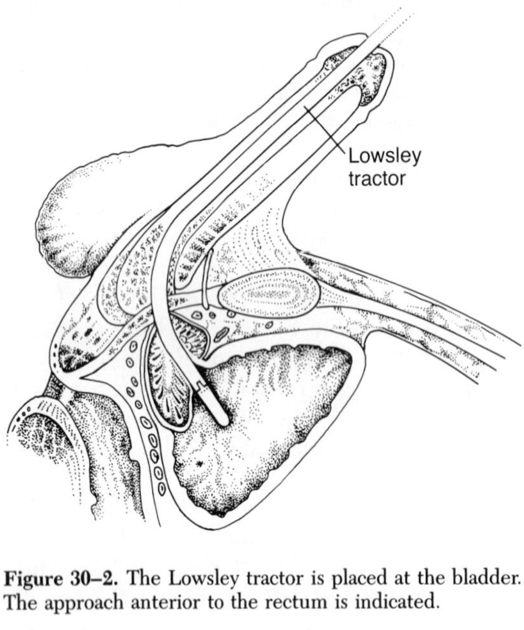

Figure 30–2. The Lowsley tractor is placed at the bladder. The approach anterior to the rectum is indicated.

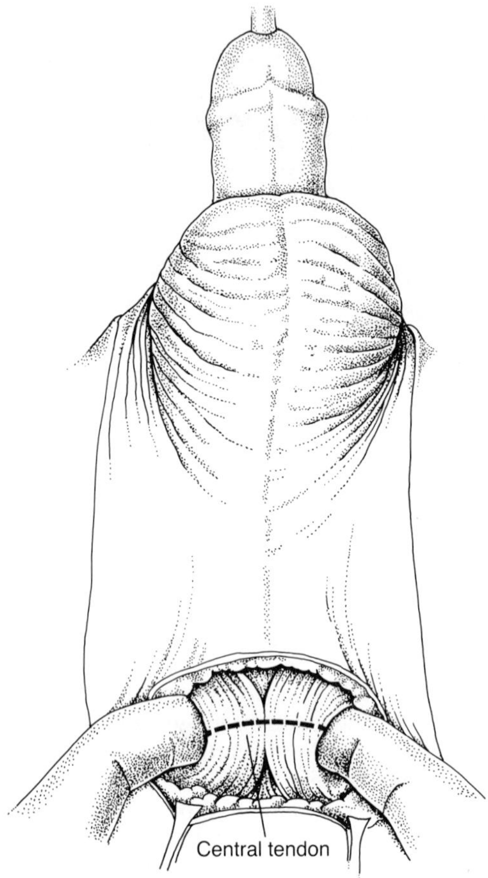

Figure 30–3. The central tendon is the muscular sheet that extends anterior to the rectum and is superficial to the external anal sphincter. Incision of the central tendon alone with the division of the projection of the external sphincter to the perineal body will permit the dissection to be carried out beneath the triangle formed by the superficial external anal sphincter.

verse perineal musculature to the anal sphincter and can be divided transversely using the cutting cautery (Fig. 30–3). Following division of the central tendon, the rectal sphincter is visualized as an arch overlying the rectum. The anterior rectal fascia is evident beneath and appears as a glistening white fascial sheath (Figs. 30–4 and 30–5).

A retractor is then placed beneath the rectal sphincter, and the sphincter fibers are elevated. Using the fascia of the rectum as a guide, the rectum can be followed to the prostatic apex with alternating sharp and blunt dissection. The rectourethralis is identified during the course of this dissection. At the apex of the prostate, the rectum makes a sharp right-angle turn because it is tented anteriorly by the rectourethralis (Fig. 30–6). The rectourethralis can be divided

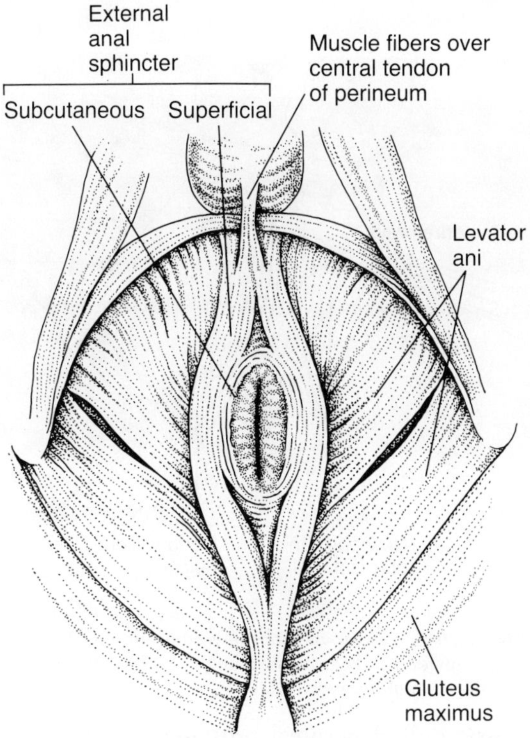

Figure 30–4. The insertion of the external anal sphincter into the transverse perineal muscle (perineal body) can be severed for a suprasphincteric approach, or a retractor can be placed in the triangle formed by the external anal sphincter just before their joining and the muscles stretched and separated for a subsphincteric approach.

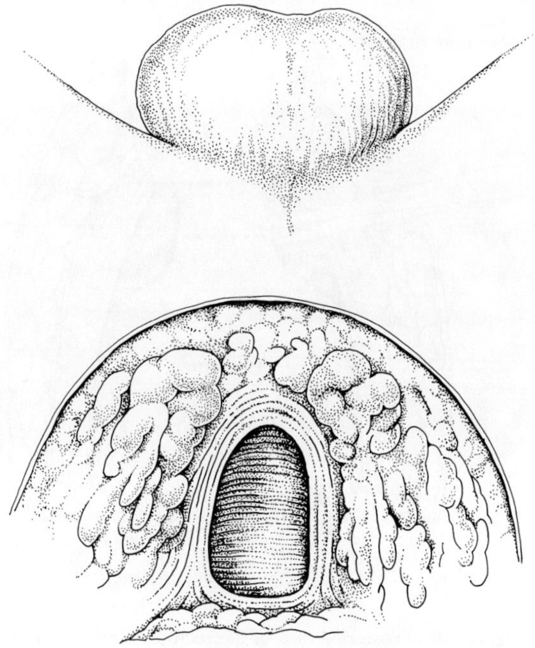

Figure 30–5. The anterior retractor has been removed for this diagrammatic representation of the subsphincteric approach. The anterior rectal fascia can be followed to the level of the rectourethralis.

sharply with scissors, allowing the rectum to be displaced posteriorly (Figs. 30–7 and 30–8). The rectum is then separated from the posterior surface of the prostate using blunt dissection between the prostate and its fascial investments anteriorly and the anterior rectal wall posteriorly. Following posterior displacement, the rectum should be protected with moist gauze and the displacement maintained with a weighted posterior retractor. During dissection of the rectum to the level of the prostate and during division of the rectourethralis, it is reasonable to place a finger into the rectum to identify the level of dissection and to protect the rectum. Blunt dissection now permits exposure of the lateral and anterior margins of the prostate (Fig. 30–9).

Following exposure of the prostate in this manner, the radical perineal prostatectomy may be accomplished in a standard manner, termed the classic perineal prostatectomy. Alternatively, the physician can utilize wide-field dissection techniques, which incorporate the periprostatic fascia. The classic perineal prostatectomy has the potential to preserve the investing neurovascular fascia and thus provide the opportunity to preserve both the innervation of the corporal tissues and erectile function. The wide-field perineal prostatectomy, which sacrifices the periprostatic fascia and the incorporated neurovascular plexus, ensures destruction of the corporal innervation. It is important to briefly describe both techniques in order that

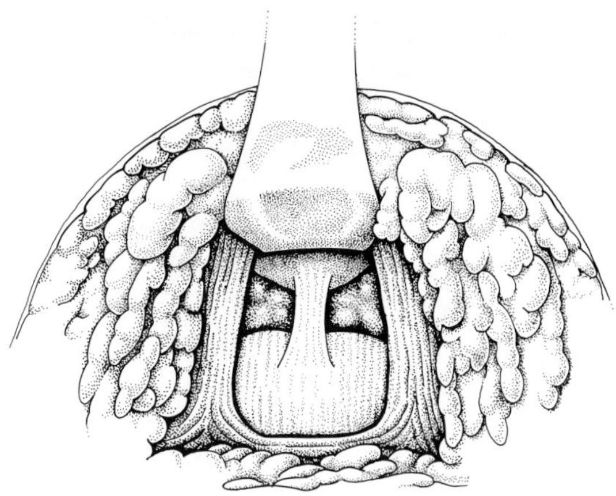

Figure 30–6. With the sphincter retracted superiorly (lateral retractor can be placed beneath the muscle to produce additional exposure), the rectourethralis can be visualized. The extent of development of this muscle is variable.

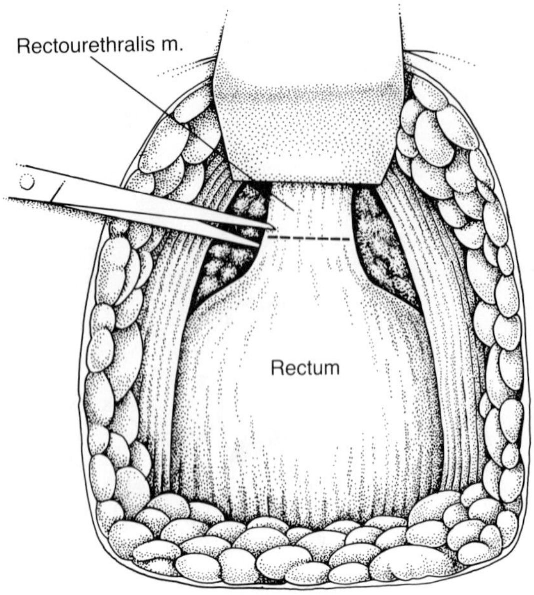

Figure 30–7. Posterior view of the rectourethralis with the rectum identified. Division of this muscle drops the rectum posteriorly and permits access to the prostate.

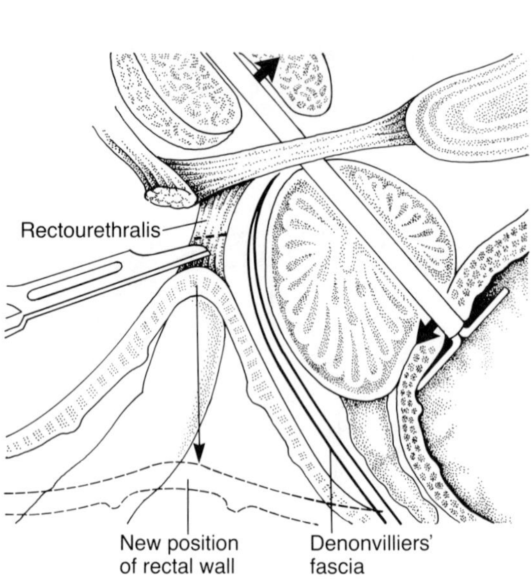

Figure 30–8. Lateral view of the rectourethralis. The surgeon's finger has been placed in the rectum to assist in identification of the rectal wall.

the attendant complications can be adequately discussed.

THE CLASSIC PERINEAL PROSTATECTOMY

The exposed prostate is surrounded by a multilayered fibrovascular fascial covering. This encircles the prostate posteriorly and laterally and is carried superiorly onto the bladder itself. Lateral to this fibrovascular covering is the muscular sling of levator ani fibers. To accomplish the classic radical perineal prostatectomy as originally described, the surgeon incises this fascial covering from left to right at the apex of the prostate. Recognizing the distribution of the nerves that innervate the corpora, it is seen that such an incision will divide the nerves that provide innervation. When the incision is made in a left-to-right manner, the lateropelvic fascia (the fibrovascular fascia) is swept aside (Figs. 30–10 and 30–11), and the apex of the prostate and the vascular supply to the prostate at the right and left bases are identified. A curved clamp may be placed around the membranous

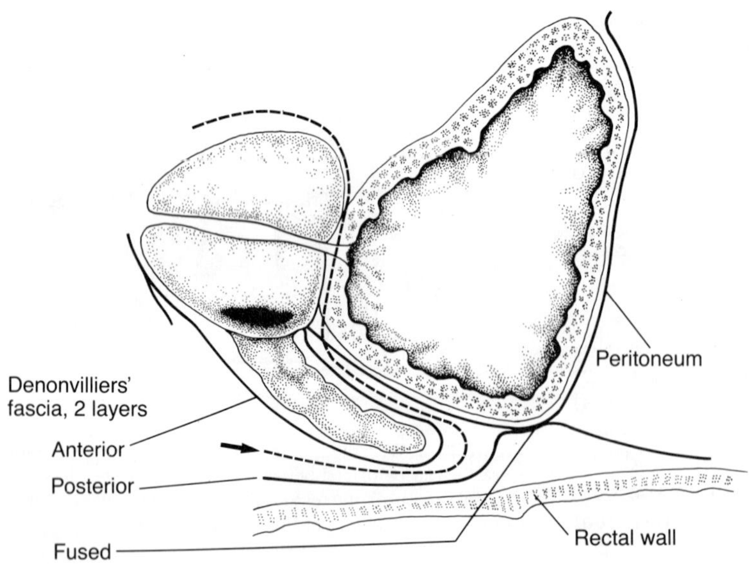

Figure 30–9. Limits of dissection for the radical prostatectomy.

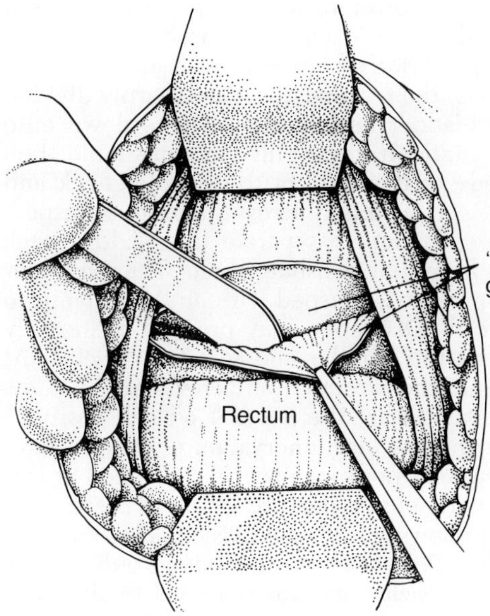

Figure 30–10. Incision of the overlying fascia (the "pearly gates") to expose the true capsule of the prostate.

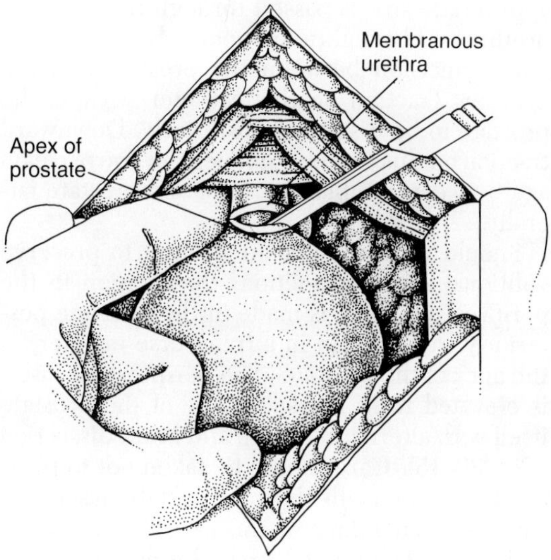

Figure 30–12. The apex of the prostate is identified and the membranous urethra sharply divided.

urethra just distal to the prostatic apex, the Lowsley retractor removed, and the urethra sharply divided (Fig. 30–12).

The Young prostatic tractor, or Foley catheter, is now passed through the prostatic urethra into the bladder and the blades extended (or balloon inflated). By applying pressure on the tractor to displace the prostate posteriorly and with blunt dissection, a plane is developed beneath the venous plexus and between the bladder and the prostate anteriorly (Fig. 30–13). As the prostate is displaced from the bladder neck anteriorly, a "horse collar" of bladder neck fibers at the bladder neck between the 10 and 2 o'clock positions is identified (Fig. 30–14). The bladder is entered beneath these fibers at the 12 o'clock position, and the incision is carried from the 12 to the 2 o'clock position and from the 12 to 10 o'clock position, preserving continuity of these bladder neck fibers. At this point, the Young catheter is withdrawn, and a Foley catheter of

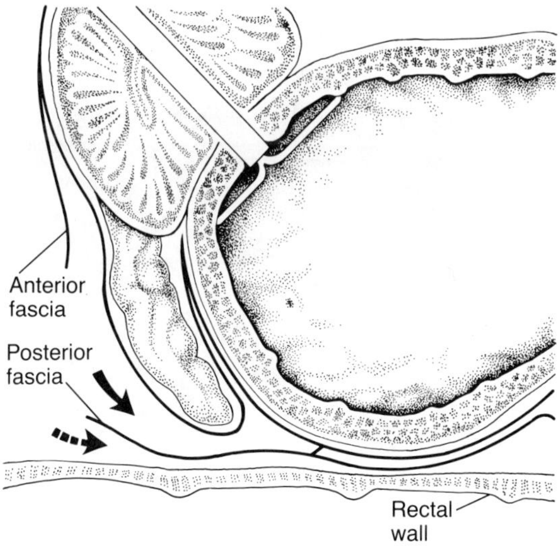

Figure 30–11. The solid arrow identifies the preferred plane of dissection above the anterior rectal fascia (the posterior fascia of Denonvilliers) and the fascia of the rectovesical septum (the anterior layer of Denonvilliers' fascia). The broken arrow indicates a line of dissection beneath the rectal fascia.

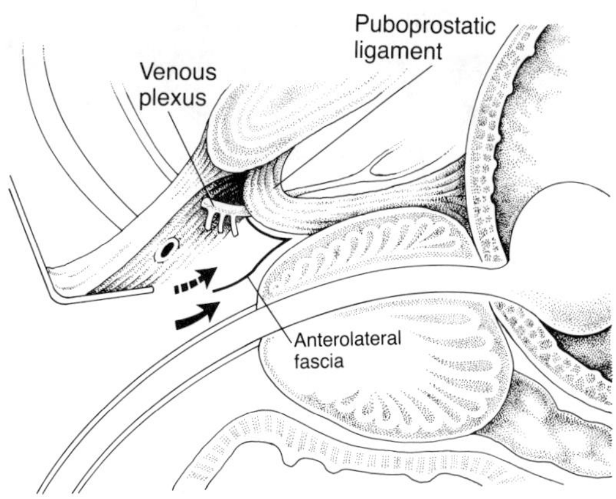

Figure 30–13. The solid arrow indicates the proper plane of dissection beneath the anterolateral fascia and beneath the venous plexus. Dissection above this fascia (dotted arrow) carries the hazard of disruption of the venous sinus and troublesome bleeding.

appropriate size is passed through the prostatic urethra and brought out superiorly through the line of incision between the prostate and the bladder. Traction on this catheter permits the prostate to be displaced posteriorly. Downward traction on this catheter defines the line of cleavage between the bladder neck and prostate laterally.

Should it be decided to attempt to preserve volitional erectile function, the incision in the periprostatic fascia is made in the mid-line posteriorly, rather than in a transverse manner, at the apex of the prostate. The periprostatic fascia is elevated from the substance of the prostate itself with alternating sharp and blunt dissection (Fig. 30–15). Care should be taken not to place a retractor beneath the periprostatic fascia because stretch injury of the neural innervation will occur. The prostate may be mobilized beneath the periprostatic fascia in a manner similar to the procedure described above. A right-angle clamp can be passed around the apex of the prostate, the membranous urethra divided at the apex, and the prostate displaced posteriorly as described above. The prostate is separated from the bladder as described and the prostate mobilized.

After the prostate has been separated from the bladder neck and is secured only by the tissue posteriorly between the 5 and 7 o'clock positions, the trigonal fibers are sharply divided at the bladder neck as they course down onto the prostatic urethra. This incision should then be made at the level of the bladder neck and may be carried totally across the posterior aspect of the specimen to separate the bladder neck fibers from the prostate itself. The posterior bladder neck is grasped with an Allis clamp to elevate it. Dissection may proceed posteriorly between the bladder and seminal vesicles. At this time, the prostate is attached only by a few fibers laterally at the 5 and 7 o'clock positions and at the vascular innervation of the prostate. The vascular pedicles may be controlled at this point with either ligature or metallic surgical clips. Following bilateral division of the vascular pedicles, the specimen is retained only by the seminal vesicles and vas deferens, which may be mobilized with alternating sharp and blunt dissection. The specimen may then be removed.

THE WIDE-FIELD RADICAL PERINEAL PROSTATECTOMY

In this procedure, the investing periprostatic fascia with the incorporated neurovascular

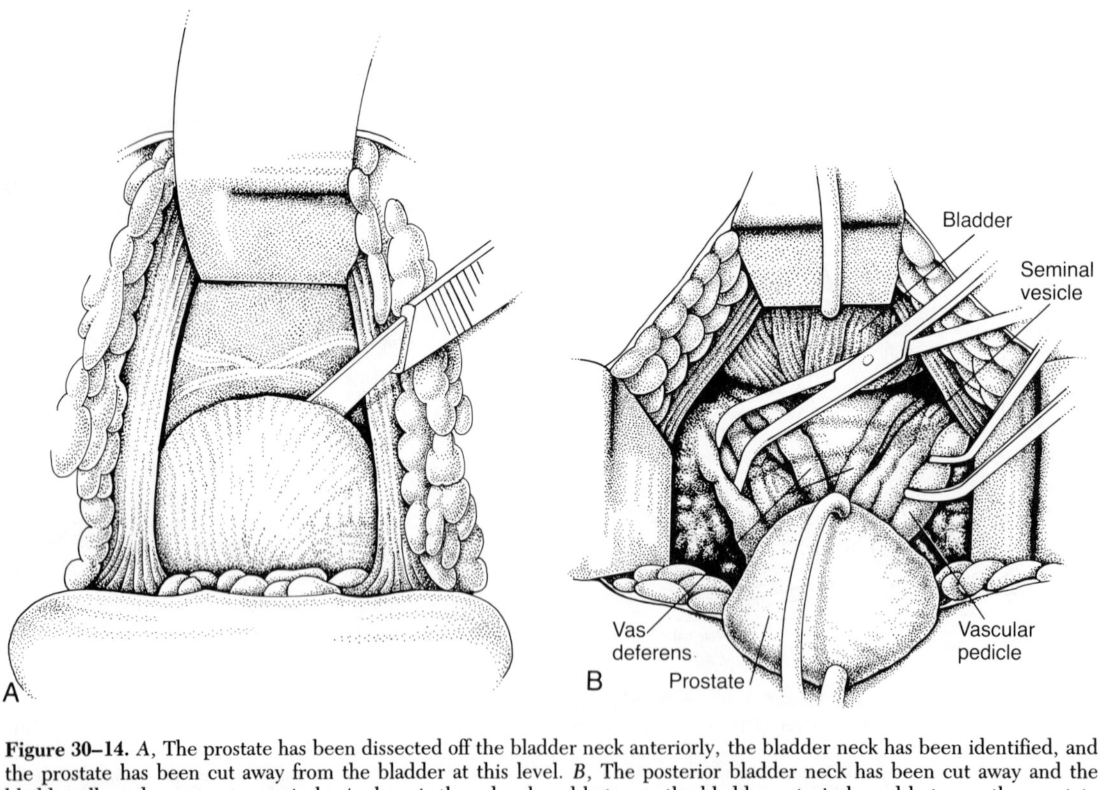

Figure 30–14. *A*, The prostate has been dissected off the bladder neck anteriorly, the bladder neck has been identified, and the prostate has been cut away from the bladder at this level. *B*, The posterior bladder neck has been cut away and the bladder allowed to retract superiorly. A plane is then developed between the bladder anteriorly and between the prostate and seminal vesicles posteriorly.

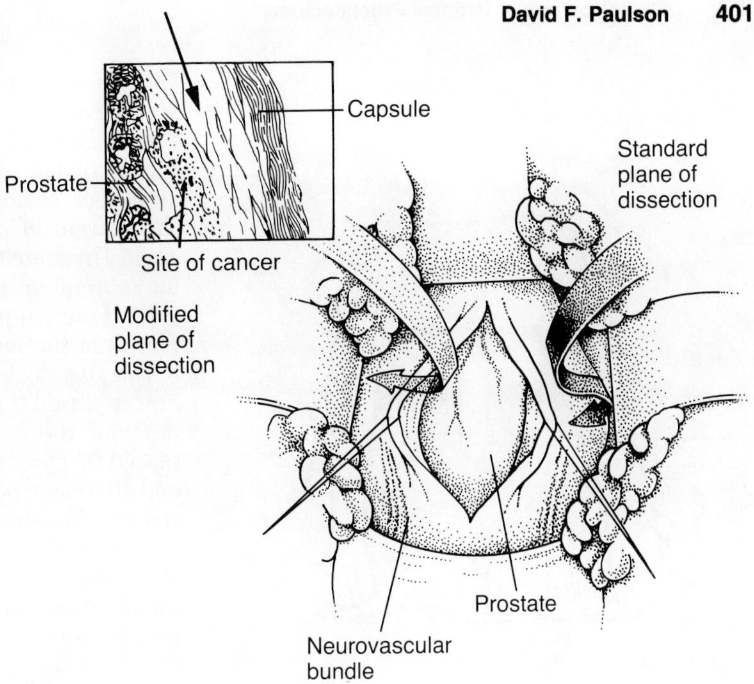

Figure 30–15. Note that dissection can be carried beneath or lateral to the tissue that has been described as the lateral pelvic fascia. When the dissection is carried beneath the lateral pelvic fascia, the operation is established as originally described. When the dissection is carried lateral, the neurovascular bundle is sacrificed; however, the margins of the procedure are increased by the width of the tissue encompassed in the surgical specimen.

plexus is sacrificed with the prostate itself. This is performed in an attempt to establish tumor-negative margins, and to provide an additional surgical margin that does not exist in the operative procedure described above. Following exposure as previously described, the prostate is covered by the fibrovascular periprostatic fascia (see Fig. 30–15). This fascia contains the neurovascular plexus associated with volitional erectile function. No attempt is made to separate the periprostatic fascia from the prostatic substance itself; instead the line of dissection is carried laterally to the periprostatic fascia, the most lateral structure now being the levator sling. A right-angle clamp is passed around the apex of the prostate but lateral to the periprostatic fascia as it sweeps onto the apex of the prostate. Although venous bleeding may be encountered when the distal margin is transected, this can be controlled under a curved retractor, or it may be left uncontrolled until the prostate is removed, at which time the bleeding spontaneously ceases. As the prostate is taken off the bladder neck anteriorly and laterally, the fibrovascular fascia will have to be sharply divided from its point of reflection onto the bladder itself. This can be performed sharply with surgical clips to control vasculature on the patent side. The prostate is mobilized from the bladder itself as described above. However, posteriorly and posterolaterally, there are two layers of fascia that cover the seminal vesicles and the vascular pedicles. With the prostate elevated in the perineum, the seminal vesicles are palpated and the two posterior layers of fascia incised in order to expose the seminal vesicles in their mid-portion. This dissection is then carried laterally and anteriorly, surrounding the seminal vesicles until they are free. This dissection will also release the specimen and provide enhanced mobility. The vascular pedicles are identified independently and controlled with absorbable suture or surgical clips. The seminal vesicles are mobilized as described above, and the specimen is removed.

Attention is now turned to reconstruction of the vesicle neck. Every attempt should be made to reconstruct the bladder neck in such a way as to provide for normal bladder neck function in the postoperative period. The vesicle neck is reconstructed, and continuity is established between the bladder neck and the membranous urethra by direct anastomosis between the reconstructed bladder neck and the membranous urethra, with identified vest sutures being used to reduce tension from this anastomosis. The bladder neck is closed moving from the 6 to 12 o'clock position with interrupted 0 chromic catgut sutures (Fig. 30–16). This permits the vesicourethral anastomosis to be placed superiorly at maximum distance from the ureteral orifices and reduces the risk for occlusion of the orifices.

The closure can be performed by moving from the 12 o'clock to the 6 o'clock position and making the vesicourethral anastomosis inferiorly. However, this rolls the posterior bladder neck, trigone, and ureteral orifices into a tube, and it

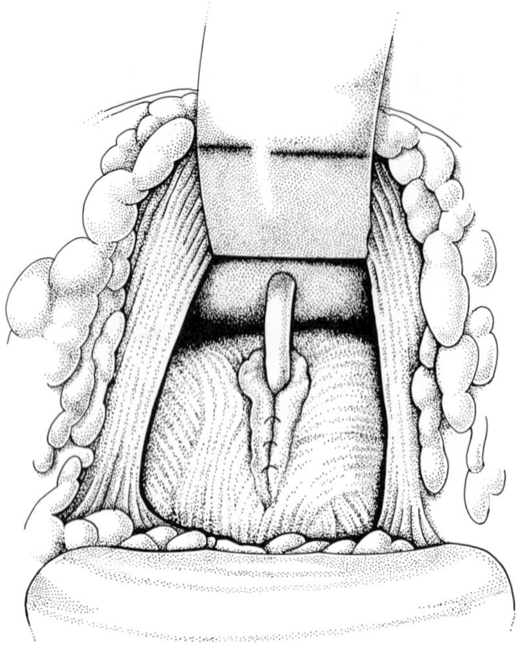

Figure 30–16. Closure of the bladder neck from 6 o'clock.

is possible to occlude the ureteral orifices by the draining Foley catheter or to incorporate the ureteral orifices in the bladder closure.

The closure of the bladder neck is accomplished by moving from the 6 to 12 o'clock position until the reconstructed bladder neck fits snugly around an 18 French (Fr.) Foley catheter

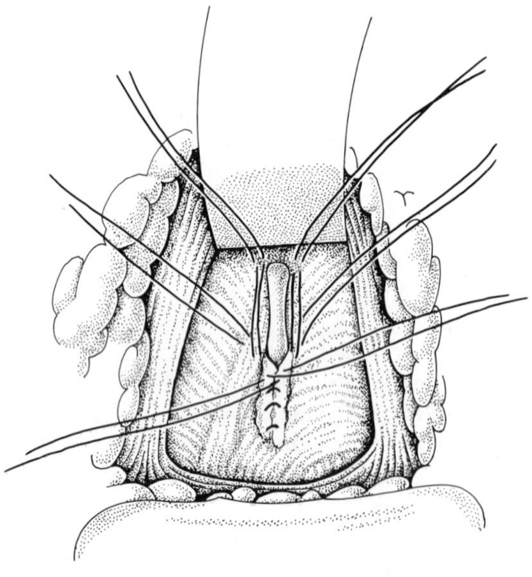

Figure 30–17. Placement of the Vest sutures at 2, 5, 8, and 10 o'clock using 0 chromic catgut. Placement of the sutures is used for the direct anastomosis.

(Fig. 30–17). At this point, the Foley catheter is removed from the bladder, and mattress sutures of 0 chromic catgut are placed about the reconstructed bladder neck at the 2, 5, 7, and 10 o'clock positions, approximately 5 mm from the margin of the newly constructed bladder neck. These are tied loosely and left long to allow for subsequent placement beneath the perineal skin. Four sutures of 00 chromic catgut are placed in the membranous urethra at the 2, 4, 8, and 10 o'clock positions. An 18 Fr. Foley catheter is passed through the urethra into the bladder and the balloon inflated. The previously placed 00 chromic catgut sutures at the 2, 4, 8, and 10 o'clock positions are placed in the reconstructed bladder neck in identical proximate positions. As these sutures are secured, the reconstructed bladder neck is brought to the membranous urethra. The 0 chromic catgut traction sutures, previously placed about the bladder neck, are then drawn through each side of the perineal body, parallel to the urethra and tied beneath the subcutaneous tissues in the perineum to support the direct anastomosis between the bladder neck and urethra.

COMPLICATIONS OF APPROACH TO THE PROSTATE, PERINEAL PROSTATECTOMY, AND THEIR MANAGEMENT

Loss of Anatomic Landmarks During Approach to the Prostatic Apex and Prostate

Following completion of the inverted U incision, the physician must be certain that the central tendon is mobilized and completely divided. The rectum can be palpated beneath the central tendon, and with blunt dissection, a tunnel approximately 2 cm anterior to the anal verge should be created beneath the central tendon and anterior to the rectum. The central tendon is then divided using the cutting cautery. Following division of the central tendon, the surgeon will usually identify the anal sphincter muscle and the anterior rectal fascia. It is important that every attempt be made to identify the anterior rectal fascia because this provides the path to the prostatic apex and prostate. Failure to identify this anatomic landmark will often cause the surgeon to carry the dissection too far anteriorly into the perineum itself, injuring either the bulbocavernosus or the membranous urethra itself.

When the anterior rectal surface cannot be identified with certainty, the surgeon should place a finger into the rectum and, with sharp dissection conducted toward the rectal surface, sharply cut away the perineal musculature until the anterior rectal surface is identified. Once this is accomplished, the dissection can be carried without difficulty to the prostatic apex. The rectourethralis is variously developed and may be only some rudimentary fibers between the apex of the prostate and the rectum, or it may be a band of several centimeters in length in the midline. In order to permit proper identification of the rectourethralis, the dissection along the anterior rectal surface should be carried just to the left and right of the midline. This can be accomplished with blunt dissection and even conducted to such an extent that the rectum may be bluntly separated from the prostate and its investing fascia prior to division of the rectourethralis.

Control of Bleeding from the Periprostatic Venous Plexus

Significant venous bleeding may be encountered during dissection at the apex of the prostate or after division of the membranous urethra when the prostate is being separated from the bladder anteriorly and anterolaterally. Although it is tempting to stop the dissection to control the venous bleeding, it is best to provide temporary control of the bleeding by pressure behind a curved narrow Deaver until the prostate is separated from the bladder neck anteriorly and anterolaterally. Once the prostate is so separated, most of the venous bleeding will spontaneously cease. Any troublesome persistent bleeding may be controlled by use of a 4 × 8 sponge wrapped around a curved narrow Deaver at the level of the anterior bladder neck.

The line of incision at the posterior bladder neck must be carried in a transverse manner between the 5 and 7 o'clock positions in order to separate the prostate from the bladder. This line of incision should be carried posteriorly until the fascia that overlies the seminal vesicles is identified. Failure to carry the incision directly posterior will result in thinning of the posterior bladder neck fibers and compromise subsequent bladder neck reconstruction. Further, if the dissection is not carried posteriorly until the fascia that surrounds the seminal vesicles is identified, subsequent blunt dissection in the purported plane between the seminal vesicles and bladder neck may result in fragmentation of the detrusor musculature and also compromise subsequent reconstruction.

The presence of a large median lobe may complicate separation of the prostate from the posterior bladder neck. If the median lobe is pedunculated and can be delivered through the bladder neck into the operative field, the incision should be proximal to the pedunculated median lobe in such a manner that the bladder neck fibers are sharply cut away and the prostatic tissue is delivered into the operative field. As previously, the dissection should be carried sharply posteriorly until the fascia surrounding the seminal vesicles is identified. If the median lobe cannot be delivered through the bladder neck into the operative field, it may be sharply amputated, to be removed following completion of the radical prostatectomy. This can be accomplished without fear of seeding tumor because the incidence of involvement of median lobe tissue by malignancy is minimal.

Problems in Reconstruction of the Bladder Neck

Problems most commonly occur when the posterior margin of incision has been carried so close to the ureteral orifices as to compromise their drainage. When there is concern regarding bladder neck closure and occlusion of the ureteral orifices, two maneuvers may prevent difficulty. Frequently, as the bladder neck is closed from the 6 to 12 o'clock positions, the posterior portion of the closure can be accomplished by placing the sutures in the detrusor musculature only, not incorporating the bladder mucosa. This provides the opportunity to bring the detrusor musculature together while keeping the suture line at a distance from the ureteral orifices. Should such a maneuver produce discomforture, the orifices may be catheterized and the ureteral catheters brought out through the perineum to be removed on the 5th and 7th postoperative days.

Inability to Void Following Catheter Removal

This is usually a transient phenomenon, most commonly reflecting edema at the site of the urethrovesicle anastomosis. When this occurs, we attempt to pass a catheter retrograde through the urethra and across the anastomosis into the bladder. If this cannot be accomplished, a trocar-introduced suprapubic cystotomy is placed and the patient undergoes cystostomy drainage for several additional days. The cystostomy catheter is then clamped and the patient encouraged to void per urethra. In no instance have we found the patient unable to do so. Aggressive attempts to pass a catheter retrograde through the urethra across the fresh anastomosis frequently produce disruption of the anastomosis with postoperative incontinence.

Urinary Drainage Through the Perineal Incision

Urinary leakage always stops. If the patients leak only when they void, the leak is distal to the reconstructed bladder neck. In these instances, the Foley catheter is not replaced and the patient is allowed to go home but is instructed to void only when seated or in the shower. With time, these leaks will close, and the patient will maintain perfect continence. If the patient drains continually through the perineal incision, the catheter is replaced and the patient left with the catheter in place. In all instances, this has provided cessation of the urinary leakage. It is important that the Foley catheter be in the most dependent portion of the bladder. Failure to so place the Foley catheter puts the drainage holes sufficiently high in the bladder so that the newly formed urine lies in the most dependent portion of the bladder and will continue to leak through the defect. If leakage continues to occur with the Foley catheter in place, a gentle cystogram should be performed to determine the placement of the Foley catheter. If it can be determined that the Foley catheter is not seated deep in the reconstructed bladder neck, it should be so placed. With such appropriate positioning of the Foley, the leakage will cease.

Stricture at the Urethrovesical Anastomosis

Three forms of obstruction will occur at the urethrovesical junction. These may be classified as immediate, early, and late. The immediate obstruction occurs at the time the Foley catheter is removed, and this problem has been addressed previously.

Early obstruction at the urethrovesical anastomosis usually appears within several months after the radical prostatectomy, and, although the onset of the obstruction may be gradual, the patient will usually present with progressive decrease in the size and force of the stream and with the necessity to strain to void, often to the point of dribbling. This usually reflects postoperative cicatricial stricture and is best handled by gentle dilatation, usually with a filiform instrument to ensure that the sound is not misdirected. Preferably, the dilatation is done with an instrument not larger than 18 to 20 Fr. Repeated dilatation may be necessary. However, we have found it seldom necessary to dilate the patient more than twice. On occasion, when the structure has not responded well to gentle dilatation, direct vision internal urethrotomy, cutting only in one position, may provide the ability to void without difficulty.

Late stricture, appearing several years after the operative procedure, usually heralds local recurrence. Similarly, local recurrence should be suspected when dilatation is accomplished, and the patient is unable to void in the immediate postdilatation period. When local recurrence is suspected, every effort should be made to confirm or deny its presence. If local recurrence is identified, the stricture is managed in a very conservative manner, the most gentle dilatation being accomplished to permit reasonable voiding until such time as the local recurrence has been managed either by radiation therapy or by androgen deprivation. Because any one of these treatments may impact upon the local recurrence, ablating the cause of the obstruction, aggressive incision, or dilatation may result in incontinence following definitive treatment of the cause for recurrence.

Urinary Incontinence

Urinary incontinence may be divided into early and late incontinence. Although the incidence of postoperative incontinence is reported to be between 10 and 18 percent, this most probably reflects the lack of experience of many in the reported series. In the hands of individuals who are skilled in radical prostatectomy, the actual incidence of incontinence is probably less than 2 percent. Therefore, the comments that follow reflect my experience in dealing with individuals accrued from elsewhere.

Early urinary incontinence may be either functional or mechanical. Functional incontinence is characterized by urgency and frequency with a stream of adequate caliber. When this is encountered in the early postoperative period, the patient is best managed with antispasmodics, usually oxybutynin hydrochloride (Ditropan) at a dose level of 5 mg, two to three times daily.

This form of functional incontinence is due probably to residual inflammation from the surgery. It may persist for several months, but gradually the patient will recognize that the antispasmodic is no longer necessary and will abandon use of this drug.

Mechanical incontinence occurs as a result of damage to the distal sphincteric mechanism or from failure to reconstruct the bladder neck adequately. These patients may be persistently wet in the early postoperative period. However, as time passes, they will demonstrate a pattern of continence early in the day, with some leakage, usually exacerbated by stress, beginning in the early or late afternoon as they tire. Although Ornade spansules, once or twice daily, may provide some relief, I am not convinced that this is a reasonable long-term therapeutic modality. These patients are best treated with encouragement and tincture of time. Those who demonstrate this pattern will usually become continent with time. The patient who presents with persistent incontinence usually has mechanical damage, which was inflicted at the time of surgery. This is most difficult to manage, and these patients usually have to undergo some form of artificial sphincter placement to establish continence. The scarring produced by the previous surgery often necessitates that the artificial sphincter be placed around the bulb of the urethra. Although previous prostatic surgery may have partially compromised blood supply in this area, we have not found erosion to be a major problem with delayed activation of the sphincter.

Loss of Potency

Despite the most careful attempts to preserve erectile function, a patient may experience lack of erectile potency in the postoperative period. Restoration of potency should be in response to patient demand. Our current feeling is that placement of a prosthetic device at the time of primary prostatic surgery is not appropriate. When voluntary erectile function is lost as a result of the operative procedure, the patient and partner should participate in the decision to restore erectile function. A considerable number of patients will not seek restoration of sexual function either because they have found alternative means for sexual gratification or because intercourse is no longer important to them or their partner in the maintenance of their relationship. Furthermore, the current climate in which erectile function may be restored by either prosthetic or pharmaceutical means provides the patient and his partner with considerable flexibility in choosing the mechanism by which potency is to be restored.

Careful attention to the principles inherent in the conduct of any surgery will reduce the incidence of complications directly related to the surgical procedure itself. Those problems that are attendant to the specific nature of the surgery can be thoughtfully managed without risk to the patient and with every likelihood of a succesful outcome.

References

Carlton CE Jr, Dawoud F, Hudgins P, et al: Irradiation treatment of carcinoma of the prostate: a preliminary report based on 8 years of experience. J Urol 108:924, 1972.

Golimbu M, Morales P, Al-Askari S, et al: Extended pelvic lymphadenectomy for prostatic cancer. J Urol 121:617, 1979.

Paulson DF, Lin GH, Hinshaw W, et al: Radical surgery vs. radiotherapy for adenocarcinoma of the prostate. J Urol 128:502, 1982.

Paulson DF: The prostate. In Paulson DF, ed: Genitourinary Surgery. New York, Churchill Livingstone, 1984.

Paulson DF: Management of prostatic malignancy. In de Kernion JB, Paulson DF, eds: Genitourinary Cancer Management. Philadelphia, Lea & Febiger, 1987.

Walsh PC, Lepor H, Eggleston JC: Radical prostatectomy with preservative of sexual function: anatomical and pathological considerations. Prostate 4:473, 1983.

COMPLICATIONS OF INTERSTITIAL RADIOTHERAPY IN THE TREATMENT OF CARCINOMA OF THE PROSTATE

31

Clanton B. Harrison • Peter T. Scardino

Radiotherapy for the treatment of prostate cancer has evolved since its therapeutic value was established in the early 1960s. The modern era of definitive external beam irradiation therapy was pioneered by Bagshaw.[1] Today, more patients are treated for localized prostate cancer with radiotherapy than with any other individual form of therapy.[2] From the beginning, investigators have worked toward alternative techniques of definitive radiotherapy that would be more target-specific. With time, it has become clear that doses of radiation in the upper range of clinical tolerance (7000 rads) are necessary for control of the local tumor in most patients. Interstitial radiotherapy has been developed to maximize the radiation dose to the cancer and minimize the complications associated with injury to adjacent normal tissues (Fig. 31–1). Several forms of interstitial radiotherapy of the prostate have emerged. The most popular are those using radioactive gold seeds and iodine seeds.

Implantation of ^{198}Au seeds is followed by low-dose external beam radiation. The ^{198}Au seeds provide local high-dose radiation with a relatively short half-life (T½). This allows the dose of radiation to the prostate to be greater than that with conventional external beam radiotherapy, but with less damage to surrounding structures. ^{125}I seeds are also utilized as an interstitial radioactive source. These ^{125}I seeds are placed in the prostatic tissue to provide rad delivery equivalent to that of external beam radiotherapy. Because their half-life is longer than that of ^{198}Au seeds, external beam therapy is not needed. Again, the goal is to reduce the radiation to adjacent structures and to increase the dose of radiation to the cancer.

Implantation of both ^{198}Au and ^{125}I seeds requires an open surgical procedure for placement of the radioactive materials so that the dose of radiation to the prostate is maximized. At the time that the interstitial seeds are placed, a pelvic lymph node dissection is performed so that the prostate cancer can be more accurately staged. Although pelvic lymph node dissection has been shown statistically to be of no therapeutic value in prostate cancer,[3] it can help in the choice of treatment and offer useful prognostic information.

Each form of radiotherapy has been associated with the morbidity that one would expect from radiation injury to normal surrounding structures. External beam radiotherapy and its complications are discussed in Chapter 23.

The complications of interstitial radiotherapy include proctitis, rectal stenosis, rectal ulcers, cystitis, urethral strictures, incontinence, and impotence as well as genital edema, peripheral edema, lymphocele, and hematoma. These complications are interrelated and difficult to sepa-

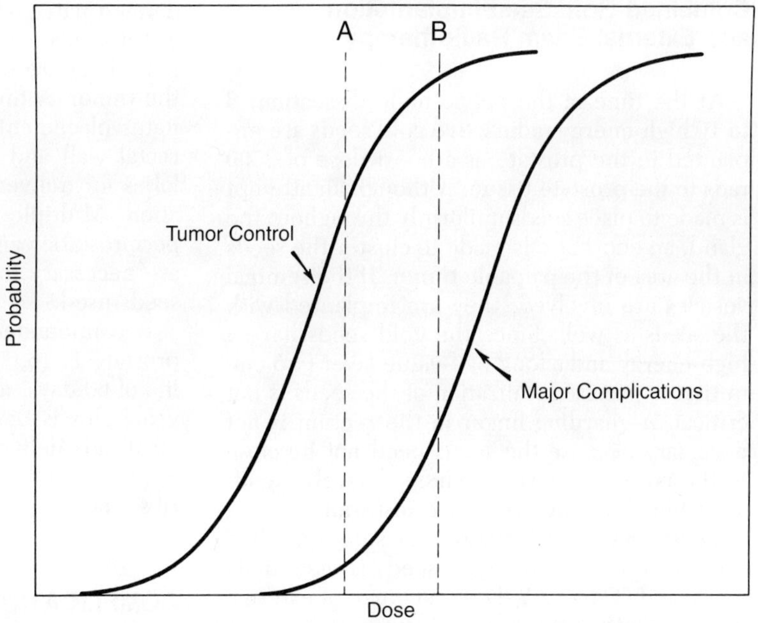

Figure 31–1. The "therapeutic index" for radiotherapy for localized prostate cancer is narrow. As the dose is increased (from A to B) to provide 90 percent local control, the complication rate increases substantially. Interstitial radiotherapy was developed to widen the gap by shifting the complication curve to the right.

rate because the surgery and radiation therapy are performed at the same time. Complications may occur either intraoperatively or in the early postoperative period, or they may occur late in the postoperative period. This chapter outlines the incidence of these complications and some techniques for their management and prevention.

OVERVIEW

The complications associated with interstitial radiotherapy result from a combination of surgical and irradiation factors. The relative frequencies of major complications, hematomas, blood loss requiring transfusion, lymphocele, lymphedema, and impotence associated with ^{198}Au and ^{125}I therapy are listed in Table 31–1. The only significant difference between the modes of interstitial radiotherapy appears to be blood loss. This seems to be directly proportional to the number of seeds implanted by needle through the periprostatic veins into the prostate. The surgical complications and their relationship to irradiation cannot be completely avoided; however, meticulous surgical technique, careful seed placement, precise computation of radiation dose, and detailed knowledge of the anatomy can help to reduce their incidence.

Table 31–1. COMPLICATIONS OF INTERSTITIAL RADIOTHERAPY

	Gold seed[a] (510 patients) (%)	Iodine seed[b,c] (415 patients) (%)
Major complications	10	3–13
Intestinal	2	3–5
Urinary	2	3–7
Lymphocele/hematoma/abscess	4	3–10
Genital/leg edema		
With PLND[d]	1	3
Without PLND	—	—
Impotence[e]	29	25
Hemorrhage requiring transfusion	1	42–50

[a]Carlton (1988)
[b]Fowler et al (1979)
[c]Schellhammer et al (1985)
[d]PLND, pelvic lymph node dissection
[e]Assessed subjectively by questionnaire.

Combined Gold Seed Implantation and External Beam Radiotherapy

At the time of the pelvic node dissection, 6 to 10 high-energy radioactive gold seeds are implanted in the prostate as a boost dose of 3500 rads to the prostate tissue. Although an attempt is made to place seeds uniformly throughout the gland, an effort also is made to cluster the seeds in the area of the palpable tumor. If the seminal vesicles are involved, they are implanted with the seeds as well. Since the gold seeds have a high-energy and a long half-value layer (4.5 cm) in tissue, precise localization of the seeds is not critical. A guarding finger in the rectum is not necessary because the seeds need not lie close to the posterior capsule. There is rarely significant blood loss or need for transfusion.

Beginning 14 to 21 days after surgery, when the radiation from the gold seeds is essentially exhausted ($T\frac{1}{2}$ = 2.7 days), a course of external beam radiotherapy is begun, using a liner accelerator and the protocol shown in Table 31–2.

A rotational technique is used to deliver 4500 rads at 225 rads per day, 4 days per week, to the prostate only when the pelvic lymph nodes are negative for metastasis. If the pelvic lymph nodes are positive, 5000 rads are delivered through opposing anterior and posterior portals to the full pelvis and the prostate. The course is split into two parts with a 2-week rest after 3 weeks of therapy. An additional 400 rads are given to the prostate alone. These courses can be altered or extended if symptoms of irradiation toxicity are severe.

Radioactive Iodine Implants

These implants also are placed immediately following a staging pelvic lymphadenectomy. Low-energy ^{125}I seeds are implanted in a rigidly defined pattern because the half layer of value of ^{125}I seeds is only 1.7 cm, and seeds must be placed homogeneously to avoid cold spots within the tumor. A finger placed in the rectum facilitates placement of seeds far enough from the rectal wall and close enough to the posterior lobes for delivery of tumoricidal doses of radiation. Multiple needle punctures through the periprostatic veins and substance of the prostate are necessary for implantation of the 40 to 70 seeds used.

Recommended dose to the periphery of the prostate is 16,000 rads because ^{125}I has a half-life of 60 days, and the dose is delivered over 1 year. This is biologically equivalent to 7500 to 8000 rads delivered by external beam therapy. Supplemental external beam radiotherapy carries a high risk of rectal complications.[4]

COMPLICATIONS

The complications associated with interstitial radiotherapy and the combined interstitial and external beam radiotherapy are similar and can occur both intraoperatively and postoperatively. Intraoperative complications include those associated with pelvic lymph node dissection and hemorrhage. Postoperative complications include proctitis, rectal ulcers, rectal stenosis, cystitis, urethral strictures, incontinence, impotence, genital and peripheral edema, lymphocele, and infection. Postoperative complications are subdivided into early onset (less than 6 weeks after surgery) and late onset (more than 6 weeks after surgery). Symptoms of postoperative complications are discussed as "mild to moderate" and "severe." Mild to moderate symptoms are treatable with medication and usually resolve with the completion of radiation therapy. Resolution of severe complications requires hospitalization and/or surgery. Some-

Table 31–2. TREATMENT PROTOCOL FOR LOCALIZED PROSTATE CANCER USING COMBINED INTERSTITIAL GOLD SEEDS PLUS EXTERNAL BEAM RADIOTHERAPY FOR PATIENTS EXPERIENCING NO EVIDENCE OF METASTASES, 1966–1979

	Pelvic Lymph Nodes	
	Negative	*Positive*
Gold seed implantation	2500–3000 r (3500 r)	2500–3000 r (3500 r)
External beam radiotherapy (begun 18–21 days later)	4000 r to prostate (4500 r)	5000 r to prostate (5400 r)
Total rads	7000 (8000)	8000 (8900)

Figures in parentheses indicate increased dose employed since 1980.

times the severity can be reduced, but the complication cannot be resolved.

Complications of pelvic lymph node dissection and their prevention and management are discussed in detail in Chapter 22.

Intraoperative Complications

Hemorrhage

Intraoperative hemorrhage is a direct result of surgical technique. Interstitial radiotherapy is associated with periprostatic hemorrhage secondary to placement of the interstitial "seeds" by the radiotherapist. The periprostatic veins are traversed with the implant needles for placement of the radioactive material. With ^{198}Au seeds, 6 to 10 seeds are placed and venous bleeding is minimal. Among 510 patients treated at Baylor College of Medicine, blood loss averaged 257 ml.[5] Blood transfusions were rarely needed.

^{125}I seed implantation requires placement of 40 to 70 seeds, and thus the number of needle punctures is greater. Fowler and associates reported an average blood loss of 1024 ml, with 42 percent of the patients requiring intraoperative or postoperative blood transfusion.[6] Schellhammer and associates reported blood losses averaging 400 ml and a 50 percent transfusion rate.[7]

A direct relationship appears to exist between the multiple needle punctures and blood loss. Persistent venous bleeding can be controlled with pressure or figure 8 chromic sutures into the venous plexus. At a time when blood transfusion is not completely safe from contamination, every effort must be made to keep blood loss to a minimum.

Postoperative Complications

Proctitis

Proctitis is caused by radiation injury to the rectum. It can result from interstitial or external beam radiation. Symptoms may vary in severity and may or may not require treatment. The placement of the ^{125}I seeds is very important because the seeds must be placed close enough to the cancer but not too close to the rectal mucosa. The technique of placing a finger within the rectum to allow palpation of the prostate while the seeds are being placed greatly reduces the incidence of proctitis. Late complications severe enough to require other than medical treatment reportedly develop in no more than 10 percent of patients.[7,8]

The incidence of proctitis with gold seed implantation, when combined with external beam radiotherapy, is similar to that with ^{125}I.[5,7] A 7 percent incidence of proctitis has been reported at Baylor College of Medicine; however, all of these cases were considered mild to moderate and required only medical management. Steroid suppository preparations, sitz baths, and stool softeners have been utilized successfully in the conservative management of proctitis.

Rectal Ulcers and Rectal Fistulas

The overall incidence of rectal ulcers and fistulas is relatively low. However, when these complications do occur, they can be difficult to manage. Iodine implants have been associated with an incidence of 1 to 2 percent of rectal ulcers.[7] The incidence following gold seed implantation is similar.[5] When medical measures have failed to provide satisfactory relief of symptoms, colostomy may be indicated. About 50 percent of rectal ulcers will respond to colostomy.[9] The remaining 50 percent and the rectal fistulas will require surgical removal and closure with gracilis muscle flaps to provide healthy tissue for healing. Biopsy of the ulcer and fistula may be indicated prior to colostomy or fistula repair to rule out recurrent carcinoma. Severe, late rectal complications of ^{125}I interstitial radiotherapy occur with a significant incidence when the interstitial therapy is followed by external beam therapy. Ross and associates reported a 26 percent incidence of severe radiation complications, and 2 of 57 patients required colostomy.[4]

Cystitis

Prevention of irritative bladder symptoms is difficult when the area receiving radiation therapy includes the pelvis. The bladder and its rich network of sensory receptors are easily irritated. As expected, ^{125}I and ^{198}Au seeds seem to cause fewer problems than external beam radiotherapy. Minor, early symptoms occur in 10 to 50 percent of the interstitial radiotherapy group.[6] These symptoms usually abate with time or with a rest period in the adjunctive external beam therapy. Late and severe complications are much less common. Irritative symptoms and intermittent hematuria present for more than 6 months can be treated symptomatically. Rarely, the diagnosis of radiation cystitis can be made. Intractable hematuria and irritative symptoms may require supravesicle diversion and/or cystectomy.

Urethral Strictures

Urethral stricture disease is another complication associated with radiation injury to normal adjacent structures. Symptoms include straining to void, a decrease in the force of stream, frequency, and nocturia. Urinary retention may also be a presenting complaint. If urethral strictures occur, they usually are in the bulbous membranous urethra and are short. They occurred in 5.2 percent of the patients described by Pilepich and colleagues[10] in a review of a large number of patients treated with external beam radiotherapy. The incidence of urethral strictures was lower with gold seeds plus external beam radiotherapy. At Baylor College of Medicine, an incidence of 2.5 percent was reported.[5]

^{125}I interstitial radiation was associated with even fewer complications associated with urethral strictures. No strong correlation was shown between transurethral resection of the prostate and the development of stricture disease.[10]

Management of urethral strictures secondary to radiation is similar to management of strictures secondary to infection or trauma; primary optical urethrectomy will usually resolve the process. Occasionally, dilatation may be necessary to keep the urethral stricture from recurring. Only rarely is open urethroplasty necessary.

Incontinence

Injury to the external sphincter mechanism and the bladder neck can cause incontinence. The reported incidence of stress and urgency incontinence is about 2 to 4 percent regardless of the type of radiation.[7] Encrustation and calcification of the prostatic urethra and external sphincter are postulated as etiologic factors by Schellhammer.[7] A correlation with previous transurethal resection has also been proposed. All cases reviewed in the Baylor experience were mild and were treated with medication or resolved spontaneously. No additional surgery was required.[5]

Late onset of incontinence may signal the recurrence of progression of local prostate cancer. A thorough investigation of this possibility is warranted. The placement of an artificial urinary sphincter around the bulbar urethra may be indicated for patients with total incontinence if local tumor progression is ruled out.

Impotence

Erectile dysfunction following pelvic lymph node dissection and interstitial irradiation has been difficult to evaluate. The preoperative erectile status, psychologic factors, and long-term effects (more than 5 years) complicate assessment. Pelvic radiation has been associated with development of pelvic vascular ischemia, Leydig cell dysfunction, and pelvic neuropathy.[11] Advancing age may also play a role. Interstitial radiation with ^{125}I appears to have a 5 percent early association and a 20 percent to 25 percent late association with impotence, and a similar incidence is associated with gold seeds combined with external beam irradiation. The incidence of impotence following external beam radiotherapy alone ranges from 25 to 50 percent.[11] A major etiologic factor associated with external beam therapy is the development of small vessel insufficiency.

The number of treatment options increases daily. Currently, the penile implant is considered the standard by which others are measured. Intracorporeal injections of papaverine are associated with inconsistent results.

Lymphocele and Hematoma

Prevention of lymph and blood collections in the pelvis following lymphadenectomy is a function of meticulous surgical technique. It is important because lymph and blood are excellent culture media for bacteria, and the continued existence of such collections results in the formation of abscesses. Fortunately, the incidence of these complications is low. A review of 510 patients who received ^{198}Au revealed only four lymphoceles requiring therapy and only three pelvic abscesses.[5] Studies of patients who received ^{125}I therapy revealed a similar incidence.[6,7]

Management can vary according to the size of the collection and the severity of the associated symptoms. Percutaneous drainage of small collections, marsupialization, and open surgical drainage of large or infected collections are options to be considered. Persistent lymph drainage can be bothersome and may require sclerosing therapy.

Genital and Lower Extremity Edema

Obstruction at the level of the pelvic and periprostatic lymphatics will result in decreased lymphatic drainage of the lower extremities and of the genitalia. The lymphatic obstruction may be secondary to excessive surgical occlusion intended to prevent lymphatic leakage and collection. It can also occur because of radiation damage to the same lymphatics. Persistent or recurring cancer may occlude the lymphatics, most likely at the level of the lymph nodes.

Prevention of excessive surgical obstruction is accomplished with a modified pelvic lymph node dissection as described by Whitmore and coworkers.[12] The modified methods of dissection provide for prognostic sampling of the lymph nodes of the prostate without complete occlusion of the lower extremity and genital lymphatics. When this technique was used, genital edema was reported in 6 percent of patients, and lower extremity edema was reported in 6.5 percent. These figures also reflect the effects of interstitial and external beam radiation on lymphatic obstruction. The reported incidence of lower extremity edema with ^{125}I interstitial implants ranges from 1.6 to 6.9 percent.

Most reported cases of genital and lower extremity edema were mild to moderate in severity and did not require treatment; however, support stockings were necessary in more severe cases. Persistent, long-term edema of the lower extremities is a complication in a few of these patients.

SUMMARY

Urologists and patients who make therapeutic decisions should fully understand the pros and cons of their choices. Physicians must seek a balance between the need for adequate treatment of the cancer and the risk of complications resulting from injury to normal tissues. Interstitial radiotherapy was developed to compete with external beam radiotherapy in this regard, the goal being to provide a more effective treatment without increasing the morbidity associated with the treatment. Gold seed and iodine interstitial implants are widely used and do not appear to differ with regard to number and kind of associated complications. Whether interstitial radiotherapy is more effective than external beam therapy is a question that remains unanswered at the present time.

References

1. Ray GR, Bagshaw MA: The role of radiation therapy in the definitive treatment of adenocarcinoma of the prostate. Annu Rev Med 26:567–568, 1975.
2. Schmidt JD, Mettlin CJ, Natarjan N, Peace BB, Beart RW Jr, Winchester DP, Murphy GP: Trends in patterns of care for prostate cancer, 1974–1983: Results of surveys by The American College of Surgeons. J Urol 136:416–421, 1986.
3. Gervasi LA, Mata JA, Scardino PT: Prognostic significance of the extent of nodal metastases in prostatic cancer. J Urol 133:203A, 1985.
4. Ross G Jr, Borkon WD, Landry LL, Edwards FM, Weinstein SH, Abadik R: Preliminary observations on the results of combined ^{125}iodine seed implantation and external irradiation for carcinoma of the prostate. J Urol 127:699–703, 1982.
5. Carlton CE Jr, Scardino PT: Long-term results after combined radioactive gold seed implantation and external beam radiotherapy for localized prostatic cancer. In Coffey DS, Resnick M, Dorr F, Karr JP (eds): A Multidisciplinary Analysis of Controversies in the Management of Prostate Cancer. New York, Plenum Publishing Corp, pp 109–121, 1988.
6. Fowler JE Jr, Barzell W, Hilaris BS, Whitmore WF Jr: Complications of ^{125}iodine implantation and pelvic lymphadenectomy in the treatment of prostatic cancer. J Urol 121:447–451, 1979.
7. Schellhammer PF, El-Mahdi AM: Pelvic complications after definitive treatment of prostate cancer by interstitial or external beam radiation. Urology XXI:451–457, 1983.
8. Jordan GH, Lynch DF, Warden SS, McCraw JD, Hoffman GC, Schellhammer PF: Major rectal complications following interstitial implantation of ^{125}iodine for carcinoma of the prostate. J Urol 134:1212–1214, 1985.
9. Anseline PF, Lavery IC, Fazio VW, Jagelman DG, Weakley FL: Evaluation of surgical treatment. Ann Surg 716–723, 1981.
10. Pilepich MV, Perez CA, Walz BJ, Zivnuska FR: Complications of definitive radiotherapy for carcinoma of the prostate. Int J Radiat Oncol Biol Phys 7:1341–1348, 1981.
11. Goldstein I, Feldman MI, Deckers PJ, Babayan RK, Krane RJ: Radiation-associated impotence: a clinical study of its mechanism. JAMA 251:903–910, 1984.
12. Whitmore WF: Interstitial I^{125} implantation in the management of localized prostatic cancer. In Kurth KH, deBruyne FMI, Schroeder FH, et al (eds): Progress and Controversies in Oncological Urology. New York, Alan R. Liss, pp 513–527, 1984.

COMPLICATIONS OF RADICAL CYSTECTOMY

32

Michael M. Lieber

Radical cystoprostatectomy, generally combined with bilateral pelvic lymphadenectomy and some form of supravesical urinary diversion or intestinal neobladder creation, is one of the more complex and technically difficult surgical procedures. This is particularly true when patients have undergone previous high-dose radiation therapy to the pelvis, previous pelvic surgery (such as partial cystectomy), or open prostate enucleation. It is also true for those who have had polychemotherapy in a neoadjuvant setting with agents such as *cis*-platinum, methotrexate, doxorubicin hydrochloride (Adriamycin), and vinblastine sulfate (Velban) (the M-VAC program) for treatment of a large and high-stage bladder cancer. In addition, the common conditions that require cystectomy, including muscle invasive transitional cell carcinoma, vesical sarcomas, and prostate adenocarcinoma that has failed to respond to previous radiotherapy, tend to occur in elderly patients who are generally not the best risks for major pelvic and abdominal surgery. Indeed, with the general increasing longevity of the population, urologists are now commonly called on to carry out radical cystoprostatectomy in patients in their ninth or tenth decade.

Radical cystectomy can be safely carried out even in very elderly or other high-risk patients. In most large teaching hospitals and cancer centers, the mortality rate from radical cystectomy and urinary diversion in modern series is about 1 percent or less. Such mortality rates can be achieved only if intraoperative and postoperative complications are avoided. Complications can be prevented only by the most detailed and systematic approach to the technical demands of radical cystectomy and prostatectomy. For radical cystoprostatectomy (particularly in the patient who received preoperative radiotherapy or neoadjuvant chemotherapy and then undergoes creation of a continent supravesical diversion or intestinal neobladder), operating time can be prolonged. For this reason, the surgeon's concentration can be less than ideal. This can lead to lapses in technique, which may cause postoperative complications. Therefore, in performing radical cystoprostatectomy and urinary reconstruction, the urologic surgeon must be thoroughly familiar with all associated technical details and potential intraoperative and postoperative complications so that he can prevent them in the operating room. The old surgical axiom is especially true when applied to radical cystectomy: Elderly and poor-risk patients tolerate one major operation very well, but they tolerate major complications and reoperations very poorly. Prevention of the very large variety of postoperative complications must therefore be equally considered with surgical techniques designed to optimally treat the underlying malignancy for patients undergoing cystectomy.

This chapter identifies and discusses many of the most common and general complications of radical cystectomy. (A more detailed description of operative technique is found in Reference 1.)

GENERAL CONDITION OF THE PATIENT

Most patients who undergo radical cystectomy and prostatectomy are over age 55. Most have some other medical problem unrelated to the bladder or prostate cancer that must be identified and controlled—indeed, fine tuned—prior to cystectomy. To advance this goal, careful preoperative evaluation by a skilled internist (or often, more than one internist) is necessary to identify medical problems and to get the patient in the best possible shape prior to surgery. Common medical problems of elderly patients, such as hypertension, coronary artery disease, heart failure, chronic bronchitis, emphysema, and diabetes mellitus, need to be fully delineated and the patient's medical condition optimized.

In my experience, it would not be unusual for a patient with significant coronary artery disease to undergo prior balloon angioplasty in order to reduce his risk at the time of cystectomy. Patients who have undergone neoadjuvant polychemotherapy, such as the M-VAC program, should be allowed to fully recover from the toxicity of the chemotherapy prior to undergoing surgery. If they are off protocol, waiting 4 to 8 weeks or more may allow their gastrointestinal tract, bone marrow, and kidneys to fully recover before exposure to the new insults generated by anesthesia, transfusion, and open abdominal surgery. Intensive, in-hospital preoperative pulmonary preparation may significantly aid those patients with chronic bronchitis. For many minor urologic procedures, such medical fine-tuning is sometimes not necessary. However, for radical cystectomy and urinary diversion or reconstruction, patients simply must be in the best possible medical condition before undergoing at an elective time this most major of urologic procedures.

For similar reasons, it is also quite important that the operating surgeon be in the best possible condition. Cystectomy and urinary diversion should be performed by a surgeon in the fittest condition, usually early in the morning, assisted by an experienced and capable operating team. In many centers now performing continent urinary diversion or intestinal neobladder reconstruction, the cystectomy operation is performed by one team and the urinary reconstruction often is performed by a second, separate team of surgeons. This two-team arrangement definitely has pluses in the details of neobladder construction, such as making a careful, watertight closure and a subtle anastomosis between the neobladder and membranous urethra, and reimplanting the ureters, for which a fresh surgeon in the midafternoon can make a big difference. If a second team is not available, a brief break for rest and refreshment during the procedure to keep one's concentration optimally focused must be considered as well. The surgeon simply must be sure that the patient, himself, his first assistant, and entire operating team are in as good general condition as possible for the surgery being contemplated.

ANESTHETIC AND MONITORING CONSIDERATIONS

At the Mayo Clinic and its affiliated hospitals, patients undergoing cystectomy as well as other major urologic procedures commonly are intensively monitored during the procedure. In addition to the usual electrocardiogram (EKG) and pulse oximeter monitoring, patients often have an arterial cannula inserted into the radial artery for instantaneous monitoring of their blood pressure as well as a central line inserted after general endotracheal anesthesia has been induced. Usually, an internal jugular vein or external jugular vein approach is used to place the central line. For patients with known cardiac problems, a Swan-Ganz catheter via the central line access can be placed at the same time or in the postoperative period.

In general, blood must be available in case transfusion is necessary during the surgical procedure. Autologous blood is most desirable and should be banked prior to the procedure with consideration to the patient's overall medical status and preoperative chemotherapy schedule. Most of my own patients have an epidural catheter inserted either preoperatively or immediately postoperatively for continuous infusion of a narcotic, such as morphine or fentanyl citrate, into the epidural space postoperatively. In current practice, patients generally receive epidural narcotics for the first 3 or 4 days after radical cystectomy. I believe that this reduces postoperative pulmonary complications such as atelectasis that are often seen in patients with large abdominal incisions. Most important, for patients whose epidural narcotic infusion works well, the near total or total absence of postoperative pain is significant for its obvious humanitarian value. To see the patient in the intensive care unit the day after surgery absolutely pain free and quite happy is a big change, and I believe a big advance, in the pain management of patients undergoing cystectomy and other major abdominal procedures.

INFECTION

Most postoperative infections in urology occur because the urine is not adequately sterilized preoperatively. Cystectomy is no exception. Because of prior transurethral surgical procedures or indwelling urethral catheters, the urine is commonly infected in patients about to undergo cystectomy. A valiant and informed effort to eliminate infection preoperatively should be carried out to reduce the risk of wound and intra-abdominal infections postoperatively, particularly with specific antibiotics for the infecting organism.

Almost every patient should undergo a thorough bowel preparation prior to cystectomy. Whereas this is obviously required for the patient whose right or sigmoid colon is going to be used to form a continent diversion or neobladder after cystectomy, it is also needed for the patient who is undergoing a simple Bricker-type ileal conduit urinary diversion. For every cystectomy patient, there is a finite risk of rectal injury while carrying out the cystoprostatectomy. This risk is markedly increased in patients who have had previous pelvic surgery, high-dose radiotherapy, or extensive neoadjuvant chemotherapy. If an intraoperative rectal injury occurs with a well-prepared bowel, the risks of subsequent infection are greatly reduced. My colleagues and I commonly use oral preoperative bowel lavage with the GoLYTELY bowel preparation, with or without antibiotics, for this purpose.

Prophylactic parenteral antibiotics are also generally started immediately prior to surgery and are continued for 48 hours postoperatively. It is hoped that established tissue levels of the antibiotics, commonly a cephalosporin such as Ancef, will reduce the chance of postoperative infection developing in the pelvis and wound. It is most important to remember to stop the prophylactic antibiotics a few days after surgery. There have been numerous instances in which patients treated postoperatively for many days with "prophylactic" cephalosporins have developed *Clostridium difficile* pseudomembranous colitis for no really good reason. Because postoperative cramps and diarrhea are not uncommon after urinary diversion intestinal surgery, sometimes such pseudomembranous colitis can be difficult to recognize and can become life threatening. There is no rational reason to continue the prophylactic antibiotics for more than a day or two.

HEMORRHAGE

The bladder and the prostate have a remarkably rich blood supply. Whereas this excellent blood supply is a wonderful resource for the urologist carrying out plastic procedures with the bladder such as partial cystectomy or a Boari flap, it also can be a formidable threat while performing radical cystoprostatectomy. In order to carry out cystectomy/prostatectomy safely, the operating urologist must have a detailed, practical knowledge of the arterial and venous blood supply of the pelvis and some favorite tactical system worked out for controlling it during surgery. For patients with bladder cancer who are undergoing cystectomy and who have not had extensive pelvic irradiation, bilateral pelvic lymphadenectomy is generally performed prior to cystectomy. In pelvic lymphadenectomy, the common external and internal iliac arteries and external iliac veins are generally fully delineated and serve as a well-developed road map to the smaller vascular channels that must be controlled during the bladder exenteration. Furthermore, the obturator nerve on each side of the pelvis is generally carefully dissected out during pelvic lymphadenectomy. Its visual identification should make injury to the obturator nerve most uncommon during cystectomy.

Once the main stem of the internal iliac (hypogastric) artery is identified on each side, it can be controlled to try to reduce the amount of blood loss in the subsequent pelvic dissection. If potency preservation is a consideration, and a nerve-sparing technique is going to be used, it is common to occlude the internal iliac artery on each side of the pelvis near its origin with a bulldog clamp during the procedure. It is most important to tag the clamps so that they are not left behind after the dissection is performed. If potency preservation is not an issue, the internal iliac artery on each side simply can be permanently ligated. Usually, it is best to carry this out distal to the main posterior branch of the internal iliac artery, the posterior superior gluteal artery, so that the patient will not experience "buttocks angina" from ischemia of the gluteus when exercising postoperatively. In addition, ligation of the internal iliac artery close to its origin on the common iliac artery can be difficult here because of atherosclerosis close to the origin.

After a high-quality pelvic lymphadenectomy has been performed, particularly in a thin patient, many of the arteries and veins passing to the bladder and prostate from anterior branches of the internal iliac artery and vein are usually easily visualized, and these branches can be readily controlled, ligated, and divided at the beginning of the radical cystectomy itself. These are the arteries and veins that generally lie in the same plane as the obliterated umbilical artery, which is most easy to identify. I generally use large metal clips to control the vascular pedicles to the bladder and prostate, but for certain patients (obese, irradiated), using surgical clamps and standard ligatures seems to work much better. The operating surgeon should be ready to use whatever technique seems most appropriate deep in the pelvis. Early on, during both the pelvic lymphadenectomy and initiation of the cystectomy, it is important not to drift too far laterally in the true pelvis or one can cause laceration of the internal iliac vein system. In general, there is no anatomic reason to go so far laterally from the bladder. Bleeding from the main internal iliac veins can be particularly troublesome and difficult to control. In contrast, venous and arterial bleeding from the vessels feeding radially into the bladder and prostate from the internal iliac system are relatively easy to control relatively close to the bladder and prostate.

Control of the posterior pedicle of branch arteries and veins going into the bladder and prostate from alongside the rectum generally requires establishing the plane between the bladder–seminal vesicles–prostate and the rectum. With a hand in this space, it is possible to gently push the rectum posteriorly and to identify and thin the deeper vascular pedicles so that they can be adequately and easily clipped or clamped. In order to enter this plane between the bladder and rectum, the peritoneum in the rectovesical cul-de-sac must be incised, and the plane between the bladder and seminal vesicles on the one side and the rectum on the other must be manually developed. Generally, this is a blind procedure done by tactile control. The usual error here is to stray too far anteriorly and to get into the plane between the bladder and the seminal vesicles rather than between the seminal vesicles and the rectum. In a thin patient, the vas deferens and the seminal vesicle are visible, and thus, this problem can be avoided. In the obese patient with a deep pelvis, it has to be done more by feel and intuition. When the correct plane is entered, it is easy to pass caudad immediately to feel the back surface of the prostate and to feel the catheter in the urethra. Vigorous misdirected dissection between the seminal vesicles and the bladder instead can lead to inadvertent entry into the trigone of the bladder, with the resultant spill of cancer cells into the wound. Thus, it is most important to get into the right plane initially.

A common source of blood loss during cystectomy/prostatectomy in the past has been extensive bleeding from the dorsal vein complex of the prostate when the apex of the prostate is dissected and the urethra divided. The early use of hemostatic sutures to control bleeding from the dorsal vein complex, as popularized by Walsh and others, is a very good technique that permits confident dissection in a relatively bloodless field.[2]

Recently, I have been carrying out the apical prostate dissection early in the course of cystectomy rather than immediately prior to removing the bladder and prostate from the pelvis. In this way, the early portion of the pelvic operation can be approached much like a radical prostatectomy. After the endopelvic fascia is divided on each side of the prostate and the puboprostatic ligaments are divided, several heavy sutures are placed around the dorsal vein complex, both distal and proximal to the prostate apex. The dorsal vein complex is divided, and the urethra is identified. The prostate apex is then mobilized early and separated from the rectum, using techniques such as those used for radical prostatectomy. Nerve-sparing or non–nerve-sparing techniques are performed as indicated by the patient's situation.[3] For many patients in my experience, particularly those who have undergone radiation therapy, it is much easier to safely enter the plane between the prostate–seminal vesicles–bladder and the rectum on the other side by beginning at the prostate apex than by beginning above in the cul-de-sac. Moreover, by starting at the prostate apex and working "north," one's second assisting hand also is usually more comfortably oriented to elevate the bladder and to expose the vascular pedicles during the cystectomy operation.

When the dorsal vein complex is not prospectively ligated and divided, bleeding from this venous complex can be tamponaded by a urethral catheter with a large balloon passed retrograde after the bladder has been removed. The balloon is then pulled down to tamponade the veins against the urogenital diaphragm. When this technique is used, direct suture ligation of the veins is generally not necessary. The urethral catheter is left in the pelvis on leg traction for 48 hours postoperatively and is then removed on the third postoperative day.

SPILLAGE OF CANCER CELLS

Spillage of cancer cells from the bladder into the wound should be assiduously avoided, and the possibility of this complication must be considered preoperatively. If, because of previous surgery or radiotherapy or, perhaps, attempted partial cystectomy, it is thought that the bladder may be opened intraoperatively, the surgeon should consider several days of preoperative external beam radiotherapy (approximately 1000 to 1200 cGys) to reduce the chance of tumor cell seeding and wound implantation. Another useful technique, when it is certain that the bladder will be removed, is to instill 4 to 10 percent formalin into the bladder through the indwelling urethral catheter for approximately 10 minutes after the patient is anesthetized. This should kill most superficial cancer cells and greatly reduce the chance of viable cell leakage from the bladder specimen.

Regarding surgical technique, there are two common technical problems that result in cell spillage. The first is noted in the foregoing section—that is, not getting into the correct plane between the rectum and seminal vesicles. If during dissection in the cul-de-sac, one gets between the bladder and the seminal vesicles, pushing vigorously caudad will result in entering the posterior wall of the bladder at the trigone with spillage of cancer cells. This must be avoided. The second problem, the leakage of urine that contains cancer cells, can occur when the membranous urethra is divided. It is most important to occlude the indwelling urethral catheter and the membranous urethra with a heavy clamp prior to dividing the urethra to prevent spillage. If tumor extends into the prostatic urethra and membranous urethra, en bloc urethrectomy should be considered at the time of the procedure.

RECTAL INJURY

Patients often have had previous high-dose radiotherapy to the pelvis. This commonly results from external beam radiotherapy to the prostate with curative intent (often a total dose of about 7000 cGys), followed by tumor progression, which requires cystoprostatectomy for salvage. For patients undergoing cystectomy who have a heavily irradiated pelvis, some surgeons recommend a preliminary approach through the perineum, much like the approach used for a perineal prostatectomy, in which the plane between the prostate and the rectum is formally developed prior to an abdominal incision. In my own practice, I have not used this technique; rather, I have approached a cystectomy/prostatectomy in patients with an irradiated pelvis much as I would an old-fashioned non–nerve-sparing radical prostatectomy. Usually this means sharply taking down the bladder and prostate from any adhesions to the back of the symphysis pubis, dividing the endopelvic fascia, finding the membranous urethra, and developing the plane between the prostate and the rectum at the very beginning. I find this to be easier than approaching caudad from the cul-de-sac in patients who have undergone previous radiotherapy.

Even with the best care and slow, cautious technique, rectal injuries will occur from time to time, particularly in patients who have undergone previous high-dose pelvic irradiation. A meticulous two- or three-layer closure of the rectal tear should be made. This is usually fairly straightforward in the patient who has had adequate bowel preparation and has reasonably preserved tissues. For patients who in fact have undergone previous x-ray therapy, the safest technique is usually to perform a proximal diverting sigmoid colostomy. If rectal injury occurs in a patient who has not been previously irradiated and for whom repair of the rectal injury is technically satisfactory and has had a good bowel preparation, simple primary closure of the injury without a proximal colostomy is probably a reasonable alternative.

Because major non-reparable rectal injury can sometimes occur, particularly in salvage cystoprostatectomy for radiation failure, it is often wise to consider alerting the patient that he may in fact need to undergo a total pelvic exenteration with removal of the rectum and a permanent colostomy as well. In addition, this procedure sometimes gives a much more satisfying and definitive result for the patient with prostate carcinoma who has failed radiation therapy.

ERECTILE IMPOTENCE

Until 5 years ago, erectile impotence was a near universal complication of cystectomy/prostatectomy. Walsh and colleagues at Johns Hopkins have now identified the autonomic neuroanatomy in the pelvis responsible for erection and have carefully described novel surgical techniques to prevent injury to the nerves going to the corpora during pelvic surgery.[4–6] The Walsh nerve-sparing technique for preserving potency during radical prostatectomy has been widely adopted, and the extension of this technique for patients undergoing radical cystectomy has been carefully described.[7] In brief, this involves using the same nerve-sparing technique when carrying out the prostatectomy portion of the cystoprostatectomy, with care taken at the prostate apex to preserve the neurovascular pedicles. Most important, Walsh and colleagues have identified the location of autonomic plexus on the pelvic side walls and have demonstrated that by staying quite close to the seminal vesicles during cystectomy, these nerves responsible for erection can be spared.

URINARY INCONTINENCE AND MANAGEMENT OF THE MEMBRANOUS URETHRA

Management of the membranous urethra formerly was a very straightforward aspect of radical cystectomy/prostatectomy. For most patients, as much of the membranous and proximal bulbous urethra from within the pelvis as possible was removed with the bladder/prostate specimen. By gentle blunt and sharp dissection and by telescoping the membranous urethra into the pelvis over the urethral catheter, it was generally possible to remove 5 to 6 cm of urethra along with the bladder/prostate specimen at the time of cystectomy. This is an excellent technique and should probably still be used in the vast majority of patients with transitional cell carcinoma of the bladder who undergo cystoprostatectomy. Since a fairly good length of urethra can be removed distal to the verumontanum, this technique is appropriate even for some patients with tumor at the bladder neck. In my experience, en bloc total urethrectomy at the time of cystectomy is technically much more difficult than carrying out a secondary urethrectomy several months later, when it is possible to place the patient in an exaggerated lithotomy position. Removal of the most proximal urethra at the time of the pelvic operation markedly simplifies the secondary urethrectomy. However, if there is actually tumor in the proximal urethra, in-continuity urethrectomy with the cystectomy specimen will be required.

Management of the membranous urethra has become a more delicate subject in the current era of neobladder reconstruction using large and small bowel intestinal segments. Many candidates for cystoprostatectomy, particularly young patients who are good medical risks, now seek to have a continent neobladder urinary diversion. In males, this requires leaving the membranous urethra and sphincter mechanism as intact as possible. Such a neobladder reconstruction is not advisable for the patient with transitional cell carcinoma affecting the prostatic urethra or with prostate cancer in which the prostate apex is heavily involved by carcinoma. These patients would be best served by a continent diversion of the Kock pouch variety or one of the techniques that uses elements of the right colon, such as the Indiana bladder.[8]

For the patient undergoing a neobladder reconstruction with use of the native sphincter for continence, the membranous urethra must be managed very much as is done during a radical retropubic prostatectomy. The urethra should be dissected right up to the prostate and dissected carefully out of the so-called prostatic notch.[9] In my experience, there is always a tendency in dissecting out the membranous urethra, to divide it farther distally than is necessary, generally with sacrifice of some of the sphincter area. Informed dissection of the prostate apex, using techniques outlined by Walsh and Myers, makes anatomic preservation of the sphincter zone maximal and should reduce the incidence of urinary incontinence after cystoprostatectomy and neobladder reconstruction.[3,9] These techniques involve placement of hemostatic sutures transversely to control the dorsal prostatic plexus, which in turn permits dissection of the prostate apex to be performed slowly under direct vision rather than in a pool of blood. With this technique, the urethra can be visualized directly where it enters the prostate and the maximum amount of urethra can be preserved for subsequent anastomosis.

For those patients in whom the urethra is left in situ, with or without a continent diversion, careful follow-up is essential to early detection of recurrent transitional cell carcinoma in the urethra. In Mayo Clinic practice, patients undergo urethral washings for cytology every 6 to 12 months for an indefinite period during follow-up. Patients with continent neobladders undergo cystoscopy and follow-up much as those with superficial papillary bladder tumors. Patients with diffuse, high-grade carcinoma in situ, with or without invasive bladder cancer, are at relatively high risk for developing urethral recurrence, particularly if the bladder neck and prostatic urethra have been involved by the carcinoma in situ. Use of a neobladder with urethral outlet in such patients is relatively contraindicated. If it is used, particularly careful follow-up is needed.

URETERAL TUMOR RECURRENCE

Patients with transitional cell carcinoma of the bladder requiring cystectomy, particularly those with large areas of high-grade flat carcinoma in situ, frequently show involvement of the terminal ureters when cystectomy specimens are carefully mapped pathologically. For this reason, it is generally appropriate to remove the last several inches of terminal ureter with the cystectomy specimen. Intraoperative frozen section pathologic examination of the ureteral margins should be performed so that the presence of carcinoma in situ or dysplasia can be detected intraoperatively, and a more proximal portion of the ureter can be used. Even when it is as important to save as much of the ureters as can be accomplished safely to aid in their placement into the new intestinal diversions, it is still most important to get high enough on the ureters (as controlled by frozen section) so that carcinoma in situ is not left at the margins.

MANAGEMENT OF THE VAGINAL CUFF AFTER FEMALE RADICAL CYSTECTOMY

Removal of the entire urethra and trigone for radical cystectomy in the female involves removing part of the anterior vaginal wall. Closure of the opening in the vagina must be done very carefully to promote good vaginal healing in this area, particularly in a patient who has had previous radiation therapy. Complications of peritoneal fluid leak or small bowel fistula from the vaginal cuff can be quite serious after cystectomy in the female. In the patient who will be sexually active after surgery, closure of the opening in the anterior vagina distally should be done in a longitudinal fashion. For patients with larger tumors or who have been heavily irradiated, necessitating removal of the anterior half of the vagina with the specimen, the posterior vaginal wall can be mobilized off the rectum and brought forward as a flap in an anteroposterior direction to close the opening in the vagina. Careful suturing with heavy running absorbable suture material should be carried out under direct vision to make sure that no leak of peritoneal fluid from the vaginal introitus will result. In the patient who has been irradiated, making a pedicle of the omentum and positioning it in the floor of the pelvis over the vaginal opening will also encourage healing in this area and prevent leakage and fistula formation.

COMPLICATIONS OF THE URINARY DIVERSION

Nearly all adult cystoprostatectomies require the use of small or large bowel segments to create a technically satisfactory and long-lasting urinary diversion after cystectomy. For this reason, the complications of the urinary diversion become an integral part of the considerations of complications of cystectomy as a whole.

Uninary Leaks and Small Bowel Obstruction

Postoperative urinary leak from a Bricker-type ileal conduit urinary diversion occurs at the proximal closure of the conduit or, more commonly, from a ureteroileal anastomosis. Such urinary leaks can be devastating in the immediate postcystectomy period and, in the past, have been associated with a high morbidity and mortality rate. Certain traditional techniques facilitate leak-free ureteroileal anastomosis. These include tension-free anastomosis and, most important, use of healthy ureter. Heavily irradiated or operatively traumatized ureter should not be used for the ureteroileal anastomosis. Minimal injury to the ureter during the anastomosis through careful use of forceps is advisable. Creation of interrupted or running watertight anastomoses using fine absorbable sutures and spatulation of the distal ureter is the most common technique. Personally, I use interrupted sutures of 4–0 Vicryl to perform these anastomoses. In addition, because I use the GIA stapler to divide the small intestine and to carry out the ileoileostomy, the proximal end of my ileal conduits is closed by the double layer of the GIA staples. This proximal end is not everted and, to date, I have not had difficulty with stone formation on staples at the proximal conduit closure.

Several newer techniques are recommended to reduce the incidence and severity of urinary leaks. Single-J 7 and 8.5 Fr. urinary diversion stents are now widely available, and I use them for essentially all of my ureterointestinal anastomoses. Coiling of the single-J catheter in the renal pelvis keeps it in position postoperatively, and having the stent cross the anastomosis facilitates its technical performance and eliminates the possibility of sewing the anastomosis closed. I generally leave the stents across the anastomosis until postoperative day 8 or 9, when gastrointestinal function has returned to normal, and the patient is on a regular diet. For patients with irradiated ureters, stents may be left in place significantly longer.

Suction drains, such as medium-sized Hemovac or Jackson-Pratt drains, are also left near the base of the conduit and in the pelvis. Such drains should be placed a few inches away from the ureterointestinal anastomosis itself. Nevertheless, they serve as excellent wicks to remove urine if it leaks. With such drains placed in the abdomen, a urine leak generally does not present as a surgical emergency in which the abdomen fills up with urine. With the drains in place to remove urine, stents across the ureteroileal anastomosis can be fashioned, if they are not originally present or no longer function, using either antegrade or retrograde radiographic techniques. With drains and stents in place, many patients with small urinary leaks can be managed without immediate reoperation and can attain a quite satisfactory ureteroileal anastomosis. In general, the presence of the stents may also serve to reduce the incidence of postoperative ureterointestinal stricture.

Intestinal Obstruction, Intestinal Content Leakage, Prolonged Ileus

The intestinal anastomosis in the usual cystectomy/intestinal diversion is created with healthy non-irradiated intestine, and postoperative complications at this site are quite rare if the blood supply to the intestinal margins is carefully preserved. I generally use intestinal staplers to carry out small bowel–small bowel and small bowel–large bowel anastomoses and have been very happy with this method, which is so much faster than sewing the anastomosis. It is my impression that with side-to-side stapled anastomoses, patients may "open up" a day or two earlier than with the more traditional end-to-end, two-layer, sewn, inverted anastomosis, but of course this is anecdotal and somewhat speculative.

Intestinal content leakage is much more likely to occur when the bowel has been irradiated and, for this reason, irradiated large and small bowel segments should be avoided if possible in carrying out urinary diversions. When there has been extensive pelvic irradiation, one can usually depend on the transverse colon to be radiation free, and this segment makes quite a satisfactory intestinal conduit. Only relatively short segments of proximal ureter are necessary to reach the transverse colon. The urologic surgeon must be mentally flexible and prepared to carry out this sort of diversion when operating on patients who have undergone heavy pelvic irradiation.

Prolonged ileus is also common in patients who have had previous abdominal surgery and radiation therapy to the intestines. In such patients, placement of a tube gastrostomy is generally advisable at the time of cystectomy so that prolonged use of an indwelling nasogastric tube is not necessary. In fact, I generally place a tube gastrostomy in all patients undergoing cystectomy, since an ileus for 7 to 10 days is not that exceptional, and patients are so much more comfortable without a nasogastric tube. The gastrostomy tube is the last tube removed from the abdomen (approximately 11 to 12 days postoperatively), after the ureteral stents and suction drains have been removed.

Incisional Dehiscence and Other Wound Problems

Total cystectomy is probably the most common urologic operation in which abdominal wound dehiscence occurs. This is no doubt because a long midline incision is commonly used for this procedure and because patients often have significant abdominal distention and ileus postoperatively. The best closure to use for such a midline abdominal incision remains controversial and a continuing subject of experimental studies among general surgeons. In my experience, most urologic oncologists close the anterior and posterior fascia and peritoneum as one layer, using interrupted simple or figure-of-eight sutures of heavy monofilament, nonabsorbable suture material, such as prolene, particularly when there is concern about wound healing. In the uncomplicated, well-nourished, thin patient, it is often easier to use an absorbable suture, such as PDS, or heavy Vicryl, or Dexon, which is easier to tie. If the patient is markedly obese, it is probably best to leave subcutaneous drains in place to remove any serum collection and to use retention sutures as well to hold the more superficial layers together.

Thrombophlebitis and Pulmonary Embolism

Patients undergoing radical pelvic surgery, particularly cystoprostatectomy, are at relatively high risk for developing pelvic and lower-extremity thrombophlebitis and pulmonary embolism. Historically, this has been one of the major complications, with the highest incidence statistically, and fatal pulmonary embolism has been one of the leading causes of mortality in published series of cystectomies. It seems most advisable to use those prophylactic measures that are of some value with this problem including perioperative subcutaneous heparin (for example, 5000 units subcutaneously every 8 hours begun preoperatively), intermittent compression stockings on the legs during the procedure, and early ambulation.

I have generally avoided the use of subcutaneous heparin in patients undergoing extraperitoneal radical prostatectomy because of my own experience and the reported experience of prolonged lymph drainage in such patients. This should not be a consideration for the patient undergoing cystectomy because generally the pelvic peritoneum is not reconstructed, and any lymph leaking in the true pelvis would be reabsorbed by the peritoneal contents. Patients who have a postoperative epidural catheter in place for continuous narcotic administration still can ambulate well; these patients and other cystectomy patients should be encouraged to ambulate the day after surgery, if possible. In some large series, full-dose postoperative anticoagulation therapy with warfarin (Coumadin) has been used, with the first dose administered in the recovery room. Although I have not prescribed this medication myself, even this major degree of anticoagulation therapy has been associated with a minimal morbidity in postoperative cystectomy patients.

CONCLUSION

Radical cystectomy/prostatectomy, usually with bilateral pelvic lymphadenectomy, appendectomy, some type of intestinal urinary diversion, and gastrostomy, must be considered a major urologic operative event, even when uncomplicated by a patient with no other major medical problems, previous intraperitoneal surgery, pelvic irradiation, or neoadjuvant chemotherapy. As a result of its many technical elements, there are numerous possibilities for intraoperative and postoperative problems and complications. Continuous focused concentration must be exercised by the surgeon during the procedure in order to reduce the incidence of such complications. Moreover, a very flexible intraoperative approach must be used with all patients. Not every patient will be treated with the same operative tactics, and the preferred or most familiar operation cannot always be applied. For example, patients who have had heavy preoperative radiation therapy are generally not good candidates for pelvic lymphadenectomy because the planes around the pelvic great vessels simply no longer exist. Moreover, sometimes so much scarring in the pelvis is present that the bladder and prostate just must be carved out using the cautery scalpel, staying close to the bladder wall much as one would in performing a simple cystectomy, because the pedicles leading to the bladder simply cannot be developed and sutured. Previous surgery or radiotherapy can affect the ureteral length available for postoperative diversion and the segment of intestine usable for either a standard conduit or a reservoir-type diversion. Therefore, the operating surgeon not only must be armed with an indispensable background of the usual good surgical techniques (such as atraumatic, tension-free anastomoses, careful hemostasis, and so forth), he also must be familiar with all of the tactical variables and options that can be used from case to case with consideration of the patient's size, sex, and exposure to radiation. Numerous published series have documented that radical cystectomy and even salvage cystectomy can be performed with highly acceptable morbidity and mortality rates. Each operating surgeon must strive to equal, if not do better than, these historical series! Awareness of potential complications and their usual major morbidity should motivate the entire operating team to pursue the highest quality operative performance in each individual case.

References

1. Lieber MM, Utz DC: Open bladder surgery. In Walsh PC, Gittes RE, Perlmutter AD, et al, eds: Campbell's Urology, 5th Ed, Volume 3. Philadelphia, WB Saunders Co, 1986, p 2639.
2. Reiner WG, Walsh PC: An anatomical approach to the surgical management of the dorsal vein and Santorini's plexus during radical retropubic surgery. J Urol 121:198, 1979.
3. Walsh PC: Radical retropubic prostatectomy. In Walsh PC, Gittes RE, Perlmutter AD, eds: Campbell's Urology, 5th Ed, Volume 3. Philadelphia, WB Saunders Co, 1986, p 2769.
4. Walsh PC, Donker PJ: Impotence following radical prostatectomy: insight into etiology and prevention. J Urol 128:492, 1982.
5. Walsh PC, Lepor H, Eggleston JC: Radical prostatectomy with preservation of sexual function: anatomical and pathological consideration. Prostate 34:473,1983.
6. Lepor H, Gregerman M, Crosby R, Mostofi FK, Walsh PC: Precise localization of the autonomic nerves from the pelvic plexus to the corpora cavernosa: a detailed anatomical study of the adult male pelvis. J Urol 133:207, 1985.
7. Schlegel PN, Walsh PC: Neuroanatomical approach to radical cystoprostatectomy with preservation of sexual function. J Urol 138:1402, 1987.

8. Rowland RG, Mitchell ME, Bihrle R, Kahnoski RJ, Piser JE: Indiana continent urinary reservoir. J Urol 137:1136, 1987.

9. Myers RP, Goellner JR, Cahil DR: Prostate shape, external striated urethral sphincter and radical prostatectomy: the apical dissection. J Urol 138:543, 1987.

COMPLICATIONS OF CYSTOPLASTY

33

Jeffrey A. Snyder • Shlomo Raz

The first cystoplasty was reported by Tizzoni and Foggi in 1888, when they performed an ileocystoplasty on a dog.[1] As early as the late 1890s, Mikulicz performed the first augmentation enterocystoplasty to correct diminished bladder capacity in a human.[2] Since that time, numerous investigators have utilized the small bowel, large bowel, and stomach[3] in various combinations in attempts to increase the capacity of the bladder reservoir.

The expanded use of enlargement cystoplasty has been made possible by advances in surgical technique, the use of self–intermittent catheterization (SIC), and a greater understanding of the pathophysiology of various intestinal segments. Historically, most of the procedures to augment bladder capacity were performed in patients suffering from tuberculosis or chronic cystitis. More recently, however, the main indication for cystoplasty is the inability to store urine because of bladder instability or detrusor hyperreflexia refractory to pharmacologic therapy. Social acceptance of self–intermittent catheterization for the treatment of urinary retention has permitted this change.

Reconstructive procedures of the lower urinary tract require a comprehensive knowledge of and experience in all aspects of bowel surgery. The success of any reconstruction is based on attention to surgical detail and delicate handling of tissues. Appropriate preoperative evaluation and patient selection are also critical factors that help determine the success of the surgery. Follow-up care must be continuous, with long-term care essential. The goal of cystoplasty is to provide a low-pressure reservoir that permits storage of urine for approximately 6 to 8 hours as well as protects the upper tracts from deterioration. Whether the patient voids spontaneously or by self–intermittent catheterization following the surgery depends on the cause of the problem. Regardless of the surgical indication, augmentation cystoplasty has significantly improved the quality of life, social acceptance, and the course of recovery and rehabilitation for the patient.

CONTRAINDICATIONS

A healthy residual bladder segment at the point of anastomosis is necessary for a successful enterocystoplasty. It is essential to determine that there is no evidence of carcinoma in situ (CIS) or overt carcinoma in the residual native bladder. In the rare cases in which cystoplasty is performed at the time of partial cystectomy for tumor, the free margin at the anastomosis should not be compromised to save a small segment of bladder.

Radiation to the pelvis is not an absolute contraindication to surgery. We must be aware, however, that the rate of complications from leakage at the anastomosis, fistula, and nondistensible bowel segment is much higher in patients who have undergone extensive radiation therapy. Under these circumstances, alternative urinary diversions should be considered.

Because the reconstructed bowel reservoir is in constant contact with urine, electrolyte absorption is commonplace. For patients with impaired renal function, vigilance is required to avoid worsening of the condition.[4,5] The use of cyclosporine has helped decrease mortality rates for patients undergoing renal transplantation; thus, preoperative renal insufficiency is no longer an absolute contraindication for enterocystoplasty. Following the construction of an adequate reservoir, the patient may be able to receive a renal transplant.[6,7] Patients with creatinine levels above 2.5 mg/dl and creatinine clearances below 40 ml/minute are at higher risk of electrolytic imbalance (metabolic acidosis).

Before augmentation, the integrity of the continence mechanism and the urethra must be checked. Because there is a possibility that urinary retention will develop after cystoplasty, an inability to perform self–intermittent catheterization and the existence of extensive urethral damage that precludes uncomplicated catheterization are contraindications to surgery. Any stricture of the urethra should be treated and stabilized prior to surgery. Bowel pathology, such as Crohn's disease, short-bowel syndrome, and so on, is a strong relative contraindication to enlargement cystoplasty.

Because of mucus formation after cystoplasty, young children may be unable to void or empty the bladder after surgery. With the increased use of self–intermittent catheterization, this is now only a relative contraindication to the surgery.

PREOPERATIVE PATIENT EVALUATION

The integrity of the upper and lower urinary tracts must be evaluated prior to major reconstructive surgery to ensure a successful result. Urinalysis should be done to rule out active infection and cytologic examination of the urine will identify the occasional case of CIS masquerading as interstitial cystitis. Upper and lower urinary tract imaging should be performed preoperatively to assess the patency, integrity, and anatomy of the kidneys, ureters, bladder, and bladder outlet. If the ureters are found to be dilated abnormally, a different surgical approach may be considered. Voiding cystourethrography will demonstrate bladder anatomy, point out diverticula that require repair, and identify patients with vesicoureteric reflux. Upright voiding cystourethrogram (VCUG) along with the urodynamic information will help to demonstrate sphincteric function. A significant preoperative post-void residual will identify a patient who is a candidate for postoperative self–intermittent catheterization. Voiding films will rule out any significant urethral pathology such as stricture or urethral diverticula.

Urodynamic evaluation of the lower urinary tract will provide useful and predictive information about postoperative voiding results. For example, findings of an acontractile bladder (detrusor areflexia) will indicate the need for self–intermittent catheterization after surgery; an incompetent bladder outlet must be dealt with prior to or during any reconstructive procedure; and detrusor instability or detrusor hyperreflexia unresponsive to conservative management may be the sole indication for enterocystoplasty. Evaluation may reveal intravesical voiding pressures in excess of 40 cm of water, which places the upper urinary tracts at risk for deterioration either from reflux or from hydronephrosis. Urodynamic studies will help to assess sphincteric function and to determine whether any procedure to the urethra at the time of enlargement cystoplasty is required.

Bowel integrity should be ascertained, particularly in older patients to rule out concurrent pathology. A sigmoidoscopy and barium enema are useful for this purpose. Information regarding the competency of the ileocecal valve can also be obtained, especially if an ileocecal segment is to be utilized and if the ureters must be reimplanted.

THE NATIVE BLADDER

There is a great deal of controversy about how the native bladder is best managed at the time of cystoplasty. In patients suffering from radiation-induced cystitis, most of the bladder should be resected, leaving only the smallest cuff of detrusor muscle for the anastomosis. Failure to recognize this before reconstruction may lead to a poor surgical result with an increased risk of fistula formation. This was reported in 1950 by Couvelaire[8] and confirmed by other investigators.[9,10] Gittes[11] and Zinman[12] suggested subtotal bladder resection in all enterocystoplasties. Their theory, which coincided with that of Turner-Warwick, was that an insufficiently resected detrusor would act as a source of weakness and therefore essentially be a diverticulum.[13] In contrast, Smith[4], Gow,[14] and Rizzo[15] dispute the necessity of bladder excision.

Our own philosophy is not to perform routine supratrigonal cystectomy. We do it only in rare cases of irradiated bladder and for the treatment of interstitial cystitis. Otherwise, in patients with neuropathic or unstable bladder conditions, a transverse flap of bladder is created widely along its posterior wall. This procedure does not appear to compromise spontaneous emptying of the bladder.

When augmentation is performed without partial or supratrigonal cystectomy, the incision of the bladder wall for anastomosis is important. A direct anastomosis to the open bladder dome is not appropriate because of the high incidence of hourglass stricture of the anastomotic area. A common method of bladder augmentation is the clam technique, in which the bladder is divided in a sagittal plane from trigone to trigone on the contralateral side. An alternative is to open the bladder on a longitudinal plane from the bladder neck area anteriorly to the trigone posteriorly. Our aforementioned method of choice is to make a large U incision in the posterior bladder wall to create an anterior bladder flap. The intestinal segment is anastomosed as a patch posterior to the bladder.

SELECTION OF INTESTINAL SEGMENT

The literature reflects controversy in defining the best possible bowel segment for use in augmentation cystoplasty. It has been proposed that the small intestine offers a lower pressure than the large intestine. It is further believed that the mass contraction of the descending and sigmoid colon is less advantageous than the cecum. Hradec's studies of intraluminal pressure measurements have demonstrated that pressures are lower in the small bowel than in the large bowel.[16] This was confirmed by others.[17]

In contrast to this, we believe that the choice of bowel segment, in fact, does not influence the outcome of augmentation cystoplasty. A segment of bowel that is large enough, that has a good blood supply, and that is detubularized and reconfigured will give a good surgical result regardless of its origin (sigmoid, cecum, ileum, or other). Other investigators[12,13] prefer to use the ileocecal segment because of its constant and reliable blood supply. This region can be mobilized extensively to accommodate the bladder situated deep within the pelvis. Also, the reanastomosis of colon to ileum is easily accomplished. We personally prefer the cecal segment also, because it reabsorbs less water, and after detubularization, it provides a wide patch that does not require suturing for reconfiguration as does the ileum.

The choice of bowel segment to be used depends on the surgeon's personal experience and preference as well as on the patient's particular circumstances.[17,31]

SELECTION OF CYSTOPLASTY CONFIGURATION

The shape and configuration of the cystoplasty is important to the success of the surgery. In our laboratory we have studied the impact of ileal reservoirs with and without detubularization. It is clear from the studies that detubularization of the bowel improves functional capacity by the mere geometric changes, provides better compliance, and lowers filling pressures.[33] Failure to detubularize the intestinal segment will result in a high-pressure reservoir and subsequent urinary incontinence or vesicoureteral reflux.[18] This is more common in large bowel segments than in small bowel segments because of mass contraction of the large bowel.

With the same length of intestinal segment, a cystoplasty with a spherical configuration will afford more volume than that with a tubular configuration. Volume-dependent phasic bowel contractions may occur in any augmentation (the ileum probably creates the lowest pressure contractions) and may be successfully treated by cholinolytic therapy or smooth-muscle–relaxant therapy.[6,19]

THE UPPER URINARY TRACTS

A low-pressure reservoir is essential to protect the upper urinary tracts. There is controversy as to when and where the ureters should be reimplanted at the time of augmentation cystoplasty. One concept is clear from the literature: If obstruction or reflux is present preoperatively, it must be corrected during reconstruction. Depending on the patient population and the causes necessitating augmentation, up to 80 percent of patients were found to require reimplantation to correct either obstruction or reflux of the ureters.[11] If the ureters are not obstructed, dilated, or refluxing, simple augmentation without reimplantation is appropriate.

It is our practice to perform a tunneled antireflux reimplantation in patients with mild to moderate reflux and good peristalsis of the ureters. If the bladder is compliant, thick, not fibrotic, and without trabeculae or diverticula, the ureters may be reimplanted in the native bladder. However, if the bladder wall is severely damaged, thick, or trabeculated, we prefer to reimplant the ureters in the bowel segment used for augmentation. If the ureters are very dilated, with poor peristalsis, we do not perform a tunneled reimplant because of the fear that the ureters will be unable to transfer urine through the tunnel. In this situation, we prefer to reimplant the ureters end-to-side to a segment of ileum that has no antireflux mechanism (such as in a Bricker diversion), create an antireflux nipple distal to the anastomosis (in general from the ileocecal valve), and anastomose the remaining bowel segment (cecum or ileum) to the bladder as an enlargement cystoplasty. In order to avoid ureteral obstruction from mucus, edema, or kinking, we feel that the use of double J stents at the time of ureteral reimplantation during an augmentation cystoplasty is very important.

COMPLICATIONS OF ENTEROCYSTOPLASTY

Complications may be categorized according to their typical timing of presentation. Perioperative complications can arise from the time of surgery to the first postoperative month. These may include gastrointestinal tract disorders, urinary tract bleeding, bowel or urinary fistula, upper urinary tract obstruction, wound infection, pulmonary problems, and venous thrombosis. Late complications may include bowel obstruction, electrolyte disorders, urinary incontinence or retention, vesicoureteric reflux or obstruction, mucus plugs, urinary infection, stone formation, and the late development of bowel neoplasm. Because of the scope of this chapter, our discussion is limited to late complications.

LATE COMPLICATIONS OF ENTEROCYSTOPLASTY

Electrolyte Disorders

Electrolyte imbalance may arise following augmentation cystoplasty because of absorption of urinary metabolites through the expanded absorbing intestinal surface area. The degree of disturbance generated depends on the renal function and the ability to maintain adequate electrolyte balance. In the past, renal insufficiency was considered a relative contraindication to the successful prevention of electrolyte disorders. However, the progressive deterioration of renal function has become an indication for reconstructive procedures in conjunction with renal transplant.

Various criteria have been developed to guide the surgeon to avoid this complication. A serum creatinine level greater than 2.5 mg/dl.[5] or a minimum creatinine clearance of 40 ml/minute[4,28–30] was an established level documented in the literature. The most common disturbance is metabolic acidosis (with hypokalemia and hyperchloremia). The highest-risk patients are those with borderline renal function who developed urinary retention and incomplete voiding after cystoplasty and who are not following a proper program of bladder emptying. High post-void residuals of urine and the ensuing urinary infections will enhance the tendency toward an electrolytic imbalance.

Urinary Fistula

Urinary fistula may occur to the skin, vagina, or a segment of bowel (in general to the bowel's anastomotic area, because of leakage). This is not a common complication and can be avoided with meticulous handling of tissue, multiple-layer anastomotic closures, and an omental inlay as a protective seal interposed between the reconstructed bladder and the vagina or rectum. These preventive measures have been found to be most useful in patients with previously irradiated bladder or bowel segments.

Adequate drainage of the augmented bladder must be provided. We utilize a 20 French urethral catheter, a 24 Fr. suprapubic tube, and adequate perivesical drains. (Penrose drains are our preference.) The catheters must be kept irrigated soon after surgery to prevent any clots or mucus obstruction that will result in leakage into the perivesical space. We routinely irrigate the catheters twice daily starting the first postoperative day. It has long been believed that the suprapubic tube should be brought out through the bladder wall to prevent vesicocutaneous fistulas.[26] This has not been our experience, and we have not seen an increased incidence of cutaneous or other fistulas when the suprapubic catheter is brought out through the augmented bowel segment.

Fistulas to the bowel may be treated with parenteral hyperalimentation and fasting, but in some instances, they may require surgical correction. Vaginal fistulas, when established, will require surgery. To avoid another laparotomy, a vaginal repair should be attempted.

Problems of Bladder Emptying

There is a high incidence of incomplete bladder emptying after enlargement cystoplasty. In our experience, this incidence will depend on the causes that required the cystoplasty. In patients with bladder instability who have no neurologic disease or have not undergone any surgery to correct urethral incompetence, about 10 percent are unable to adequately empty the bladder contents. In patients with bladder instability with concomitant or prior urethral surgery, the incidence is approximately 30 percent. In patients with neurologic disease and bladder external sphincter dyssynergia such as myelomeningocele, paraplegia, or multiple sclerosis, the incidence is above 90 percent. Therefore, it is essential to inform patients preoperatively of this problem and of the possibility that they may require lifelong self–intermittent catheterization.

During the first year or two following reconstruction, mucus produced within the bladder may contribute to outlet obstruction. Because of the need for repeated cystoscopic manipulations and bladder irrigations, the use of bladder augmentation in young male children should be strongly debated prior to embarking on a reconstructive procedure utilizing a bowel segment.[4] The problem does tend to subside after the second year, when the lining of the bowel segment is altered. These problems tend to be less common in the female patient.

Urinary Incontinence

Inability to store urine after cystoplasty may result from sphincteric incompetence or from poor storage capability of the enlarged bladder. This complication can be avoided in part if the bladder outlet resistance is properly evaluated prior to surgical intervention and if the bowel segment is detubularized to create a low-pressure reservoir. Despite these precautions, postoperative incontinence may result from elevated bladder pressures. An increase in pressure may have several causes. One very common cause is the hyperactivity and peristaltic contractions of the bowel segment in spite of proper detubularization. Another possibility is the continuation of uninhibited bladder contractions of the native bladder. Rarely, stricture of the native bladder to augmented bowel anastomosis may create an hourglass deformity of the reconstructed segment, leading to poor urine storage. This problem can be prevented by a proper anastomosis of a wide open patch or "clam" of the bladder with the bowel segment. Uninhibited contractions of the bowel segment can be managed with pharmacologic therapy (Lomotil, Imodium, Pro Banthine, Bentyl, and others), whereas bladder instability can be further improved with oxybutynin hydrochloride (Ditropan), imipramine hydrochloride (Tofranil), or a combination of both.

Diminished bladder capacity after cystoplasty may have organic causes. In such patients, testing under general or spinal anesthesia will reveal that the bladder capacity remains small, whereas under general anesthesia, the bladder expands easily when the cause of instability is functional. We should suspect ischemia of the bowel segment, which requires further surgery to substitute or to add another patch of bowel.

At the time of augmentation, consideration should be given to correct sphincteric incontinence. In the female, the most common procedure for anatomic stress incontinence is a Burch suspension. The lateral placement of the suspension sutures will avoid urethral obstruction. However, if the cause of sphincteric incompetence is intrinsic damage to the sphincteric unit (multiple surgeries, trauma, exposure to radiation, or neurogenic disease), a bladder neck suspension may not be sufficient to achieve continence.[35] In these patients, consideration must be given to a compression procedure such as a sling[36] or to the implantation of an artificial urinary sphincter.

In the female, we have not personally used the artificial sphincter because of the excellent result provided by the use of fascial and more recent vaginal wall slings. In the male, we have also successfully used fascial slings.[34] The insertion of an artificial sphincter at the bladder neck or bulbar urethra during the cystoplasty or later will provide continence in more than 75 to 90 percent of patients.

Vesicoureteral Reflux

Preoperative evaluation should identify those patients with vesicoureteral reflux. The caliber and peristalsis of the ureters should also be considered. The principles noted in the foregoing discussion of our approach to ureteral reimplantation apply to reflux that occurs as a complication of enlargement cystoplasty. It is a known fact that lower and upper urinary tract infections are correlated to bladder pressures. Patients undergoing self–intermittent catheterization with low-pressure reservoirs rarely have symptoms of upper urinary tract infections in spite of reflux. On the other hand, patients with high-pressure reservoirs (poor compliance or uninhibited contractions) have the highest risk for upper urinary tract infections and renal deterioration. Vesicoureteral reflux in patients after cystoplasty and in those requiring self–intermittent catheterization is well tolerated provided that compliance, capacity, and the pressures of the enlarged bladder are adequate. In these patients, there is usually no need for secondary ureteral reimplantation.

Patients who experience postcystoplasty vesicoureteral reflux with recurrent upper urinary tract infections, massive upper urinary tract dilation, kidney scarring, or loss of renal parenchyma will require secondary reimplantation. Prior to surgery, urodynamic evaluation of the enlarged bladder should be performed to rule out the presence of a high-pressure system.

If the native bladder is in good condition, the reimplantation may be performed in the bladder area without complications. However, if the bladder is thick, trabeculated, or fibrotic, we prefer to reimplant the ureters in the bowel segment. As noted in the aforementioned discussion, the decision to use an antireflux mechanism will depend on the quality of the ureters.

When utilizing a combined ileocecal segment, the valve integrity should be investigated preoperatively and reconstruction based on its competency. We have found that preoperative and intraoperative testing of the ileocecal valve is not reliable in ensuring postoperative protection against reflux. When this particular segment of bowel is used, we always reinforce or reconstruct the ileocecal valve. Our preferred method involves intussusception of the ileocecal valve with fixation of the nipple to the wall of the cecum with ureteral reimplantation directly into the proximal ileal segment. Because stone formation and recurrent urinary tract infection have occurred in a significant number of our patients when the staples were placed intraluminally and exposed to urine, we now place the staples in the outer two layers of the intussuscepted segment.

Urinary Tract Infection

De novo urinary tract infection is commonly found in patients with bladders augmented with bowel. In fact, the incidence of asymptomatic bacteriuria is probably very high, especially for patients on self–intermittent catheterization. If, however, the bladder can be maintained with low intravesical pressures and reflux can be prevented, only those patients with previous pyelonephritis or undetected ureteral obstruction should be affected. Careful postoperative vigilance using periodic cystoscopy will also identify those patients with excessive mucus production and plugs, which are prone to cause urinary tract infections.

When self–intermittent catheterization is required, a strict regimen of timed catheterization and fluid restriction should be maintained. Failure to adhere to this program will result in high bladder pressures, and symptomatic urinary tract infection will develop. Chronic suppressive antibiotics are commonly administered to these patients and very effectively prevent upper urinary tract infection and symptomatic lower urinary tract infection. Nevertheless, closely following the program of self–intermittent catheterization will also avoid symptomatic infection. We do not routinely prescribe antibiotics after enlargement cystoplasty for patients requiring self–intermittent catheterization.

Stone Formation

The incidence of bladder stone formation in patients following enlargement cystoplasty is higher than its incidence in the normal population. The causes of this complication include the presence of mucus, incomplete bladder emptying, and urinary tract infections. This complication can be avoided by close surveillance; patients voiding spontaneously, post-void residuals and urine cultures must be controlled often. Cystoscopy must be performed every 3 to 6 months, at least during the first 2 years after surgery to detect mucus accumulation and stone formation.

Neoplasms

The occurrence of carcinoma in an augmented bladder has long been thought to be very low. Whether the true incidence is, in fact, low or whether the long-term follow-up is inadequate remains a point of contention. It is not certain whether preoperative evaluation of the bowel segment with random biopsy in the previous studies was done to rule out occult disease. To date, there have only been eight reported cases of de novo carcinoma in an augmented bladder.[21–26] It is well known that the lining of the bowel segment adapts to chronic contact with the urine. Histologic changes including bowel mucosa atrophy, loss of intestinal villi, and squamous metaplasia have all been well described.[26] Six of these patients were previously diagnosed as having tuberculosis, and all six patients underwent ileocystoplasty. Four developed adenocarcinoma[21,23,25] and two developed transitional cell carcinoma.[22,23] Kirby reported a case of squamous cell carcinoma of the cervix. The patient underwent a cecocystoplasty and subsequently developed adenocarcinoma in the bowel segment eight years postoperatively.[24] Egbert reported on a 43-year-old male who developed undifferentiated sarcoma in both the bladder and the bowel segment of the augmentation ileocystoplasty after a latent period lasting 19 years.[26]

We have encountered the development of carcinoma in two additional patients in our series of 400 who underwent augmentation cystoplasty. The first patient, a 69-year-old male, underwent a sigmoid colocystoplasty and developed transitional cell carcinoma in both the bowel and the bladder segment 24 years following surgery. The second patient, a 40-year-old female, had had an ileocecocystoplasty for urinary incontinence and developed a poorly differentiated small cell carcinoma in the bladder segment after an eight-year latency period.

The lesson to be learned is that such patients will require lifelong surveillance. The possibility of carcinoma should always be considered because of the long latent period between reconstruction and its development.[28]

SUMMARY

The combination of greater surgical expertise and pathophysiologic understanding has led to the successful treatment of bladder problems through augmentation cystoplasty. Although initial short-term follow-up is extremely encouraging, we must wait to review the long-term results of bladder augmentation and bowel reanastomosis before endorsing these procedures without reservation. However, complications can be reduced significantly with meticulous handling of tissues, attention to surgical detail, expanding our knowledge of the basic pathophysiologic changes, and precise patient selection.

References

1. Tizzoni G, Foggi A: Die Wiederherstellung der Harnblase. Zentralbl Chir 26:641, 1888.
2. Mikulicz J: Zur Operation der Augeborenen Blasenspalte. Zentralbl Chir 26:641, 1899.
3. Leong CH: Use of the stomach for bladder replacement and urinary diversion. Ann R Coll Surg Engl 60:283, 1978.
4. Smith RB, VanCangh P, Skinner DG, Kaufman JJ, Goodwin WE: Augmentation enterocystoplasty: a critical review. J Urol 118:35, 1977.
5. Skinner DG: Further experience with the ileocecal segment in urinary reconstruction. J Urol 128:252, 1982.
6. Stephenson TP, Mundy AR: Treatment of the neuropathic bladder by enterocystoplasty and selective sphincterotomy or sphincter ablation and replacement. Br J Urol 57:27,1985.
7. Hendren WH: Editorial comment on Skinner, DG: further experience with the ileocecal segment in urinary reconstruction. J Urol 128:256, 1982.
8. Couvelaire R: La "petite vessie" des tuberculeaux genito-urinaires. Essai de classification place et variantes des cysto-intestino-plasties. J Urol 56:381, 1950.
9. Kerr WK, Gale GL, Peterson KSS: Reconstructive surgery for genitourinary tuberculosis. J Urol 101:254, 1969.
10. Gil-Vernet JM Jr: The ileocolic segment in urologic surgery. J Urol 94:418, 1965.
11. Gittes RF: Bladder augmentation procedures. In Zinman L, Libertino JA, eds: Reconstructive Urologic Surgery: Pediatric and Adult. Baltimore, The Williams & Wilkins Co, 1977, pp 216–226.
12. Zinman L, Libertino JA: Technique of augmentation cecocystoplasty. Surg Clin North Am 60:703, 1980.
13. Turner-Warwick RT, Ashken MH: The functional results of partial, subtotal and total cystoplasty with special reference to ureterocaecocystoplasty, selective sphincterotomy and cystocystoplasty. Br J Urol 39:3, 1967.
14. Dounis A, Abel BJ, Gow JG: Cecocystoplasty for bladder augmentation. J Urol 123:164, 1980.
15. Lunghi F, Nicita G, Selli C, Rizzo M: Clinical aspects of augmentation enterocystoplasties. Eur Urol 10:159, 1984.
16. Hradec EA: Bladder substitution: indications and results in 114 operations. J Urol 94:406, 1965.
17. Turner-Warwick RT, Handley-Ashken M: The functional results of partial, subtotal and total cystoplasty. Br J Urol 39:3, 1967.
18. Hendren WH: Urinary undiversion and augmentation cystoplasty. In Kalalis PP, King LR, Belman AB, eds: Clinical Pediatric Urology, 2nd ed. Philadelphia, WB Saunders Co, 1985.
19. Light JK, Engelmann UH: Reconstruction of the lower urinary tract: observations on bowel dynamics and the artificial urinary sphincter. J Urol 133:594, 1985.
20. Sidi AA, Gonzalez RA: Enterocystoplasty in the management and reconstruction of the pediatric neurogenic bladder. Unpublished data, 1986.
21. Stone AR, Davies N, Stephenson TP: Carcinoma associated with augmentation cystoplasty. Br J Urol 60:236, 1987.
22. Smith P, Hardy GJ: Carcinoma occurring as a late complication of ileocystoplasty. Br J Urol 43:576, 1971.
23. Leedham PW, England HR: Adenocarcinoma developing in an ileocystoplasty. Br J Urol 60:158, 1973.
24. Kirby RS, Lloyd-Davies RW: Adenocarcinoma occurring within a caecocystoplasty. Br J Urol 57:357, 1985.
25. Takasaki E, Murahashi I, Toyoda M, Honda M, Waku S: Signet ring adenocarcinoma of ileal segment following ileocystoplasty. J Urol 130:562, 1983.
26. Egbert BM, Kraft JK, Perkash I: Undifferentiated sar-

coma arising in an augmented ileocystoplasty patch. J Urol 123:272, 1980.

27. Shirley SW, Mirelman J: Experiences with colocystoplasties, cecocystoplasties, and ileocystoplasties in urologic surgery: 40 patients. J Urol 114:289, 1975.
28. Roblejo PG, Malament M: Late results of an ileocystoplasty: a 12-year followup. J Urol 109:38, 1973.
29. Kuarstein B, Mathison W: Sigmoidocystoplasty in adults with enuresis. Surg Gynecol Obstet 153:65, 1981.
30. Whitmore WF, Gittes RF: Reconstruction of the urinary tract by cecal and ileocecal cystoplasty; review of a 15-year experience. J Urol 129:494, 1983.
31. Murphy JJ, Myint MK, Scott LB, Scwegman CW: Absorption of urinary constituents from various segments of the gastrointestinal tract used as urinary conduits or reservoirs. Surg Forum 6:604, 1955.
32. Kuss R, Jardin A: Commentary on colocystoplasty. In Whitehead ED, ed: Current Operative Urology. Hagerstown, Maryland, Harper & Row Publishers Inc, 1975, pp 742–749.
33. Schimdbauer CP, Chiang H, Raz S: The impact of detubularization on ileal reservoirs. J Urol 138:140, 1987.
34. Raz S, McGuire EJ, Ehrlich RM, Zeidman EJ, Wang SC, Alarcon A, Schimdbauer C, McLaughlin S: Fascial sling to correct male neurogenic sphincter incompetence: the McGuire/Raz approach. J Urol 139:528–531, 1988.
35. Raz S, Ehrlich RM, Zeidman EJ, Alarcon A, McLoughlin S: Surgical treatment of the incontinent female patient with myelomeningocele. J Urol 139:524–527, 1988.
36. Raz S, Siegel AL, Snyder JA: Vaginal wall sling. J Urol 141:43, 1989.

COMPLICATIONS OF URETHRAL SURGERY IN THE MALE

34

Richard Turner-Warwick

Complications of Urethral Stricture Surgery and Some Ways of Preventing Them

Successful surgery is the result of anticipating and avoiding the potential complications that are inherent in every injury and every operation; clinical judgment and operative procedures are essentially developed to achieve this. The principles of preventing complications are epitomized by the evolution of the various procedures that are required for the resolution of the wide range of urethral problems that confront a urethral surgeon.

No single procedure is appropriate for all urethral reconstructions. There are other good options and it is always salutary to see contrarily conceived procedures "working" in the hands of others; nevertheless, some procedures are more prone to complications than others.

The development of procedures for urethral repair and reconstruction over the past 3 decades now offers the opportunity of restoration of efficient voiding and freedom from instrumentation to almost every patient with a urethral stricture. Standards have also changed within this time. Whereas a long-term stricture-free rate of 75 to 80 percent used to be regarded as a reasonable result of a definitive reconstruction, now a failure rate of more than 6 to 8 percent after substitution procedure and *almost any* restenosis after a one-stage anastomotic repair even of complex pelvic fracture urethral distraction defects[1,2] should cause a reconstructive surgeon to reflect upon the selection of the procedure or the technique of its performance—or both.

Internal urethrotomy is a relatively simple general urologic procedure for the management (though less often the long-term cure) of most strictures of the bulbo-penile spongy urethra; however, it is essential to recognize the limitations of this procedure because its indiscriminate use can result in complications, some of which are potentially disastrous.

The views expounded in this chapter are simply a distillate of personal experience in this intriguing subspecialist field to which many friends and colleagues have made outstanding contributions.

Bulbo-Penile Urethral Surgery

STRUCTURAL AND FUNCTIONAL CONSIDERATIONS

For definable reasons, the surgical restoration of a stable, normal-caliber urethra is by no means a simple matter. Its unique structure is a fundamental factor—both in its predisposition to the formation of strictures and in their surgical treatment.

The Spongy (Bulbo-Penile) Urethra

Microstructure. The whole length of the wall of the bulbo-penile urethral lumen is formed by its surrounding spongy erectile tissue, simply lined by a layer of uroepithelium applied almost directly to its vascular spaces. It is the healing response of this delicate spongy tissue and the consequent spongiofibrosis that are responsible for the development of strictures of the bulbo-penile urethra and that determine their nature.[3]

Macrostructure. In the penile area the lumen of the urethra is *concentrically* located within the spongy tissue, which forms its wall some 3 to 4 mm thick. However, the bulbar urethral lumen is *eccentrically* located in a dorsal position within the bulk of the bulbar spongy tissue expansion.

Thus, throughout the length of the bulbar and the penile urethra, the thickness of the spongy tissue in the dorsal, 12 o'clock, position is a uniform 3 to 4 mm (Fig. 34–1).

In the penile area, the urethra is firmly anchored to the undersurface of the corpora in the 10 to 2 o'clock sector, whereas in the bulbar area the adhesion is linear.

The relatively thin and uniform layer spongy tissue forming the roof of the urethra is relevant to the siting of an internal urethrotomy (see subsequent discussion). Furthermore, in the course of definitive bulbar urethral reconstructions, the *eccentric* posterolateral bulk of the spongy tissue generally requires a definitive spongioplasty procedure, i.e., posterior spongioplasty[1] for anastomotic procedures and posterolateral redeployment spongioplasty for the redeployment urethral roof-strip (TWARS) procedures (see subsequent discussions).

Vascularization

The retrograde distal collateral blood supply of the bulbo-penile urethra is a fundamental factor determining the extent of its surgical mobilization.[5,6]

Bulbar Urethral Emptying

The normal bulbar urethra is emptied completely after voiding by its low-pressure closure mechanism created by the combination of the vasculoelasticity of the bulbo-spongy tissue, augmented by voluntary contraction of the surrounding bulbo-spongiosus muscle. There is a natural tendency for the efficiency of the bulbar urethral emptying mechanism to diminish with age, so it is not unusual for male patients to present, about the age of 50, with a recent onset of postvoiding urethral after-drip resulting from bulbar urethral pooling of urine—a problem that is simply resolved by assisting its evacuation by finger pressure in the perineum after voiding.[7]

An increase in the efficiency of urethral emptying is necessary for procreation. The conversion of the continuous stream of an orgasmic emission into an efficient forceful ejaculation is achieved by the combination of a sustained increase in the bulbo-penile urethral closure-pressure created by the erectile engorgement of its surrounding spongy tissue and the reflex ejaculatory contractions of the surrounding spongiosus muscle compressing the consequent increase in its bulk.[6]

Definitive urethral reconstructive procedures inevitably impair the natural closure-pressure mechanisms of both the spongy tissue and its surrounding musculature. Indeed, this is often already impaired to some extent by the spongiofibrotic stricture process. Although it is sometimes possible to reconstruct some residual bulk of periurethral spongy tissue by a redeployment spongioplasty, it is obviously deficient after excision of an extensive spongiofibrosis. However, the procedure of oversewing the incised lateral margins of a urethroplasty incision in the bulbar spongy tissue, which is sometimes advocated to achieve perioperative hemostasis, is an often unnecessary sacrifice of potentially valuable overclosure tissue.

Thus it is fundamentally important that the lumen of a reconstructed bulbar urethra have a normal and even caliber and that the bulbospongiosus muscle be overclosed to support it whenever possible.

Urine retained in a sacculated reconstructed

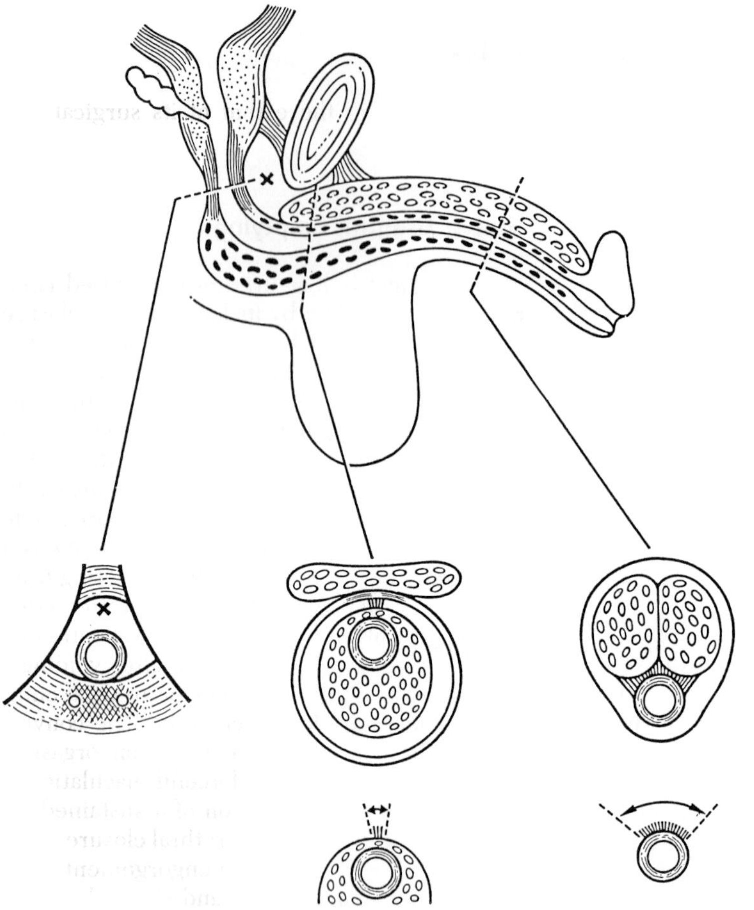

Figure 34–1. Anatomical relationships. In the penile urethra the spongy tissue is concentrically arranged; in the bulb it is dorsally eccentric. Thus, throughout the anterior bulbo-penile urethra, the thickness of the spongy tissue on its dorsal (12 o'clock) aspect is only 3 to 4 mm. The subprostatic membranous urethra relates anterolaterally to the pubo-urethral space. Posteriorly it is densely adherent to the perineal body, and posterolaterally (4 and 8 o'clock) it relates to the nervi erigentes. © 1987, Institute of Urology.

urethra is a well-recognized source of complications—the postvoiding after-discharge of a volume of urine commensurate with its capacity, infection of stagnant retentions of urethral urine, and encrustation of hairs (especially when a scrotal-skin substitution procedure has been used without effective epilation).

THE PATHOGENESIS OF STRICTURES OF THE BULBO-PENILE SPONGY URETHRA

A basic understanding of the pathogenesis of strictures of the bulbo-penile spongy urethra, their development, and the significance of spongiofibrosis is essential to their successful reconstruction and to the prevention of complications.

Partial loss of the uro-epithelial lining is the primary factor in the development of almost every spongy urethral stricture, whether it is caused by internal trauma, urethritis, or external trauma. The loss of any proportion of the circumference of the epithelial lining of the urethra generally results in commensurate narrowing of its lumen during healing because the margins of the residual epithelium are approximated by the natural urethral closure-pressure so that the unepithelialized defect forms a cleft, which tends to heal rapidly by cross-adhesion and epithelial overbridging (Fig. 34–2). The intermittent passage of urine opens these clefts, and this repeated separation and re-exposure of the vascular spongy tissue spaces leads to a gradual increase in the underlying spongiofibrosis.

Unfortunately, this complex combination of slow epithelial proliferation, cleft opening and closure, and spongiofibrosis also results in a tendency to restenosis whenever bare areas are created by the treatment of a stricture by dilatation or by internal urethrotomy. Attempts to promote early uro-epithelialization of the denuded clefts by keeping them open for a prolonged period with an indwelling catheter are generally unsuccessful.

To avoid complications, urethral surgery must particularly take into account the inherent characteristics of urethral healing that result in a

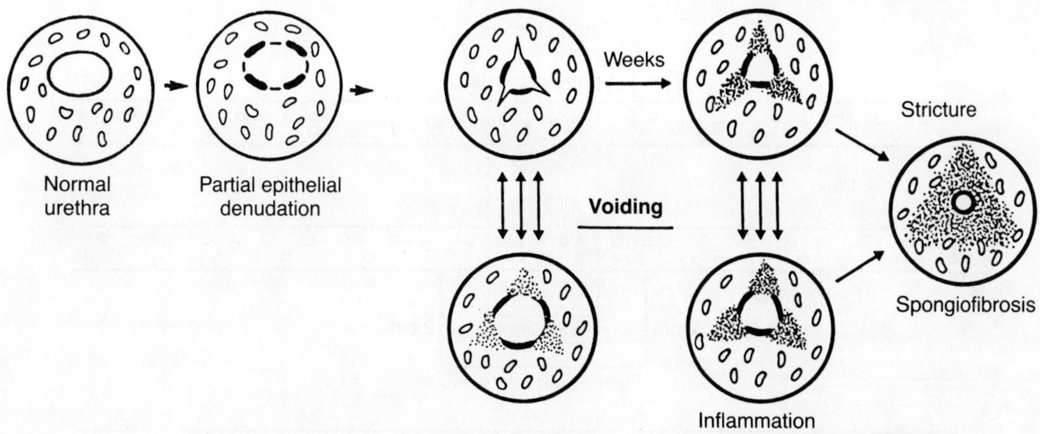

Figure 34–2. Urethral healing after partial denudation. The natural closing-pressure that evacuates the bulbo-penile urethra approximates the margins of the uro-epithelium. The intervening clefts are intermittently opened by the voiding stream, and the spongy tissue thus exposed gradually becomes spongiofibrotic. © 1987, Institute of Urology.

tendency to cross-adhesion of adjacent or opposing areas of unepithelialized tissue and suture lines. It is for this reason that the margins of an anastomotic roof-strip "combination" urethroplasty should be spread apart and anchored laterally (see subsequent discussion).

The Surgical Significance of Spongiofibrosis and the "Grey" Urethra

Proximal and distal to almost every stricture, with the exception of the rare congenital variety, the urethral lumen is surrounded by a layer of spongiofibrosis; the extent and the severity of this vary greatly, and it is particularly important to appreciate that a surgically significant longitudinal extension may surround a urethral lumen that appears quite normal radiographically.

The extent of the spongiofibrosis associated with a stricture is thus an important factor that often determines both the type and the extent of the surgical procedure that is required for its satisfactory long-term resolution (Fig. 34–3); unfortunately, failure to appreciate the stricture potential of nonstenotic spongiofibrosis is still a common cause of restenosis.[1,8]

To emphasize this stricture potential of a spongiofibrotic extension around a normal-caliber urethra, proximal and distal to a stricture, we have termed it "grey" in contradistinction to the normal urethra, which appears pink when it is opened because the vascular spongy tissue is seen through its immediately overlying translucent uroepithelial cover.[3,4,6,8]

Surgical procedures involving unstrictured spongiofibrotic "grey" urethra have a high restenosis potential unless appropriate precautions are taken to prevent this. Reanastomosis of a spongiofibrotic proximal and distal urethral segment after the excision of a short stricture commonly results in recurrent stenosis, and this has tarnished the reputation of anastomotic urethral repair, which is much the most successful reconstructive procedure when conditions are appropriate.[1]

Thus, limiting the extent of a substitution procedure to the length of the urethra that is *actually* strictured is a common cause of restenosis.[1,8]

The Primary Etiologic Characteristics of Spongiofibrosis

The proximal and distal extent of the spongiofibrosis associated with a stricture is primarily related to its etiology. Subsequently it often becomes extended in response to treatment—slowly by repeated gentle dilatations, more quickly by episodes of infection, and sometimes immediately by the healing response to urethrotomy.

When a stricture is the result of external trauma due to a simple straddle or pelvic fracture injuries, the initial longitudinal extent of the spongiofibrotic healing is generally minimal. Simple uro-epithelial denudation resulting from endoscopic instrumentation and indwelling catheters generally results in a relatively superficial inflammatory response and a thin layer of spongiofibrosis; however, an extensive inflammatory response resulting from urethral infec-

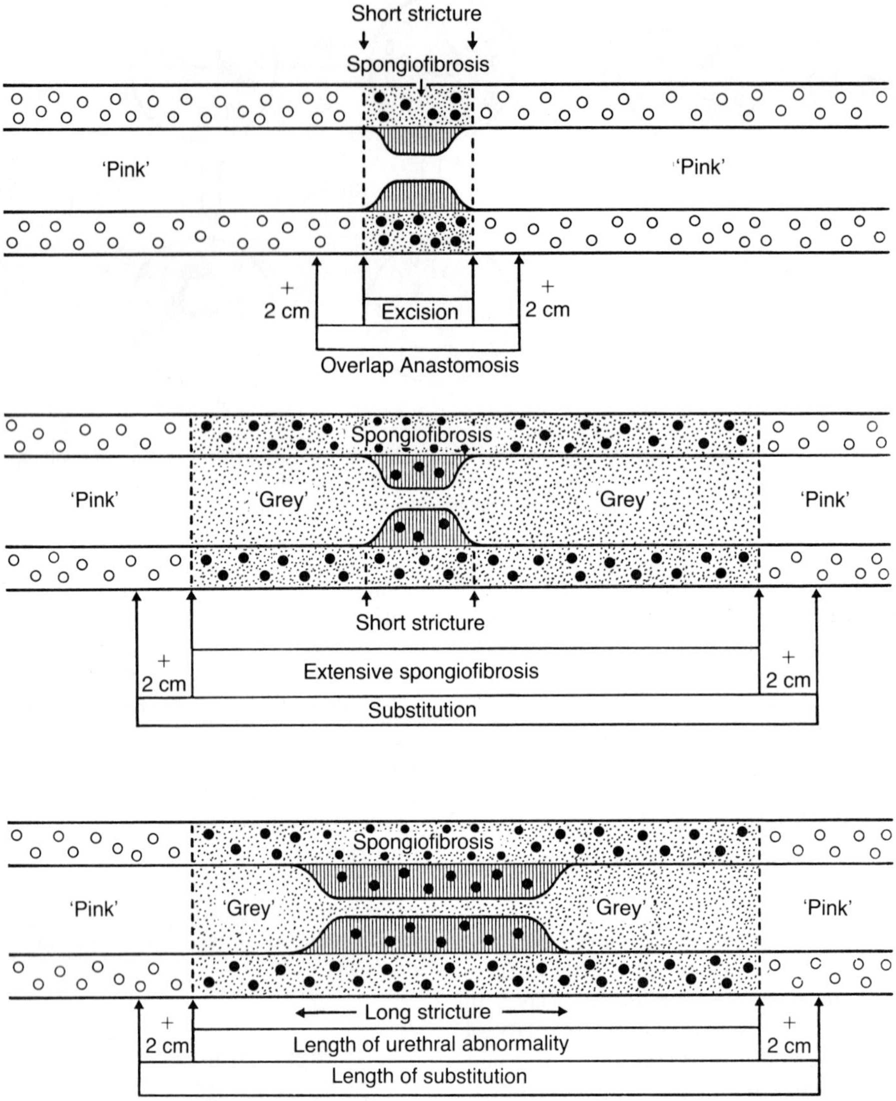

Figure 34–3. It is the extent of the spongiofibrotic urethral abnormality, not the stricture itself, that is the factor determining whether an anastomotic or a substitution repair procedure is appropriate. The lumen of "grey" spongiofibrotic urethra proximal and distal to a stricture is not stenosed, but nevertheless it has a stricture potential that is exacerbated by surgical procedures; a surgical repair should, therefore, extend into the normal "pink" urethra. © 1987, Institute of Urology.

tion urethrotomy tends to involve the spongy tissue to a greater depth.

The Identification of Spongiofibrosis

A urethral stricture only becomes palpable when it is associated with gross periurethral spongiofibrosis. Mild, but nevertheless surgically significant, spongiofibrosis may not be apparent until the urethra is opened at operation; not only is the color of its lining different, but a well-demarcated layer of subepithelial fibrosis is distinguishable from the delicate surrounding spongy tissue spaces on its transected surface. Unfortunately, this is often obscured by bleeding during operative procedures undertaken with an inappropriate anesthesia. Epidural blockade, in particular, tends to create complicating turgescence and erections (see subsequent discussion).

The true longitudinal extent of spongiofibrotic urethra is often identifiable only by critical comparison when the opening incision extends into normal "pink" urethra; however, superficial urethral scarring, the excavation of the glands of

Littre, and the greyish-yellow color associated with severe spongiofibrosis are generally obvious. Thus, to avoid complications, both anastomotic and substitution procedures should extend at least 2 cm into macroscopically normal pink urethra proximal and distal to the urethral abnormality; they should not be restricted just to the strictured segment.[1,7]

THE BASIC PRINCIPLES OF URETHRAL RECONSTRUCTION

Three distinct procedure-principles are available for the repair and reconstruction of the urethral lumen: (1) excision and anastomosis, (2) regeneration, and (3) substitution procedures.

Excision and Anastomosis. The only stricture-resolving procedure with an expectation of a long-term success rate approaching 100 percent is excision and spatulated circumferential anastomosis.[1] Unfortunately, if restenosis is to be avoided, this can only be used when the length of the urethral abnormality is sufficiently short to be excised, leaving a sufficient length of entirely normal urethra distal and/or proximal to the re-resection to enable a 2-cm overlap anastomosis to be achieved—without either tension or the subsequent development of an erection-chordee.

In practice, therefore, the indications for one-stage anastomotic repair are generally limited to congenital and external injury strictures of the *bulbar* urethra and also to subprostatic pelvic fracture urethral distraction defects (PFUDDs); this is because most strictures due to other causes are associated with a compromising extent of spongiofibrosis. Because the elastic lengthening of the *penile* urethra is almost fully extended during an erection, an overlap anastomosis in this area—even without any resection—tends to result in a curvature-chordee.

Regeneration. Regeneration procedures depend upon the completion of part of the circumference of the neourethral lining by regenerative proliferation of the uroepithelium. The long-term success of both urethral dilatation and of internal urethrotomy is entirely dependent upon whether epithelialization can occur before restenosis develops: commonly it does not.

The principle of the Denis Browne buried-strip procedure is to *induce* apposition-regeneration and thus the completion of the epithelial lining of the neo-urethra. However, although this is a valid principle as a back-up procedure in reconstructive surgery, it is no longer advocated as a solo procedure for urethral reconstruction. Implanted "mesh cages" that stent the urethra open[9] show promise of extending the use of regeneration procedures.

Substitution Procedures. All epithelial urethral substitutes and all individual techniques for their use have inherent shortcomings. Some have proved better than others, but all have a significant incidence of both early and ongoing complications and restenosis.

"Combination" Procedures. "Combination" procedures have been developed[3,4,6,10] for the resolution of bulbar strictures that are associated with a considerable extent of spongiofibrosis in order to reduce the incidence of complications associated with solo-substitution procedures. A fixed-flat roof-strip is created—preferably by urethral redeployment/anastomosis—to form about 50 percent of the neo-urethral circumference; the effect of this is to reduce the proportion of the augmentation substitution and to combine it with the back-up potential of the Hamilton-Russell–Denis Browne buried-strip principle.

In summary therefore, in the author's opinion, the small but inevitable incidence of failure of procedures involving substitution should *never* be introduced unnecessarily for the definitive resolution of strictures that are *appropriate* for repair by excision and circumferential anastomosis. However, *overstretching* the critical indications for a potentially uncomplicated anastomotic procedure results in a rapid escalation of problems that can be decimated by the use of combination procedures.

It is important to re-emphasize that fact that any urethral surgery—endoscopic or open—that fails to resolve a bulbo-penile urethral stricture is likely to complicate a subsequent definitive procedure. This can be critical; for instance, an iatrogenic urethrotomy extension of minimal spongiofibrotic scarring associated with a short traumatic stricture resulting from a pelvic fracture or straddle injury may preclude a subsequent one-stage anastomotic repair, and, of course, damage to the distal sphincter mechanism is virtually irreparable.

THE PRINCIPLES OF CATHETER DRAINAGE AFTER URETHRAL RECONSTRUCTION

Although it is commonly used, a standard-shaft balloon-retained catheter is an occasional source of predictable complications after urethral reconstruction. When the endeavor is to eradicate complications completely, this may not be acceptable.

Catheter-Balloon Complications

A catheter balloon may complicate a recently reconstructed urethra:

1. Balloon deflation may result in the premature loss of the catheter and this, or the replacement of it, can compromise reconstructive procedures.
2. Partial deflation of the balloon may result in it slipping, still oversized, into the area of a reconstruction and damaging it.
3. Inadvertent severe traction may withdraw a fully inflated balloon into the reconstructed area and disrupt it.
4. Even when fully deflated, residual corrugations on the surface of an overstretched balloon may be sufficiently rough to disturb a free skin-graft urethroplasty.

Thus, when a urethral catheter is used after a urethral reconstruction, it is most safely retained by a transvesical sling-stitch to a crush-button on the abdominal wall.

Unfenestrated Catheter-Shaft Complications

Urethral exudates are greatly increased by urethral injury or suture lines; if they accumulate in the urethral space they tend to become infected and may compromise healing. Natural passive drainage of the exudates along an empty urethra occurs when urine is drained postoperatively by a suprapubic catheter; however, there is a tendency for them to pool posteriorly after a bulbar reconstruction. Unless it is quite small,[11] the shaft of a standard fenestrated catheter indwelling in the urethra tends to obstruct the free drainage of the exudates.

Fenestrated Urethral Catheter Drainage

Positive drainage of the urethral lumen exudates is achieved by a fenestrated catheter;[1] however, this should be regarded as a urethral drain and it should always be used in conjunction with a suprapubic catheter.

Irrigation of the pericatheter space by the passage of urine along a fenestrated catheter does not compromise a urethral reconstruction, but appropriate management is essential. In particular, a fenestrated catheter should never be used for a bladder washout after a urethral reconstruction unless its fenestrations are first pushed back into the bladder so that none lies in the urethral area. Otherwise, suture line extravasation may result from the pressure of the irrigation fluid.

Postoperatively, a fenestrated catheter facilitates verification of the state of healing of a reconstruction by a "catheter-gram." Contrast introduced into a fenestrated catheter flows into the pericatheter space so that the water-tight healing of a reconstruction can be verified by the exclusion of contrast extravasation; the pressure of the instillation can be accurately controlled by elevating the suprapubic catheter drainage bag to 15 to 20 cm above the pubis. This simple fenestrated catheter-gram study avoids the potential complications of the described procedure of removing a regular shaft balloon catheter and reintroducing another if a retrograde urethrogram shows contrast extravasation at the site of a patch-plasty repair.

Fenestrated catheters are best made of plastic because the lumen of these is relatively large compared with that of silicone or rubber catheters. Size 16 F is generally appropriate for adults. The extent of the fenestrated area of the shaft should be tailored to the circumstances and does not usually extend distal to the peno-scrotal junction. Fenestrations are simply made by sharp-bending the catheter and cutting off the projecting kink-angle of the flattened fold with scissors.

Complications of Perineal Urethrostomy Catheters

The occasional complications resulting from a percutaneous perineal urethrostomy catheter, which used to be advocated for penile urethral reconstructions, are simply avoided by the routine use of a suprapubic catheter.

Thus, in the quest of *eradicating complications* completely after definitive bulbar urethral reconstructions, this author strongly advocates the routine use of a sling-stitch-retained fenestrated urethral catheter drain *and* an accurately located suprapubic catheter with an adequate lumen (18 to 20 F) to ensure that it does not become blocked (Fig. 34–4).

An adequate suprapubic catheter size is particularly important after the reconstruction of complex pelvic fracture urethral distraction defects when the catheter drainage may have to

Safe catheter management after patchplasty

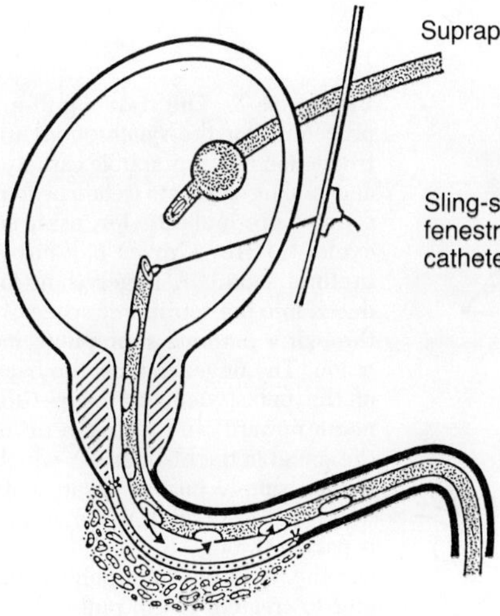

1. Positive drainage of pericatheter urethral space
2. Catheter-gram identifies extravasation
3. Sling-stitch prevents premature removal
4. No balloon risk to graft

Figure 34–4. Urine drainage after urethral reconstruction is most safely achieved by the combination of a suprapubic and a sling-stitch-retained fenestrated urethral catheter. A plastic catheter is preferable for fenestrating because its lumen is relatively large compared with that of a silicone or rubber catheter. The extent of the fenestrated area of the shaft is tailored to the circumstances; it does not usually need to extend distal to the peno-scrotal junction for a bulbar urethroplasty, and size 16 Ch is generally appropriate for an adult except where a larger one is required to stent a free-graft. The fenestrations are simply made by sharp-bending a catheter and cutting off the projecting kink-angle of the flattened fold with scissors. The fenestrations in the urethral catheter shaft ensure positive drainage of the exudates, and they also facilitate postoperative contrast studies to exclude suture line extravasation before its removal—the catheter-gram. The use of a balloon-retained urethral catheter is a source of occasional complications caused by the accidental withdrawal of an undeflated balloon or the obstructed drainage of exudates by the standard shaft and consequent pericatheter infection. © 1987, Institute of Urology.

be maintained for 3 weeks or more and a coincident urine infection with a urea-splitting organism that causes rapid encrustation may not be eradicable until the healing of the reconstruction is complete.

A simple procedure for the synchronous insertion of an accurately positioned suprapubic catheter and a fenestrated urethral drainage catheter sling suture is illustrated in Figure 34–5. Complications associated with failure of free catheter drainage must be regarded as unacceptable, especially when they are the result of poor placement or unreliable retention of catheters.

INTERNAL STRICTUROTOMY

The basic principle of internal stricturotomy is to enlarge the urethral lumen by urethrotomy incisions carried through the spongiofibrosis that surrounds a stricture. When these incisions extend into a supple tissue layer, the lumen is expanded by the pressure of the irrigating fluid, creating a bare area. The "supple layer" may be either the relatively normal spongy tissue surrounding the spongiofibrosis, or in the penile area, or the adventitial tissue outside it (Fig. 34–6).

Since optical urethrotomy became a routine general urologic procedure, restenosis has tended to be treated by repeated urethrotomy. However, when a urethrotomy fails to achieve a stable nonobstructive recalibration without frequent repetition, there are practical advantages in teaching patients to self-recalibrate with a 20 F olivary-tip plastic dilator after an accurate recalibration of the full length of the urethra to 26 to 28 F with the Otis urethrotome. Patients are instructed to repeat this self-dilatation as often as is necessary (usually 1 to 4 weeks) to ensure its easy passage and to return to the clinic if they fail to pass the whole length of the dilator into the penis so that only the distal end protrudes from the external meatus.

When an anterior urethral stricture becomes difficult to manage by urethrotomy, it can be resolved by a TWARS/PIPS reconstruction (see subsequent discussion)—usually in one stage if it is not associated with chronic infection or chordee. Urethrotomy of a subprostatic urethral defect resulting from a pelvic fracture is not generally contraindicated because the distal sphincter mechanism is already damaged by the initial injury; however, for all but the most minimal injury of this type, it is likely to prove ineffective because, unlike spongy urethral strictures, pelvic fracture urethral distraction defects are commonly associated with dense intervening hematoma-fibrosis through which an effective expansion of the lumen cannot be created by simple incision (see subsequent discussion). Furthermore, overenthusiastic attempts to create an intercommunicating urethral false passage through extensive intervening fibrosis may result in serious complications.[5,6]

Technique of Urethrotomy

The technique of Sachse optical urethrotomy is widely practiced and requires no elaboration

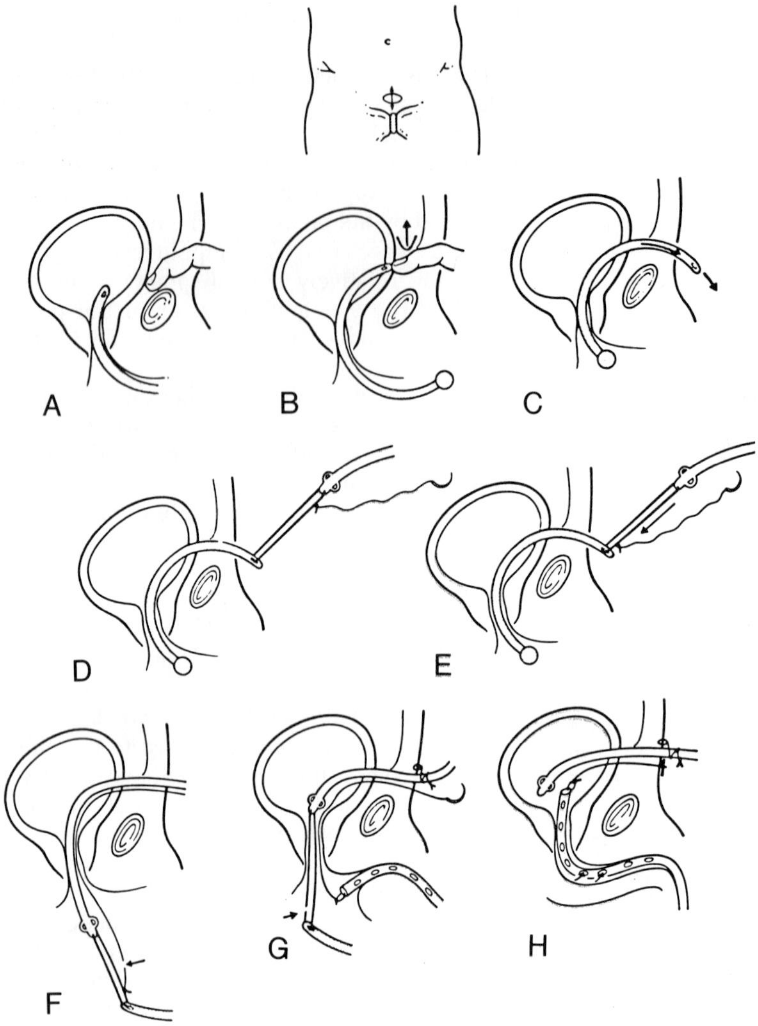

Figure 34–5. The T-W "pull-in" procedure for the synchronous introduction of a suprapubic catheter and a sling stitch to retain a fenestrated urethral catheter, using an eyelet-tip Hey-Groves half-circle urethral sound. A finger is introduced into the retropubic space (A) through a minimal suprapubic incision. The fingertip feels the back of the pubis, deflects the peritoneum upward, and feels the tip of the sound in the bladder (B), which is then simply pushed through its wall (C). A monofilm nylon suture is passed through the sound eyelet and the tip of the suprapubic catheter to create a 15-cm pull-in loop (D). The knot is pushed to the tip of the sound (E) so that the sling-stitch end of the suture is also pulled through and used to retain the fenestrated catheter. The suprapubic catheter is pulled right through the posterior urethra into the urethrostomy (F) to ensure that it is not merely invaginating the fundus of the bladder, and its tip is then pulled back to lie in the bladder base where, after checking that it drains freely, it is retained with a skin stitch. The pull-in nylon loop is cut (G) and withdrawn (H). © 1987, Institute of Urology.

apart from re-emphasizing the importance of avoiding damage to the intramural sphincter mechanism of the membranous urethra and also the potential advantages of an inferolateral direction of incision. However, a general urologic enthusiasm for the optical procedure has tended to overshadow the value of the Otis urethrotome, which is an equally effective and complementary instrument and is, in fact, easier to use when it can be passed. So far as healing is concerned, there is no significant difference between the urethrotomy incisions created by the two instruments. Indeed, the endoscopic appearances immediately after a urethrotomy by the two instruments are generally identical and undistinguishable. Thus, when it can be passed, the Otis instrument is much easier to use, especially in the anterior bulbar and penile urethra.

In practice, the atraumatic passage of the Otis instrument can be greatly facilitated by a size 7 ureteric catheter endoscopically through the stricture into the bladder. After unscrewing the tip of the Otis instrument, its male thread can be screwed directly and securely into the lumen of the catheter, which can then be used as a filiform guide (Fig. 34–7).

Complications of Urethrotomy

Although a urethrotomy incision extending into normal spongy tissue tends to extend the spongiofibrosis longitudinally, in general a subsequent definitive reconstructive procedure in the bulbar and the penile area is made only marginally more difficult by this secondary scarring. Thus, with the exception of short congenital and straddle-injury strictures that are eminently suitable for a simple and extraordinarily reliable

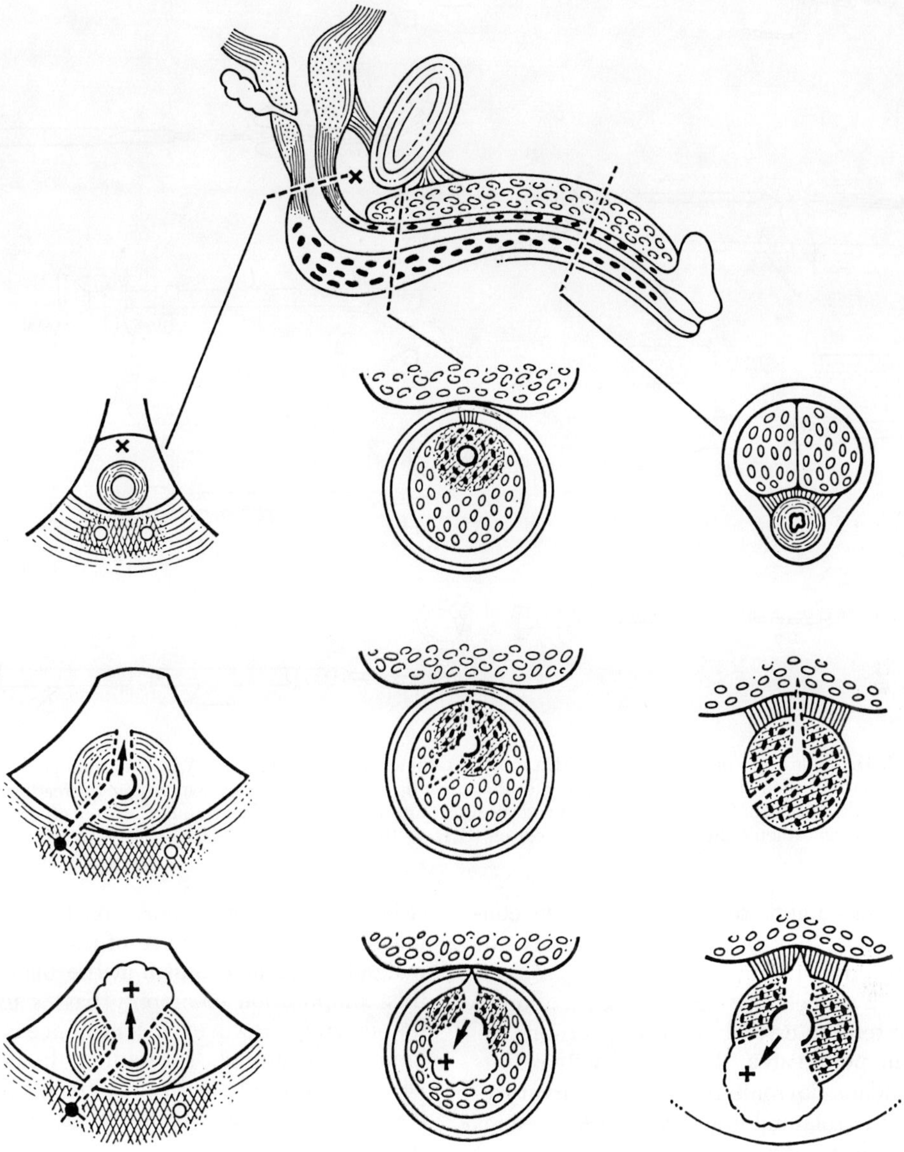

Figure 34–6. What is the optimal sector for urethrotomy? A urethrotomy that transects the 3 to 4 mm thickness of the distal sphincter in the membranous urethra commonly renders it incompetent; however, when it is required to relieve a neuropathic detrusor-sphincter dyssynergic obstruction, its direction should be anterolateral, into the pubo-urethral space, because posterolateral incisions in this area risk damage to the nervi erigentes and impotence. In the bulbo-penile spongy urethra, stricturotomy incisions in the 4 to 8 o'clock sector are more likely to extend into a supple tissue plane than in the traditional 12 o'clock site where the spongy tissue is only 3 to 4 mm thick and commonly spongiofibrotic. © 1987, Institute of Urology.

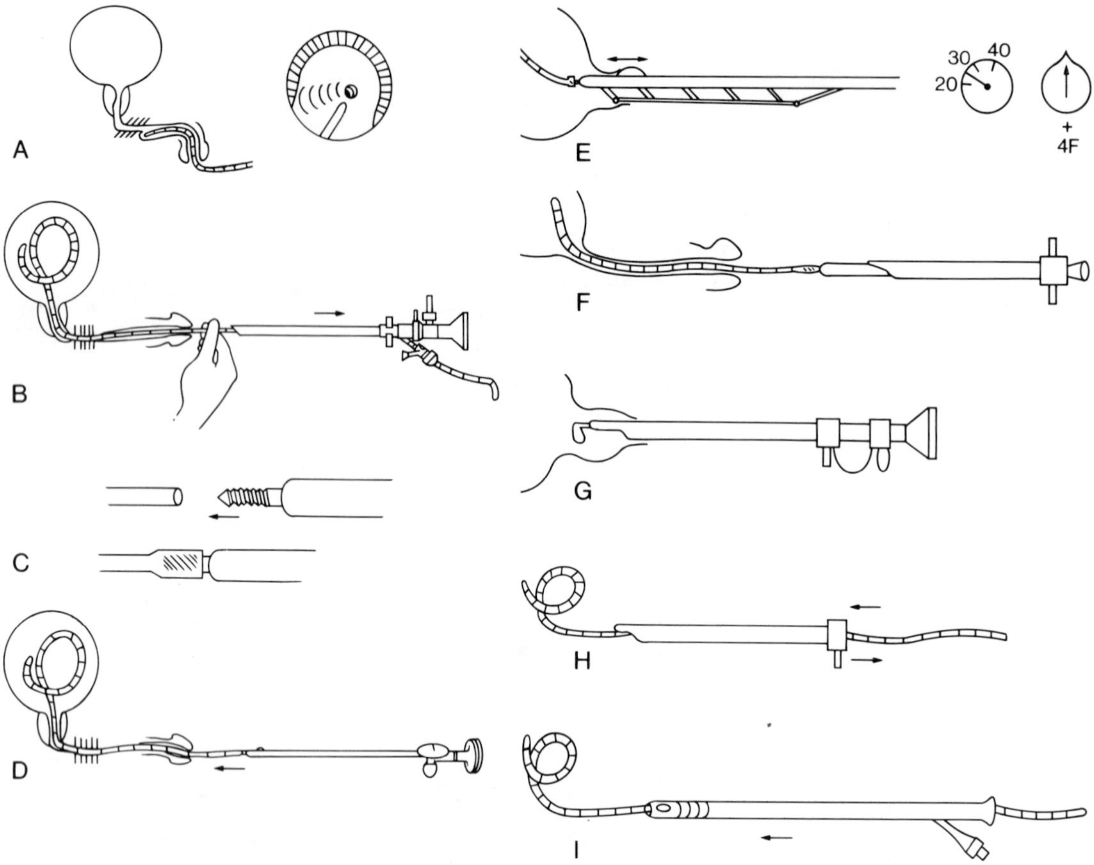

Figure 34–7. The endoscopic passage of a 6- to 7-Ch ureteric catheter through a stricture (A, B) is a useful guide of sufficient length for the introduction of (1) an Otis urethrotome, the screw-tip of which creates its own gripping-thread in the 6- to 7-Ch catheter lumen (C, D, E); (2) a resectoscope sheath using an internal plastic "follow through" dilator of appropriate size (F, G); (3) a urethral catheter after its tip has been cut off (H, I). © 1987, Institute of Urology.

one-stage anastomotic repair, there are few contraindications to a trial of urethrotomy for spongy urethral strictures.

Dorsal 12 o'clock incisions more than about 3 mm deep tend to extend into the cavernous tissue. In the penile area, this occasionally results in a secondary Peyronie-like ventral curvature-chordee. Inferolateral 4 and 8 o'clock incisions in the penile urethra may, of course, transect the full thickness of its spongy wall so that a few days of catheter drainage are then required to prevent urine extravasation. The Otis instrument is distinctly preferable to the optical for this because it avoids the risk of extravasation of the irrigating fluid during the procedure.

A bulbar urethrotomy extending posteriorly into the distal sphincter mechanism *is potentially disastrous and generally contraindicated* because of the risk that sphincterotomy of the 3- to 4-mm thickness of the intramural distal urethral sphincter will render it incompetent (Fig. 34–8). When urinary continence is maintained by the competence of the normal proximal sphincter mechanism at the bladder neck, this complication commonly passes unnoticed; immediately, however, incontinence is the common result after its subsequent functional ablation by prostatic or bladder-neck surgery unless a definitive intramural reconstructive procedure is used.[3]

TISSUE HANDLING IN URETHRAL RECONSTRUCTIONS: SUTURES AND SUTURING

Meticulous technique is critically essential to the success of reconstructive urethral surgery. Delicate tissue handling is a quality that almost all surgeons believe they practice; however, some less sensitive techniques are easily identifiable. For instance, no true reconstructive surgeon applies Allis forceps to tissues intended for

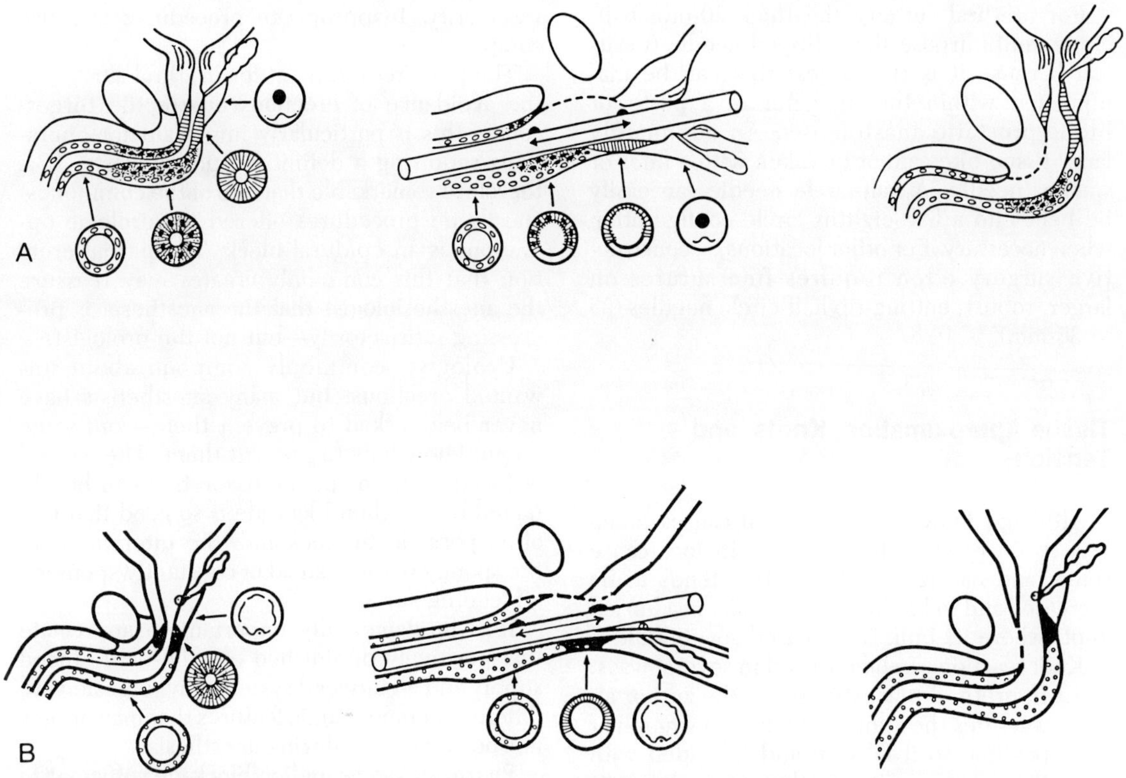

Figure 34–8. (A) The disaster of extending a posterior bulbar urethrotomy into the sphincter-active membranous urethra. Incompetence of the distal sphincter mechanism resulting from such an incision does not become apparent until incontinence develops after a subsequent prostatectomy-ablation of the bladder neck sphincter. (B) Urethrotomy of a postprostatectomy distal sphincter-stricture commonly results in the disastrous complication of incontinence. The essential of the treatment of such strictures is to preserve the function of the damaged remnants of the mechanism. © 1987, Institute of Urology.

preservation because they create nasty crush damage—a simple test of delicacy is whether an instrument can be clip-closed on one's finger without discomfort. In terms of tissue handling, no instrument is more tissue-sensitive than one's fingers, and instruments that are used for reconstruction should be delicate extensions of the fingers.

Sutures and Suturing

Suturing technique is also fundamentally important. Surgery owes much to the pioneer development of synthetic absorbable polyglycolic acid Dexon suture material by Davis and Geck in 1970. Several years passed before any other became available.

There are great advantages of PGA sutures over catgut sutures:

1. Their absorption causes minimal tissue reaction.
2. Their tensile strength is much greater so that the equivalent of a catgut suture gauge is 2 or 3 sizes smaller.
3. Their tensile strength lasts much longer.

The shortcomings of catgut as a suture for urinary tract reconstruction caused the author to abandon it long before the introduction of PGA sutures.[12] Indeed, one of the reasons why the two-stage skin-inlay procedure was preferred at that time was that nonabsorbable, nonreactive sutures could be used for the critical first-stage because they could be removed during an interval procedure.

In practice, 4 × 0 PGA sutures provide reliable strength for most anastomotic urethral procedures, and smaller sizes are sufficient for substitution procedures. However, it is not always possible to use ideally fine sutures because, at the time of this writing, they are not generally available outside North America on suitably robust needles of appropriate size for suturing the tough scarred tissue that is often encountered in reconstructive urinary tract surgery.

For urethral surgery the thick 20-mm half-circle multipurpose sharp-tipped needle is critical because it is the largest that can be manipulated within the diameter of a posterior bulbo-prostatic anastomosis. An adequately large tissue bite cannot be taken with a finer or smaller needle. A half-circle needle can easily be bent into a five-eighths circle configuration when necessary. For other locations, reconstructive surgery often requires fine sutures on larger, robust, cutting-tip half-circle needles (25 to 35 mm).

Tissue Approximation, Knots, and Tension

Although PGA suture material causes much less tissue reaction than cutgut, it does cause some, and naturally, this reaction tends to be increased and to last longer at the site of a buried knot, where its bulk is increased several-fold.

Knot reaction can be reduced in several ways:

1. In urethral reconstructions, the author always ties the knot on the lumen whenever possible so it falls off and is voided with the urine as soon as the suture loses its tensile strength (about the fifth postoperative week). This is contrary to some traditional precepts, but it works well, and no relevant complications, encrustation, or stone formation have been noted over approximately 20 years.
2. The number of knots on a long suture line can be reduced by continuous run of five or more tissue bites tied head-to-tail without tension and again with the knots on the lumen.

Although PGA sutures themselves cause relatively little tissue reaction, it is easy to cause a great deal by overtightening and thus strangulating the tissue enclosed within their bite.

Great care must be taken to avoid such strangulation when tightening the "throws" of a knot. Similarly, the author does not usually allow an assistant to "follow" a continuous suture opposing a critical tissue-line, because using it as a "retractor" inevitably overtightens it.

HEMOSTATIC AND HEMORRHAGIC ANESTHESIOLOGIC PROCEDURES

Appropriate anesthesiologic procedures can greatly improve the operative field for definitive urethral reconstruction by reducing the local vascularity. Inappropriate procedures can also complicate it.

The basic requirement for urethral surgery is the avoidance of erections or erectile turgescence; this is particularly important for operations requiring a definitive spongioplasty. It is therefore remarkable that one of the commonest anesthetic procedures offered for urologic operations is an epidural block. The partial erection that this commonly creates may reassure the anesthesiologist that the anesthesia is progressing satisfactorily—but not the urologist.

Urologists commonly complain about unwanted erections, but many anesthetists have never been asked to prevent them—and some do not know how to prevent them. The control of bleeding from spongy tissue that can be obtained by ganglion blockade is so good that it is often possible to "look into the interstices" of the spongy tissue instead of constantly sponging a bleeding surface.

It is fundamentally important to appreciate that positively diminished erectile-tissue blood supply and an induced systemic hypotension are different hemodynamic features that may or may not be coincident during anesthesia.

Pharmacologic ganglion blockade sufficient to cause dilatation of the pupils induces a specific reduction in the vascular circulation of the erectile tissue before it significantly reduces the systolic blood pressure; however, effective systemic hypotension induced, for instance, by sodium nitroprusside is relatively ineffective in reducing spongy tissue bleeding. It is remarkably difficult to obtain pharmacologic control of a passive erection already induced by epidural anesthesia, although control may be obtained by a more extensive local blockade.

Systemic hemostasis achieved by bradycardic anesthesia[13] is particularly important for long operations such as an abdominoperineal repair of a complex pelvic fracture stricture, especially in children.

Patient Positioning and Surgical Approach for Bulbo-Membranous and Penile Surgery

A simple midline perineal incision, with the patient in a standard lithotomy position, provides excellent exposure for bulbo-membranous surgery. If an anterior observational scroto-urethral inlay proves necessary, it is easily achieved by the Turner-Warwick drop-back procedure.[8,12] No surgical assistants are required if an appropriate ring-retraction system is used, and certainly none should intervene between the seated surgeon, the low instrument table, and the seated scrub nurse. When there is any likelihood of need for a synchronous perineoabdominal approach, the position is appropriately modified (see subsequent discussion on PAPA procedure).

The exaggerated lithotomy position provides no advantage for an anterior approach to the prostato-membranous urethra through the subpubo-urethral space. Indeed, the posterior prerectal approach to the prostato-membranous urethra that it facilitates involves some risk to potency.

The classic posterior horseshoe incision limits the anterior exposure. It is awkward to extend, and it compromises an observational inlay urethrostomy unless it is primarily modified to create a posteriorly based scroto-perineal flap,[14,15] a procedure that is unnecessarily complicated unless a questionable preoperative decision has been made to use a scrotal skin substitution procedure (see subsequent discussion).

The Principles and Techniques of Bulbo-Bulbar Anastomotic Urethroplasty

The feasibility of a circumferential anastomotic repair of a radiographically "short" urethral stricture is critically dependent upon the assessment of the extent of the associated spongiofibrosis at the time of operation.

The factor limiting the length of a bulbar urethral abnormality that can be resolved by anastomosis is the extent of the elastic lengthening that can be achieved by mobilizing the residual bulbar urethra proximal and distal to the stricture. This is naturally somewhat compromised by the associated bulbar scarring so that, in practice, it is rarely possible to excise a segment of bulbar urethral abnormality longer than about 1.0 cm and still obtain a 2-cm spatulated overlap anastomosis without risking a chordee (Fig. 34–9).

The bulbar urethra is mobilized from the base of the penis back to the membranous urethra in the subpubo-urethral space. The urethral lumen is opened inferiorly over a distance of about 2 cm immediately *distal* to the stricture. Both its lining and the cut edge of the spongy tissue are inspected critically to determine the anterior extent of the associated spongiofibrosis. The appropriate siting of the incision into the bulbar urethra *proximal* to the stricture is dependent upon this finding. If the anterior extent of the spongiofibrosis is minimal, the spatulating incision into the proximal bulbar urethra should be *superior* so that a fixed-flat spatulated posterior/anterior overlap anastomosis can be achieved; however, when the extent of the spongiofibrosis distal to a short bulbar stricture precludes a circumferential overlap anastomotic repair, the urethra proximal to it is spatulated *inferiorly* for the creation of the redeployment fixed-flat roof-strip element of a bilaterally pedicled island penile-skin (BIPIPS) "combination" urethroplasty.

To avoid cross-adhesion and restenosis, the lateral margins of a spatulated anteroposterior (not laterolateral) anastomosis are spread-fixed laterally to the undersurface of the penile crura. Penile curvature-chordee is obviated by avoiding any mobilization of the penile urethra, and angulation-chordee is reduced by relaxing the suspensory ligament (see page 471). Tension-relieving sutures along the superior surface of the mobilized bulbar urethra prevent erection-traction on the anastomosis postoperatively.[3]

Postoperatively, the combination of suprapubic catheter urine drainage and sling-stitch-retained fenestrated urethral catheter drainage of the urethral exudates is advised (see Fig. 34–4) (the author never uses a balloon-retained catheter in a reconstructed urethra). The urethral catheter is removed about the eighth or ninth postoperative day if a contrast cathetergram has shown satisfactory urethral healing without suture-line extravasation.

Any instance of restenosis after an anastomotic urethroplasty should cause a surgeon to reflect upon either the technique or the choice of procedure—or both.

THE PRINCIPLES OF SUBSTITUTION URETHROPLASTY

No substitute for the urethra is as good as the urethra itself; some substitutes are much better than others, but all have inherent shortcomings and, consequently, a commensurate incidence of early and ongoing late restenosis.

"Wet" and "Dry" Skin

"Wet" epidermal surfaces, such as those of the urethra, the foreskin, the mouth, the vagina, and the labia, are specifically adapted to their

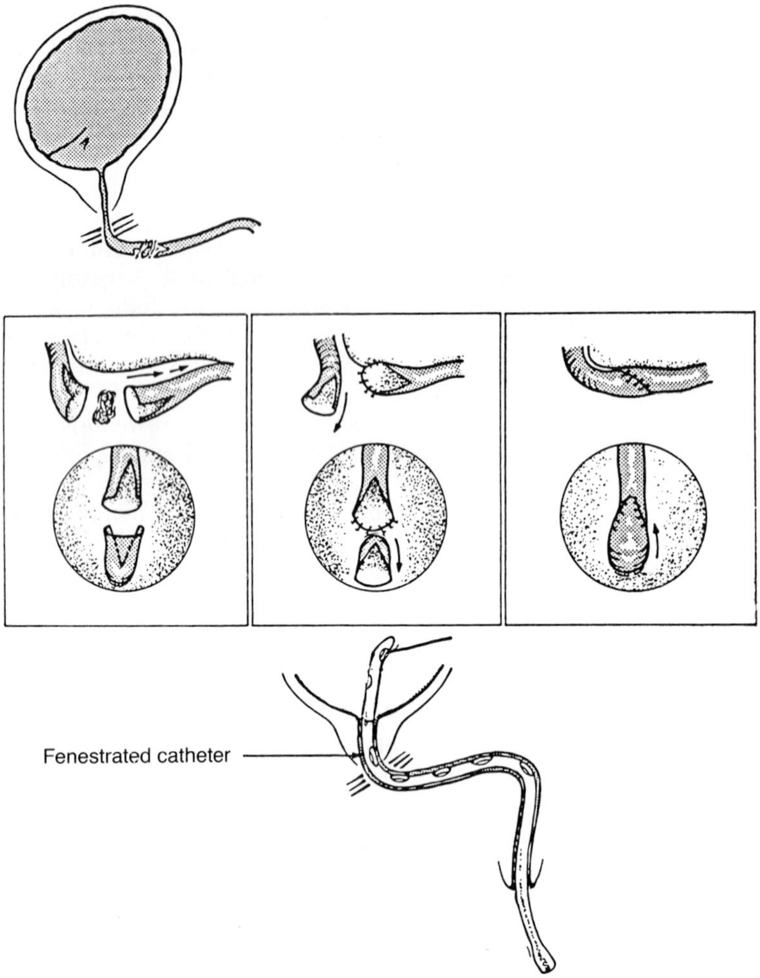

Figure 34–9. Anastomotic repair of a short traumatic bulbar stricture associated with minimal spongiofibrosis. The 2-cm overlap anastomosis between the spatulate ends of the normal proximal and distal must be arranged urethra anteroposteriorly, not side-to-side, so that the margins of the anastomosis can be suture-anchored laterally to avoid restenosis resulting from cross-adhesion. © 1987, Institute of Urology.

moist environment. "Dry" surface skins, such as those of the scrotum, the thigh, and the abdomen, tend to become inflamed and eczematous when constantly urine-soaked.[3,5,6] Thus, some donor skin areas are particularly inappropriate for urethral substitution.

Penile skin, however, can be regarded as "semi-dry"—somewhat intermediate between wet and dry skin. It is distinctly moisture-resistant and relatively hairless compared with the scrotal skin and has been long preferred for hypospadiac urethral substitution, where it has stood the test of time.

We are far from understanding the microbiologic characteristics that distinguish these epithelia, but microscopic features, such as a thick dermis, subcutaneous fat, and hair follicles, certainly augment the incidence of the potential complications involved in the *pedicled* transposition of a "dry" skin into a "wet" environment.

Free-Graft Urethroplasty

The pioneer work of Horton and Devine established that full-thickness skin grafts are superior to split skin for urethral substitution. They advocate their use as either a partial circumference patch-plasty or a circumferential "tuboplasty." Full-thickness skin grafts are generally based "unsupported" on the surrounding adventitial tissue.

However, the paraurethral spongy tissue provides a particularly good graft-bed and, in fact, this represents the nearest approximation to the re-creation of a normal urethra in which the uroepithelium is applied virtually directly to the vascular spaces of the spongy tissue. Patch-spongioplasty is particularly appropriate for the recreation of a near-perfect glans-neo-meatoplasty on a two-stage basis—a procedure that is particularly important for hypospadiac "retrievoplasty."[16] Patch-spongioplasty is also a useful technique for augmenting a bulbar urethral roof-strip after a lateral redeployment spongioplasty.

A free-graft of buccal skin is useful for relatively small areas of urethral substitution such as hypospadiac glans meatoplasty corrections. Bladder urothelium can also be used on a free-graft basis for anterior urethral substitution, but it tends to become protuberant and "sticky" if it is exposed at a neo-meatus.

Pedicle-Graft Substitution Procedures

Scrotal Skin

Although the mobility of the scrotal skin facilitates its use on a pedicled basis, both for a scroto-urethral inlay and as an island skin graft, scrotal skin has two major inherent shortcomings that seriously compromise its use as a urethral substitute:

1. It is a "dry surface" skin, which is particularly prone to developing eczematous and inflammatory reactions (stenosing scrotitis) when urine-sodden.
2. It is hair-bearing.

In fact, occasional hairs growing in the lumen of a urethral substitution reconstruction of appropriate and even caliber do not usually cause problems; however, in association with a sacculated bulbar urethral reconstruction they tend to become encrusted in stagnant urine pockets. This commonly results in stone formation and infection.

Thus, in general, hair-bearing skin is best avoided for urethral reconstruction and, in the event that it is necessary, it is advisable to epilate the neo-urethral area meticulously during the interval stage of a two-stage procedure.[8] Inability to do this in children, before pubertal hair development, results in a significant incidence of late complications when scrotal skin is used for perineal hypospadiac urethral reconstruction.

Thus, we do not advocate the use of one-stage pedicled island scrotal skin urethral substitution procedures, because they do not provide the opportunity for effective epilation and revision; neither do we advocate *circumferential* scrotal skin substitution, even on the two-stage drop-back inlay basis that provides direct access for interval procedures.

Nevertheless, for some specific purposes scrotal skin is invaluable. An observational scrotourethral inlay is an essential component of two-stage "combination" augmentation roof-strip procedures for complex bulbo-urethral reconstructions, and a rotation flap of scrotal skin is generally the best penile shaft skin substitution.

PENILE URETHROPLASTY

Reconstruction of the penile urethra is relatively simple compared with the problems involved in the glans-meatus distally and the bulbar urethra proximally: success is simply dependent upon the creation of a stricture-free tube because it is pendulous and free draining, so that any saccular irregularities of the reconstructed urethra do not retain urine. (Were it otherwise, Denis Browne's classic buried-skin-strip procedure would not have achieved even passing acceptance.)

Penile urethral reconstruction is generally facilitated by the fact that the immediately overlying penile skin provides a good substitute that is relatively well-adapted to a wet environment and is virtually hair-free. Furthermore, because it is well vascularized by its uniquely mobile subcutaneous tissue, it is relatively easy to use on a pedicled island-skin graft (PIPS) basis.[8,12,17]

Thus the whole circumference of the penile urethra can be reconstructed from a 3-cm wide (30 mm = 30 F) in-rolled strip of penile skin on its lateral vascular pedicle—or any proportion of it in combination with a fixed-flat roof-strip—(the laterally pedicled island penile-skin [LAT-PIPS] procedure) (Fig. 34–10). The introduction of *any* incidence of complications resulting from inevitable occasional partial "failure-of-take" of a full-thickness skin graft is particularly difficult to justify in the penile urethral area when the same skin is generally available on a more reliable pedicled basis.

However, both the natural mobility and the vascular reliability of the penile skin are seriously compromised by a previous surgical mobilization, and the extent of this impairment is not easy to estimate reliably at the time of operation. For this reason, when undertaking a hypospadiac "retrievoplasty" or "diasterplasty" after the failure of multiple previous surgical endeavors, there is often a paucity of well-vascularized penile skin appropriate for a one-stage reconstruction so that a two-stage procedure may be advisable, using part of the available skin as a full-thickness (rather than a pedicled) graft to form a 2-cm wide fixed-flat urethal roof-strip because this procedure is less likely to result in an overextensive loss of critical skin than an un-

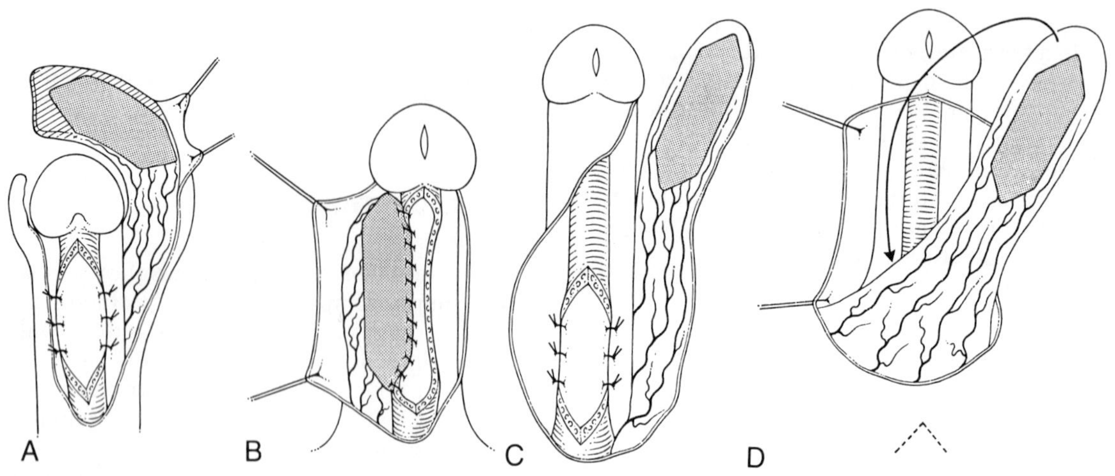

Figure 34–10. One-stage pedicled island skin urethral substitution procedures. (A) The unilateral pedicled island foreskin (UNIPIFS) graft for urethral substitution for distal penile and glans-neomeatal urethral reconstruction—single- or double-sided. (B) The lateral pedicled island penile-skin (LATPIPS) graft for penile urethral substitution. (C) The unilateral pedicled island penile-skin (UNIPIPS) substitution for anterior bulbo-penile urethroplasty. (D) The bilaterally pedicled island penile-skin (BIPIPS) substitution, our preferred procedure for bulbomembranous urethral substitution—partial TWARS or circumferential. Complications resulting from the shortcomings of scrotal skin compromise its use on a one-stage pedicled island basis because this provides no opportunity for interval stage revision and epilation. © 1986 Institute of Urology.

predictable failure of a precarious blood supply.

Scrotal Skin-Flap Substitution of the Penile Shaft Skin

Although scrotal skin is relatively unsuitable for urethral substitution, a scrotal flap provides a very satisfactory substitute for penile shaft skin when this has been used for urethral substitution. To reduce the risk of complications due to skin loss, however, it is important to recognize that the collateral blood supply of the scrotal skin across the median raphe is relatively poor. Thus the scrotal flap should either be mobilized and advanced on a 180-degree rotation and a unilateral pedicle basis (Fig. 34–11) or, if its elasticity and length permit, as a bilaterally based advancement (which has the advantage of avoiding a tendency to penile rotation in the early postoperative period owing to tethering by a unilaterally based scrotal rotation flap—although this tends to resolve by natural stretching in the course of time).

The Prevention of Fistulas by Underlap-Overlap Overclosure

The commonest complication of penile urethral reconstruction is the development of a closure-line fistula. Some incidence of this may be almost inevitable after a one-stage procedure, but a significant incidence after a two-stage reconstruction is much less acceptable. The most successful fistula-preventing procedure is wide separation of the urethral closure and overlying skin closure suture lines. The best way of achieving this is wide lateral separation by an extended underlap-overlap of the subcutaneous tissue layer. Hence, the width of the subcutaneous tissue of a scroto-penile overclosure flap should considerably exceed the width of the skin replacement (Fig. 34–12).

PENILE-SKIN-SUBSTITUTION BULBAR URETHROPLASTY

When available, the foreskin is the natural source of pedicled (UNIPIFS) grafts of wet skin for glans-meatoplasty and for anterior bulbo-penile urethral reconstruction.[18] The unilaterally pedicled island penile-skin (UNIPIPS) principle of urethral reconstruction can be extended to the bulbo-membranous area but, because the unilateral vascular pedicle becomes increasingly extended even when carefully mobilized, its blood supply sometimes becomes precarious and may result in graft failure.

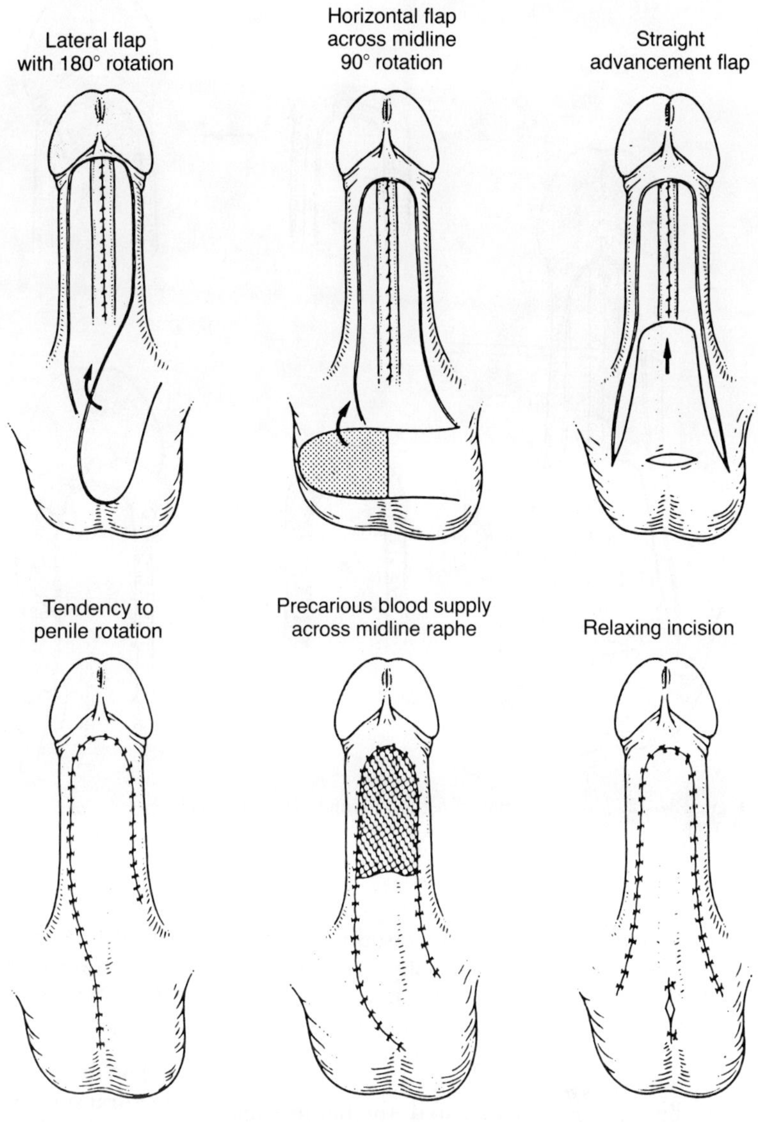

Figure 34–11. Scrotal-flap substitution of penile skin. © 1986, Institute of Urology.

Bilaterally Pedicled Island Penile-Skin (BIPIPS) Bulbar Urethroplasty

The bilaterally-based pedicled island penile-skin (BIPIPS) procedure for bulbo-membranous urethral reconstruction (Fig. 34–13)[10] was the natural development of the unilaterally-based island-graft procedure that we have used for bulbo-penile urethroplasty for many years.[6] Even when patients have been circumcised, the ventral penile skin, from the glans to the scrotum, is sufficient to replace the whole length of the bulbo-membranous urethra when it is mobilized on a bilaterally-based subcutaneous vascular pedicle; this is due to the combination of the extraordinary mobility of the subcutaneous vascularization of the penile skin, which is easily demonstrated by the fact that only minimal traction on the tip of the penis is required to enable it to reach back as far as the anus.

Thus pedicled penile skin is our much preferred substitute for both the penile and the bulbar urethra. It has proved distinctly more reliable for urethral reconstruction than any other skin that is locally available on a pedicled basis.

The BIPIPS procedure has become our procedure of choice for the one-stage augmentation of our roof-strip TWARS bulbar urethroplasty procedure.[10] Its particular advantages are as follows:

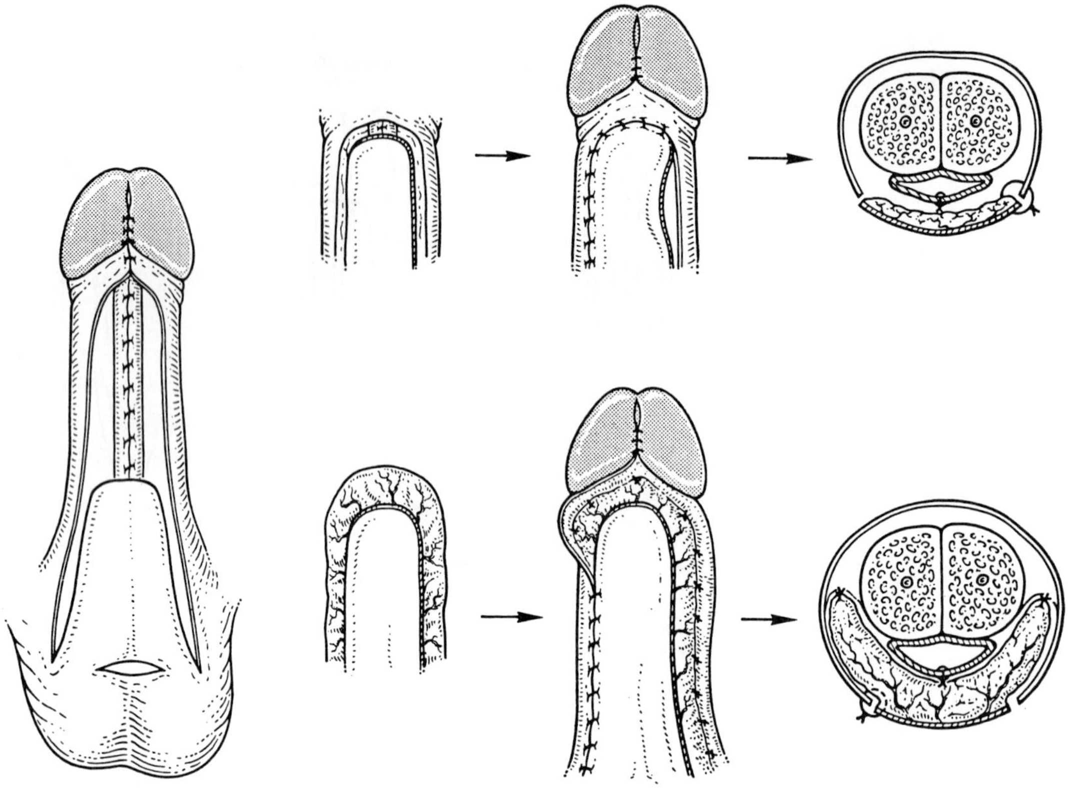

Figure 34–12. The prevention of fistulas by underlap/overlap overclosure of scrotopenile rotation flap subcutaneous tissue. © 1986, Institute of Urology.

1. It can be used in circumcised patients.
2. The penile skin is virtually hairless.
3. Its broad bilateral subcutaneous pedicle provides a more reliable blood supply than a unilateral pedicle when it is extensively mobilized.
4. Retrogradely invaginated, the hairless distal apex of the pedicle penile skin island easily reaches the membranous and the supramembranous urethra.
5. The retrograde paraurethral course of the PIPS pedicle enables overclosure of a posterolateral redeployment spongioplasty to be achieved (when it is available) and of the bulbo-spongiosus muscle. This support helps to prevent sacculation of the substitution-reconstruction and may even restore postvoiding evacuation and ejaculation.
6. The ventral penile skin defect is readily closed by a scrotal rotation-flap,[8] the vascular pedicle of which is naturally separate from that of the penile skin and is consequetly unimpaired by the combination of the two mobilization procedures.

Hemi-Substitution: The Principle of the Augmented-Roof-Strip (TWARS) "Combination" Urethroplasty Procedures

The incidence of complications resulting from urethral substitution-graft failures can be further reduced by limiting the proportion of their contribution to the neo-urethral circumference, i.e., using them in "combination" to avoid a circumferential substitution whenever possible.

The combination procedure was originally developed as a two-stage procedure to enable the healing of bulbo-prostatic anastomotic restoration of urethral continuity after pelvic fracture urethral injuries to be observed[8]; this augmentation proved unnecessary, and the "combination" anastomotic principle was adopted for the one-stage resolution of complex bulbar strictures.[1]

The basic principle of a "combination" bulbo-urethroplasty is the creation of a fixed-flat roof-strip 1.5 to 2 cm wide to form about half the neo-urethra circumference. The remaining part is completed by a substitution graft—usually on

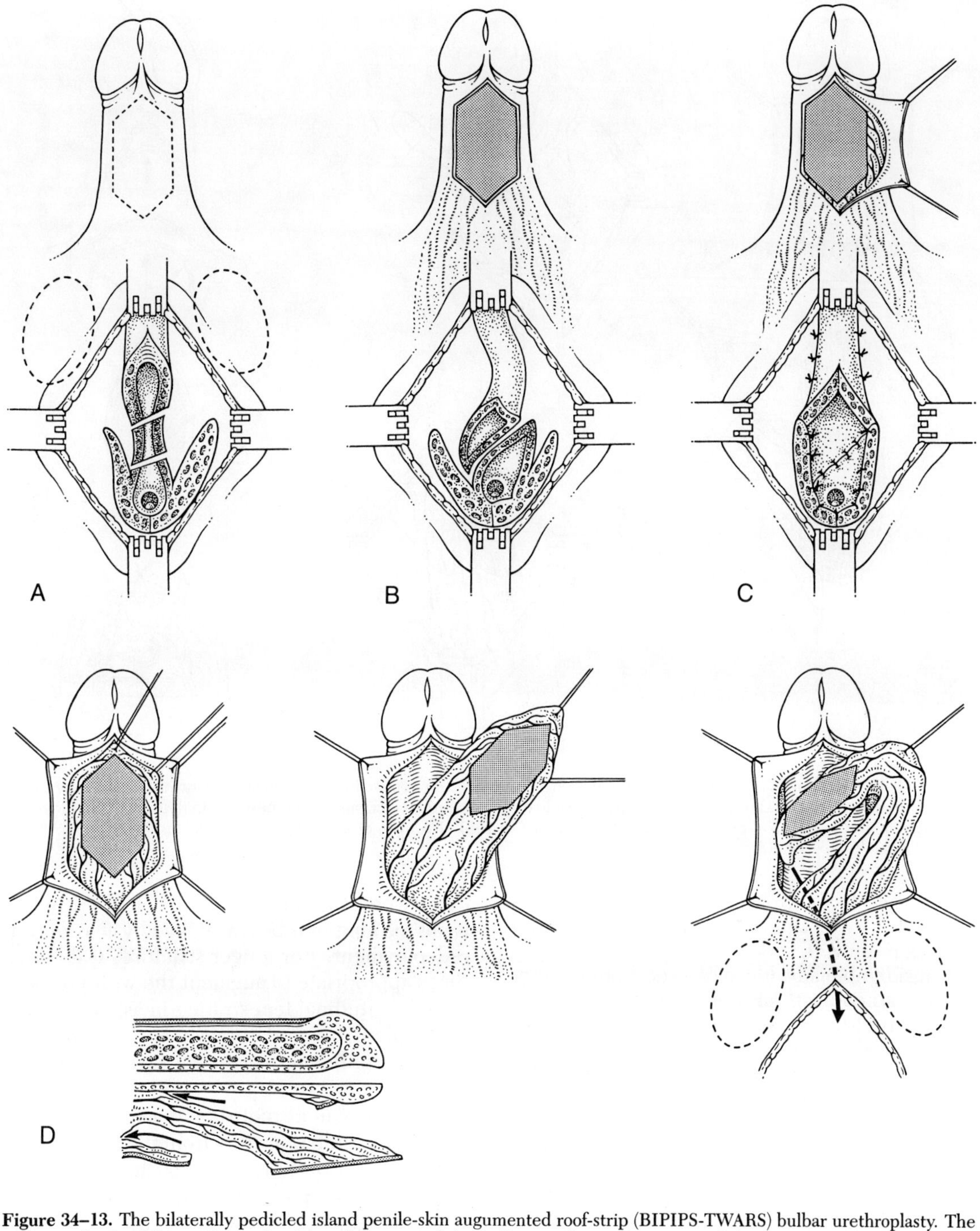

Figure 34–13. The bilaterally pedicled island penile-skin augumented roof-strip (BIPIPS-TWARS) bulbar urethroplasty. The creation of a fixed-flat roof-strip by (A) mobilization of the bulbar urethra and excision of the stricture; (B) restoration of urethral roof-strip continuity by an oblique reanastomosis with a lateral redeployment spongioplasty; (C) mobilization of an island of penile skin, based proximally on a broad bilaterally vascularized subcutaneous pedicle; (D) redeployment of the BIPIPS graft by retrograde inversion.

Illustration continued on following page

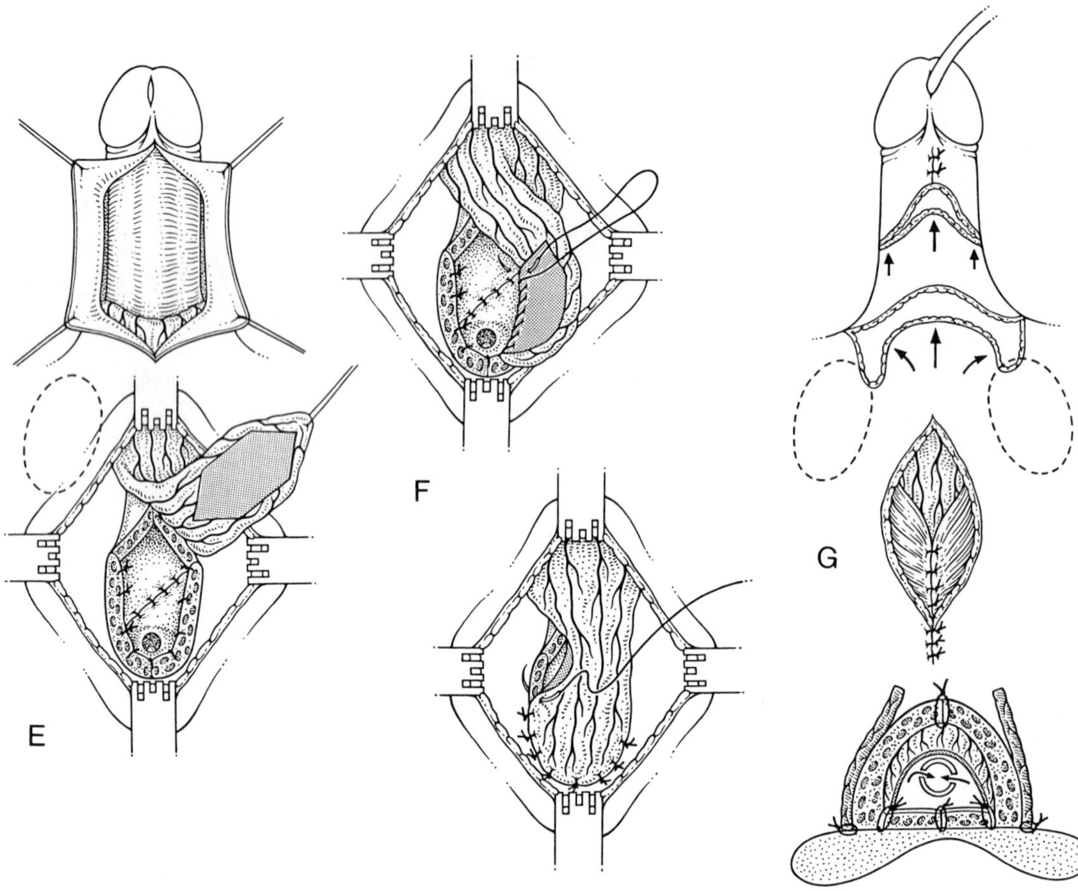

Figure 34–13 (continued). (E) BIPIPS augmentation of the urethral roof-strip with fenestrated urethral and suprapubic catheter drainage; (F) overclosure of spongiosus and bulbar muscles; and (G) closure of the penile skin defect by redeployment of uncircumcised penile skin or scrotal flap advancement. © 1987, Institute of Urology.

a one-stage basis with a PIPS graft, but sometimes on a two-stage basis when local circumstances require it.

Considerable advantages accrue from the creation of a neo-urethral roof-strip:

1. A fixed-flat roof-strip is unlikely to develop secondary narrowing if it survives, provided its lateral margins are properly suture-anchored, laterally.
2. Even if part of the augmenting neo-urethral overclosure graft should fail, it is relatively unlikely to result in restenosis because, on the Denis Browne principle, tissue closure over an established epithelial roof-strip tends to epithelialize by regeneration.

The Creation of a Bulbar Urethral Strip

A neo-urethral roof-strip in the bulbar area can be created by a variety of procedures; however, when the length of the strictured lumen is not too long, it is best achieved by anastomotic redeployment. For longer strictures it is sometimes appropriate to augment the width by strategic longitudinal fenestrating incisions that are "held open" by the lateral anchoring sutures so that the epithelial defects can heal by regeneration.

A redeployment roof-strip is achieved by mobilizing the bulbar urethra from the bulbo-membranous junction to the base of the penis, transecting it at the point of maximum narrowing of the lumen and increasing the width of the roof-strip by a side-to-side overlap anastomosis (Fig. 34–14). Because the urethral lumen is dorsally eccentric within the bulb, a definitive "lateral redeployment spongioplasty" of the posterolateral bulk of the spongy tissue is an essential component of this.[3]

The posteriorly based flaps of the excess

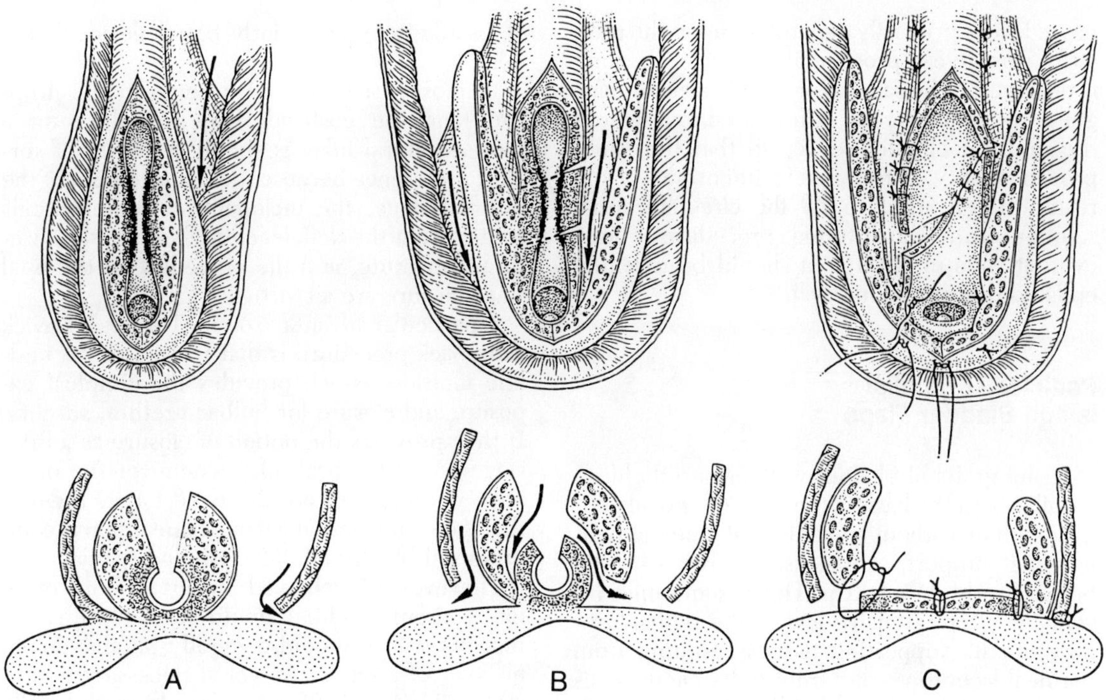

Figure 34–14. A lateral redeployment spongioplasty is required to achieve a fixed-flat roof-strip by anastomotic redeployment in the bulbar area owing to the dorsal eccentricity of its lumen within the spongy tissue: (A) the lumen of the mobilized bulbar urethra is opened and the midline origin of the bulbo-spongiosus muscle detached; (B) the excess bulk of the lateral spongy tissue is dissected away, preserving its posterior blood supply and leaving a layer 3 to 4 mm around the urethral lumen for its vascular support; (C) the continuity of the urethral roof-strip is restored by an oblique anastomosis, and it is fixed flat by lateral anchor sutures.

Note the posterior extent of the angle of the spongioplasty dissection that enables the proximal lumen of the subsphincteric bulbar urethra to be spread open by anchor sutures to avoid the development of a restenosis at the posterior end of the augmenting skin graft. © 1987, Institute of Urology.

spongy tissue are reflected by sharp dissection, and areas of spongiofibrosis within these spongy flaps must be carefully excised. Any normal supple spongy tissue that remains can be preserved on the basis of its main posterior blood supply and redeployed lateral to the fixed-flat roof-strip for subsequent overclosure support.

There is an important additional maneuver that reduces the risk of posterior stenosis when a bulbar stricture extends close to the sphincter mechanism. The incision separating the spongioplasty flaps is extended posteriorly so that the bulbo-membranous junction can be circumferentially "funnelled open" by anterolateral anchoring (see Fig. 34–14) sutures and posterior transfixion sutures through the posterior bulbar tissue flap.

Substitution-Augmentation of Bulbar Roof-Strip "Combination" Urethroplasty

The completion of the neo-urethral circumference overclosing a roof-strip can be achieved either on a one-stage basis or deferred to a second stage.

1. *One-Stage.* Our much preferred procedure for the one-stage augmentation of a fixed-flat bulbar-urethral roof-strip is the bilaterally pedicled island penile-skin (BIPIPS) procedure whenever the quality of both the roof-strip and the penile skin is appropriate. The BIPIPS graft is, in fact, the only substitution procedure that the author uses for circumferential bulbar urethral reconstruction.
2. *Two-Stage.* When the quality of a redeployment roof-strip is dubious and unlikely to be offset by the quality of a BIPIPS graft—and particularly when there is a potentially complicating residual local infection—a two-stage procedure is advisable, using the drop-back scroto-urethral inlay.[8] This provides access for the direct observation of the healing of the roof-strip and for any subsequent arrangement that may be necessary.

Because the success of a two-stage TWARS

procedure is primarily dependent upon the roof-strip, closure can proceed as soon as its healing is observed to be satisfactory. Only a small margin of the inlaid scrotal skin is used to augment the urethral circumference, so that the time-proven quality of this is less important to the result that it used to be for circumferential scroto-urethral substitution procedures; however, its neo-urethral area should be carefully epilated during the interval.

Pedicled Urothelial Island Bladder Flaps

Island grafts of bladder wall and urothelium, mobilized on the basis of the inferior vesical pedicle, with or without an additional omental pedicle graft support, can be used to re-create the bulbar urethral roof-strip. This is sometimes invaluable after extensive loss of the bulbar urethra and its supporting tissues resulting from perineal lacerations and from ischemic necrosis after inappropriate overmobilization of the bulbar penile urethra in misguided attempts to restore urethral continuity after pelvic fracture injuries.[5,18]

Pedicle Grafts of Local Skin

Attempts to reconstruct the anterior urethra with pedicled tube grafts of dry surface skin from the lower abdomen, the inner thigh, and the perineum are described in reconstructive surgical texts; however, they are generally unsatisfactory as a result of the inflammatory response in the inappropriate epidermis and the thick dermis and also the chronic induration that tends to develop in the subcutaneous fat.

Principles of Two-Stage Scroto-Urethral Inlay Urethroplasty

The wide, posteriorly placed scroto-urethral funnel was developed[12] to overcome the disadvantages of Johannson's subperineal scrotal-invagination tunnel procedure, which failed to provide direct access to overcome the inherent shortcomings of the use of scrotal skin as a urethral substitute by appropriate interval procedures. Such a posteriorly placed scroto-urethral inlay can be achieved either by a scrotal drop-back procedure[12] or by a posteriorly based perineo-scrotal flap,[14,15] which was a development of Leadbetter's posteriorly based perineal skin inlay.[19]

In most cases the choice between the drop-back and the posterior flap procedure for a scroto-urethral inlay is simply a matter of surgical preference because the management of the interval stage, the incidence of complications arising from the deficiencies of scrotal-skin urethral substitute, and the procedure of the final stage closure are all virtually identical.

A particular advantage of the Turner-Warwick drop-back procedure is that it is based on midline incision, which provides the simplest exposure and closure for bulbar urethral surgery. It thus provides the option of closure as a first-stage scroto-urethral inlay whenever the operative findings indicate the need for it. Indeed, this is the only option when perineal skin is compromised by chronic infection and fistulas.

However it is achieved, in this author's opinion a circumferential scroto-urethral substitution procedure should generally be abandoned in favor of a one-stage—or if necessary a two-stage—TWARS/PIPS procedure because penile skin is much more reliable. Nevertheless, there are a few remaining indications for a simple scroto-urethral inlay—particularly after the *en bloc* excision of the spongy urethra and its surrounding tissues required for a classic "water-can" stricture associated with infection and fistulous tracts and also for the treatment of anterior urethral tumors by ureterectomy. In such cases the lack of supporting urethral overclosure tissue generally precludes a final-stage urethral closure.

The Turner-Warwick Scrotal Drop-Back Procedure

The Turner-Warwick scrotal drop-back procedure is described in detail elsewhere;[8,18,20] however, a few important technical points help to avoid complications.

The drop-back of the scrotum, which ensures direct vision access to the prostato-membranous urethra, is achieved by incising the otherwise obstructing perineal skin in the midline and closing this incision horizontally. It is particularly important to ensure that the bulk of the inter-testicular subcutaneous tissue behind the peno-scrotal junction is mobilized by appropriate relaxation so that it drops back behind the inlay to provide a well-vascularized skin-bridge posteriorly. The secondary incision into the invaginated scrotal drop-back is appropriately sited and sutured with 4 × 0 PGA sutures (Fig. 34–15).

The Management and Duration of the Interval Stage

The term "two stage" applied to a scroto-urethral inlay is technically a misnomer because it fails to emphasize that the key to success of a reconstruction of the more complex bulbo-membranous strictures is the meticulous management of the *interval* stage. The prime purpose of such an inlay is to provide access for

1. Direct observation of the healing of the fixed-flat roof-strip of a "combination" procedure (see previous discussion).
2. The local rearrangement of the inlay or regrafting of the roof-strip.
3. Hair follicle destruction in any part of the inlay that is required for the closure completion of the circumference of the neo-urethra.

The duration of the interval between the first stage and the final closure is dependent upon the time that it takes to establish a stable, time-proven, stricture-free inlay. Long-term success is dependent upon this.

When the success of a scrotal inlay was entirely dependent upon the survival of a circumferential scrotal-skin substitution, an interval stage of at least 6 to 8 months was required to evaluate its stability. The interval can be considerably reduced in the two-stage augmented roof-strip "combination" procedures because the success of these is primarily dependent upon the establishment of a satisfactory roof-strip, and the stability of this is apparent more quickly. Nevertheless, it is wise to allow time for the healing reaction to complete and for the margin of the inlaid scrotal skin to establish its vascular connections before proceeding to closure.

Thus, it is most important to explain the principles of a two-stage procedure to a patient before undertaking it and to emphasize that the

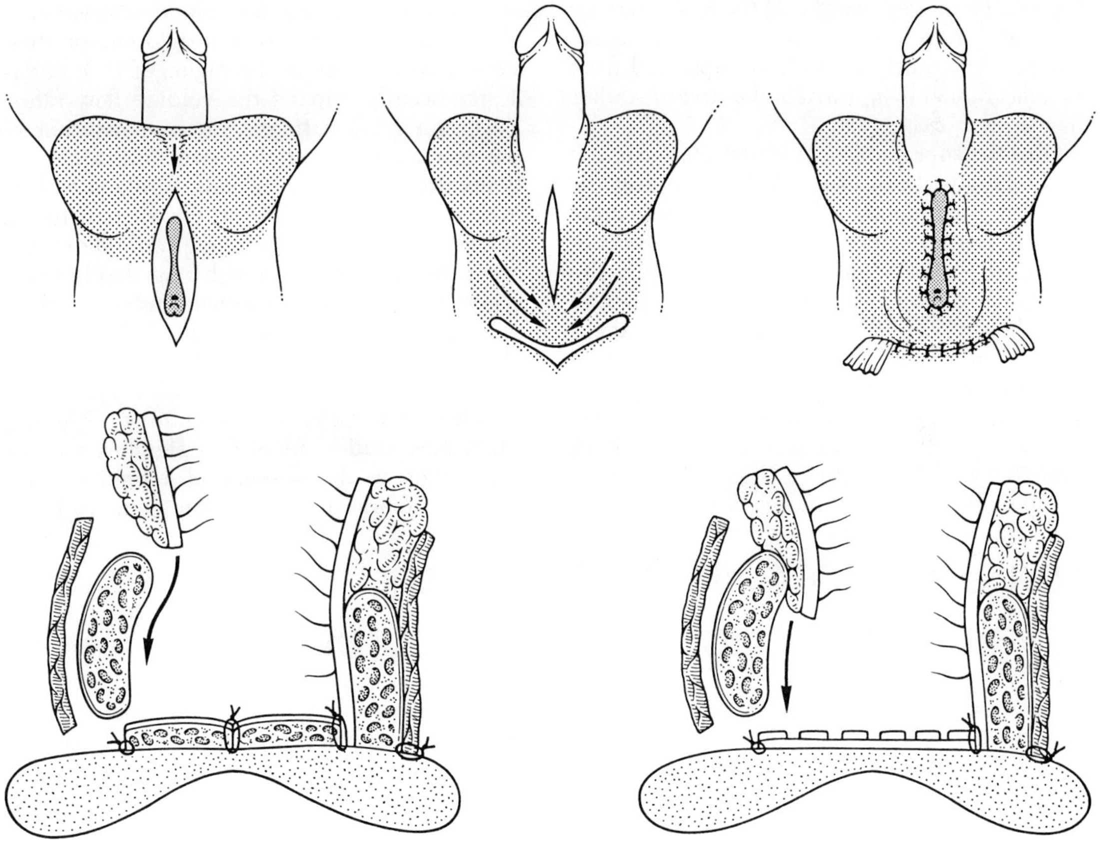

Figure 34–15. The Turner-Warwick scrotal drop-back procedure. After a primary midline incision, a first-stage scroto-urethral inlay urethrostomy is simply achieved by the drop-back procedure when it is necessary to observe the healing of a precarious redeployment or free-graft roof-strip bulbar urethral reconstruction before proceeding to the final stage. © 1987, Institute of Urology.

situation should be reviewed, as an inpatient interval procedure, under anesthesia some 3 to 4 months after the first stage to enable adjustments and epilation to be undertaken. Only then it is possible to predict the timing of the final-stage closure of an inlay urethroplasty.

Closure of a Scroto-Urethral Inlay

The successful closure of a scroto-urethral inlay urethroplasty requires meticulous attention to detail. It should be covered by a combination of suprapubic and fenestrated catheter drainage (see previous discussion).

The scroto-urethral inlay funnel is circumcised, taking care not to cut the skin "on the stretch" and thus leaving a neo-urethral strip that is less than 3 cm (30 mm = 30 F). In practice it is best to incise the inlay skin on one side and to separate it completely before proceeding to the other side.

Because a scroto-urethral inlay is invaginated through the incised margins of the bulbo spongy tissue and muscle, to preserve these for overclosure, they must be carefully separated from the inlay funnel by *upward* and *outward*, rather than inward, dissection.

After the suprapubic and fenestrated urethral catheters have been inserted, the neo-urethral skin strip is trimmed to size. In the penile area, the neo-urethra is tube-closed with a loose continuous 4 × 0 PGA suture approximating the subdermal tissues rather than the skin margin itself; however, in the bulbar area, when there is sufficient spongy tissue for effective overclosure, the margins of the neo-urethral tube are simply approximated by including the subdermal tissues in the bite of interrupted 3 × 0 PGA spongio-overclosure sutures (Fig. 34–16).

The bulbo-spongiosus muscle is overclosed in an endeavor to restore bulbar urethral evacuation. The closure of the perineal subcutaneous tissue is achieved by dead-space encircling sutures, which divide the subcutaneous tissue space into compartments, each of which drains efficiently onto the surface so that no drainage tubes are required.

The Evaluation of Urethral Stricture Surgery Calibration Versus Uro-Flow Rate

Two distinct criteria—that commonly may indicate quite different long-term results—are used for the evaluation of the results of operative procedures for urethral strictures. A truly successful urethral reconstruction should re-create a stable tube of even caliber that calibrates to normality (22 to 24 F). Such a state of affairs cannot be proved urodynamically because, while a recording flow meter is an important instrument for the evaluation of patients both before and after urethral reconstruction, it is only a screening test for the identification of bladder outlet obstruction; a rigid stricture can stenose to a caliber in the region of 10 F before it significantly impairs the voiding flow rate.[21] Furthermore, a patient's stricture may not be the only cause of outlet obstruction. Many patients attending stricture clinics are dilated with increasing frequency for an obstruction that is in fact the result of increasing prostatic enlargement, and a few patients with long-standing dyssynergic bladder-neck mechanisms prove never to have had a urethral stricture at all. This emphasizes the importance of retrograde urethrography in the diagnosis and the follow-up and also of video-voiding-cystourethrography, especially when flow studies identify a significant outlet obstruction in the absence of a rigid urethral stenosis calibrating to less than about 14 F.

The Sphincter Mechanisms and the Treatment of "Sphincter-Strictures"

The whole length of the posterior urethra, from the internal meatus to the membrano-bulbar urethral juncture, is sphincter-active. The feasibility of many posterior urethral procedures, such as the resolution of prostatic obstruction and the repair of sphincter-strictures and pelvic fracture urethral distraction injuries, depends upon the independent function of the proximal and the distal sphincter mechanism. Normally each of these is competent and independently capable of maintaining continence in the absence of the other, provided it has sustained no injury.[22] An accurate knowledge of the sphincter anatomy is, therefore, essential.

The Sphincter Mechanisms of the Prostato-Membranous Urethra

The bladder-neck sphincter is functional from the internal meatus down to the level of the

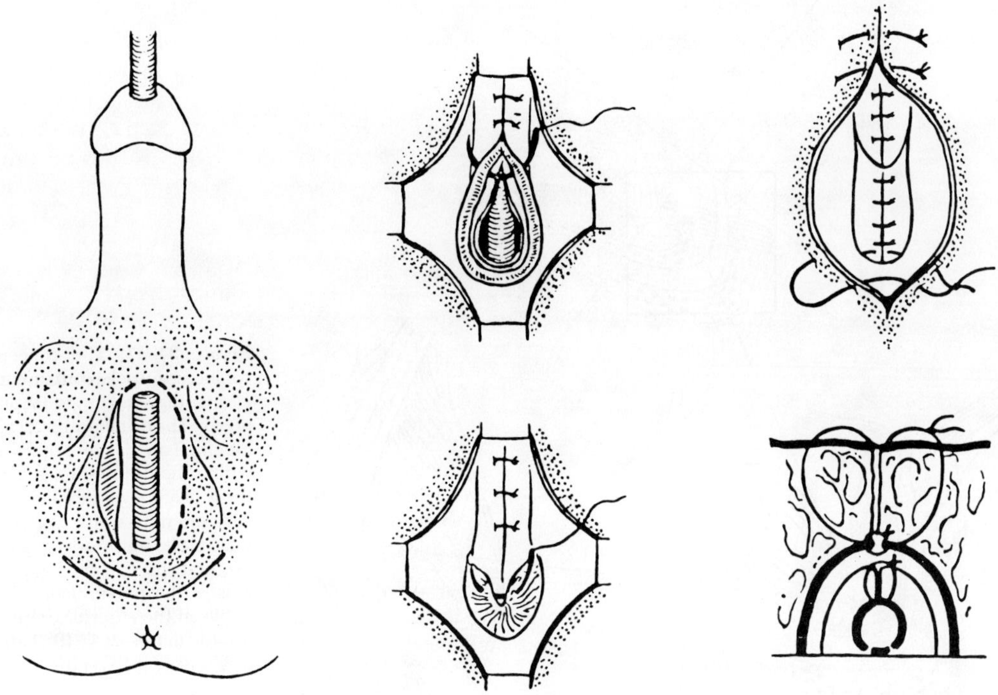

Figure 34–16. The basic principle of urethral closure (one- or final-stage) is the creation of a 3-cm width of neo-urethra to form the epithelial circumference of a 30 mm = 30 Ch urethral lumen. when available, overclosure of redeployed normal spongy tissue and the bulbar muscles supports the reconstruction and helps to prevent the development of secondary sacculation. The subcutaneous tissue is closed by dead-space-encircling sutures, which divide it into vertical compartments, each of which drains efficiently onto the surface so that no drainage tubes are required. © 1987, Institute of Urology.

verumontanum, and it is normally competent in the male, provided it is not rendered incompetent by unstable detrusor contractions.[22,23]

The 2- to 3-cm length of the distal urethral mechanism extends from the verumontanum down through the apical prostatic capsule to the membrano-bulbar urethral junction. Its functional occlusion is entirely dependent upon the two layers of smooth and striated muscle that form the whole 3- to 4-mm thickness of its wall. There is no periurethral "external" sphincter mechanism "external" to it anterolaterally, and the midline fusion of the pelvic floor musculature behind it is incapable of maintaining a sustained occlusion of the urethra except in spastic neuropathy.[24]

The Pubo-Urethral Space: The Urogenital Hiatus of the Pelvic Levator Diaphragm and the Myth of the Urogenital Diaphgram

The common description of a urogenital diaphragm enclosing a bulk of striated external sphincter muscle encircling the membranous urethra is totally inaccurate. It is readily apparent in the course of bulbo-membranous urethral reconstructions that there is no significant sphincter musculature immediately anterior or lateral to the membranous urethra.[22,24,25,26]

Turner-Warwick emphasized[25] that in the supposed location of the mythical anterior urogenital diaphragm there is, in fact, a pubo-urethral space created by the urogenital hiatus in the pelvic floor levator diaphragm into which, after minimal mobilization of the bulbar urethra from a perineal approach, a fingertip can be inserted between the membranous urethra and the subpubic arch, up to the level of the pubo-prostatic ligamentous bundle (Fig. 34–17). This pubo-urethral space is highly relevant to many surgical procedures in this area and to the variations in both the site of subprostatic urethral rupture and the extent of the associated hematoma in pelvic fracture urethral injuries. It can also be used for the location of the balloon of an inflatable incontinence prosthesis as an alternative to an encircling periurethral cuff.[25]

Detailed anatomic studies[26] confirm that the only muscles of the pelvic floor that relate directly to the membranous urethra are the pos-

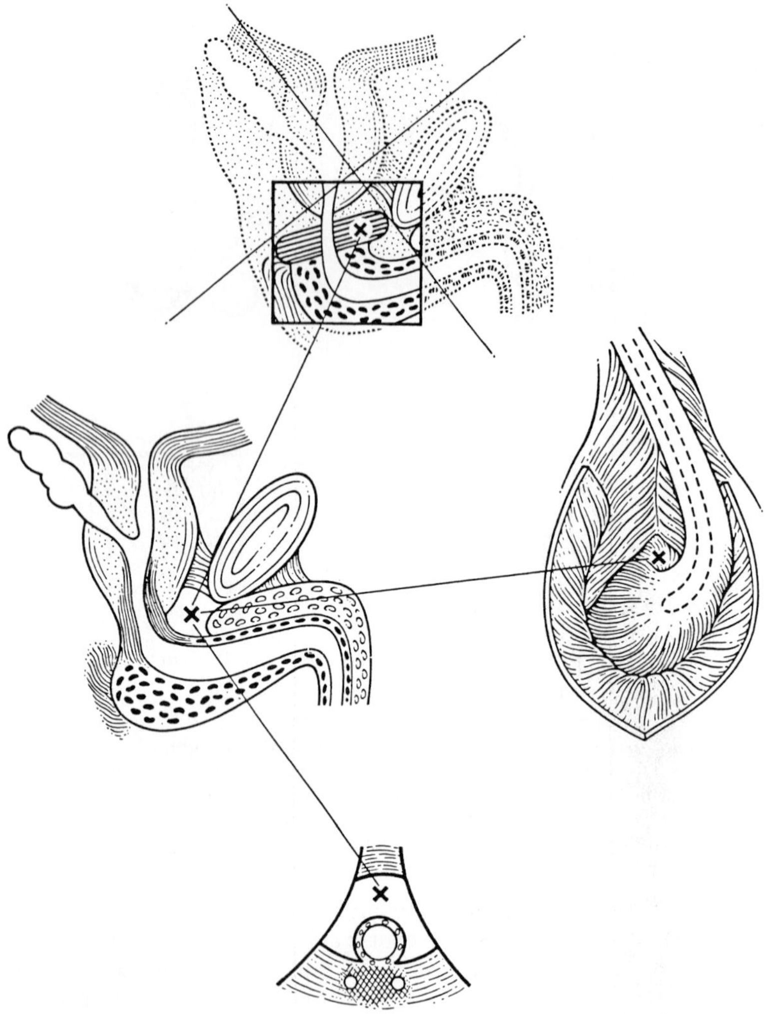

Figure 34–17. The concept of a sphincter-muscle-containing "urogenital diaphragm" is totally erroneous. The distal urethral sphincter mechanism is located entirely within the 3- to 4-mm thickness of the wall of the membranous and the supramembranous urethra, and this relates anteriorly to the pubo-urethral space in the urogenital hiatus of the pelvic floor diaphram, between the anterior origins of the levator muscles. © 1987, Institute of Urology.

teriorly located pubo-urethral elements of the pelvic levators and the transverse perineii that insert into the perineal body, which is adherent to its posterior surface.

Because the functionally effective muscular elements of the distal urethral sphincter mechanism are located entirely within the 3- to 4-mm thickness of the wall of the membranous and the supramembranous urethra, its functional competence is easily damaged or destroyed by longitudinal transection resulting from internal urethrotomy by surgical procedures such as prostatectomy or bulbo-membranous urethroplasty and by pelvic fracture injuries.[22,24,25] Thus, because urinary continence is entirely dependent upon the competence of the distal sphincter mechanism after functional ablation of the bladder neck mechanism during prostatectomy, great care must be taken to avoid unnecessary surgical injury to the subprostatic urethra.

The nervi erigentes, innervating the erection mechanism of the penile corpora, lie in close posterolateral relationship to the membranous urethra. Injury to them may result in impotence, and they are particularly at risk during sphincter-relaxing urethrotomy incisions in the 4 and 8 o'clock positions and also during a posterior pre-rectal surgical exposure of the membranous urethra in the exaggerated lithotomy position.

The Principles of the Management of Postprostatectomy Sphincter-Strictures

Postprostatectomy strictures involving the distal sphincter mechanism are much the most difficult of all strictures to resolve satisfactorily because they are located in the only sphincter mechanism that remains after prostatectomy, whether transurethral or enucleation. The unsatisfactory prostatectomy that created the stricture by damaging the sphincter-active urethra also damaged its functional competence to a varying extent.

The Significance of the Distinction Between Supple and Rigid Sphincter-Strictures

There is a wide variation in the extent of sphincter damage associated with sphincter-strictures. On one extreme the sphincter mechanism may be almost undamaged and supple, the stricture being the result of simple denudation of the epithelial lining. On the other, densely fibrotic sphincter-strictures are associated with severe sphincter damage. There are, of course, all variations between these extremes.[27]

Even a minimal recalibration of a rigid sphincter-stricture to 16 to 18 F, by the passage of dilators, may be sufficient to render it incompetent and a patient incontinent. On the other hand, the oversized dilatation of a supple stricture associated with minimal sphincter damage to a caliber of 36 F is no significant diminution of urinary control. The safest method of treating the more rigid sphincter-deficient stricture is by frequent self-recalibrating dilatation. Often this is best achieved by teaching the patient to pass a soft olive-tipped plastic dilator once or twice a week.

Sphincter-Strictures

The primary consideration in the management of a postprostatectomy sphincter-stricture is the preservation of the residual sphincter function, rather than the eradication of the stricture itself. The options for this are discussed elsewhere[27]; however its management by internal urethrotomy, Otis or endoscopic, carries a potentially disastrous risk of damage to the precarious residual function of its sphincter mechanism, which is already damaged to a variable extent by the stricture-generating injury (see Fig. 34–17).

Pelvic Fracture Urethral Injuries and Urethral Distraction Defects

Fortunately, pelvic fractures are not common—the urethra is ruptured in only about 10 percent of cases, and only the minority of the end results are "complex." The usual location of the urethral rupture in the adult is within 2 cm of the sphincter-active subprostatic urethra, where it is relatively unsupported because it relates anteriorly to the pubo-urethral space described by Turner-Warwick[24,28]—not to a fictitious "urogenital diaphragm" enclosing an imaginary sphincter mechanism "external" to the so-called membranous urethra. In the child, before the prostate matures, the site of injury is less predictable, and it is not unusual for it to occur at the level of the bladder neck mechanism.

MEMBRANOUS URETHRAL STRICTURES: THE IMPORTANT DISTINCTION BETWEEN SPHINCTER-STRICTURES AND PELVIC FRACTURE URETHRAL DISTRACTION DEFECTS

A circumferential rupture of the subprostatic sphincter-active urethra associated with a pelvic fracture creates a *distraction defect,* and this generally destroys the functional competence of the distal sphincter mechanism. It is quite distinct from a *continuity stricture* of the sphincter-active membranous urethra in its etiology, its functional effect, and its management.[27]

A pelvic fracture urethral distraction defect (PFUDD) may be short or long, and it may be simple or complex. It commonly becomes occlusive unless communication between the prostatic urethra proximally and the bulbar urethra distally is maintained by dilatation of a *false passage* through the dense intervening hematoma/hematoma-fibrosis. Although a PFUDD almost always results in functional incompetence of the intrinsic distal urethral sphincter,[8,29] on evaluation by voiding cystourethrography this deficiency is sometimes masked because an intact pubo-urethral sling element of the pelvic floor levator diaphragm can achieve a "stop-test" occlusion of the voiding stream—albeit only momentarily and insufficiently to maintain continence.[29]

Simple membranous urethral strictures are commonly the result of internal urethral injury (prostatic surgery, instrumentation, catheter or tumor invasion). They are better conceived as sphincter-strictures because although the intrinsic distal urethral sphincter mechanism is intact its function is generally impaired to a variable extent, and this is the important factor in their management.[27]

Thus, although both PFUDDs and sphincter-strictures are commonly referred to as membranous urethral strictures—in the sense that they both involve the subprostatic "membranous" urethra—the principles of their management are entirely different, and failure to make this distinction is, in itself, a potential source of complications. The essential treatment of a sphincter-stricture resulting from prostatic surgery is to preserve the residual function of the distal sphincter mechanism, because continence is entirely dependent upon it after the ablation of the bladder neck mechanism.[27] However, because the distal sphincter is generally functionally ablated as a result of a PFUDD injury, continence depends upon the bladder neck mechanism; excisional reconstruction is not contraindicated.[8,29]

COMPLICATIONS OF THE INITIAL INJURY

Hemorrhage, Hematoma, and Hematoma-Fibrosis

Pelvic fracture injuries invariably result in the development of a pelvic floor hematoma, the size of which varies from minimal to massive and lethal. The extent to which the bulk of this hematoma is absorbed or replaced by contracted *hematoma-fibrosis* is also very variable and somewhat unpredictable.

In the absence of a coincident lower urinary tract injury, even an extensive eventual hematoma-fibrosis resulting from a pelvic fracture injury is of little or no clinical consequence; however, when it is associated with a urethral distraction injury, even a small hematoma-fibrosis may critically complicate its surgical resolution. Nevertheless the significance of hematoma-fibrosis is rarely discussed and is often underestimated.

The location and the extent of the secondary hematoma-fibrosis that complicates the resolution of established urethral distraction defects naturally relates to the origin of the hematoma and how it was confined. An understanding of the potential variations of this is important[10] (Fig. 34–18).

Pelvic Floor Hematoma Without Urethral Injury. Pelvic floor hematoma-fibrosis surrounding the bladder base and prostate may impair the functional contraction of the bladder neck sphincter and compromise its competence, but otherwise it rarely affects the urinary tract. Apart from reflux-emission, incompetence of the bladder neck is generally asymptomatic so long as distal mechanism is functional.

Localized Hematoma Associated With A Subprostatic Urethal Injury. When the local hematoma associated with a minimal subprostatic urethral injury is confined by the boundaries of the pubo-urethral space, the extent of the consequent hematoma-fibrosis is limited.

Coincident Independent Hematoma. The localized subprostatic hematoma fibrosis associated with a urethral distraction defect may be quite separate from the retropubic hematoma-fibrosis that complicates its resolution by compromising the function of the only residual sphincter mechanism at the bladder neck.

Confluent Hematoma. More extensive prostato-urethral dislocation injuries result in a confluent paraurethral/pelvic-floor hematoma, and the ultimate extent of the hematoma-fibrosis intervening between the distracted ends of the subprostatic urethral rupture may be considerable.

The Natural Progress of Healing and the End-Result Complication

The less severe subprostatic urethral distraction injuries are generally appropriately treated initially by simple suprapubic catheter drainage. When this is discontinued, 3 or 4 weeks later, the patient commonly voids through the urethral-distraction hematoma cavity, which gradually shrinks, reducing the prostato-bulbar urethral gap and the lumen of the intervening false passage (Fig. 34–19). The end result is a considerable reduction in the volume of the hematoma—but usually a significant residual extent of dense hematoma-fibrosis. The time that this process takes to complete varies from a few months to a year or so, according to the volume of the hematoma that has to become organized, and it is this that determines the timing of a delayed repair. When the local healing reaction to a subprostatic urethral injury is complete, 4 to 12 months after a pelvic fracture accident, there are a number of possible end results (Fig. 34–20).

Incomplete injuries sometimes heal without

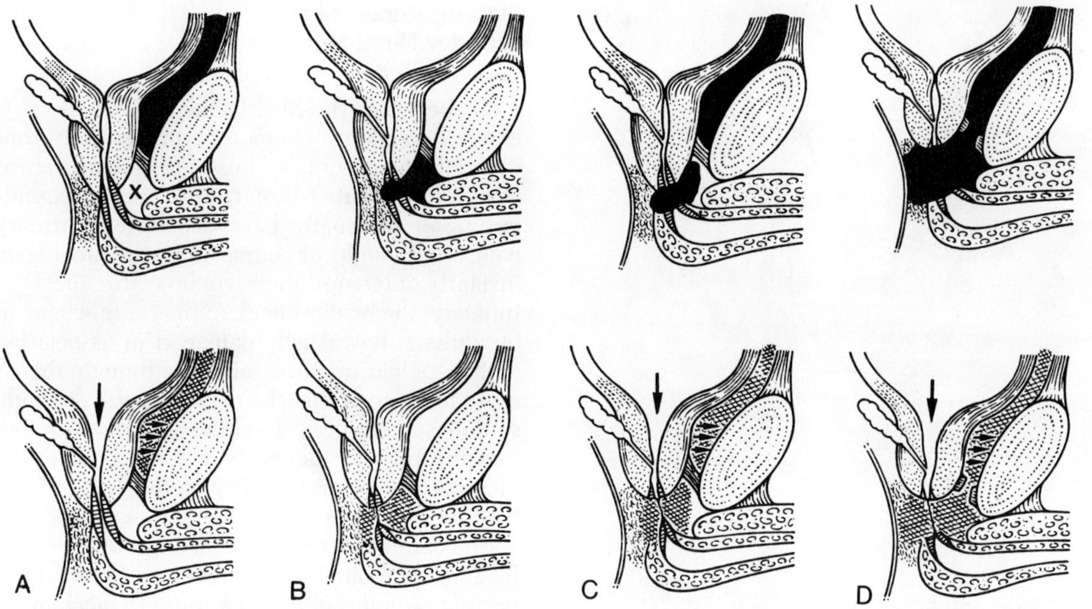

Figure 34–18. The development and the results of healing of the hematoma resulting from pelvic fracture injuries. (A) Hematoma-fibrosis resulting from the resolution of a pelvic floor hematoma commonly tethers a normal bladder neck mechanism to the inner aspect of the pelvis, pulling it open as it retracts and thus rendering it incompetent. (B) Minor degrees of subprostatic urethral rupture can result in the development of a hematoma confined to the pubo-urethral space; this commonly results in a short distraction defect and localized hematoma-fibrosis. (C) The combination of a pelvic floor hematoma, (A) and a pubo-urethral space hematoma (B) naturally tends to result in the combination of an incompetent bladder neck mechanism and a short subprostatic urethral defect associated with minimal fibrosis. (D) A confluent retropubic-subprostatic hematoma associated with rupture of the puboprostatic ligaments results in a complex urethral defect associated with extensive hematoma-fibrosis. © 1986, Institute of Urology.

causing either stenosis or distal sphincter incompetence. Occasionally the competence of the distal sphincter mechanism may be lost without the development of a stenosis. If this complication is suspected, it can be identified; however, all too often it does not become apparent until a patient becomes incontinent after a subsequent prostatic resection that destroys the only residual sphincter mechanism at the bladder neck.

Pelvic Fracture Urethral Distraction Defects

Simple. The commonest end-result of a subprostatic urethral injury is the development of a relatively short prostato-bulbar urethral gap associated with a minimally extensive hematoma-fibrosis. Such a *simple* short-gap end-result defect can be resolved by a relatively simple perineal-approach anastomotic repair. This can be regarded as an acceptably uncomplicated outcome of the management of the initial injury.

Complex. A complex pelvic fracture urethral distraction defect generally requires a perineo-abdominal approach to resolve one or more of its features:

1. Extensive retropubic hematoma-fibrosis.
2. A long prostato-bulbar urethral gap.
3. Side-tracking false passages into the retropubic space or osteomyelitic cavities.
4. Fistulas into the rectum, the bladder base, the perineum, or the suprapubic area.
5. Coincident incompetence of the bladder neck sphincter mechanism due to either intrinsic damage or peripheral hematoma-fibrosis retraction.

Thus the need for a perineo-abdominal procedure for the repair of a urethral distraction defect is often predictable from the complexities revealed by the preoperative radiographic appearances. Although these complications may not always be preventable, it is their development that the urological management of the initial injury should endeavor to avoid.

Sphincter Mechanism Injury and Urinary Incontinence

The whole length of the posterior urethra, from the internal meatus down to the membra-

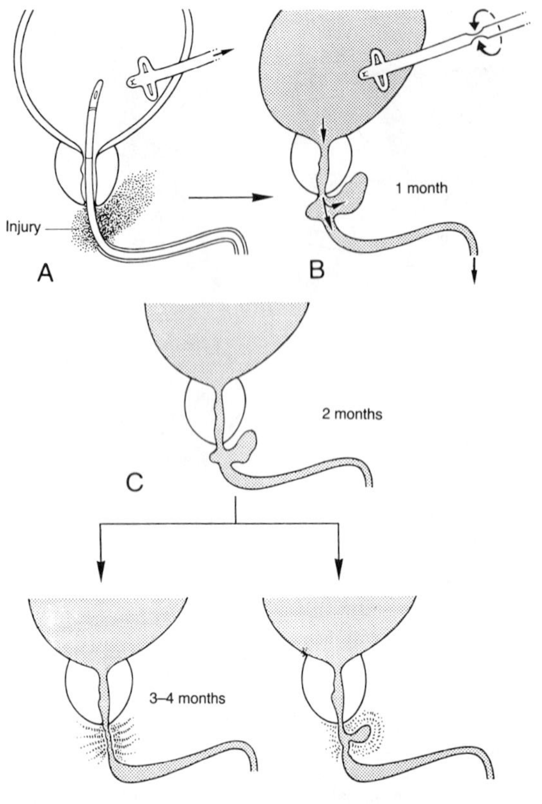

Figure 34–19. The progress of the healing of a subprostatic urethral-disruption hematoma. (A) An indwelling standard-shaft urethral catheter should not be used because it obstructs the natural drainage of the hematoma and exudates. Suprapubic catheter drainage is advocated. (B) When the suprapubic catheter is clamped 3 to 4 weeks after the accident, the patient voids through the hematoma cavity between the distracted ends of the ruptured urethra. In the course of the subsequent weeks, the false passage through the intervening fibrosis tends to stenose or occlude. (C) The stenotic false passage may be associated with the formation of epithelialized sacculations in which calculi commonly accumulate. © 1973, Institute of Urology.

nobulbar junction, is sphincter-active. The feasibility of most surgical procedures involving the posterior urethra depends upon the independent function of the two sphincter mechanisms proximal and distal to the verumontanum. Normally each of these is competent and independently capable of maintaining continence in the absence of the other, provided it has sustained no injury.[8,22,25]

Thus, after a prostate operation involving the bladder neck mechanism, continence is maintained by the distal urethral sphincter. When the distal sphincter function is destroyed by a subprostatic urethral distraction injury, continence is dependent upon the bladder neck mechanism.

Incompetence of the Bladder Neck Mechanism

In the male, the bladder neck mechanism is generally reliably competent unless it is rendered incompetent by unstable detrusor contractions; patients whose continence is dependent upon it usually have satisfactory urinary control although, of course, they are unable to instantly interrupt their voiding stream. Fortunately, the bladder neck sphincter mechanism of adults is not usually damaged in association with a pelvic fracture injury, although this is more likely to occur when injury results in wide symphysial diastasis. In children, however, before the prostate develops and protects it, the incidence of primary injury at the level of the bladder neck is considerably higher.

The commonest cause of incompetence of the bladder neck after a pelvic fracture injury is the *peripheral tethering of an uninjured mechanism* by the natural shrinkage-replacement of an extensive pelvic floor hematoma by hematoma-fibrosis.[5,10] In such cases its functional competence is usually restored by simple mobilization, achieved by removing the dense anchoring retropubic fibrosis anteriorly. The reliability of this procedure is dependent upon preventing secondary fibrotic re-immobilization by occluding the consequent para-prostatic dead-space cavity with a supple omental pedicle graft, which ensures the continued functional mobility of the sphincter mechanism.

Iatrogenic Injuries and the Bladder Neck

Unfortunately the majority of damaged bladder neck mechanisms found at the time of definitive repair of pelvic fracture urethral injuries are the result of iatrogenic mismanagement complications:

1. Primary reduction of a prostatic dislocation by traction on a urethral balloon catheter with a consequent pressure or expansion injury of the bladder neck mechanism.
2. Creation of false passages into the bladder base close to the bladder neck mechanism by the misguided passage of urethral sounds.
3. Overenthusiastic optical urethrotomy in an ill-conceived and misguided attempt to create an intercommunicating false passage by "dead reckoning" through the dense hematoma-fibrosis intervening be-

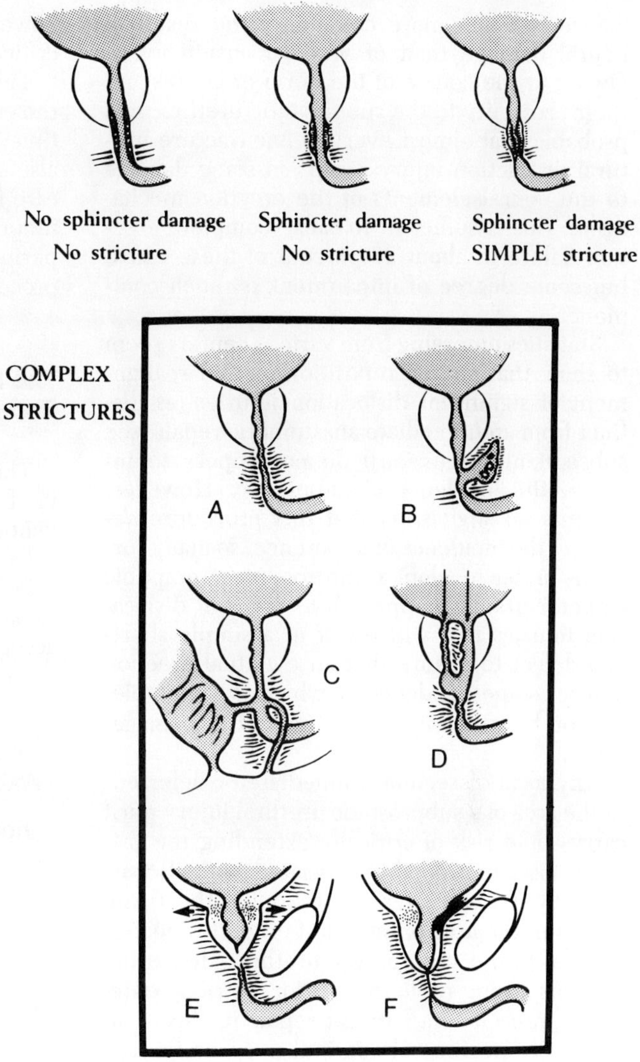

Figure 34–20. The end results of pelvic fracture urethral injuries. Subprostatic urethral injuries commonly destroy distal urethral sphincter function and result in the development of a 'simple' stricture that can usually be resolved by a perineal-approach repair. Complex strictures require an abdominoperineal-approach repair to resolve. (A) A long distraction defect. (B) A distraction sacculation. (C) Fistulas into the rectum, perineum, thigh, or lower abdomen. (D), Incompetence of the only remaining sphincter mechanism at the bladder neck may be due to hematoma-fibrosis retraction (E) or to sphincter damage (F). © 1973, Institute of Urology.

tween the distracted ends of the prostatic and the bulbar urethra.

4. Erroneous endoscopic loop resection of the bladder neck mechanism, supposing it to be contributing to persistent bladder outlet obstruction. When the need for relaxation of a urodynamically proven dyssynergic bladder neck obstruction is necessary, it should be achieved by endoscopic incision in the 12 o'clock position because this is relatively simple to reconstruct in the event of subsequent need.[22]

Impotence

Impotence is a major and disastrous complication of pelvic fracture injuries—it can occur in the absence of urinary tract injury, but the incidence is higher when the subprostatic urethra is ruptured, and higher still when this is associated with a major prostato-vesical dislocation. It is important to recognize that erection, ejaculation, and the achievement of a satisfactory orgasm are three separate and independent functions. The sensation of orgasm is rarely damaged by a pelvic fracture injury, and ejaculation is commonly restored after reconstitution of the urethral continuity. The great majority of patients experience a failure of their erection mechanism for days or weeks after a pelvic fracture injury, but most recover satisfactory erections—some up to a *year or more* after their injury.

The advent of the investigation and treatment of impotence by intracorporal papaverine injections has shown that the pelvic fracture erection failure is much more commonly the result of neural damage than of vascular insufficiency. Owing to the course of the nervi erigentes and their proximity to the subprostatic urethra, it is probable that almost every pelvic fracture urethral distraction injury results in some damage to the neural elements of the erection mechanism. This is sufficient to cause complete erection failure in about 20 percent of these cases, but some degree of impairment is much commoner.

Statistics emerging from various centers seem to show that simple repositioning and realignment of significant dislocation injuries (as distinct from an immediate anastomotic repair [see subsequent discussion]) do not appear to increase the incidence of impotence. However, there is no suggestion that this procedure *decreases* the incidence of impotence, so many surgeons prefer to adopt a conservative suprapubic catheter drainage approach to *minimal* dislocation injuries that will result in a simple short-gap defect to ensure that an eventual erection failure, some incidence of which is inevitable, cannot be attributable to the initial management.

Any local dissection, immediate or deferred, in the area of a subprostatic urethral injury must carry some risk of critically extending the primary local neuropathy associated with it, particularly if it involves separation of the tissue planes in the area of the nervi erigentes posterolateral to the subprostatic urethra. Hence the author's strong preference is for a strictly *anterior* approach to a surgical repair in this area, using the perineo-abdominal progression-approach (PAPA) operating position and procedure (see subsequent discussion), carefully avoiding any disturbance or mobilization of retroprostatic tissue plane.

However, the normal posterolateral relationship of the neural pathway to the subprostatic urethra is often grossly disturbed by severe urethral dislocation injuries, and furthermore, they become secondarily incarcerated by scar tissue or hematoma-fibrosis. These features introduce an unpredictable factor in relation to the survival of any functionally intact neurons after subsequent surgery. Even if direct injury can be avoided by an anterior approach, a distortional effect could be critical when a mechanism is precariously innovated. This seems to be borne out in practice because the incidence of secondary impotence after a delayed anterior-approach repair is very low when a fully functional erection mechanism has survived the initial accident; however, an impaired mechanism is occasionally critically affected by any local surgery.

The crural branches of the pudendal artery to the erection mechanism of the corpora are sometimes damaged by the initial injury, but they are also at risk during anastomotic repair; special care is necessary to avoid injury to them on the inner aspect of the subpubic rami during both perineal- and total pubectomy-approach repair procedures.

The Prevention of Complex End-Result Complications

The primary aim of the management of a pelvic fracture urethral injury should be the prevention of the development of complex end results, most of which stem from an unreduced dislocation and the eventual extensive hematoma-fibrosis. A "simple" distraction defect is an acceptable outcome, provided its achievement has not increased the risk of impotence.

Reduction Realignment and the TWESSAR Procedure

Routine early reduction realignment of prostatic urethral dislocation injuries has been strongly advocated for many years. The Turner-Warwick procedure[7,10] of the simple elastic sling-suture-aligned reduction (TWESSAR) (Fig. 34–21) overcomes the shortcomings of the vest suture. The advantages of this are as follows:

1. It is quick and easy to perform, so that a relatively inexperienced surgeon can achieve it in a matter of minutes in the course of a complicated abdominal operation for other major injuries.
2. It is reliable because the approximation of the ruptured ends of the prostato-membranous urethra is maintained by sustained isotonic elastic-band traction, which maintains the reduction in spite of some movement associated with an inadequately immobilized unstable fracture of the pelvis.
3. Urethral alignment is achieved by a sling-suture-retained fenestrated shaft catheter, which also ensures the drainage of serosanguinous exudates that otherwise accumulate at the site of the subprostatic urethral rupture.
4. The procedure requires no tissue dissection apart from the simple division of any residual prostatic tethering to a dislocated pubic bone fragment; thus, there is min-

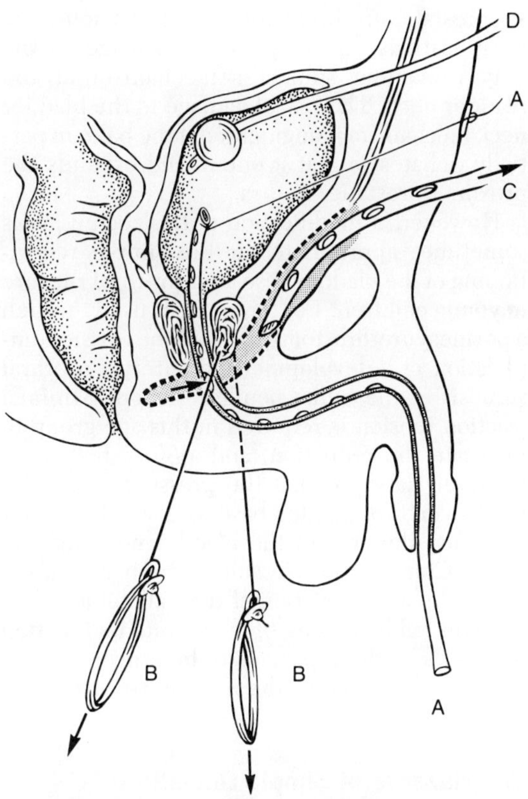

Figure 34–21. The TWESSAR (Turner-Warwick elastic sling-suture-aligned reduction) procedure for the early operative reduction of severely dislocated pelvic fracture urethral injuries after retropubic evacuation of hematoma. A sling-stitch is used to retain the fenestrated catheter drain used for urethral alignment. (A) Elastic band traction on a nylon prostatoperineal reduction sling-stitch. (B) Retropubic suction drainage. (C) Suprapubic catheter. (D) The elastic bands are anchored to the thigh by traction (one-way-stretch) adhesive tape. © 1973, Institute of Urology.

imal risk of increasing the natural incidence of neural or vascular impotence.

The TWESSAR procedure usually ensures that any residual urethral defect is short and simple; sometimes the urethral healing is stricture-free. However, the fenestrated alignment catheter used for the TWESSAR procedure must be inserted with care and delicacy. This is easy when the prostate is grossly dislocated, but when it has some residual tetherings to the pelvic floor, it is most important not to disturb these and any residually intact elements of the nervi erigentes within them; the term "railroading" that is sometimes used to describe this maneuver has certain unfortunate rough handling connotations.

It is generally advisable to treat minimal dislocation subprostatic ruptures by simple suprapubic catheter drainage without a urethral catheter; however, the TWESSAR procedure has proved so simple, reliable, and uncomplicated that its use can be advocated whenever there is a significant distraction.

Immediate Anastomotic Repair of Subprostatic Urethral Distraction Injury

When the pelvic fragments are stable and the urethral injury is not complicated by contraindicating polytrauma, the alternative to a simple reduction realignment procedure may be early anastomotic repair using either a perineal or retropubic approach. This sometimes proves difficult, but some satisfactory stricture-free results have been claimed, although a number require a subsequent revision repair, which may prove more complicated as a result of the primary procedure.

It is claimed that the incidence of impotence is not significantly increased by an immediate anastomotic procedure; however, until this is confirmed, many surgeons prefer a simple reduction realignment procedure such as the TWESSAR, which definitively avoids any dissection or suturing in the area of the already disturbed nervi erigentes in the region of the apex of the prostate—thus avoiding any suspicion that if impotence supervenes it is a complication of the accident and not of the intervention (see page 461). The probable need for a secondary perineal-approach anastomotic repair of a "simple" distraction defect can be regarded as a reasonable price to pay for this assurance because loss of potency is the only urogenital complication of a pelvic fracture injury for which there is no truly satisfactory subsequent surgical solution in the event that spontaneous recovery does not occur.

THE POTENTIAL COMPLICATIONS AND SHORTCOMINGS OF SOME URETHRAL INJURY MANAGEMENT PROCEDURES

The Hazards Of Urethral Catheters

The use of a Foley balloon catheter in the management of urethral injuries can result in serious complications.

Catheter Shaft Complications

Quite apart from the possibility of catheter-material toxicity, which has now been virtually eliminated, the simple presence of an indwelling 18- to 20-F catheter shaft tends to obstruct the free urethral drainage of exudates that are greatly increased as a result of traumatic injury and surgical suture lines. It seems clear that the development of paraurethral infection is much more relevant to this than to its introduction at the time of catheterization; after urethral injury it is generally best to avoid any indwelling standard-shaft urethral catheter, and this principle is widely accepted.

The Advantages of Fenestrated-Shaft Catheter Drainage

Positive drainage of the pericatheter space can be achieved by using a catheter with fenestrations in that part of the shaft that lies in the bulbar urethra.[7] Urethral secretions and exudates drain directly into the lumen of the catheter, and the space around it is washed clean by the flow of urine. It is always advisable to use a suprapubic catheter drainage in conjunction with a fenestrated catheter, which of course, should never be used to irrigate the bladder unless it is pushed in so that all the fenestrations lie within its cavity.

Furthermore, monitoring the progress of the healing of a ruptured or reconstructed urethra is simplified by radiographic fenestrated-catheter contrast studies. During these, the intraurethral pressure can be precisely controlled by elevating the suprapubic catheter bag above the pubis, thus creating an intravesical pressure of, say, 15 to 20 cm above the pubis before introducing aqueous contrast into the fenestrated catheter. Complications resulting from forceful urethrographic extravasation and premature removal of the catheter are thereby eliminated.

Thus a fenestrated catheter is particularly valuable for the reduction realignment of a ruptured urethra, and the author routinely uses it for the drainage of urethral exudates after a urethral reconstruction procedure.

Catheter Balloon Complications

The passage of the full length of a catheter into a ruptured urethra does not indicate that it has entered the bladder; increasing the urethral distraction damage by distention of its balloon at the site of a rupture is a well-recognized complication.

Unfortunately the discredited traditional maneuver of sustained traction on a balloon catheter to reduce the dislocation associated with a subprostatic urethral rupture is still a source of complications due to pressure damage to the only remaining sphincter mechanism at the bladder neck. The risk of damage to the bladder neck mechanism is augmented if the balloon partially deflates so that it enters and expands the proximal prostatic urethra.

However, a modification of this technique is sometimes appropriate for the simple repositioning of the bladder base after urethral rupture in young children. For boys, this is used through a perineal urethrostomy to avoid the classic complication of a development of anterior urethral stenosis at the bulbo-penile junction. Minimal traction tension is required in this age group to maintain the reduction, and a 30-cc balloon is relatively large so that the pressure is distributed over the bladder base as a whole, rather than just the area of the bladder neck mechanism. Complications resulting from an unrecognized partial deflation of the balloon are simply avoided by adding blue dye into its inflation fluid—the sudden passage of blue urine always seems to be noted in the nursing records.

The Hazards of Simple Dilatation

If a curved metal dilator is used in the early stage of healing in an attempt to maintain the passageway between the distracted ends of the urethra, it is a matter of luck whether it finds the distracted prostatic urethra in the retropubic hematoma-cavity or passes up in front of the prostate. It is remarkably easy to create an anterior false passage into the bladder base when its wall is softened by the local tissue healing response and incontinence may result from the consequent bypassing of the only remaining sphincter mechanism at the bladder neck.

The Hazards of Internal Urethrotomy

A trial of urethrotomy may be appropriate in some *minimal* subprostatic pelvic fracture urethral injuries. Although the treatment of a sphincter-stricture of the membranous urethra by urethrotomy is generally inadvisable because of the risk of damage to its mechanism (see subsequent discussion), this is not a consideration when its function has already been destroyed by the accident/disruption.

However, a urethrotomy is only likely to *succeed* when the incision can be extended into a supple expandable tissue plane. Unfortunately the pubo-urethral space is characteristically obliterated by dense hematoma-fibrosis after all but the most minimal pelvic fracture urethal injuries, and a simple incision into this tends to close immediately. Hence it is most unlikely that any but the most minimal pelvic fracture urethral distraction defects (PFUDDs) will respond to internal urethrotomy; however, if a trial of it is decided upon, it is essential to avoid inappropriate procedures that can result in complications:

1. Incisions in the posterolateral sector are contraindicated by the proximity of the nervi erigentes and the consequently increased risk of secondary impotence.
2. Distal extension of the incision into the spongy tissue of the bulbar urethra can result in spongiofibrosis, which may foreshorten its available length and compromise a subsequent anastomotic repair.
3. Dorsal incisions extending into the normal bulbar urethra distally transect the relatively thin layer of spongy tissue in its 12 o'clock sector, thus dictating a dorsal, rather than the usual ventrally located, spatulating incision for an anastomotic repair and consequently requiring a 180-degree rotation of the mobilized bulbar urethra.
4. An extended blind incision with an optical urethrotome endeavoring to enter the prostatic urethra by dead reckoning creates a false passage that can sometimes greatly complicate the situation by entering the rectum or damaging the bladder neck sphincter as it enters the bladder base (see Fig. 34–20).

The Shortcomings of Substitution Procedures

It is almost invariably possible to achieve an anastomotic repair of a PFUDD when the bulbar urethra is normal, and the long-term stricture-free reliability of this procedure is so good that, in the author's opinion, substitution procedures should never be introduced (unless there is a specific indication in an individual case), because of the inevitable incidence of inherent complications associated with them.

Thus in a personal series of more than 400 PFUDD repairs, a substitution procedure has been used only in the small number of cases in which the spongy element of the bulbar urethra was abnormal as a result of the original accident, a previous incidental stricture, or the failure of a previous attempt at its surgical resolution. The complications associated with the various substitution procedures have been discussed.

THE IMMEDIATE MANAGEMENT OF THE UROLOGIC COMPLICATIONS OF PELVIC FRACTURE URETHRAL INJURIES

The basic principles of the immediate management of urinary tract injuries are (1) the treatment of the urologic complications and the mitigation of the consequences; and (2) the avoidance of any further complications as a result of treatment. Maintaining a balance between these principles naturally requires fine judgment.

The Role of the Urologist

The relative importance of the urologist in the management of patents with a pelvic fracture urethral injury changes remarkably within a week of their emergency admission. The immediate consideration is to preserve life, which is sometimes gravely at risk. This essentially involves the restoration of the circulating volume and the emergency treatment of any coincident intracranial, intrathoracic, and intra-abdominal complications.

"While there may be other serious orthopaedic problems, those related to the fractured pelvis itself are much less likely to create a long-term cripple than the complications resulting from an associated urethral injury; it is the urologist who will have to share the burden of any residual disability resulting from this with the patient when the thoracic, the abdominal, and even the orthopaedic aspects are probably long forgotten."[30]

Apart from any associated hemorrhage, the urinary tract injuries themselves are not an urgent priority at the time of a patient's admission, so that the establishment of an appropriate urinary drainage system needs to be integrated with other priority complications, especially the intra-abdominal and the orthopedic stabilization of a mobile pelvic fragmentation. However, "this can in no way justify the delegation of the primary urological responsibility out of hand, to a traumatologic team; even the apparently simple insertion of a urethral catheter in such cases can generate serious complications and the primary urologic duty is to determine immediately whether there is or there is not a significant urinary tract injury by the simplest appropriate means."[10]

A Simple Routine for the Immediate Evaluation of Urinary Tract in Pelvic Fracture Urethral Injuries

Intravenous urographic contrast is given as soon as the pelvic fracture patient is admitted to the emergency room. Thirty to 40 minutes later the patient is positioned for a kidney, urethra, and bladder film and, immediately before this is taken, an additional 20 ml of dilute aqueous urocontrast is injected into the urethra using a standard 20-ml syringe with its nozzle held into the meatus so that the fluid does not escape around it. A single film is then usually sufficient to show (Fig. 34–22) whether (1) the anterior and posterior urethra is intact or the contrast agent is extravasating; (2) the bladder is round and low (indicating little or no dislocation or pelvic hematoma), compressed by a pelvic hematoma into a pear shape (with or without dislocation), or round and high (indicating a major bladder-base dislocation); (3) both kidneys are excreting and draining normally; and (4) the ureters and bladder are intact.

If the absence of periurethral extravasation proves the urethra to be intact, a small-caliber nursing-convenience urethral catheter can be inserted with impunity, and the urologist can retire from the fray. If any urinary tract abnormality is demonstrated, further appropriate urologic action is obviously essential.

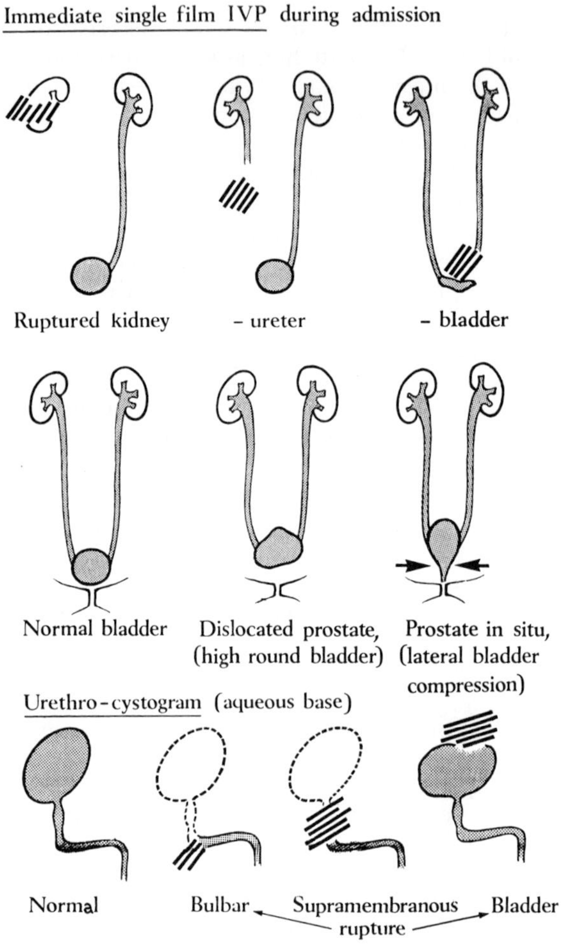

Figure 34–22. The immediate single-film urogram with synchronous retrograde urethrogram to demonstrate or exclude urinary tract injuries associated with a pelvic fracture accident. © 1973, Institute of Urology.

THE QUEST FOR A COMPLICATION-FREE DEFERRED ANASTOMOTIC BULBO-PROSTATIC RESTORATION OF URETHRAL CONTINUITY

When the bulbar urethra is normal, it is almost always possible to restore stricture-free urethral continuity after a distraction injury by a deferred one-stage spatulated overlap bulbo-prostatic anastomosis; the potential long-term reliability of this procedure is so good that the cause of any complications must be sought with a view to their prevention.

The progression-approach bulbo-prostatic anastomosis procedure that we use[1–3,5,10] differs in significant detail from that described by Waterhouse and colleagues.[31] Furthermore, because it is, in reality, a multiprocedure operation, it is not possible to describe it as a single entity—only by outlining the principles of the various individual component procedures that may or may not be required according to the findings at the time of operation.

Although it may take many hours, it must be one of the most cost-effective complex operations because there is an extraordinarily high expectation that a suprapubic-catheter–dependent urologic cripple will be discharged from the hospital within 3 to 4 weeks—voiding freely with satisfactory urinary control without the need for any further routine urethral instrumentation or long-term follow-up supervision. The following observations are based upon a personal series of more than 400 one-stage multiprocedural repairs of the pelvic fracture urethral distraction defects. In the space available it is possible only to highlight some of the principles that seem particularly important to the prevention of complications.

The Timing of a Definitive Repair Procedure

A definitive anastomotic repair is generally best postponed until the local healing reaction is complete and the hematoma has contracted to dense hematoma-fibrosis. The time that this takes is naturally determined by the bulk of the residual hematoma that remains after the initial treatment—generally at least 3 to 4 months, but longer if the hematoma is large.

The Progression-Approach Anastomotic Repair Procedure

Four approach options are available for the restoration of urethral continuity by the Turner-Warwick progression-approach anastomotic repair (PAAR) procedure: the perineal approach and three perineo-abdominal approach procedures, the retropubic, the partial pubectomy, and the total pubectomy (Fig. 34–23). Further details of these are recorded elsewhere.[1–3,5,10,28]

The Advantages of the Perineo-Abdominal Progression-Approach (PAPA) Operating Position

The use of the Turner-Warwick PAPA operating position (Fig. 34–24), which was originally developed for the reliable repair of complex vesicovaginal fistulas,[28,32,33] is essential for the four-option progression-approach anastomotic repair of subprostatic urethral distraction defects.

Irrespective of the apparent preoperative simplicity or complexity of the urethral injury and of the anticipated extent of the procedure, the patient is positioned on the operating table for a synchronous abdominoperineal procedure and prepped and draped with a single operating field. This facilitates the progression from a perineal to a perineo-abdominal approach, with or without partial or total resection of the pubic bone according to the findings as the operation proceeds (see Fig. 34–24). One assistant is quite enough—the surgeon can reposition from the

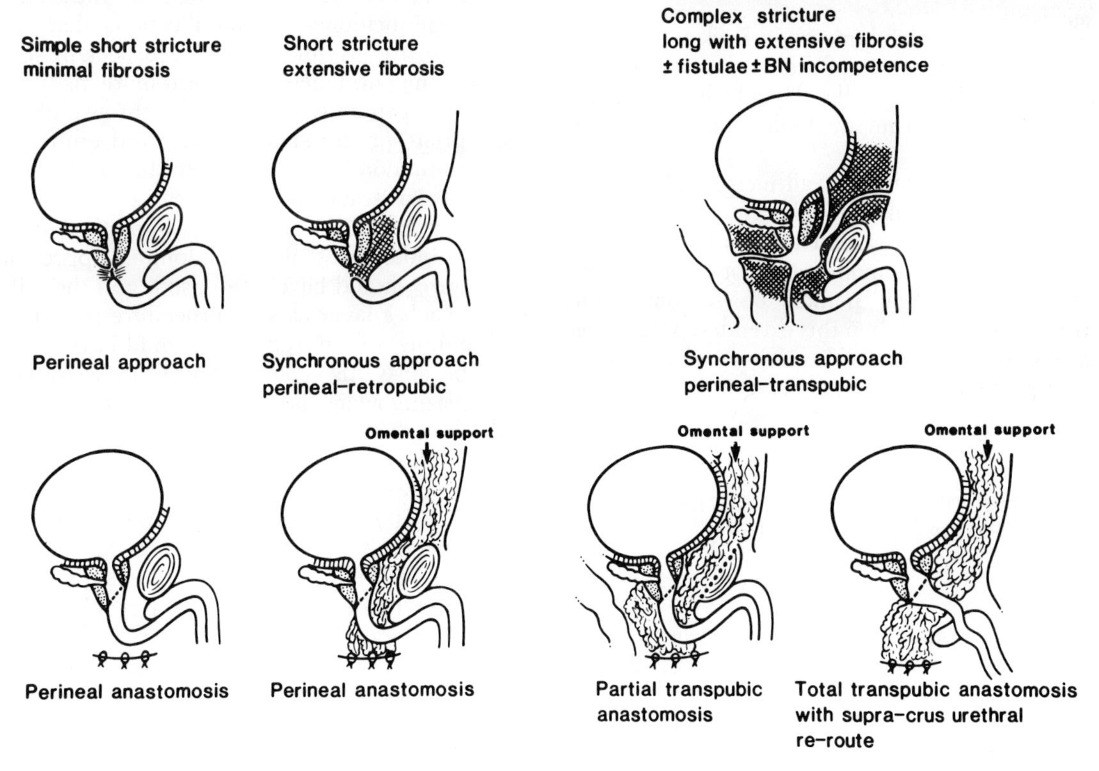

Figure 34–23. The Turner-Warwick four-option perineo-abdominal progression-approach (PAPA) procedure for the resolution of urethral distraction defects following pelvic fracture according to the findings at operation. © 1975, Institute of Urology.

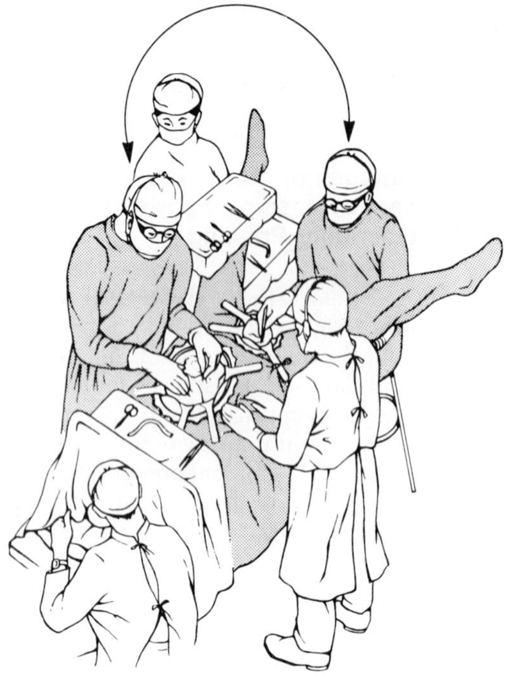

Figure 34–24. The operating position for the Turner-Warwick perineo-abdominal progression-approach (PAPA) for complex pelvic surgery. One surgeon with appropriate ring retraction minimizes the need for an assistant. © 1967, Institute of Urology.

perineum to the abdomen and back as often as required in the course of the operation, with no more disturbance to the layout than walking around the instrument table and the scrub nurse.

A midline abdominal wall incision should always be used for abdominal access because it is often necessary to extend this up to the xiphisternum to achieve mobilization of the right gastroepiploic vascular pedicle of the omentum from the stomach when this extended procedure is required to enable a short-apron omentum to be repositioned in the pelvis.[5,10,32,33]

The Shortcomings of the Limited-Option Perineal and Pubectomy Approach Procedures

In many centers the choice of access for the repair of pelvic fracture urethral defects is limited to two antipodal approach procedures—the simple perineal and the formal total pubectomy (transpubic)—without intermediate options that extend an inadequate exposure on the one hand and avoid unnecessarily extensive bone resection and its occasionally attendant complications on the other.

This disadvantage is often augmented by the use of different operating positions for these procedures—the exaggerated lithotomy and the frog-leg—which are singularly ill adapted to perioperative interconversion when the need for this becomes apparent in the course of the operation.

Consequently it is necessary for a surgeon using these either/or approach procedures to elect, preoperatively, which to use—although sometimes the factors upon which the decision should be properly based cannot become apparent until they are revealed in the course of the operation.

The Complications of Inappropriate Perineal-Approach Procedures

A number of reports have claimed that a perineal-approach procedure can be used for the great majority of pelvic fracture urethral distraction defects; however, some of these also record an incidence of complications that we would regard as unacceptable, especially restenosis, incontinence, and anastomotic fistulas, which are generally avoidable by the use of an appropriate progression-approach procedure.

The situation is comparable to that of the closure for vesicovaginal fistulas because almost any incidence of failure after a vaginal-approach procedure indicates that an abdominal-approach procedure should have been used, and the failure of such a layer-closure procedure indicates that an omental interposition should have been used because this is almost always successful—emphasizing again the importance of the PAPA procedure.[28,32,33]

Thus, however "simple" a short-gap pelvic fracture urethral defect appears to be, it is advisable to allocate an appropriate reservation of operating time, surgical experience, and cross-matched blood to enable a perineal-approach procedure to be extended into a synchronous abdominal-approach procedure. Only thus can one avoid the occasional disastrous failure to achieve a satisfactory anastomotic repair that is stricture-free in the long term because of an unexpected encounter with an extensive solid block of hematoma-fibrosis "concrete" around a beguilingly short-gap defect.

The Evaluation of Pelvic Fracture Urethral Distraction Defects Before a Definitive Delayed Repair

Cystourethrography

A normal urethrographic appearance of the lumen of the anterior spongy urethra generally excludes an abnormality such as a bulbo-penile stricture that is likely to contraindicate a one-stage anastomotic repair; however, it may not reveal a compromising associated extension of secondary spongiofibrosis resulting from complications of previous surgical procedures such as internal urethrotomy (an anastomotic repair involving a spongiofibrotic bulbar urethra prone to restenosis).

Cystographic failure to demonstrate the prostatic urethra is often regarded as a nuisance because it precludes measurement of the prostato-bulbar urethral gap; however, in reality this is generally reassuring evidence of competence of the bladder neck because a mechanism that remains open at all stages of bladder filling clearly indicates that it is incompetent (either as a result of intrinsic damage or traction-tethering by retropubic hematoma-fibrosis).

A synchronous cystogram and retrograde urethrogram—the "up-and-downagram"[5,10,28]—is a most important component of pre-repair investigation because it may reveal abnormalities such as fistulous tracks and false passages that are highly relevant to the extent of the reconstructive procedure but that may be difficult or even impossible to identify at operation. This is particularly important in short-gap defects that might otherwise appear, from the findings at operation, to be suitable for a simple perineal-approach repair.

Thus, although a preoperative up-and-downagram reveals most of the features that identify pelvic fracture urethral defects as complex and consequently requiring a synchronous perineo-abdominal-approach repair, it is fundamentally important to appreciate that *the radiographic demonstration of a short-gap prostato-bulbar urethral defect is not a valid basis for a surgical assumption that it is appropriate for a simple perineal-approach repair;* this can only be accurately determined by the operative findings at the time of reconstruction. Because the length of a gap is immaterial to the planning of a Turner-Warwick progression-approach procedure,[5,10,28] radiographic and instrumental "gapometry" is irrelevant to this.

Computed Tomography

Although a CT scan may reveal an unexpectedly extensive hematoma-fibrosis associated with a short-gap defect and thus give additional forewarning of the need for a perineo-abdominal procedure, a negative scan does not necessarily indicate that a short-gap defect is *appropriate* for a simple perineal-approach repair.

Cystourethroscopy

When an occlusive short-gap urethral defect has been treated by long-term indwelling suprapubic catheter drainage, suprapubic catheter-track cystourethroscopy is essential to exclude secondary catheter calculi because failure to detect and remove these can result in their complicating urethral impaction after a perineal-approach repair. Endoscopic evaluation of an incompetent bladder neck is important to determine whether this is the result of sector damage.

THE BASIC COMPONENTS OF THE TURNER-WARWICK PROGRESSION APPROACH ANASTOMOTIC PROCEDURE AND THE PREVENTION OF COMPLICATIONS

The basic essential for the avoidance of postoperative complications is to anticipate them, and an essential feature of this is the surgeon's inclination and ability to adapt a procedure according to the actual findings at the time of operation—many of which cannot be predetermined however detailed the preoperative evaluation. Hence the basic principles of the TITBAPIT (Take It To Bits And Put It Together) and the progression-approach procedures.[1,5,10,28]

Excision of Hematoma-Fibrosis and False Passages

The meticulous and complete excision of all the paraurethral and retropubic hematoma-fibrosis is a particularly emphasized component of a complication-free restoration of prostato-bulbar urethral continuity.

If the paraurethral fibrosis associated with a short-gap defect is minimal, it can be removed and the anastomosis completed through a perineal approach. The simple retropubic option of the four progression-approach procedures was developed[3,5,10] for the reconstruction of the short-gap defects that prove to be associated with unexpectedly extensive hematoma-fibrosis; it enables the rigid-walled dead space that results from its excision to be occluded by the transposition of an omental pedicle flap (see the following discussion). The perineo-retropubic approach is also used for the mobilization and omental wrapping of a hematoma-incarcerated incompetent bladder neck. In this procedure, the anastomotic restoration of urethral continuity is usually achieved from the perineum.

The prospect of the resection of an extensive paraprostatic hematoma-fibrosis may appear formidable, but it is simplified by the realization that it was formed in the manner of pre-mixed concrete so that when it has been meticulously carved away by what is perhaps best described as a "Michelangelo procedure" the dis-encased prostate and the lateral paravesical tissues are found to be quite normal and supple. Furthermore, although hemostasis in the lateral sulcus can be somewhat troublesome, the preprostatic venous plexus is long since obliterated. False passages and fistulous tracts associated with hematoma-fibrosis must of course be meticulously excised.

Tension-Free Approximation of the Mobilized Bulbar Urethra to the Prostate

No useful reduction of the prostato-bulbar gap can be achieved by mobilization of the prostate in a deferred repair because of its posterior fibrotic anchorage and, when the erection mechanism has survived the initial injury, it is particularly important to limit the exposure for the restoration of urethral continuity to the *anterior* aspect of the prostate to reduce the risk of secondary impotence due to disturbance of the residual intact elements of the nervi erigentes behind its apex. The importance of this consideration may call to question the use of the exaggerated lithotomy position and the posterior perineal-approach procedure, which is specifically avoided by the Turner-Warwick PAPA procedure (see p. 467).

Mobilization of the Bulbar Urethra

After division of the bulbar urethra immediately below the subprostatic hematoma-fibrosis, its mobilization to the base of the penis generally achieves 4 to 5 cm of elastic lengthening, which is sufficient to achieve a tension-free 2-cm spatulated overlap anastomosis with the apical prostatic urethra after bridging a gap of 2.0 to 2.5 cm or so (Fig. 34–25).

When the prostato-bulbar gap is longer than 2 to 3 cm as a result of a high dislocation of the prostate, or when the available elongation of the mobilized bulbar urethra has been foreshortened by damage secondary to previous surgical complications, it may be advisable to re-route the mobilized bulbar urethra transpubically, over the penile crus on one side, to enable it to reach the high-lying prostate directly. This requires a total resection of the pubis to prevent complication of secondary bone incarceration, especially in children before bone growth ceases. With the exception of the rare coincidence of pubic osteomyelitis, the occasional need for supracrural urethral re-routing is virtually the only indication for a total pubectomy approach in the Turner-Warwick four-option progression-approach procedure. It is almost never necessary to remove the whole of the pubis simply to gain access for a bulbo-prostatic anastomosis because a partial resection of the posterior margin with a Capener's gouge is generally sufficient.[1,3,5,10,28]

The Complications Resulting From an Overextended Mobilization of the Bulbar Urethra

The endeavor to obtain additional length for tension-free approximation of the bulbar urethra to the prostate by an extended mobilization of the penile urethra is generally contraindicated because of the risk of both proximal ischemia and chordee.

1. The bulbar spongy tissue normally receives its main blood supply from the posterior bulbar vessels. When these are divided by a proximal urethral transection, the retrograde blood supply along the normal bulbo-penile spongy tissue derived from its distal collateral communications is usually sufficient (Fig. 34–26). However, this may be critically impaired by an overextensive mobilization of the urethra onto the penile shaft, by the coincidence of a hypospadiac deformity in which there is no continuity of the penile spongy urethra with that of the glans, and by extensive spongiofibrosis resulting from previous urethritis or urethral surgery.
2. Because the available longitudinal elasticity of the penile urethra is extended during

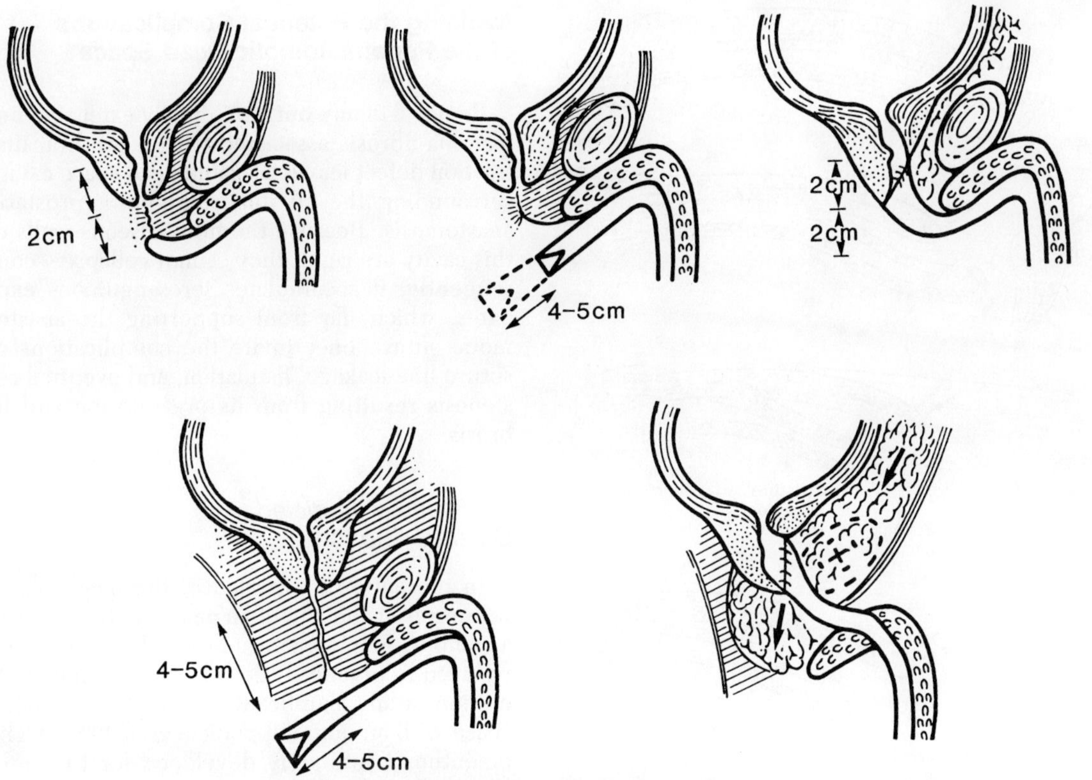

Figure 34–25. The principles of achieving tension-free approximation of the bulbar urethra to the apex of the prostate for the anastomotic restoration of urethral continuity of end-result pelvic fracture urethral injuries. The natural elasticity of the normal bulbar urethra generally provides 4- and 5-cm lengthening after mobilizing it to the base of the penis, thus enabling a subprostatic gap of 3 cm or more to be bridged with a 2-cm overlap anastomosis. An extended mobilization into the penile shaft should never be undertaken to gain additional length. Longer gaps may require supracrural transpubic rerouting. © 1973, Institute of Urology.

an erection, any attempt to gain extra urethral length by mobilizing the penile urethra is likely to result in a curvature chordee of the penile shaft[3,5,10,28] (Fig. 34–27).

3. When the suspensory ligament of the penis is tight, mild tension on a bulbar urethra that is mobilized to the base of the urethra can result in a base-angulation chordee. This fulcrum effect created by the suspensory ligament can be minimized by dividing its superficial element so that the base of the penis slides back a little. The loss of a centimeter or two of penile length creates a relatively insignificant disability. Division of the suspensory ligament is a natural consequence of a total pubectomy approach and is easily achieved through a midline perineal incision by simple dissection around one side of the base of the penis anteriorly.[1,3,5,10,28]

The Complications of an Incisional Extension of the Crural Bifurcation

The procedure of an incision into the angle of the crural bifurcation and a resection of the margin of the subpubic arch to foreshorten the course of a mobilized urethra and thus achieve a tension-free bulbo-prostatic anastomosis provides only a limited extension, and the mobilized urethra then lies in direct contact with the exposed cavernous tissue, where it is at some risk of erosion by a penile prosthesis if this subsequently proves necessary.

The Fixed-Flat Spatulated Bulbo-Prostatic Anastomosis

The inherent tendency of a spongy urethral anastomosis to contract and restenose can be

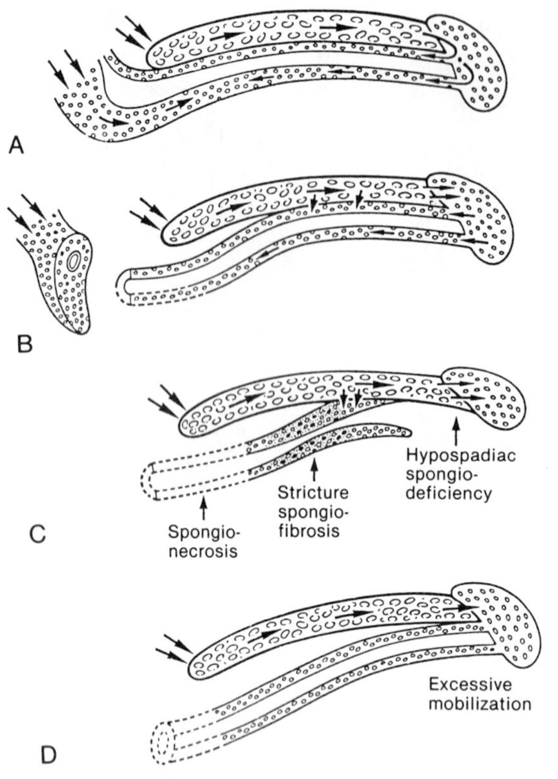

Figure 34–26. The vascular principles of urethral mobilization. After division of the main posterior bulbar arteries, vascularization of the proximal end of the mobilized bulbar urethra is dependent on the retrograde blood supply along its spongy tissue (A, B). Ischemic necrosis of the proximal end of the mobilized urethra may result when the retrograde blood supply is compromised by hypospadiac maldevelopment (C), incidental spongiofibrosis, or division of distal collateral vessels by mobilization of the penile urethra (D). © 1983, Institute of Urology.

prevented by the combination of an overlap spatulation and lateral spread-flat fixation. Because the subverumontanal urethra is commonly concentric within the apical tissue of the prostate, a wedge-shaped resection of the anterolateral sector of this is commonly required to achieve the necessary fixed-flat spatulation (Fig. 34–28). Because the normal caliber of both the apical prostatic urethra and the posterior bulbar urethra is in the region of 25 F, the eventual caliber of an efficient overlap anastomosis should be 25 + 25 = 50 F. This short segment of augmented caliber should persist as a small localized bulbar dilatation shown by follow-up urography—positively excluding any question of the complication of recurrent anastomotic stenosis.

Avoiding the Potential Complications of the Perianastomotic Dead Space

Removal of any but a minimally extensive hematoma-fibrosis associated with a urethral distraction defect leaves a sizable dead space cavity surrounding the all important bulbo-prostatic anastomosis. Because the fibro-osseous walls of this cavity are rigid, they cannot collapse—consequently, it accumulates serosanguinous exudates, which, far from supporting the anastomotic suture line, invite the complications of suture line leakage, fistulation, and eventual restenosis resulting from its organization and fibrosis.

The Value of Pedicled Omental Support

In the author's experience, the incidence of restenosis at the site of an anastomotic repair of a complex pelvic fracture urethral defect can be reduced to practically zero by the routine obliteration of any significant perianastomotic dead space with an omental pedicle graft.[1,3,5,10,32] The omentum is uniquely developed for the resolution of local inflammatory processes, not only because of its blood supply, but also because of its abundant lymphatic drainage, which absorbs inflammatory cell debris and macromolecular protein exudates that would otherwise result in a purulent accumulation. Furthermore, once an inflammatory situation has resolved, the omentum always regains its suppleness—consequently, it ensures the freedom of the functional movement of any part of the urinary tract that it envelops so that it is not impaired by the secondary fibrosis that otherwise develops in retropubic and periuretric fat. Thus, omental wrapping not only greatly reduces the incidence of complications after the surgical repair and reconstruction of the urinary tract, but it is fundamental to the success of complex refunctional procedures such as sphincteroplasty.

One of three definitive omental pedicle-mobilization procedures is required to enable the omental apron to reach the perineum; these are detailed elsewhere.[5,10,32]

Avoidable Causes of Failure of Omental Pedicle Graft Repairs

An omental pedicle graft repair of a fistula or prevention of dead-space complications in the pelvis is so reliable that complications and fail-

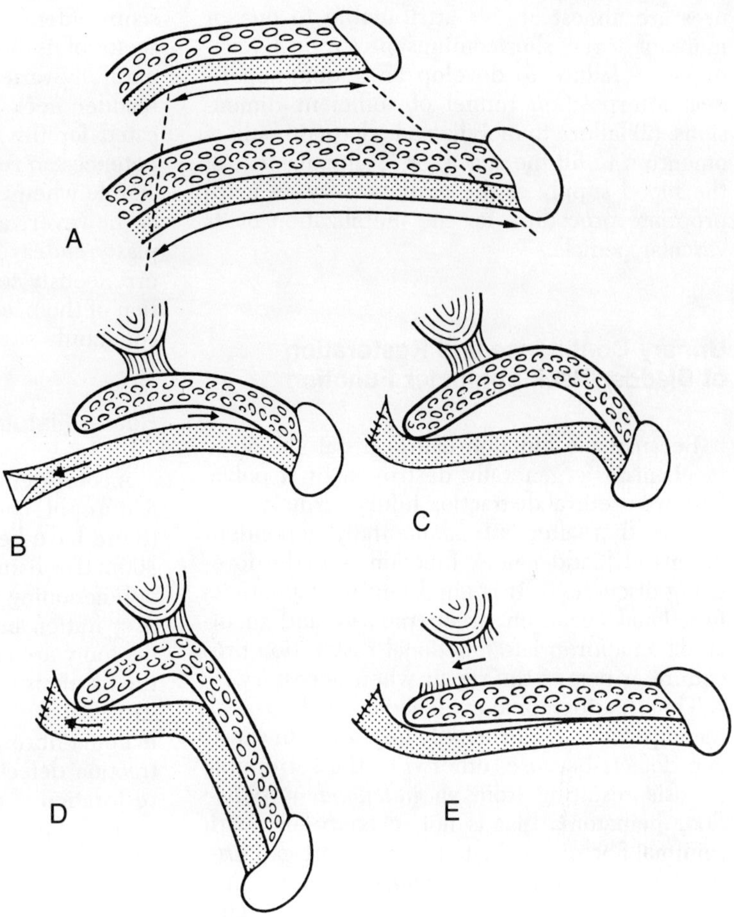

Figure 34–27. The mechanical principles of anterior urethral mobilization. (A) The available elastic lengthening of the penile urethra is naturally somewhat stretched during an erection. Endeavors to obtain additional urethral length for an anastomotic repair by mobilizing the penile urethra (B) result in penile curvature chordee (C). Angulation chordee after bulbar urethral mobilization (D) can be reduced by division of the angulating fulcrum created by the suspensory ligament (E); this does not result in any significant disability. © 1983, Institute of Urology.

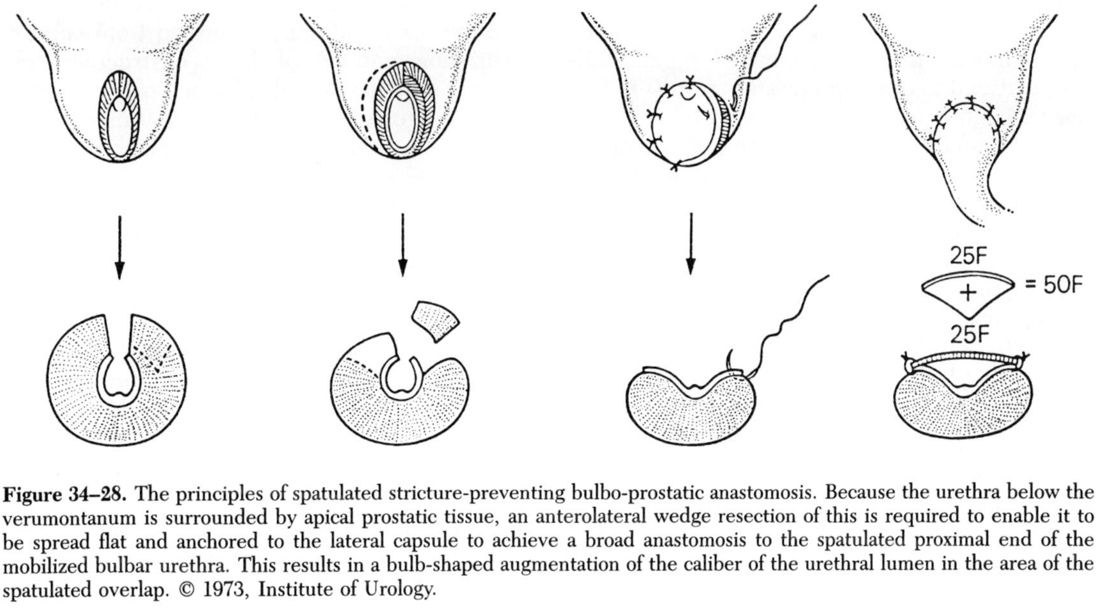

Figure 34–28. The principles of spatulated stricture-preventing bulbo-prostatic anastomosis. Because the urethra below the verumontanum is surrounded by apical prostatic tissue, an anterolateral wedge resection of this is required to enable it to be spread flat and anchored to the lateral capsule to achieve a broad anastomosis to the spatulated proximal end of the mobilized bulbar urethra. This results in a bulb-shaped augmentation of the caliber of the urethral lumen in the area of the spatulated overlap. © 1973, Institute of Urology.

ures are almost always attributable to one or more of three shortcomings of surgical technique:[5,32] failure to develop an abdominoperineal interposition tunnel of sufficient dimensions; (2) failure to mobilize an adequate bulk of omentum to fill the space; or (3) impairment of the blood supply of the omentum by an inappropriate procedure for the mobilization of its vascular pedicle.

Urinary Continence and Restoration of Bladder-Neck Sphincter Function

Because the function of the distal sphincter mechanism is generally destroyed by a pelvic fracture urethral distraction injury, urinary continence thereafter is fundamentally dependent upon the bladder-neck function (see the foregoing discussion). It is important to evaluate its functional occlusion preoperatively and to include an appropriate functional-restoration procedure as part of the repair when necessary.

Thus, cystographic evidence of bladder-neck incompetence is particularly important in short-gap defects because, otherwise, the retropubic fibrosis resulting from an *independent* pelvic floor hematoma that is not in continuity with minimal fibrosis associated with a short-gap urethral lesion may not be recognized during a simple perineal repair (see the foregoing discussion).

The cystographic demonstration of an incompetent bladder-neck mechanism is, in itself, a definitive indication of the need for a synchronous lower-abdominal exploration, even if the urethral distraction defect is otherwise apparently suitable for perineal-approach repair. Failure to attend to this appropriately results in urinary incontinence.

The commonest cause of incompetence of the bladder-neck sphincter after a pelvic fracture is external circumferential tethering of a normal uninjured mechanism by the contraction of a retropubic hematoma-fibrosis (see the foregoing discussion). The endoscopic appearances of this are those of a fixedly open, but otherwise normally circular, bladder-neck mechanism; its simple mobilization, by resection of the fibrosis anteriorly and laterally, together with its replacement by a supple omental pedicle wrap, is usually all that is necessary to restore its competence.

Incompetence of the bladder neck may also result from a segmental injury of the mechanism itself; this is generally indicated by the endoscopic identification of a notched scar in one sector of its circumference, the location of which naturally varies according to its cause. A formal bladder neck sphincter reconstruction is indicated for this, and satisfactory sphincter competence can result.[5] This procedure is relatively simple when the defect is anterior, as it usually is; however, a posterior reduction sphincteroplasty endeavoring to restore the function of an erroneously conceived transurethral loop resection of the bladder neck is a formidable and less commonly successful procedure.

Rectal Fistula

A coincident rectal fistula is not an uncommon feature of complex fracture urethral injuries (there have been more than 30 in our series of 400). If a fistula is not already protected by a defunctioning colostomy, a preoperative bowel preparation and a perioperative temporary loop-ileotomy are required. In the majority of cases, the fistulous track into the rectum is quite small so that, after appropriate resection of the hematoma-fibrosis associated with the urethral distraction defect down to the rectal wall and the restoration of urethral continuity, simple occlusion of the dead space by the omental pedicle graft is generally sufficient to occlude the fistula orifice without a formal suture closure (Fig. 34–29).

CONCLUSION

The advances in definitive reconstructive procedures have naturally stemmed from subspecialization, and few of the reconstructive techniques that have evolved can be regarded as general urologic procedures. A urologist specializing in them should have appropriate personal experience with some of the relevant techniques of plastic surgery, of video-urodynamic evaluation of the functional behavior of the lower urinary tract, and adequate training in colorectal surgery. Furthermore, reliable success is fundamentally dependent not only upon meticulous technique and personal experience, but also upon an instinctive surgical inclination to adopt and to adapt procedures according to the unpredictable findings at the time of operation. For complex problems, an endeavor to select a particular operative procedure preoperatively is generally inappropriate. In reconstructive surgery, the TITBAPIT principle is often critical to success.

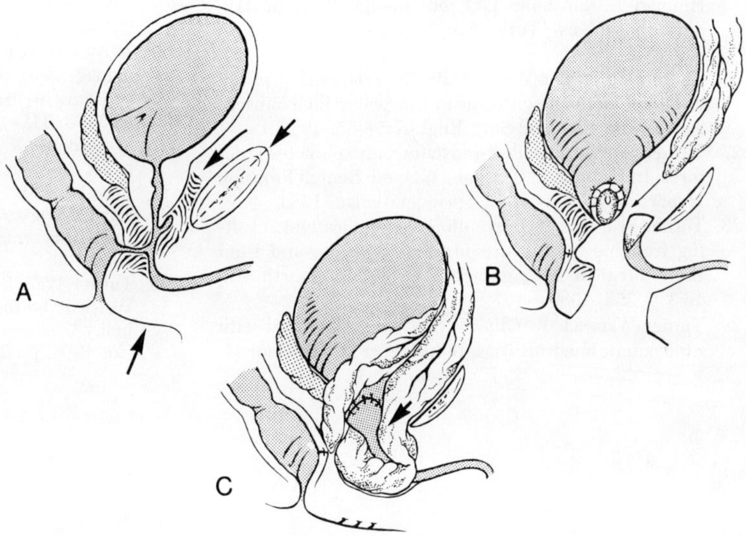

Figure 34–29. A prostato-rectal fistula associated with a pelvic fracture injury (A) is reliably resolved by the Turner-Warwick omentum-supported bulbo-prostatic anastomotic repair (B, C). © 1973, Institute of Urology.

Surgeons with general urologic training who do not have special additional experience in reconstructive procedures, and a particular aptitude for them, must be advised that "having a go" at the definitive resolution of a difficult stricture problem is unlikely to be in the best interests of their patients, because any failed attempt, however well intended and however meticulously performed, almost inevitably complicates a subsequent "retrievoplasty." The importance of this should not be overlooked.

References

1. Turner-Warwick R: Observations on the treatment of traumatic urethral injuries and the value of the fenestrated urethral catheter. Brit J Surg 60:775–781, 1973.
2. Turner-Warwick R: Complex traumatic posterior urethral strictures. J Urol 118:564–574, 1977.
3. Turner-Warwick R: Urethral stricture surgery. In Glenn I, Boyce G, eds: Urologic Surgery, 3rd ed. Philadelphia, Lippincott, 1983, pp 689–719.
4. Turner-Warwick R: The principles of functional reconstruction of the lower urinary tract. In Bevan PG, ed: Reconstructive Procedures in Surgery. Oxford, Blackwell Scientific Publications, 1982, pp 193–233.
5. Turner-Warwick R: The principles of urethral reconstruction. In McDougal S, ed: Rob Smith's Operative Surgery (Urology). London, Butterworth, 1985, pp 480–520.
6. Turner-Warwick R: Urethral stricture surgery. In Glenn JF, et al., ed: Urologic Surgery, 4th ed. Philadelphia, Lippincott, 1989.
7. Arnold EP: The urodynamic significance of minor problems. Urol Clin North Am 6:193–197, 1979.
8. Turner-Warwick R: The repair of urethral stricture in the region of the membranous urethra. J Urol 100:303–314, 1968.
9. Milroy EJG, Chapple CR, Eldin A, Wallsen N: A new treatment for urethral strictures—a permanently implanted stent. J Urol 141:1120–1122, 1982.
10. Turner-Warwick R: Urethral stricture surgery. In Mundy AR, ed: Current Operative Urology. 1989, pp 160–218.
11. Gibbon N: A new type of catheter for urethral drainage of the bladder. Br J Urol 30:1–7, 1958.
12. Turner-Warwick R: A technique of posterior urethroplasty. J Urol 83:416–419, 1960.
13. Pallister WKP: Rheostasis: Reduced bleeding without sustained hypotension by minimal ganglion blockade. Report of 6th European Congress of Anaesthesia, 1982, p 2.
14. Gil Vernet JM: Un traitement des stenoses traumatiques et inflammatoires de l'uretre posterieur. Nouvelle methode d'uretoplastie. Journal d'Urologie et de Nephrologie 72:97–108, 1966.
15. Blandy JP, Singh M, Tressider GC: Urethroplasty by scrotal flap for long urethral strictures. Br J Urol 40:261–267, 1968.
16. Turner-Warwick R: Observations upon techniques for reconstruction of the urethral meatus, the hypospadias glans deformity of the penile urethra. Urol Clin North Amer 6:643–655, 1979.
17. Orandi A: One stage urethroplasty—a four-year follow-up. J Urol 107:977–980, 1972.
18. Turner-Warwick R: The use of pedicle grafts in the repair of urinary tract fistulae. Br J Urol 44:644–656, 1972.
19. Leadbetter GW: A simplified urethroplasty for strictures of the bulbous urethra. J Urol 83:54–59, 1960.
20. Turner-Warwick R: Repair of urethral sutures in the male. In Rob C, Smith R, eds: Operative Surgery: Urology, 3rd ed. London, Butterworth, 1977, pp 315–342.
21. Smith J: The measurement and significance of the urinary flow rate. Br J Urol 38:701–706, 1966.
22. Turner-Warwick R, Whiteside CG: Clinical urodynamics. Urol Clin North Am 6(1):13–30, 1979.
23. Bates CP, Whiteside CG, Turner-Warwick R: Synchronous cine pressure-flow cystourethrography. Br J Urol 42:714–723, 1970.
24. Turner-Warwick R: The sphincter mechanism—the avoidance of post-prostatectomy incontinence. In Weber W, Jonas D, eds: Die Post Operative Harninkontinenz des Mannes. Internationales Symposium, Frankfurt am Main. Stuttgart, Thieme, 1979, pp 17–33.
25. Turner-Warwick R: The sphincter mechanisms: their relation to prostatic enlargement and its treatment. In

Hinman F, Chisholm GD, ed: Benign Prostatic Hypertrophy. New York, Springer Verlag, 1983, pp 809–828.
26. Chilton C, Turner-Warwick R: The relationship of the distal sphincter mechanism to the pelvic floor musculature. Ann Roy Coll Surg Engl 67:54–55, 1985.
27. Turner-Warwick R.: Post-prostatectomy sphincter-strictures. In Hinman F, Chisholm GD, ed: Benign Prostatic Hypertrophy. New York, Springer Verlag, 1983.
28. Turner-Warwick R: Prevention of complications resulting from pelvic fracture urethral injuries—and from their surgical management. Urol Clin North Am 16:335–358, 1989.
29. Turner-Warwick R: Clinical problems associated with urodynamic abnormalities. In Lutzeyer W, Melchior M, eds: Urodynamics 1. Berlin, Springer-Verlag, 1973, pp 237–263.
30. Turner-Warwick R: A personal view of the immediate management of pelvic fracture urethral injuries and subsequent urethral strictures. Urol Clin North Am 4:81–93, 111–124, 1977.
31. Waterhouse K, Abrahams JI, Gruber H, et al: The transpubic approach to the lower urinary tract. J Urol 109:486–490, 1973.
32. Turner-Warwick R: The use of the omental pedicle graft in urinary tract reconstruction. J Urol 116:341–347, 1976.
33. Turner-Warwick R: Urinary fistula in the female. In Walsh P, Gittes RF, Perlmutter AD, et al, eds: Campbell's Urology, Edition 5. Philadelphia, WB Saunders Co, 1986, pp 2718–2738.

COMPLICATIONS OF URETHRAL VALVE SURGERY

35

W. Hardy Hendren

Urethral valves vary greatly in degree of severity.[1] An example of the most severe is the valve in the neonate that results in almost complete obstruction of the urethra. This causes great hypertrophy of the bladder, often with cellules and diverticula. Also, there is usually bilateral hydroureteronephrosis. In some of these severely affected infants, there is bilateral massive vesicoureteral reflux. However, others have dilated, tortuous megaureters without reflux. In still others, there may be massive reflux on only one side where there is a unilateral dysplastic kidney. Interestingly, it is more often the left kidney that is affected rather than the right kidney.[2] Massive unilateral reflux may have a protective effect on the opposite kidney by providing a "pop off" for high pressures in the bladder that is obstructed by ureteral valves.[3] Two other "protective factors" that have been noted are large congenital diverticula of the bladder seen in some of these cases and/or urinary extravasation, with or without urinary ascites.

An example of less severe valves are those in the older boy who has voiding disturbances such as frequency, urgency, uncontrolled wetting, and even bed-wetting.[4] There are many gradations in the clinical picture of urethral valves between the two extremes. This chapter discusses the variety of urethral valves, complications that valves can cause, and complications that can result when valves are treated by various means. There are many recent reports of large series of urethral valves in boys with long-term follow-up.[5–17] These reports illustrate the considerable controversy over treatment of the common problems of urethral valves and emphasize the fact that valves can cause death, depending on how much function is present when the diagnosis is made, and whether surgical management preserves that function or results in continuing loss of function from obstruction, reflux, and infection.

ANATOMY OF VALVES

There are small ridges or folds in the normal male urethra that are readily visible endoscopically. Most urethral valves are an accentuation of these folds. Seventy years ago, Young and associates described the principal types of urethral valves (Fig. 35–1).[8] Type I valves are by far the most common. They arise from the urethral crest, distal to the verumontanum. In some of these, the crest is short so that the leaflets are close to the verumontanum. In others, the crest is elongated so that the leaflets are considerably distal to the verumontanum. In mild cases, the leaflets occlude only the lower half of the urethral lumen as viewed through the endoscope. In more severe cases, however, they encircle the urethra to join at the 12 o'clock position, forming a diaphragm. There can be a slit-like opening in the diaphragm and almost complete urethral obstruction.

Type II valves are extremely rare; in fact, some surgeons doubt their existence. It is common to see small type II folds from the verumontanum to the bladder neck in cases of severe type I valves. Usually, they are not significant. However, we have seen several examples of type II valves that appeared to be significant in

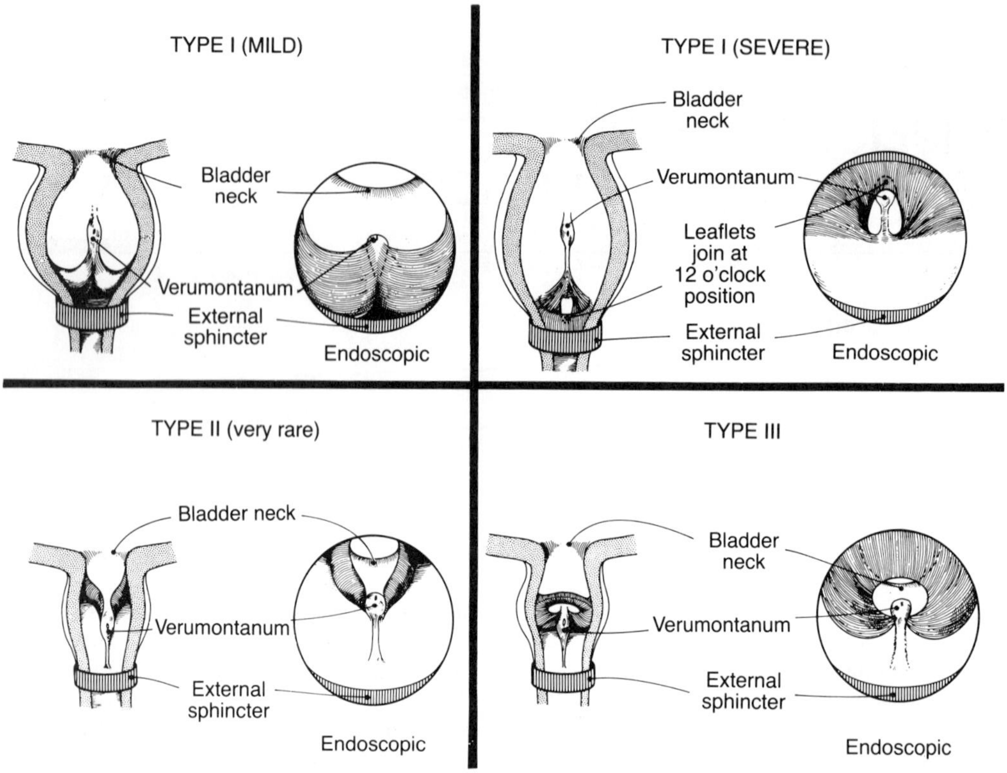

Figure 35–1. Types of urethral valves. *A,* Mild type I valves, common in boys with voiding disturbances and infection. These are often missed radiographically and endoscopically. *B,* Severe type I valves in which the leaflets encircle the urethra and join at the 12 o'clock position, forming a diaphragm. This is usually associated with severe upper urinary tract changes. *C,* Type II valves, which are extremely rare. They are more often seen in association with severe type I valves. *D,* Type III valve with diaphragm-like configuration, occurring usually at the level of the verumontanum but sometimes more distally. Some valves are hybrid in their appearance, i.e., intermediate between types I and III.

association with type I valves but only two cases in which type II valves existed alone.

Type III valves differ in that they present as a diaphragm, most often located at the level of the verumontanum, but occasionally occur elsewhere. They can be located distal to the external urethral sphincter and are then referred to as anterior urethral valves.[19] Anterior urethral valve-like obstruction has been described as being situated as far distal as the fossa navicularis, just inside the urethral meatus.[20] The anatomy of an anterior urethral valve usually differs from valves seen in the posterior urethra because the defect is essentially a urethral diverticulum in which the distal rim obstructs the flow of urine. In the posterior urethra, it is not uncommon to see valves that are a hybrid form, having an appearance that is intermediate between type I and type III.

SYMPTOMS

The symptoms caused by urethral valves vary with the severity of urethral obstruction. In a review of our own cases, patients were divided into four groups.[1] Group 1 had small urethral valves, which were demonstrable endoscopically and radiographically, but had no secondary anatomic changes such as paraureteral diverticula or vesicoureteral reflux. The upper urinary tracts were normal. Group 2 had minor secondary changes, including small diverticula and reflux, but upper urinary tracts were still normal. Group 3 had larger diverticula, more severe reflux, and upper urinary tract damage from urinary infection. Group 4 had severe upper urinary tract damage, hydronephrosis, megaureters, and, often, uremia.

The majority of the severe cases presented in the first year of life. It is not uncommon, however, for a boy with serious upper urinary tract decompensation to be clinically silent until there is a urinary infection at 6 to 8 years of age. In order of frequency of occurrence, symptoms in boys with valves include bed-wetting, urinary infection, day-wetting, poor stream, frequency, dribbling, hematuria, and acute urinary retention. A poor stream is generally thought to be the hallmark of urethral valves; however, in the majority of cases, this is an unreliable sign. Preoperatively, parents will often believe that the boy's urinary stream is adequate. Postoperatively, the same parents will volunteer that the stream is much more forceful and that previously, they really did not appreciate that it was abnormal.

We encountered one octogenarian who presented with urethral valves and retention.[21] He had been unaware of a voiding problem previously. We also recently treated a 20-year-old patient with severe valve obstruction that was discovered when he was evaluated for hypertension caused by massive hydronephrosis secondary to urethral valves. Unsuspected valves have been discovered in adults undergoing dialysis and/or renal transplantation.[22] An obstructing urethral valve has been described in a female but this is very rare.[23]

Residual urine is not always seen in boys with urethral valves. Any hollow viscus, including the bladder, can compensate for a certain degree of obstruction by muscular hypertrophy, which allows emptying despite obstruction. Measuring intravesical voiding pressures by suprapubic insertion of a needle into the bladder will disclose that voiding is accomplished in some of these children with pressures of 80 to 100 mm Hg, i.e., 3 to 4 times higher than normal. Urodynamic study of the bladder in some cases after valves have been destroyed will demonstrate that the bladder is noncompliant and continues to have high intravesical pressure.[24,25] Augmentation cystoplasty using bowel can help in some of these cases.[26]

ROENTGEN DIAGNOSIS OF VALVES

The frequent use of antenatal ultrasonography allows many infants with hydronephrosis from urethral valves and other pathologic states to be diagnosed before they are born.[27–29] The antenatally diagnosed cases can be especially problematic because there is often oligohydramnios, resulting in pulmonary hypoplasia.[30] Intrauterine decompression of the fetal urinary tract has been described by both open operation and percutaneous catheter decompression.[31,32] Antenatal intervention carries risk and does not always result in benefit.[33] We believe that the main value of intrauterine diagnosis today is that it enables the surgeon to initiate appropriate treatment soon after birth.

After birth, a male with urinary infection, abnormality of voiding, or failure to thrive should be screened for urethral valves. The isolated symptom of bed-wetting is seen in some boys with mild urethral valves. We do not screen all bed-wetters for valves at a young age, however, unless there are other symptoms, such as daytime frequency, urgency, dribbling, or a history of infection. If a boy has bed-wetting beyond 7 or 8 years of age, it is reasonable to exclude the possibility that urethral valves exist before placing him on various medications or referring him for psychiatric consultation, which we have seen done for several boys with valves.

Roentgenographic evaluation should include intravenous pyelography (IVP), renal ultrasonic examination, and voiding cystourethrography. The IVP results can be perfectly normal in mild cases, or they can show extreme hydronephrosis in more severe cases. Cystourethrography should be performed using dynamic technique; a single static cystogram is valueless. Cinecystography was used over 20 years ago and monitored the entire act of voiding. Today, multiple spot films are taken during fluoroscopic monitoring of voiding in the oblique position. This limits radiation exposure and gives better anatomic detail.

The accuracy of the radiographic diagnosis of urethral valves is in direct proportion to the experience of the radiologist. It is helpful when there is a close collaboration between the radiologist and the surgeon, who has the opportunity to observe the anatomy through the endoscope. The most common complication we have seen in urethral valves is the failure to diagnose them, both radiographically and endoscopically. This is true not only in mild cases, but also in very obvious severe urethral valves. Indeed, we have seen many patients with severe valves who had undergone major surgery for reflux and megaureters when the primary problem was unrecognized urethral valve obstruction. To illustrate this, the author made a motion picture in 1975 showing multiple examples of urethral valves.[34]

Radiographically, quite a different picture can be seen in patients who have almost identical anatomic findings through the endoscope (Figs. 35–2 through 35–4). Generally, there is some elongation and widening of the prostatic urethra. There is usually indentation of the prostatic urethra just at or proximal to the external sphincter in type I urethral valves and at the level of the verumontanum in type III urethral valves. The bladder neck is usually hypertrophied. In some

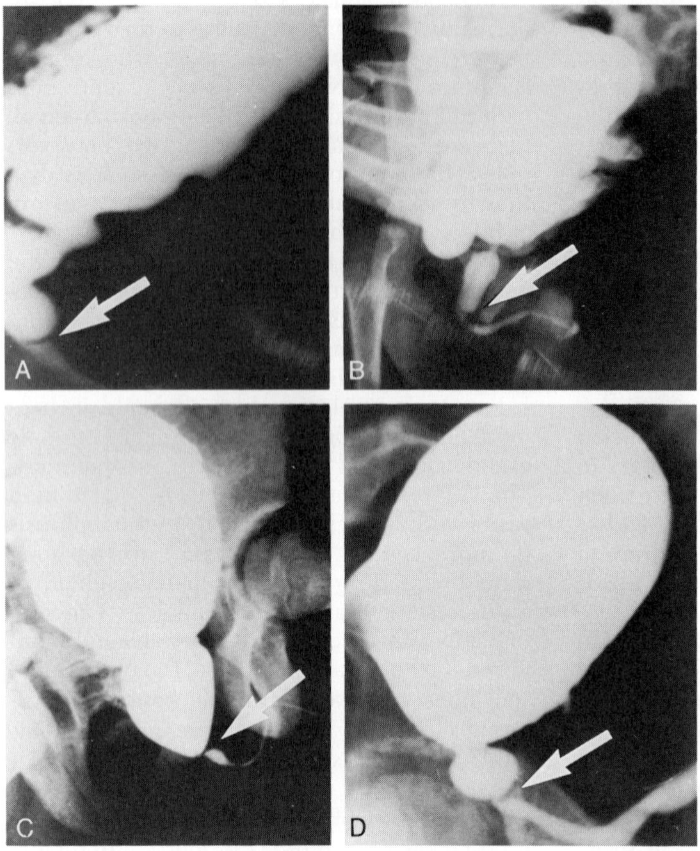

Figure 35–2. Cystourethrograms of four boys with posterior urethral valves. Note that although all four patients had urethral valves, no two x-rays are alike. *A*, Voiding study of 3-month-old boy who had urinary tract infection. Arrow points to level of obstruction from type I urethral valves. The posterior bladder neck is very prominent. There is cellule formation in the trigone and no reflux. *B*, 5-year-old boy presenting with urinary tract infection. Arrow points to the level of obstruction, distal to the verumontanum and proximal to the external sphincter. There is elongation and widening of the prostatic urethra and marked secondary hypertrophy of the bladder neck. There is also massive vesicoureteral reflux. *C*, An 8-year-old boy studied for bed-wetting. As in *A* and *B*, this is also a type I urethral valve, with marked obstruction just proximal to the external urethral sphincter. There is marked widening of the prostatic urethra, but the shape is entirely different from that shown in *A* and *B*. *D*, Type III urethral valve—a diaphragm obstructing at the level of the verumontanum—in a 5-year-old boy with bed wetting, day wetting, and urinary frequency.

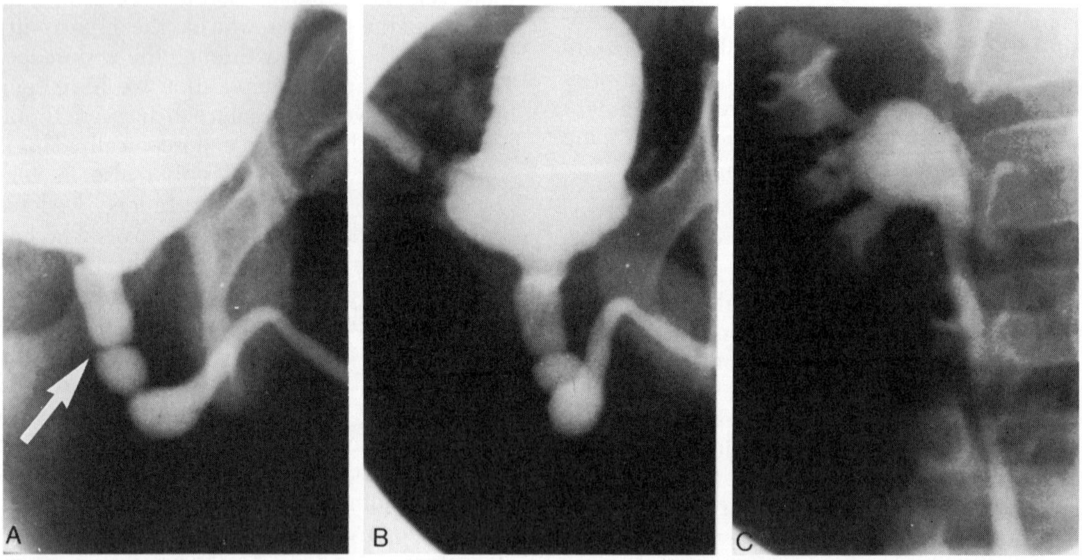

Figure 35–3. Nine-year-old boy with chief complaints of bed-wetting and daytime urgency. *A*, Collar-like indentation (arrow) of a small type I urethral valve, just distal to verumontanum (arrow) and 1 cm proximal to the external sphincter. *B*, *C*, Moderate right vesicoureteral reflux. Valves were resected with Bugbee electrode, a transient admission. Bed wetting and daytime urgency disappeared immediately. The patient then noted a heavier stream that was easier to initiate. Originally, voiding had been considered normal. Reflux was minimal and confined to the lower ureter on 2-year follow-up. Reflux of this degree will disappear in about 50 percent of cases after valves are removed.

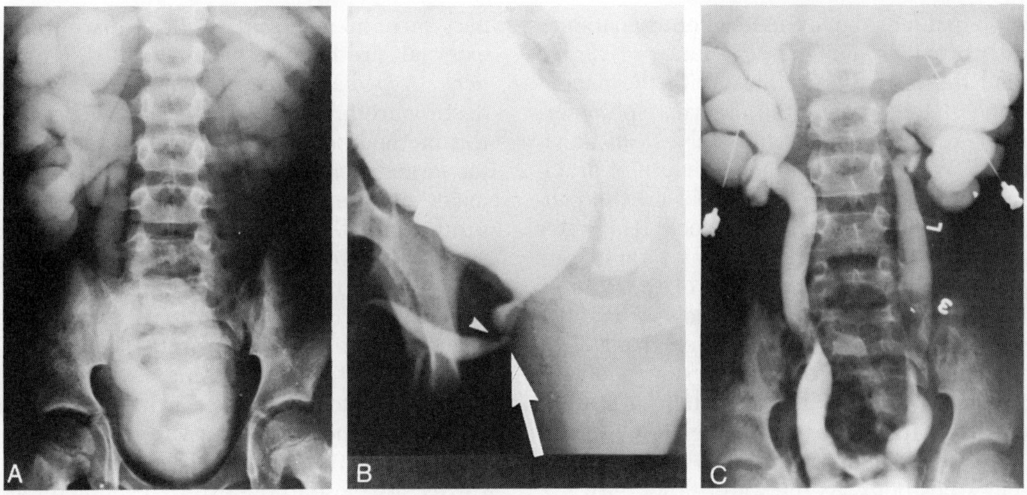

Figure 35–4. Six-year-old boy referred to the Endocrinology Service for "diabetes insipidus." The history included urinary frequency, day and night wetting, and polyuria. *A,* IVP showing severe bilateral hydronephrosis. Blood chemical values included a blood urea nitrogen level (BUN) of 40 mg per 100 ml; creatinine, 1.3 mg per 100 ml; and creatinine clearance, 44 L absolute per day. *B,* Voiding cystourethrogram. White arrow points to valve obstruction. The bladder is large and trabeculated, and reflux is noted in the dilated right ureter. Notice that although these are classic type I urethral valves, the appearance of this prostatic urethra is quite different from the cases shown in Figure 35–2. The prostatic urethra is slightly dilated but not elongated. Valves arise from a very short crest at the inferior margin of the verumontanum. Moderate bladder neck hypertrophy is evident. The stream apparently was satisfactory on this examination. Voiding pressures were 50 mm Hg, at a rate of only 2.5 ml per second. *C,* Preoperative antegrade perfusion pressure dynamic study. There is a No. 22 spinal needle inserted into each renal collecting system. The bladder is emptied by an inlying catheter. Opening pressure was only 3 ml of dye on each side, and pressures did not rise after perfusing with 10 ml per minute for 9 minutes.

patients, this is an actual hypertrophy, but in others, it is an accentuation of a relatively normal bladder neck by the dilated prostatic urethra. Paraureteral diverticula and vesicoureteral reflux are common. In subtle cases the elongation and dilatation of the prostatic urethra may be minimal. The bladder is generally trabeculated, varying from minimal to severe, with multiple sacculations. During voiding, the stream can be hesistant, with intermittent trapping of contrast in the prostatic urethra. However, some may void with good force by exerting high bladder pressure.

Voiding films can be obtained in two ways. We most often insert a small (No. 3.5 or 5.0 French) feeding catheter through the urethra into the bladder, filling the catheter with a contrast medium until the child voids. We then remove the catheter during micturition. We have found this catheter technique to be entirely satisfactory; it does not distort valve anatomy. Alternatively, if the bladder is palpable, one can insert a No. 22 French needle suprapubically, infusing contrast under fluoroscopic control to obtain appropriate films during micturition. We have not encountered any complication from the insertion of a suprapubic needle.

ENDOSCOPIC VISUALIZATION OF VALVES

The modern fiberoptic endoscopes have greatly facilitated diagnosis of urethral valves, even in young infants. Miniature endoscopes (No. 7.5 French) are available from several companies. Considerable endoscopic experience in treating young males is necessary to gain familiarity with normal and abnormal endoscopic findings. Today's miniature video cameras represent a great step forward in recording urethral valve pathology, for teaching purposes, and for permitting multiple viewers to observe valve destruction.

Infant urethral sounds should be used very gently in calibrating the male urethra to determine the appropriate endoscope size. Too large an instrument can create severe trauma and must never be used. Urethras of newborn males will generally accept the No. 7.5 French endoscope, which gives an excellent view of the anatomy. Some newborns will accept a number 10 sheath; larger sizes are used in older boys. Endoscopy, like radiography, should be dynamic in order to evaluate prostatic urethral anatomy. Maintaining the water-irrigating reservoir 3 to 4 feet above the level of the patient's bladder provides enough hydrostatic pressure to distend the prostatic urethra. With the panendoscope at the level of the external sphincter, which is readily recognizable, valves can be visualized. We generally attach a length of drainage tubing to one of the stopcocks on the panendoscope. Opening this stopcock lets water flow toward the panendoscope at a rapid rate because of the siphoning effect of the tubing. This simulates micturition and shows what folds or valves look like when the patient voids.

Only the most severe grades of valves actually occlude the view when the prostatic urethra is distended. Much more often, the view is about 50 percent occluded, from the 3 o'clock to the 9 o'clock positions. As the water flows outward, however, leaflets that are not very prominent can balloon impressively into the urethral lumen. Hypertrophy of the bladder neck is usual in these cases. In some, the endoscope must be pointed toward the ceiling to pass over the posterior rim of the bladder neck and into the bladder. Some degree of bladder trabeculation is to be expected. This should not be misinterpreted, however; distending the bladder of a normal neonate gives the impression of slight trabeculation. This emphasizes the need for the surgeon to be thoroughly familiar with normal structures before attempting to interpret abnormal structures.

The interureteric ridge is often hypertrophied. Ureteral orifices can be normal, or they may be extremely patulous. A paraureteral diverticulum just above the ureteral orifice is a common finding. In extreme cases, a ureteral orifice may lie on the lower rim or back wall of a diverticulum. Some urethral valve leaflets are filmy, and passage of the endoscope may tear a valve, particularly a type III diaphragm or the diaphragm formed by severe type I valves. Other urethral valves are quite thick.

SURGICAL DESTRUCTION OF URETHRAL VALVES

As the anatomy of urethral valves varies greatly, so does the treatment of these patients. Many years ago, open resection was commonly practiced, splitting the symphysis pubis and resecting valves under direct vision because suitable endoscopic equipment was not available.[35] This technique is mentioned only to stress that it is outmoded. Open resection is not only unnecessary, it is likely to result in permanent urinary incontinence as a result of disrupting the external urethral sphincter and the bladder neck. A pediatric resectoscope can be used to destroy urethral valves; however, we do not use this method because a pediatric resectoscope is too large to pass transurethrally in most young males. Its use may, therefore, require perineal urethrostomy, which should be avoided if possible. We have seen both urethral stricture and disruption of the external urethral sphincter result from perineal urethrostomy, which is performed in the bulbous urethra close to the external sphincter. While using a resectoscope, it is tempting to bring the cutting loop or hook toward the operator to cut valve leaflets. These leaflets, particularly those of severe type I valves, are close to the external sphincter at the 12 o'clock position. Thus it is important to cut from below and upward against the distal edge of the valve leaflet to destroy it without injuring the nearby external sphincter. This is true no matter what method is used.

Cendron and coworkers showed that prolonged urethral catheter drainage can erode valves, but there are complications of long-term catheter drainage that are best avoided.[36] We have seen a number of cases, nonetheless, in which the original films showed urethral valves that were partially destroyed by pressure necrosis of a catheter.

Johnston demonstrated that valves can be visualized directly by using an otoscope through a perineal urethrostomy.[37] The Nd:Yag laser has been used for destroying valves.[38] Valves have been cut by passing a hooked electrode in the nonanesthetized patient, engaging the valve with fluoroscopic control and cutting it with diathermy.[39,40] I cannot subscribe to that technique, however, because it risks cutting the adjacent sphincter. Another method that has been used is avulsing the leaflets by drawing an inflated Fogarty embolectomy balloon catheter through them.[41]

I firmly believe that all of the relatively blind methods are not as good as visualizing valves accurately through an endoscope of proper size and fulgurating them under direct vision using a miniature electrode.

Some have described endoscopic visualization of valves via a suprapubic cystostomy site.[42] However, in my experience, the natural curve of the male urethra beneath the symphysis pubis makes it difficult to accurately visualize the diaphragm-like confluence of the valves at the 12 o'clock position. Vesicostomy should be considered in the very small premature infant with urethral valves whose urethra is too small to accept even the No. 7.5 French endoscope.[43,44] That will decompress the upper urinary tracts and allow endoscopic valve ablation several weeks later when the infant is larger.

In my opinion, the surgeon who treats young infants with valves should have a No. 7.5 French endoscope with an operating channel available. The electrode I prefer is the wire stylette of a #3 woven ureteral catheter to which a Bovie electrode cord is attached. There must be no side holes in the catheter sheath or the current arc will cross the endoscope lens and burn it. A larger endoscope sheath can be used in older patients which allows better water flow. In Figs. 35–4 and 35–5 are shown typical type I valves and their ablation.

The wire is wrapped around a Bovie electrode and advanced or withdrawn into the catheter sheath by an assistant, so that only 3 to 4 mm of wire are exposed. Cutting current is used, applied in very brief bursts, with water alternately flowing toward the bladder or downward toward the panendoscope to wash away bubbles. Plastic tubing attached to one of the stopcocks on the endoscope drains the outflow water into a bucket on the floor. This provides a siphoning effect, which speeds the drainage.

In severe valves that form a diaphragm dorsally, the first incision is made at the 12 o'clock position, from below and moving upward, after first accurately visualizing the location of the external urethral sphincter.[45] Indeed, the 12 o'clock incision in the diaphragm formed by the confluence of type I valve leaflets is the most essential part of the procedure. Some surgeons do only that. (Sphincter fibers that extend upward along the prostatic urethra will contract when valves are being fulgurated, especially if the current is too great.) In addition, I prefer to destroy the center of each lateral leaflet by cutting the left leaflet at the 5 o'clock position and the right leaflet at the 7 o'clock position. Alternatively, the surgeon can pierce the center of a

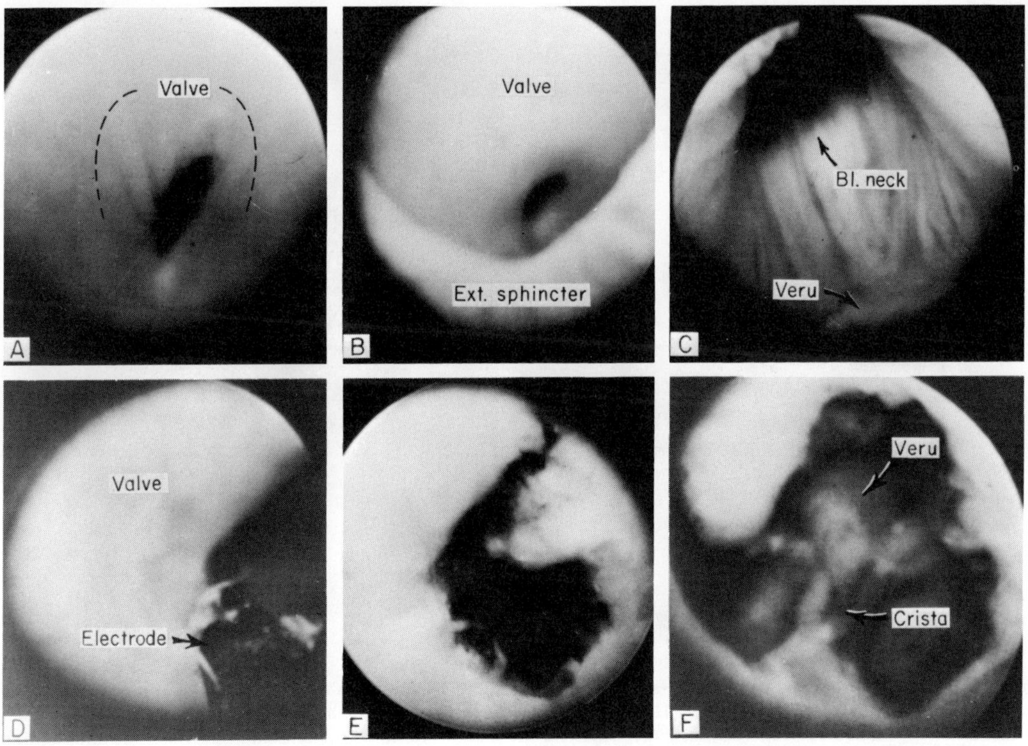

Figure 35–5. Endoscopic photographs of patient whose roentgenograms are shown in Figure 35–4. *A*, Close up view of type I valves forming diaphragm. *B*, Scope is pulled slightly more distally to show position of external sphincter. Valves are bulging downward as water is allowed to run toward panendoscope. *C*, Moderately hypertrophied bladder neck. *D*, Electrode is in place and is about to cut left valve leaflet. *E*, Electrode has cut the diaphragm confluence of two valves at the 12 o'clock position and the left valve leaflet from the 3 to 5 o'clock position. Right valve leaflet is still intact. *F*, Right valve leaflet is similarly destroyed. Note cloverleaf opening where valves were. There is a clear view of the verumontanum. External sphincter, about 1 cm distally, remained intact (not shown in this illustration).

leaflet from below, and avulse it by pushing the panendoscope and electrode together up into the bladder.

After cutting severe type I valves, there should be a clear view of the verumontanum and the external sphincter (Figs. 35–5 through 35–7). Destruction of valves by an electrode in this manner should not produce injury to the surrounding urethra, the verumontanum, or the sphincter. In our experience, no patient of any age has developed stricture from this precise method of destroying many valves.

It is important to leave the bladder neck intact, except in very rare circumstances. A Y-V-plasty or endoscopic incision of the bladder neck can cause incontinence, especially if the external sphincter is not intact 2° to injury during endoscopic resection or perineal urethrostomy. Cutting the bladder neck can also cause retrograde ejaculation. Rarely, the hypertrophied bladder neck does not allow good bladder emptying, despite satisfactory resection of valves. We may then cautiously incise it *just a little* to open it (Fig. 35–7).

In general, the bladder neck is rarely revised or cut today, whereas two decades ago this was often performed. If there is secondary bladder neck obstruction after valve ablation, treatment with phenoxybenzamine, an alpha-adrenergic blocking agent, may be helpful.[46] Special mention should be made regarding valve ablation in the urethra of patients who have undergone prior diversion (vesicostomy, ureterostomy, and so on). Endoscopic valve destruction in these cases, in which there is a "dry urethra," is very apt to cause stricture.[47] Under such conditions, valve ablation should be followed by placement of a Silastic catheter until the patient begins to

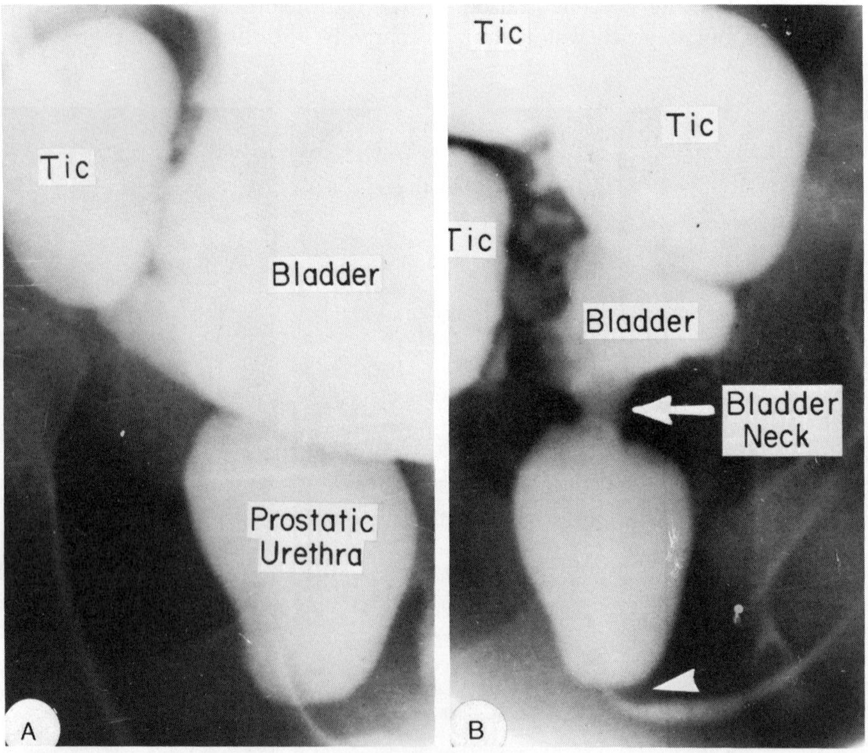

Figure 35–6. Nine-year-old boy with 2-year history of day and night wetting and a weak stream. No problem noted in earlier years. *A*, At beginning of micturition; *B*, Halfway through micturition. Note the multiple large diverticula, satisfactory contraction of the bladder during voiding, hypertrophy of the bladder neck, a widely dilated prostatic urethra, and abrupt cutoff of dye at level of external sphincter by type I valves. Although IVP showed very poor visualization bilaterally, with massive hydronephrosis, BUN was only 30 mg per 100 ml. Creatinine was 1.1 mg per 100 ml and clearance was 60 L absolute per day. Renal pelvic pressures measured 10 cm initially, but rose to 25 cm after 6 minutes of perfusion at the rate of 10 ml per minute. Classic type I valves were removed, using a cutting electrode. A study 3 months later showed no valves, but voiding pressures were still elevated (50 mm Hg), and voiding rate was still only 3.5 ml per second. The bladder neck was therefore secondarily incised just a little, and the patient immediately begin voiding much more forcefully. Renal perfusion studies improved greatly at this time, measuring 8 cm baseline and rising to 10 cm with perfusion. One must be very cautious when incising the bladder neck.

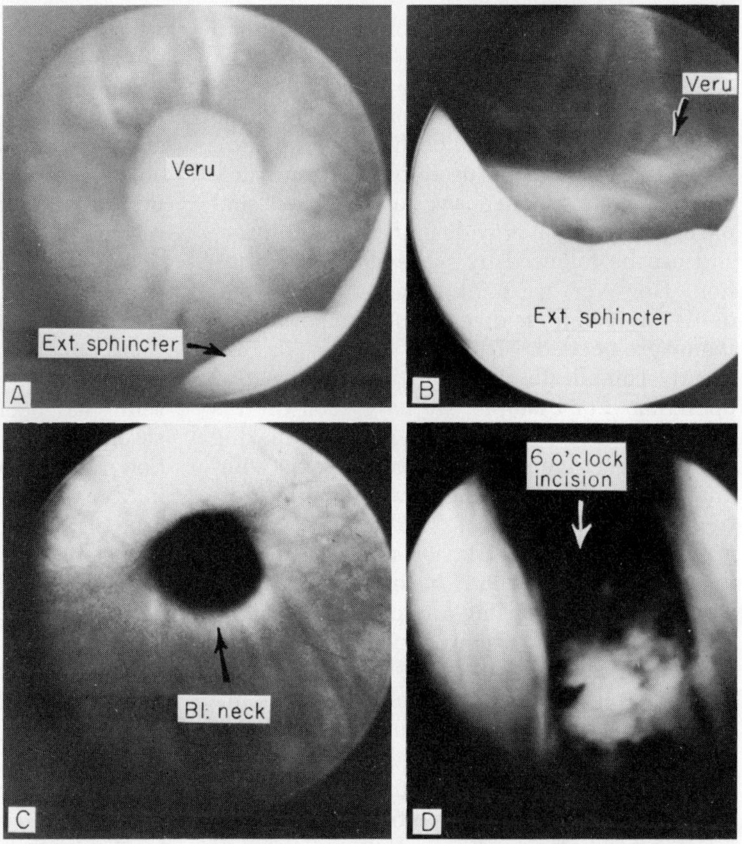

Figure 35–7. Photographs at cystoscopy, 3 months after TUR of valves, seen in Figure 35–6. *A*, Scope at level of external sphincter, which is clearly shown, with good view of verumontanum and no valve tissue arising from it. (Original appearance had been identical to that shown in Figure 35–5*A*, *B*.) *B*, Scope pulled further distally to show more of external sphincter. *C*, The bladder neck is highly contracted, particularly in relation to the still greatly dilated prostatic urethra. *D*, Incision of a bladder neck at 6 o'clock position, which immediately improved voiding.

void (i.e., bladder function is restored). Avoiding the development of urethral stricture is an important consideration in treating males with valves.[48]

Boys with urethral valves who have normal or nearly normal upper urinary tracts and who have lesser degrees of secondary changes, such as reflux, generally require only endoscopic resection of their valves. This is done on an outpatient basis, i.e., as a transient admission with the procedure performed under brief general anesthesia. The patient goes home 2 hours later and does not require a urethral catheter. Formerly, a week of catheter drainage was employed, and these patients had much greater discomfort than do patients today. Most patients have dysuria for several days. They are maintained on prophylactic, suppressive antimicrobial therapy, such as sulfisoxazole or nitrofurantoin. Only rarely has any problem developed, such as bleeding or urinary retention, that required readmission.

TREATMENT OF SEVERE VALVE CASES

In contrast to mild cases, there are infants with uremia, acidosis, dehydration, and, often, sepsis in the first month or two of life. Occasionally, there is extravasation of urine from a point of rupture in the urinary tract of an infant with valves, sometimes accompanied by urinary ascites.[49,50] Drainage must be employed to stop the leak. There is considerable disagreement among experienced surgeons as to how these cases are best managed, although all agree that these young infants are at great risk. It should be emphasized that there is more than one way to manage certain surgical problems and to gain a satisfactory outcome. Preference for one method does not deny the merit of another technique. Furthermore, better nephrologic management of these patients has made certain practices that did not work well 20 years ago more successful today.

Certain points should be made regarding these babies. First, each one represents a challenge in terms of judgment and technical skill. The best results are achieved in centers where enough complex pediatric uropathology is treated to enable a surgeon to acquire the necessary skills. Second, this area of surgery is still developing. Although the principles of many urologic procedures have changed little in the past 20 years, much *has* changed and is still changing in the management of severe urethral valves.

Temporary diversion of the urinary tract in these infants was once widely practiced.[51–56] The use of this technique has declined. Various diversions, such as loop ureterostomy, end ureterostomy, and cutaneous vesicostomy, are simple to perform, can provide immediate drainage, and can be followed by successful reconstruction. However, we think that by today's standards, more of these diversions were performed than were needed. "Temporary diversions" can greatly complicate an eventual reconstructive operation. For example, we have seen ureters tethered upward by loop ureterostomy, making it impossible to reimplant the lower ureter without simultaneously taking down the ureterostomy. This is a formidable task.[57] Since various types of temporary diversion are easy to perform, the surgeon who is inexperienced in the complexity of managing these babies can be tempted to perform a temporary diversion in the belief that subsequent reconstruction will be easier. In our experience, reconstruction is difficult no matter how it is managed.

A small infant with urethral valves and severely dilated upper urinary tracts should first be given vigorous supportive treatment. A No. 5 French plastic feeding catheter is passed through the urethra to drain the bladder. Appropriate broad-spectrum antibiotics are administered if there is urosepsis. Dosage of drugs is adjusted appropriately when nephrotoxic agents, such as kanamycin or gentamicin, are used to allow for diminished renal function. Acidosis and dehydration are treated with appropriate intravenous solutions. Often, the infant will improve dramatically.

It should be emphasized that catheter drainage in these patients is short-term. It is used for a few days and it should not be prolonged beyond a week or two at the most. This procedure should not be compared with prolonged suprapubic tube drainage that was used years ago and has since fallen into disrepute. If the infant does not improve rapidly despite satisfactory metabolic management, we then prefer temporary percutaneous nephrostomy drainage. This can be performed in a few minutes by inserting a small plastic catheter through a needle with ultrasonic control. Only rarely is open nephrostomy necessary today.

After appropriate metabolic management, the patient's valves are then resected endoscopically, except in the case of a premature baby who is too small for this to be feasible. In some cases, endoscopic resection is all that is needed; hydronephrosis as well as ureteral dilatation and tortuosity can improve. If the patient shows improved renal function, an absence of bacilluria, and a generally thriving condition, it is reasonable to wait; some patients will not require further treatment. Others will need an elective reconstructive procedure later to correct diverticula, reflux, or ureteral obstruction. Although the view has been expressed that reflux that persists should not be surgically corrected because those upper urinary tracts are irreversibly damaged, I do not subscribe to that view.[58] Persistent reflux has been correlated with end-stage disease, and even sterile reflux with outlet obstruction can be shown to cause interstitial nephritis in primates.[59,60] Therefore, if a considerable degree of reflux persists despite relief of ureteral obstruction, particularly if there is infection, we perform an antireflux operation. Antireflux surgery in these cases is much more difficult than reimplanting fairly normal ureters into a normal bladder. Also the rate of complications is higher in hypertrophied valve bladders.

Some wide ureters without reflux will become narrower after valve ablation; however, others do not. Some of these ureters are histologically abnormal and will drain better if the lower ureter is shortened, tapered, and reimplanted.[61] This is a difficult procedure in a "valve bladder." Generally, we follow these patients for months or years to determine whether the upper urinary tracts are improving. This can be done with serial IVP, or, more recently, by ultrasonography or DPTA scintigraphy.[62]

Antegrade pyelography with perfusion pressures can help to differentiate between dilated ureters that have ureteral vesical obstruction and ureters that drain well despite radiographic evidence of dilatation.[63,64] When additional reconstructive surgery is necessary, ureters can be shortened, tapered, and reimplanted.[65,66]

In treating boys with severely damaged urinary tracts accompanied by markedly reduced renal function, massive reflux, ureterovesical obstruction, and similar disorders, we have been inclined to proceed early with a direct reconstructive procedure.[67,68] Several points should be emphasized about this, however. First, reconstructive procedures are performed selectively on only the worst cases. Second, it is undertaken only after satisfactory metabolic repair has been accomplished, and the child is fully able to withstand 3 to 4 hours of anesthesia. Third, it is a major surgical undertaking that should be performed only by surgeons who operate frequently on small babies. Finally, it requires skilled pediatric anesthesia and postoperative management. Although endoscopic fulguration of urethral valves in an older child can be a routine procedure performed in a community hospital setting, management of severe cases requires the general experience and expertise of a major medical center that treats a volume of these cases.

ILLUSTRATIVE CASES

The following brief case presentations illustrate certain points of importance regarding urethral valves.

CASE 1 (Fig. 35–8). A 13-year-old boy developed acute urinary retention after being struck in the lower abdomen by a basketball. There was no previous history of any urinary complaints. A catheter was passed, which emptied the bladder, and the patient was referred for investigation. A voiding cystourethrogram showed remarkable dilatation of the prostatic urethra and a typical type I urethral valve proximal to the external urethral sphincter. There was moderate vesicoureteral reflux. Both lower ureters were slightly dilated. A cystoscopy revealed that the bladder was trabeculated, the bladder neck was hypertrophied, and the ureteral orifices were slightly patulous. The valves were resected endoscopically. The patient subsequently voided, in his own words, "like a firehose." He had not realized previously that his stream was less forceful than normal. Vesicoureteral reflux subsequently disappeared. There has been no further urinary complaint during a 17-year follow-up.

COMMENT. Our experience has shown that moderate reflux will disappear in about 50 percent of cases, excluding cases of massive reflux.

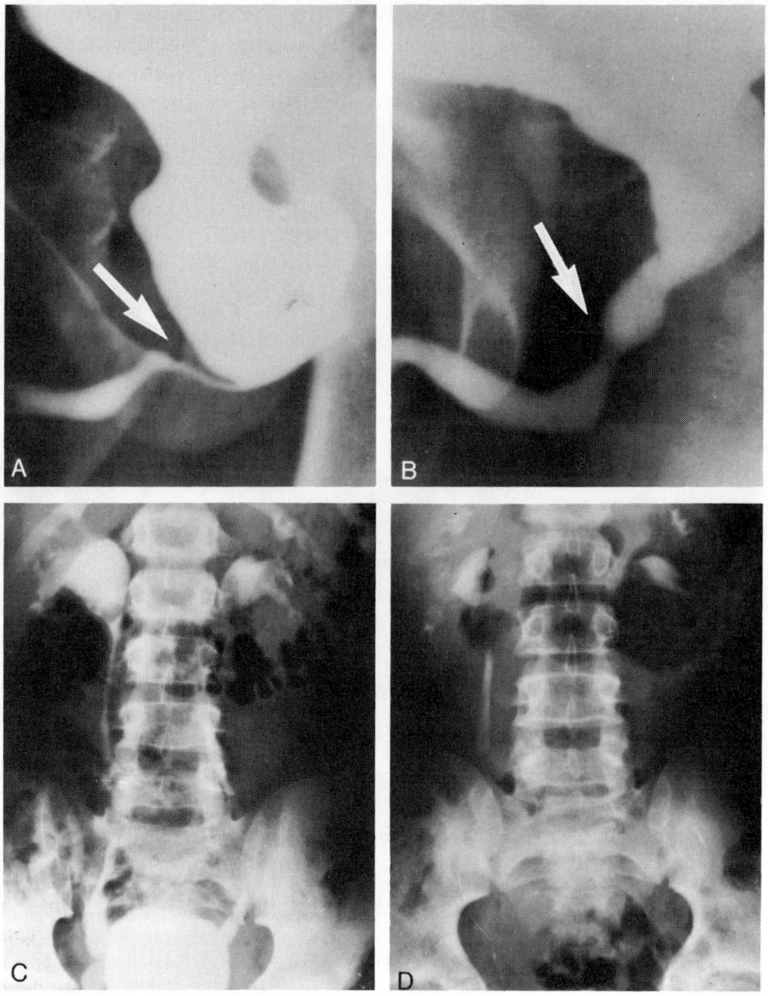

Figure 35–8. *A*, Preoperative voiding cystourethrogram with obvious type I valves (arrow) obstructing prostatic urethra. Note very dilated prostatic urethra. *B*, Voiding study, 2½ years after TUR of valves. *C*, Preoperative IVP. Note mild dilation of both lower ureters. There was moderate reflux bilaterally, which disappeared on later study. *D*, IVP 2½ years after TUR. Normal upper urinary tracts and ureters are evident.

The likelihood that reflux will disappear spontaneously is improved if ureteral orifices do not have a "gopher hole" appearance and if there is no adjacent paraureteral diverticulum, which usually indicates the absence of muscle behind the ureter. If the upper urinary tracts are reasonably normal, no bacilluria is present, and the anatomy of the ureterovesical junction is not grossly abnormal, we follow reflux nonoperatively in boys with uretheral valves. We intervene surgically if infection occurs or the reflux persists after long-term observation.

CASE 2 (Figs. 35–9 and 35–10). A week-old infant presented with gram-negative septicemia. The bladder and kidneys were palpable. Catheter drainage with a No. 5 French plastic feeding catheter, antibiotic administration, and intravenous therapy led to remarkable improvement in the infant. Intravenous pyelogram showed severe bilateral hydronephrosis and poor renal visualization. One week after admission, the valves were resected endoscopically. Retrograde pyelograms at the time delineated the upper urinary tract anatomy. The patient thrived while under close observation. There was persistent partial obstruction of the right ureter at both the ureterovesical and ureteropelvic junctions, and massive reflux was evident on the left side. A reconstructive procedure was performed at 1 year of age to correct these problems. When last seen at age 12, the patient was well.

COMMENT. This patient responded very well to catheter drainage, followed by endoscopic resection of valves. No further surgical procedure was done initially, but he was followed closely during the next year. Because there was no change in the partial obstruction on the right or in the reflux on the left, repair was elected. If the initial function studies had shown borderline function or the clinical response had been less than ideal, a reconstructive procedure would have been performed earlier.

CASE 3 (Fig. 35–11). A 3-month-old infant was referred for treatment of a weak urinary stream. Cystography disclosed typical type I urethral valves and severe bladder trabeculation. There was no reflux. Intravenous pyelogram showed massive bilateral ureteral tortuosity. Valves were resected by open technique (now outmoded), and a Y-V plasty was performed on the bladder neck, which, however, would not be done today. Nothing more was done at that time. Cinefluorography 3 months later showed bilateral ureterovesical obstruction. Ureteral peristalsis was active, but the contrast churned back and forth in the ureters, emptying poorly into the bladder.

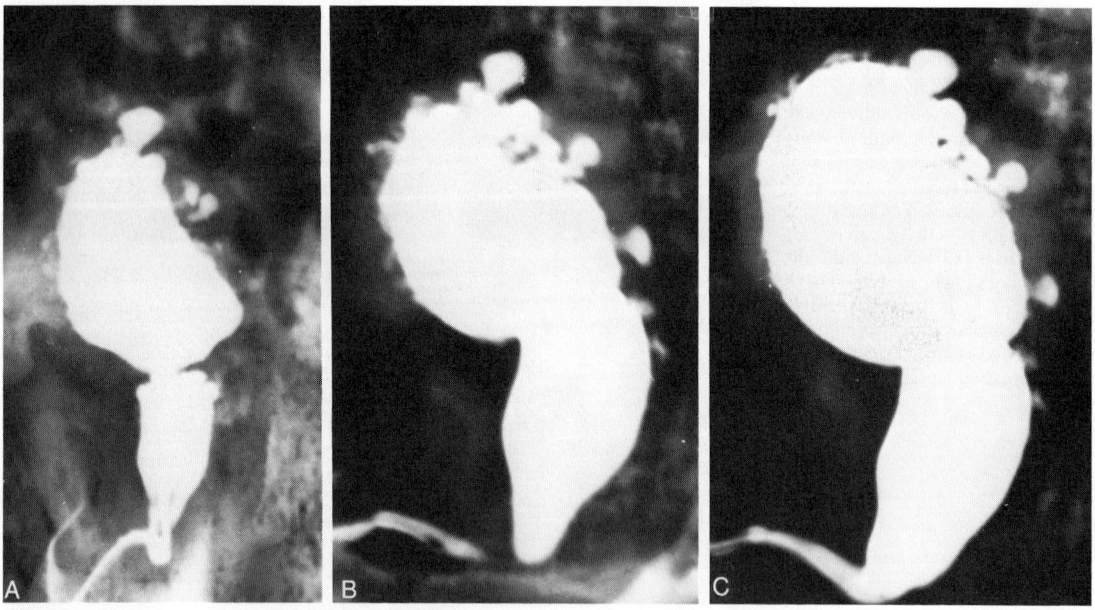

Figure 35–9. Voiding cystourethrogram at age 1 week. There is a No. 5 feeding catheter in the urethra, through which the bladder was filled to the point of distention, initiating voiding. Note the variable appearance of valvular obstruction, membranous urethra, and bladder neck, which is hypertrophied. Multiple cellules are evident. After 1 week of catheter drainage, rehydration, and antibiotic therapy, the valves were destroyed. Reconstructive operation was performed later, at 1 year of age.

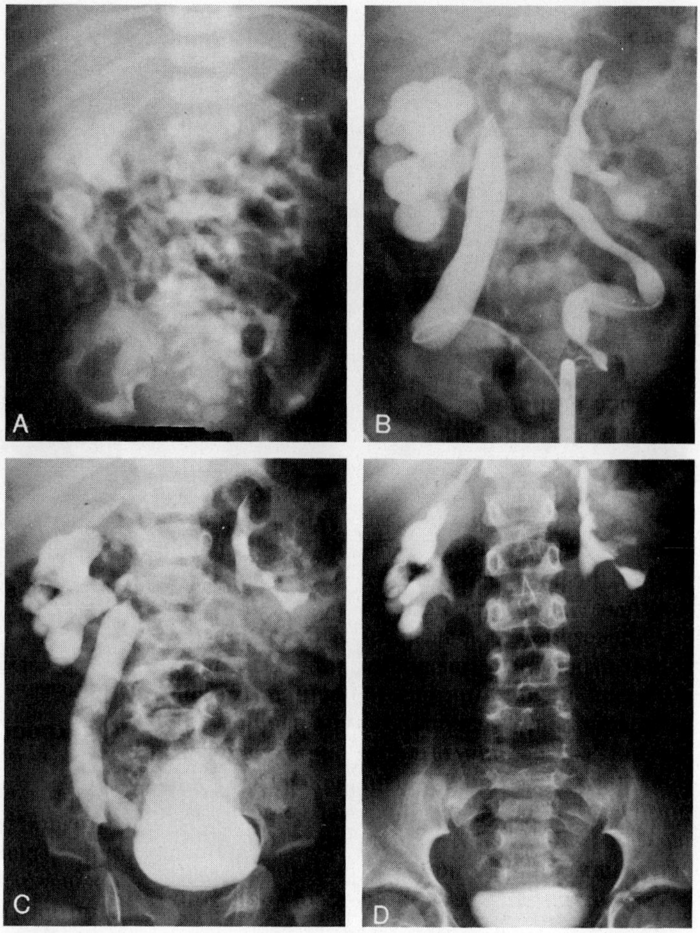

Figure 35–10. Representative roentgenograms. *A*, IVP, on admission, at age 1 week, with poor bilateral function and hydronephrosis. *B*, Retrograde pyelogram at time of TUR, showing bilaterally dilated, tortuous ureters. *C*, IVP, at age 5 months. Considerable left-sided reflux and partial obstruction at both ends of right ureter remained; therefore, a reconstructive operation was performed at 1 year of age.

Staged reconstruction of the ureters was undertaken. Both dilated, nonrefluxing ureters had a narrow terminal ureteral segment typical for primary obstructive megaureter. They were tapered and reimplanted into the bladder. The left side remained obstructed, and reoperation was successful. Upper ureteral tortuosity was straightened also.

Subsequent studies showed normal ureteral emptying and no reflux. The patient was very well, and his upper urinary tracts remained normal. At age 11, the bladder neck and prostatic urethra were narrowed, via a symphysis split exposure, to correct stress incontinence caused by the open resection of the urethral valves and Y-V plasty to the bladder neck performed in infancy. The patient was a completely normal young man until he met his death in an automobile accident at age 19.

COMMENT. When we first saw this baby, we thought that a urinary diversion would probably be needed, particularly when no change occurred in the upper urinary tracts after resection of the urethral valves was performed. Some previous successes with extensive repair of megaureters in infants led us to attempt this procedure. This case illustrates how open valve resection and widening of the bladder neck can cause stress incontinence. (Neither of those modalities are in use today, 24 years later.) Reoperation via a symphysis split corrected that iatrogenic complication.[69] The case also illustrates that some nonrefluxing megaureters do not improve spontaneously after valve resection and may require resection, tapering, and reimplantation just as would be performed for primary obstructive megaureter. Serial IVP examinations and/or ultrasonic follow-up, sometimes with antegrade pressure perfusion, can help decide which cases need ureteral surgery. We have not found radionuclide study with furosemide (Lasix) washout very helpful in a very dilated system.

CASE 4 **(Fig. 35–12).** A 3-month-old infant was referred with acute urinary infection. His blood urea nitrogen (BUN) level was 70 mg per 100

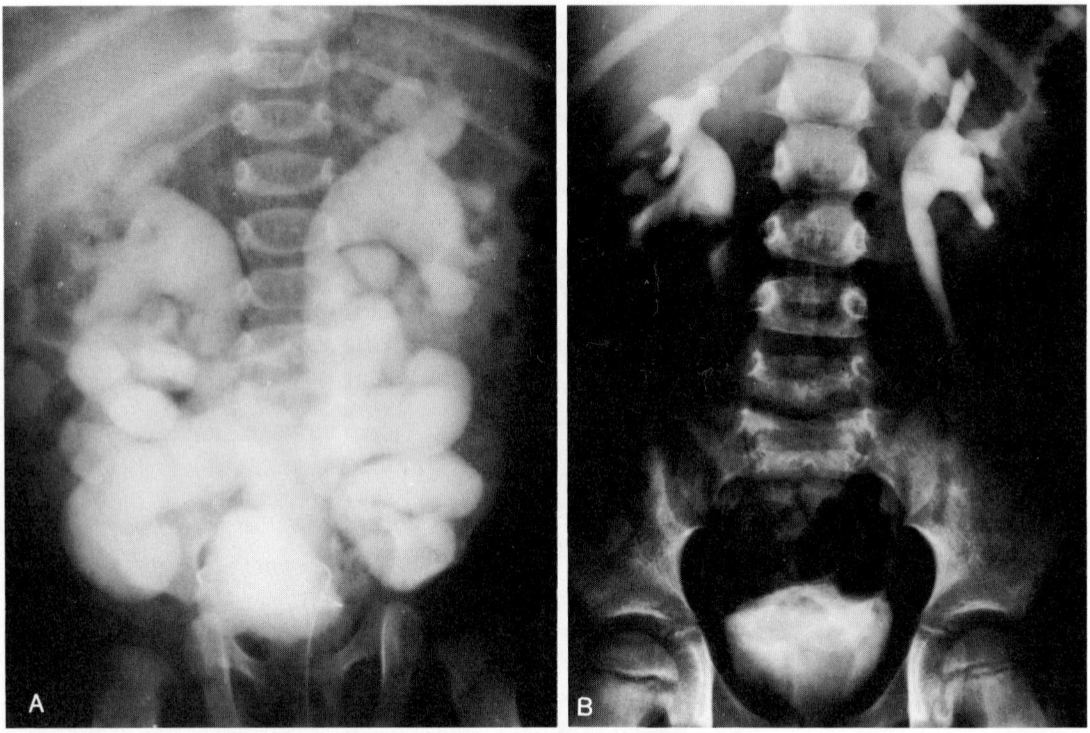

Figure 35–11. *A*, IVP, at age 3 months, showing massive ureteral tortuosity. *B*, IVP, at age 12 years. (All films had approximately this same appearance in the previous 10 years since reconstruction was performed.)

ml, and his creatinine was 3.6 mg per 100 ml. An IVP showed poor visualization bilaterally, and a cystogram revealed typical urethral valves with massive reflux. His condition improved dramatically during 4 days of catheter drainage and vigorous supportive therapy with fluids and antibiotics. A cystoscopy revealed that the ureteral orifices were widely dilated, thus confirming that massive reflux would persist despite endoscopic resection of valves. Accordingly, in addition to resecting the valves transurethrally, the lower ureters were shortened, tapered, and reimplanted. The massively dilated and tortuous upper ureters were repaired 6 weeks later. He is now 20 years old, 6 feet, 3 inches tall, weighs 202 pounds, and is a star collegiate basketball player. BUN is 9 mg per 100 ml, and serum creatinine is 1.4 mg per 100 ml. Creatinine clearance is 144 L absolute or 66 L per square meter of body surface area.

COMMENT. A direct reconstruction was performed in this case because the anatomy observed through cystoscopy would have predictably resulted in continued massive reflux, which the patient could ill afford. Repeated urosepsis would have destroyed the already damaged and extremely hydronephrotic upper urinary tracts. This particular case is presented because two complications occurred, neither of which precluded a good end result. First, there was partial obstruction of the first left lower ureter when the catheter stents were removed 2 weeks after the lower ureters were shortened, tapered, and reimplanted. This required short-term nephrostomy drainage on the left side. Shortening and tapering of the upper urinary tracts were performed somewhat sooner than usual. Second, a postoperative nephrostogram showed a small leak from the left upper ureteral suture line. This sealed during an additional week of temporary nephrostomy drainage.

Upper ureteral surgery has not been used in the majority of these cases. However, in ureters that remain dilated, with ineffective peristalsis and persistent tortuosity of the ureteropelvic junction (which can cause partial obstruction) we do not hesitate to attempt surgical repair. This task is much easier than repairing the lower ureter. However, there are two reasons why upper ureteral surgery should never be undertaken prior to operating on the lower ureter. First, correcting the lower ureter first usually obviates the need for upper ureteral surgery. Second, in each of the few cases in which we encountered ischemia of the lower ureter while performing a lower ureteral reconstruction procedure, the

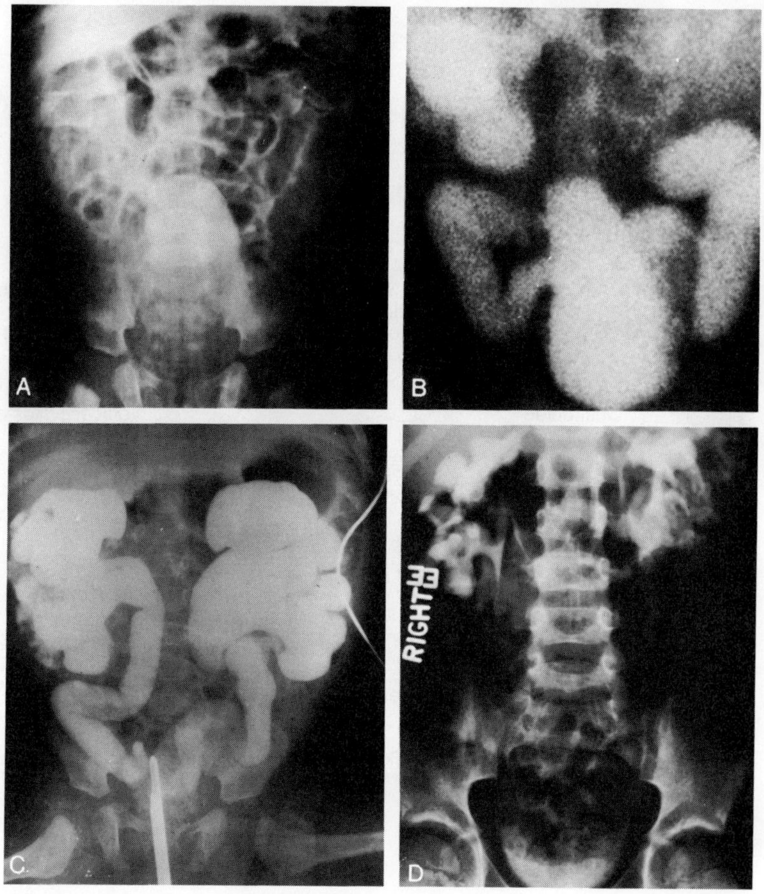

Figure 35–12. *A*, Preoperative IVP showing large bladder and poor visualization of upper urinary tracts. Patient was referred with this film, *B*, Preoperative cystogram showing massive reflux, tortuous ureters, and hydronephrosis. Urethra showed typical valves. Doing the cystogram first will often obviate the need for an IVP to visualize the upper urinary tracts if there is reflux. *C*, Retrograde study at time of valve resection and lower ureter repair, which is seldom done immediately and only in very severe cases. *D*, IVP, at age 8 years. Appearance is the same on a recent study at age 20 years.

upper ureter had been previously operated on, which had reduced its collateral blood supply.

The abnormal x-rays when the patient was a critically ill 3-month-old infant were ominous. We credit early complete repair with salvage of his urinary tract. It stopped obstruction and reflux early, preventing further infection and deterioration of his very hydronephrotic upper urinary tracts. He is a normal adult with a creatinine clearance two thirds of that in normal adult valves.

CASE 5 (Figs. 35–13 and 35–14). A one-year-old infant was referred for further reconstructive urinary tract surgery. Dribbling was noted at one month, and type I urethral valves were diagnosed. They were destroyed endoscopically. Anuria occurred 5 days later, and, therefore, left cutaneous ureterostomy was performed in the mid-left ureter, with subsequent improvement. There was never evidence of function on the right side; right nephroureterectomy was performed. The left ureterostomy was then closed, followed by left ureteral reimplantation to correct reflux. Obstruction occurred, and left nephrostomy was performed. Nephrostomy drainage was maintained for 5 months until the time of referral. A nephrostogram showed high implantation of the ureter into the dome of the bladder and marked narrowing of the terminal ureter. Reoperation was performed.

The kidney and ureter were mobilized through an extensive transabdominal exposure, and care was taken to preserve the blood supply. The left lower ureter was not viable, owing to extensive scarring from previous surgery and previous exteriorization of the mid-ureter. There was no alternative but to discard the lower half of the left ureter. Fortunately, mobilizing the left kidney and pexing it downward, together with cautiously straightening the upper ureter (being very careful to preserve its blood supply) gave enough length to implant the ureter after it had been tapered appropriately. This was performed as a cross-trigone reimplant in order to achieve adequate tunnel length in this small, scarred, trabeculated trigone. Now at age 14, the patient is well.

COMMENT. This infant was first managed in a

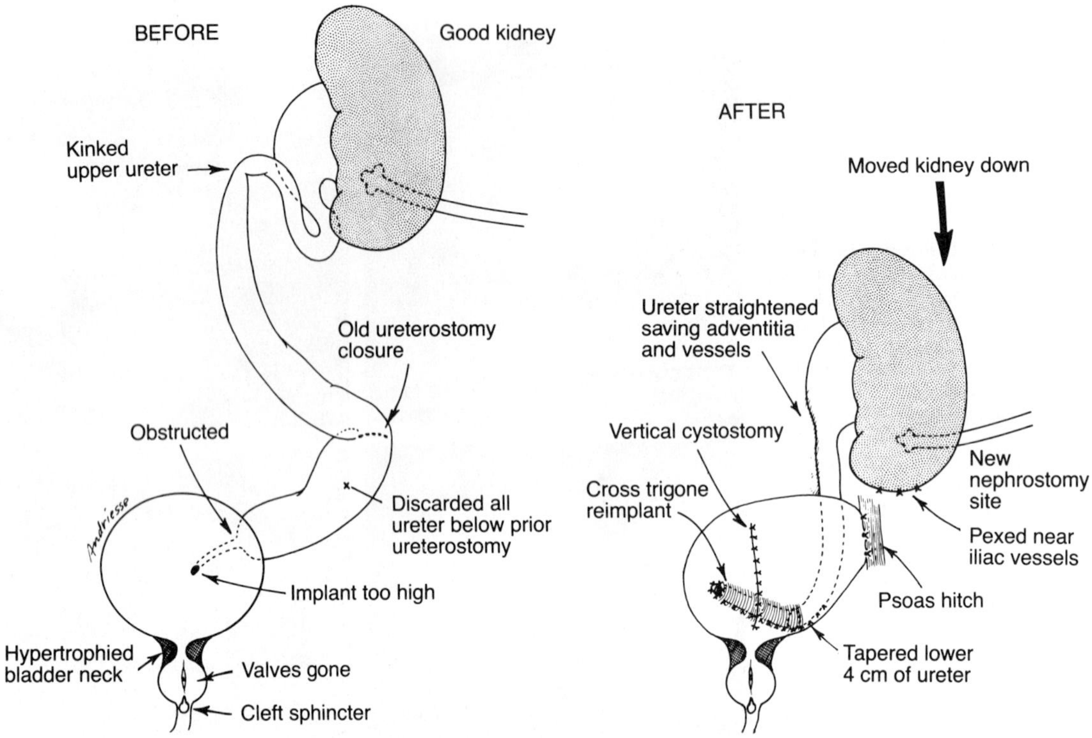

Figure 35–13. Diagram of prereconstruction and postreconstruction anatomy.

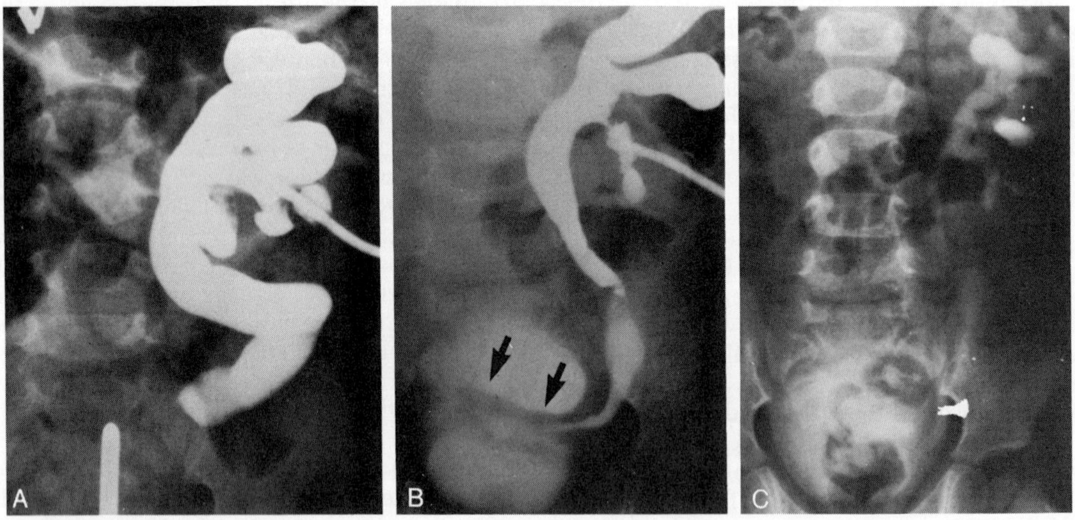

Figure 35–14. *A*, Nephrostogram taken at time of referral, at age 1 year. Patient had obstruction at ureteral vesical junction. *B*, Nephrostogram taken 2 weeks after reconstructive procedure. Arrows show cross trigone ureteral reimplantation, outlined by edema surrounding ureter. Nephrostomy tube was removed the following day. *C*, IVP, at age 14 years.

community hospital, where there was no previous experience in caring for a case of this complexity. The initial endoscopic resection of valves injured the external urethral sphincter at the 12 o'clock position; such an injury can easily occur because type I valves often lie so close to the external sphincter. With an intact bladder neck, the youngster is nonetheless continent.

Anuria occurring after transurethral resection in a child who initially had no ureteral obstruction is almost certainly caused by dehydration resulting from inadequate fluid replacement during postobstructive diuresis. These infants require expert nephrologic management. Their kidneys concentrate poorly, which can result in very rapid salt and water depletion after relief of valve obstruction.

Ureterostomy was probably unnecessary in this particular patient. Doing a ureterostomy in the mid-ureter greatly complicated the subsequent reconstruction because it required discarding all of the ureter from that point downward. If ureterostomy is elected, it is important to place it high, preferably near the ureteropelvic junction, in order to provide satisfactory drainage of the kidney while leaving enough ureter distally to work with should a reconstructive procedure be necessary. When the lower ureter was reimplanted, it was placed in the dome of the bladder. Experience has shown that obstruction and reflux are best prevented by placing the ureter in the trigone posteriorly, not in the side wall or dome of the bladder.

This infant was destined to have right nephroureterectomy because the right kidney was a dysplastic shell from the outset, which is not uncommon in infants with valves. This case poignantly demonstrates many of the problems that can be encountered. These can be avoided as the surgeon becomes more experienced, which is possible only if there is an opportunity to treat many patients with difficult conditions.

Case 6 (Figs. 35–15 through 35–17). A 9-week-old infant was referred with acute urinary infection and marked bilateral hydronephrosis. A small catheter passed through the urethra curled up in a urethral diverticulum. Needle stick voiding cystourethrogram showed a typical urethral diverticulum with valve obstruction of the urethra by its distal lip. There was massive reflux into dilated megaureters. Urethral obstruction was relieved by transurethral resection, using a small wire electrode through a No. 10 French endoscope sheath. Both ureteral orifices were greatly dilated. Accordingly, a re-

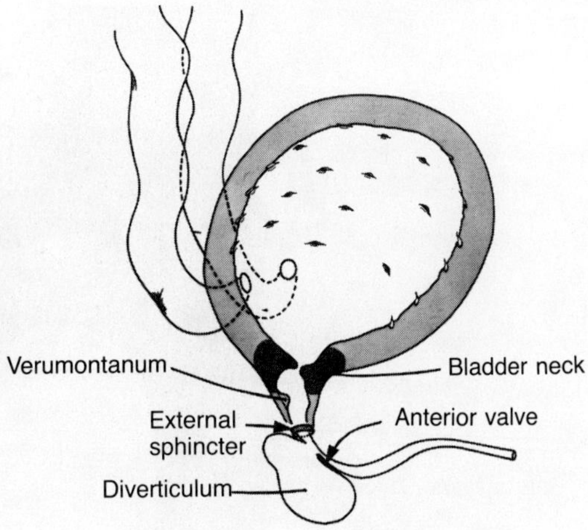

Figure 35–15. Diagram showing anatomy of urethral diverticulum causing valve-like obstruction of the anterior urethra, distal to the external sphincter.

constructive procedure was performed under the same anesthesia to shorten, taper, and reimplant the ureters. The infant's course was uneventful. At age 13 years, serum BUN was 15 mg per 100 ml; creatinine, 0.7 mg per 100 ml; and creatinine clearance, 100 L per square meter of body surface area. He is now 17 years old and well.

Comment. We have found it possible to correct the valvular obstruction in such cases by endoscopic resection of the distal rim of these diverticula. Open repair is also possible. Like posterior urethral valves, these cases can vary in severity.

Although urethral valves are almost exclusively a disease of males, their rare occurrence in females should be mentioned. We have seen two girls with high-grade obstruction of the urethra by valve-like folds that arose at the bladder neck and projected down into the urethra, similar to type I valves. In one of these patients, bilateral ureteral reimplantation for reflux had been carried out twice before without success, and eventually right nephrectomy was performed. The overlooked valves were undoubtedly a major factor in the failure of her ureteral reimplantations. Valve resection and a third reimplantation of the left ureter were successful.

Valves in females can be identified by bending a silver malleable probe into a "shepherd's crook" and passing it into the urethra alongside the panendoscope. By pulling it along the floor of the distal trigone, bladder neck, and urethra, it is possible to hook a valve leaflet. This maneuver should be performed in any female whose bladder is trabeculated and in whom ure-

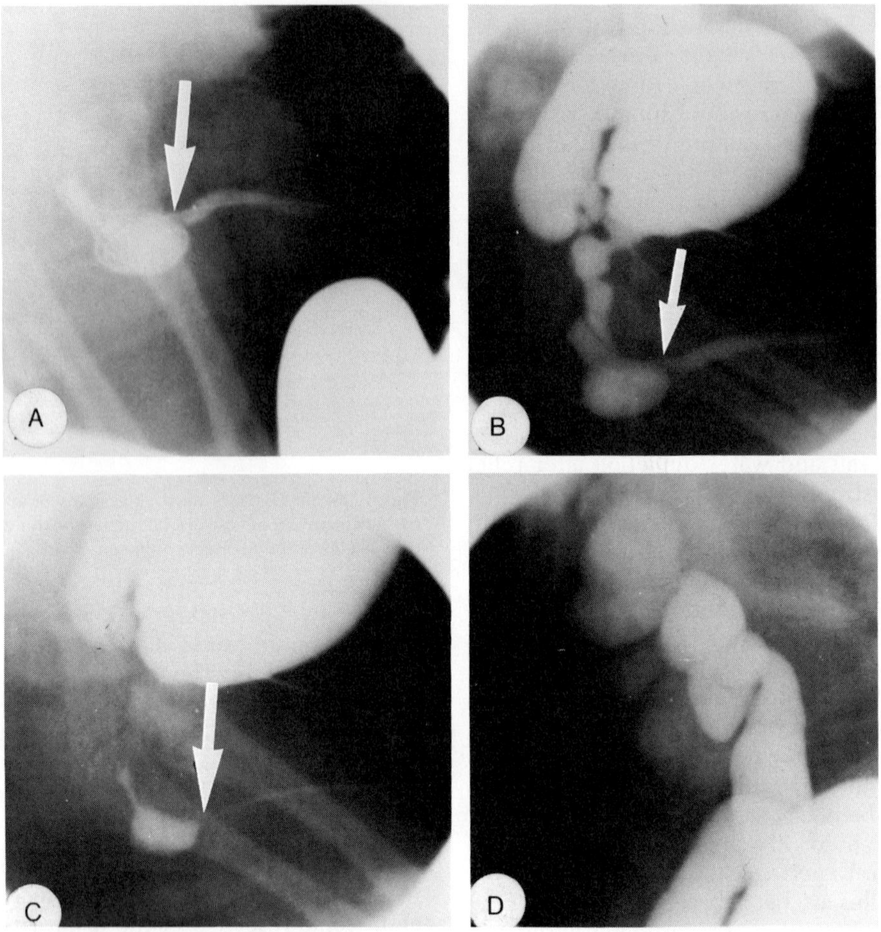

Figure 35–16. Preoperative cystograms. *A*, No. 5 plastic feeding catheter curled up in the diverticulum (arrow). *B*, Voiding study obtained by suprapubic needle stick of bladder to infuse contrast medium. Note valve-like obstruction from distal rim of diverticulum (arrow). *C*, Contrast retained in diverticulum. *D*, Massive bilateral reflux.

thral obstruction seems to be present without good cause.

The most common valve-like obstructions we have seen in females, however, are those caused by incompletely resected ectopic ureteroceles. If the distal lip of a ureterocele remains, it can form a cul de sac during micturition that fills with urine and partially obstructs the urethra. This can be identified by using the "shepherd's crook" technique. The ureterocele remnant is destroyed endoscopically. If there is a muscle defect in the bladder, it should be repaired.

URINARY TRACT "UNDIVERSION"

There are many boys living today with urinary diversion that was performed because the patients originally had urethral valves with hydronephrosis. To date, I have "undiverted" 177 children and young adults.[70–73] Sixty-three of these patients were boys with urethral valves. The most common type of diversion is the ileal conduit procedure, which is illustrated in the following cases.

CASE 7 (**Figs. 35–18 and 35–19**). An 11-year-old boy was referred in January 1974 for possible undiversion. Urinary infection occurred at 3 months of age. Cystography showed massive reflux and hydronephrosis. Suprapubic cystostomy was performed. Bilateral renal calculi were removed later. At 3 years of age, an ileal conduit was performed, and a second left nephrolithotomy was required. A cystogram showed a small bladder, typical of many years of nonuse. The ileal loop was taken down from the abdominal wall, tapered, and reimplanted into the bladder, using the antirefluxing tunnel technique. Normal urinary control and capacity followed, the

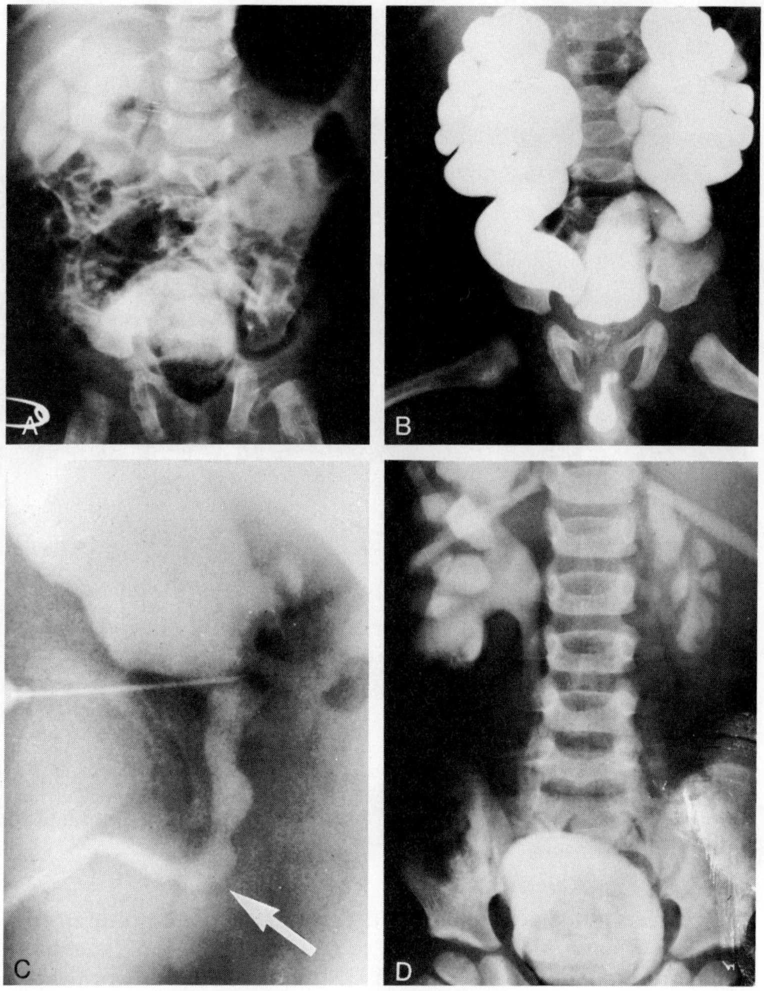

Figure 35–17. Representative roentgenograms. *A*, Preoperative IVP, at age 9 weeks. Massive bilateral hydronephrosis, with poor visualization of left side. *B*, Preoperative cystogram showing massive reflux and hydronephrosis. This infant was managed by direct reconstructive surgery. *C*, Voiding study, using suprapubic needle stick technique, 6 months following reconstructive procedure. Arrow points to previous site of diverticulum, now almost normal in appearance following endoscopic resection. There was no reflux in the ureters, which had been shortened, tapered, and reimplanted. *D*, IVP at age 3½ years.

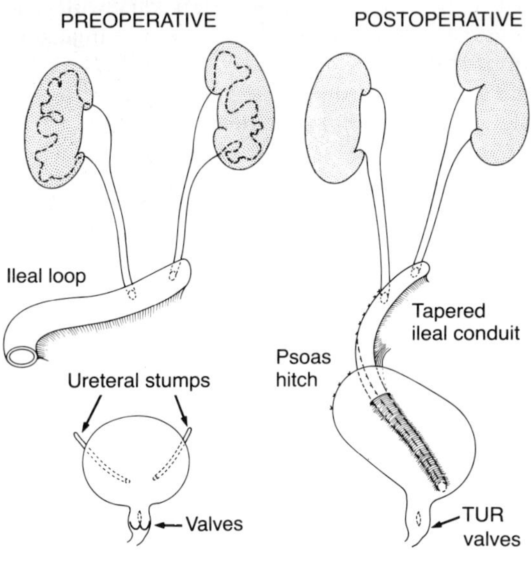

Figure 35–18. Preoperative and postoperative "undiversion."

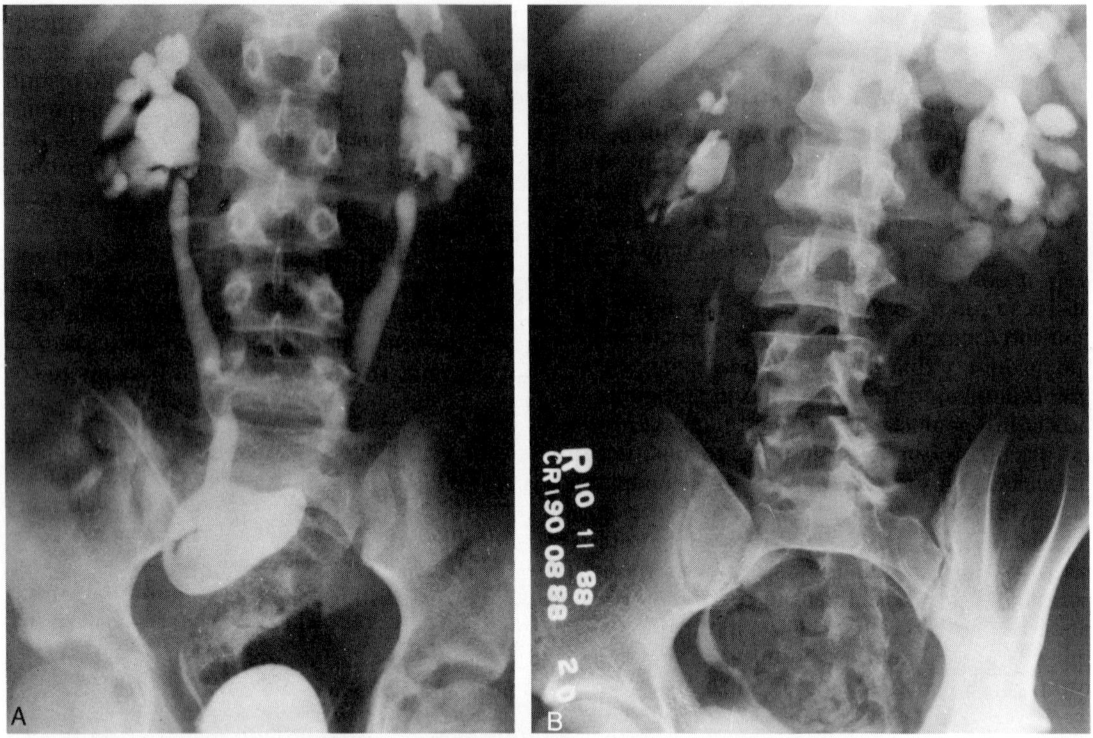

Figure 35–19. *A*, Preoperative simultaneous cystogram and loopogram when patient was referred at age 11 years. Note small bladder, which attained normal capacity after undiversion. Many long defunctioned bladders required augmentation with bowel. *B*, IVP, at age 26 years, 15 years following undiversion procedure. Upper urinary tracts are stable, and the patient is well.

upper tracts remained stable, and there is no reflux or urinary infection.

The patient is now age 26. The BUN is 20 mg per 100 ml, serum creatinine is 1.8 mg per 100 ml, and creatinine clearance is 48 L per square meter of body surface area. He is 6 feet 3 inches tall, married, and living a normal life. Renal function will be followed despite his being well 15 years postoperatively.

COMMENT. There are hundreds of youngsters and young adults whose upper urinary tracts have been previously diverted and who have a normally innervated bladder that could be refunctionalized. Indeed, many myelodysplastic bladders can be undiverted, often by narrowing the bladder outlet, augmenting the bladder, and emptying by intermittent self-catheterization. In our experience, this approach has had many advantages. Psychologically, the quality of life improves without the need for a collecting bag, despite the fact that there are many patients who manage reasonably well wearing an appliance when it is absolutely necessary. We have found that the maintenance of a sterile urinary tract is much easier after undiversion that it is while exteriorized to the surface. We consider urinary diversion in these patients to be a complication of urethral valves. In light of the success of recently developed reconstructive techniques, many of them deserve further consideration.

CONCLUSION

Urethral valves are much more common than it is generally appreciated. They vary widely in severity; some are small, causing minimal urethral obstruction, whereas others are large, causing massive hydronephrosis in the newborn. Unskilled management of these patients can lead to many serious complications, most of which can be avoided.

References

1. Hendren WH: Posterior urethral valves in boys: a broad clinical spectrum. J Urol 106:298, 1971.
2. Hoover DL, Duckett JW Jr: Posterior urethral valves, unilateral reflux and renal dysplasia: a syndrome. J Urol 128:994, 1982.
3. Rittenberg MH, Hulbert WC, Snyder HM III, et al: Protective factors in posterior urethral valves. J Urol 140:993, 1988.
4. Arnold SJ, Ginsburg A: Radiologic and photoendoscopic studies in posterior urethral valves in enuretic boys. Urology 4:145, 1974.
5. Duckett JW Jr: Current management of posterior urethral valves. Urol ClinNorth Am 1:471, 1974.

6. Rabinowitz R, Barkin M, Schillinger JF, et al: Upper tract management when posterior urethral valve ablation is insufficient. J Urol 122:370, 1979.
7. Krueger RP, Hardy BE, Churchill BM: Growth in boys and posterior urethral valves: primary valve resection vs. upper tract diversion. Urol Clin North Am 7:265, 1980.
8. Kurth KH, Alleman ER, Schroder FH: Major complications of posterior urethral valves. J Urol 126:517, 1981.
9. Mollard P, Sarkissian J, Tostain J: Management of the upper urinry tract in boys with posterior urethral valves (65 cases) (Author's transl). Chir Pediatr 22:411, 1981.
10. Egami K, Smith ED: A study of the sequelae of posterior urethral valves. J Urol 127:84, 1982.
11. Atwell JD: Posterior urethral valves in the British Isles: a multicenter B.A.P.S. review. J Pediatr Surg 18:70, 1983.
12. Churchill BM, Krueger RP, Fleisher MH, et al: Complications of posterior urethral valve surgery and their prevention. Urol Clin North Am 10:519, 1983.
13. Aaronson IA: Posterior urethral valve: a review of 120 cases. S Afr Med J 17:418, 1984.
14. Glassberg KI: Current issues regarding posterior urethral valves. Urol Clin North Am 12:175, 1985.
15. Scott JE: Management of congenital posterior urethral valves. Br J Urol 57:71, 1985.
16. Burbige KA, Hensle TW: Posterior urethral valves in the newborn: treatment and functional results. J Pediatr Surg 2:165, 1987.
17. Parkhouse HF, Barratt TM, Dillon MJ, et al: Long-term outcome of boys with posterior urethral valves. Br J Urol 62:59, 1988.
18. Young HH, Frontz WA, Baldwin JC: Congenital obstruction of the posterior urethra. J Urol 3:289, 1919.
19. Tank ES: Anterior urethral valves resulting from congenital urethral diverticula. Urology 30:467, 1987.
20. Scherz HC, Kaplan GW, Packer MG: Anterior urethral valves in the fossa navicularis in children. J Urol 138:1211, 1987.
21. Nieh PT, Hendren WH: Obstructing urethral valves in octogenarian. Urology 13:412, 1979.
22. Mueller SC, Marshall FF: Spectrum of recognized posterior urethral valves in the adult. Urology 22:139, 1983.
23. Cherrie RJ, Leach GE, Raz S: Obstructing urethral valve in a woman: a case report. J Urol 129:1051, 1983.
24. Bauer SB, Dieppa RA, Labib KK, et al: The bladder in boys with posterior urethral valves: a urodynamic assessment. J Urol 121:769, 1979.
25. Campaiola JM, Perlmutter AD, Steinhardt GF: Noncompliant bladder resulting from posterior urethral valves. J Urol 134:708, 1985.
26. Gearhart JP, Albertsen PC, Marshall FF, et al: Pediatric applications of augmentation cystoplasty: the Johns Hopkins experience. J Urol 136:430, 1986.
27. Cremin BJ, Aaronson IA: Ultrasonic diagnosis of posterior urethral valve in neonates. Br J Radiol 56:435, 1983.
28. Thomas DF, Irving HC, Arthur RJ: Prenatal diagnosis: how useful is it? Br J Urol 57:784, 1985.
29. Brown T, Mandell J, Lebowitz RL: Neonatal hydronephrosis in the era of sonography. Am J Roentgenol 148:959, 1987.
30. Nakayama DK, Harrison MR, deLorimier AA: Prognosis of posterior urethral valves presenting at birth. J Pediatr Surg 21:43, 1986.
31. Harrison MR, Golbus MS, Filly RA, et al: Fetal surgery for congenital hydronephrosis. N Engl J Med 306:591, 1982.
32. Manning FA, Harrison MR, Rodeck C: Catheter shunts for fetal hydronephrosis and hydrocephalus: report of the International Fetal Surgery Registry. N Engl J Med 315:336, 1986.
33. Sholder AJ, Maizels M, Depp R, Firlit CF, et al: Caution in antenatal intervention. J Urol 139:1026, 1988.
34. Hendren WH: Urethral valves: diagnosis and endoscopic resection (Film). Eaton Film Library and the Film Library of the American College of Surgeons, 1975B.
35. Gross RE: The Surgery of Infancy and Childhood. Philadelphia, WB Saunders Co, 1953, p 736.
36. Cendron J, Deburge JP, Karlaftis C: Valvulae of the posterior urethra. J Urol Nephrol 75:15, 1969.
37. Johnston JH: Posterior urethral valves: an operative technic using an electric auriscope. J Pediatr Surg 1:583, 1966.
38. Ehrlich RM, Shanberg A, Fine RN: Neodymium: YAG laser ablation of posterior urethral valves. J Urol 138:959, 1987.
39. Bruce J, Stannard V, Small PG, et al: The operative management of posterior urethral valves. J Pediatr Surg 22:1081, 1987.
40. Whitaker RH, Sherwood T: An improved hook for destroying posterior urethral valves. J Urol 135:531, 1986.
41. Diamond DA, Ransley PG: Fogarty balloon catheter ablation of neonatal posterior urethral valves. J Urol 137:1209, 1987.
42. Zaontz MR, Firlit CF: Percutaneous antegrade ablation of posterior urethral valves in infants with small caliber urethras: an alternative to urinary diversion. J Urol 36:247, 1986.
43. Arap S, Monti P, Nahas WC, et al: Vesicostomy: a temporary urinary diversion in childhood. J Urol 91:429, 1985.
44. Rushton HG, Parrott TS, Woodard JR, et al: The role of vesicostomy in the management of anterior valves of neonates and infants. J Urol 138:107, 1987.
45. Parkkulainen KV: Posterior urethral obstruction: valvular or diaphragmatic? Endoscopic diagnosis and treatment. Birth Defects 13:63, 1977.
46. McGuire EJ, Weiss RM: Secondary bladder neck obstruction in patients with urethral valves: treatment with phenoxybenzamine. Urology 5:756, 1975.
47. Crooks KK: Urethral strictures following transurethral resection of posterior urethral valves. J Urol 127:1153, 1982.
48. Myers DA, Walker RD, 3rd: Prevention of urethral strictures in the management of posterior urethral valves. J Urol 126:655, 1981.
49. Tank ES, Carey TC, Seifert AL: Management of neonatal urinary ascites. Urology 16:270, 1980.
50. Greenfield SP, Hensle TW, Berdon WE, et al: Urinary extravasation in the newborn male with posterior urethral valves. J Pediatr Surg 17:751, 1982.
51. Johnston JH: Temporary cutaneous ureterostomy in the management of advanced congenital urinary obstruction. Arch Dis Child 38:161, 1963.
52. Leape LL, Holder TM: Temporary tubeless urinary diversion in children. J Pediatr Surg 5:288, 1970.
53. Perlmutter AD, Patil J: Loop cutaneous ureterostomy in infants and young children: late results in 32 cases. J Urol 107:655, 1972.
54. Sober I: Pelvioureterostomy-en-Y. J Urol 107:473, 1972.
55. Williams DI, Cromie WH: Ring ureterostomy. Br J Urol 47:789, 1975.
56. Dwoskin JY: Management of the massively dilated urinary tract in infants by temporary diversion and single-stage reconstruction. Urol Clin North Am 1:515, 1974.

57. Hendren WH: Complications of ureterostomy. J Urol 120:269, 1978.
58. Johnston JH: Vesicoureteric reflux with urethral valves. Br J Urol 51:100, 1979.
59. Tejani A, Butt K, Glassberg K, et al: Predictors of eventual end-stage renal disease in children with postoperative urethral valves. J Urol 136:857, 1986.
60. Mendoza JM, Roberts JA: Effects of sterile high-pressure vesicoureteral reflux on the monkey. J Urol 130:602, 1983.
61. Hanna MK, Jeffs RD, Sturgess JM, et al: Ureteral structure and ultrastructure. Part III: the congenitally dilated ureter (megaureter). J Urol 117:24, 1977.
62. Gordon I, Ransley PG, Hubbard CS: 99mTc DTPA scintigraphy compared with intravenous urography in the follow-up of posterior urethral valves. Br J Urol 60:447, 1987.
63. Whitaker RH: Methods of assessing obstruction in dilated ureters. Br J Urol 45:15, 1973.
64. Whitaker RH: The ureter and posterior urethral valves. Br J Urol 45:395, 1973.
65. Hendren WH: Operative repair of megaureter in children. J Urol 101:491, 1969.
66. Hendren WH: Complications of megaureter repair in children. J Urol 113:238, 1975.
67. Hendren WH: A new approach to infants with severe obstruction: early complete reconstruction. J Pediatr Surg 5:184, 1970.
68. Bjordal R, Eek S, Knutrud O: Early reconstruction of wide ureter in children. Urology 11:326, 1978.
69. Peters CA, Hendren WH: Splitting the pubis for exposure in difficult reconstructions for incontinence. J Urol 142 (Pediatric Supplement): 1989, p 527.
70. Hendren WH: Reconstruction of previously diverted urinary tracts in children. J Pediatr Surg 8:135, 1973.
71. Hendren WH: Urinary tract refunctionalization after prior diversion in children. Ann Surg 180:494, 1974.
72. Hendren WH: Urinary undiversion and augmentation cystoplasty. In Kelalis P, King LR, Belman AB, eds: Clinical Pediatric Urology, 2nd ed. Philadelphia, WB Saunders Co, 1985, p 620.
73. Hendren WH: Urinary undiversion (refunctionalization of the previously diverted urinary tract). In Walsh PC, Gittes RF, Perlmutter AD, Stamey TA, eds: Campbell's Urology, 5th ed. Philadelphia, WB Saunders Co, 1986, p 2137.

COMPLICATIONS OF FEMALE ANTI-INCONTINENCE SURGERY

36

David R. Staskin

The successful surgical management of urinary incontinence in the female patient demands an accurate diagnosis and the selection and skillful performance of the appropriate surgical procedure.

In order to make an accurate diagnosis, the surgeon must understand the pathophysiology of the urinary loss by efficiently choosing and accurately interpreting the diagnostic procedures that can clearly identify the underlying problem. A history, physical examination, radiographic study, urodynamic evaluation, and endoscopic evaluation may be necessary to identify the site and mechanism.

Selection of the optimal surgical approach is based on several factors. The surgical procedure should be generally accepted for its ability to correct, compensate for, or circumvent the cause of the incontinence. The surgeon must be qualified in the performance and postoperative management of the procedure. The surgery must be individualized to the patient, who must medically tolerate the procedure; understand the risks, benefits and alternatives; and be able to manage her postoperative condition.

This chapter reviews the pitfalls associated with the diagnosis and surgical correction of incontinence per urethra.

DIAGNOSIS

The diagnosis of "genuine stress incontinence" (GSI) is mandatory before a procedure is performed on the female bladder outlet. The degree to which the lower urinary tract should be evaluated prior to surgery for GSI is controversial. The controversy surrounds the necessity, usefulness, and cost-effectiveness of various tests aimed at the following:

1. The objective demonstration of GSI.
2. Diagnosing bladder dysfunctions, which may mimic the symptoms of GSI.
3. Documenting bladder dysfunction coincident with GSI.
4. Differentiating between pure anatomic support problems of the bladder neck and intrinsic urethral dysfunction.

Urinary loss per urethra may result from bladder or bladder outlet dysfunction, alone or in combination (Table 36–1). Identification of the underlying mechanism for urinary incontinence must be understood before surgical therapy is begun.

The performance of various urodynamic, radiographic, or endoscopic studies, alone or in combination, following the standard history and physical examination has been advocated.

History

There is general acceptance that the diagnosis of GSI cannot be made by symptoms alone. The association of the symptoms of "stress incontinence" with outlet pathology and "urge incontinence" with detrusor pathology has introduced inaccuracies into the diagnosis and therapy of female incontinence.

The differential diagnosis of "incontinence with physical stress or activity" may be inaccu-

Table 36–1. URINARY LOSS PER URETHRA

Detrusor Dysfunction (Elevated Intravesical Pressure, with or without Outlet Dysfunction)

1. Overactive detrusor
   a. Uninhibited contractions
      (1) Bladder instability
         (a) Idiopathic
         (b) Irritation
         (c) Obstruction
      (2) Bladder hyperreflexia (neurologic lesion)
         (a) Suprapontine
         (b) Suprasacral
   b. Non-compliant detrusor
      (1) Fibrosis
         (a) Radiation
         (b) Inflammation
         (c) Connective tissue disease
      (2) Neurogenic (peripheral denervation)
2. Underactive detrusor
   a. Peripheral denervation
   b. Smooth muscle decompensation
   c. Pharmacologic (anticholinergics or smooth muscle relaxants)

Outlet Dysfunction ("Genuine Stress Incontinence"; Decreased Urethral Resistance, with or without Detrusor Dysfunction)

1. Anatomic support (types I and II)
2. Intrinsic urethral closure defect (type III)
3. Total urethral destruction

rate as a result of the similar presentations of various underlying conditions. Common conditions associated with stress activities and the differences in etiology and therapeutic approach are presented in Table 36–2. Many patients with stress incontinence have uninhibited contractions provoked by increased activity and do not have GSI. As many as one third of patients with GSI have urgency, and a similar percentage of patients with uninhibited bladder contractions lose urine during physical activity without the "urge" to void.

Classification of patients by grading the volume (small = stress or urethral incontinence and large = urge or bladder incontinence), persistence (constant leakage = total urethral incompetence), time of day (nighttime problems or wetting in bed = urge incontinence), and activity level (urinary loss with coughing and straining = GSI) may direct the physician, but it is not sufficient to proceed with surgery. Based on the history alone, even with extensive questioning, the physician can expect to be wrong at least 20 percent of the time about the etiology of the incontinence.[1]

In addition to questions concerning urinary incontinence, a complete urologic history is essential. A prior history of lower urinary tract surgery on the bladder (e.g., vesicostomy, augmentation, or reduction cystoplasty) or bladder neck–urethra (e.g., urethral dilations, internal urethrotomy, bladder neck resection or revision, diverticulectomy, and bladder neck suspension) or a history of a chronic indwelling catheter should be specifically explored because of the effects on both bladder and urethral functions.

The Simplified Examination (Urologic Diagnostic Procedures)

A simplified evaluation of stress incontinence is presented in Table 36–3.

Flow

The urinary flow rate is a reflection of bladder emptying. An indication of bladder outlet interaction is obtained. A low or interrupted flow rate suggests poor bladder contractility, voiding by abdominal straining, or the presence of outflow obstruction; it should be considered an indication for further urodynamic evaluation before surgery is undertaken. Patients with poor bladder emptying may be predisposed to urinary retention following surgery. A normal flow rate does not always ensure adequate detrusor function, as many patients with overflow incontinence may generate a good flow with abdominal straining. A "super" flow has been described in patients with GSI and is attributed to decreased outflow resistance, but it should not be considered pathognomonic of GSI.

Post-void Residual

A post-void residual (PVR) is recommended in every patient as a further indication of emptying function. Placement of the catheter should be coordinated with a cath-culture and the performance of cystometry.

An elevated PVR may be the result of a noncontractile bladder or outlet obstruction. The suspicion of outlet obstruction should increase with a prior history of bladder neck surgery. Patients with poor preoperative emptying of the bladder, unless the underlying cause is outlet obstruction or a large cystocele that is repaired during the procedure, are prone to increased emptying problems when the bladder outlet resistance is increased. If an areflexic neurogenic bladder is the underlying cause, preoperative intermittent catheter training is recommended.

Table 36–2. DIFFERENTIAL DIAGNOSIS IN "STRESS INCONTINENCE"

Genuine Stress Incontinence (GSI)

Urethral resistance is overcome as a result of a deficit in urethral closure pressure. Urinary loss occurs during elevations of intravesical pressure. The increases in intravesical pressure are not a result of bladder contractions but are secondary to increases in intra-abdominal pressure that are transmitted to the bladder during physical activity.

The *decreased urethral resistance* may be due to a problem with *anatomic support* of the posterior bladder neck (type I) or to the bladder neck and urethra (type II). Hypermobility of the bladder neck permits posterior extra-abdominal intravaginal rotation of this area, predisposing to unequal pressure transmission between the bladder and the proximal urethral continence mechanism. *Decreased urethral resistance* may also result from a deficit in the *intrinsic urethral closure mechanism* (type III). The decrease in urethral coaptation or compression may result from multiple surgical procedures, trauma, denervation, radiation therapy, or severe postmenopausal mucosal-submucosal urethral atrophy. Multiple surgical procedures or a chronic indwelling catheter may cause total urethral destruction.

From a surgical standpoint, type I and type II GSI responds to "bladder neck suspension" procedures, which restore anatomic relationships. Type III GSI requires procedures that provide increased urethral compression (fascial or vaginal wall slings, periurethral injection of polytef (Teflon) or collagen, or an artificial sphincter). Total urethral destruction may respond to a sling, urethral plication, or bladder-flap reconstruction, or bladder neck closure with suprapubic tube placement or urinary diversion may be needed.

Stress-Induced Uninhibited Bladder Contractions

Urethral resistance is overcome by a *true bladder contraction*, which is triggered by physical activity. The etiology of the bladder instability may be neurologic (*detrusor hyperreflexia* from a cerebral or spinal lesion) or idiopathic (detrusor instability). This condition is classically referred to as "urge incontinence."

After establishing the absence of other lower urinary pathology, uninhibited bladder contractions should be treated with anticholinergic therapy.

Stress-Provoked Overflow Incontinence

Urinary retention secondary to a noncontractile bladder or secondary to outlet obstruction predisposes to the acute "overflow" loss of urine associated with increased physical activity. The noncontractile bladder may be a low-pressure (compliant) bladder or a high-pressure (noncompliant) bladder.

Overflow incontinence may resolve with acute therapy directed at the underlying cause. If the condition is chronic, intermittent catheterization may be required for bladder emptying. Anticholinergic therapy or bladder augmentation may be necessary for the establishment of a low-pressure "reservoir" if the bladder is chronically noncompliant. Genuine stress incontinence may be coexistent. If denervation is the cause for the noncontractile bladder, type III stress incontinence should be suspected.

Complicated GSI

1. GSI with uninhibited bladder contractions
2. Combined types II and III
3. GSI with overflow incontinence
4. GSI with coexistent prolapse (cystocele)
5. Total urethral destruction

Table 36–3. SIMPLIFIED EVALUATION OF STRESS INCONTINENCE*

1. Patient presents to the office with a full bladder. Voids in private into commode with flowmeter.†
2. Patient is placed into the lithotomy position. The bladder is catheterized with a plastic disposable catheter. Post-void residual (PVR) and urine culture are obtained.†
3. The bladder is filled to 250 to 300 ml as cystometry is performed. The plastic catheter is used to illustrate urethral hypermobility with coughing and straining.
4. The catheter is removed. If the patient has immediate urinary loss (characteristically a "spurt") with coughing and straining, which disappears with careful elevation of the bladder neck (care is taken to not compress the urethra), genuine stress incontinence (GSI) is presumed. (Note: uninhibited contractions may coexist with GSI.)‡
5. A physical examination is performed with specific attention to identifying associated anterior (cystocele, uterine) or posterior (enterocele or rectocele) pelvic prolapse or unrelated pelvic pathology. A bimanual pelvic examination is performed. An assessment of levator tone, rectal tone, and a sensory evaluation of the S2, S3, and S4 dermatomes should be accomplished at this time. A repeat examination with the patient in the standing position may be indicated to evaluate uterine prolapse or enterocele formation. A rectal examination is performed. At the termination of the examination, a single dose of oral antibiotic may be elected.†

*Evaluation includes history, flow, PVR, Q-tip test, cystometry, Marshall test, and physical examination.

†If the patient demonstrates an abnormal flow rate, elevated PVR urine, negative or nonclassic Marshall test result, a history of neurologic disease, or previous unsuccessful surgery for incontinence, additional urodynamic, radiographic, or cystoscopic studies are considered.

‡If the patient fails to demonstrate urinary loss or is possibly losing urine from an extraurethral source, a "pad-tampon test" is considered.

Urinalysis and Culture

Urinary tract infections have been known to precipitate sensory urgency, but have not been documented to cause uninhibited bladder contractions or GSI. Regardless, a sterile urine is required preoperatively. The presence of hematuria requires complete urologic evaluation prior to the consideration of incontinence surgery.

Cystometry

If a cystometer is available, carbon dioxide or water cystometry should be utilized to assess bladder sensation, capacity, and compliance and to document the presence or absence of uninhibited bladder contractions. Fast filling rates, coughing, and straining may provoke uninhibited bladder contractions. Simple cystometry, performed by incremental filling of the barrel of a 60-cc syringe attached to the catheter, has been advocated, but it does not provide a "hard copy" recording and may not be as sensitive in assessing low-level detrusor contractions or noncompliance. If cystometry is performed with a catheter without a balloon, care should be taken during cystometry to observe for small amounts of urinary loss around the catheter that may occur during uninhibited contractions. Bladder contractions that are accompanied by urinary leakage around the catheter may not be recorded as elevations of intravesical pressure because of the low outlet resistance. When uninhibited contractions with urinary loss around the catheter are suspected, it may be necessary to occlude the urethra or to utilize a Foley catheter to demonstrate the increases in detrusor pressure.

The indications for cystometry are controversial. As a screening test for all preoperative patients, cystometry allows confirmation of a stable compliant reservoir. Although approximately 30 to 40 percent of females do not demonstrate a voluntary bladder contraction, in those who do, the incidence of prolonged postoperative urinary retention is extremely rare. In the absence of a cystometrically demonstrated bladder contraction, a normal flow rate and a minimal PVR are usually indications that the absence of a demonstrable voluntary contraction may be a result of the testing environment. In patients with poor flow rates and elevated urinary residuals, the incidence of postoperative retention or poor bladder emptying is more common.

The etiology of incontinence may be multifactorial (see Table 36–1). Although establishing the presence of GSI is sufficient to proceed with surgery in the majority of cases, underlying bladder dysfunction may be missed by performing a stress test alone. Cystometry should be performed in any patient with a suspected or established neurologic lesion, a history of prior unsuccessful surgery, or severe urgency symptoms. The cost-effectiveness of cystometry is apparent if one compares the cost of cystometry versus the cost of unnecessary or unsuccessful surgery. The morbidity associated with cystometry is negligible if it is performed at the time of obtaining a urinary PVR.

Physical Examination

Bladder and Bladder Outlet

The observation of urethral hypermobility, the demonstration of the objective loss of urine during stress maneuvers, and the identification of the site and volume of urinary loss have been demonstrated utilizing the "Q-tip," Marshall, and "pad-tampon" tests.

Q-Tip Test. A surgical procedure aimed at elevating and supporting the bladder neck ideally should be performed after establishing the presence of the anatomic defect and its relationship to the urinary loss. A semirigid plastic catheter (adapted for cystometry) may be utilized to observe hypermobility (Q-tip test), to record the PVR, and to perform the cystometrogram (CMG). In most cases, the urethral hypermobility is obvious and a separate instrumentation is not required. Practitioners should be cautioned against using a wooden stick with cotton because this may cause a foreign body to be left in the urethra.

Marshall Test. An immediate "spurt" of urine during straining or coughing, which resolves with careful elevation of the bladder neck or trigone (taking care not to compress the urethra), has classically been associated with stress incontinence.[2,3] Multiple provocative stress maneuvers may cause an uninhibited bladder contraction, which results in small-volume urinary loss, and may confuse the results of this stress test.

The objective demonstration of urinary loss is a prerequisite for the proper diagnosis and surgical therapy of incontinence. In the majority of patients, the identification of urinary loss by a careful physical examination is not a problem. Some patients with GSI may show negative Marshall test findings because of small volumes within the bladder, or they may demonstrate positive stress test findings only in the standing position. Filling the bladder to a minimum of 300 ml and re-examining the patient while she is standing are recommended. A voiding cystourethrogram (VCUG) with fluoroscopy is helpful for confirming urethral hypermobility and the objective loss of urine in the standing position.

A "complication" of surgery can be the successful performance of a suspension procedure on a patient who is subjectively "wet," who may be wet from fluid other than urine, or who is losing urine from another source other than the urethra (Fig. 36–1). Therefore, when the physical examination does not reveal the site of the urinary loss, every patient who complains of "wetness" must be methodically evaluated for the source, type of fluid, and relative quantity. The spectrum of wetness is presented in Table 36–4.

Pad Test. A "pad test" may be performed by the patient at home or during the office visit. A vaginal tampon and external pad are placed, and the patient performs activities that are associated with wetness. The pad test can be performed in conjunction with a preadministered urinary coloring agent, e.g., oral phenazopyridine (Pyridium). The pad and tampon are visually examined and weighed. This technique can differentiate urine from other fluids by color, site (urethra versus vagina by the distribution of staining), and quantity (weight in gm = ml) of urinary loss.

The pad test can be very informative to the physician who is puzzled by these findings:

1. A "negative examination" for urinary loss (subjective wetness by the patient and a negative stress test in the lithotomy and standing positions).
2. A patient's complaints of wetness out of proportion to that noted on the physical examination (minimal or infrequent incontinence).
3. A history of prior pelvic surgery or trauma (fistula).
4. A congenital abnormality (ureteral ectopia).

In some patients a voiding cystourethrogram (vesicovaginal fistula), intravenous urogram (ureterovaginal fistula, ureteral ectopia), or cystoscopy may be necessary for a definitive diagnosis.

Coexistent Pelvic Pathology

Coexistent vaginal pathology must be noted prior to proceeding with surgery. Atrophic vaginitis may be treated preoperatively with estrogens to improve tissue pliability and blood supply. Anterior vault (cystocele or uterine) prolapse should be recognized and repaired at the time of surgery. Elevation of a cystocele may be necessary to unmask incontinence during the stress test. Postoperative support of the anterior vaginal wall may accentuate pre-existing posterior pelvic weakness, and a pre-existing enter-

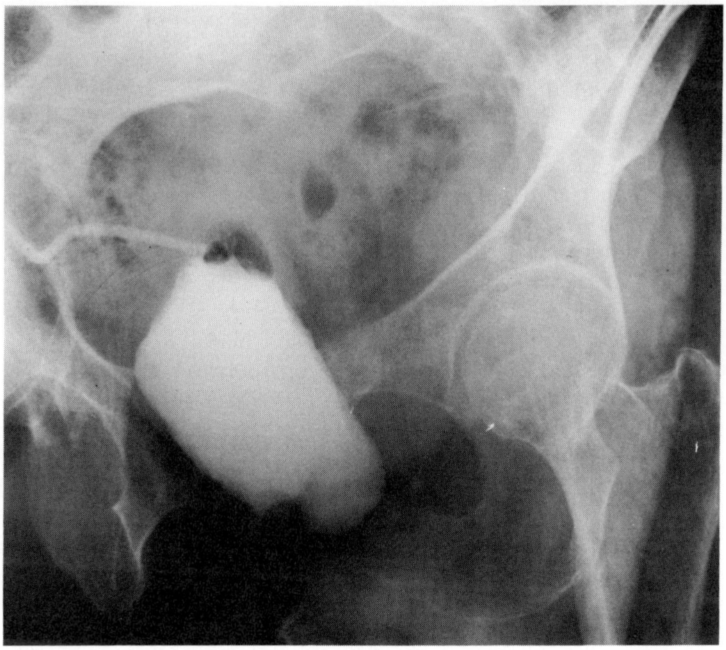

Figure 36–1. Cystogram through suprapubic tube of a patient with three previous bladder neck suspension failures. In addition to the presence of total urethral incompetence, a vesicovaginal fistula can also be observed. Functional bladder capacity due to severe fibrosis was 125 ml. As a result of the patient's age and medical conditions, a transvaginal closure of the bladder neck with suprapubic tube placement was performed.

Table 36–4. SPECTRUM OF WETNESS

Urinary	Nonurinary
Extraurethral Leakage	Vaginal (transudate or exudate)
Vaginal fistula	
Urethral	Rectal
Vesical	Perspiration
Ureteral	Subjective (not wet)
Ureteral ectopia	
Vaginal voiding	
Urinary Loss per Urethra*	

*See Table 36–1.

ocele may be accentuated. An assessment of levator tone by having the patient "squeeze" the examining fingers placed against the levator musculature may be combined with a review of Kegel exercises for patients with mild symptoms. A bimanual pelvic examination is performed. An assessment of rectal tone and the S2, S3, and S4 dermatomes is performed to rule out sensory or motor deficits. A rectal examination is performed to exclude a rectocele or rectal mass and to heme-test the stool. A physical examination in the standing position is often necessary to evaluate uterine prolapse or enterocele formation and to elicit GSI.

When there is a history of abnormal vaginal bleeding, a Papanicolaou (PAP) smear and a preoperative evaluation for uterine pathology are required. A hysterectomy is not indicated for improving the results of incontinence surgery but should be considered only if there is appropriate uterine pathology. Gynecologic referral may be indicated for a combined procedure.

Additional Testing

Voiding Cystourethrography

Historically, radiologic studies have provided significant insight into understanding the anatomic defect and the results of surgery in patients with GSI.[4–7] Lateral cystourethrography with a radiopaque catheter or beaded chain performed at rest, and with provocative maneuvers, has been utilized to examine the relationship of the urethra, urethrovesical junction, and bladder base to the bony structures of the pelvis (Fig. 36–2). Loss of the posterior urethrovesical (PUV) angle alone (Green type I) (Fig. 36–3) and loss of the PUV angle with combined loss of the vertical urethral axis (Green type II) (Fig. 36–4) have been described and classified. Type I and type II incontinence are manifested by posterior and inferior rotational movements of the bladder neck and proximal urethra to a dependent position with respect to the bladder. "Funneling" of the bladder neck as urine enters the posterior urethra is associated with a loss of the baseplate of the bladder.[8,9] Patients with type III incontinence classically demonstrate funneling of the bladder neck and an open proximal urethra at rest (Fig. 36–5). Videofluoroscopy is superior to static films. Objective loss of urine can be demonstrated, and the study may be considered the "physical examination" in the standing position.

Objections to the "angle concept" derive from the absence of abnormal angles in 20 percent of patients with stress incontinence, and the presence of abnormal angles in 20 percent of women who do not have stress incontinence.[6] The absence of urinary loss in patients with bladder neck hypermobility represents compensation at the distal urethral mechanism.

The observation of bladder diverticula suggests elevated intravesical pressure, usually associated with uninhibited bladder contractions in the presence of voluntary sphincter inhibition, or functional or anatomic outlet obstruction. Observation of a vesicovaginal or proximal urethral fistula is also possible (see Fig. 36–1). In uncomplicated cases, cystography is not recommended for screening for these conditions.

The primary criticism of cystography is the failure to measure intravesical pressure during the study. When the cystogram is performed with a double-lumen catheter, which allows simultaneous monitoring of the intravesical pressure during filling and provocative maneuvers, uninhibited contractions and poor bladder compliance can be recognized (Fig. 36–6). Overflow incontinence associated with poor bladder compliance and stress-induced uninhibited bladder contractions mimicking GSI may be misinterpreted on a radiographic report.

Videocystography with simultaneous cystometry may be indicated in patients with prior unsuccessful surgery for stress incontinence, especially when the observation of poor urethral support is not apparent.[10,11]

Cystoscopy

The role of cystoscopy in the diagnosis of stress incontinence is limited. Although endoscopy may be advocated to exclude coexistent urethral or bladder disease, preoperative cystoscopy for routine observation of the urethra does not seem to add significant information for the diagnosis of GSI. The presence of coexistent hematuria or severe irritative symptoms must be evaluated on their own merit, with the ap-

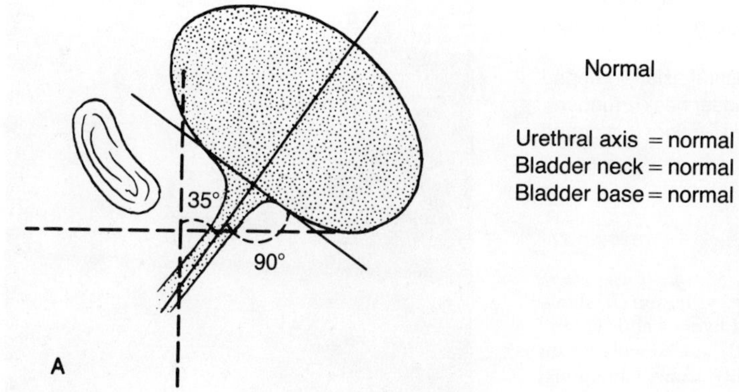

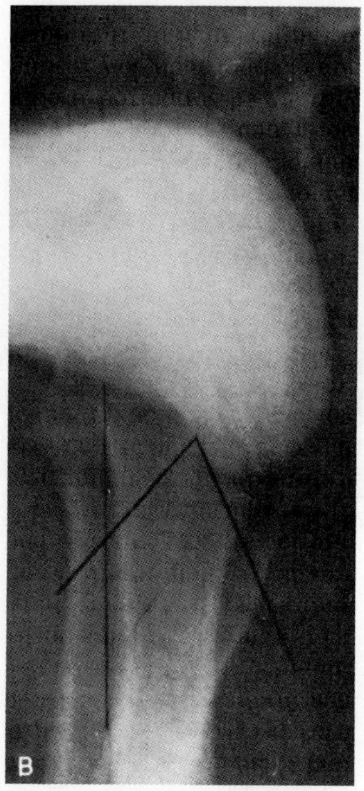

Figure 36–2. Diagram *(A)* and lateral straining cystogram *(B)* showing normal urethral axis (well supported urethra), normal urethral trigonal angle (competent bladder neck), and the base of the bladder above the inferior ramus of the pubis.

propriate radiographic, cytologic, and endoscopic studies.

Pressure-Flow Studies

Pressure-flow studies are indicated only when the suspicion of outlet obstruction exists as a result of an obstructed flow rate and elevated PVR. Obstruction in the female patient without a history of urethral surgery, inflammatory disease, multiple sclerosis, or spinal cord trauma is rare. The diagnosis of outlet obstruction in the female patient is difficult to make on physical examination, sounding of the urethra, or cystoscopy. The VCUG may indicate poor urethral opening during "voiding," but the true intravesical pressure is not known. Although isometric contractions (cystometry performed with an obstructing Foley catheter) may be associated with significant intravesical pressure, most female pa-

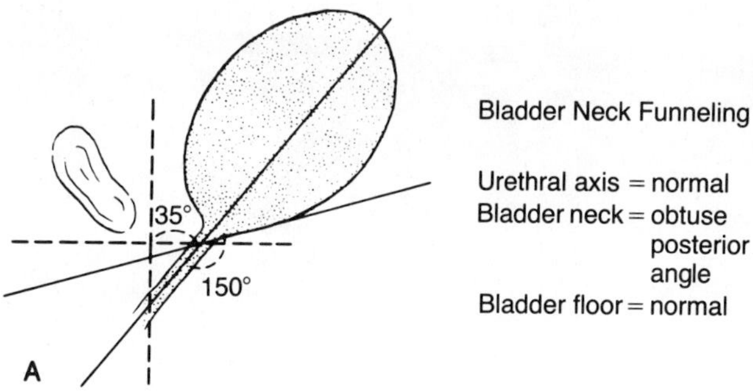

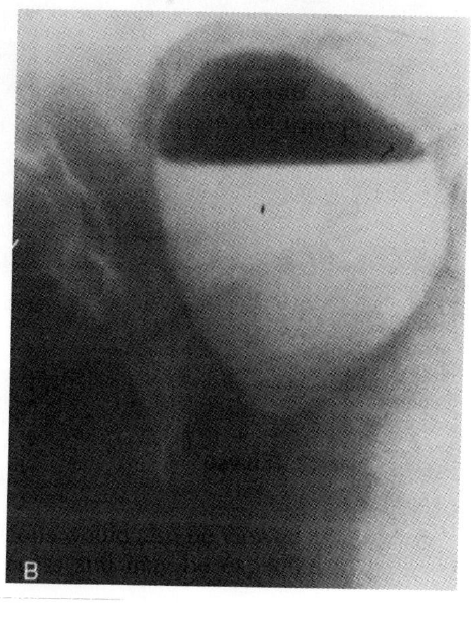

Figure 36–3. *A*, Diagram showing the increase of the urethrotrigonal angle (funneling of the bladder neck) without cystocele or urethral hypermobility (type I). *B*, Oblique straining cystogram showing the bladder neck in a dependent position (funneled and open).

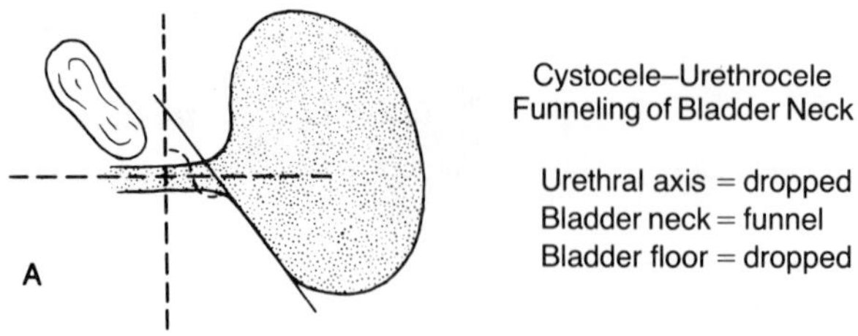

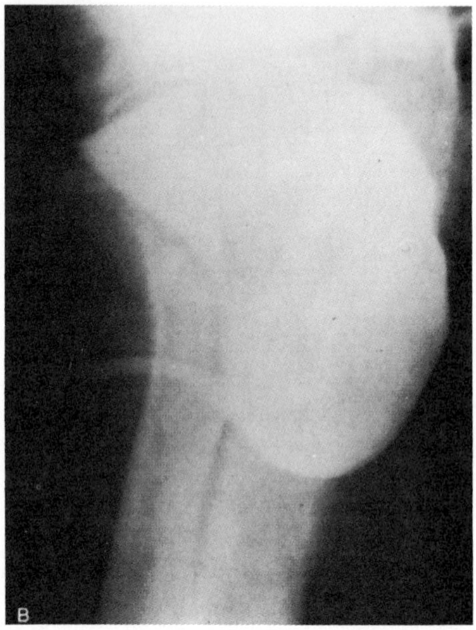

Figure 36–4. Diagram *(A)* and lateral straining cystogram *(B)* showing the increase in the urethral axis (urethral hypermobility), and increase in the urethral trigonal angle (type II). A cystocele is also present. Repair of the urethral hypermobility alone (abdominal vesicourethropexy) may obstruct the bladder neck by leaving a large cystocele. Repair of the cystocele alone may leave the urethra in a dependent position and may increase the tendency toward stress incontinence.

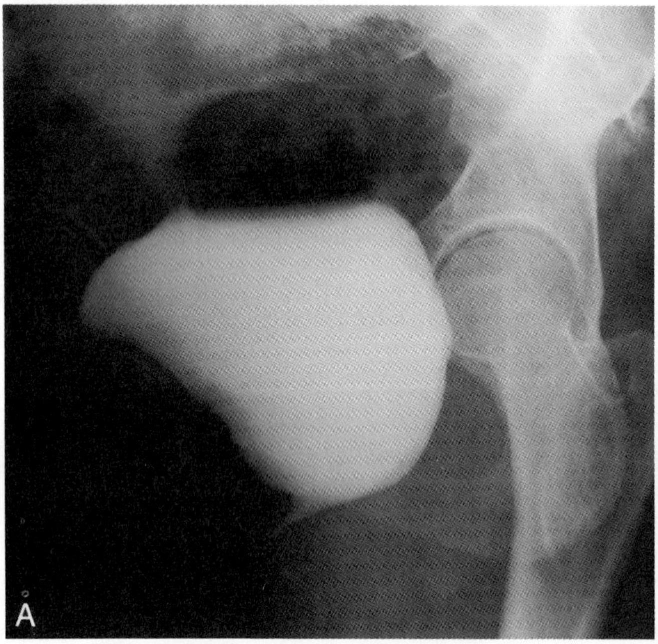

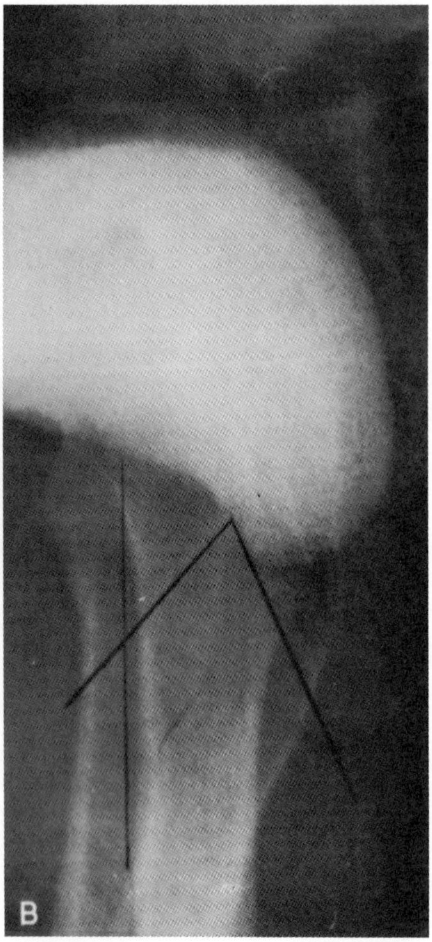

Figure 36–5. *A*, Cystogram demonstrating an open bladder neck at rest in a patient with good anatomic support following unsuccessful bladder neck suspension surgery (type III stress incontinence). Urethral profilometry demonstrated a proximal urethral closure pressure less than 10 cm of water. *B*, Stress incontinence in the same patient during abdominal straining. A simultaneous cystometrogram demonstrated the absence of detrusor dysfunction.

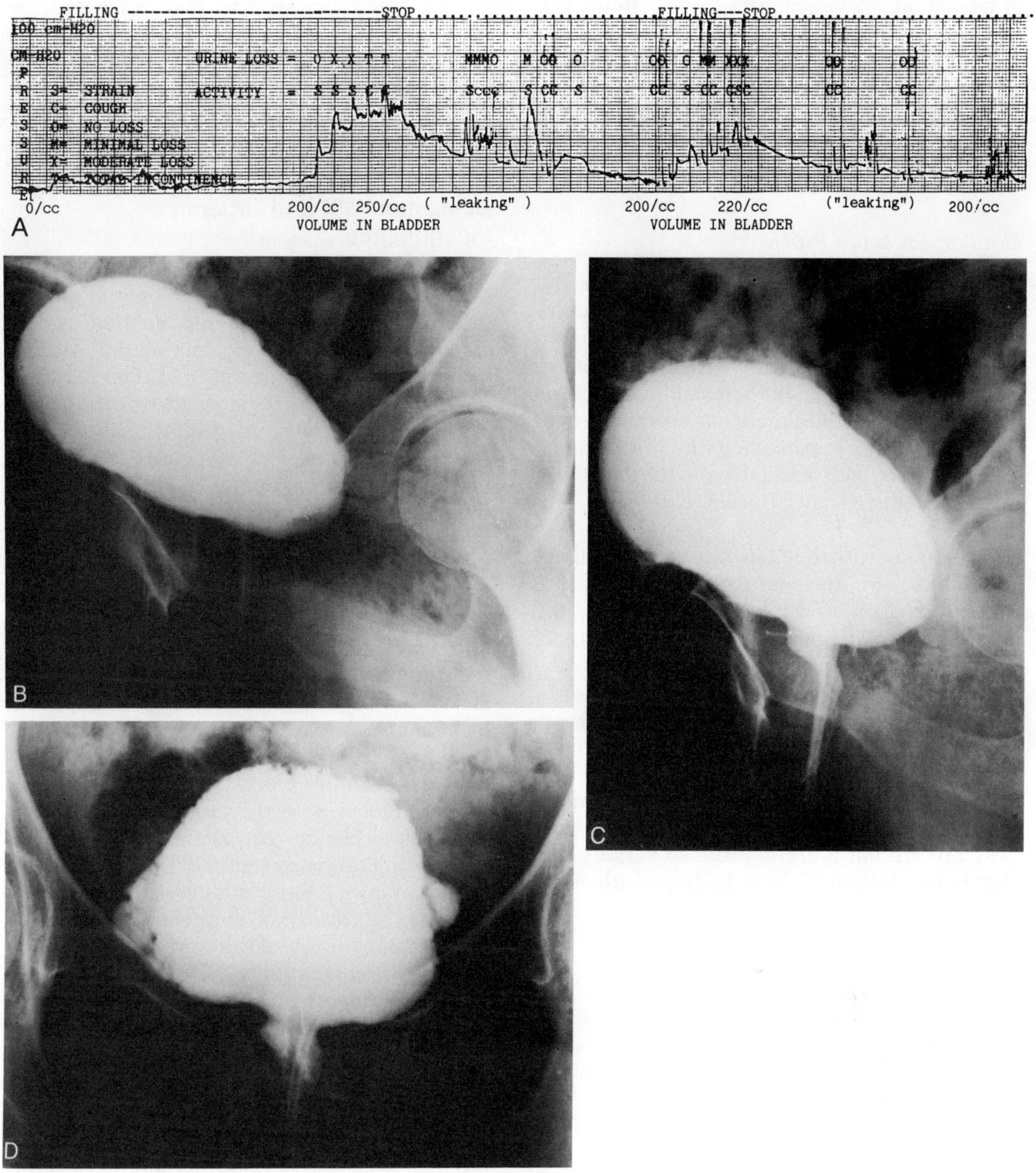

Figure 36–6. *A*, Cystometrogram from simultaneous voiding cystometrogram-vesicourethrogram (CMG-VCUG) (6 Fr double-lumen catheter) in a patient with two prior unsuccessful bladder neck suspensions, revealing the intravesical pressure associated with bladder filling to 250 ml with accompanied provocative maneuvers. Poor bladder compliance was observed between 200 and 250 ml. The observed stop in intravesical pressure elevation with cessation of filling is consistent with the diagnosis of noncompliance. (A bladder contraction would demonstrate continued elevation of intravesical pressure without bladder filling.) Coughing (C) and straining (S) are indicated as well as the degree of urinary loss, none (0), minimal (M), moderate (X), and total incontinence (T). At low bladder volumes and low pressures, the patient is continent. Elevation of the intravesical pressure increases the degree of urinary loss until total incontinence is observed. After the patient coughs and leakage occurs, bladder volume is reduced and the pressure approaches baseline. Incremental filling confirms the initial impression. A combined bladder augmentation and fascial sling were performed.

B, Cystogram (oblique) at 175 ml, demonstrating a closed bladder neck with coughing at baseline pressure. (See *A*.)

C, Cystogram (oblique) at 225 ml, demonstrating opening of the bladder neck during coughing with increased intravesical pressure. (See *A*.)

D, Cystogram (anteroposterior) at 250 ml, demonstrating total urethral incontinence with minimal provocation. (See *A*.)

tients void with low detrusor pressures because of low outlet resistance. To diagnose outlet obstruction, an elevated intravesical pressure and a low flow rate must be demonstrated. In patients who void with significant abdominal straining, subtracted detrusor pressures (intra-abdominal pressure minus intravesical pressure) may be necessary.

Urethral Pressure Profile

The measurement of static (resting) or dynamic (comparison of urethral versus bladder pressure increase during provocative maneuvers) is seldom indicated in the incontinence evaluation. Although both maximum urethral closure pressure and functional urethral length tend to be lower in patients with GSI, so much overlap exists with normal patients that these measurements cannot be used as reliable indicators.[12,13]

In women with demonstrable "urethral incontinence," (1) the resting posterior closure pressure is significantly lower than the resting anterior aspect (opposite findings in controls), (2) the transmission of bladder pressure to the urethra during coughing is significantly lower than controls, and (3) endoscopic suspension enhances transmission throughout the length of the urethra.[14–16]

Despite these findings, preoperative measurements of urethral length and transmission pressure are not a prerequisite to surgery and the demonstration of these findings without simultaneous radiographic (fluoroscopy) or clinical demonstration of incontinence is not an indication for surgery.[14] In patients with clinical lower motor neuron disease, and in those with GSI with a well-supported urethra, the demonstration of abnormally low resting closure pressures in the proximal urethra during fluoroscopically monitored profilometry is useful for establishing the diagnosis of type III incontinence.[10]

Electromyography

Sophisticated neuropysiologic studies have demonstrated selective damage to the pudendal nerve innervation of the striated urethral sphincter by needle electromyography,[17] and an increase in sacral evoked potential latency times in patients with stress incontinence.[18] Despite these findings, the use of electromyography of the pelvic floor and external sphincter is not indicated prior to routine surgery. However, a clinical history or physical findings of pelvic floor denervation (peripheral neuropathy or cauda equina syndrome) may be associated with intrinsic urethral dysfunction and should raise the suspicion of type III stress incontinence.

PREOPERATIVE CONSIDERATIONS

Coexistent GSI and Urgency Incontinence

The prognostic significance of the symptom of urinary urgency and the preoperative urodynamic demonstration of uninhibited bladder contractions on the outcome of bladder neck suspension procedures remains controversial.

The conclusions from studies analyzing the success of bladder neck suspension procedures in patients with preoperative urinary urgency must be interpreted carefully. The criteria used for selection of the patients, the application of the terms "urge" and "stress" incontinence, and the analysis of the etiology of the incontinence in the patients who failed to respond to surgery differ among the various studies. In some of the studies, anti-incontinence surgery was performed on patients with "stress-provoked urge incontinence," mixed incontinence, or pure urge incontinence without any element of GSI. Several of the studies failed to correlate the symptom of urgency with the urodynamic finding of uninhibited bladder contractions and therefore did not differentiate "sensory" from "motor" urgency. Many of these studies failed to define whether the resolution of urgency was a sensory change or the result of the conversion of a bladder with preoperative urodynamically demonstrated bladder instability to a postoperative urodynamically demonstrated "stable" bladder. The etiology of the surgical failure (abnormal detrusor behavior versus failure to correct the deficit in outlet resistance) is often unclear.

Several authors have proposed that preoperative sensory urgency and uninhibited bladder contractions may both resolve following suspension of the bladder neck.[1,11] The etiology of the preoperative urinary urgency has been related to the entrance of urine into the proximal urethra during the descent and opening of the bladder neck.[10,19–21]

If one accepts this theory, a major problem is that of distinguishing *detrusor instability* that is causally related to an open bladder neck from *idiopathic detrusor instability* that does not respond to surgical correction of the anatomic defect. Although surgical correction of the anatomic defect for GSI is often accompanied by the resolution of urgency, support of the bladder neck for urgency incontinence alone, without associated GSI, has not met with equal success. According to some authors, provocative cystometry in the standing position may give some prognostic information.[20,21] Fifty-five percent of patients with cough-provoked instability versus 14 percent of those with spontaneous uninhibited contractions were continent following surgery in one study.[22] Other authors differentiated patients by observing the maximal detrusor pressure during uninhibited contractions. When detrusor pressures were greater than 25 cm of water[23] or 35 cm of water,[24] prognosis for incontinence following surgery was poor.

One certainly cannot dispute the philosophy that bladder neck suspension procedures will correct the GSI component of the problem, and the expectations for the resolution of urgency symptoms are somewhat justified by clinical experience. The argument can be strengthened by considering the possible clinical outcomes of surgical intervention for GSI with associated "urge" symptoms.

Urgency (Sensory) with GSI

The presence of preoperative "sensory" urgency may be expected to resolve; if it does not, sensory urgency is rarely associated with urinary loss and the surgery for "incontinence" would be successful. Cystometry may be useful in identifying patients with urgency but without true uninhibited bladder contractions. Urinary urgency may persist postoperatively, and patients should be advised of this problem prior to surgery.

Urgency (Motor-Uninhibited Bladder Contractions) with GSI

Failure of conventional anti-incontinence procedures to correct incontinence in patients with a preoperative diagnosis of uninhibited bladder contractions has been reported by several authors.[22,23,25–31] Conversely, other authors have reported a substantial number of patients with uninhibited bladder contractions who respond well to bladder neck suspension procedures.[1,11,32–34]

Correction of the GSI component and complete resolution of uninhibited contractions would be ideal results and may be expected in a small percentage of patients. The persistence of urodynamically demonstrable but clinically asymptomatic low-level uninhibited bladder contractions would also be viewed as a total surgical success and may be expected in patients with low-pressure uninhibited contractions.[23,31] In one series, approximately two thirds of the patients with preoperative detrusor instability had no postoperative urgency symptoms.[11]

The correction of GSI with persistent symptomatic uninhibited contractions that are responsive to anticholinergic therapy would also provide total continence, but a patient may be troubled by persistent frequency and urgency. Correction of the GSI component with persistent incontinence secondary to uninhibited contractions may be interpreted as improved, unchanged, or worse, depending on the frequency and volume of urinary loss. Patients with high-pressure uninhibited contractions are most likely to have symptomatic incontinence. In approximately 10 percent of patients, urodynamically demonstrable detrusor instability developed in the postoperative period.[11] These patients were presumed to be a mixed group, who had instability that was not demonstrated despite provocative preoperative cystometry, and a group in whom instability developed following the surgery.[11] The etiology of the development of postoperative instability is unknown and may be only a reflection of subclinical preoperative instability. Regardless of the interpretation of these results, *there is little evidence to support bladder neck suspension procedures for bladder instability without GSI.*

Urgency (Motor-Detrusor Hyperreflexia) with GSI

The surgical repair of GSI in the presence of detrusor hyperreflexia (uninhibited contractions secondary to a demonstrable neurologic lesion) must be considered separately. Detrusor hyperreflexia that does not respond preoperatively to anticholinergic therapy would not be expected to resolve with correction of the GSI. In these patients, preoperative anticholinergic therapy is indicated in order to assess the relative contribution of the separate pathophysiologic entities. If high-pressure detrusor hyperreflexia is present, correction of the GSI component of the incontinence is not indicated unless it is the major component of the patient's clinical incontinence. A pad test performed while the patient is receiving anticholinergic therapy may help to quantitate and differentiate the GSI and detrusor hyperreflexia contributions to the urinary loss.

Combined Type II and Type III Incontinence

Multiple urethral surgeries, especially prior failed urethropexies; a history or physical examination consistent with somatic or autonomic peripheral neuropathy; a positive Marshall test with a well-supported urethra; or a cystogram demonstrating an open and funneled bladder neck at rest, with or without urethral hypermobility, should increase the suspicion of isolated type III or combined type II and type III incontinence due to a deficiency in the intrinsic urethral closure mechanism (see Fig. 36–5). Accepted bladder neck suspension procedures may occasionally provide continence by creating a fulcrum of compression at the bladder neck. It is difficult, however, to achieve continence with standard bladder neck suspension procedures, without obstructing the urethra. Fascial sling strips, fascial patch slings, or anterior vaginal wall patch slings provide compression pressure along the urethra in addition to urethral elevation and should be strongly considered.[19,35–37] Periurethral injection of inert paste materials may also provide increased urethral resistance.[38] Artificial sphincter implantation may also be utilized; however, this is technically difficult and is subject to mechanical problems as well as urethral and vaginal cuff erosion.[39,40]

GSI with Overflow Incontinence

Overflow incontinence secondary to a noncontractile bladder without GSI may respond to intermittent catheterization alone. Acute bladder outlet obstruction requires intermittent catheterization and observation, with consideration of cutting the suspending sutures if the patient fails to void for a prolonged period of time while demonstrating good bladder contractility. Chronic postoperative obstruction necessitates urethral remobilization and resuspension. A bladder neck suspension for GSI associated with a noncontractile bladder and elevated urinary residuals may lead to total retention. Preoperative intermittent catheterization training is recommended. If the bladder has a low functional capacity, urinary frequency and urgency may be severe. If the bladder shows a significant loss of compliance, upper tract deterioration may result secondary to the increased intravesical pressures obtainable following the surgically produced increase in urethral resistance. Anticholinergic therapy may be successful in many cases, but bladder augmentation may be required in severe cases.

In patients with peripheral denervation (myelomeningocele, infrasacral cord tumors, radical pelvic surgery) or bladder fibrosis (chronic infection, chronic indwelling catheter), stress incontinence may result from a mixture of urethral incompetence and chronically elevated intravesical pressure secondary to noncompliance. The increases in intravesical pressure at high bladder volumes "opens" the bladder neck and defunctionalizes the proximal urethral continence mechanism. This may occur with or without coexistent urethral denervation or injury (see Fig. 36–6).

Some patients with long-standing total incontinence may demonstrate noncompliance on cystometry that resolves postoperatively with bladder distention. Fast filling rate cystometry (100 to 125 ml/minute) may accentuate noncompliance, and slow filling rate cystometry (10 to 20 ml/minute plus urine output) may be utilized to achieve a volume of 300 ml, allowing assessment of preoperative functional bladder volumes and pressures.

GSI with Cystocele

The postoperative development of incontinence after the repair of a cystocele in a previously continent individual is distressing to both the patient and physician. Explanations for the preoperative "masking effect" of the cystocele include the accentuation of the urethral vesical angle (kinking) with coughing and straining and the ability of the cystocele to transmit intra-abdominal pressure out through the vagina rather than to the bladder outlet.

Caution should also be given to the practice of urethral suspension without cystocele repair. Elevation of the bladder neck without support of the bladder base will result in "kinking" of the bladder neck, resulting in outlet obstruction.

Total Urethral Destruction

Patients who have undergone multiple urethral procedures or in whom a chronic indwelling catheter has been placed eventually suffer from total urethral destruction. A patulous urethra is evident on physical examination. Often these patients have neurologic deficits that have allowed nonpainful traction on the Foley balloon with urethral erosion.

Plication or bladder flap reconstruction of the urethra is often difficult because of excessive scarring and tissue destruction. Sling procedures may provide adequate compression or obstruction of the urethra.

In patients with neurologic deficits and the inability to tolerate intermittent catheterization, bladder neck closure by a transvaginal[41] or transabdominal route[42] with suprapubic tube placement or urinary diversion may be necessary.

SIGNIFICANT NON-UROLOGIC HISTORY

Medical History

The general medical evaluation prior to considering anti-incontinence surgery is not reviewed. Many conditions that may complicate the surgical treatment of genuine stress incontinence can be elicited in a careful history.

Neurologic History

Specific questions must be asked with regard to neurologic conditions that may affect bladder or urethral function. Common cerebral lesions (e.g., stroke, Parkinson's disease, brain tumor) and suprasacral spinal lesions (e.g., trauma, transverse myelitis) may be associated with an upper motor neuron pattern of detrusor hyperreflexia. Infrasacral and peripheral neuropathies (e.g., lumbar disc/laminectomy, radical pelvic surgery, diabetes) are associated with bladder areflexia. Peripheral denervation is frequently associated with a loss of bladder compliance. Multiple sclerosis and spina bifida may manifest an upper or lower motor neuron presentation.

Neurogenic urethral dysfunction may be the result of spinal cord injury or peripheral denervation. Spinal cord injury may result in detrusor-sphincter dyssynergia (uninhibited bladder contractions with external sphincter contraction during the bladder contraction), causing problems with both urine storage and emptying. Infrasacral or peripheral lesions are associated with intrinsic and external sphincter denervation, resulting in sphincteric incompetence.

Surgical/Radiation History

A prior history of radical pelvic surgery (gynecologic or general) or of pelvic fracture or gynecologic trauma should raise the suspicion for bladder, urethral, or pelvic floor denervation or fistula formation. Neurosurgical procedures may affect bladder or urethral function. Pelvic radiation therapy may affect innervation, blood supply, bladder capacity, and urethral coaptation and may also prevent tissue mobilization during surgery and healing in the postoperative period.

Medical Conditions

Medications that inhibit bladder contractility, specifically anticholinergics or smooth muscle relaxants, may be required for chronic pain or for cardiac, pulmonary, or gastrointestinal conditions. Pulmonary disease associated with a chronic cough should be addressed preoperatively so that abrupt high-pressure increases in intra-abdominal pressure can be limited in the immediate postoperative period. Diabetes may be associated with cerebrovascular disease, peripheral neuropathy, and polyuria. Coagulopathies and anticoagulant therapy are contraindications to surgery. Back or hip conditions that would necessitate special intraoperative positioning should be recognized. Decreased manual dexterity, obesity, or other factors that might limit self-catheterization (if required) should be addressed prior to the surgical procedure. Many women have occupations that require heavy lifting, and they may need to limit activity for 3 to 6 months following the surgery.

CHOICE OF SURGICAL PROCEDURE

It is generally accepted, as Marshall has stated, that any one of the established operations that repositions the "vesical neck up away from the introitus toward the umbilicus should correct ordinary stress incontinence . . . greater than 90 percent of the time." Although the proponents of *abdominal* versus *vaginal* approaches, *periurethral* versus *paraurethral* suture placements; and *large* versus *small*, *horizontal* versus *vertical*, and *one*, *two*, or *"no"* incisions may debate the merits of their respective procedures, the results for the generally accepted methods of bladder neck suspension are essentially equal. Prospective, randomized long-term studies performed by the same group of surgeons, who historically do not advocate a specific procedure, are limited.[43]

Abdominal versus Vaginal Approach

The most convincing indication for selecting either an abdominal[44,45] or vaginal;[37,46–49] approach is the presence of coexistent pathology, which would necessitate simultaneous repair. Certainly, a patient requiring a urethral diverticulectomy, cystocele or rectocele repair, or vaginal hysterectomy would benefit from a vaginal approach. An abdominal hysterectomy or other lower abdominal procedure provides access to the lithotomy position because back problems, hip disorders, or leg contractures suggest an abdominal approach. The ability to perform endoscopic-needle suspension procedures under a local anesthetic with sedation would favor this approach in patients who prefer or require limited anesthesia.

Patients with a prior history of failed bladder neck surgery may sometimes have a bladder neck that is fixed in a dependent position, and remobilization of this area is required in order to achieve the best results with resuspension. Patients with outlet obstruction secondary to oversuspension also require remobilization of the bladder neck area. When these conditions are encountered, access to the bladder neck area is possible but may be difficult through a repeat abdominal approach. Remobilization of the bladder neck area can be directly accomplished with a modified Pereyra-Raz approach or abdominal approach but not with other forms of endoscopic-needle bladder neck suspensions.

In the case of type III stress incontinence, in which a "sling" suspension is required, a fascial patch or vaginal wall patch procedure through a vaginal approach allows direct access to the proximal urethral area without the need for extensive dissection in the retropubic space and tedious dissection of the urethra from the anterior vaginal wall.[19,35–37]

A decreased operating time and shortened hospital stay[50] have been attributed to the vaginal approach, with some authors advocating an outpatient or 24-hour stay with vaginal procedures. The surgeon's preference and familiarity with the procedure, as well as the patient's preference for a "smaller" incision, should be taken into consideration.

Periurethral versus Paraurethral Suture Placement

Marshall-Marchetti (abdominal) and Stamey suspension (vaginal) techniques, which place sutures periurethrally, as opposed to paraurethral suture placement during the Burch or Tanagho (abdominal) and modified Pereyra-Raz (vaginal) procedures, have been debated with respect to postoperative bladder instability, urethral trauma (vascular or neurogenic), and the ability to provide adequate culposuspension.[51]

Postoperative continence results do not seem to differ with respect to periurethral or paraurethral sutures, and controlled urethral function studies that would favor one approach over another have not been performed. There is a suggestion of increased postoperative bladder instability with periurethral procedures, but the implications are not clear. The ability of paraurethral suture placement to provide superior colposuspension suggests their use in patients with small or moderate cystoceles or decreased anterior vaginal wall mobility.

Vaginal Approach

Anterior colporraphy alone often fails to provide adequate support to the urethra (maximal elevation 1 to 1.5 cm) and is associated with a decreased success rate compared with abdominal and vaginal bladder neck suspension procedures. Type I incontinence, which affects approximately 25 percent or fewer of patients with GSI, would be expected to respond to anterior culporraphy, which addresses the urethrovesical angle; however, type II incontinence, which presents with significant urethral hypermobility, has demonstrated a less than 50 percent rate secondary to inadequate elevation of the bladder neck.[8,9,25,52,53]

The modified Pereyra-Raz procedure differs from other endoscopic-needle bladder neck suspension procedures in the dissection of the anterior levator muscle from the inferior surface of the pubic bone and entrance into the retropubic space. An increased ability to achieve adequate colposuspension is achieved by freeing the levator muscles during access to the retropubic space. Remobilization of the urethra and the ability to guide the suspension needle under finger guidance through the retropubic space are afforded. As a result of the universal success of most procedures, however, the modified Pereyra-Raz technique does not appear to afford superior surgical results for initial surgery. In repeat procedures, access to the retropubic space for remobilization of the bladder neck may be an advantage of this approach.

INTRAOPERATIVE COMPLICATIONS

Hemorrhage

Intraoperative bleeding may be of venous or arterial origin. When the abdominal approach is used, the most troublesome bleeding is encountered in the perivesicular venous plexus. Cauterization and chromic suture ligatures are appropriate, with the primary caution being adequate exposure and identification of tissues. Cauterization near the urethra is ill advised because of tissue damage. Non-absorbable sutures are avoided because of the potential for stone formation in the urinary tract. Venous bleeding usually subsides with packing and patience, but bleeding that is due to suspension suture placement often responds simply to tying of the sutures. Although adequate hemostasis is mandatory before closing, placement of a vaginal pack often provides adequate tamponade. This may be performed intraoperatively for observation.

Bleeding during a vaginal approach usually occurs secondary to inadvertent entrance into the medial portion of the labia and during the modified Pereyra-Raz procedure at the edge of the levator muscle, which has been freed from the inferior surface of the pubic bone. Labial bleeding may be avoided with careful attention during the initial incision and dissection to the internal labial border, which forms the lateral portion of the anterior vaginal wall. As a result of the vascularity of this area, suture ligation is necessary when there is persistent bleeding.

Bleeding at the dissected edge of the levator muscle is more troublesome because of decreased exposure. Placement of the proline suspension sutures and elevation of the bladder neck are advised in order to observe whether hemostasis is obtained solely by this maneuver. Placement of additional chromic sutures at the edge of the levator may be necessary.

Bleeding during cystocele repair may be avoided by careful dissection of tissues in the vesicovaginal space away from the posterior surface of the anterior vaginal wall epithelium. Intraoperative injection of sterile saline within the vesicovaginal space aids in this dissection. The use of epinephrine is of minimal benefit, and careful monitoring is required. During cystocele repair, additional vascularity is encountered laterally at the edge of the levator and posteriorly at the edge of the peritoneum if a hysterectomy has been performed. The tying of sutures placed for the repair; the placement of additional suture ligatures, with care to avoid deep bites in the area of the ureters; and a vaginal pack constitute appropriate measures.

Vaginal bleeding through a pack signifies uncontrolled bleeding. In cases of severe bleeding, when the source cannot be identified, the umbrella pack of Mikulicz[54] or an intravaginally placed Foley catheter, inflated to 50 to 60 ml and wrapped in gauze, may be necessary.

Urethral, Bladder, and Ureteral Injuries

Injury to the urethra or bladder during abdominal urethropexy requires closure with absorbable suture and adequate postoperative drainage of the bladder and retropubic space. Ureteral injury is rare, although incorporation of the ureter into a misplaced suspension suture may occur. If injury is suspected, the bladder should be opened and retrograde catheterization of the ureters should be performed. Immediate deligation should be sufficient. Stent placement is reassuring even if the ligation time is short and additional tissue was incorporated within the suture, which normally "protects" the ureter. The stent can be cystoscopically removed at the first postoperative visit (2 weeks).

Transvaginal entrance into the urethra or bladder requires careful attention to avoid fistula formation. Repair with absorbable suture is indicated. A two-layer closure is preferable. Adequate bladder drainage must be maintained postoperatively for 10 days to 2 weeks if a large defect is apparent. Placement of a suprapubic tube is helpful for long-term bladder drainage. Entrance into the bladder neck or bladder during passage of the suspension needle rarely necessitates special attention. Careful cystoscopy is required to prevent this problem. Entrance into the bladder neck or bladder during retropubic space dissection during the modified Pereyra-Raz procedure may require an abdominal incision to close a large defect. In addition to primary closure, the retropubic space should be adequately drained and a suprapubic tube should be placed to allow prolonged bladder drainage (10 days to 2 weeks). A cystogram should be performed prior to removal of the catheter.

Ureteral injury may be suspected during a cystocele repair. The routine use of intravenous indigo carmine to observe ureteral efflux is often reassuring. In cases of suspected injury, a retrograde ureterogram may be indicated. Immediate deligation is indicated and is often the only treatment necessary; however, retrograde stent placement may be elected.

POSTOPERATIVE COMPLICATIONS

Infection

The prevention of infection is the first step in management. The urine must be sterile preoperatively. An antibacterial vaginal douche, in addition to the intraoperative preparation, is recommended the morning of the procedure. A first-generation cephalosporin is adequate for intravenous prophylaxis.

Despite the frequent use of vaginal and suprapubic pledgets during endoscopic-needle suspensions, the incidence of infection is rare. Local treatment is initially advisable, but re-exploration and removal of the offending foreign body may be necessary. The use of endoscopic-needle suspensions, in which a small suprapubic incision is required, may be of benefit in severely obese patients in order to avoid a large abdominal incision. Irrigation of the wound with antibiotic solution has been performed routinely in many series.

A Penrose or Hemovac drain has been utilized for retropubic drainage during some abdominal approaches but does not seem to have influenced postoperative infection rates.

Suprapubic Pain

The problem of osteitis pubis, a culture-negative inflammatory condition affecting the pubic bone, occurs in approximately 2.5 percent of patients undergoing retropubic vesicourethropexy. Pain in the area of the pubic symphysis, confirmed by bone films that reveal increased density or mottled rarefaction, constitutes the presenting symptom. Placement of the suspending sutures into the cartilaginous midline rather than the periosteum may prevent this problem. Postoperative analgesics and anti-inflammatory agents are equally sufficient postoperative therapy. The disease is usually self-limited, but in rare instances wedge resection of the pubic bone is required.

Suprapubic pain following endoscopic-needle suspension may be secondary to sutures that are close to the pubic bone, to excessive tension on the rectus muscle during activity, or to nerve entrapment. Anchoring of the suspension sutures on the pubic bone may improve rectus pain but also may result in an increased incidence of pubic bone problems. To alleviate chronic pain, it may be necessary to cut the sutures via the suprapubic incision. At 3 months postoperatively, cutting the sutures rarely causes recurrence of the incontinence due to retropubic scarring, but patients should be informed of this risk.

Thrombophlebitis and Pulmonary Embolism

Early ambulation and elastic stockings have replaced the use of anticoagulant therapy in patients undergoing bladder neck suspension procedures.

Persistent Incontinence

For the patient with persistent incontinence following suspension, a review of the principles applied to the preoperative evaluation is mandatory. A urinary flow rate, PVR, and CMG should be performed in addition to the Marshall test. Immediate failure to attain continence is usually associated with inadequate support of the urethra, with bladder instability, or with overflow incontinence.

The Marshall test, administered to a patient with a full bladder, may reveal persistent urethral hypermobility attributable to suture failure. Erosion of the sutures from the periurethral tissues is the most common cause. The tissue that is utilized for the suspension, the mobility of the anterior vaginal wall, the tension at which the sutures are tied, and the activity level of the patient (especially chronic coughing or straining during lifting or bowel movements) are contributory factors to suture failure.

The use of colposuspension techniques, which utilize paravaginal rather than periurethral tissue, can often provide better tissue, especially during repeat surgery.[55] The ability to free the levator from the pubic bone in the modified Pereyra-Raz procedure also allows bladder neck suspension with less tension on the sutures. During the abdominal or vaginal approach, placement of the fingers in the vagina during tying of the suspension sutures aids the surgeon in judging at which point "maximum suspension" is obtained with the "minimum tension" on the sutures. Tying any suspension "as tightly as possible" may be counterproductive if the extra elevation obtained is not significant and the erosion rate of the suture through the tissue is increased.

Support of the mid-urethra without support of the bladder neck is a result of either poor needle passage during endoscopic suspensions or improper identification of the bladder neck during the abdominal approach. If the mid-urethra is supported without bladder neck support, persistent incontinence and urethral obstruction may result. Palpation of the Foley balloon during needle passage, endoscopic visualization of the placement of the needles, and confirmation of support at the level of the bladder neck during suture elevation are critical in endoscopic suspensions. Identification of the Foley balloon, dissection at the bladder neck level, and, according to some authors, opening of the bladder during surgery to visualize the bladder neck are appropriate precautions during an abdominal approach for accurate suture placement.[45] Regardless of the number and location of periurethral or bladder sutures placed during abdominal procedures, success with endoscopic suspensions has enforced the principle that the suture at the level of the bladder neck is the most critical, and essentially the only, support that is necessary.

Persistent incontinence with a well-supported urethra should raise the suspicion of type III stress incontinence. A cystogram that reveals funneling at the level of the bladder neck at rest or a urethral pressure profile that demonstrates poor proximal urethral closure pressure is confirmatory.

Overflow incontinence should be treated with intermittent catheterization until postoperative pain and urethral irritation have resolved. The patient's medications should be reviewed, with specific attention to pain medications or anticholinergics that may be affecting bladder contractility.

Bladder instability should be treated with anticholinergic therapy (oxybutynin, 2.5 to 5.0 mg taken by mouth four times daily). The urine should be cultured and an appropriate antibiotic prescribed. Bladder instability that was not present preoperatively should alert the physician to the possibilities of outlet obstruction, sutures within the bladder or urethra, or a persistent urinary tract infection.

Non-absorbable sutures have been found within the bladder and have been attributed to inaccurate intraoperative suture placement or erosion of the suture into the bladder postoperatively. Endoscopic removal of the offending suture has rarely affected continence and is necessary to prevent continued bladder irritability, infection, and stone formation.

Materials utilized for sling surgery or an artificial sphincter cuff may also be found within the urethra or bladder. Intraoperative dissection through the urethra during abdominal approaches or erosion is the most common cause. The offending material must be removed. The success of autologous materials (facial patch and facial strip slings) and the high erosion rate of artificial materials (artificial mesh) should be taken into consideration when the sling material is chosen.

Urinary Retention

Prolonged urinary retention following bladder neck suspension is one of the most troublesome complications. The incidence of prolonged retention with the abdominal approach (Marshall-Marchetti) has been reported at 6 percent. Endoscopic suspensions with a periurethral suture placement (Stamey) required from 1 to 120 days for adequate bladder emptying. In this series, half of the patients voided by the seventh day and fewer than 7 percent required more than 30 days of bladder drainage (Stamey).[49] Correction by the modified Pereyra-Raz procedure revealed adequate bladder drainage in half the patients by 3 days and retention greater than 2 weeks in fewer than 10 percent of patients.

Several methods have been used to ease the period of difficult emptying in these patients. The most beneficial appears to be the placement of a suprapubic cystocath at the time of surgery, which allows the assessment of urinary residual and temporary management after discharge, without requiring indwelling or intermittent urethral catheterization. If patients require bladder drainage for extended times following surgery, they are instructed in intermittent catheterization at the first office visit (2 to 3 weeks) when postoperative urethral discomfort is minimized.

While the endoscopic bladder suspension is being performed, individual passage of the suture strands and ipsilateral tying of the sutures, followed by tying the sutures over the midline, provide the opportunity to loosen the suspension by cutting the sutures tied across the midline. This will loosen the suspension without totally affecting the integrity of the support. Cutting the sutures across the midline is usually reserved for patients who are in urinary retention for approximately 4 to 6 weeks following the surgery and who exhibit a good bladder contraction. Success of bladder neck suspension procedures that utilize absorbable sutures suggests that cutting of the non-absorbable sutures used in endoscopic suspensions should not affect the integrity of the surgery after the retropubic scarring has occurred. In patients with a documented bladder contraction and inability to void, obstruction may be presumed and cutting of one suture may be adequate to "release" the suspension.

Retention following sling surgery is more common and is related to the higher degree of urethral obstruction. Usually, a patient with good preoperative bladder contractility will void to completion after the bladder has been allowed to compensate for the increased outflow resistance. When a neurologic entity is responsible for a noncontractile bladder and poor urethral closure (type III stress incontinence), intermittent catheterization should be anticipated and taught preoperatively. If a frequent high-pressure detrusor hyperreflexia or a noncompliant detrusor is present, high storage pressures between intermittent catheterizations may predispose the patient to upper tract problems. A full urodynamic evaluation is essential before increasing outlet resistance in these patients (e.g., spinal cord injury, spina bifida, following radiation, and following radical hysterectomy).

SUMMARY

The diagnosis and therapy of incontinence in the female patient should be approached in a simple and orderly fashion. The majority of patients are easily diagnosed and treated by current techniques. Patients who present with a complex history, an abnormal simplified examination, or a history of unsuccessful prior surgery require additional meticulous evaluation. The selection of therapy should be based on an accepted procedure that addresses the underlying pathophysiology, is commensurate with the skills of the surgeon, and provides a successful result for the patient.

References

Cited References

1. Shortliffe L, Stamey TA: Urinary incontinence in the female. In Walsh PC, Perlmutter AD, Gittes RF, Stamey TA, eds: Campbell's Urology, 5th ed. Philadelphia, WB Saunders Co, 1986, pp 2680–2711.
2. Marshall VF, Marchetti AA, Krantz KE: Correction of stress incontinence by simple vesicourethral suspension. Surg Gynecol Obstet 88:590, 1949.
3. Marchetti AA: Urinary incontinence. JAMA 162:1366, 1956.
4. Jeffcoate T, Roberts H.: Stress incontinence of urine. J Obstet Gynecol 59:685, 1952.
5. Hodgkinson CP: Stress urinary incontinence in the female. Surg Gynecol Obstet 102:595, 1965.
6. Greenwald SW, et al.: Cystourethrography as a diagnostic aid in stress incontinence. Obstet Gynecol 29:324, 1967.
7. Tanagho EA: Simplified cystography in stress urinary incontinence. Br J Urol 46:295, 1974.
8. Green TH, Jr: The problem of urinary stress incontinence in the female: an appraisal of its current status. Obstet Gynecol Surv 23:603, 1968.
9. Green TH, Jr: Urinary stress incontinence: pathophysiology, diagnosis and classification. In Buchsbaum HJ, Schmidt JD, eds: Gynecologic and Obstetric Urology. Philadelphia, WB Saunders Co, 1978.
10. McGuire EJ: Combined radiographic and manometric assessment of urethral sphincter function. J Urol 118:632, 1977.
11. McGuire EJ, Lytton B, Kohorn EI, Pepe V: The value of urodynamic testing in stress urinary incontinence. J Urol 124:256, 1980.
12. Massey A, Abrams P: Urodynamics of the female lower urinary tract. Urol Clin North Am 12(2):236, 1985.
13. Constantinou CE, Govan DE: Spatial distribution and timing of transmitted and reflexly generated urethral pressures in healthy women. J Urol 127:964, 1982.
14. Constantinou CE: Resting and stress urethral pressures as a clinical guide to the mechanism of continence in the female patient. Urol Clin North Am 12(2):247, 1985.
15. Hilton P, Stanton SL: Urethral pressure measurements by microtransducer: the results in symptom-free women and in those with genuine stress incontinence. Br J Obstet Gynaecol 90:919, 1983.
16. Toews HA: Intraurethral and intravesical pressures in normal and stress-incontinent women. J Obstet Gynecol 29:613, 1967.
17. Smith ARB, Warrell DW: Proceedings of the International Continence Society, 1985, p 300.
18. Fanciullacci F, Sandri S, Politi P, et al: Sacral evoked potential in normal women and women with stress incontinence. Neurol Urodynamics 6(4):321, 1987.
19. Karlson S: Experimental studies on the functioning of the female urinary bladder and urethra. Acta Obstet Gynecol Scand 32:285, 1953.
20. Laval KU, Lutzeyer W: Stress-incontinence as a stimulus for detrusor hyperreflexia. Proceedings of the ICS, Rome, 1979, pp 197–200.
21. Mahoney DT, Laferte RO, Blais DJ: Incontinence of urine due to instability of micturition reflexes. Urology 15:229, 1980.
22. Lose G, Jorgensen L, Johnsen A: Predictive value of detrusor instability index in surgery for female urinary incontinence. Neurourology and Urodynamics 7:141, 1988.
23. Lockhart JL, Vorstman B, Politano VA: Anti-incontinence surgery in females with detrusor instability. Neurourology and Urodynamics 3:201, 1984.
24. Pou-Song JM, Lockhart JL, Suarez A, Lansman H, Politano VA: Female urinary incontinence: Preoperative selection, surgical complications, and results. J Urol 136:831, 1986.
25. Hodgkinson CP: Stress urinary incontinence—1970. Am J Obstet Gynecol 108:1141, 1970.
26. Arnold EP, Webster JR, Loose H, Brown ADG, Turner-Warwick RT, Whiteside CG, Jequier AM: Urodynamics of female incontinence: factors influencing the results of surgery. Am J Obstet Gynecol 117:805, 1973.

27. Bates CP, Whiteside CG, Turner-Warwick RT: Synchronous cine-pressure flow cystometry with special reference to stress and urge incontinence. Br J Urol 42:714, 1970.
28. Stanton SL, Cardozo L, Williams JE, Ritchie D, Allan V: Clinical and urodynamic features of failed incontinence surgery in the female. Obstet Gynecol 51:515, 1978.
29. Jørgensen L, Lose G, Mølsted-Pederson L: Vaginal repair in female motor urge incontinence. Eur Urol 13:382, 1987.
30. Jørgensen L, Lose G, Mortensen SO, et al: The Bursh colposuspension for urinary stress incontinence in patients with stable and unstable detrusor function. Neurolol Urodyn, in press.
31. Wilkie, DHL, Stanton SLS, Barzilai M: Combined stress incontinence and detrusor instability: Does colposuspension help? Proceedings of the ICS, 16th Annual Meeting, Boston, 1986, pp 618–620.
32. Beck RP, Arnusch D, King C: Results in treating 210 patients with detrusor overactivity incontinence of urine. Am J Obstet Gynecol 125:593, 1976.
33. Meyhoff HH, Walter S, Gerstenberg TC, Olesen KP, Nordling J, Pedersen PH, Hald T: Incontinence surgery in female motor urge incontinence. Acta Obstet Gynecol Scand 62:365, 1983.
34. Wheelahan JB: The pressure-volume plot and prediction of treatment outcome in female incontinence. Br J Urol 58:514, 1986.
35. McGuire EJ, Lytton B: The pubovaginal sling in stress urinary incontinence. J Urol 119:82, 1978.
36. Nichols DH: The sling operations. In Cantor EB, ed: Female Urinary Stress Incontinence. Springfield, Ill, Charles C Thomas, 1979.
37. Raz S: Modified bladder neck suspension for female stress incontinence. Urology 17:82, 1981.
38. Lewis FI, Lockhart JL, Politano VA: Periurethral polytetrafluorethylene injections in incontinent female subjects with neurogenic bladder disease. J Urol 131:459, 1984.
39. Bruskewitz R, Raz S, Kaufman JJ: Treatment of urinary incontinence with the artificial sphincter. J Urol 126:469, 1981.
40. Scott FB: The use of the artificial sphincter in the treatment of urinary incontinence in the female patient. Urol Clin North Am 12(2):305, 1985.
41. Zimmern P, Hadley R, Leach G, et al: Transvaginal closure of the bladder neck and placement of a suprapubic catheter for destroyed urethra after long term indwelling catheter. J Urol 134:554, 1985.
42. Reed R, Snyder K, Fruchtman B: Closure of the bladder neck in patients undergoing continent vesicostomy for urinary incontinence. J Urol 120:40, 1978.
43. Stanton SL: The choice of surgery for incontinence. Br J Urol 54:74, 1982.
44. Burch JC: Cooper's ligament urethrovesical suspension for stress incontinence. Am J Obstet Gynecol 100:764, 1968.
45. Lee RA: Correcting recurrent stress incontinence. Contemp Ob/Gyn 12:33, 1978.
46. Pereyra AJ, Lebherz TB: Combined urethrovesical suspension and vaginourethroplasty for correction of urinary stress incontinence. Obstet Gynecol 30:537, 1967.
47. Hadley HR, Zimmern PE, Staskin DR, Raz S: Transvaginal needle bladder neck suspension. Urol Clin North Am 12(2): 291, 1985.
48. Stamey TA: Endoscopic suspension of the vesical neck for urinary incontinence. Surg Gynecol Obstet 136:547, 1973.
49. Stamey TA: Endoscopic suspension of the vesical neck for urinary incontinence in females: report on 203 consecutive patients. Ann Surg 192:465, 1980.
50. Loughlin KR, Bittes RF, Klein LA, Whitmore WF III: The comparative medical costs of two major procedures available for the treatment of stress urinary incontinence. J Urol 127:536, 1982.
51. Hodgkinson CP, Stanton SL: Retropubic urethropexy or colposuspension. In Stanton SL, Tanagho EA, eds: Surgery of Female Incontinence. New York, Springer-Verlag, 1980.
52. Drukker BH: Anterior colporrhaphy. In Buchsbaum HJ, Schmidt JD, eds: Gynecologic and Obstetric Urology. Philadelphia, WB Saunders Co, 1978.
53. Green TH, Jr: Vaginal repair. In Stanton SL, Tanagho EA, eds: Surgery of Female Incontinence. New York, Springer-Verlag, 1980.
54. Burchell C: The umbrella pack to control pelvic hemorrhage. Conn Med 32:734, 1968.
55. Stanton SL, Cardozo L: Results of colposuspension operation for incontinence and prolapse. Br J Obstet Gynecol 86:693, 1979.

Uncited Reference

Burch JC: Urethrovaginal fixation to Cooper's ligament for correction of stress incontinence. Am J Obstet Gynecol 100:768, 1961.

COMPLICATIONS OF SURGERY FOR MALE URINARY INCONTINENCE

37

J. Keith Light

INTRODUCTION

Urinary incontinence in the adult male is most often secondary to prostatectomy. Although it is estimated to develop in approximately 1 percent of patients who undergo transurethral resection for benign prostatic hypertrophy, the figure is higher for patients who undergo radical prostatectomy. The precise incidence of patients requiring surgery for severe urinary incontinence following radical prostatectomy is unknown at present, but previous reports indicate that it ranges from between 2 and 15 percent.[1,2] Lesser degrees of stress incontinence occur more frequently, with the reported incidence being as high as 87 percent.[3] Trauma and neurologic diseases may also result in urinary incontinence. The patient today has a much greater chance of maintaining urinary continence than previously. Frequently, a combination of approaches is necessary to achieve this. Each patient needs to be assessed individually prior to surgery.

Surgical procedures to correct male urinary incontinence can be divided into three broad groups as follows:

1. Reconstruction of a new sphincteric mechanism, in which the patient's own tissues, usually the bladder neck, are used to reconstruct a new sphincteric mechanism.
2. Substitution for the damaged sphincteric mechanism, which usually entails compression of the tissues with a device, e.g., an artificial sphincter.
3. Compression of tissue, which is accomplished with injected materials, such as Teflon, or the use of a fascial sling.

RECONSTRUCTION OF A NEW SPHINCTERIC MECHANISM

Inherent to the success of this procedure is the normality of the bladder muscle; the tissue must be supple with normal vascularity and intact innervation. Reconstruction of the bladder neck to form a new functioning sphincter utilizes either the anterior or the posterior (i.e., trigone) bladder wall.

The trigonal tubularization described by Young and Leadbetter is seldom applicable to adult males, as incontinence in this group usually follows prostatectomy.[4,5] The majority of prostatectomies are now performed transurethrally, which results in scarring of the trigone secondary to the resection, rendering the tissues rigid and unsuitable for reconstruction. More recently, Tanagho and associates have described reconstructing a new sphincter using the anterior bladder wall.[6] This method avoids the scar tissue caused by the prostatectomy. In essence, a tube is formed from the anterior bladder wall, which is anastomosed to the prostatic capsule.

The main drawback to attempted reconstruction of a new sphincteric mechanism is the low success rate. The failure rate with the Tanagho anterior bladder tube ranges from 30 to 50 percent.[7] Leadbetter recently reported a 43 percent failure rate in adults after a 10- to 20-year follow-up using his technique.[8] Other complications include stenosis of the reconstructed tube, resulting in obstruction. It is, therefore, not uncommon to see patients who develop a combination of urinary incontinence and urinary retention following this type of reconstruction.

The initial reconstruction stands the best chance of success. Multiple operations to reconstruct the bladder neck are to be avoided.

SUBSTITUTION OF THE SPHINCTERIC MECHANISM

Substitution for a damaged or nonfunctioning sphincteric mechanism implies the use of a device. Essential to the success of this approach are the normal vascularity of the tissue and the use of compression forces less than the systolic blood pressure to avoid ischemic necrosis.

In 1961, Berry described the use of an acrylic block placed under the bulbocavernosus muscle to compress the bulbar urethra.[9] Kaufman, from 1968 to 1974, described several models of a silicone gel prosthesis designed to achieve continence by passive compression of the bulbous urethra.[10] At best, the long-term results were only moderate, with a 61 percent success rate. The reasons for failure were infection, urethral erosion as the pressure was not satisfactorily controlled, and recurrent incontinence, probably secondary to pressure atrophy of the tissue beneath the device. Neither the Berry nor the Kaufman device is in widespread use today.

Rosen introduced his prosthesis in 1976.[11] The device was inflated by means of a pump-reservoir located in the scrotum. The device was connected to an inflatable "cuff," which was placed around the bulbar urethra and held in place with two prongs. Although initial results were encouraging, late complications were common. These included infection and, particularly, urethral erosion. The latter complication occurred because the pressure in the "cuff" was controlled by the patient and not by the device. The patient continued to fill the cuff under pressure until continence was achieved. Unfortunately, this was at the expense of urethral viability. This device, as those described above, now belongs in the archives.

The AMS800 Artificial Urinary Sphincter

The first AMS artificial urinary sphincter was implanted by Scott in 1973.[12] Numerous refinements have resulted in the current device, the AMS800 series (Fig. 37–1). The main advantages of this device over previous devices are

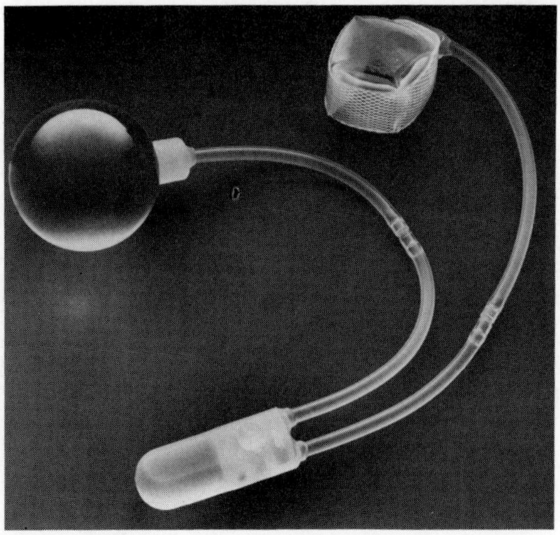

Figure 37–1. AMS 800 Artificial urinary sphincter. (Courtesy of American Medical Systems, Inc., Minnetonka, Minnesota.)

1. Pressure regulation by the balloon and not by the patient
2. Prevention of stress incontinence with placement of the balloon in the submuscular, extraperitoneal position
3. Application to sphincteric incontinence of diverse etiology
4. Implantation at the bladder neck in both sexes or bulbar urethra in males
5. The ability to activate and deactivate the device without surgery
6. Unobstructed urination

This device has proved to be the most reliable method thus far for restoring urinary continence in males. However, two factors have emerged that place the patient in a high-risk category. Both adversely affect the vascularity of the tissue at the cuff site and thus increase the risk of ischemic necrosis with compression. Previous radiation to the pelvic area invariably diminishes the blood supply to the urethra and bladder neck. The incidence of cuff erosion in this group of patients is therefore increased. Previous urethral damage, e.g., stricture or reconstruction, similarly impairs the blood supply and also increases the risk of erosion. Although the bladder neck is the preferred site for the cuff placement, this is seldom possible in the adult male because an operative procedure or trauma has previously involved this site. The bulbous urethra is used to place the cuff if the bladder neck is unsuitable.

With the new artificial urinary sphincter, the incidence of cuff erosion is definitely related to the balloon pressure and tissue vascularity. With normal vascularity, a 61 to 70 cm balloon is used for a bulbar sphincter and a 71 to 80 cm balloon for a bladder neck sphincter. However, if the tissues appear unsuitable at the time of surgery, lower pressure balloons are recommended. It should be remembered that the artificial urinary sphincter is used to treat urinary incontinence secondary to sphincteric weakness, not abnormalities of bladder function. Appropriate urodynamic evaluation is therefore essential prior to surgery to characterize bladder function. The success with the artificial urinary sphincter is directly related to the type of bladder function present.[13]

Standardization of the surgical technique and improved reliability of the device have significantly decreased the complications. Problems may still occur, however, and can prove frustrating to both physician and patient. In the author's series of 37 patients treated with the artificial sphincter for post-prostatectomy incontinence, the success rate was 94.5 percent. However, 20 percent of these patients who underwent preoperative radiotherapy developed cuff erosion.

An understanding of the device mechanism is important when considering the causes of malfunction. The control-pump assembly contains the fluid resistors, one-way valves, and poppet valves. The balloon pushes fluid across the resistors, first to fill the pump and then to fill the cuff. It takes approximately 10 minutes for the cuff to become fully pressurized in vivo for any given balloon pressure. Upon squeezing the pump, fluid passes easily and immediately to the balloon. Upon releasing the pump, fluid is siphoned from the cuff to immediately refill the pump. Thus, repeated pumping deflates the cuff. When the cuff is empty, the pump no longer re-expands and stays "flat." Automatic refilling of the pump and then the cuff occurs because of the pressure differential between the balloon and cuff.

The following clinical and surgical protocol is used by the author to diagnose complications resulting from the artificial sphincter.

Clinical Protocol (Fig. 37–2)

Examination and manipulation of the pump is the single most important aspect of the clinical evaluation. The most common problem occurring postoperatively is urinary incontinence. There are two basic causes for persistent or recurrent urinary incontinence following insertion of the artificial sphincter. The first involves the device itself, and the second is related to abnormal detrusor behavior.

A urine culture is also performed to ensure that the urine is sterile. If not, the appropriate antibiotic treatment is given.

Device Failure

A decrease in the closing pressure of the cuff accounts for most instances of device failure. The two most common causes for this are a leak in the device and pressure atrophy of the tissue

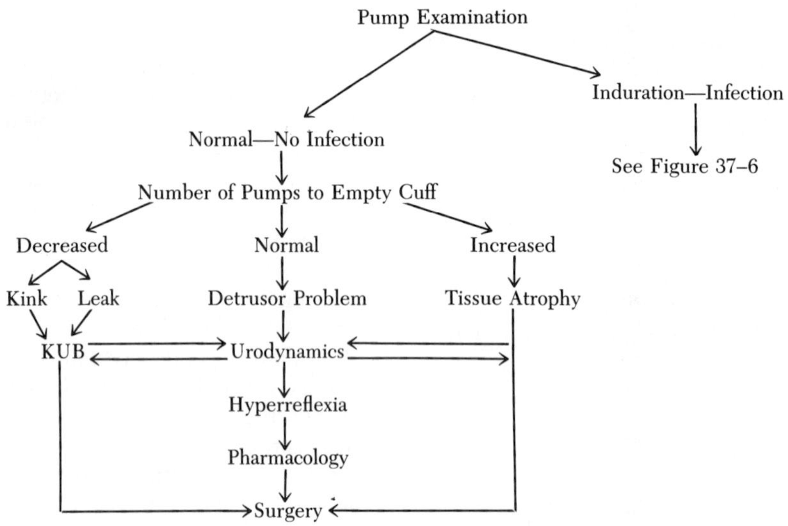

Figure 37–2. Trouble shooting—clinical protocol.

beneath the cuff. Other problems include tube kinks, debris in the system, and a restrictive sheath around the reservoir.

Leak in the Device. The fluid loss may be gradual or sudden, depending on the size of the leak, and may occur at any stage following implantation of the device. Characteristically, the patient notes that the number of pumps required to empty the cuff has decreased or that the pump does not refill, i.e., it stays "flat." This can be easily confirmed on clinical examination of the pump. A plain x-ray of the pelvis may show total absence of dye within the system or a decrease in the balloon shape. It should be remembered, however, that a balloon volume of only 10 ml may look radiologically normal. Radiologically, a normal-appearing balloon does not exclude the presence of a slow leak.

In the past, the cuff was the most common site for a leak, followed by the balloon. In previously reported series in which repeat surgery was required for a mechanical problem, a cuff leak was responsible in 56 percent of instances of a leak and a balloon leak in 13 percent.[14] The introduction of the silicone-coated cuff in 1983, however, has sharply diminished the incidence of cuff leaks by preventing friction between its inner soft backing and outer firm backing. The author has implanted the silicone-coated cuff in 75 patients of various ages since 1983. The follow-up has ranged from 4 to 60 months with a mean of 36 months. No leak has occurred to date in any of the device components, indicating a significant improvement in its mechanical reliability compared with that in earlier series. The site of the leak is determined at surgery.

Pressure Atrophy. A variable degree of pressure atrophy inevitably occurs beneath the cuff, the severity of which is related to the balloon pressure. This problem is now the most frequent reason for sphincter revision. The pressure-volume relationship of the balloon is sigmoid shaped. The pressure, therefore, will drop sharply for a relatively small decrease in volume below a critical balloon volume of approximately 14 ml. Significant pressure atrophy will decrease the cuff closing pressure by "siphoning" fluid from the balloon, thus decreasing the pressure. In an attempt to compensate for this decrease in balloon volume and, therefore, pressure, the manufacturers have recommended increasing the amount of fluid initially placed in the balloon from 16 to 22 ml. This additional fluid has minimal effect on the final balloon pressure. There is a limit, however, on the ability of the cuff to transfer adequate pressure to the tissue in the presence of significant atrophy, and eventually, the cuff becomes inefficient although the balloon volume and pressure are normal.

The AMS800 control pump assembly expresses approximately 0.75 ml of fluid with each pump. This is in contrast to the AMS791/2, which has a pump volume of 0.50 ml. Assuming that no leak exists, the number of pumps required to empty the cuff gives a reasonably accurate estimate regarding cuff volume to be made. Generally, a snug-fitting cuff will contain 0.75 to 2.0 ml depending on the position, i.e., in bulbous urethra or bladder neck, respectively. A 4.0-ml volume pump (5 pumps) for a bladder neck cuff or 3.0-ml (4 pumps) for a bulbar urethral cuff usually indicates that the cuff is too large. This can be determined clinically by counting the number of pumps required to empty the cuff.

In a reported series, these two problems—a leak in the device and pressure atrophy—were responsible for 88 percent of the malfunctions that resulted in repeat surgery following inserting of the artificial sphincter.[14] It is, therefore, possible to diagnose 88 percent of the possible mechanical malfunctions that result in the need for further surgery simply by clinical examination of the pump. If doubt is still present, urodynamic evaluation can be performed to confirm that the cuff is inefficient.

Debris. Occasionally, debris within the system can simulate a leak in the device. The patient, however, usually reports that the number of pumps required to empty the cuff varies, as does the continence status, because of the intermittent obstruction to the resistors caused by the debris. This obstruction prevents full cuff pressurization. Primary malfunction of the control assembly is extremely rare, and it follows, therefore, that the introduction of debris occurs at the time of surgery or following a leak.

Kink. A kink in the tubing causing incomplete refilling of the cuff or pump may also simulate a leak. A straight x-ray of the pelvis will often identify the site of the kink as well as show dye within some components of the system. The specific abnormality found on pump manipulation will depend on the site of the kink. If it occurs between the cuff and pump, the pump will refill very slowly following the first manipulation. If, however, the kink lies between the pump and balloon, difficulty will occur when the device is initially manipulated.

Restrictive Reservoir Sheath. Occasionally, a restrictive sheath forms around the reservoir postoperatively. This results in the inability of the reservoir to distend to accept all the fluid from the cuff. Characteristically, the first couple of pumps are easy, followed by a progressive increase in resistance as the elasticity of the sheath is exceeded. The significance of a restrictive sheath is that it may prevent complete cuff deflation and therefore interfere with adequate urination. Urinary incontinence associated with this problem is usually an overflow type secondary to incomplete bladder emptying. This can be avoided by ensuring that the patient completely empties the cuff on a regular basis in the postoperative period.

Abnormal Tissues

If there is no change in the pumping characteristics of the device, the reason for the incontinence usually lies within the tissues, i.e., the bladder. Detrusor hyperreflexia and poor bladder compliance are two common causes. Both conditions result in an increase in intravesical pressure at variable volumes. If this exceeds the cuff pressure, fluid will move out of the cuff, resulting in a decrease in the closing pressure and, therefore, urinary leakage. Urodynamic evaluation is essential to diagnose this problem. Cystometry is now routinely performed postoperatively in this situation to categorize bladder function.

Detrusor function may change following insertion of the device. This occurs most commonly in patients in whom the cause of incontinence is neuropathic and is probably related to the increased sensory stimuli from detrusor distention. Altered detrusor function is in no way related to the mere presence of the device but to the effects of bladder outlet occlusion resulting in probable increased sensory input from increased bladder distention. Frequently, preoperative hyperreflexia is initially aggravated or detrusor instability precipitated by the surgery, and both conditions are treated initially with anticholinergics. Flow rate and post-void residual tests are also performed to exclude the presence of an outflow obstruction and/or inefficient bladder emptying. An overflow type of incontinence can thus be excluded.

Static urethral pressure profilometry with the cuff open and closed is no longer recommended to assess cuff efficiency. A more accurate estimate can be obtained using retrograde perfusion "sphincterometry," in which a catheter is placed into the distal penile urethra, which is then manually occluded against the catheter. Fluid is then perfused through the catheter at 60 ml/minute using a continuous infusion pump. A simultaneous pressure tracing is obtained. The pressure at which the graph becomes horizontal is the "opening pressure" of the cuff. This should be equal to or higher than the lowest range of the balloon pressure for the cuff to be considered effective. If this "opening pressure" is much lower than the balloon pressure, the cuff is inefficient.

Profilometry with the cuff open is a general measure of outflow resistance and may indicate an inadequate sphincterotomy or poor cuff opening. Pressure-flow studies with simultaneous video cystourethrography performed transurethrally are an excellent means of confirming abnormal detrusor function or outlet obstruction as a cause for the urinary leakage.

Surgical Protocol (Fig. 37–3)

The first step in surgical protocol is to perform retrograde gas sphincterometry to determine the "opening pressure" of the cuff. This correlates well with the results obtained using water as a medium and is quicker during the surgery. The same rationale applies as described above; this measurement also serves as a baseline for comparison following "corrective" surgery (Fig. 37–4). Cystoscopy is performed to assess the cuff site and exclude an erosion.

The electrical test is performed following exposure of the device connectors to determine the presence or absence of a leak. If a leak is found, the damaged component is exchanged and the system refilled. In the absence of a leak, the balloon volume is measured. With significant pressure atrophy around the bladder neck, this volume will be significantly less than the original volume inserted. Finally, the cuff volume is measured. The total volume of the cuff and balloon should equal the original volume inserted if the inefficient cuff is secondary to pressure atrophy and not secondary to a leak. A smaller cuff will correct the problem, and repeat gas sphincterometry will show the expected increase in the "opening pressure" (Fig. 37–5).

In the presence of urinary incontinence secondary to pressure atrophy, a smaller cuff is required to restore continence. The mere addition of fluid to the balloon without exchanging the cuff is contraindicated in this situation. Provided the balloon pressure is kept constant, progressive atrophy does not occur. Multiple operations to repeatedly replace a smaller and smaller cuff are, therefore, unnecessary. Rarely will the total volume have decreased in the absence of a leak.

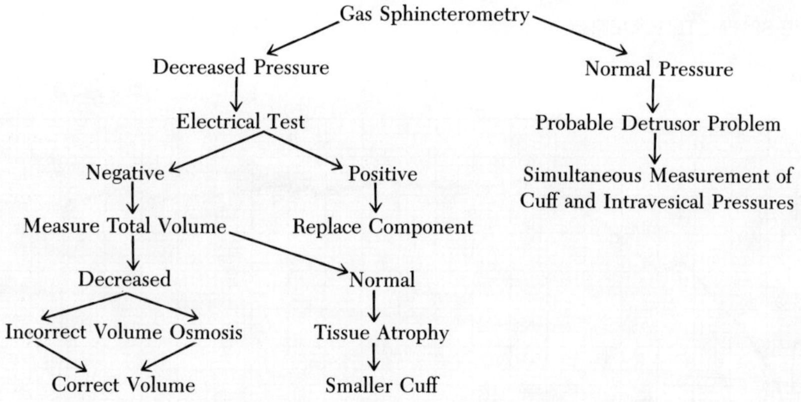

Figure 37–3. Trouble shooting—surgical protocol.

Original insertion of the incorrect volume is one possible cause of incontinence, whereas fluid loss secondary to osmosis from a hypo-osmolar mixture is another. Replacement of the fluid will solve the problem. In the event that the opening pressure is normal, the problem will usually involve the bladder. This, however, should have been suspected on preoperative evaluation. An augmentation cystoplasty may be necessary with poor bladder compliance or uncontrolled hyperreflexia.

Infection (See Fig. 37–6)

Infection involving the artificial sphincter is a serious complication, and removal of the device is inevitable. Any induration around the pump, local skin hyperemia, or pain with manipulation suggests infection. The sudden onset of pain and swelling around the pump suggests cuff erosion. In addition, a persistent, burning pain in the perineum in the presence of a bulbar cuff points to an impending cuff erosion.

In the presence of a suspected infection, exclusion of a cuff erosion is imperative. This is best achieved with a cystoscopy in the operating room, with arrangements being made to proceed with removal of the device if necessary. A urethrogram is contraindicated because this may contaminate a sterile erosion or fail to show extravasation if the erosion is small. Only the cuff may have to be removed if a sterile erosion of

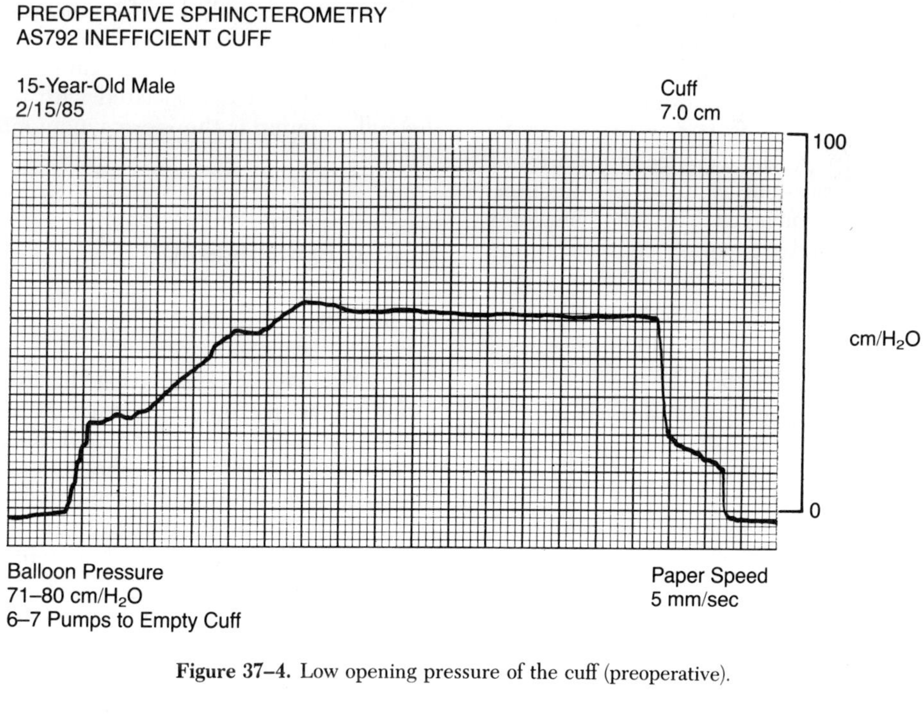

Figure 37–4. Low opening pressure of the cuff (preoperative).

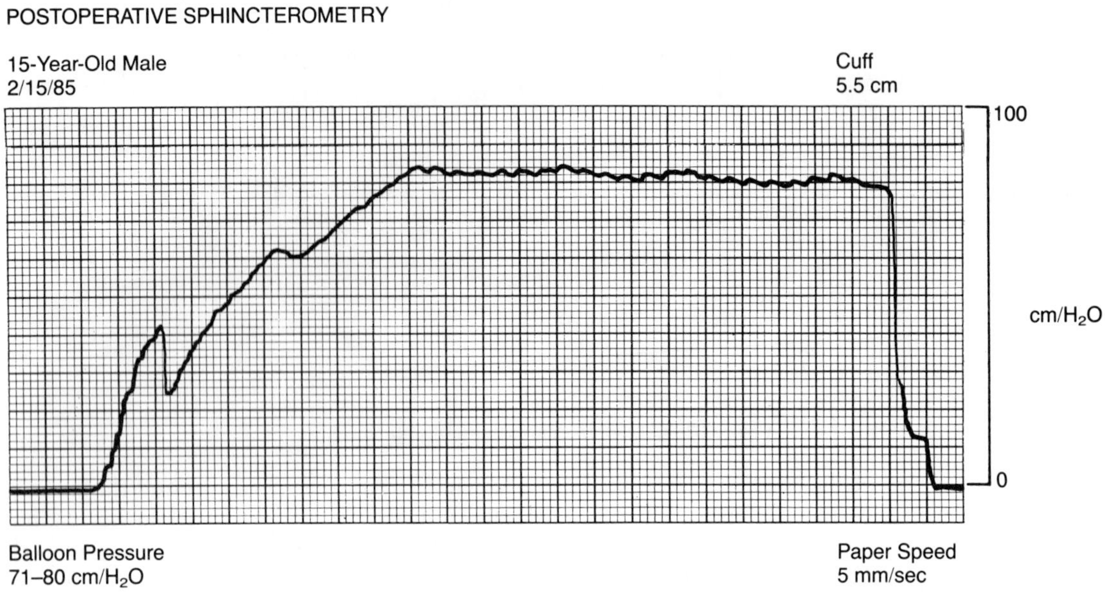

Figure 37–5. Increase in cuff opening pressure following repair surgery.

the bladder neck exists, or it may be relocated, if possible, with a bulbar sphincter. Removal of the entire device is necessary, however, with an erosion in the presence of infected urine. Cystoscopy may reveal mucosal edema at the cuff site without an apparent erosion. In this situation, the device should be deactivated and a full course of intravenous and oral antibiotics given. Repeat cystoscopy should be performed 6 weeks later to ensure that a small erosion has not been missed. The device may then be activated if the mucosa overlying the cuff site appears healthy, and oral antibiotics are continued for several months.

Patients with an infected device rarely present with the usual systemic signs of an infection, e.g., leukocytosis or fever. The key symptoms and signs described are usually confined to the pump area. If the infection is left untreated, eventual erosion of the pump or cuff will occur.

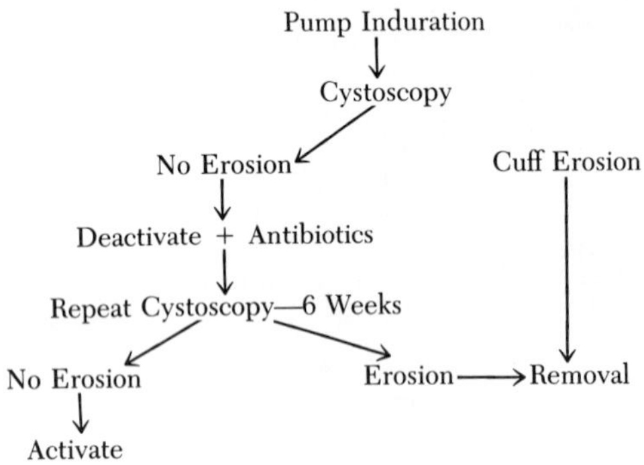

Figure 37–6. Infection protocol.

Several methods have been attempted to salvage a known infected device; they include long-term antibiotic treatment, irrigation of the prevesical space with the appropriate antibiotic solution, and exchanging the infected device. This author, however, has not succeeded in salvaging a known infected device using all three of these methods and, therefore, has abandoned this approach for the artificial sphincter. An infected device that does not respond to antibiotic treatment or that is associated with erosion of the cuff or pump is therefore synonymous with removal.

TISSUE COMPRESSION

Injections

In 1963, Sachse reported on the use of sclerosing injections to cure urinary incontinence, but the procedure was abandoned owing to the occurrence of pulmonary emboli.[16] Politano refined this technique by injecting Polytef paste (Teflon) around the urethra to increase outflow resistance. Success rates of 73 percent in males have been reported.[17] Frequently, however, more than one injection is required. Although the simplicity of the procedure is indeed attractive, the occurrence of emboli to distant organs has been reported, the clinical significance of which at present is unsettled. Other complications have been few and limited to infection, low grade fever, and prolonged urinary retention. Contrary to popular belief, however, insertion of the artificial urinary sphincter following a failed Teflon injection almost always fails. Two reasons account for this: (1) presence of a subclinical infection at the injection site that contaminates the artificial urinary sphincter at insertion and (2) difficulty in defining tissue planes for accurate placement of the cuff because of the fibrosis or the amount of Teflon present.

Fascial Sling

Whereas fascial slings have been used with success in female patients, this method is not applicable to male patients with post-prostatectomy incontinence. Scarring of the bladder neck renders placement of the fascial sling extremely difficult, and the rigid nature of the tissue prevents adequate occlusion of the lumen. Although reports attest to the successful use of fascial slings for males with neuropathic urinary incontinence secondary to a decentralized bladder, continence is achieved at the expense of requiring intermittent self-catheterization.[18] Owing to the now significant improvement in the reliability of the artificial urinary sphincter, the author prefers insertion of the device to the use of the fascial sling. Previously, the main objection to the artificial sphincter was the relatively high reoperation rate for device malfunction. The silicone-coated cuff has now proved to be very reliable, with a follow-up of 5 years revealing no malfunction. The ability to urinate per urethra allows for more comprehensive restoration of lower urinary tract function and therefore patient satisfaction.

CONCLUSION

The adult male with urinary incontinence has a far greater chance of achieving continence now than ever before. The surgical procedure to be performed must be meticulously chosen after consideration of all the complications and success rate.

References

1. Walsh PC: Radical prostatectomy for treatment of localized prostatic cancer. Urol Clin North Am 7:583, 1980.
2. Nichols RT, Barry JM, Hodges CV: Morbidity of radical prostatectomy for multifocal Stage I adenocarcinoma. J Urol 117:83, 1977.
3. Rudy DC, Woodside JR, Crawford ED: Urodynamic evaluation of incontinence in patients undergoing modified Campbell radical retropubic prostatectomy: a prospective study. J Urol 132:708, 1984.
4. Young HH: An operation for the cure of incontinence of urine. Surg Gynecol Obstet 28:84, 1919.
5. Leadbetter GW Jr: Surgical correction of total urinary incontinence. J Urol 91:281, 1964.
6. Tanagho EA, Smith DR, Meyers FH, et al: Mechanism of urinary incontinence, Volume II. Technique for surgical correction of incontinence. J Urol 101:305, 1958.
7. Tanagho EA: Bladder neck reconstruction for total urinary incontinence: 10 years of experience. J Urol 125:321–326, 1981.
8. Leadbetter GW Jr: Surgical reconstruction for complete urinary incontinence: 10- to 22-year followup. J Urol 133:205, 1985.
9. Berry JL: A new procedure for correction of urinary incontinence: preliminary report. J Urol 85:771, 1961.
10. Kaufman JJ: Treatment of post-prostatectomy incontinence using a silicone-gel prosthesis. Br J Urol 45:646, 1973.
11. Rosen M: A simple artificial implantable sphincter. Br J Urol 48:675, 1976.
12. Scott FB: Treatment of urinary incontinence by implantable prosthetic sphincter. Urology 1:252, 1973.
13. Light JK, Scott FB: Use of the artificial urinary sphincter in spinal cord injury patients. J Urol 130:1127, 1983.
14. Light JK, Scott FB: The artificial urinary sphincter in children. Br J Urol 56:54–57, 1984.
15. Webster GD, Sikelnich SA: Troubleshooting the malfunctioning Scott artificial urinary sphincter. J Urol 131:269, 1984.
16. Sachse H: Sclerosing therapy in urinary incontinence: indications, results, complications. Urol Int (Basel) 15:225–244, No. 4, 1963.
17. Politano VA: Periurethral Teflon injection for urinary incontinence. Urol Clin North Am Volume 5, No 2, pp 415–422, 1978.
18. Raz S, McGuire EJ, Ehrlich RM, Zeidman EJ, Wang SC, Alarcon A, Schmidtbauer C, McLaughin S: Fascial sling to correct male neurogenic sphincter incompetence: The McGuire/Raz Approach. Urol 139:528–531, 1988.

COMPLICATIONS OF SCROTAL SURGERY

38

(Including Vasectomy, Vasovasostomy, and Orchiopexy)

Mark B. Sender • Martin A. Koyle • Jacob Rajfer

The risks and complications of scrotal surgery and the prevention and management of these complications require an understanding of the normal anatomy and function of the scrotum. Most of these concerns are related to the surgical incision as well as to general postoperative problems such as hemorrhage, infection, and edema.

ANATOMY

Generally, the scrotum is a pouch that holds the testes below the penis and pubic symphysis. A median septum partitions the testes, which are anchored to the scrotal sac inferiorly by the gubernaculum. The scrotal tissue is composed of an overlying layer of skin, a subcutaneous dartos muscle, and extensions from the anterior abdominal wall musculature, including the external spermatic fascia and muscle, the internal spermatic fascia and muscle (cremaster), and, occasionally, an extension of peritoneum, such as the tunica vaginalis.[1]

Within each scrotal compartment are the testis, epididymis, and spermatic cord. The blood supply to the scrotum is derived from the external pudendal artery, the internal pudendal artery, and branches of the vasal and testicular arteries. The blood supply to the scrotum courses from the lateral aspect of the scrotum toward the median raphe. Thus, in order to avoid unnecessary blood loss during surgery, transverse scrotal incisions parallel to these vessels should be made or, alternatively, incisions in the median raphe itself should be performed. The venous channels are usually parallel to the arterial supply. The lymphatic drainage is primarily to the superficial inguinal nodes so that scrotal infections may lead to tenderness and enlargement of these nodes. The rich blood supply and elasticity of the scrotal tissue allow for excellent healing, but its distensibility, anatomic dependency, and the existence of potential third spaces between the scrotal wall and the testes deprive the scrotum of the ability to confine hemorrhage or to prevent edema.

PRINCIPLES OF SCROTAL SURGERY

Consideration should be given to several general principles of scrotal surgery. The rich vascular network throughout the skin and dartos demands meticulous attention to hemostasis. To avoid postoperative hemorrhage, the method of closure utilized should also be meticulous, with attention to at least a two-layer closure that incorporates the dartos muscle in one layer and the skin in the other. A variety of compression and elevation techniques have been proposed to circumvent or minimize edema and hemorrhage in the postoperative period. Among these are bulky compression dressings, with or without scrotal support, suturing the most inferior part of the scrotum to the lower abdominal wall over gauze dressings,[2] and the turban compression technique,[3] which is what we utilize exclusively. We do not recommend the routine use of drains for primary, clean trans-scrotal surgeries such as hydrocelectomies.

Assessment and management of postoperative hemorrhage requires attention to the size and distribution of the hematoma, the evaluation of baseline bleeding studies, scrotal elevation, and patient immobilization. Serial physical examinations are necessary to rule out continued expansion of the hematoma. Typically a non-expanding, stable hematoma represents bleeding within the dartos, and exploration will seldom be required, or for that matter successful, in the evacuation of the hematoma. Similarly, there is a risk of introducing infection if one explores a non-infected hematoma. Exploration should be reserved for expanding hematomas and may be performed via the initial incision, although at times it may be necessary to enlarge the incision to better identify and control the sites of hemorrhage. With adequate hemostasis, a small rubber drain is recommended, followed by a careful two-layer closure and scrotal compression. The drain may be removed within the first 24 to 48 hours postoperatively. Considerable ecchymosis and edema with generalized discoloration of the scrotum and penis is almost inevitable and may last for several weeks.

It is not surprising that infectious complications may occur following scrotal surgery when one considers the pathogenic bacteria found in the perineum. However, the scrotum seems to be relatively resistant to postoperative infection, probably owing in part to its rich vascular supply as well as to some enhanced local tissue resistance to infection. When an infection does occur, it is usually superficial and managed with simple drainage and local wound care. Infection within the scrotum itself may occur after surgery or trauma to the scrotal contents. This usually requires incision and drainage of the scrotum. Should a large postoperative hematoma become infected, drainage may be prolonged and merit surgical debridement and excision of the infective source.

Infections in the scrotum can be minimized by adherence to a few simple surgical principles. First, shaving of the scrotal skin should be performed just prior to surgery rather than the day before. Second, prophylactic antibiotics should be given in the operating suite just prior to initiation of the surgical incision. Finally, it has been our experience that the use of braided sutures such as silk anywhere in the scrotum leads to a high incidence of infection, and this has precluded the use of such material in our clinic. There are instances in which surgical hemostasis is suboptimal or drainage is necessary; in such a setting, a small rubber drain placed in the most dependent portion of the scrotum is advisable to prevent intrascrotal collections.

On the surface, the attendant morbidity from scrotal surgery may not seem considerable unless one takes into account the expectation of the return to work soon after what is usually a minor surgical procedure as well as the attendant pain and discomfort that can prevent normal activity, often for many weeks.

COMPLICATIONS OF SURGICAL PROCEDURES

Orchiopexy

Cryptorchidism is a relatively common abnormality. Most surgical procedures (orchiopexy and, occasionally, orchiectomy) for this disorder are performed primarily in the pediatric population. The customary orchiopexy incision is made in the inguinal area, but the scrotal pouch (subdartos), which is created for the placement of the testis, is usually placed in the most dependent part of the scrotum. Occasionally, a subdartos pouch is also created to anchor the testis to the scrotum.[4] Besides scrotal pain, edema, hemorrhage, and infection, the complications from an orchiopexy are usually related to the testis itself. Some of these are: (1) loss of testicular viability as a result of poor mobilization of the spermatic cord or excessive tension on the testis after it is anchored to the scrotal wall, and (2) long-term complications such as infertility and testicular malignancy. If a malignancy occurs in a patient who has undergone an orchiopexy earlier in life, the nodal drainage of the scrotum may be altered, allowing for wider dissemination of lymphatic metastases.[5]

In the majority of patients who have undergone an orchiopexy for cryptorchidism, a patent processus vaginalis is usually found. This potential hernia sac is usually ligated during the procedure. Although rare, complications such as an ileus, a bowel injury, or bowel obstruction may occur from this part of the procedure. Occasionally, a true hernia is found during the orchiopexy, and a herniorrhaphy is indicated. Compromise of the testicular vasculature may occur during an orchiopexy because of excessive tightness of the internal inguinal ring, and this may ultimately lead to testicular infarction. This is most commonly due to compromise of the venous return of the spermatic vessels and, clinically, presents as a painful enlargement of the testis postoperatively. If this complication is not recognized early, particularly if it is bilateral, it may lead to testicular atrophy and hypogonadism. Every so often, particularly in the pediatric patient, a vas is accidentally excised with the hernia sac during an orchiopexy but more commonly during a hernia repair. If the complication is recognized at the time of injury, a microscopic attempt to attach the two ends of the vas may be feasible. Other rare complications of inguinal orchiopexy/hernia repair have included inadvertent bladder perforation or even partial cystectomy.

In certain boys whose testes are located intra-abdominally, a microscopic autotransplantation of the testis is required.[6] This involves anastomosis of the testicular artery and vein to the inferior epigastric artery and vein and placing the testis into the scrotum. In this procedure, the vas with its arterial supply is left undisturbed. Related complications may develop in the testis (infarction, edema), the scrotum (edema, hemorrhage, infection), or the abdomen (ileus, bowel obstruction).

Prosthetic Surgery

Remarkable advances have been achieved in the development of implantable, externally controlled continence and impotence devices. Control pump mechanisms have been designed for implantation within the scrotal compartment; however, infection remains one of the most serious complications of prosthetic surgery. The hallmark of control of infection lies in attention to good preoperative, operative, and postoperative care. Preoperatively, this includes verifying that the urine is sterile, taking a shower with a surgical scrub the day before and the morning of surgery, and removal of hair in the operating room immediately prior to the 10-minute surgical preparation. In addition, the patient should be draped with impermeable plastic or paper. Antibiotic or povidone-iodine (Betadine) irrigation should be used liberally to bathe the wound and prosthesis prior to implantation. Meticulous attention should be given to hemostasis and wound closure. The use of non-braided suture material is recommended. Preoperative prophylactic antibiotics should be administered and there is some support for their use into the postoperative period.[7] Urethral catheters, if used, should be removed in the recovery room if at all possible. If a penile prosthetic device becomes infected, drainage and removal of the device is the safest management. Occasionally, if the infection is not severe, treatment with intravenous antibiotics may salvage some of the devices. Most commonly encountered organisms are *Staphylococcus epidermidis*, *Pseudomonas aeruginosa*, and *Proteus* species.[7,8] A Gram stain of the wound may help in the identification of the organism, and appropriate antibiotic therapy may be initiated prior to laboratory identification of the offending organism.

Another complication that may occur with these prosthetic devices is implantation of the pump in the hemiscrotal compartment that is not on the patient's dominant side. Occasionally, this may necessitate repositioning the device. Erosion of a penile or anti-incontinence prosthesis universally requires removal of the device. If a semi-rigid penile prosthesis erodes through the glans or shaft of the penis, the device may be removed in the office. If any prosthetic device erodes through the urethra, removal of the device and urinary diversion, by either a urethral or preferably by a suprapubic tube, is indicated. A urethrogram should be performed 2 to 4 weeks after the eroded device is removed to determine the integrity of the urethra because urethral strictures are common in this setting.

Kinking of the tubing of these devices used to be a common problem before kink-proof tubing was developed. In addition, in the early models of inflatable penile prostheses, cylinder erosion and aneurysmal formation in the penis and cylinders were almost a certain end result because of the types of material used in the construction of these cylinders. Weakness in the cylinders at the site the tubing entered the cylinders resulted in rupture of the device and leakage of the fluid. These problems have generally been corrected by the use of stronger bioinert materials such as Gore-Tex.

Testicular prostheses, though non-physiologic, are cosmetically and psychologically enhancing therapeutic options for patients with an empty hemiscrotum with Klinefelter's syndrome, in which the testes are pea-sized and barely palpable. These devices may be inserted at the time of or following the orchiectomy. The device may be inserted via a scrotal or an inguinal approach.[9,10] One contraindication is the presence of an infection near the site of the implantation.[11] For young boys, the size of the prosthesis may need to be changed as the child ages because of expected growth of the normal testis and scrotum. We have observed extrusion of testicular prostheses through the scrotal wall and feel this is mainly due to aggressive dissection of a subdartos pocket. If the testicular prosthesis is not placed in the most dependent portion of the scrotum, a revision may be necessary. In patients with Klinefelter's syndrome, it is not necessary to perform an orchiectomy prior to inserting the testicular prosthesis. For some patients, retention of the testes will obviate the need for exogenous androgen therapy.

Vasectomy

Bilateral vasectomy is among the most commonly performed surgical procedures.[12] In general, it is safe, efficient, and economical in its goal to produce elective sterility in men. The operative procedure can be performed under local anesthesia as an outpatient in an office setting. To save time, the patient's scrotal hair should be shaved before he comes to the office. To facilitate the vasectomy and to help ensure potential reversibility, the vas remote from the epididymis in the mid-scrotum should be selected. The bilateral vasectomy can be performed through one midline or two separate scrotal incisions.

Occasional complications may occur following a vasectomy, but in general these are relatively minor. Scrotal discomfort and edema are treated by analgesia, scrotal support, and ice packs. Postoperative hemorrhage and subsequent hematoma are best contained by careful hemostasis with the cautery during the procedure and by use of a turban dressing for the first 24 hours after the procedure. Occasionally, incision and drainage of a hematoma are required. Epididymitis is reported to occur in 0.4–6.1 percent of patients and is probably the result of epididymal engorgement as a result of the vas ligation.[13] Symptomatic short-term therapy with non-steroid, anti-inflammatory drugs usually resolves the condition. Non-resolution of symptoms may herald sperm granuloma formation in the epididymis, which we feel is the result of epididymal blowouts. These usually lead to epididymal obstruction. Unremitting pain is usually responsive to vasovasostomy or vasoepididymostomy; however, because the vasectomy was initially performed to achieve sterility, epididymectomy is an alternative to cure this unremitting epididymal pain.

Rates of sperm granuloma formation at the site of the vasectomy (vasitis nodosa) exceed rates for all other complications of vasectomy, occurring in up to 15 percent of patients.[14] These are usually non-symptomatic. The condition represents a granulomatous inflammatory response to extravasated sperm into the perivasal tissues, and may present during the perioperative period or later on.

Infectious complications are rare following a vasectomy. Usually the skin sutures may develop a superficial infection, and this responds to local care and a mild antibiotic. Deep wound infections are usually rare and are associated with the use of braided suture material. Incision and drainage of the wound with removal of any such suture material are required to resolve this situation.

The most severe complication is failure of the operation to result in sterility, and this is seen in approximately 1 in 200 to 400 patients. Presence of sperm in the semen analysis may represent too few ejaculations, failure to cut both vasa, or spontaneous recanalization. Spontaneous recanalization is seen in less than 1 percent of patients, usually within the first 3 months. Increased rates of recanalization occur with the formation of sperm granulomas, removal of less than 1 cm of vas, incomplete stripping of tissues from around the vas, deep abscess formation, and cautery of only one end of the vas during vasectomy as performed in open-end vasectomies. Steps to avoid this complication include cauterization of both ends of the cut vas, interposition of the perivasal tissues between cut ends, redirection of the ends of the vasa, and ligation without strangulation of the vasal stumps. Each of these steps certainly renders a future vasavasostomy problematic. Should the patient not become azoospermic following the vasectomy, a repeat bilateral vasectomy is the required treatment, since it is impossible to determine which side has recanalized. The operation should be performed at a new site on the vas, well away from the scarring from the previous vasectomy, if possible.

Vasovasostomy and Vasoepididymostomy

Among the population of men who undergo vasectomy for sterilization, a significant percentage seek to regain fertility for a variety of reasons.[12] Other patients in whom infertility resulting from epididymal or vasal obstruction secondary to congenital or infectious disease has ocurred may desire surgical reconstruction. Microscopically and macroscopically assisted operative techniques have been devised to reanastomose the cut ends of the vasa or, less commonly, the epididymis to the vas.[15] Patency rates in the range of 90 percent have been achieved in patients who have undergone this procedure.[15,19] Pregnancy rates, however, are between 40 and 70 percent. The exact reasons for this discrepancy are not known but seem to relate to the length of time since vasectomy and to unrecognized epididymal blowouts that cause epididymal obstruction.[15]

Almost all patients will experience some discomfort and edema following the procedure. Like other scrotal surgical procedures, analgesia, scrotal elevation, and placement of ice packs will alleviate most of these complaints. Depending on the type of dissection performed, these symptoms may last for up to 3 weeks. Infections, both superficial and deep, following vasovasostomy or vasoepididymostomy are rare.

A vasovasostomy or vasoepididymostomy may fail because of technical problems such as inadvertent occlusion of the lumen from the sutures, leakage of sperm at the anastomotic site with resultant scar formation (sperm granuloma) and obstruction of the vasal lumen, anastomotic disruption, and ischemia of the end of the cut vas and subsequent obstruction. All of these conditions lead to azoospermia or severe oligospermia with poor motility either immediately or within the first 6 months after the operation.

There is some evidence that the high incidence of anti-sperm antibodies as measured in the semen of patients who have undergone a vasectomy reversal may influence sperm motility postoperatively and inhibit normal fertilization. The use of high-dose steroids to decrease these anti-sperm antibodies carries with it the risks of aseptic necrosis of the femoral head, weight gain, hypertension, and development of Cushing's syndrome. To date, very little efficacy has been shown with steroid therapy.[16–18]

Ligation of Spermatic Veins

A varicocele is defined as an abnormal dilation of veins of the pampiniform plexus that surround the testis and spermatic cord. Clinically, a varicocele may present as groin pain or may be found incidentally in men with abnormal seminal parameters. In the pediatric age group (puberty to 18 years of age), a varicocele may be found in as many as 15 percent of the boys. It is usually seen on the left side, but in 15 to 20 percent of cases it is bilateral.[19] Unilateral right-side varicoceles occur rarely. When an adult presents with the acute onset of a varicocele, it may suggest occlusion of the renal vein or inferior vena cava. Methods of treatment involve ligation or occlusion of involved veins.[20] This can be accomplished via surgery or radiologic techniques. With surgery, two types of surgical approaches are used; one is high ligation in the retroperitoneum, whereas the other involves ligation of the spermatic veins in the inguinal canal.

An obvious complication with surgery is failure to ligate all of the involved veins, yielding persistence of the varix. This may be confirmed with a venogram in the postoperative period. In the pediatric age group, it has been recommended that an intraoperative venogram be performed to identify any residual veins.[21] Another complication is accidental occulsion of the testicular artery. This may be prevented if careful dissection of the veins is performed and if a Doppler flowmeter is used intraoperatively. Because of the rich anastomoses between the vasal and testicular arteries, accidental occlusion of the testicular artery will not result in testicular atrophy unless the patient's vasal artery is occluded (such as following a vasectomy). Scrotal swelling and discomfort tend be more prominent with an inguinal dissection than with the high retroperitoneal approach to treat a varicocele. If surgical ligation is performed for an abnormal semen parameter or for pain, it should be explained to the patient that reversal of this seminal defect may not be achieved or that pain may not diminish even though the procedure is technically successful.

Epididymectomy

Seldom should epididymitis require surgical intervention. Occasionally, a patient with recurrent chronic or suppurative epididymitis may be relieved of symptoms by excision of the epididymis or complete epididymo-orchiectomy. Partial epididymectomy for painful adenomatoid tumors or diagnostic dilemmas of indurated epididymides may be indicated.

The major complication of epididymectomy is injury to the blood supply to the testis. The testicular artery and vein exit the cord at the junction of the epididymis and testis, sending off small branches to both structures. Dissection begun at the lower pole of the testis and carried toward the cord permits identification of the vascular pedicle at the junction of the middle and upper thirds along the epididymis, and allows preservation of the main blood supply to the testis. Should the spermatic vessels be injured, the testis should be observed for viability because its survival may be maintained by collaterals alone.

If an epididymectomy is performed because of pain such as that experienced following a vasectomy, the patient should be advised that the pain may not be totally relieved.

Orchiectomy

Scrotal orchiectomy is indicated in the surgical treatment of recurrent recalcitrant epididymo-orchitis and for castration in patients with advanced prostatic carcinoma. The major risk of an orchiectomy is hemorrhage from the transected spermatic cord. Attention to detail, separate ligation and division of the spermatic vessels and vasa deferentia, and adequate scrotal compression are the guidelines to reduce the risk of developing this complication. If hemorrhage occurs, exploration may be necessary to drain the hematoma. We recommend that non-braided sutures be used to ligate the spermatic cord to reduce the chance of the sutures becoming infected.

Patients who undergo a bilateral orchiectomy may experience hot flashes and impotence. Both of these side effects are related to the hypogonadism that results from the bilateral orchiectomy. In our practice, treatment with clonidine (0.1 to 0.2 mg orally twice a day) sometimes lessens the severity of the hot flashes.

Spermatocelectomy

Spermatoceles are single or multiple cysts arising from the rete testis, ductuli efferentes, or epididymis that are filled with opalescent fluid and spermatozoa. They are akin to weaknesses in the wall of these structures with diverticular formation. Like hydroceles, they typically transilluminate. Diagnosis rests upon the presence of sperm or sperm fragments in the fluid. Spermatoceles merit surgical treatment for pain or cosmesis. However, surgery should not be performed if the patient is still in his reproductive years because there is a high incidence of occlusion of the ductal system following this procedure. Scrotal pain and possible recurrence of spermatoceles may occur following surgical excision.

We frequently see small spermatoceles in men who have had a prior vasectomy, which suggests the possibility of a pressure phenomenon in the epididymal lumen as the cause of their development. If a spermatocele is found during a vasectomy reversal, it should be left alone because of the possibility and probability of epididymal obstruction following an attempt to excise its wall.

Scrotal Trauma

The scrotum may be involved either in blunt or in penetrating trauma. Penetrating scrotal trauma usually requires exploration to ascertain the degree of injury, whether the scrotal contents have been violated, and to identify and control intrascrotal hemorrhage. If the testis is fractured, debridement and closure of the tunica albuginea are necessary.

Blunt trauma to the scrotum may manifest as hematocele or ruptured testis. Consideration should be given to torsion of the spermatic cord and epididymitis when evaluating the patient who presents with the clinical history of some minor scrotal trauma. Differentiation also rests upon the urinalysis and physical examination. At our institution, the finding of a hematocele usually requires surgery because non-invasive techniques (such as ultrasound, nuclear scanning, and even magnetic resonance imaging) to better define the pathology have proved to produce inaccurate results.

Scrotal skin avulsion results most commonly from industrial or large machinery accidents. Less than complete loss of skin (as little as 20 percent remaining) will allow adequate coverage of the scrotal contents. Careful cleansing and debridement should be employed before a primary closure is attempted. Insufficient scrotal skin for closure mandates mobilization of the testis to adjacent areas for coverage. The ideal solution is a thigh pouch superficial to the subcutaneous fat. Avoiding tension on the cord when it is placed on the abdominal wall and positioning the testes at different heights to avoid possible friction while walking are important caveats.

Testicular injuries should command immediate repair. Delay promotes loss of spermatogenesis as well as hormonal functions. Repair involves debridement of devitalized tissues including extruding seminferous tubules, meticulous hemostasis, and repair of the tunica albuginea. Inspection of the testis may reveal complete testicular devascularization and may indicate the need for orchiectomy. Bilateral traumatic testicular amputation may be managed aggressively with microsurgical replantation techniques. No thought should be given to the placement of a testicular prosthesis until complete healing has occurred, and a separate inguinal approach may be performed. Gangrenous infection remains the most feared complication associated with scrotal trauma, and prophylactic antibiotics are suggested.

Hydrocelectomy

Hydroceles occur in both the pediatric and the adult age groups. In the former, it is associated with a patent processus vaginalis and migration of peritoneal fluid into the tunica vaginalis. Most of these will close off within the first year of life, and the hydroceles will resolve spontaneously. If they do not, it usually indicates that a potential hernial sac is present that needs to be ligated during the procedure, which should be approached from an inguinal incision. In the adult population, hydroceles occur because of an imbalance between secretion by the tuncia albuginea of the testis and resorption of this fluid by the parietal layer of the tunica vaginalis. In these cases, obliteration of the hydrocele sac alone is indicated, and this can be done via a transscrotal approach.

Complications in the pediatric age group are related to incisional pain, infection, and ligation of the hernia sac (see section on orchiopexy in cryptorchidism). In the adult, hemorrhage, swelling, and pain are the most common complications. The use of a turban dressing helps tamponade any troublesome bleeding. If a hematoma fails to stop enlarging, it may need to be drained surgically. Recurrences are rare in hydrocelectomies and are usually due to incomplete obliteration of the hydrocele sac. Occasionally, the epididymis may be accidentally ligated with the suture used to obliterate the hernial sac regardless of whether the bottleneck or Lord's procedure[22] is performed. We have seen this complication lead to subsequent vasoepididymostomies in two individuals.

Torsion of Testis (Appendages)

Torsion or twisting of the spermatic cord results in ischemia to the gonad. It is one of the most common surgical emergencies for males from infancy to the third decade of life. Its peak incidences are at birth and during the pubertal age group. Surgery is the treatment of choice; this involves salvage of the affected gonad and an orchiopexy of both the ipsilateral and the contralateral gonads.[23]

Necrosis of the testis may occur unless torsion is immediately considered and surgery performed within 6 to 8 hours of the onset. Necrosis is universally found in neonates with testicular torsion, and for this reason, surgery may not be warranted. Because neonate torsion is extravaginal, contralatral orchiopexy may not be necessary, although there is some debate regarding this.[24] In the pubertal patient, nuclear scanning is usually the most reliable test to help make the diagnosis of a testicular torsion. If a testis does not look or appear viable either by using fluorescein and a Wood's lamp, by incising the tunica albuginea and observing for brisk bleeding, or by measuring tissue oxygen levels with a surface oximeter, orchiectomy should be performed. A contralateral orchiopexy should still be performed. There is some evidence that retention of the ischemic testis in the scrotum following torsion may lead to secondary changes in the contralateral testis that may affect subsequent fertility.

Acute scrotal pain may also involve torsion of the appendix epididymis and/or appendix testis. These appendages should be excised if operated on. There are no sequelae from misdiagnosing a torsion of the appendage, but most of the time it is difficult to differentiate clinically a torsion of the appendage from a torsion of the gonad.

References

Cited References

1. Grant, JCB, ed: An Atlas of Anatomy, 5th ed. Baltimore, Williams & Wilkins, 1962.
2. Orecklin J, Dale G: A simplified form of scrotal compression dressing. Presented at meeting of the American Urological Association, Western Section, Honolulu, April 1973.
3. Manson A, MacDonald G: Turban: scrotal dressing. J Urol 137:238, 1987.
4. Rajfer, J: Technique of orchiopexy. Urol Clin North Am 9:421–427, 1982.
5. Klein FA, Whitmore WF Jr, Sogani C, Batata M, Fischer H, Herr HW: Inguinal lymph node metastases from germ cell testicular tumors. J Urol 131:497, 1984.
6. Silber SJ: The intra-abdominal testis: microvascular autotransplantation. J Urol 125:329, 1981.

7. Montague D: Inflatable penile prostheses. Semin Urol 2:145, 1984.
8. Furlow WL: The prosthetic management of urinary incontinence. Semin Urol 2:138, 1984.
9. Lattimer JK, Vakil BF, Smith AM, Morishima A: A natural testicular prosthesis. J Urol 110:81, 1973.
10. Abbassian AA: Testicular prosthesis: a new insertion operation. J Urol 108:436, 1972.
11. Rosen JS, Benson RC: Testicular prostheses. Semin Urol 2:176, 1984.
12. Goldstein M, Feldberg M: The Vasectomy Book. Los Angeles, JP Tarcher, 1982.
13. Ball TP, Epididymitis. In Kaufman, JJ, ed: Current Urologic Therapy. 2nd ed. Philadelphia, WB Saunders Co, 1986.
14. Schmidt SS, Morris RR: Spermatic granuloma: the complication of vasectomy. Fertil Steril 24:941, 1973.
15. Silber SJ: Vasectomy and vasectomy reversal. Fertil Steril 29:125, 1978.
16. Hendry WF, Stedronska J, Hughes L, et al: Steroid treatment of male subfertility caused by antisperm antibodies. Lancet 2:498, 1979.
17. Hargreave TB, Elton RA: Treatment with intermittent high dose methylprednisolone or intermittent betamethasone for antisperm antibodies: preliminary communication. Fertil Steril 38:586, 1982.
18. Haas GG, Manganiello P: A double blind placebo-controlled study of the use of methylprednisolone in infertile men with sperm-associated immunoglobulins. Fertil Steril 47:295, 1987.
19. Saypol DC: Varicocele. J Androl 2:61, 1981.
20. Dubin L, Amelar RD: 986 cases of varicocelectomy: a 12 year study. Urology 10:446, 1977.
21. Levitt S, Gill B, Katlowitz N, Kogan SJ, Reda E: Routine intraoperative post-ligation venography in the treatment of the pediatric varicocele. J Urol 137:716, 1987.
22. Lord PH: A bloodless operation for the radical cure of idiopathic hydrocele. Brit J Surg 51:914, 1964.
23. Harrison RH: Torsion of the Spermatic Cord, Testis, and Vestigial Appendages. New York, Harcourt Brace Jovanovich, 1982, pp 54–59.
24. LaQuaglia MP, Bauer SB, Eraklis A, Feins N, Mandell J: Bilateral neonatal torsion. J Urol 138:1051, 1987.

Uncited References

Cottle GF: Avulsion of scrotum, left testicle and sheath of penis. US Nav Med Bull 20:457, 1924.

Dale GA: Complications of scrotal surgery. In Smith, RB, Skinner DG, eds: Complications of Urologic Surgery. Philadelphia, WB Saunders Co, 1976, pp 395–407.

COMPLICATIONS OF PENILE SURGERY

39

Aaron Kirkemo

COMPLICATIONS OF CIRCUMCISION

Over 1.25 million circumcisions are performed annually in the United States.[1] The bulk of the nonreligious circumcisions are performed as prophylactic procedures in the ill-founded hopes of decreasing the incidence of penile cancer, ensuring adequate penile hygiene, preventing the transmission of venereal disease, and preventing phimosis. This really represents a sociological phenomenon because many countries in which routine circumcisions are not performed have equivalent incidences and death rates from penile carcinoma.[2] An ad hoc committee of the American Academy of Pediatrics addressed the cancer-risk issue as well as the presumed benefits of circumcision and concluded that "there is no absolute medical indication for routine circumcision of the newborn."[3]

Clear medical indications for circumcision are phimosis (with or without episodes of balanitis) and paraphimosis. Circumcision may be considered as a prophylaxis against paraphimosis in certain males receiving penile prostheses. Routine neonatal circumcision is contraindicated in any abnormality that may necessitate future penile reconstruction, such as hypospadias, epispadias, megalourethra, or webbed penis.[4] Any medical or surgical condition that puts the child at risk should also be considered before performing a routine circumcision.

Neonatal Circumcision

A majority of neonatal circumcisions are performed using mechanical aids, such as the Plastibell device and the Gomco clamp. Procedures involving these two devices result in approximately the same incidence of complications.[5] Both employ the same principle of crushing the preputial skin over a bell-shaped anvil, which accomplishes both division of the skin and hemostatic compression of the preputial vessels (Fig. 39–1). In neonatal circumcision, the adhesions between the glans and the prepuce are lysed with a small probe. If these are not completely lysed, epithelial skin bridges or smegma inclusion cysts may form. A dorsal slit is then made to allow the anvil to be seated over the glans. Iatrogenic epispadias can be inadvertently created if the glans is not carefully visualized before the incision is made. To ensure that an appropriate amount of preputial skin is taken, an incision line is marked on the penile shaft skin where it expands over the corona of the glans before the clamp is placed. Once the prepuce is pulled over the bell, it is secured with a crushing Gomco clamp or tied with a Plastibell device to produce hemostasis. The redundant prepuce is then excised.

Any incisional bleeding that occurs should be treated with pressure or ligation, using absorbable suture material. Application of vasoconstrictive agents should be discouraged because of the possibility of systemic side effects if the material is absorbed. Electrofulguration should also be avoided because of the potential of penile necrosis.[6] A sterile circumferential dressing may be applied along with an antibiotic salve. Care must be taken not to apply the dressing so tightly that an iatrogenic paraphimosis develops. Re-

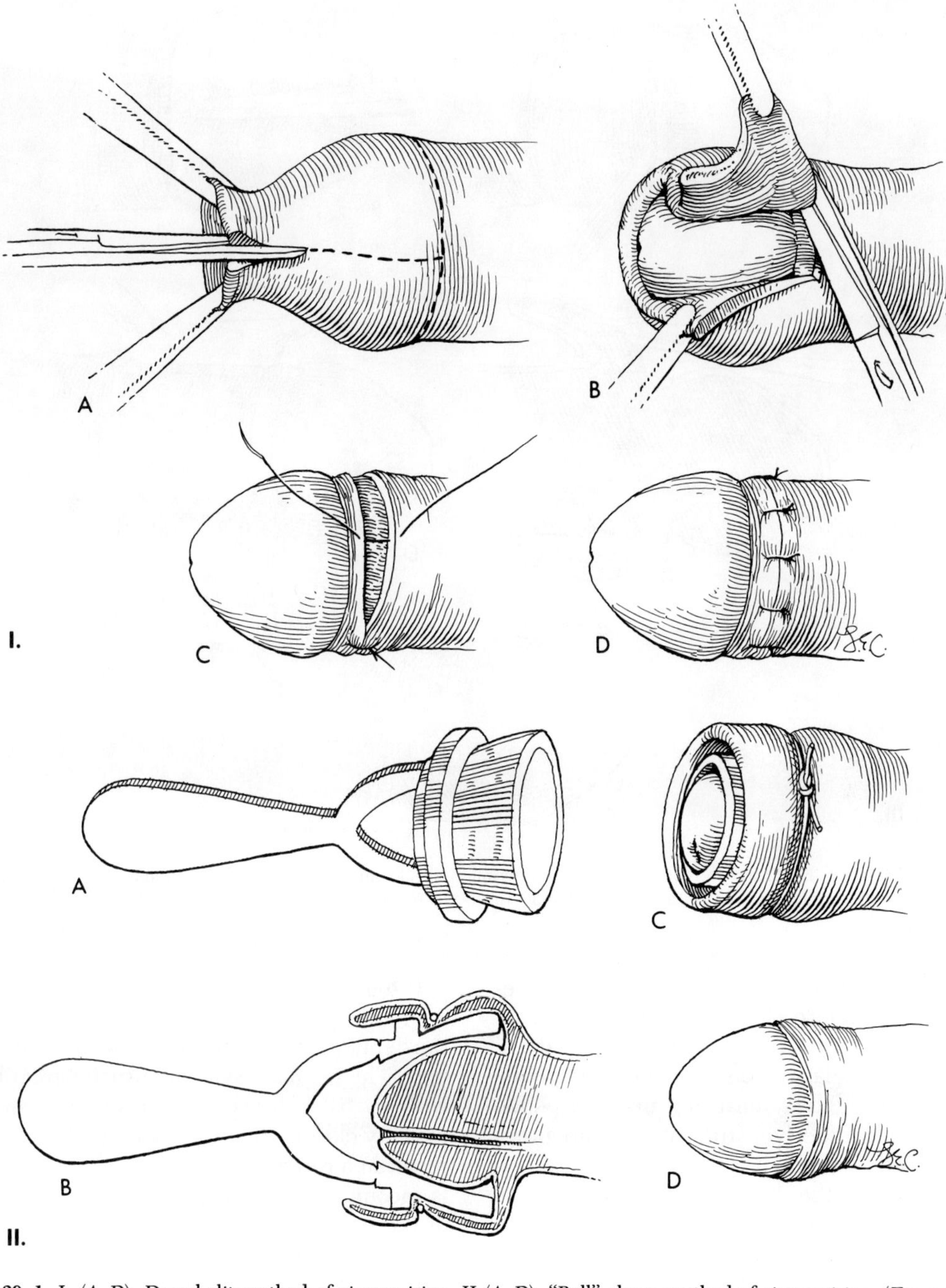

Figure 39–1. I. (*A–D*), Dorsal slit method of circumcision. II (*A–D*), "Bell" clamp method of circumcision. (From Peters PC: Complications of penile surgery. In Smith RB, Skinner DG, eds: Complications of Urologic Surgery: Prevention and Management. Philadelphia, WB Saunders Co, 1976, p 410.)

ports of penile necrosis have been reported from too tight a dressing.[7]

The Plastibell anvil is allowed to drop off within 5 to 8 days, whereas the Gomco clamp is removed immediately. Parents should be instructed to seek medical care if the Plastibell anvil migrates or has not fallen off within the allotted time. Migration or retention of the bell can result in an iatrogenic paraphimosis with ulceration and erosion of the glans, penile shaft, or urethra.[8]

Most child and adult circumcisions are accomplished using the dorsal slit or sleeve resection method (Fig. 39–2). Essentially, the same precautions must be exercised as with the neonatal circumcision. Special care must be taken while

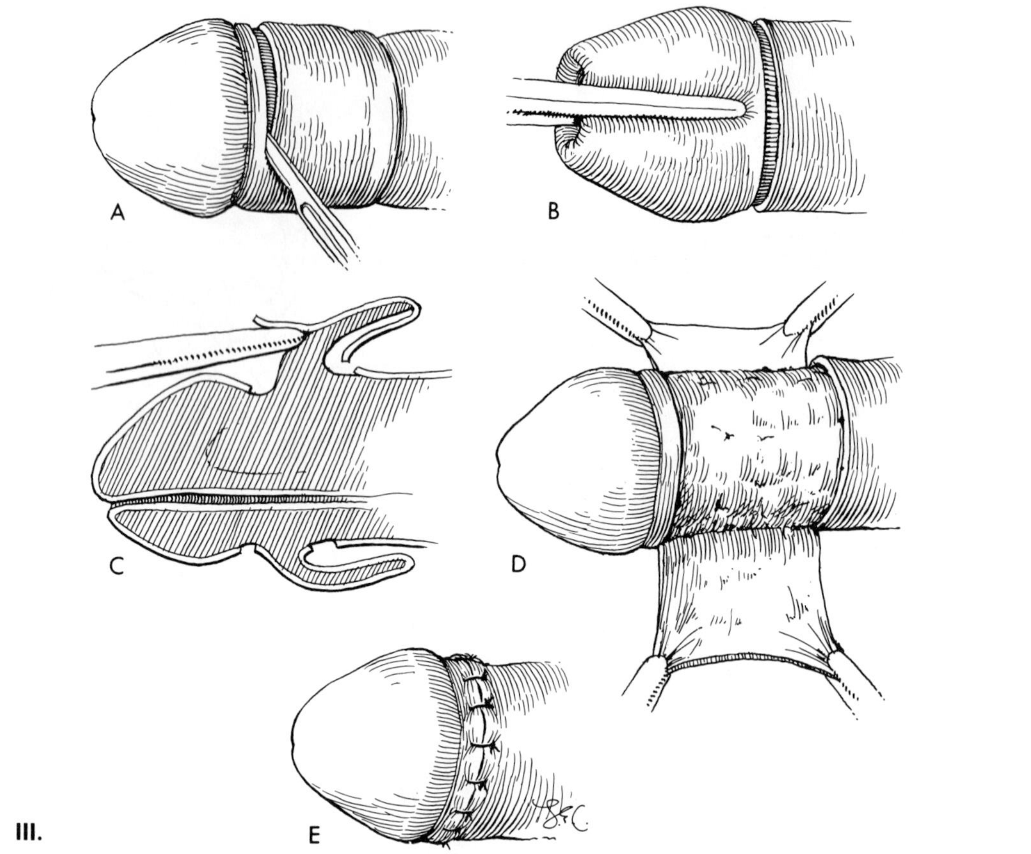

Figure 39–2. III. (*A–E*), Sleeve resection method of circumcision. (From Peters PC: Complications of penile surgery. In Smith RB, Skinner DG, eds: Complications of Urologic Surgery: Prevention and Management. Philadelphia, WB Saunders Co, 1976, p 411.)

excising the prepuce ventrally to prevent urethral injury. Before closure, meticulous hemostasis must be carried out, paying special attention to the frenular vessels. Prevention of penile torsion is avoided by ensuring that the penile shaft skin and underlying tunical layers are properly aligned. Placement of several chromic quadrant sutures in the dartos-Buck layers helps to maintain proper alignment and relieve tension on the cutaneous suture line. Plain catgut sutures may then be used for the skin closure, which eliminates the "railroad-track" scarring that is frequently seen. Inclusion cysts are avoided by proper skin eversion during closure.

Should skin bridges develop after a circumcision, they may be easily treated with simple excision of the skin tag. The proximal and distal incision sites are best closed with plain catgut sutures to minimize scarring. The sebaceous inclusion cysts caused by retained smegma in the incision line may be handled with simple excision.

If too much penile shaft skin is taken during a circumcision in the infant, it is best to treat the denuded penis with simple wet-to-dry dressings. The neonatal skin will usually granulate in with a satisfactory cosmetic result.[9] Attempts at primary closure of a large penile skin defect can result in a retracted or buried penis. When this is encountered, it may be treated with degloving of the penis and placement of a split-thickness skin graft over the distal exposed portion of the penis. Radhakrishnan describes a technique in which two opposing U-shaped skin flaps are made just superior to the base of the penis (Fig. 39–3).[10] The superior U-shaped flap is based on the anterior abdominal wall. The inverted flap extends down between the pubic mons and the base of the scrotum. Mobilization of the inferior flap at the base of the penis allows for it to be freed, as well as providing coverage of the distal shaft. Coverage of the base of the penis is provided with lateral flaps.

If a cicatricial phimosis develops, the circum-

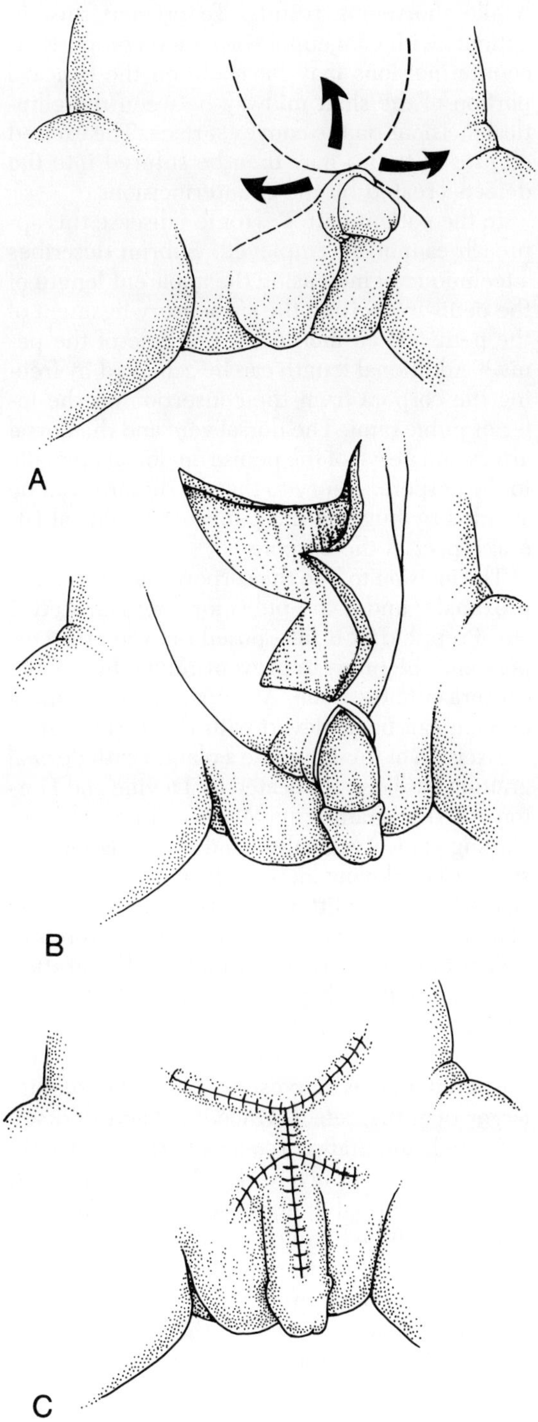

Figure 39–3. *A*, Opposing U flaps created. *B*, Mobilization of flaps. *C*, Coverage of penis with flap.

cision should be repeated. When this complication is associated with penile regression, Kaplan recommends that a circumferential incision be made immediately proximal to the cicatricial band rather than using a dorsal slit.[4] This minimizes loss of skin that may be used for coverage of the penile shaft.

Urethrocutaneous fistulas can be managed in the same fashion as those encountered post hypospadias repair.

Meatal stenosis secondary to meatal ulceration is commonly encountered after infant circumcisions. The poorly cornified glanular skin is very sensitive to ammonia dermatitis and mechanical irritation from diapers and results in scarring of the meatus. This can be prevented by protecting the newly exposed glans with petroleum salve and by frequent diaper changes.[11] Should it occur, a standard meatotomy may be performed.

Amputation of the penis or glans may be treated with immediate replantation, discussed later in this chapter.

MANAGEMENT OF PENILE CURVATURE

Management of congenital curvature of the penis related to hypospadias and epispadias is discussed elsewhere. Peyronie's disease and the rare disorder congenital corporal disproportion are the most frequent adult etiologies of penile curvature. The surgical approach to penile curvature must be tailored to the patient's condition. If the curvature is secondary to congenital disproportion of the corpora, a Nesbit procedure is most appropriate. It should also be performed following puberty because this condition is thought to be secondary to disproportionate corporal growth. Too early an attempt at correction may necessitate reoperation.[12]

Peyronie's disease with associated impotence is best treated with plaque incision and placement of a penile prosthesis. The potent patient with Peyronie's disease may be treated with plaque excison and grafting or with any of the aforementioned options. Before embarking on surgical correction of Peyronie's disease, the caveat must be emphasized that the process may arrest and spontaneous regression can occur.[13] The patient with impotence, painful erections, or curvature that precludes satisfactory intromission warrants surgical consideration. It is prudent to wait until a growing plaque has stabilized before proceeding with surgery.

The Nesbit procedure was originally described for treatment of congenital corporal disproportion[13a] (1979). It may also be applied to the potent patient with Peyronie's disease.[14] A circumcision incision is made and the penis is degloved, staying on a plane deep to Buck's fascia. This is particularly important in the patient with Peyronie's disease in order to be able to visualize the dorsal neurovascular bundle and avoid injury to it during subsequent mobilization. An artificial erection is then created by injecting saline intracorporally after placing a Penrose tourniquet at the base of the penis (Gittes' test).[15] Elliptical wedges of tunica albuginea are excised opposite the concavity. All spongy tissue beneath the tunica should be preserved. The ellipses should not exceed 1 cm by one-half to one-third the circumference of the corporal body, to preserve a smooth shaft. Closure of the defect is accomplished with a running suture of polyglycolic acid (Dexon), PDS, or permanent monofilament. (Buried knots should be used with permanent sutures to prevent painful subcutaneous lumps.)[16] A repeat Gittes' test should be performed. If needed, additional ellipses of tunica may be taken and the procedure repeated until satisfactory correction of the curvature is achieved.

Peyronie's plaques are most frequently found dorsally. Therefore, the Nesbit procedure requires ventral ellipse excisions. The urethra may have to be mobilized if large ellipses need to be taken. A Foley catheter should be placed prior to development of the plane between the corporal bodies and the spongiosum, to prevent injury to the urethra. If a urethral injury is recognized at the conclusion of this procedure, a flap of Buck's fascia should be interposed between the spongiosum and the corpora after the urethra has been closed with absorbable sutures. The catheter should be left in place for 7 to 10 days to allow for adequate healing of the urethra.

Ventral curvature of the penis requires mobilization of the dorsal neurovascular bundle before making the ellipses. To prevent injury to the bundle, dissection should begin over the normal corpora and, once a plane is found, carried out into the region of the plaque. A portion of plaque can be left with the neurovascular complex. Electrocautery should be used judiciously to prevent glandular anesthesia from thermal injury to the nerve. Impotence has been seen occasionally after this procedure.[17] In these instances, placement of a penile prosthesis is suggested.[16]

A disadvantage of the Nesbit procedure is that penile shortening results. To prevent this, in patients with congenital corporal disproportion, counterincisions may be made on the concave portion of the shaft midway between the elliptical incisions on the convex surface. The excised ellipses of tunica may then be sutured into the defects created by the counterincisions.

In the patient with Peyronie's disease this approach cannot be employed. Subrini describes a technique of increasing the apparent length of the penis by incising the suspensory ligament of the penis via an incision at the base of the penis.[18] Additional length can be achieved by freeing the corpora from their insertion on the inferior pubic rami. The dorsal vein and the dorsal artery and nerve of the penis run dorsal medially to the corpora. Injury to these structures can be avoided by hugging the pubis on the dorsal lateral aspect of the corpora.

The incision to free the corpora may be carried proximally under the pubis for approximately 7 cm. Prepubic fat is interposed between the corpora and the pubis to prevent reinsertion of the corpora onto the bone. An apparent lengthening of 3 cm can be achieved with this maneuver.

Excision of the Peyronie's plaque with dermal grafting has been advocated by Devine and Horton.[19] Other grafting materials can be used, including tunica vaginalis[20] and rectus fascia.[21] A standard degloving incision deep to Buck's fascia is made and a Gittes' test is performed. The plaque is identified and marked out. Mobilization of the neurovascular bundle and/or urethra is carried out if they overlie the plaque. Stay sutures are placed at the quadrants, and the defect is stretched to assess the size of the graft. The graft that is harvested should be slightly larger than the defect. Once it is harvested and prepared, the graft is secured with running absorbable sutures such as 4–0 PDS or Vicryl. If a defatted dermal graft is used, it is mandatory that the graft be totally de-epithelialized to prevent the creation of epidermal inclusion cysts. It should be only 1 mm thick (if too thin, aneurysmal dilation results, if too thick, scarring and graft contracture result).[22] A watertight closure and correction of the deformity are assured by repeating the Gittes' test. Buck's fascia and the skin are then closed with absorbable sutures. A compressive gauze fluff dressing is carefully applied so that it is not so tight as to cause pressure necrosis of the skin. Impotence after the procedure is a well-recognized complication.[23,24] Alternative therapies should be considered if there is impotence distal to the plaque, if the plaque is larger than several centimeters in any direction, or if it extends deeply into the intracorporal septum. Prior irradiation or history of steroid use is a relative contraindication, also.

The patient with Peyronie's disease with total or partial impotence or severe fibrosis with large or multiple plaques and the patient who does not want to risk impotence should be managed with a penile prosthesis. A semirigid prosthesis may be placed via a degloving incision. This may correct the deformity. Should it fail, the plaque can be incised transversely until adequate correction is achieved. Buck's fascia is then secured over the defect using absorbable sutures. The skin is closed in standard fashion.[25] Inflatable penile prostheses may also be used to correct the deformity.[26]

COMPLICATIONS OF PENILE PROSTHESES

Since the first edition of this text was published, there has been a dramatic change in the technology of penile prostheses. The national experience with inflatable prostheses was in its infancy 15 years ago. Since then, the number of devices, both semirigid and inflatable, has grown dramatically. Reliability of the inflatable devices has continued to improve with changes in implantation techniques as well as with improvements in the materials and devices themselves. At present there are six available noninflatable penile prostheses available in the United States. Six inflatable penile prostheses are on the market, of which two are self-contained units. A mechanical chain-link adjustable rigidity device is also in production.

Discussion of the evaluation of the impotent patient is beyond the scope of this text. However, once the decision is made to implant a penile prosthesis, certain factors must be taken into consideration to ensure a satisfactory outcome.

Mechanical failure of any of the devices can occur. Fractures of all the different noninflatable penile prostheses, although rare, have been reported.[27,28]

The intrinsic and surgically related mechanical failure rate of the inflatable devices is appreciably higher, as would be expected. Even with perfect technical success, failure of the prosthesis to meet the expectations of the patient and his partner is distressingly high.[29,30] The patient must be made aware that these devices afford, at best, only a close approximation to the natural erection. In addition to the standard risks, he should be informed of the relative risk of reoperation for correction of mechanical failure of the device. The complications that lead to the dissatisfied patient can be prevented if he is given enough information to intelligently participate in the choice of the prosthesis.

Infection in Penile Prosthetic Surgery

Implantation of prosthetic material into a vascular organ will carry an obligate risk of infection. Penile prosthetic surgery is associated with an infection risk of approximately 2 to 7 percent.[31–34] Surgery should be performed only if cultures indicate that the urine is sterile. A povidone-iodine shower should be given the night before surgery. The shave preparation of the patient should be deferred until just before surgery to diminish colonization of preparation-induced skin lacerations.

Staphylococcus epidermidis is found in 60 percent of penile prosthetic infections. To minimize prosthetic infection, parenteral prophylactic antiobiotics must be given 1 to 2 hours preoperatively to ensure adequate levels of drugs in the tissue. They should provide coverage against *S. epidermidis, S. aureus,* and the common gram-negative organisms seen in the perineal region. This can be accomplished with an aminoglycoside and a cephalosporin such as cefoxitin. Vancomycin may be used in the penicillin-allergic patient. Postoperative chemoprophylaxis should be continued for 72 hours.

Use of the surgical isolation bubble system with the high energy particulate air (HEPA) filter is being advocated to diminish the infection rate, though no clinical trials have been published yet.

Implantation Techniques

The choice of the type of incision used is dictated by the prosthesis and by needs for ancillary penile surgery. The self-contained inflatable and semirigid penile prostheses may be implanted via a suprapubic, penile shaft, circumcising, penoscrotal, or perineal approach. Either a suprapubic or a penoscrotal incision may be used for the inflatable penile systems.

Unless dictated by the need for extensive penile shaft surgery or for a circumcision, the most universal incision is the penoscrotal approach.

Contact with the neurovascular bundle and many lymphatics is avoided by this incision, which reduces the risk of glandular anesthesia, penile ischemia, or edema.[35] Direct visualization of the corpora spongiosum helps to minimize urethral injury. Extension of the incision is possible, allowing for penile shaft surgery.

A median raphe incision is made at the penoscrotal junction 3 to 4 cm into the scrotum. The bluish corpora spongiosum is visualized after incising Buck's fascia. Lateral subfascial dissection then exposes the tunica albuginea of both corpora. Paired stay sutures are placed 4 to 5 mm lateral to the urethra, and a longitudinal corporotomy is made. If an inflatable system is to be inserted, the incision should be made proximal to the plane of the penile–abdominal-wall junction.[36] This allows the cylinder tubing to exit from the distal edge of the corporotomy. Tunica closure is carried out over the solid portion of the cylinder, decreasing cylinder injury and wear erosion.

Dilation of the corpora is produced using either Hagar dilators or the Dilamezinsert. Nothing smaller than a No. 7 Hagar dilator should be used. Urethral injury is avoided by hugging the lateral wall of the corpora and keeping the penis on stretch. A single pass should be made in each direction to prevent creation of false channels that may hinder passage of the prosthesis. If marked fibrosis is encountered at the start of dilation, careful lateral subtunica dissection with Metzenbaum's scissors can be used initially.

Distal dilation must be carried to the septum of the corpora and glans to prevent the Supersonic Transport (SST) glans deformity once the prosthesis is placed.[37] Too vigorous distal dilation can result in a urethral-cutaneous fistula. This is more likely to occur in spongiosal fibrotic conditions such as diabetic or postpriapism impotence. Inadequate proximal dilation can lead to undersizing of the prosthesis with ultimate loss of erection as the prosthesis migrates proximally. Cylinder wear and failure may also occur if the tubing of inflatable prostheses is drawn intracorporally.[38] Migration of the cylinders can occur if overzealous proximal dilation causes an unrecognized crural perforation.

As dictated by the type of device, sizing of the prosthesis is carried out. The corpora are irrigated with an antibiotic solution such as genitourinary (GU) tribiotic solution. Placement of the prosthesis is then performed. If guiding sutures are included with the device, either the Furlow introducer[39] or the Dilamezinsert may be used. Both corpora should be dilated and the guide sutures made before inserting the inflatable prosthesis. This reduces the risk of cylinder damage should the septum be perforated with either the dilator or the Keith needle. Preplacement of tunica closure sutures is recommended for inflatable prostheses. Corporotomies should be closed with absorbable sutures to prevent inflatable cylinder wear.[34,40] Twists in the inflatable cylinders must be avoided during insertion to prevent wear failure. The tubing of the inflatable systems must exit the proximal portion of the corporotomy to avoid cylinder contact. Wear failure from failing to do this was commonly seen until the advent of rear-tip extenders, which have diminished the incidence of this complication.[41,42]

If mechanical prostheses have been inserted, they should be serially inflated and deflated to assess the quality of the erection, the occurrence of any cylinder kinks, and the ease of fluid flow into and out of the system.

The reservoir of the inflatable systems should then be inserted into the space of Retzius. This may be done either through the inguinal canal or above the pubis. Placement of the reservoir outside the pelvis should be considered if there is concern of significant pelvic fibrosis or scarring secondary to radiation, infection, or multiple pelvic surgeries.[43] This can prevent the erosion of the reservoir into bladder or bowel.[44]

The barrel reservoir inserter makes inguinal insertion quite simple. After the bladder is emptied, the external inguinal ring is palpated, and the transversalis fascia of the inguinal floor is bluntly perforated. Avulsion of the inferior epigastric vessels can occur unless the finger hugs the pubic tubercle. A potential space for the reservoir is then created retropubically, using blunt finger dissection along the pubis. Bleeding is ruled out by examining the space using a long beaked nasal speculum. The reservoir inserter is then passed through the fascial defect using the index finger as a lateral guide. The reservoir is delivered into the retropubic space and filled according to the instructions of the manufacturer. To prevent hernia formation, the inflated reservoir should be pulled down so that the reservoir dome occludes the floor defect. Any weakness of the floor should be corrected with a formal inguinal incision where a herniorrhaphy can be performed after reservoir placement.

A dependent subdartos scrotal pouch is then created ipsilateral to the patient's dominant hand using blunt dissection. After the pouch is irrigated with antibiotic solution, the filled device pump is placed, and the tube going to the contralateral cylinder is passed through the medial wall of the pouch and scrotal septum. The pouch is then closed with a running absorbable suture. These two maneuvers prevent cephalad migration of the pump, which has been a major cause for tubing kink in the past.[31] Mating of the respective tubes is then accomplished using special sutureless connectors once the tubing has been trimmed to ensure that no kinking will occur. The device should be inflated and deflated several times to ensure satisfactory function, absence of leaks, and so on.

Once the wound has been irrigated with antibiotic solution, the subcutaneous layer is closed with 3–0 Vicryl sutures. The skin is approximated with an intradermal 4–0 Vicryl suture followed by collodion. The cylinders are left partially inflated for 48 to 72 hours and then are totally deflated. After placement of a Foley catheter, a gentle compressive scrotal dressing is applied. Both are removed the next day.

Complications of Prosthesis Implantation

Several potential complications can be avoided by adequate postoperative instruction. Regardless of prosthesis type, the patient should wear loose-fitting clothes to reduce pressure on the penis and glans. He should refrain from sex for 4 to 6 weeks postoperatively and then resume sexual activity only if pain free. Cycling of the inflatable devices at least every 2 days is mandatory to prevent cicatricial sheath formation around the components. The reservoir of the Hydroflex prosthesis lies in the proximal crura. If this device or the inflatable prosthesis system is kept partially inflated during the initial weeks, spontaneous erections may ultimately occur. This results from decreased compliance of the reservoir due to constricting scar buildup. Cylinder aneurysm formation can be diminished by instructing the patient to inflate the device only enough to achieve an erection satisfactory for intromission.

The corporal septum should be closed with absorbable sutures if it is perforated during dilation. This minimizes wear failure of inflatable cylinders. If not technically feasible, cycling of the device can be deferred for several weeks in the hope of allowing spontaneous closure of the defect.

Urethral perforation should be treated with placement of a Foley catheter and termination of the procedure. If the contralateral prosthesis is in place, that portion of the device may be left in situ. At least 6 months should be allowed before replacing the cylinder, although even then, risk of reperforation is high. In many instances, a satisfactory erection can be achieved with a single cylinder.[45]

Perforation of the crura of the corpora during dilation can be treated by creation of a neotunica using woven Dacron sheeting. The sheeting is folded over the proximal portion of the prosthesis and the sides are approximated using a running 2–0 Prolene suture. After the "sock" is trimmed, it is passed into the proximal crus using a Hagar dilator.[45a] It is secured to the tunica with multiple mattress sutures. The prosthesis is then seated into this shortened crus. Only the rear tip extenders should touch any of the neotunica, in order to prevent cylinder wear (Fig. 39–4).

Occasionally, it is not possible to dilate the corpora secondary to severe corporal fibrosis. Sharp scissor dissection through extended corporotomies may be needed. Injury to the urethra is avoided by performing this dissection with a Foley catheter in place. If adequate tissue cannot be resected to accommodate a prosthesis, an augmentation corporoplasty with Gore-Tex can be done. Longitudinal corporotomies ending 1 to 2 cm short of the glans are made, and the fibrotic spongy tissue is debulked using sharp dissection. A pocket deep enough to seat the distal end of the prosthesis is dissected out sharply. Extrusion of the prosthesis can result if this distal pocket is not made. If proximal dilation is not possible, the same process should be carried out. The appropriate-size noninflatable prosthesis is placed into the newly created corporal grooves. A split Gore-Tex graft is then used to close the defect, using a running 3–0 Prolene suture with buried knots.

A floppy, poorly supported glans (SST deformity) may occur despite adequate distal seating of the prosthesis. The glans is plicated to the corpora using horizontal mattress sutures placed through a dorsal subcoronal incision. The Vicryl sutures should be placed dorsolaterally to avoid injury to the neurovascular bundle.

If a patient complains of inability to inflate or deflate the device, a radiograph should be obtained. This will help define the nature of the problem. Kinks are easily seen and often may be repaired under local anesthesia. Once the skin incision has been made, all further dissection should be carried out with electrocautery to prevent inadvertent laceration of the tubing.

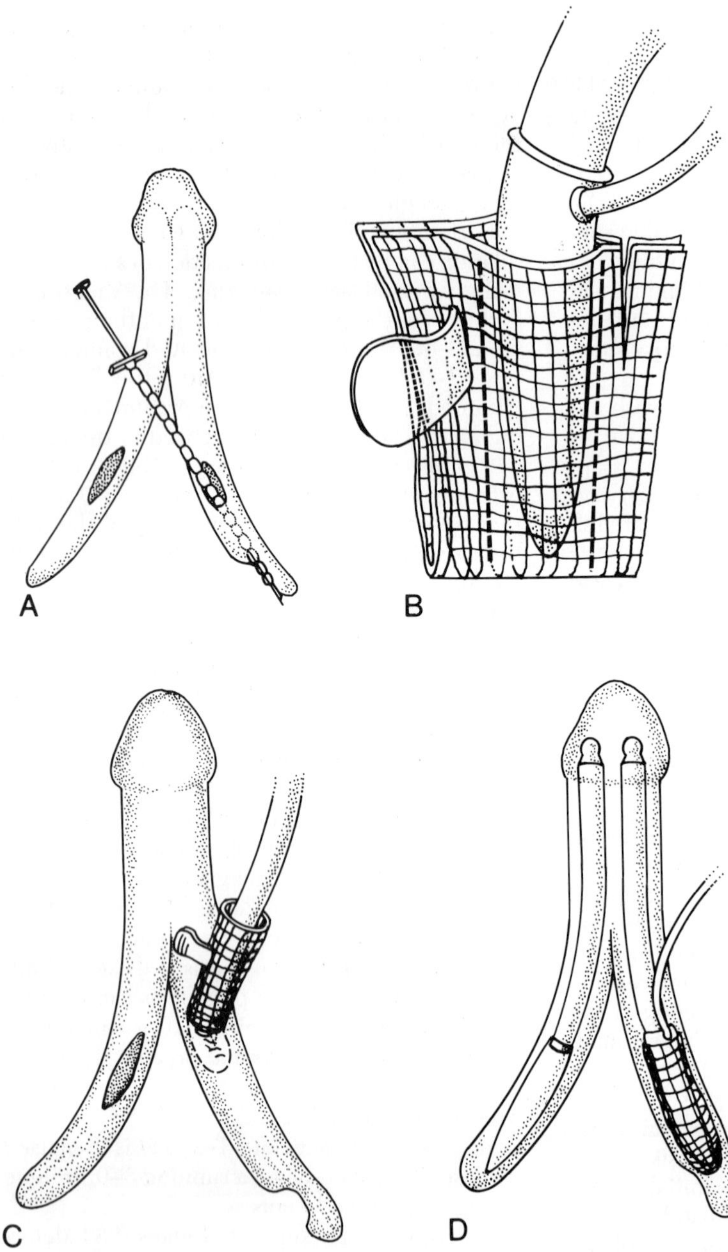

Figure 39–4. *A*, Perforation of proximal crus by Furlow inserter. *B*, Creation of Dacron "sock." *C*, Sock is passed into proximal crura, then secured to the tunica with multiple 2–0 Prolene mattress sutures. *D*, Prosthesis positioned in Dacron neotunica cup.

The kink is isolated, and the redundant tubing is excised and a new connector placed. Both straight and right-angled connectors are available to address various tubing geometries.

Should no contrast be seen on the plain film, an obvious leak exists. Cylinder failure is the most likely cause.[46,47] The connectors should be explored first. If these are intact, all connections are taken down. The ground of a sterile ohmmeter is then attached to the patient. Each component should be filled with saline using a blunt-tip metal needle connected to the other lead of the ohmmeter. A leak in the component will be manifested by a drop in resistance from infinity to less than infinity (i.e., conductance of current through the leak point). Once all components have been checked, the defective portions may be replaced.[34]

Asymmetric cylinder filling and aneurysm formation, with and without rupture, have been seen in all inflatable systems.[48] Radiographic determination of the aneurysm extent is helpful; exploration needs to be carried out. If the aneurysm is due to disruption of the suture line, simple replacement of the involved cylinder and closure of the defect are needed. Most often, there is an associated aneurysmal weakening of the tunica. Simple replacement of the affected cylinder is prone to failure unless the attenuated tunica is resected back to normal tissue and closed primarily. If this results in significant loss of corporal diameter, it is best to trim the most attenuated tissue back and either place a nondistensible inflatable cylinder such as the American Medical Systems Model 700 CX cylinder[41] or replace both corporal bodies with noninflatable prostheses.

Asymmetric filling can also result from corporal fibrosis around the cylinders. This frequently does not respond to dilation. In these instances, the fibrosed spongy tissue is incised with an Otis urethrotome. A small transverse incision is made in the distal penile shaft extending through the tunica. The urethrotome is passed through the proximal incision and brought out through the distal corporotomy. Progressive incisions of the fibrotic tissue are made dorsolaterally in the 10 o'clock position (Fig. 39–5).[49]

If an inflatable system becomes infected, treatment is complete removal of the system because it is surrounded by a pseudocapsule that forms a single communicating sinus through which bacteria can track. In the case of the other devices, it may be possible to treat a single infected cylinder with removal of the involved side. This is usually manifested as extrusion of one of the cylinders. Such treatment should be contemplated only if the devices have been in place for at least several months. By that time, a pseudocapsule should have formed around the contralateral device and hence excluded it from the vascular system. Obviously, broad-spectrum antibiotics to cover *S. epidermidis* and gram-negative organisms should be given pending the results of appropriate cultures.

Superficial penile tissue loss that does not extend deep to the tunica can be treated with antibiotics and local mechanical or chemical debridement. If there is concern of cavernitis, the device must be removed. There are reports of gangrene of the glans and penis[50,51] as well as penile erosions,[51,52] which need to be treated with removal of the prosthesis, cultures, antibiotics, and appropriate debridement. The penoscrotal approach, which stays away from the dorsal neurovascular bundle, should help minimize the risk of glans necrosis. Delayed erosions that are not related to infection tend to be seen primarily in patients experiencing spinal cord disorders.

Penile prostheses should not be placed in patients with chronic indwelling Foley catheters because of the high incidence of urethral erosion in this population. This is seen in both inflatable and noninflatable systems. If intermittent catheterization is used instead, the risk is greatly diminished.[53] Patients with spinal cord problems should also be cautioned to wear loose-fitting clothing and to watch carefully for any early decubitus-type penile skin changes. Additional pressure-relieving measures should be taken or erosions will result.[54]

If corporal tissue is lost, prosthetic corporoplasties, as described for treatment of severe corporitis, may be employed. This procedure should not be performed until all wounds have completely granulated in and epithelialized.

Occasionally, extensive skin loss is encountered. If there is satisfactory corpora beneath the skin loss, the split-thickness skin grafts may be considered. When there has been significant loss of corpora and skin, a well-vascularized skin flap will be needed to cover the prosthetic neocorpora. This is accomplished by resurfacing the penile skin defect using the technique that Cecil described for covering a neourethra with a scrotal skin flap.[55]

Protracted penile pain is also encountered postoperatively. Intracorporal injections with lidocaine (Xylocaine) may be tried in patients with noninflatable prostheses. Pain lasting longer than 2 to 3 months is usually caused by an oversized prosthesis. Replacement with either a smaller girth or a shorter prothesis may be offered if all conservative measures fail.

COMPLICATIONS OF PENILE AMPUTATION

Penile amputation is an uncommon injury. The majority of cases are secondary to self-mutilation, criminal acts, and industrial accidents. There are reports of iatrogenic amputations secondary to circumcision, and herniorrhaphy.[56]

Psychiatric consultation should be obtained immediately in cases of self-mutilation in order to help manage the acute psychotic behavior both preoperatively and postoperatively. Bleeding is controlled with pressure dressings until the patient can be stabilized and taken to the operating room. The amputated segment should be transported on ice after being wrapped in saline-soaked gauze. All organs should be considered for replantation. Successful replantations have been accomplished in penises retrieved from septic tanks and with delays of up to 8 hours.[57]

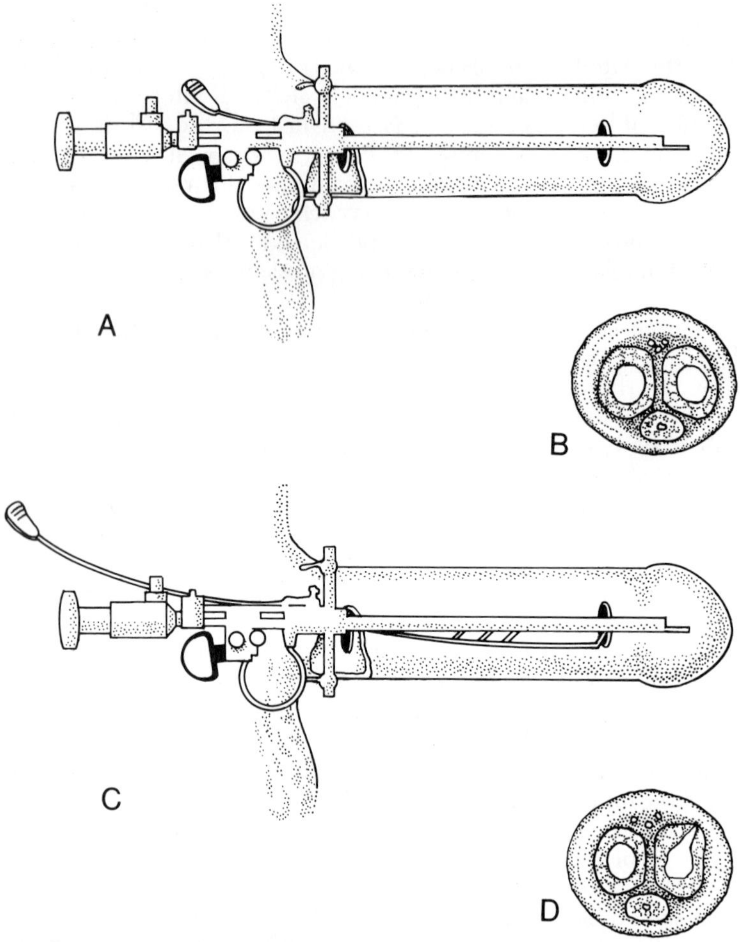

Figure 39–5. *A*, Positioning of urethrotome. *B*, Strictured left corpus with prosthesis removed. *C*, Incision of fibrotic spongy tissue. *D*, Incised stricture.

Upon taking the patient to surgery, the penis is washed with iced Ringer's lactate containing heparin and broad spectrum antibiotics. The dorsalis penis and profunda arteries are cannulated and irrigated with the same iced solution until the effluent from the dorsal vein has cleared.[58]

Once the patient has been anesthetized and prepared and draped for surgery, a Penrose drain tourniquet is applied to the proximal stump for hemostasis. Both stumps are debrided as necesssary. A two-layered spatulated anastomosis of the corpora spongiosum is carried out using interrupted 4–0 Vicryl sutures. This is stented with a Foley catheter. Approximation of the tunica albuginea is accomplished with 2–0 interrupted Vicryl sutures. Closure of Buck's fascia clockwise from 2 to 10 o'clock with 4–0 Vicryl sutures brings the dorsal neurovascular bundle into apposition. Microscopic anastomosis of the deep dorsal vein, the dorsal penile nerves, and one or two of the dorsal arteries is done with interrupted 8–0 or 9–0 Prolene sutures. Additional absorbable sutures are placed dorsally in Buck's fascia and Colles' fascia to relieve tension at the microvascular anastomoses. The skin is then closed with 4–0 nylon sutures. A suprapubic cystostomy tube is placed.

Should it be impossible to carry out a microvascular repair, replantation should still be attempted because penile necrosis rarely occurs.[57] In an extensive review by Carroll and associates,[58a] repair of only the corpora and urethra resulted in restoration of erections in all viable replants, although the incidence of stricture formation was higher.

Skin necrosis occurs almost uniformly regardless of replantation technique. Glans necrosis is also very common.[59] Once all necrotic tissue has been debrided, split-thickness skin grafts may be applied. Because of the high incidence of skin loss, some authors recommend excision of the penile skin at the time of initial surgery. The denuded penis is buried in a subcutaneous tunnel on the anterior scrotum.[60] Two to 3 months later, the penis with its overlying skin is mobilized from the scrotum. The penile and scrotal skin edges are closed with absorbable sutures. This modification of the Cecil technique may be used in lieu of skin grafting if delayed excision of necrotic penile skin is necessary, especially if a urethral fistula must be repaired.

Necrosis of the glans can be treated with debridement and coverage with a skin graft or by burying the necrotic glans in the scrotum along with the penis. Urethral strictures are handled with dilation or visual urethrotomy as indicated.

Should the amputated portion of the penis be lost, the stump should be handled using the same methods as for penile carcinoma (Fig. 39–6). Despite satisfactory creation of a new urethral meatus, spraying of urine from penile regression may occur. Placement of a semirigid penile prosthesis can rectify this problem.[61]

COMPLICATIONS OF PENILE SKIN LOSS

Isolated penile denudation results from avulsion injuries, burns, and skin necrosis from other causes. Distal skin loss is treated with placement

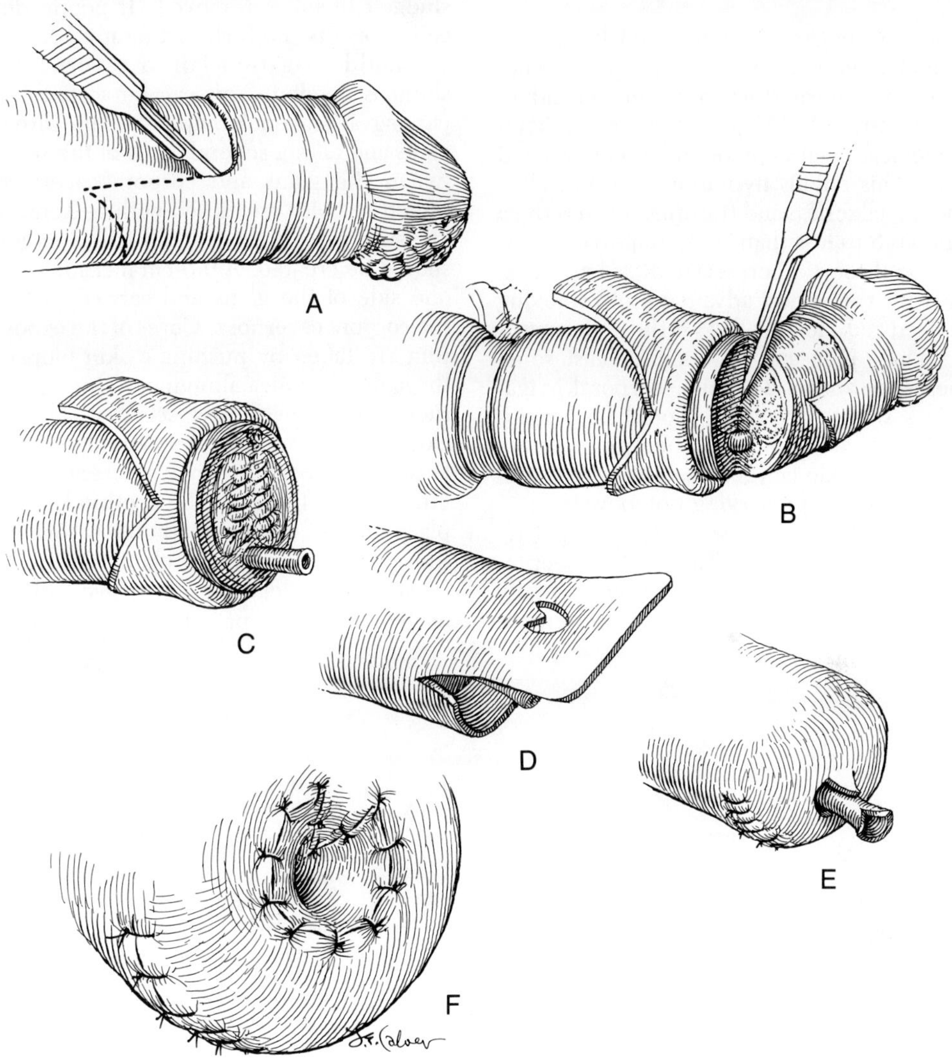

Figure 39–6. Partial amputation of the penis. *A*, Incision of skin of dorsum to extend 1 to 1½ inches below ventral aspect of incision. *B*, Amputation of involved area with 2 cm of healthy tissue. *C*, Urethra projecting 1 cm beyond cut edge of corpora. *D*, Buttonhole on skin for new meatus. *E*, Closure of ventral skin. *F*, Anastomosis of mucous membrane to skin to include wedge of skin in circumference. (From Peters PC: Complications of penile surgery. In Smith RB, Skinner DG, eds: Complications of Urologic Surgery: Prevention and Management, Philadelphia, WB Saunders Co, 1976, p 413.)

of a split-thickness skin graft. Small noncircumferential defects may be treated with primary closure after debridement and undermining of the edges. Management is more difficult if the skin loss occurs only proximally. Severe distal skin lymphedema will result if a significant skin bridge does not exist.[58] Circumferential skin loss must be treated with excision of all distal skin up to the coronal sulcus. Resurfacing with a split-thickness skin graft is then carried out (Fig. 39–7).

COMPLICATIONS OF PRIAPISM MANAGEMENT

Priapism management is dictated by its etiology. Radiation therapy or appropriate chemotherapy is indicated for priapism secondary to tumor infiltration.[62] Most authors recommend initial medical treatment of sickle cell–related priapism. This entails hydration, oxygen, alkalinization, analgesics, and transfusions to reduce hemoglobin S to less than 30 to 40 percent. Automated erythrocytopheresis facilitates rapid exchange with the added advantage of removing only sickled red blood cells.[64] If these measures fail to reduce pain and produce at least some detumescence within 24 hours, corporal irrigation and a shunt procedure should be considered.[65] Conservative medical therapy in young patients with sickle cell disease has been especially successful in preserving potency.[66]

Drug-related priapism secondary to papaverine and phentolamine (Regitine) injection therapy for impotence should be treated initially with intracavernous injections of norepinephrine. A concentration of 10 μg in 10 ml of normal saline is injected into the corpora cavernosa at a rate not to exceed 15 ml (15 μg) over 5 to 10 minutes. This avoids systemic side effects.[66a]

Corporal irrigation should be carried out initially in patients experiencing spontaneous priapism as well as in those with sickle cell disease who fail to respond to medical therapy. This may be done under general, spinal, or local anesthesia. Local anesthesia is accomplished by injecting 1 percent lidocaine into the glans and distal corpora. Then 16-gauge angiographic catheters are passed through the glans into both corpora cavernosa. Saline is flushed through one needle and drained through the other until all the sludged blood is removed. If penile detumescence results, no further therapy is needed.

Should irrigation fail, a cavernoglandular shunt is needed. This can be accomplished by passing a Travenol biopsy needle through the glans and taking several cores of the septum between the glans and corpora cavernosa. The puncture holes are closed with 5–0 chromic catgut sutures.[67] If this should fail, a larger shunt should be created. A 0.5-cm incision is made on one side of the glans and carried to the tip of the corpora cavernosa. Cores of the exposed septum are taken by pushing a skin biopsy punch through the tunica albuginea. The septal plug is then excised with iris scissors. The glans is closed with a running 5–0 Vicryl suture. If this fails, the procedure may be repeated on the other side.[68] Injury to the urethra is avoided by placement of a Foley catheter before either of these procedures. The glans closure stitches must be superficial in order to avoid obliteration of the shunt. Compressive dressings should not

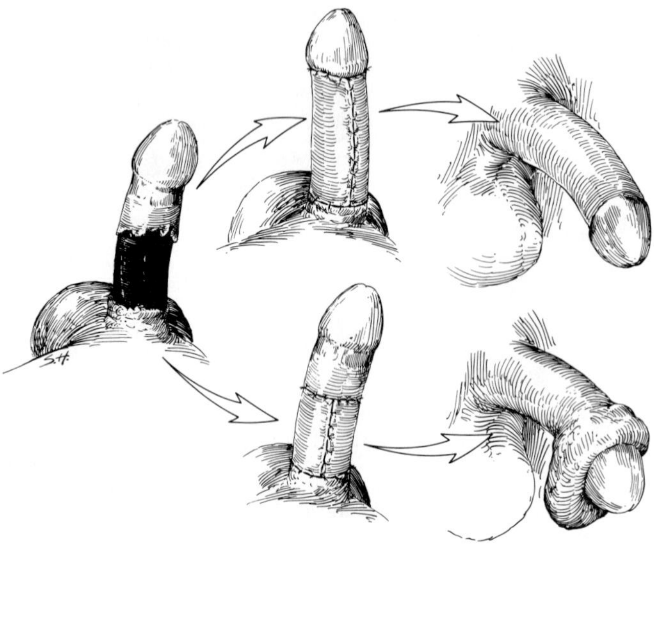

Figure 39–7. Inferior portion of figure: lymphedema resulting from an attempt to save distal penile skin. Superior portion of figure: Proper method of treating avulsion injuries of penile skin. Skin is removed completely to coronal sulcus and replaced with split-thickness graft to the point of proximal injury. A good result without lymphedema is shown as the final step in the superior portion of the figure. (From Peters PC: Complications of penile surgery. In Smith RB, Skinner DG, eds: Complications of Urologic Surgery: Prevention and Management. Philadelphia, WB Saunders Co, 1976, p 420.)

be used because they may close the shunt and can cause skin or penile necrosis.[69]

Failures of the cavernoglandular shunts have been treated successfully with the side-to-side cavernospongiosal shunt.[70] Bilateral shunts are sometimes needed. This procedure carries a risk of urethrocutaneous fistula, urethrocavernous fistula, and stricture formation.[71] A cavernosaphenous shunt[72] may also be utilized, although it is a much more involved procedure and uses a saphenous vein that may be needed for other purposes in the future. Pulmonary emboli from thrombosis of this graft have also been reported.

Impotence is a recognized complication of priapism and its therapy. Some cases of impotence are related to persistent venous leak after shunting procedures. Infusion cavernosography should be carried out unless the patient's penis feels woody and noncompliant. If a patent shunt is demonstrated, a surgical closure of the defect can restore potency.[73] Penile prosthesis placement should be performed in the other cases.

References

1. Wallerstein E: Circumcision. Urol Clin North Am 12:123, 1985.
2. Wallerstein E: Circumcision: an American Health Fallacy. New York, Springer Publications, 1980.
3. Thompson HC, King LR, Knox E: Report of the ad hoc task force on circumcision. Pediatrics 56:610, 1975.
4. Kaplan GW: Complications of circumcision. Urol Clin North Am 10:543, 1983.
5. Gee WF, Ansell JS: Neonatal circumcision: a ten year overview: with comparison of the Gomco clamp and the Plastibell device. Pediatrics 58:824, 1976.
6. Pearlman CK: Reconstruction following iatrogenic burn of the penis. J Pediatr Surg 11:121, 1976.
7. Sterenberg N, Golan J, Ben-Hur N: Necrosis of the glans penis following neonatal circumcision. Plast Reconstr Surg 68:237, 1981.
8. Datta NS, Zinner NR: Complication from Plastibell circumcision ring. Urology 9:57, 1977.
9. Sotolongo JR, Hoffman S, Gribetz ME: Penile denudation injuries after circumcision. J Urol 133:102, 1985.
10. Radhakrishnan J, Reyes HM: Penoplasty for buried penis secondary to "radical" circumcision. J Pediatr Surg 19:629, 1984.
11. Klauber GT, Sant GR: Disorders of the male external genitalia. In Kelalis PP, King LR, Belman AB, eds: Clinical Pediatric Urology. Philadelphia, WB Saunders Co, 1985, pp 825–863.
12. Belman AB: Anomalies of the urinary tract—urethra. In King LR, Kelalis PP, Belman AB, eds: Clinical Pediatric Urology. Philadelphia, WB Saunders Co, 1985.
13. Williams J, Thomas GG: The natural history of Peyronie's disease. J Urol 103:75, 1970.

13a. Nesbit RM: Congenital curvature of the phallus: report of three cases with description of corrective surgery. J Urol 93:230, 1979.

14. Benson RC, Patterson DE: The Nesbit procedure for Peyronie's disease. J Urol 130:692, 1983.
15. Gittes RF, McLaughlin AP: Injection technique to induce penile erection. Urology 4:473, 1974.
16. Coughlin WF, Culley CC, Paulson DF: Surgical correction of Peyronie's disease: the Nesbit procedure. J Urol 131:282, 1984.
17. Pryor JP, Fitzpatrick JM: A new approach to the correction of the penile deformity in Peyronie's disease. J Urol 122:622, 1979.
18. Subrini L: Surgical treatment of Peyronie's disease using penile implants: survey of 69 patients. J Urol 132:47, 1984.
19. Devine CJ, Horton CE: Surgical treatment of Peyronie's disease with a dermal graft. J Urol 111:44, 1974.
20. Das S: Peyronie's disease: excision and autografting with tunica vaginalis. J Urol 124:818, 1980.
21. Bruschini H, Mitre AI: Peyronie's disease: surgical treatment with muscular aponeurosis. Urology 5:505, 1979.
22. Devine CJ, Horton CE: Commentary on Peyronie's disease In Whitehead E, Leiter E, eds: Current Operative Urology. Philadelphia, Harper and Row Publishers. 1984, pp 1218.
23. Melman A, Holland TF: Evaluation of the dermal graft inlay technique for the surgical treatment of Peyronie's disease. J Urol 120:421, 1978.
24. Mauro PG, Luis RR, Spence CR: Peyronie's plaque: excision and graft versus incision and stent. J Urol 127:55, 1982.
25. Raz S, Dekernion JB, Kaufman JJ: Surgical treatment of Peyronie's disease: a new approach. J Urol 117:598, 1977.
26. Malloy TR, Wein AJ, Carpiniello VL: Advanced Peyronie's disease treated with the inflatable penile prosthesis. J Urol 125:327, 1981.
27. Agatstein EH, Farrer JH, Raz S: Fracture of semirigid penile prosthesis: a rare complication. J Urol 135:376, 1986.
28. Benson RC, Patterson DE, Barrett DM: Long-term results with the Jonas malleable penile prosthesis. J Urol 134:899, 1985.
29. Kaufman JJ, Boxer RJ, Boxer B, Quinn MC: Physical and psychological results of penile prosthesis: a statistical survey. J Urol 126:173, 1981.
30. Krauss DJ, Bogin D, Culebras A: The failed penile prosthetic implantation despite technical success. J Urol 129:969, 1983.
31. Montague DK: Experience with semirigid rod and inflatable penile prostheses. J Urol 129:967, 1983.
32. Keesler R: Complications of inflatable penile prostheses. Urology 18:470, 1981.
33. Furlow WL: Inflatable penile prosthesis: Mayo Clinic experience with 175 patients. Urology 13:166, 1979.
34. Scott FB, Fishman IJ, Light JK: A decade of experience with the inflatable penile prosthesis. World J Urol 1:244, 1983.
35. Merrill DC: Clinical experience with Scot inflatable penile prosthesis in 150 patients. Urology 22:371, 1983.
36. Malloy TR, Wein AJ, Carpiniello VL: Revised surgical technique to improve survival of penile cylinders for the inflatable penile prosthesis. J Urol 130:1105, 1983.
37. Summers JL, Malament I: The length of the corpora cavernosa in man and its relationship to penile prosthetic implants. J Urol 127:443, 1982.
38. Fallon B, Gerber WL: New complication of inflatable penile prothesis. Urology 18:405, 1981.
39. Furlow WL: Inflatable penile prosthesis: new device for cylinder insertion. Urology 12:447, 1978.
40. Barry JM, Giesy JD, McDuffie R: Actuarial survivals of

inflatable and flexible, hinged penile prostheses. Urology 209:605, 1982.
41. Furlow WL, Barrett DM: Inflatable penile prosthesis: new device design and patient-partner satisfaction. Urology 24:559, 1984.
42. Malloy TR, Wein AJ, Carpiniello VL: Improved mechanical survival with revised model inflatable penile prosthesis using rear-tip extenders. J Urol 128:489, 1982.
43. Riemenschneider HW: Epigastric placement of reservoir for inflatable penile prosthesis. Urology 17:79, 1981.
44. Leach GE, Shapiro CE, Hadley R, Raz S: Erosion of inflatable penile prosthesis reservoir into bladder and bowel. J Urol 131:1177, 1984.
45. Gaur DD: Single implants in the treatment of erectile impotence. J Urol 126:745, 1981.
45a. Fritzler M, Flores-Sandoval FN, Light JK: Dacron "sock" repair for proximal corporal perforation. Urology 28:524, 1986.
46. Fallon B, Rosenberg S, Culp DA: Long-term followup in patients with an inflatable penile prosthesis. J Urol 132:270, 1984.
47. Joseph DB, Bruskewitz RC, Denson RC: Long-term evaluation of the inflatable penile prosthesis. J Urol 131:670, 1984.
48. Fein RL, Needell MH: Early problems encountered with the Mentor inflatable penile prosthesis. J Urol 134:62, 1985.
49. Diokono AC: Asymmetric inflation of the penile cylinders: etiology and management. J Urol 129:1127, 1983.
50. McClellan DS, Masih BK: Gangrene of the penis as a complication of penile prosthesis. J Urol 133:862, 1985.
51. Rossier AB, Fam BA: Indication and results of semirigid penile prostheses in spinal cord injury patients: long-term followup. J Urol 131:59, 1984.
52. Chaikin L, Carrion H, Politano V: Complications of the Small-Carrion penile prosthesis: long-term followup. J Urol 126:44, 1981.
53. Light JK, Scott FB: Management of neurogenic impotence with inflatable penile prosthesis. Urology 17:341, 1981.
54. Van Arsdalen KN, Klein FA, Hackler RH, Brady SM: Penile implants in spinal cord injury patients for maintaining external appliances. J Urol 127:331, 1981.
55. Cecil AB: Repair of hypospadias and urethral fistula. J Urol 56:237, 1946.
56. Hanash KA: Plastic reconstruction of partially amputated penis at circumcision. Urology 18:291, 1981.
57. Bhanganada K, Chayavatana T, Pongnumkul C, Tonmukayakul A, Sakosatayadorn P, Komaratat K, Wilde H: Surgical management of an epidemic of penile amputations in Siam. Am J Surg 146:376, 1983.
58. McDougal WS, Persky L: External genital injuries. In Libertino J, ed: International Perspectives in Urology, Vol I. Baltimore, Williams and Wilkins Co, 1981, p 39.
58a. Carroll P, Lue T, Schmidt R, Trengrove-Jones G, McAnnich J: Penile replantation: Current concepts. J Urol 133:281, 1984.
59. Mendez R, Kiely WF, Morrow JM: Self-emasculation. J Urol 107:981, 1972.
60. McRoberts JW, Chapman WH, Ansell JS: Primary anastomosis of the traumatically amputated penis: case report and summary of literature. J Urol 100:751, 1968.
61. Burkholder GV, Newell ME: Amelioration of problems of partial penile amputation. J Urol 122:562, 1979.
62. Nelson JH, Winter C: Priapism: evolution of management in 48 patients in a 22-year series. J Urol 117:455, 1977.
63. Baron M, Leiter E: The management of priapism in sickle cell anemia. J Urol 119:610, 1978.
64. Walker EM, Mitchum EN, Rous SN, Glassman AB, Cannon A, McInnes BK: Automated erythrocytophoresis for relief of priapism in sickle cell hemoglobinopathies. J Urol 130:912, 1983.
65. Kinney TR, Harris MB, Russell MO, Duckett J, Schwartz E: Priapism in association with sickle hemaglobinopathies in children. J Pediatr 86:241, 1975.
66. Seeler RA: Intensive transfusion therapy for priapism in boys with sickle cell anemia. J Urol 110:360, 1973.
66a. Lue, TF, Hellstrom WJG, McAnnich JW, Tanagho EA: Priapism: A refined approach to diagnosis and treatment. J Urol 136:104, 1986.
67. Winter CC: Cure of idiopathic priapism. Urology 8:389, 1976.
68. Datta NS: A new technique for creation of a cavernoglandular shunt in the treatment of priapism. J Urol 136:602, 1986.
69. Weiss JM, Ferguson D: Priapism: the danger of treatment with compression. J Urol 112:616, 1974.
70. Wasmer JM, Carrion HM, Mekras G, Politano VA: Evaluation and treatment of priapism. J Urol 125:204, 1981.
71. Robbins DM, Crawford EG, Lackner HL: Late development of a urethrocavernous fistula after cavernospongiosum shunt for priapism. J Urol 133:126, 1984.
72. Grayhack JT, McCullough W, O'Connor VJ, Trippel O: Venous bypass to control priapism. Invest Urol 1:509, 1964.
73. Ebbehoj J: Insufficient penile erection due to abnormal drainage of cavernous bodies. Urology 13:507, 1979.

Reference

Jonas U, Gunther HJ: Silicone-silver penile prosthesis: description, operative approach and results. J Urol 123:865, 1980.

COMPLICATIONS OF HYPOSPADIAS REPAIR

40

Jack S. Elder • John W. Duckett

During the past 25 years, numerous changes in the repair of hypospadias have occurred. For example, reconstruction of mid-penile or penoscrotal hypospadias with chordee that was previously performed in multiple-stage procedures with hospital stays of 1 week is now performed routinely in a single stage with magnification, often in an outpatient setting or with a single night's hospital stay. Furthermore, the goals of reconstruction have been refined, with increasing emphasis not only on the functional result but on the cosmetic appearance as well. It is widely recognized that the successful repair is likely to be more a matter of experience and ability of the surgeon than of the technique employed.

The goals of hypospadias repair include (1) resection of chordee; (2) construction of a hairless urethra of sufficient diameter and length; (3) construction of a urethral meatus at the tip of the glans; (4) allowing the patient to void in a straight stream without significant splaying or deflection; (5) molding a conical glans; and (6) rearrangement of the dorsal skin to provide a uniform ventral skin cover. Familiarity with the techniques of hypospadias reconstruction and good surgical technique are essential if the surgeon expects to achieve good cosmetic results.

There are numerous potential pitfalls that may prevent a successful hypospadias repair, and a thorough understanding of the types of complications that may occur as well as their predisposing factors is essential. Even more important is that the surgeon should understand why a particular complication occurred and know how to manage it to ensure a satisfactory outcome.

Toward this end, this chapter focuses primarily on the management of complications of a variety of one-stage hypospadias repairs and reviews the approach to a failed hypospadias repair. Description of the type of hypospadias will refer to the location of the meatus following correction of any fibrous chordee.

APPROACH TO THE CHILD WITH HYPOSPADIAS

In general, six different one-stage procedures are preferred for the correction of hypospadias. This is not meant to imply that there is a cookbook approach to hypospadias repair but simply to identify the principles involved in this surgery. Since there are many individual variations with each patient, the surgeon operating on children with hypospadias cannot have a limited experience and repertoire of procedures and expect to achieve optimal results.

The meatal advancement and glanuloplasty (MAGPI) procedure may be useful in as many as 60 to 70 percent of patients. It reconstructs the glanular or coronal hypospadias in which there is a shallow urethral groove and transverse skin bridge just distal to the meatus (Fig. 40–1).[1] Patients in whom this occurs require correction because of ventral deflection of the urinary stream. It is important that the meatus be compliant and that the ventral skin on the distal penile shaft be well vascularized. Thus, some patients with coronal hypospadias should not undergo the MAGPI repair. While MAGPI usually results in a normal-appearing circumcised phal-

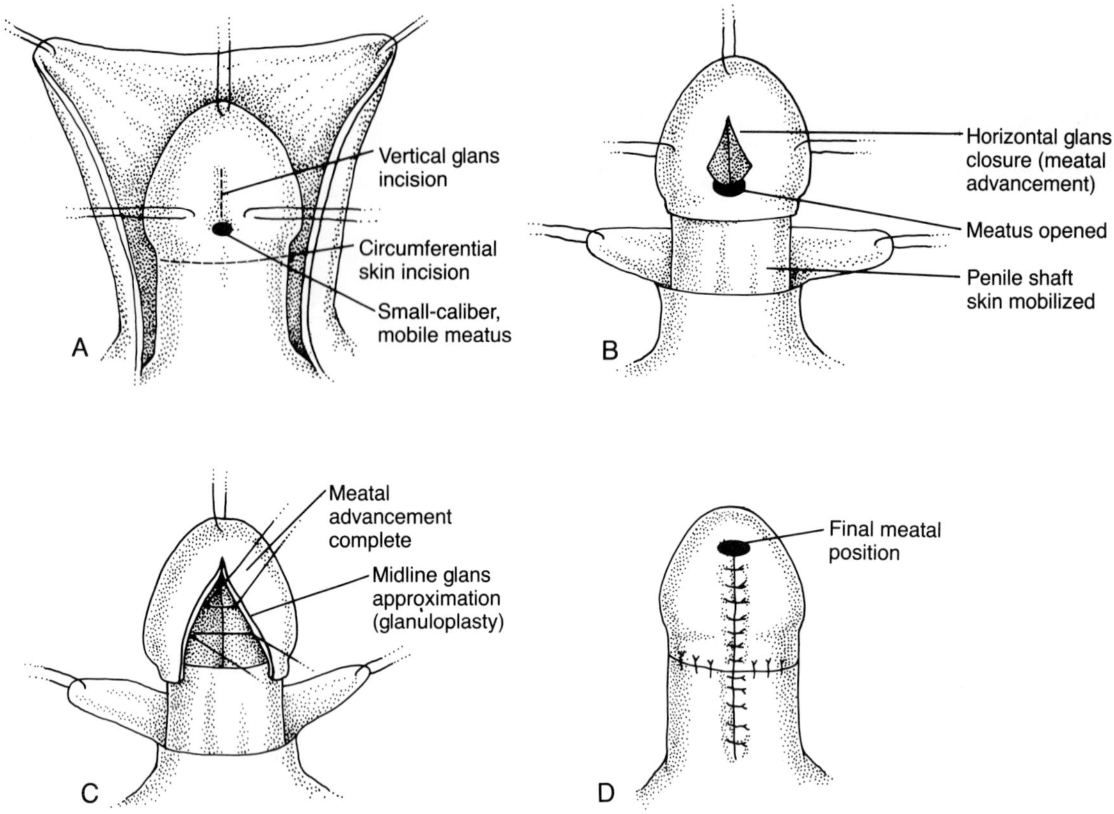

Figure 40–1. Meatal advancement and glanuloplasty (MAGPI). *A*, Coronal or subcoronal meatus. Incision of ridge of tissue between meatus and tip of urethral groove, and circumferential subcoronal incision 8 mm proximal to meatus and corona. *B*, Transverse Heineke-Mikulicz closure of dorsal meatal edge to distal glanular groove. *C*, Traction toward the tip of the glans allows approximation of the edges of the glans. *D*, Vertical mattress closure of glans. Sleeve resection of redundant prepuce with midline skin closure. (Reproduced with permission from Sheldon CA, Duckett JW: Hypospadias. Pediatr Clin North Am 34:1259, 1987.)

lus, a modification has been developed that allows preservation of the foreskin with an uncircumcised appearance.

If the meatus is subcoronal but compliant and not associated with chordee, an "extended MAGPI" procedure may be considered. When the meatus is subcoronal and a MAGPI is attempted, the meatal advancement may result in significant deformity of the glans. Furthermore, there tends to be greater stress on the glansplasty, increasing the possibility that separation of the glans may result postoperatively. These factors must be considered in choosing the type of operation to perform on a child with subcoronal hypospadias.

If the meatus is too proximal for a MAGPI but has a good ventral blood supply, or if there is a meatal variant such as a fish-mouth or noncompliant meatus, the Mathieu flip-flap procedure is preferable (Fig. 40–2).[2] When performing the meatal-based flap, it is important to preserve as much of the blood supply to the flap as possible.

In mid-penile hypospadias or distal penile hypospadias with divergent corpus spongiosum or poorly vascularized ventral skin, the onlay island flap may be used (Fig. 40–3).[3] In this procedure, which is a variant of the tubularized transverse preputial island flap, a rectangular flap of the ventral prepuce is isolated, sutured to the intact urethral plate, and covered by glans wings.

If fibrous chordee is present, the urethral plate distal to the meatus must be incised in order to straighten the penis before proceeding with the urethroplasty. In general, the transverse preputial island flap technique is preferred if a single-stage urethroplasty is to be performed (Fig. 40–4).[4] If there is considerable ventral skin deficiency following complete resection of chordee tissue, the dorsal foreskin may be left with the ventral preputial island flap and used as a ventral skin cover, called the double-faced island flap (Fig. 40–5). This prevents overlapping suture lines in the repair and in most cases has yielded a nice cosmetic result.

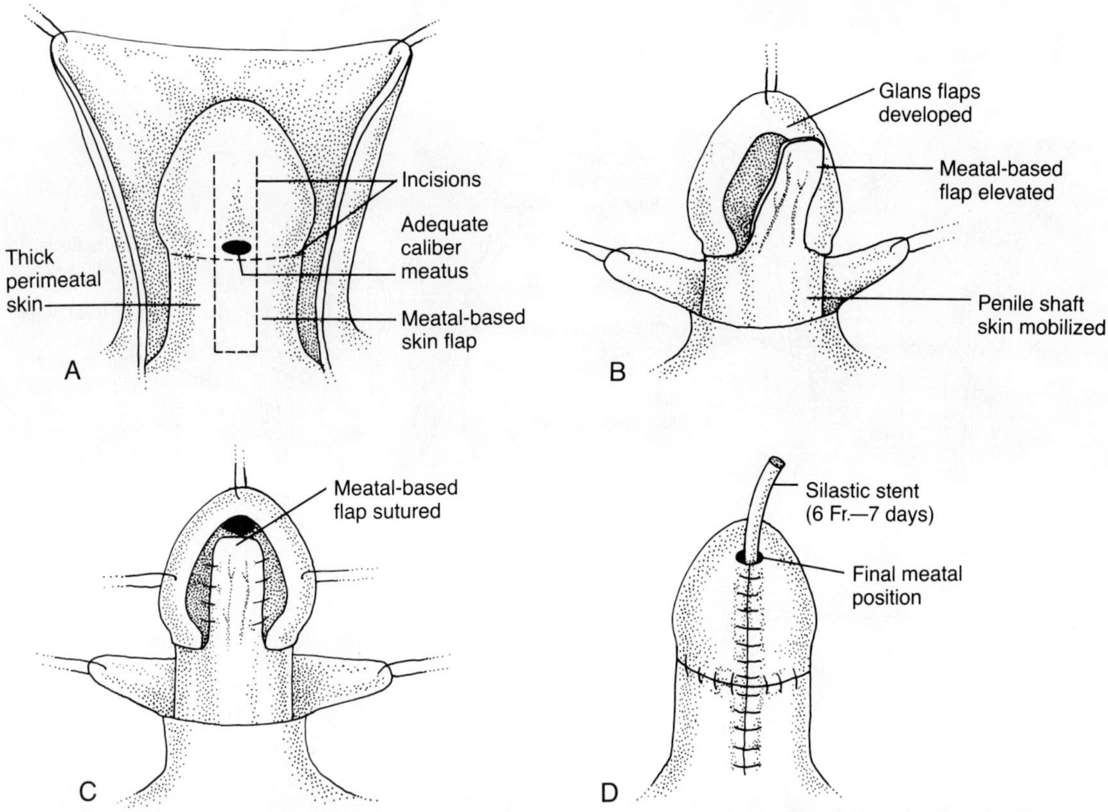

Figure 40–2. Mathieu (flip-flap) hypospadias repair. *A*, Coronal or subcoronal hypospadias with deep urethral groove and well-vascularized ventral skin. Dotted lines outline skin flaps. *B*, The meatal-based flap is mobilized, and the lateral glans wings are developed. *C*, Anastomosis of flap to urethral plate, creating neourethra. *D*, Glans flaps cover the neourethra. Excess preputial skin is excised with midline skin closure. (Reproduced with permission from Sheldon CA, Duckett, JW: Hypospadias. Pediatr Clin North Am 34:1259, 1987.)

In patients with perineal hypospadias, the midline scrotal skin may be tubularized using a Thiersch-Duplay technique because the skin is hairless and connected to the standard tubularized island flap (Fig. 40–6).

In general, if significant engulfment of the penis is present, scrotoplasty is deferred and performed as a separate procedure in order to minimize the possibility of devascularizing the preputial flap.

In urethral reconstruction, it is important to maintain the lumen of the neourethra at the appropriate size, generally 12 to 14 French. Furthermore, one must be certain that the tube is not too long when it is sutured to the glans.

The glans channel technique allows one to construct a meatus of normal caliber positioned at the tip of the penis. The channel itself is calibrated at 16 to 18 Fr. Splitting the glans in order to mobilize glanular wings is discouraged because the tissue bulk of the island flap neourethra tends to cause dehiscence of the glanular closure.

Ideally, hypospadias repair should be performed when the child is 6 to 18 months old. Children are at particular risk for separation anxiety between 15 and 24 months and may develop fears of genital injury or multilation between 3 and 6 years.[5] Performing the hypospadias repair by 18 months on an outpatient basis is thought to obviate these psychiatric concerns. The mean stretched penile length increases by only 0.8 cm between 1 and 3 years of age,[6] and complications are not higher in children under 1 year of age.[7] Ultimately, the child should have no recollection of the surgical procedure and the parents will be reassured that their child is normal.

All procedures, even the most complicated hypospadias reconstructions, can be performed safely on an outpatient basis. The following important features have contributed to success with this approach:

1. At the beginning of the procedure, a dorsal penile block is performed using 0.5 percent bupivicaine hydrochloride with a

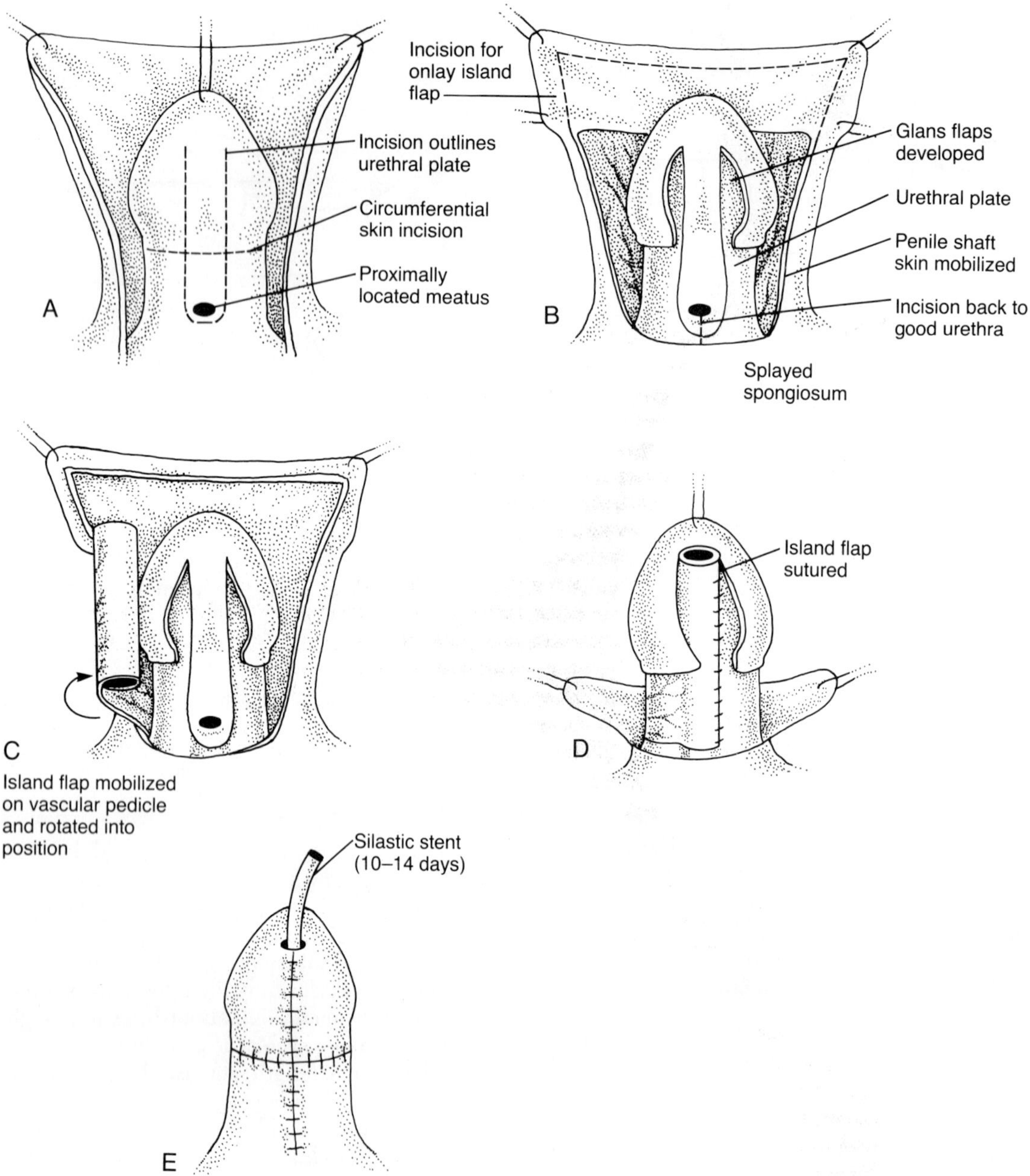

Figure 40–3. Onlay island flap. Mid-penile hypospadias or distal penile hypospadias with poorly vascularized ventral skin. *A*, Dotted lines outline skin flaps. *B*, Urethral plate defined with incision of urethra backed proximally to well-vascularized tissue. Glans wings developed. Onlay island flap outlined in ventral preputial skin. *C*, Island flap mobilized and brought ventrally. *D*, Anastomosis of onlay flap to urethral plate. *E*, Completed repair. (Reproduced with permission from Sheldon CA, Duckett JW: Hypospadias. Pediatr Clin North Am 34:1259, 1987.)

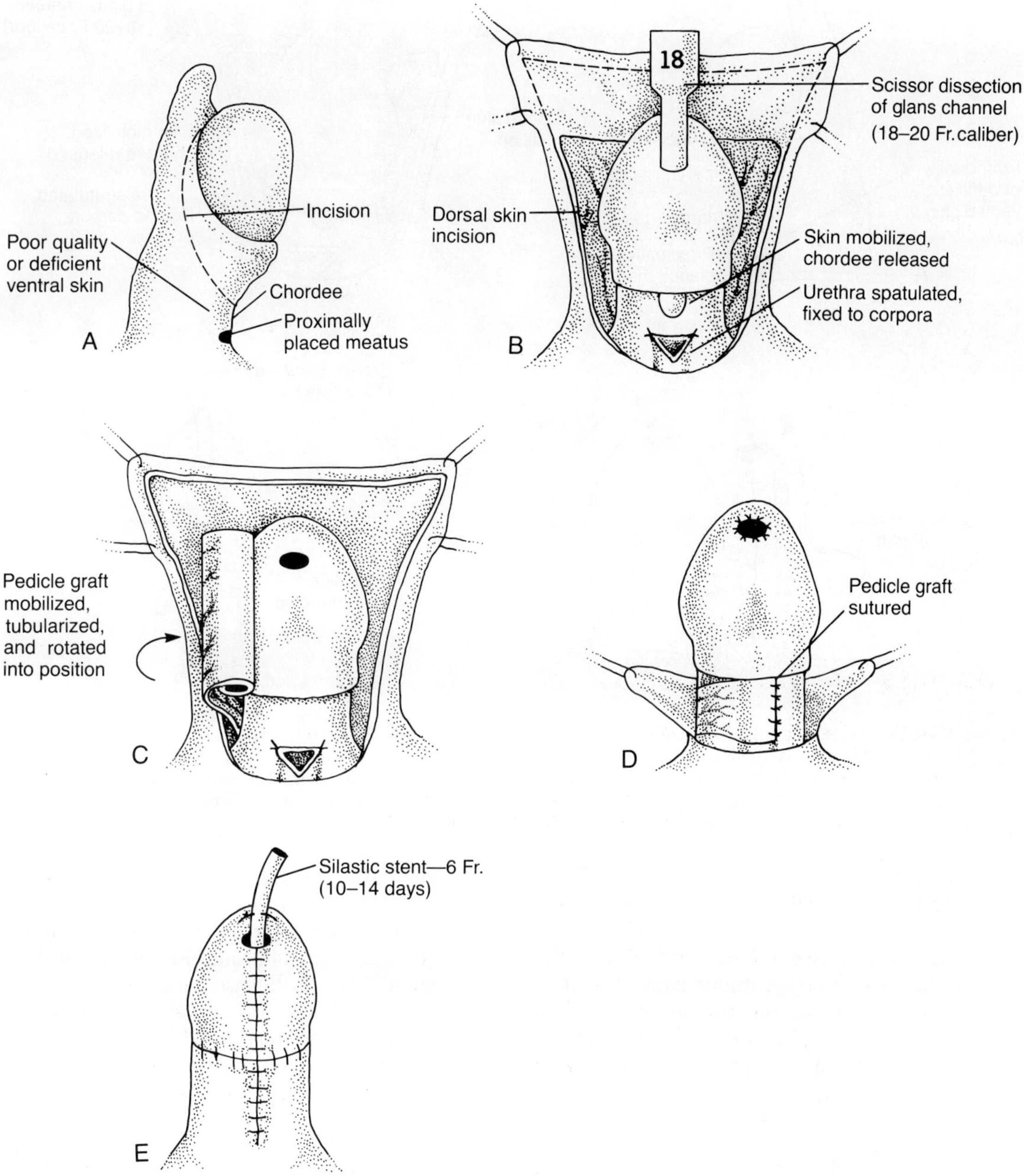

Figure 40–4. Transverse preputial island flap hypospadias repair. *A*, Penoscrotal hypospadias with fibrous chordee. Circumferential incision 8 mm proximal to corona and distal to urethral meatus. *B*, Chordee released. Glans channel created. Island flap outlined on ventral preputial skin. *C*, Pedicle flap mobilized and rotated to ventrum of penis. *D*, Urethral and meatal anastomoses completed. *E*, Midline ventral skin coverage. (Reproduced with permission from Sheldon CA, Duckett JW: Hypospadias. Pediatr Clin North Am 34:1259, 1987.)

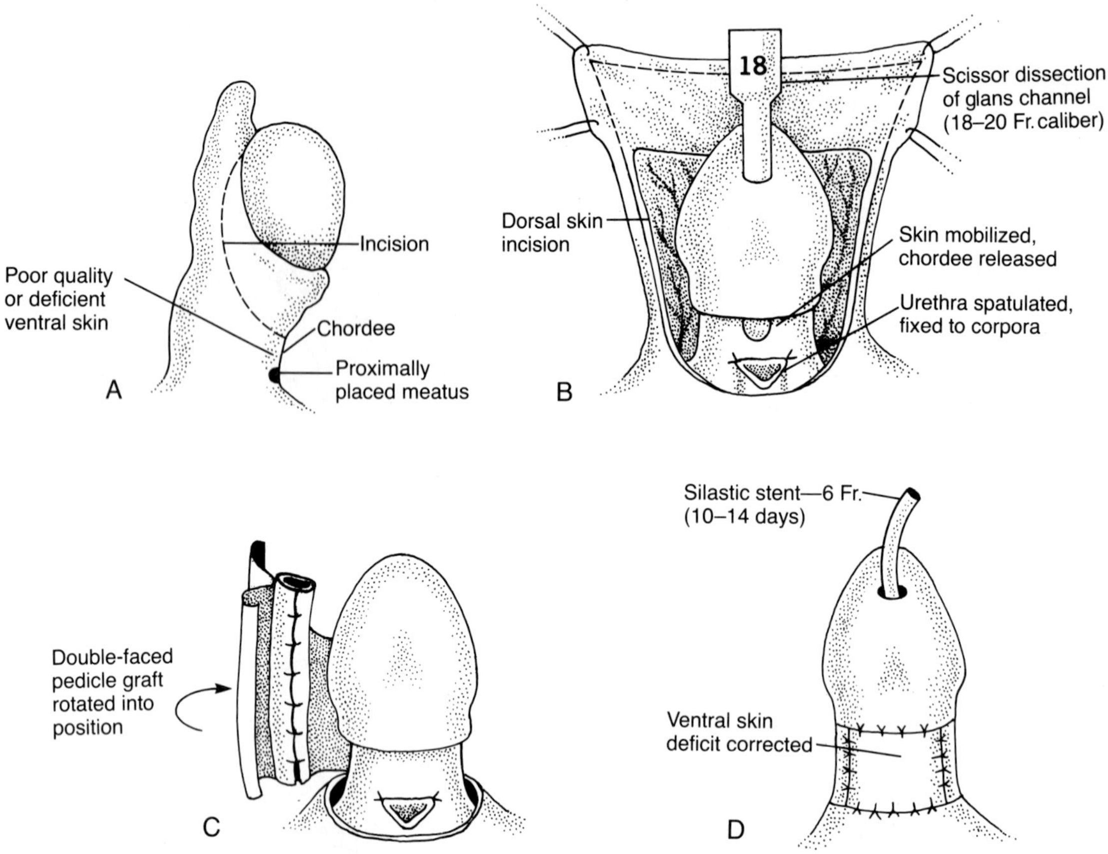

Figure 40–5. Double-faced transverse preputial island flap hypospadias repair. Penoscrotal hypospadias with fibrous chordee and deficient ventral skin. *A*, Penoscrotal hypospadias with fibrous chordee. Circumferential incision 8 mm proximal to corona and distal to urethral meatus. *B*, Chordee released. Glans channel created. Island flap outlined on ventral preputial skin. *C*, Dorsal prepuce is left attached to tubularized ventral foreskin. *D*, Completed repair. (Reproduced with permission from Sheldon CA, Duckett JW: Hypospadias. Pediatr Clin North Am 34:1259, 1987.)

maximum dosage of 2 mg/kg. This allows lower concentrations of inhalational anesthetic agents to maintain general anesthesia, prevents erections, and allows the child to wake up without pain. An alternative to this is the caudal block. If an erection develops during the procedure, it is usually an indication that the bladder is full.

2. At the beginning of the procedure, 1 percent lidocaine hydrochloride with 1:100,000 epinephrine (maximum dosage 5 mg/kg) is infiltrated into the areas where the incisions will be made. This minimizes intraoperative bleeding and obviates the need for a penile tourniquet. Tissue ischemia does not result, and the hemostatic effect remains intact throughout the duration of most procedures. When epinephrine is used, it is essential to inform the anesthesiologist because halothane, a common inhalational anesthetic used in pediatric anesthesia, sensitizes the heart to catecholamines, and ventricular arrhythmias may result. Often, enflurane (Ethrane) or isoflurane (Forane) is used instead. The cardiovascular effects of bupivicaine and lidocaine are additive. Bleeding vessels are cauterized with low current after grasping the tip of the vessel delicately. Neither suture ligatures nor drains are used routinely.
3. At the end of the reconstruction, the repair is tested with a small amount of saline. When a vascularized flap is used, the bladder is drained with a 6 Fr. silicone urethral stent, which is passed into the bladder. The stent may be obtained from ventriculoperitoneal shunt tubing. This is passed into the bladder and sutured to the glans with 5–0 monofilament sutures and drains continuously into a diaper. An alternative is the "splent" described by Mitchell and Kulb,[8] which is a 13 Fr. silicone tube with

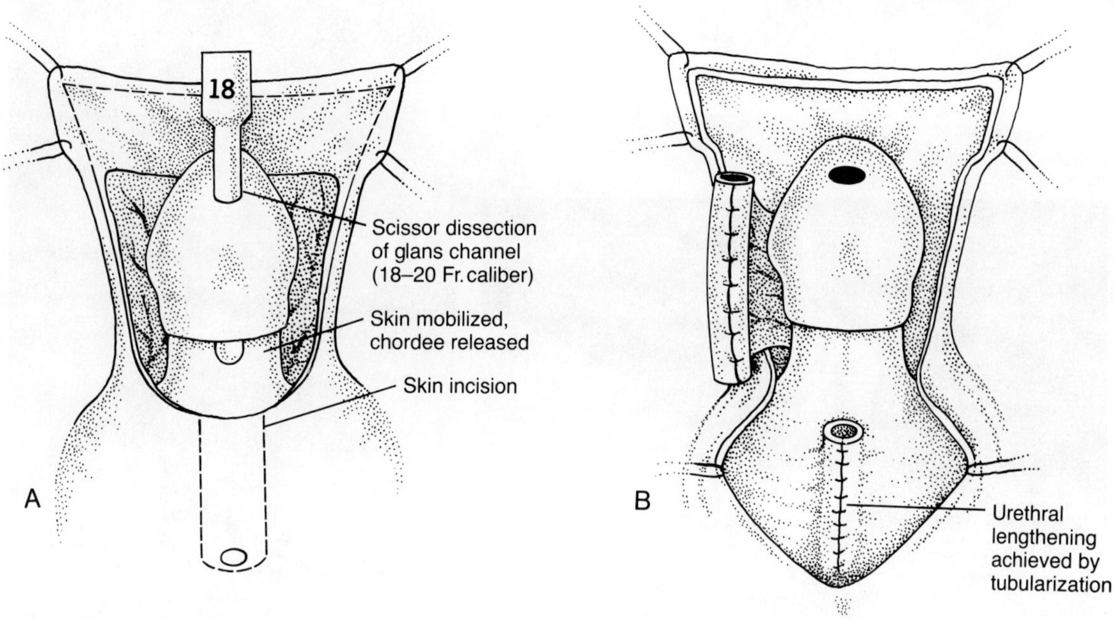

Figure 40–6. Perineal hypospadias with bifid scrotum; island flap repair. *A*, Outline of incisions allowing generous paraurethral flap of non–hair-bearing skin. Island flap outlined. *B*, Tubularization of proximal skin tube to penoscrotal junction and mobilization of tubularized island flap. (Reproduced with permission from Sheldon CA, Duckett JW: Hypospadias. Pediatr Clin North Am 34:1259, 1987.)

a longitudinal strip removed that is passed 1 cm proximal to the neourethra. This allows the child to void through the urethra immediately following urethroplasty. Disadvantages of the splent include dysuria and urinary extravasation if the repair is not completely watertight, potentially resulting in fistula, diverticulum formation, or wound infection.

4. When a stent is used, a compressive dressing is applied, either a Silastic elastomer[9] or a transparent occlusive dressing such as Opsite or Bioclusive (Fig. 40–7).

Using the approach outlined above, during a 1-year period, 97 percent of boys undergoing a MAGPI and 92 percent of those undergoing a vascularized flap procedure were discharged the same day. Reasons for hospital admission included observation for hematoma, completion of the procedure late in the afternoon, an adjunctive surgical procedure requiring hospitalization, and suspected malignant hyperthermia.

Postoperatively, boys in whom the MAGPI repair is performed undergo dressing removal in 1 or 2 days and void through the repair. In contrast, with vascularized flaps and an indwelling urethral stent, half-dose trimethoprim/sulfamethoxazole is used as long as the stent is in place. In children under 2 years of age, only acetaminophen is used for analgesia. Bladder spasms are controlled with one quarter of a belladonna and opium (B & O) suppository every 6 hours. The child is seen in the office several times during the first 2 weeks. The dressing is removed after 5 to 7 days, and the urethral stent is removed after 12 to 14 days. When the stent is removed, a urine or stent culture is obtained because 10 percent of patients produce a positive urine culture.

Late postoperative care includes assessment of the urethral meatus and wound at periodic intervals as necessary. For complex cases, the meatus is assessed in the office by passing an 8 or a 10 Fr. tapered-tip Hodgson sound, which is manufactured by Greenwald.[10] These instruments are used simply for calibration and not dilation. Although some parents are asked to dilate their child's meatus daily with the plastic tip from a tube of ophthalmic ointment, this is not routine because families fear hurting the child or damaging the repair.

COMPLICATIONS

The frequency of complications is directly related to the complexity of the repair (Tables 40–1 and 40–2) and the experience of the surgeon.[11] With an appropriately selected patient, the complication rate from a MAGPI repair should be

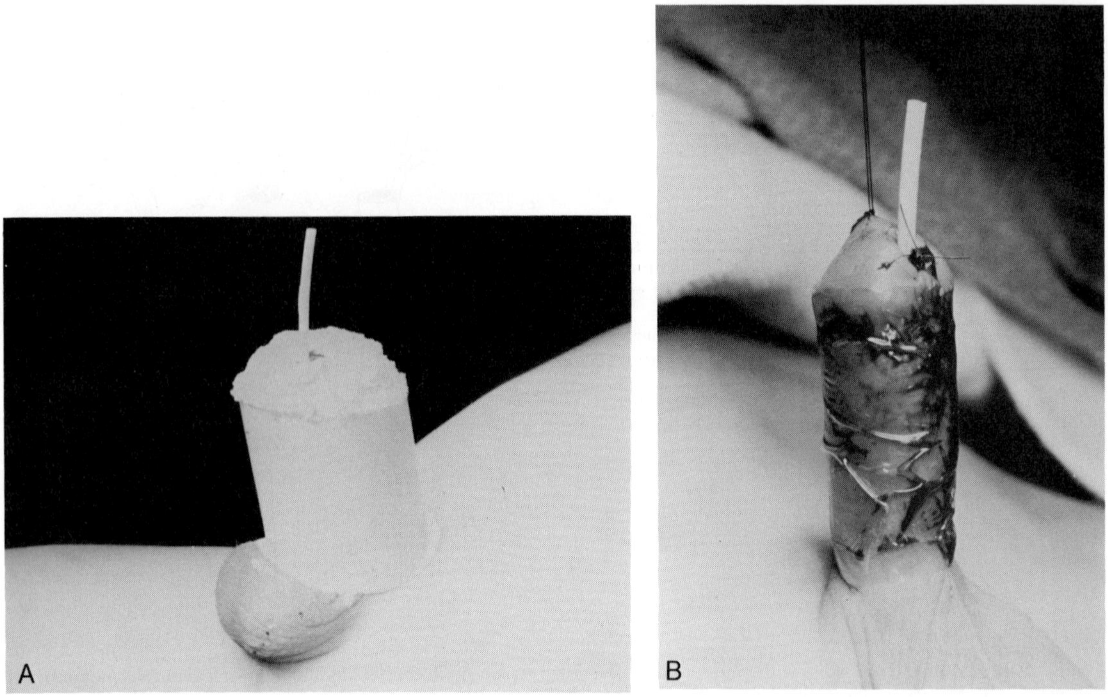

Figure 40–7. Dressings for vascularized flap hypospadias repairs. *A*, Silicone foam elastomer. *B*, Transparent adherent dressing. A 6-French silicone urethral stent is sutured to the glans, allowing continuous egress of urine.

less than 2 to 3 percent. With a Mathieu flip-flap or onlay island flap procedure, the complication rate generally is 10 percent or less. When a tubularized island flap is used, however, the complication rate tends to increase to 15 to 20 percent or more.[12] In two reviews of island flap repairs, the overall complication rate was 33 to 50 percent[13,14] One may be dissuaded by these seemingly high complication rates in centers with accumulated experience. However, in a number of instances, the problems may be managed successfully in the office or with a short outpatient surgical procedure such as a urethral dilation.

The keys to managing these problems are to (1) prepare for them and to be aware that the particular complication may develop, (2) recognize them early in order to lessen the chance of an unsuccessful surgical outcome, and (3) determine why the problems occurred to decrease the possibility that they will develop in future patients. One should not perform hypospadias surgery if he or she is unable or unwilling to manage these complications.

Acute Complications

Hematoma

A hematoma in the immediate postoperative period can be avoided with an effective external compressive dressing to tamponade the bleeding. On occasion, the child may need to return to the operating room to irrigate out the accumulated blood. If the hematoma is not recognized until several days following the surgery, one should consider removing some of the skin sutures to allow evacuation of the hematoma. Use of dressings soaked with half-strength hydrogen peroxide helps dissolve the adherent blood clots. If the hematoma is large, the vascularity of the pedicle flap or free skin graft used for urethral reconstruction may be impaired. Furthermore, fibrosis of the clot may result in postoperative chordee. Therefore, if there is concern about bleeding at the end of the operative procedure, a ¼-inch Penrose drain should be left in the subcutaneous space.

Wound Problems

Although severe wound infection in hypospadias repair is rare, mild or localized wound infections and delayed healing are possible because of compromised vascularity as well as the moist environment and proximity to the potentially unsanitary perineum. Several things can be done that may reduce the chance of infection. On the night prior to surgery, the patient's genitalia should be scrubbed with povidone-iodine or pHisoHex soap, especially in the pubertal

Table 40–1. REPORTED COMPLICATIONS OF ONE-STAGE HYPOSPADIAS REPAIRS

Series	Number of Patients	Complications (%)	Fistula (%)	Meatal Stenosis (%)	Anastomotic Stenosis (%)
	MAGPI				
Duckett, 1981[1]	200	1 (0.5)			
Hensle et al, 1983[48]	25	1 (4)	1 (4)		
Arap et al, 1984[49]	10	1 (10)			
Livne et al, 1984[50]	66	2 (3)	0	0	
Shapiro, 1984[11]	55	4 (7)	2 (4)	1 (2)	
Man et al, 1986[14]	46	4 (9)	2 (4)	1 (2)	
	Mathieu (Flip-Flap)				
Mills et al, 1981[32]	15	5 (33)	3 (20)	1 (7)	
Wacksman, 1981[51]	20	2 (10)	1 (5)	1 (5)	
Gonzales et al, 1983[52]	63	5 (8)	3 (5)	1 (2)	
Woodard & Cleveland, 1982[53]	76	19 (25)	10 (13)	8 (11)	1 (1)
Hanna, 1983[54]	21	2 (10)	1 (5)	1 (5)	
Redman, 1983[55]	60	26 (43) 17 (28)	17 (28) required reoperation	13 (22)	
Shapiro, 1984[11]	72	9 (12)	4 (6)	2 (3)	
Man et al, 1986[14]	4	2 (50)	0	1 (25)	
Elder et al, 1987[3]	34	2 (6)	0	1 (3)	
	Island Flap Techniques ***Onlay Island Flap***				
Elder et al, 1987[3]	50	3 (6)	1 (2)	0	0
	Transverse Preputial Island Flap				
Duckett, 1981[4]	100	10% required secondary surgery			
Man et al, 1986[14]	33	11 (33)	6 (18)	0	3 (9)
Barraza et al, 1987[13]	50	25 (50)	7 (14)	2 (4)	11 (22)
	Double-Faced Transverse Preputial Island Flap				
Wacksman, 1986[57]	37	3 (8)	2 (5)	1 (3)	0
	Other Techniques				
Belman, 1981[41] (Broadbent)	16	10 (63)	7 (44)	0	
Kim & Hendren, 1981[58] (tubularized meatal-based flap with mobilized glans wings)	50	2 (4)	0	2 (4)	
Koff, 1981[59] (urethral mobilization)	10	1 (10)	0	1 (10)	
Belman, 1982[42] (Mustarde)	30	5 (17)	3 (10)	2 (7)	
Chang, 1984[64] (urethral mobilization)	11	0			
Nasrallah & Minott, 1984[60] (MAGPI & urethral mobilization)	28	0			
Man et al, 1986[14] (Mustarde urethral advancement)	9 3	3 (33) 0	3 (33)	0	

Table 40–2. REPORTED COMPLICATIONS OF FREE GRAFT TECHNIQUES IN HYPOSPADIAS REPAIR

Series	Source of Graft	Number of Patients	Complications (%)	Fistula (%)	Meatal Stenosis (%)	Anastomotic Stenosis (%)
Hendren & Crooks, 1980[61]	Penile skin	69	6 (9)	1 (1)	1 (1)	3 (4)
Woodard & Cleveland, 1982[53]	—	28	14 (50)	11 (39)	3 (11)	2 (7)
Hanna, 1983[54]	Preputial/penile skin	27	5 (19)	4 (15)	1 (4)	0
Redman, 1983[55]	Penile skin	10	3 (30)	3 (30)		
Burbige et al, 1984[22]	Inner arm or buttock	11	4 (36)	2 (18)	0	2 (18)
Shapiro, 1984[11]	Prepuce or inner arm	15	3 (20)	2 (13)	1 (7)	0
Shapiro, 1986[62]	Penile skin or inner arm	14	2 (14)	1 (7)	0	0
Vyas et al, 1987[63]	Preputial skin—most cases	33	13 (39)	6 (18)	0	7 (21)
Coleman et al, 1981[44]	Bladder mucosa	9	7 (78)	0	6 (67)	1 (11)
Li et al, 1981[45]	Bladder mucosa	64	19 (30)	12 (19)	6 (9)	1 (2)
Hendren & Reda 1986[46]	Bladder mucosa	35	6 (17)	0	0	0

male. Intraoperatively, attention to gentle atraumatic technique is crucial. For example, the use of skin hooks or small holding sutures for skin flaps is preferred to grasping the flap with forceps. Furthermore, the smallest and least reactive suture material should be used.

Although perioperative antibiotics have not been demonstrated to alter the risk of wound infection, if an open stent is used for urinary diversion, postoperative antimicrobial therapy is necessary. Urinary infection must be monitored when using diversion. Urine cultures should be performed 2 to 3 weeks after the stent is removed if the child is still having irritative voiding symptoms. If infection persists, one should suspect that a utricle is present.

If a major postoperative infection occurs, it should be recognized and treated promptly. The incision should be opened to establish drainage and a wound culture obtained. Appropriate antibiotics should be administered, and necrotic tissue should be debrided. Tub baths are helpful in promoting debridement. If there is disruption of the urethra so that the child is voiding into the open wound, urinary diversion should be instituted, with either a urethral or suprapubic catheter.

Wound separation may be caused by infection, edema, hematoma, erections, insufficient blood supply to the tissues, weakened or frayed suture material, and vigorous removal of the dressing. In addition, it may result from tension on the skin closure. If the defect in the wound is small, it will granulate and epithelialize in rapidly if it is clean. On the other hand, if the defect is more than 5 mm in size, and there is no infection, Steri-Strips may be used to try to reapproximate the skin edges loosely. In general, the placement of additional sutures to try to close the defect is counterproductive. Devitalized tissue should be removed because it is more vulnerable to bacterial infection than vascularized tissue.

In the vascularized pedicle flap procedures, necrosis of the preputial skin flaps used for skin cover may occur. Ideally, this possibility should be recognized during the hypospadias surgery itself, because the devascularized portion of the skin flaps will appear cyanotic. Application of a dressing that is too tight or a hematoma also may devascularize flaps with marginal viability. In such cases, an eschar usually forms with gradual epithelialization of the defect. Grafting is usually unnecessary. In most cases, the pedicle flap will remain intact, and a satisfactory result may occur without reoperating. On the other hand, if glanular wings are used to cover the neourethra, as used in an onlay island flap or Mathieu flip-flap repair, localized wound infection may occur, resulting in breakdown of the glans closure.

Fistula

If a fistula is recognized shortly after removal of the urethral or suprapubic catheter, passing a feeding tube back through the repair into the bladder to divert the urine a little longer should be considered. However, there is little evidence that this is more likely to result in fistula closure than by simply allowing the patient to void on his own. If the fistula is small, and there is no inflammation or meatal stenosis, the fistula has a reasonable chance of closing spontaneously. It may be necessary to dilate the urethra with the tip of an ophthalmic ointment tube periodically to ensure an adequate meatal caliber.

Chronic Complications

Following an unsuccessful single-stage hypospadias repair, it is important to evaluate the patient carefully in planning the secondary surgical procedure. Often, multiple problems necessitate correction such as a fistula with concurrent meatal stenosis or a urethral diverticulum at the site of a fistula. A urethra that is too long may kink at the anastomosis. Secondary surgery in boys with hypospadias can present a tremendous operative challenge. The variety of potential complications attests to the necessity of careful attention to each detail in the initial operative procedure.

Urethrocutaneous Fistula

The most common postoperative complication is a urethrocutaneous fistula. The incidence of this complication varies between centers but clearly is highest in more extensive urethral reconstructive procedures (Tables 40–1 and 40–2). In some cases, the fistula is associated with meatal stenosis or a distal urethral stricture, resulting in higher urethral pressure during voiding and a "blowout" of the urethral repair. In most cases, a fistula results from a combination of factors including wound infection, failure to create a watertight anastomosis, delayed healing because of devitalized tissue, apposing suture lines, failure to invert the epithelium of the neourethra, or a poorly vascularized neourethra. If a suprapubic tube is used in the initial reconstruction, one should be certain to remove meatal crusting before allowing the child to void in order to prevent high urethral pressure.

Operative management of the fistula necessitates experience in a variety of plastic surgical principles including the use of a variety of skin flaps.[15–20] Intraoperatively, the urethra distal to the fistula must be assessed for narrowing. If an 8 or a 10 Fr. bougie à boule can be passed to the fistula, there is neither concomitant stenosis nor distal stricture. It is useful to inject saline retrograde into the urethra to determine whether another fistula or possibly an associated diverticulum exists. A small lacrimal duct probe is passed through the apparent fistulous tract(s) to identify its path; occasionally, these tunnel obliquely in the subcutaneous tissue several millimeters. Furthermore, passing the probe distally through the fistula may reveal an obstructing flap or valve. Before proceeding with excision of the fistula, an artificial erection should be induced if one suspects that chordee is present.

The fistula is circumscribed in an elliptical manner and carefully dissected with the metal probe in place to its connection with the urethra. It is then cut flush with the urethra and the fistula is closed with a running 7–0 polyglycolic acid (Dexon) or polydioxanone (PDS) suture, turning the mucosal edges into the lumen. One should ensure that the closure is watertight by filling the urethra with saline in a retrograde manner and compressing the proximal urethra. A second subcutaneous layer may be closed perpendicular to the initial suture line to avoid overlap, although this is not critical. Skin closure is performed with 6–0 chromic sutures. Superglue is applied to the closed wound for dressing. In most cases of simple fistula repair, urinary diversion is unnecessary. These procedures may be performed in an outpatient setting, and the success rate is approximately 90 percent.[12] If the fistula is 5 mm or larger, or if there is an associated problem, urinary diversion with a silicone stent is preferable. In large fistulas, the "pants-over-vest" (Durham Smith) technique of skin closure is helpful to ensure a successful result.[16]

The incidence of urethral fistula formation following primary hypospadias repair may be reduced with the use of a scrotum-based flap of tunica vaginalis, which is used to cover the reconstructed urethra, as advocated by Snow.[21] This may also be a useful adjunct to the difficult fistula closure.

Urethral Stricture

The second most common complication following hypospadias repair is urethral stricture. In general, these occur at the site of the proximal anastomosis following tubularized urethral reconstructive procedures. In most cases, the stricture becomes evident during the first 2 or 3 months following hypospadias repair, either by diminished force of the urinary stream or by straining to void, or it may become apparent during postoperative calibration of the neourethra. The etiology of the stricture can vary, depending on the type of repair performed. In an island pedicle flap, the stricture may be functional, secondary to angulation at the proximal anastomosis. This may be avoided by fixing the lateral edges of the proximal urethra to the tunica albuginea of the corporal bodies before performing the anastomosis. In addition, generous spatulation of the urethra and proximal flap is helpful. In other cases, the stricture may result simply if the neourethra is too narrow.

Free grafts of full-thickness preputial or penile skin are best for urethral reconstruction because they are thin and will revascularize well. However, we have found that thicker free grafts harvested from the groin skin or inner upper arm do not function as well. Thick induration around the graft lasts for months, and a diffuse stricture of the entire neourethra requires frequent dilation and ultimately replacement in some cases. Thick split-thickness grafts may be a better urethral replacement[22] but we have not used them. If a free graft is used, a cicatricial scar is more likely to develop at the anastomosis.

The management of the stricture depends upon its severity. In one series, 15 of 23 (65 percent) of strictures responded to a single dilation under anesthesia.[13] If this is unsuccessful, however, direct vision urethrotomy with the 11 Fr. pediatric resectoscope may be effective. Urinary diversion should be performed with a silicone stent passed into the bladder and sutured to the glans. Concomitant injection of a steroid solution directly into the incised stricture may be helpful in preventing recurrence.[23] Repeated dilations or urethrotomies should not be performed; rather, these should be managed by direct repair of the stricture, generally by excision and reanastomosis, a vascularized pedicle onlay island to bridge the strictured area, or a free patch graft.

Urethral Diverticulum

When the tubularized island flap urethroplasty is used, a diffuse urethral diverticulum may form and has been reported in 10 percent of patients (Fig. 40–8).[24,25] A significant diver-

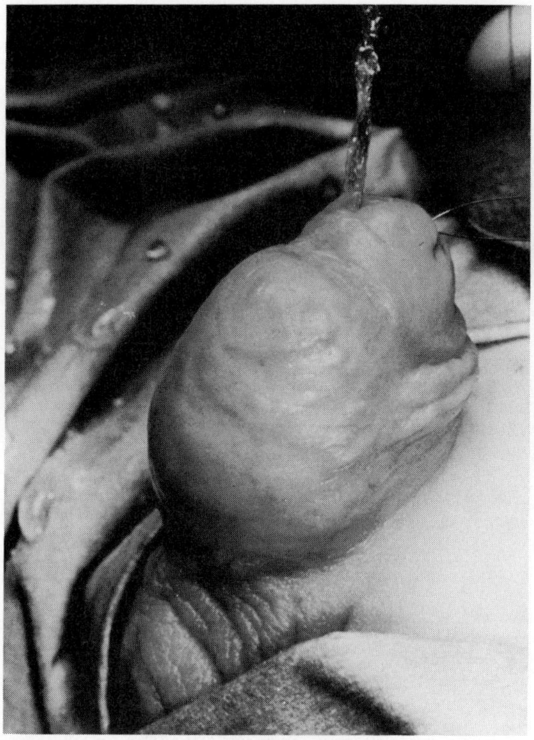

Figure 40–8. Urethral diverticulum in an 18-month-old child, 6 months following double-faced transverse preputial island flap repair. (Reproduced with permission from Elder JS, Duckett JW: Urethral reconstruction following an unsuccessful one-stage hypospadias repair. World J Urol 5:19, 1987.)

ticulum was present in 11 percent of boys who had undergone multiple failed hypospadias repairs.[26] Several factors appear to be contributory, including:

1. creation of a urethra with a caliber that is too large.
2. urinary extravasation from the neourethra secondary to wound disruption resulting in an epithelialized sac which allows urinary stasis.
3. an increase in outlet resistance (such as meatal stenosis) that develops following wound healing. This results in gradual dilatation of the neourethra, similar to an aneurysmal dilatation, because of a lack of supporting corpus spongiosum.
4. a neourethra that is too long, resulting in kinking at the level of the glans channel.

Usually the diverticulum is not apparent until 3 to 6 months following urethroplasty. These boys produce a weak urinary stream with post-void dribbling and often experience ballooning of their ventral penile shaft. They are prone to urinary tract infections because of urinary stasis.

An intraoperative retrograde urethrogram is helpful in delineating the extent and severity of the diverticulum and in detecting associated problems (Fig. 40–9). Distal urethral caliber must be assessed with the bougie à boule. In some cases, the diverticulum may be excised and reduced in a longitudinal fashion. A circumcising incision is made and the penile skin is dropped back to the penoscrotal junction in this situation. If a localized proximal diverticulum exists near the penoscrotal area, an incision in the scrotum pulled over the repair site allows the diverticulum to be closed without overlapping suture lines. One should look for an associated fistula adjacent to a diverticulum. For cases of distal urethral narrowing, a variety of flaps have been described utilizing the diverticular tissue to bridge the strictured area (Figs. 40–10 and 40–11).[27] Clearly, an understanding of flaps in plastic surgery and creative use of these flaps are helpful. After resection of a diverticulum, the urine should be diverted for 7 to 10 days.

Meatal Stenosis

Another long-term problem is meatal stenosis. With careful and frequent follow-up in a child in whom it is suspected, this complication often can be prevented. If the meatus is small, the parents are asked to dilate the child's meatus daily with the tip of an ophthalmic ointment tube. Intraoperatively, the chances of meatal stenosis may be minimized by ensuring that the meatal caliber is adequate at the completion of the procedure. In the preputial island flap procedure, the glans channel is created by excision and incision of glans tissue rather than by simply forcibly dilating the channel to the desired size.

If the stenotic meatus is refractory to postoperative dilatation, a variety of options are available. If the surgeon thinks that the meatus should be closer to the tip of the glans, a dorsal meatotomy may be sufficent, as performed during the MAGPI procedure. More frequently, a dorsal glans flap must be elevated, its underlying scar excised, and the gap bridged with the flap, completing a Y–V-plasty. In more severe cases, a more extensive glanulomeatoplasty may be necessary. In such cases, a ventral flap is developed and folded into the split glans,[28] or a ventral transverse onlay island flap may be used and covered with glans wings.[29]

A complicating feature that sometimes occurs is the development of balanitis xerotica obliterans (BXO). This idiopathic condition is charac-

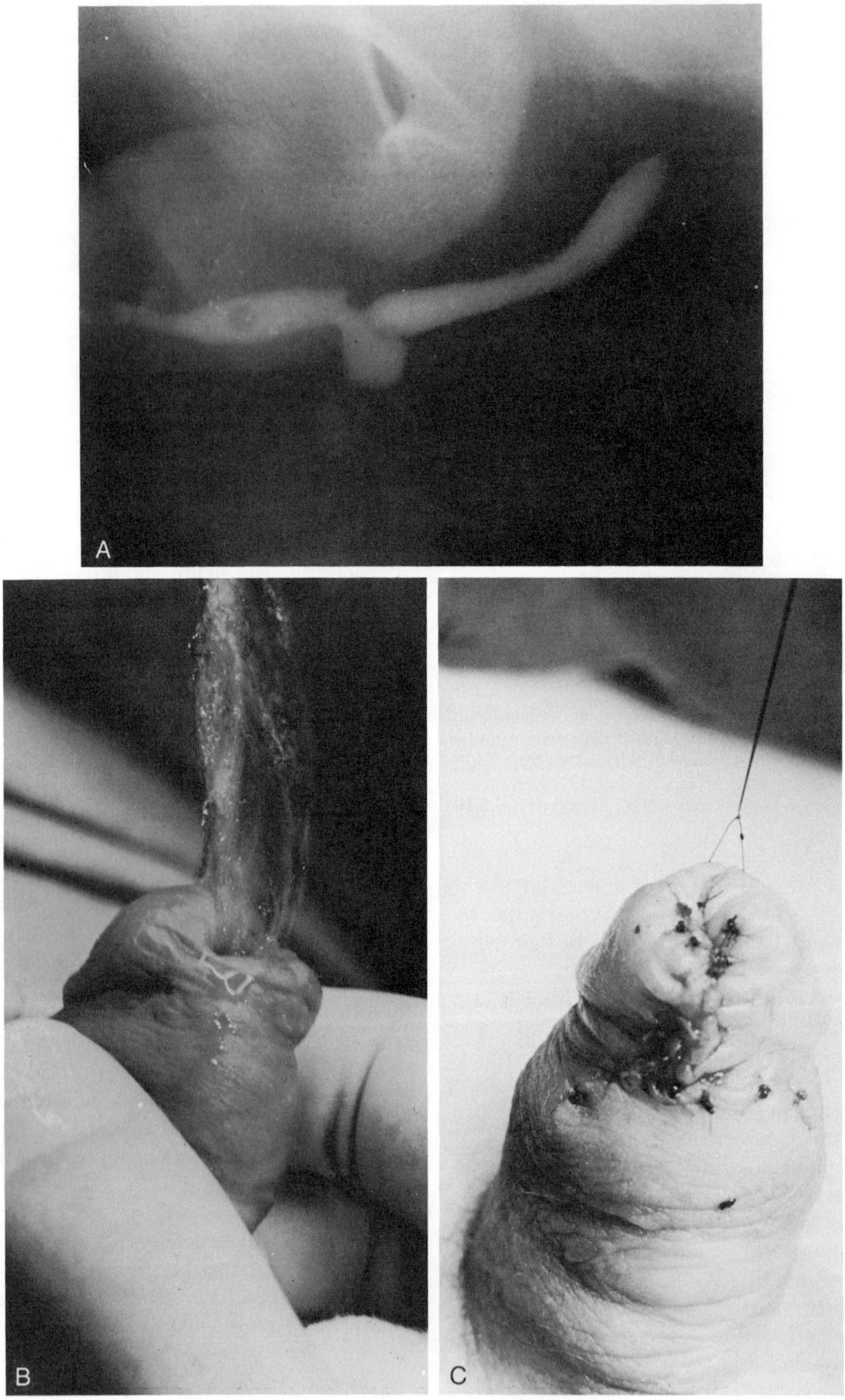

Figure 40–9. *A*, Retrograde urethrogram demonstrating small diverticulum and fistula in a boy with two previous hypospadias repairs. *B*, Antegrade injection of saline through a catheter in the bulbous urethra demonstrates substantial splaying of the urinary stream. *C*, Meatal advancement and glanuloplasty (MAGPI) has been performed to reconstruct the urethral meatus and glans. Diverticulum and fistula have also been repaired. The patient now voids with a normal urinary stream. (Reproduced with permission from Elder JS, Duckett JW: Urethral reconstruction following an unsuccessful one-stage hypospadias repair. World J Urol 5:19, 1987.)

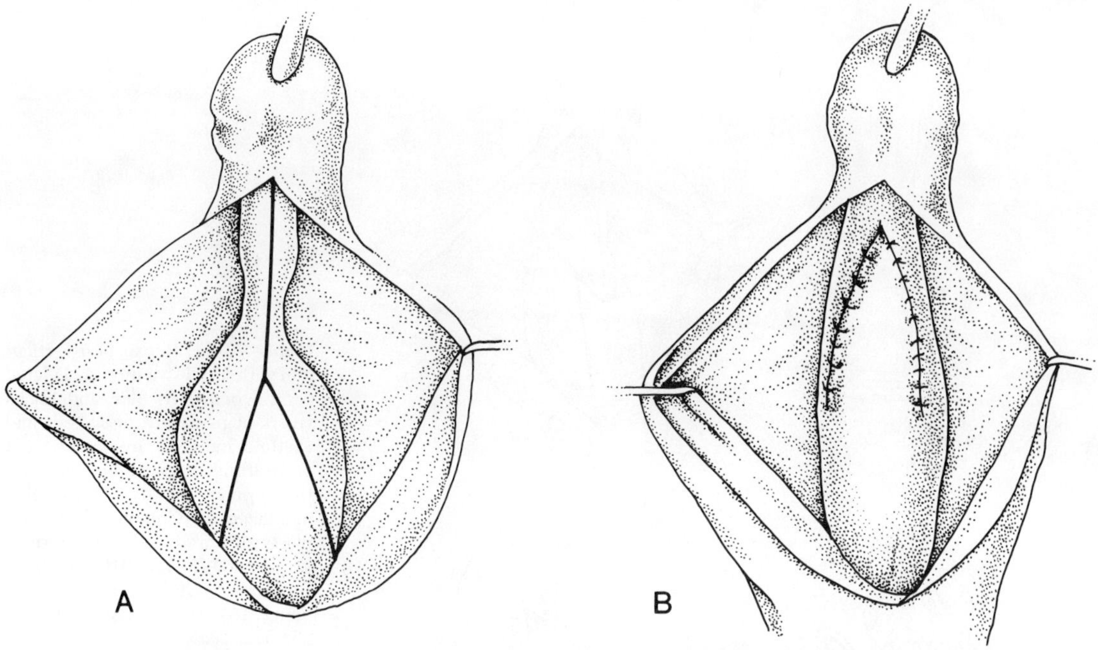

Figure 40–10. Repair of urethral diverticulum with distal stricture. *A*, Urethral incisions for Y-V repair. *B*, Completed urethroplasty. (Reproduced with permission from Winslow BH, Vorstman B, Devine CJ Jr: Urethroplasty using diverticular tissue. J Urol 134:552, 1985.)

terized by a chronic inflammatory infiltrate in the dermis and hyperkeratosis and is recognized by a pale halo circumscribing the meatus. In patients whom a tubularized flap has been created or a graft performed, the condition seems to involve primarily the ventral preputial skin and thus may result in diffuse induration of the neourethra with puckering of the meatus.[30] Meatal stenosis tends to recur in patients with BXO who have undergone meatoplasty. Steroid injections may be helpful in diminishing the severity of BXO, but most patients require excision of the affected area and reconstruction.

Chordee

With the widespread application of the technique to produce artificial erection, persistent postoperative chordee is uncommon. In primary hypospadias repair, it is imperative that the penis be straight before the urethroplasty is performed. In patients with penoscrotal or perineal hypospadias, even following excision of the fibrous chordee tissue, the penis may still have significant ventral tethering. Occasionally, a vertical incision between the corpora will allow it to straighten. More often, dorsal plication is necessary. When performing dorsal plication, the surgeon must be careful to avoid the neurovascular bundle. Rather than excising ellipses of the tunica on each side, simple plication is performed with 4–0 Tevdek or Ticron sutures, which are soft, permanent braided suture materials. These sutures are preferred to polypropylene because the cut ends of the latter suture are hard and can be noticeable subcutaneously.

In secondary surgical procedures, if an artificial erection demonstrates chordee, a subcoronal circumferential incision should be made with the penile skin mobilized. In most cases, the chordee is mild and can be corrected with dorsal plication as discussed previously. If the ventral scarring is severe, excision of the tunica albuginea may be necessary with a patch graft of dermis or tunica vaginalis. At times, one also may find a disturbing degree of glanular tilt. This may be corrected by using plicating sutures under the dorsum of the glans. One should remember that the blood supply to the glans penis is usually via a single dorsal artery;[31] therefore, significant mobilization of the dorsal aspect of the glans risks devascularization.

Other Meatal Complications

A retrusive meatus is an occasional complication of a MAGPI or Mathieu flip-flap repair in which the glansplasty has broken down. The urethra may not have been sufficiently compliant to allow the meatal advancement, the distal

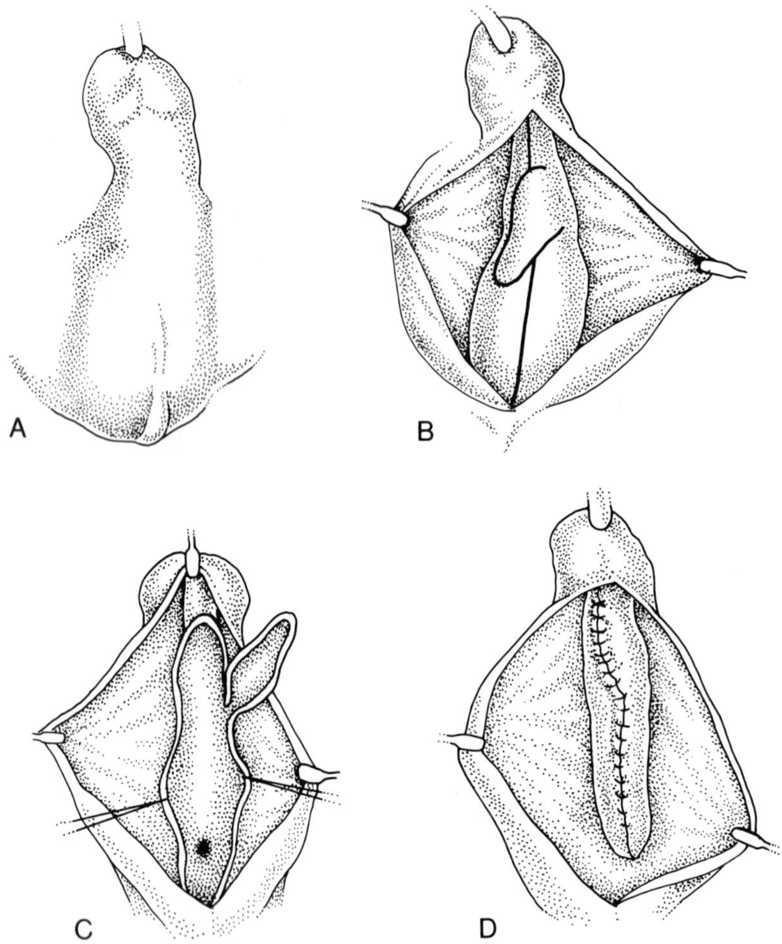

Figure 40–11. Repair of diverticulum with distal stricture. *A*, Dilated ventral penis. *B*, Skin and fascial layers of penis are dissected, and urethral incisions are marked out on urethral diverticulum. *C*, Urethra open with diverticular flap mobilized. *D*, Completed urethroplasty. (Reproduced with permission from Winslow BH, Vorstman B, Devine CJ Jr: Urethroplasty using diverticular tissue. J Urol 134:552, 1985.)

penile skin for the flip-flap may have been too thin, or infection may have resulted in premature dissolution of the glansplasty sutures. In these cases, the deformity is primarily cosmetic and not functional; that is, often, the stream is not significantly distorted. However, if there is significant splaying or deflection of the urinary stream, secondary reconstruction is advised. In general, a Mathieu flip-flap procedure is effective. Attempts to achieve an apical meatus in all cases of hypospadias result in a higher complication rate and can be considered "the price of perfection."[32] Nevertheless, a meatus at the tip of the glans is the desired cosmetic result and this goal is encouraged.

Splaying of the stream occurs either with a retrusive meatus or with an unsatisfactory coronal meatus following hypospadias repair. In a series of 33 patients undergoing the Denis Brown operation, 39 percent complained of significant splaying, although the peak urinary flow rate was normal.[33] In a series from the Mayo Clinic in which most patients had undergone a multiple-stage procedure, 20 percent experienced significant splaying during voiding.[34] With current techniques that emphasize construction of a glanular meatus, this complication is not as common. For example, in a series of boys undergoing the MAGPI procedure, only 4.5 percent reported significant splaying of the stream.[35] Often meatal revision, either with a MAGPI procedure or with a Mathieu flip-flap repair, corrects the problem (Fig. 40–9). At the beginning of the procedure, the stream should be evaluated by compression of the full bladder or by injecting saline antegrade through a #18 angiographic catheter inserted percutaneously into the urethral lumen at the level of the penoscrotal junction.[36] Sometimes the glans channel meatus has redundant skin forming a doughnut-like appearance that requires excision to improve stream quality.

Other Urethral Problems

If there is hair in the urethra, complications such as infection and calculi formation may occur, but these are infrequent. This problem usually is seen following the older multiple-stage procedures in which hair-bearing scrotal skin was used for urethral reconstruction. If complications develop, the stones and incrustation can be cleaned out during urethroscopy. In a severe situation, the urethra may be replaced with a free patch graft or a short island pedicle flap.

Some boys have long-term problems with recurrent urinary tract infections. These may be secondary to a urethral diverticulum or a redundant urethroplasty that permits stasis of urine. A voiding cystourethrogram should be performed to determine whether a prostatic utricle is present. In 50 percent of boys with perineal hypospadias and in 10 percent with penoscrotal hypospadias, an enlarged utricle is present.[37] The utricle may be a source of urinary stasis predisposing to chronic urinary tract infections, but most likely a distal stenosis is present. Very rarely should a patient with hypospadias in whom a utricle develops require excision.

Psychiatric Concerns

Psychosexual consequences have been recognized in a number of men who have undergone hypospadias repair. In a series of adults (mean age 27 years) who underwent hypospadias correction at a mean age of 5 years, 38 percent had had limited or no sexual experience, and the overall group tended to have fewer coital partners and were older at initiation of sexual activity compared with an age-matched control group.[38] Furthermore, double-blinded independent assessment suggested that the men were less secure with their masculinity and had higher anxiety and hostility levels and lower self-esteem and capacity for interpersonal relations.[39,40] Most of the men had undergone two or three operative procedures for hypospadias correction. For these reasons, and those outlined at the beginning of this chapter, ideally, correction of hypospadias should be performed by 18 months of age.

RECONSTRUCTION FOLLOWING MULTIPLE FAILED HYPOSPADIAS REPAIRS

Patients who have undergone multiple unsuccessful hypospadias repairs represent one of the greatest challenges to pediatric urologists.[26] These patients have been termed "hypospadias cripples." This term should be abandoned not only because of the disparaging connotation but also because of the potential litigious implications of the term. These patients generally have multiple problems that need to be corrected. Although the physician performs a surgical procedure on these patients with a plan in mind, often the procedure must be modified considerably to accommodate intraoperative findings.

In general, it is worthwhile to perform a retrograde urethrogram or voiding cystourethrogram to assess the urethral anatomy (Fig. 40–9). The primary problem in many patients is to bridge a long urethral defect. In some patients, there is sufficient residual penile skin to perform a repeat island pedicle flap—either tubularized or as an onlay—depending on the situation. An alternative is the Broadbent repair, in which a skin flap is created distal to the meatus and carried obliquely around the shaft, which is then tubularized and brought through a glans channel.[41] If the meatus is somewhat distal and there is residual chordee, a Mustarde repair may be performed, in which a proximal meatus-based skin flap is tubularized and brought through a glans channel after excision of the residual fibrous chordee.[42]

If these measures fail, a free graft is necessary. In the past, a free skin graft has been obtained from a non–hair-bearing site such as the penis, the medial aspect of the upper arm, or the thigh. A full-thickness skin graft is preferable to a split-thickness graft because the latter contains very little or no dermis and contracture will occur. However, a thick split-thickness skin graft is probably satisfactory;[22] these have been cut with a dermatome and contain a thick portion of the dermis. Thus, they are probably closer to full-thickness grafts than to split-thickness grafts. An important surgical consideration is that skin thickness varies depending on the donor site. Free grafts rely on vascularity from the recipient site. The split-thickness skin graft requires a less vascularized recipient bed than a full-thickness graft because of the greater number of blood vessel openings on the split-thickness graft undersurface. In a reoperative situation in which the vascularity of the recipient field may be compromised, this consideration is important. We have abandoned the use of groin or inner arm full-thickness grafts owing to the thickness of the skin.

We have been pleased with the free bladder mucosal graft.[43–47] Although this type of graft has been used in primary hypospadias reconstruction,[44,45] we have reserved it for the patient who

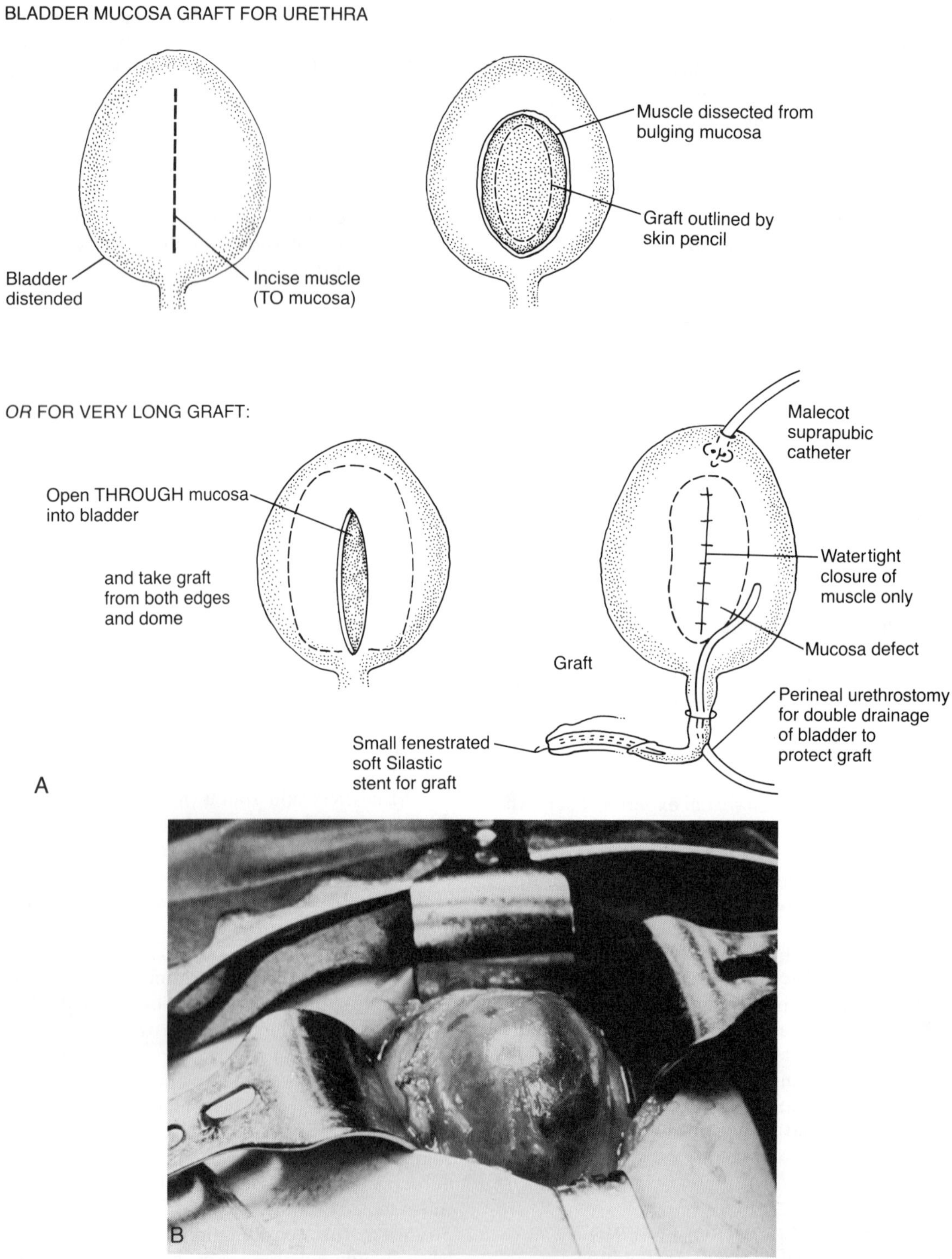

Figure 40–12. Bladder mucosa graft. *A*, Operative procedure for obtaining bladder mucosa graft. (Reproduced with permission from Hendren WH, Reda EF: Bladder mucosa graft for construction of male urethra. J Pediatr Surg 21:189, 1986.) *B*, Intraoperative view of exposed bladder mucosa in preparation for free graft. (Reproduced with permission from Elder JS, Duckett JW: Urethral reconstruction following an unsuccessful one-stage hypospadias repair. World J Urol 5:19, 1987.)

has had a previous unsuccessful repair. Before harvesting the graft, as much of the penile surgery should be performed as possible. Following exposure of the distended bladder, the bladder muscle is incised vertically with the cautery to expose the mucosa, which will protrude (Fig. 40–12). At this point, one can bluntly dissect the muscle and submucosa off the mucosa to expose a large section from which to obtain a graft. After the graft is harvested, it is tubularized over a suitable-sized catheter. The graft should be kept moist with cool saline during its preparation. One end of the graft is then spatulated and sutured to the patient's urethra (all previous urethroplasties should be removed). The graft is brought out through a glans channel and sutured to the tip of the penis with interrupted 6–0 chromic sutures. The graft should be trimmed so that it is not too wide or too long. In addition, the suture line on the graft should be kept dorsal so that it lies against the corporal bodies of the penis.

Following penile reconstruction, a suprapubic tube and silicone urethral stent are used. Postoperatively, the meatus should be kept moist with an antibiotic ointment for 2 to 3 weeks. In preparing the bed for the graft, it is important that all previous scar tissue be excised in order to allow maximum vascularization of the graft. In addition, the use of suction drains for 48 hours will ensure proper tissue approximation for revascularization of the bladder mucosa graft. The primary long-term complication with these grafts has been meatal stenosis, occurring in a significant number.[44] Postoperative meatal dilation by the parents should be routine for several months.

References

1. Duckett JW: MAGPI (meatoplasty and glanuloplasty): a procedure for subcoronal hypospadias. Urol Clin North Am 8:513, 1981.
2. Gibbons MD, Gonzales ET, Jr: The subcoronal meatus. J Urol 130:739, 1983.
3. Elder JS, Duckett JW, Snyder HM: Onlay island flap in the repair of mid and distal penile hypospadias without chordee. J Urol 138:376, 1987.
4. Duckett JW: The island flap technique for hypospadias repair. Urol Clin North Am 8:503, 1981.
5. Klykylo W, Schultz J: Genital surgery timing: psychological and surgical aspects. Dial Ped Urol 6(May):3, 1983.
6. Schonfeld WA, Beebe GW: Normal growth and variation in the male genitalia from birth to maturity. J Urol 48:759, 1942.
7. Manley CB, Epstein ES: Early hypospadias repair. J Urol 125:698, 1981.
8. Mitchell ME, Kulb TB: Hypospadias repair without a bladder drainage catheter. J Urol 135:321, 1986.
9. DeSy WA, Oosterlinck W: Silicone foam elastomer: a significant improvement in postoperative penile dressing. J Urol 128:39, 1982.
10. Hodgson NB: Urethral sounds. Soc Pediatr Urol Newsletter. May 16, 1986.
11. Shapiro SR: Complications of hypospadias repair. J Urol 131:518, 1984.
12. Duckett JW: Hypospadias. In: Gillenwater JY, Grayhack JT, Howards SS, Duckett JW, eds: Adult and Pediatric Urology, Vol 2. Chicago, Year Book Medical Publishers, 1987, p 1880.
13. Barraza MA, Roth DR, Terry W, Livne PM, Gonzales ET Jr: One-stage reconstruction of moderately severe hypospadias. J Urol 137:714, 1987.
14. Man DWK, Vordermark JS, Ransley PG: Experience with single stage hypospadias reconstruction. J Pediatr Surg 21:338, 1986.
15. Horton CE, Devine CJ, Graham JK: Fistulas of the penile urethra. Plast Reconstr Surg 66:107, 1980.
16. Dennis MA, Walker RD III: The repair of urethral fistulas occurring after hypospadias repair. J Urol 128:1004, 1982.
17. Singh AK, Chandra R: Closure of urethral fistula by rhombic flap. Br J Urol 57:112, 1985.
18. Lau JTK, Ong GB: Subglandular urethral fistula following circumcision: repair by the advancement method. J Urol 126:702, 1981.
19. Geltzeiler J, Belman AB: Results of closure of urethrocutaneous fistulas in children. J Urol 132:734, 1984.
20. Moscona AR, Govrin-Yehudain J, Hirshowitz B: Closure of urethral fistulae by transverse Y-V advancement flap. Br J Urol 56:313, 1984.
21. Snow BW: Use of tunica vaginalis to prevent fistulas in hypospadias surgery. J Urol 136:861, 1986.
22. Burbige KA, Hensle TW, Edgerton P: Extragenital split thickness skin graft for urethral reconstruction. J Urol 131:1137, 1984.
23. Noe HN: Endoscopic management of urethral strictures in children. J Urol 125:712, 1981.
24. Pfister RR: Apparent diverticulum formation in island graft hypospadias repair. Soc Pediatr Urol Newsletter, May 17, 1985.
25. Aigen AB, Khawwand N, Skoog SJ, Belman AB: Acquired megalourethra: an uncommon complication of the transverse preputial island flap urethroplasty. J Urol 137:712, 1987.
26. Stecker JF Jr, Horton CE, Devine CJ Jr, McCraw JB: Hypospadias cripples. Urol Clin North Am 8:539, 1981.
27. Winslow BH, Vorstman B, Devine CJ Jr: Urethroplasty using diverticular tissue. J Urol 134:552, 1985.
28. Brannen GE: Meatal reconstruction. J Urol 116:319, 1976.
29. Jordan GH: Reconstruction of the fossa navicularis. J Urol 138:102, 1987.
30. Filmer RB: Balanitis xerotica obliterans in children and teenagers. Soc Pediatr Urol Newsletter, February 14, 1986.
31. Juskiewenski S, Vaysse PH, Moscovici J, Hammoudi S, Bouissou E: A study of the arterial supply to the penis. Anat Clin 4:101, 1982.
32. Mills C, McGovern J, Mininberg D, Coleman J, Muecke E, Vaughan ED Jr: An analysis of different techniques for distal hypospadias repair: the price of perfection. J Urol 125:701, 1981.
33. Svensson J, Berg R: Micturition studies and sexual function in operated hypospadiacs. Br J Urol 55:422, 1983.
34. Glassman CN, Machlus BJ, Kelalis PP: Urethroplasty

for hypospadias: long-term results. Urol Clin North Am 7:437, 1980.
35. MacMillan RDH, Churchill BM, Gilmour RF: Assessment of urinary stream after repair of anterior hypospadias by meatoplasty and glanuloplasty. J Urol 134:100, 1985.
36. Horton CE, Winslow BH, Vorstman B: Intraoperative stream evaluation. Soc Pediatr Urol Newsletter, Nov. 1, 1985.
37. Devine CJ Jr, Gonzalez-Serva L, Stecker JF Jr, Devine PC, Horton CE: Utricular configuration in hypospadias and intersex. J Urol 123:407, 1980.
38. Berg R, Svensson J, Astrom G: Social and sexual adjustment of men operated for hypospadias during childhood: a controlled study. J Urol 125:313, 1981.
39. Berg G, Berg R: Castration complex. Acta Psychiatr Scand 68:143, 1983.
40. Berg R, Berg G: Penile malformation, gender identity and sexual orientation. Acta Psychiatr Scand 68:154, 1983.
41. Belman AB: The Broadbent hypospadias repair. Urol Clin North Am 7:483, 1981.
42. Belman AB: The modified Mustarde hypospadias repair. J Urol 127:88, 1982.
43. Memmelaar J: Use of bladder mucosa in a one-stage repair of hypospadias. J Urol 58:68, 1947.
44. Coleman JW, McGovern JH, Marshall VF: The bladder mucosal graft technique for hypospadias repair. Urol Clin North Am 8:457, 1981.
45. Li Z-C, Zheng Y-H, Sheh Y-X, Cao Y-F: One-stage urethroplasty for hypospadias using a tube constructed with bladder mucosa: a new procedure. Urol Clin North Am 8:463, 1981.
46. Hendren WH, Reda EF: Bladder mucosa graft for construction of male urethra. J Pediatr Surg 21:189, 1986.
47. Elder JS, Duckett JW: Urethral reconstruction following an unsuccessful one-stage hypospadias repair. World J Urol 5:19, 1987.
48. Hensle TW, Badillo F, Burbige KA: Experience with the MAGPI hypospadias repair. J Pediatr Surg 18:692, 1983.
49. Arap S, Mitre AI, De Goes GM: Modified meatal advancement and glanuloplasty repair of distal hypospadias. J Urol 131:1140, 1984.
50. Livne PM, Gibbons MD, Gonzales ET Jr: Meatal advancement and glanuloplasty: an operation for distal hypospadias. J Urol 131:95, 1984.
51. Wacksman J: Modification of the one-stage flip-flap procedure to repair distal penile hypospadias. Urol Clin North Am 8:527, 1981.
52. Gonzales ET Jr, Veeraraghavan KA, Delaune J: The management of distal hypospadias with meatal-based, vascularized flaps. J Urol 129:119, 1983.
53. Woodard JR, Cleveland R: Application of Horton-Devine principles to the repair of hypospadias. J Urol 127:1155, 1982.
54. Hanna MK: Single-stage hypospadias: techniques and results. Urology 21:30, 1983.
55. Redman JF: Experience with 60 consecutive hypospadias repairs using the Horton-Devine techniques. J Urol 129:115, 1983.
56. Elder JS, Duckett JW, Snyder HM: Onlay island flap in the repair of mid and distal penile hypospadias without chordee. J Urol 138:376, 1987.
57. Wacksman J: Use of the Hodgson XX (modified Asopa) procedure to correct hypospadias with chordee: surgical technique and results. J Urol 136:1264, 1986.
58. Kim SH, Hendren WH: Repair of mild hypospadias. J Pediatr Surg 16:806, 1981.
59. Koff SA: Mobilization of the urethra in the surgical treatment of hypospadias. J Urol 125:394, 1981.
60. Nasrallah PF, Minott HB: Distal hypospadias repair. J Urol 131:918, 1984.
61. Hendren WH, Crooks KK: Tubed free skin graft for construction of male urethra. J Urol 123:858, 1980.
62. Shapiro SR: Free graft patch 1-stage procedure to repair penile hypospadias unsuitable for the flip-flap procedure: indications and experience. J Urol 136:433, 1986.
63. Vyas PR, Roth DR, Perlmutter AD: Experience with free grafts in urethral reconstruction. J Urol 137:471, 1987.
64. Chang T-S: Anterior urethral advancement: a one-stage technique for hypospadias repair. Br J Plast Surg 37:530, 1984

COMPLICATIONS OF EXSTROPHY AND EPISPADIAS SURGERY

41

John P. Gearhart • Robert D. Jeffs

The surgical management of classic exstrophy presents one of the greatest challenges facing the urologist. Many reconstructive techniques have been described to repair classic bladder exstrophy. Today, however, there is a unified approach to the surgical management of this disorder. The staged approach to the functional closure of bladder exstrophy has provided an increasingly successful result over the last several years.[1–3] The method of treatment is bladder closure immediately after birth or as soon thereafter as possible, and may include a penile lengthening procedure and bilateral iliac osteotomy.[2]

Bladder neck reconstruction along with an antireflux procedure is usually performed at the age of 3 years, when the patient has achieved satisfactory bladder capacity. The epispadias repair is then completed by the age of 4 to 5 years. However, this repair may precede bladder neck–plasty as a maneuver to add outlet resistance when the bladder is slow to adapt to an adequate capacity.[4]

This chapter identifies the complications of exstrophy and epispadias treatment and defines methods to avoid many of the problems commonly experienced by patients treated in the past. Historically, patients with bladder exstrophy were managed with urinary diversion. Treatment options included ureterosigmoidostomy, ureterotrigonosigmoidostomy, cutaneous ureterostomy, ileal conduit, Heitz-Boyer-Hovacque procedure, and colon conduit. All of these procedures have been plagued with significant complications. Furthermore, even earlier attempts at initial bladder closure did not offer any better results than the aforementioned procedures. Johnston and Kogan, in their review of the literature in 1974, found only a 15 to 20 percent overall success rate in patients who underwent functional bladder closure.[5]

In the early 1970s, both Jeffs and Cendron introduced a staged approach to functional closure of bladder exstrophy.[6–7] In the first stage, the everted bladder is turned in, and the abdominal wall defect is closed. This converts the bladder exstrophy into a complete epispadias with incontinence. The second procedure is performed when the bladder achieves a capacity of 50 to 60 ml. At this time, the bladder neck reconstruction with correction of vesicoureteral reflux is performed. Epispadias repair is done either at the same time as bladder neck reconstruction, or if necessary, as a separate procedure. If the bladder capacity has not reached 60 ml by the time the child is approximately 3 years of age, epispadias repair is performed before bladder neck reconstruction. (This is discussed later in the chapter in the section on the treatment of the small bladder associated with exstrophy.)

The success of the staged approach has been most encouraging. A 92 percent continence rate in patients who were managed in this manner has been reported by Jeffs.[4] Mollard, utilizing a similar technique in 16 patients, reported a continence rate of 69 percent.[3]

The authors' review of the complications associated with classic exstrophy and epispadias repair included 144 patients who were treated at the Johns Hopkins Hospital between 1975 and 1985. Of these children, 51 (35 percent) were referred to our pediatric urology service before any surgical reconstruction had been performed, and 93 (65 percent) had undergone the initial surgical intervention elsewhere and were referred to us for further therapy.

HISTORIC PERSPECTIVES OF FUNCTIONAL BLADDER RECONSTRUCTION

Thiersch, Trendelenburg, and Young were among the first to attempt a one-stage surgical closure of bladder exstrophy.[8–10] Marshall and Muecke reviewed 329 procedures of functional bladder closure reported in the literature between 1906 and 1966 and determined that urinary continence and preservation of renal function was achieved in only 16 patients.[11] The incidence of abdominal wall and bladder dehiscence, urinary fistulas, and incontinence with reflux and pyelonephritis frequently led to urinary diversion. Over the past 20 years, modifications in the management of functional bladder closure have contributed to a dramatic increase in the success of this procedure. Significant modifications have been: (1) defining criteria for selection of patients suitable for functional closure; (2) staging the reconstruction procedures; and (3) performing bilateral iliac osteotomies at the time of bladder closure.

The reconstructive procedures have been staged as follows: (1) early closure of the bladder with no attempt to achieve continence, (2) closure of the pelvic rim with or without iliac osteotomy, (3) epispadias repair in advance of continence procedure, if needed to produce increased bladder capacity, and (4) bladder neck–plasty with ureteroneocystostomy.

CURRENT EXSTROPHY TREATMENT

The successful treatment of exstrophy by way of functional closure demands that the needs of each child be carefully considered at birth. Bladder size and the functional capacity of the detrusor muscle are important factors in the ultimate outcome of functional closure. It is easy to confuse apparent bladder size with potential bladder capacity; only under anesthesia can one accurately evaluate true bladder size. The bladder may appear small, yet under anesthesia it may demonstrate an acceptable capacity, indenting easily when pushed inward by a gloved finger.

If the initial bladder capacity is felt to be 5 ml or more after closure, one can expect the bladder to develop adequate size and capacity following successful closure. The bladder is turned in and removed from surface irritation and repeated trauma so that it will enlarge and gradually increase its capacity. On the other hand, a small fibrotic bladder patch without elasticity or contractility cannot be selected for the usual closure procedure. Other conditions that have prevented a successful initial closure include ectopic bowel, hypoplasia of one side of the bladder, penile scrotal duplication, or severe hydroureteronephrosis at birth.

Many patients with small bladders are now undergoing closure, and some will obtain a volume that can give a satisfactory dry interval. Small bladders in other patients can be used to create a urethra when cystoplasty is subsequently performed to increase bladder capacity in the Arap manner. Also, a small bladder can be used as a template in later bladder augmentation if adequate capacity is not eventually achieved. Likewise, the genital anomaly associated with exstrophy may be so severe as to preclude successful genital reconstruction and continence in these patients. The epispadiac penis may be so short and broad that a change to female sex of rearing should be considered. However, in our group of 144 patients, only one patient has had a penis that was so rudimentary that female sex of rearing was advised and chosen. The change, however, did not preclude bladder closure, and the patient is continent following staged reconstructive repair.

The main complications of bladder exstrophy closure are bladder prolapse, outlet obstruction, bladder calculi, renal calculi, and wound dehiscence.[12] However, our results suggest a significant decline in their occurrence. Efforts to avoid the occurrence of these complications are discussed under the following three categories: (1) initial bladder closure, (2) the incontinent interval, and (3) the bladder neck reconstruction.

INITIAL BLADDER CLOSURE

The technique for initial primary bladder closure previously described and diagrammed[2] is

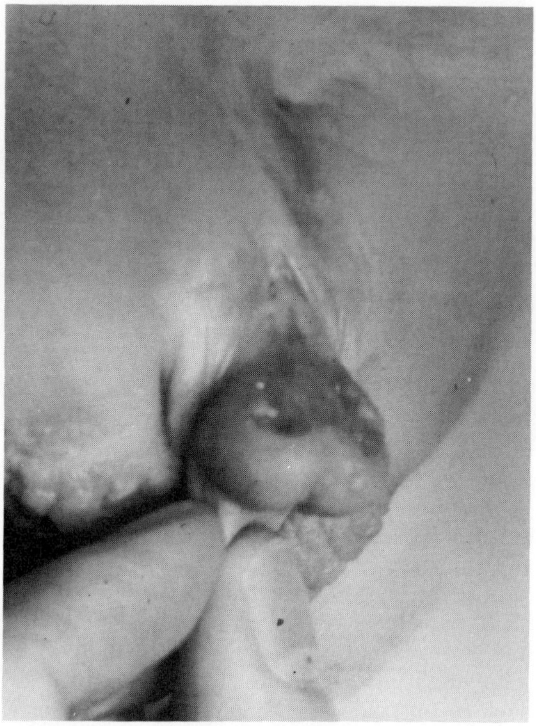

Figure 41–1. A closed exstrophy. The urethral meatus exists at the level of the symphysis pubis at the base of the penis. This is due to the posterior urethra not being placed adequately within the pelvic ring under a well-closed pubic arch.

to close the bladder, bladder neck, and proximal posterior urethra in a secure manner to allow free egress of urine following healing. For later reconstruction and eventual attempt to achieve continence, it is important to place the bladder and bladder neck within the pelvic ring to allow the urethra to drain under a well-closed pubic arch. This placement makes it possible for the pelvic musculature to act on the urethra to interrupt the urinary stream. Tailoring of the bladder neck and the suspension of the vesicoureteral angle is more easily achieved when the bladder neck is within the pelvic ring; it is more difficult when the bladder is covered merely by skin and fascial flaps and when there is continued mobility of tissue between the pubic bones. Furthermore, this difficulty frequently occurs if the exit from the bladder is at the level of the upper border of the symphysis, which further complicates the creation of a bladder neck and reconstruction of the urethra (Fig. 41–1).

The distance from the anal verge to the umbilicus is shortened in exstrophy; therefore, deeper structures are crowded into a smaller space. By freeing the transverse bar of tissue that represents the urogenital diaphragm from the pubic symphysis and inferior ramus of the pubis, one enables the urethra to exit from the pelvis more posteriorly. At the same time, sectioning of the suspensory ligament tissue and anterior attachments of the corpora cavernosa of the penis to its anterior ramus corrects most of the dorsal chordee and allows the penis to gain length and a more dependent angle. In the male and sometimes in the female, the urethral groove is lengthened by transecting the mucosa distal to the prostatic or posterior urethra, allowing the bladder neck to recede into the pelvis. The subsequent gap produced in the urethral groove or between the urethra and the vagina is filled with rotation flaps of paraexstrophy skin. Formerly, these flaps were made somewhat long; however, they are now reduced in size to small bilateral rotation flaps to ensure a better blood supply.[2] Also, in male patients who have a fairly straight penis and good urethral groove, the urethral mucosa is maintained and not transected, thus preserving tissues best suited for later urethral reconstruction.

The dissection described and an excision of the triangle of tissue (including the umbilicus) have normally allowed for an increase in length from the umbilical area to the urethral exit. If this line still appears to be short, and dorsal chordee appears to pull on the urethra, elongation is accomplished with additional releasing incisions or Z-plasties. The aforementioned closure would appear more easily accomplished if it were performed in a sterile field and with tissues that could be immobilized during the healing period and brought into apposition without tension. Tension, infection, and movement can cause slight dehiscence and exposure of deeper holding sutures, resulting in subsequent minor or major degrees of bladder prolapse (Fig. 41–2). In a series of 20 patients in whom a repeat closure of an exstrophy of the bladder was performed following dehiscence after the initial closure, the two most common complications were wound infection (42 percent) and bladder prolapse (46 percent).[13]

PREVENTION OF COMPLICATIONS

Infection

To minimize the possibility of infection, the bladder is closed as soon as possible after birth, and in the interval between birth and bladder closure, the bladder should be protected with a

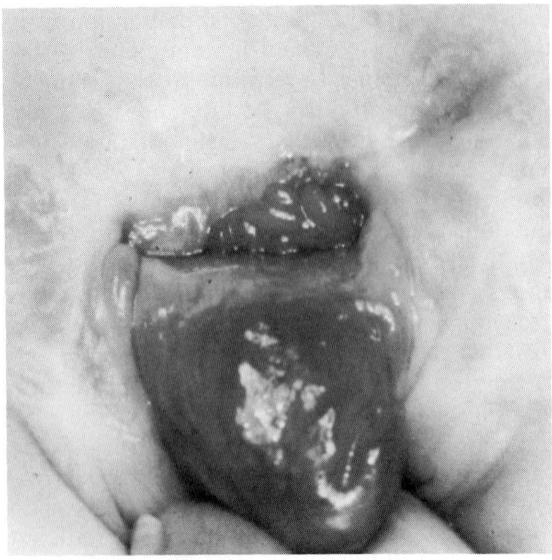

Figure 41–2. Bladder prolapse following exstrophy closure. Initial bilateral iliac osteotomy was not performed, but was performed later at the time of secondary posterior urethra and bladder neck closure.

plastic film such as Saran Wrap to prevent petroleum jelly, gauze, or the diaper from denuding the mucosa and removing the epithelium and natural surface antibodies. Urine should be rinsed off frequently with water or baths at body temperature. All efforts should be made to minimize diaper rash and ammoniacal burns that occur in this area from contamination with urea-splitting organisms.

At the time of the initial closure, preoperative antibiotics are usually given in the form of ampicillin and gentamicin and are continued for 5 to 7 days after surgery. Antibiotics are an important adjunct to successful bladder closure because following exstrophy, bladders and surrounding tissues become contaminated and antibiotic therapy is an effort to convert a contaminated area into a clean surgical wound. The local area is thoroughly washed and cleansed with povidone-iodine (Betadine), and the bladder and its interstices are liberally soaked. The preparation at the initial closure includes the area from the nipples to the knees and from the base of the scapula, downward to the buttocks and behind the leg to the popliteal fossa posteriorly. The entire area is draped into the operative field at the time of surgery. This allows access to the posterior body wall when manipulating the pelvic ring to provide a stable anterior midline closure. Also, the osteotomy incision is covered with a surgical adhesive dressing. Finally, gauze or an adhesive surgical covering is inserted in or applied to the anus to prevent stool contamination during the procedure.

Tissue Mobility and Wound Tension

The other factors in wound dehiscence other than infection are mobility and wound tension. They are handled by firm anterior fixation of the two sides of the pubis following either neonatal molding or pelvic osteotomy. The authors agree with Ansell and others that neonatal closure 48 to 72 hours after birth should be considered, and a successful result can be accomplished if the pubic bones are easily brought into apposition with lateral pelvic compression.[14] However, some patients have a very wide diastasis owing to delayed closure for a number of days and will require bilateral iliac osteotomy. In patients who are not treated immediately after birth, osteotomy is necessary to get a good midline closure, and it is felt that this is helpful in achieving continence in the subsequent bladder neck reconstruction. Osteotomy provides for a more secure anterior and midline wound closure in those patients who are not treated at birth and in whom there is wide separation of the pelvic ring.

Iliac osteotomy can be performed close to and parallel to the sacroiliac joint. However, our recent experience with the anterior sector osteotomy has led us to adopt this procedure because of decreased blood loss and operating time. When done in this position, anterior apposition is achieved without flattening of the pelvis and thus, without drawing the penis inferiorly under the pubic closure. Therefore, penile length is enhanced rather than decreased by the osteotomy procedure. Movement in a healing wound usually results in excess moisture, eventual infection, and subsequent distraction or dehiscence.

It is felt that fixation of the wound is a very important part of initial healing, and a three-part plan is recommended to obviate the problem of movement. First, an attempt is made to provide good fixation of the coapted pubic bones by heavy horizontal mattress sutures tied on the outside of the closure. Once completed, it is quite easy to place other heavy nylon sutures in the rectus fascia, which is now closer to the midline. Sutures used in the past almost always broke and were more likely to come through the skin. The pubic stitch is usually of a very large caliber (#2 nylon) to give the initial strength required. The same caliber stitch is also used in interrupted sutures above the pubic closure in the rectus fascia.

Second, the external fixation for the closed pelvic ring is carried out by modified Bryant's traction (Fig. 41–3) for a period of 3 weeks in neonates and for 4 weeks in older children. In some older children with failed closures who have even undergone previous iliac osteotomy, the iliac osteotomy is repeated, and the patient is left in modified Bryant's traction for 5 to 6 weeks to achieve a successful closure. External fixation, plaster casts, wrapping of the legs, and so forth have been tried, but it is felt that the distracting muscular forces are minimized more effectively by modified Bryant's traction than by other measures. Admittedly, this necessitates a prolonged hospital stay, but because it helps provide primary healing in a potentially contaminated wound and is especially effective in the older child with a previous failed repair, the time is certainly well worth any added expense.

The third important feature of wound fixation is to control the muscular activity of the child. This necessitates a team effort among the physicians, nurses, and parents, who must pamper the child to ensure that pain, frustration, hunger, and muscle spasms do not produce undue or prolonged activity that defeats attempts to prevent wound mobility.

Mothers are encouraged to nurse and cuddle their babies while they are in traction and to assist the nursing staff when the child appears to be agitated. When the mother is not present during the procedure, recorded tapes of her heart sounds are sometimes used in an attempt to simulate the restful intrauterine environment. In addition, analgesics, antispasmodics, and tranquilizers are used liberally to help provide a reasonably calm postoperative course.

In an attempt to prevent wound infection, non-reactive absorbable polyglycolic acid (Dexon) sutures are used. In the symphysis, the preferred stitch is #2 nylon, and the skin stitches are also of monofilament nylon of smaller size. The use of these sutures appears to be an improvement over the earlier use of catgut, braided, or silk sutures. Also, Dexon mesh has been used in one patient in whom it was felt that the anterior rectus fascia was not of good quality. The wound healed nicely, and at the time of bladder neck reconstruction, the rectus fascia was opened and was found to be well healed with good fascial coaptation.

Complications of Osteotomy

We firmly believe in performing iliac osteotomies because 90 percent of the children re-

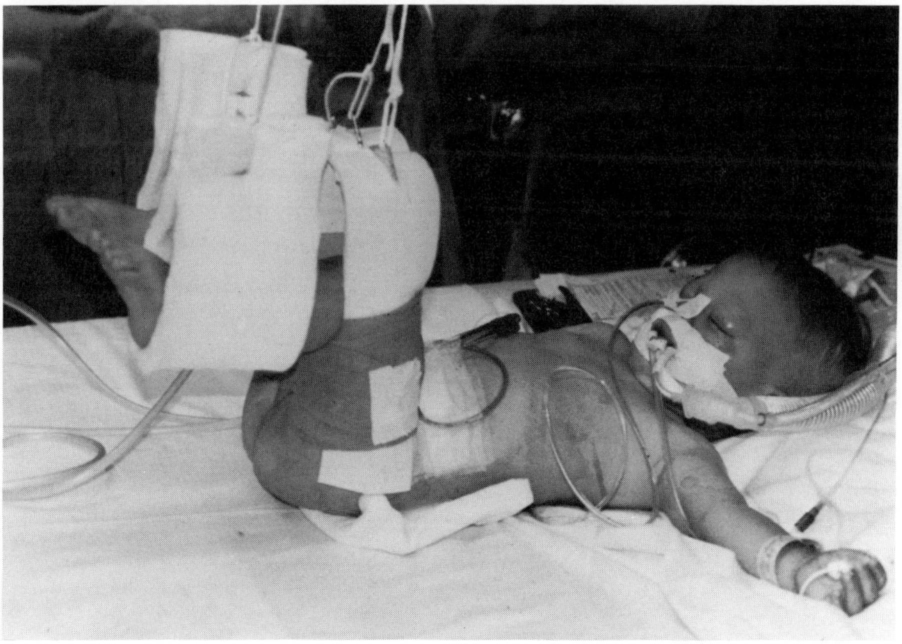

Figure 41–3. Modified Bryant's traction in a 2-year-old child who underwent secondary exstrophy closure. Careful padding and support of the popliteal fossa are essential, as is proper suspension of the feet. The child's buttocks should be off the bed just enough to slide a diaper underneath.

ferred to our institution following partial or complete bladder dehiscence had not undergone prior osteotomy.[13] For example, two children who were referred to our institution for reclosure after wound dehiscence had undergone prior osteotomy. Although the osteotomies were successful, neither child was left in modified Bryant's traction for an extended period. In fact, after being taken out of Bryant's traction at the end of 2 weeks, each day more of the bladder could be visualized through the dehisced lower abdominal wound (Fig. 41–2). Exteriorization of the pubic stitch does occur in approximately 20 to 30 percent of patients who have been seen. However, should the suture become loose or cut through the tissues during subsequent healing, the anterior placement of a knot in a horizontal mattress suture ensures that it will not erode into the urethra or interfere with the bladder or urethral lumen.

Osteomyelitis was seen in patients in the past when pins were used to suspend the legs before the current use of skin traction. However, pins still may be required in the older child in whom skin traction would put undue tension on the superficial skin layers (Fig. 41–4). Perineal nerve palsy has occurred occasionally because of inadequate padding of the popliteal fossa when the knees are slightly bent when the patient is in modified Bryant's traction. (This has not been a problem in the newborn patient because the knees are not bent, and the legs are completely extended.) Undue loss of blood has not been a problem with iliac osteotomy even in the very young patient. Nevertheless, osteotomy wounds sometimes do ooze fairly freely for 3 to 4 days postoperatively. As noted in the foregoing discussion, these osteotomy wounds are covered with adhesive surgical dressings, which are not removed. They usually separate from the wound in 7 to 10 days. It should be mentioned, however, that in some patients who have had failed closures and underwent repeat iliac osteotomies, blood loss can be more extensive. Two patients in the past have required transfusions for this. However, the added benefit of closures performed with repeat iliac osteotomy is worth the slight increase in operative blood loss.

A complication that has been encountered only once was described by Fowler in Melbourne, Australia: the occurrence of rotation at the osteotomy site while the patient was in traction, which led to a lumbar lordosis when the patient subsequently healed and assumed the erect position. The absence of this problem in our experience is attributed to the technique of osteotomy, which divides the posterior periosteum and both tables of iliac wing and leaves the anterior periosteum intact as a hinge that

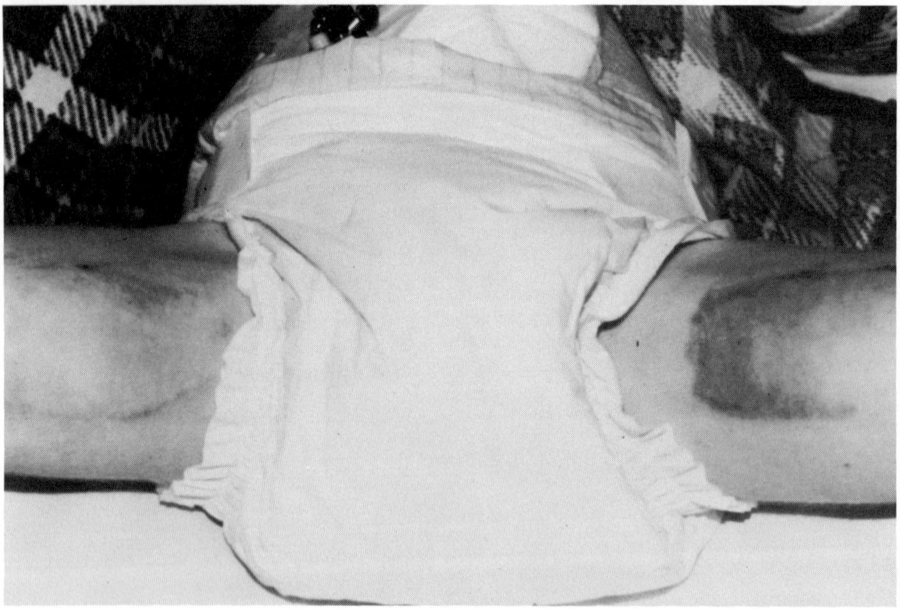

Figure 41–4. Superficial burns of the inner aspect of the thigh, secondary to traction in an older child who may have benefited from placement of Steinmann pins to suspend the extremities. However, these burns did heal nicely with topical measures only.

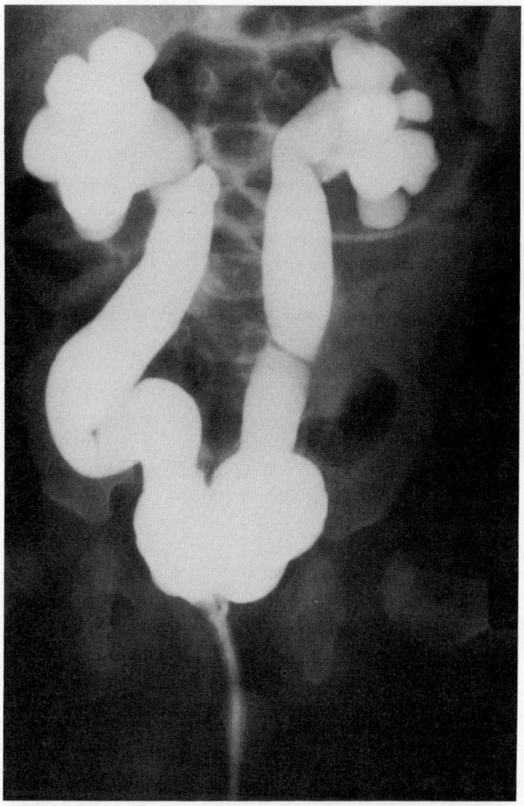

Figure 41–5. Massive hydroureteronephrosis in a child in whom a stricture developed at the junction of posterior and penile urethras subsequent to penile lengthening. Revision of the bladder outlet was required.

should prevent the rotation described. The patient in whom this occurred was a 5-year-old-boy who had undergone repeat iliac osteotomy because of a complete dehiscence of the bladder anteriorly.

Other Complications

Urethral stricture has occurred at the juncture of the posterior and penile urethra subsequent to penile lengthening. Most of these have responded to dilatation or minor urethrotomy and have not required operative revision. However, one patient referred to this institution developed a severe stricture at this juncture, which resulted in massive hydronephrosis and reflux (Fig. 41–5). Multiple procedures were required to correct this problem.

Penile lengthening procedures must not be taken lightly because of the bleeding that may occur in mobilizing the prostatic plate in the male and because of the possible damage to the corpus spongiosum that can occur in the very young child. Care must be taken when dissecting over the corporal bodies, especially between the lower edge of the urogenital diaphragm, the urethral plate, and the top of the corpora cavernosa. In one patient referred to us, corporal damage has resulted in the inability to achieve erection in the corpus on one side. It appears that this condition is permanent and will seriously interfere with erections and sexual function (Fig. 41–6).

The complications of hypertension and oliguria are of major concern in patients undergoing initial bladder closure. Early in this senior author's first series, patients developed alarming postoperative hypertension, and it proved to be associated with a degree of oliguria and acute bilateral hydronephrosis.[6] The problem can be completely eliminated by ureteral intubation begun at the time of closure, and remaining 5 to 7 days postoperatively. Drainage is then accomplished by suprapubic Malecot catheter. However, if these tubes are draining well, and if the child will be in traction for 3 to 4 weeks, often we do not remove these stents for up to 2 weeks.

A commonly seen complication of ureteral intubation is blockage of the small ureteral stents. Normally, the stents are No. 3.5 Fr. pediatric feeding tubes that have small perforations at the end. These are easily clogged by debris or small blood clots, and we simply excise the ends of the tubes to make one large hole that is easier to irrigate through to dislodge clots. The tubes are secured to the suprapubic tube at the skin line with Steri-Strips to keep them in position and to prevent inadvertent removal. The stents along the suprapubic tube are irrigated at regular intervals to ensure patency.

To prevent complications after the period of immobilization, it is recommended that the adequacy of the bladder neck outlet be tested by injecting a small amount of saline into the suprapubic tube to ensure easy access to the urethra. Calibration or dilatation of the urethra or bladder neck outlet is performed to permit free drainage. An abbreviated intravenous pyelogram (IVP) just prior to the patient's discharge has proved invaluable to check for adequate bilateral function and drainage. After IVP, the suprapubic tube is routinely clamped and several residual urine determinations are taken. If these residuals are low, the suprapubic tube is removed. A culture from the bladder is taken through the suprapubic tube prior to removal, to ensure that the bladder urine remains sterile. In addition to the administration of antibiotics,

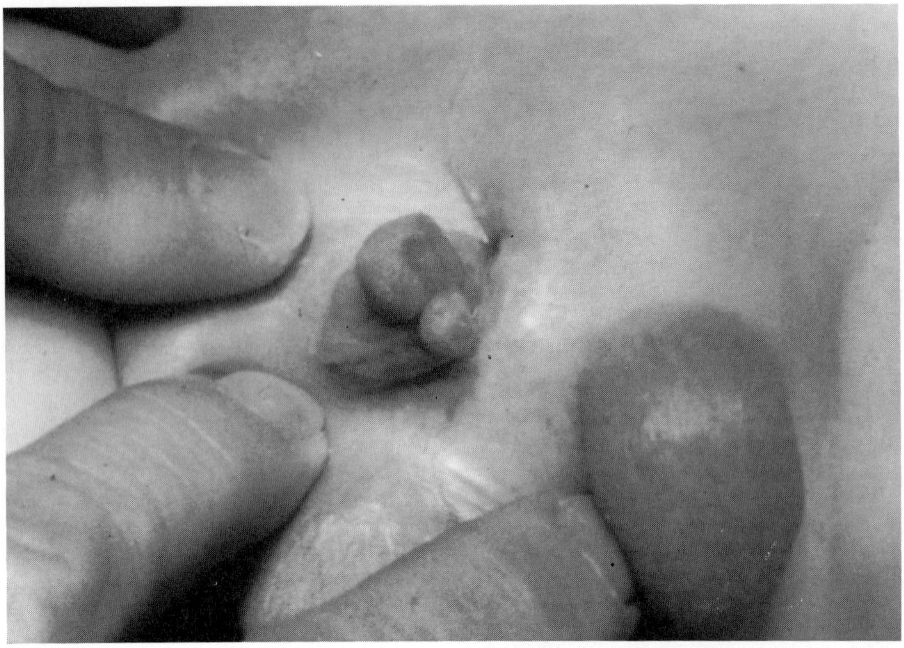

Figure 41–6. A small corporal body on the left secondary to vascular embarrassment at the time of corporeal mobilization.

antibiotic bladder irrigation has been used when contamination occurs, and amphotericin B solution can be used topically to treat yeast colonization in the bladder or urethra.

At the time of discharge as well as throughout the period of hospitalization, parents are cautioned about the complications that can occur, particularly those associated with infection and retention. They are also cautioned to be alert to periods of dry interval after the initial closure. Low-pressure drainage from the urinary tract is expected. Patients are placed on suppressive medication postoperatively, the effectiveness of which is monitored regularly through cultures taken with an eye dropper from the area of the bladder neck during follow-up office visits. Repeat IVP is obtained at about 4 to 6 months after initial closure to ensure that upper urinary tract drainage remains satisfactory and that obstruction or reflux is not causing any undue change. However, if the results of the IVP performed prior to discharge look relatively normal, an ultrasonogram is now used in place of the 4-month postoperative IVP.

Finally, in handling the initial surgery and convalescence, it should be emphasized that bladder closure is a significant procedure and requires a good neonatal team of pediatricians, pediatric anesthesiologists, nurses, and social workers in addition to the surgical team itself. The procedure of bladder closure should not be taken lightly and should be considered only when a concentrated team effort can be organized and when the team is comfortable with managing postoperative exstrophy complications and is prepared to perform continence procedures at a later date.

THE INCONTINENT INTERVAL

Even though a patient has had a successful first-stage closure and is free of obvious complications, he still must have detailed follow-up care to detect complications. Normal bladder closure converts a child with exstrophy into one with a complete epispadias and incontinence. An ultrasonogram or IVP is repeated at intervals during the next 2 to 3 years to detect any upper urinary tract change that can cause reflux or infection. Antibiotics should be continued at least through the first 6 months and as necessary thereafter. Normally, the child is continued on suppressive antibiotic therapy throughout the incontinent interval. Should bladder outlet resistance cause urine to be retained within the bladder, leading to reflux and ureteral dilatation with infected urine, it may be necessary to dilate the urethra or to occasionally resort to intermittent catheterization. If bladder outlet resistance persists, an antireflux procedure may be required as early as 6 months to 1 year after the initial bladder closure. If a continent interval has resulted unexpectedly from the initial closure, no further procedures to achieve continence may be required. However, in our experience this is somewhat rare.

Should infection persist in spite of adequate antibiotic treatment, endoscopy may be required to detect the presence of a stone, which usually forms on the stitch nidus. Parents should be informed that if the child has a significant dry interval, it may indicate inadequate low-pressure drainage and should be reported to the physician.

Following bladder closure and at the time of bladder neck–plasty later in the course of treatment, no stent, drain, or catheter is left in the urethra. It seems sufficient to have an intact urethral mucosal strip to maintain the adequacy of the urethra. The presence of a stenting catheter or drain appears to induce infection so that partial wound dehiscence in the urethra or bladder neck frequently occurs. Instrumentation of the urethra should be avoided for a period of 3 to 4 weeks during the initial closure stage and for a definite 3 weeks after the bladder neck–plasty.

In the conversion from exstrophy to complete epispadias with incontinence, the bladder capacity gradually increases and inflammatory changes in the mucosa resolve. Cystograms at 2 to 3 years postoperatively will indicate bilateral reflux in nearly 100 percent of patients and will provide an estimate of bladder capacity. Even in the completely incontinent patient, bladder capacity gradually increases to the point at which it can be distended at cystography to a capacity of 60 ml. Some patients have very small bladders, and it may require 4 to 5 years to achieve acceptable capacity (Fig. 41–7).

A tight bladder closure, untreated urinary tract infection, and reflux may cause uncontrollable ureteral dilatation (Fig. 41–5). Judgment is required to know when to abort attempts at functional closure and to turn to urinary diversion as a means of preserving renal function. The change of plan is seldom necessary if a wide outlet has been constructed during the initial closure and if careful attention has been given to the details of follow-up care.

At the age of 3 to 5 years, if the bladder has achieved a capacity of 50 to 60 ml when distended, treatment of the incontinence and reflux is instituted. Cultures and radiologic studies should indicate sterile urine and good ureteral drainage in the distended bladder. The rationale for performing bladder neck reconstruction

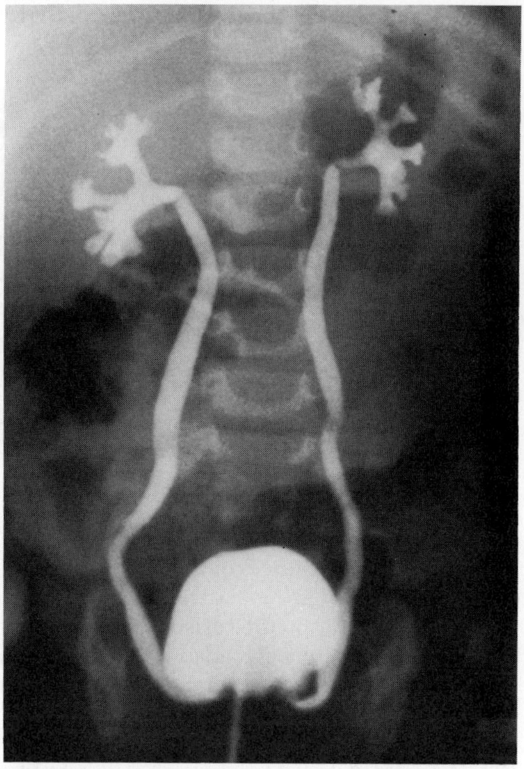

Figure 41–7. A bladder with a capacity of 70 ml in a 4-year-old child. Completion of bladder neck reconstruction was considered.

prior to urethral reconstruction is that iatrogenic damage to the reconstructed urethra may result if instrumentation is required for urinary retention immediately following the bladder neck reconstruction. However, if by the age of 3 years, the bladder capacity has not reached 50 ml, epispadias repair is performed and bladder neck reconstruction is postponed until bladder capacity increases. Construction of a neourethra usually adds resistance to urine outflow and therefore contributes to increasing bladder capacity.

COMPLICATIONS OF BLADDER NECK RECONSTRUCTION

Incontinence

Incontinence is a complication of exstrophy that our procedures are designed to correct. When incontinence persists after corrective surgery, the complication becomes a surgical one. An attempt is made to obtain continence by creating a narrow bladder neck and an elongated posterior urethra in the Leadbetter manner.[15] The reflux is corrected by transtrigonal reimplants, which are also necessary to move the ureters away from the bladder neck repair so that the trigonal tissue may be used to create the bladder neck. In the past, the Cohen transtrigonal reimplant was used.[16] However, our preference is for a more cephalic course for the ureters, which involves using the same hiatus but constructs the submucosal tunnel in a cephalic position. This brings the ureteral meatus from each ureter together near the midline of the bladder. This maneuver works quite well with the ureters positioned onto the upper aspect of the trigone and away from the neo–bladder neck. The bladder neck is suspended in the Marshall-Marchetti-Kranz manner to create angulation between the urethra and the bladder floor.[17]

The degree of tightness of the urethra and the continence length are measured by intraoperative profilometry, and the resistance of the bladder neck is measured after bladder closure. Our results indicate that a urethral closure pressure of 70 to 100 ml of water over a length of 2.5 cm is necessary to achieve a successful outcome.[18] Finally, a Marshall-Marchetti-Kranz bladder neck suspension is performed to increase further the continence length and the urethral closure pressure.[17] This repair must be allowed to heal for 3 weeks without placement of an indwelling stent and with use of a suprapubic tube before voiding.

Thirty-nine patients have undergone initial bladder neck reconstruction at our hospital between 1975, when primary bladder closure was first performed at this institution, and 1985. Urinary continence in a series of patients with classic exstrophy following bladder neck reconstruction is difficult to assess, and perfect urinary control would not be expected in any age-matched control group of patients. Urinary continence in our patients who underwent exstrophy repair has been assessed by parental reporting of average daytime dry interval. Achievement of an average daytime dry interval of more than 3 hours is considered an excellent surgical result. In our group of patients, 92 percent achieved an excellent surgical result when assessed by the criteria cited.[4] Five percent of patients had a dry interval of 1 to 3 hours, and 3 percent of patients had a dry interval of less than 1 hour.[4] It is noteworthy that in the same review of patients, 11 of whom had undergone unsuccessful primary closure, an excellent result was obtained in only 55 percent of patients, a 1- to 3-hour dry interval was obtained in only 18 percent, and 27 percent had a daytime dry interval of less than 1 hour.

A number of factors certainly account for a high continence rate. Leadbetter considered the length of the bladder neck to be the most significant factor contributing to achieving continence, and therefore we follow his recommendation to construct a bladder neck approximately 3 cm in length.[15] In addition, bilateral iliac osteotomies performed at the time of closure permit placement of the urethra within the pelvic ring. This maneuver allows for the levator ani and puborectalis muscles to aid in voluntary urinary control. Bladder neck suspension aids in preventing static and stress incontinence. The effectiveness of the bladder neck suspension has been demonstrated intraoperatively, using urethral pressure profilometry.[18]

It is also imperative that the mechanism for achieving urinary continence does not compromise renal function. Upper urinary tract evaluations in our patients have been obtained following bladder neck reconstruction, utilizing IVP. In 50 patients reviewed, 49 had a follow-up IVP available for review. Forty-three (88 percent) had normal upper urinary tracts.[4] Three children (6 percent) had persistent grade II vesicoureteral reflux after bladder neck reconstruction with bilateral Cohen reimplantation, whereas six (6 percent) demonstrated varying degrees of hydronephrosis in follow-up studies. Patients responded to appropriate management, which included repeat bilateral ureteroneocystostomy in four patients and augmentation cystoplasty in two.

Complications following bladder neck reconstruction are rare. In a series of consecutive bladder neck reconstructions in 25 patients, postoperative urinary retention developed in eight. Bladder outlet obstruction resolved in all eight patients following dilatation, prolonged suprapubic catheter drainage, or intermittent self-catheterization.

Obstruction to the flow of urine occurring at the end of the 3-week healing period may be managed by further treatment with suprapubic drainage, by gentle dilation of the urethra, or by intermittent self-catheterization. For example, a young female patient in our practice underwent bladder neck reconstruction after secondary bladder closure. Obstruction of urine flow through the neourethra occurred, and the neourethra could not be passed with a cystoscope. Utilizing interventional radiologic techniques, a guide wire was placed through the

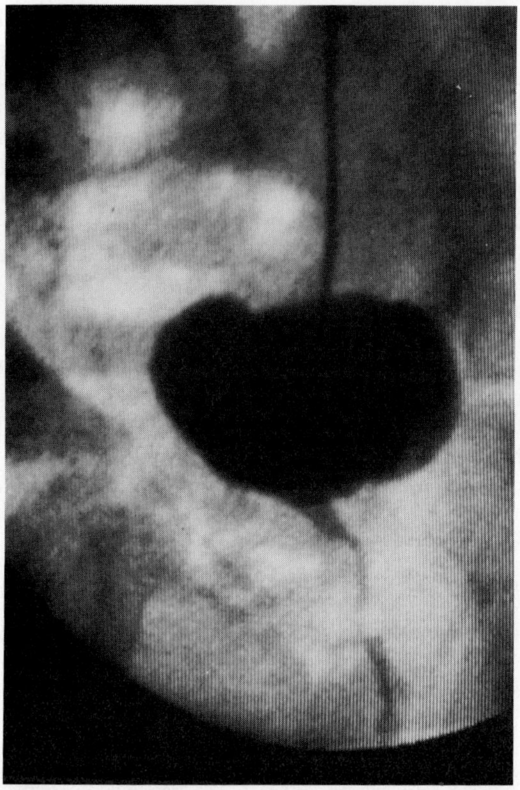

Figure 41–8. Fluoroscopic bladder neck reconstruction in a young female child who had undergone the operation approximately 6 weeks prior to the study. Stricture was demonstrated in the mid-urethra and could not be reversed from below. Therefore, with the use of interventional radiologic techniques, a guide wire was placed through this. Gentle dilation was performed, and a catheter was then placed into the bladder. The child is now dry for 3 hours during the day and is also dry at night.

suprapubic tract and into the bladder neck and out through the urethra (Fig. 41–8). Gentle balloon dilatation of the neobladder neck and urethra was then performed without difficulty. The child currently has a 3-hour dry interval and is dry at night.

As indicated from the results of our studies, urinary continence with a long dry interval does not occur immediately after bladder neck reconstruction and can take as long as several years to achieve. In some series, the interval between bladder neck reconstruction and urinary continence ranged from 1.5 to 2.8 years, depending on the success or failure of the patient's primary closure.[4] The bladder must also adjust to a new environment and new constraints. In addition, and probably more important, the patient must learn for the first time to recognize bladder filling and must be able to initiate voluntary detrusor contractions. With cooperation and time, urinary continence can be achieved in 92 percent of patients who have had a successful initial bladder closure.

If stress incontinence or dribbling is still present 3 or 4 weeks after bladder neck reconstruction, the chance of obtaining good control is relatively small. As noted, some patients gain continence with time, usually by increasing their bladder capacity and dry interval rather than by achieving better closure of their outlet. In the male, growth of the prostate may help produce control, but in general, postoperative evidence of continuous dribbling incontinence is a sign that further adjustment with some type of intervention may be required. A small series of patients with an inadequate dry interval have benefited by the injection of collagen at the bladder neck area to supplant outlet resistance and to achieve an adequate dry interval. Also, in another small series of young adult patients, ultrasonographers utilizing transrectal ultrasound techniques were able to identify what they thought was prostate tissue in only one of six young men. Therefore, growth of the prostate may not be as important a factor in attaining eventual continence as formerly thought.

The timing of the bladder neck–plasty depends on the capacity of the bladder as determined during the incontinent interval. The very small bladder closed shortly after birth does indeed become soft and pliable and increases in volume despite the absence of any degree of continence. At approximately 2 years of age, a capacity of 50 ml, measured at the time of cystogram, is expected. If this capacity is not achieved and if there seems to be a reasonable chance that it will increase, the penile epispadias is then repaired (Fig. 41–9). This adds some resistance to the outflow of urine, and frequently the capacity will increase to 50 ml or more, and one can proceed with bladder neck–plasty. In another series of patients with small capacities after initial closure, epispadias repair prior to bladder neck reconstruction increased the mean bladder capacity by an additional 70 ml.[4] Hydronephrosis following bladder neck–plasty and reimplantation can persist. Careful follow-up to provide adjustment for partial retention and infection must be undertaken to prevent this complication. If hydronephrosis occurs and small bladder capacity persists, bladder augmentation can be performed to protect the upper urinary tracts and to help achieve improved continence (Fig. 41–10).

In a review of 12 patients who experienced failed exstrophy reconstruction and required

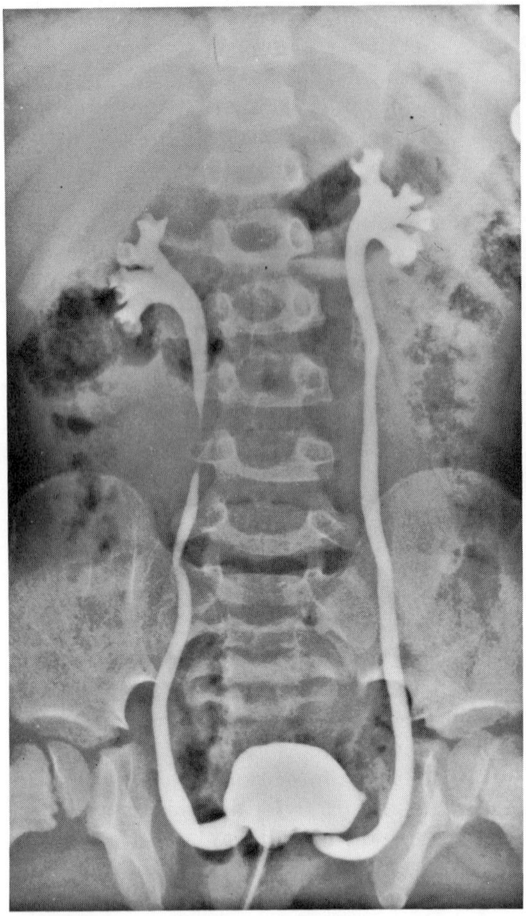

Figure 41–9. Vesicoureterogram (VCUG) in a child with a very small bladder capacity of approximately 35 ml. At this juncture, an epispadias repair was accomplished in an effort to increase outlet resistance and, hopefully, to improve bladder capacity.

bladder augmentation, eight had dehiscence after initial bladder closure and nine had undergone at least one prior unsuccessful bladder neck procedure.[19] Five patients had inadequate bladder volume after initial or subsequent closure and epispadias repair, but the bladder did not accommodate a volume of 50 ml or greater. Seven patients failed to improve bladder capacity after bladder neck–plasty, but they had small-capacity bladders and persistent incontinence. Adjunctive procedures were performed at the time of augmentation and included a bladder neck–plasty in three patients, one of whom underwent a repeat procedure, another of whom had a transureteroureterostomy and psoas hitch. The third patient underwent a Mitrofanoff procedure in association with ileal augmentation and bladder neck closure.

In three patients, an artificial urinary sphincter was placed for continence. These included one patient for an undiversion, in which the sphincter was placed around the tubularized bladder. In a second patient who underwent a bladder exstrophy variation, the sphincter was placed at the upper prostatic level after two ectopic ureters were removed from the posterior urethra. The third patient received the sphincter around a failed bladder neck–plasty at 5 years of age. Eleven of these 12 patients are continent, although nine require intermittent self-catheterization. There were no major complications in this group of patients. Therefore, it is felt that in the failed exstrophy reconstruction, augmentation cystoplasty provides prolonged stability of the upper urinary tracts and continence and has proved to be a successful alternative to diversion

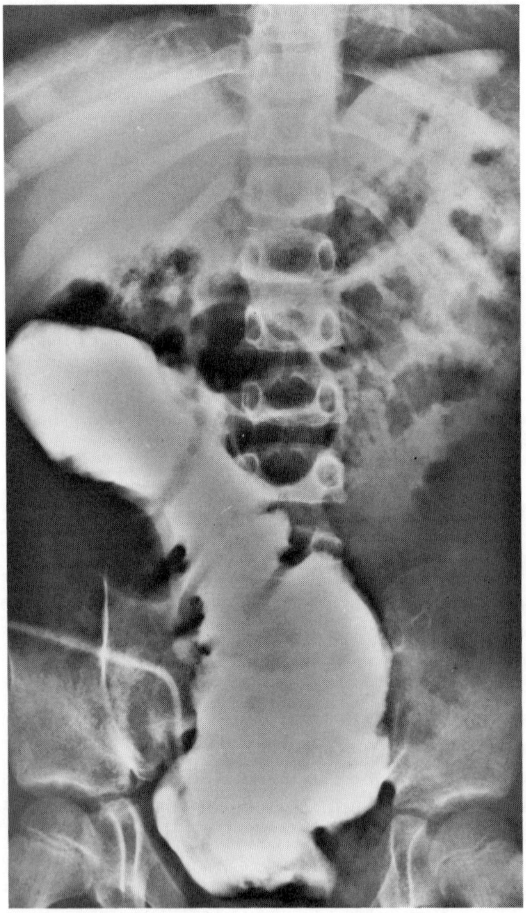

Figure 41–10. The same patient as in Figure 41–9 after epispadias repair and bladder neck reconstruction. The bladder remained small, and incontinence persisted. Bladder augmentation along with a Mitrofanoff procedure was accomplished, and the patient is currently "dry" on intermittent catheterization.

in this select group of patients who experienced exstrophy repair failures.[19]

EPISPADIAS REPAIR

Construction of the neourethra and further penile lengthening and dorsal chordee release are usually performed approximately 1 year following bladder reconstruction, unless earlier repair was required to increase the bladder capacity. At either time, a modified Young urethroplasty is performed when there is sufficient penile skin for construction of the urethra and coverage of the neourethra and when the dorsal urethral groove has sufficient length. Full-thickness grafts are reserved for when penile skin is unavailable to perform a modified Young urethroplasty. Again, a pedicle tube constructed from ventral preputial tissue may also be used to bridge the defect between the prostatic and glandular urethra (Montfort; personal communication, 1985).

As noted, the surgical technique for the Young urethroplasty[20] is performed by placing a nylon suture through the glans, which provides traction for the penis. Incisions are made over two parallel lines marked previously on the dorsum of the penis to outline an 18 mm strip extending from the prostatic urethral meatus to the tip of the glans. Triangular areas of the dorsal glans are excised adjacent to the urethral strip, and glandular flaps are constructed. Glandular flaps need to be made quite thick and incised deeply to cover the urethra thoroughly and to provide a very dependent urethral meatus. Lateral skin flaps are then mobilized, and a Z-plasty type incision is made over the suprapubic area. The Z-plasty incision allows exposure and division of the suprapubic suspensory ligaments and of any old scar tissue. Also at this time, the corporal bodies may be mobilized a bit on each side to gain a slight amount of extra length and a bit more dependency of the phallus. The urethral strip is simply closed in a linear manner from the prostatic opening to the glans over a 10 Fr. feeding tube using 6–0 Dexon sutures. The subcutaneous layer is closed with two separate layers of 6–0 Dexon sutures. The skin is normally reapproximated with interrupted 5–0 Dexon sutures. The glans is reapproximated with vertical mattress sutures of 4–0 prolene, and small segments of vascular loop are interposed between the loops of the vertical mattress suture. This aids in the easy removal of these vertical mattress sutures after several days and helps to prevent unsightly scars in the glans penis from these sutures. A #8 Silastic stent is normally left in the neourethra, along with a suprapubic cystostomy tube.

Complications of Epispadias Repair

The most common complication of epispadias repair is a urethrocutaneous fistula. In a series from this institution, fistulas developed in nine of 24 patients with urethroplasty.[1] In four of the nine patients, the fistulas resolved spontaneously, and the other five patients required surgical intervention. Of the fistulas that required surgical repair, four occurred near the corona and the fifth occurred at the mid-shaft area. The corona is the area of the penis that is most deficient in circumferential penile skin, and therefore multiple layers of closure are difficult to achieve. In the proximal shaft, the skin is more redundant, and distally the glandular flaps cover the neourethra and heal quickly, usually without fistula. The area of the corona is at risk after repair. All fistulas that were closed surgically in patients in the series remained healed, and all were closed in multiple layers.

All possible factors have been evaluated in the past to try to determine whether osteotomy, sequence of bladder neck–plasty, and epispadias repair, when the initial repair was done, equal the number of bladder closures and whether preoperative androgen stimulation affects the rate of fistula formation.[1] Of these factors, only prior osteotomy appeared to decrease the rate of fistula formation that required fistula closure (15 percent in patients who had undergone osteotomy compared with 67 percent who had not). Other factors did not appear to be significant.

When the parents of these children were questioned about the current status of the genital reconstruction, they noted the flaccid penis when standing was directed downward to horizontal in 83 percent of the children. When erection was observed, the penis was reported as directed upward in 47 percent, horizontally in 47 percent, and downward in 6 percent. The parents were extremely satisfied with the cosmetic appearance of the penis, but almost all expressed some concern as to whether the penis would achieve adequate size for sexual intercourse after puberty.

RESULTS OF EXSTROPHY SURGERY

Penile Appearance

The majority of patients in our series of cases have not yet reached adulthood and therefore, may develop problems that occur only in older patients. However, older patients have been seen at Johns Hopkins sporadically with a variety of problems pertaining to exstrophy repair. Most of these young adults handle their problems well; however, the most severe problems are encountered in the group that had undergone diversion previously.

Certainly, penile size and shape have been a problem for a number of these patients. Although many make good and imaginative use of their short phallus, others have voiced concern over its short, broad appearance. Interestingly, only a few have complained of residual chordee. Some have been counseled and have learned to live with their problems, and others have undergone surgery, depending on their emotional status and degree of complaint.

The penile lengthening procedure as proposed by Johnson can be performed to achieve a more dependent penile position, especially in the patient who has undergone previous diversion.[21] Sometimes this group of patients can obtain greater length by a repeat penile lengthening procedure, if carefully performed. Likewise, the procedure of inward corporeal rotation as described by Koff has been of benefit in selected patients.[22] In this procedure, surgery is performed on the ventrum of the penis, away from previous suture lines and scars.

Repeat iliac osteotomy has been proposed by Schillinger as a way to achieve greater penile length, and in our opinion, it is not worth the risk in the older patient.[23] If dorsal curvature remains a problem after the aforementioned measures have been attempted, revision of the urethra with interposition of a bridging tube may be necessary to allow for correction of the chordee and short urethra. Also, a corporal substitution procedure with dura mater, such as recommended by Woodhouse, could be helpful in achieving a straight penile length if there is disproportion to the size and length of the corporal bodies.[24]

A very small number of patients have been treated who are almost sexually disabled from their diminutive penile size. These patients may have very well benefited from a change in gender when they first presented with their exstrophy problem. Otherwise, several patients have complained not only of shortness but also of penile shape. They are counseled that this is the nature of their defect, and many learn to live with it. However, others are found to object to scarred and unsightly suture lines from previous surgery (Fig. 41–11). Thick creases of skin on the penis may lead to painful intercourse. Corrective procedures can be developed to improve penile appearance, even if skin grafts are required. Proper placement of the skin grafts can make the penis more pendulous and less a part of the scrotum.

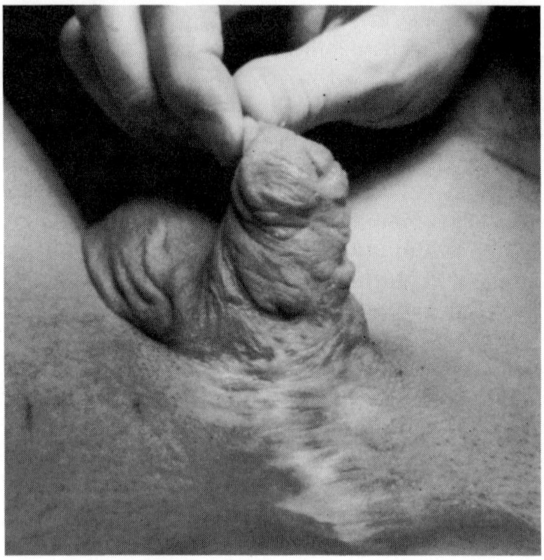

Figure 41–11. Exstrophy with multiple penile reconstruction in an 18-year-old who had been unhappy about the cosmetic appearance of the penis mainly because of the wrinkled skin and multiple suture lines. A good portion of the redundant, scarred skin was excised, and a skin graft was applied with improvement in his cosmetic appearance.

Ejaculatory and Introital Difficulties

Another problem encountered in the older group of patients is ejaculatory dysfunction. Again, many of those who underwent previous diversion surgery have a seminal fistula located in the mons area or at the base of the penis. If an ejaculatory tube can be constructed close to the end of the penis, this problem can sometimes be obviated. In adolescent and young female patients, the anterior location of the vaginal introitus can cause difficulty with intercourse. Often, an episiotomy can be performed to make intromission easier.

Stomal Complications

Finally, stomal problems continue to occur in the adolescent and young adult years. A number of young people have difficulty tolerating the stoma because of its effect on their self image. All of these patients have undergone diversion, and a number have had previous cystectomy. Some of these patients require psychological counseling, and others may benefit from a continent urinary diversion.

Many of these young adults have multiple problems that require hours of discussion just to get them comfortable enough to voice their concerns. If the surgeon involves himself in exstrophy work, he must be prepared to spend a great deal of time with these patients and their families as well as with the exstrophy support team.

FERTILITY, PREGNANCY, AND MALIGNANCY

Reconstruction of the male genitalia and preservation of fertility were not primary objectives of early surgical management of bladder exstrophy. Many accounts of pregnancy and the initiation of pregnancy by males with bladder exstrophy have been reported. Shapiro's review revealed that of 2500 patients who had undergone exstrophy and epispadias repair, 38 males who had fathered children and 131 females who had borne offspring were identified.[25] A retrospective analysis has been done in patients who have undergone primary closure and in patients who have undergone urinary diversion. A normal sperm count was found in only one of eight men following functional bladder closure and in four of eight men following urinary diversions. The most likely difference for this observed fertility potential is iatrogenic damage to the verumontanum or ejaculatory ducts in functional closure or the possibility of retrograde ejacuation.

Libido in patients who have had exstrophy repair remains quite high. The erectile mechanism in patients who have undergone epispadias repair appears intact because 87 percent of young boys in our series have a witnessed erection following epispadias repair,[20] and as noted, female patients with exstrophy have borne offspring.[25] Complications following surgery have been cervical and uterine prolapse, and these young women must be informed of the likelihood of uterine and cervical prolapse following pregnancy. Birth by cesarean section is recommended for women who have undergone functional bladder closure and bladder neck reconstruction to alleviate stress on the pelvic floor and to avoid traumatic injury to the surgically constructed urinary sphincter mechanism.

The inherent malignant potential of the closed exstrophied bladder has not been determined, since long-term follow-up of a large number of bladder exstrophy patients without urinary tract infection, obstruction, and chronic irritation has not been assembled. Until the malignant potential of the noninfected, nonobstructed closed exstrophy bladder is determined, a high index of suspicion should be maintained for potential malignant degeneration. Three epithelial malignancies have been reported in patients with closed exstrophy, and these bladders were not closed at birth. Exstrophy bladders that are left everted are predisposed to develop squamous cell carcinoma secondary to repeated trauma.[26] Published case reports and other sources have found rhabdomyosarcoma in three individuals with bladder exstrophy.[27]

Adenocarcinoma of the colon adjacent to the ureterointestinal anastomosis in ureterosigmoidostomy has been well reported.[28] The mean latency time is approximately 10 years between the creation of the ureterointestinal anastomosis and the diagnosis of intestinal tumor. Although not commonly performed at this time, patients who undergo ureterosigmoidostomy should be evaluated periodically by barium enema or sigmoidoscopy because they are indeed at greater risk for development of cancer.

INITIAL ADJUSTMENT

Adequate social adjustment of the patient with bladder exstrophy has been well documented. These patients in previous reviews were strikingly normal and well adjusted. The main objective of surgical intervention in bladder exstrophy repair is to enable the patients to achieve normal social interactions with their family and community. With the excellent results of the staged functional approach to bladder exstrophy, it is gratifying that great progress has been achieved toward the realization of this goal.

CONCLUSION

This review of the complications of the treatment of bladder exstrophy emphasizes the complexity of reconstruction of the bladder in exstrophy repair. In experienced hands, the surgical results following primary bladder closure, bladder neck reconstruction, and epispadias repair are quite acceptable. In a review of staged functional closure of bladder exstrophy by Oesterling and Jeffs, it was demonstrated that secure abdominal wall closure, urinary continence with preservation of upper urinary tracts, and a cosmetically acceptable penis can be achieved in patients with a successful primary closure and in a fairly high percentage of patients who have undergone an unsuccessful primary bladder closure.[4] Likewise, in a review by Gearhart and Jeffs of 12 patients who experienced failed staged exstrophy reconstruction, 11 are doing well following bladder augmentation and further continence procedures.[19] Therefore, although complications such as dehiscence, deterioration of renal function, and fistula do occur, with careful attention to surgical detail and frequent follow-up, these patients can have normal childhoods and develop as contributing members of society.

References

1. Lepor H, Jeffs RD: Primary bladder closure and bladder neck reconstruction in classical bladder exstrophy. J Urol 130:1142, 1983.
2. Jeffs RD: Exstrophy. In Walsh PC, Gittes RF, Perlmutter AD, Stamey TA, eds: Campbell's Urology, 5th ed. Vol. 2, Philadelphia: WB Saunders Co, 1985, p 1882.
3. Mollard P: Bladder reconstruction in exstrophy. J Urol 124:515, 1980.
4. Oesterling JE, Jeffs RD: The importance of a successful initial bladder closure in the surgical management of classical bladder exstrophy: analysis of 144 patients treated at the Johns Hopkins Hospital between 1975 and 1985. J Urol 137:258, 1987.
5. Johnston JH, Kogan SJ: The exstrophic anomalies and their surgical reconstruction. Curr Prob Surg, August 1974, pp 1–39.
6. Jeffs RD, Charrois R, Mani M, Juriansz AR: Primary closure of the exstrophied bladder. In Scott R, ed: Current Controversies in Urological Management, Philadelphia, WB Saunders Co, 1972, pp 226–242.
7. Cendron J: Treatment of bladder exstrophy. Central Problem. Ann Chir Infant 12:974, 1982.
8. Thiersch C: Ueber die entstehungswetse und operative behandling der epispadie. Arch der Hieckunde 10:20, 1869.
9. Trendelenburg R: The treatment of ectopia vesicae. Ann Surg 44:281, 1906.
10. Young HH: Exstrophy of the bladder: the first case in which a normal bladder and urinary control have been obtained by plastic operation. Surg Gynecol Obstet 74:729, 1942.
11. Marshall VF, Muecke EC: Congenital abnormalities of the bladder. In: Handbuck der Urologie. Malformations. Berlin: Springer-Verlag, Vol 7, Part 1. 1968, p 165.
12. Jeffs RD: Complications of exstrophy surgery. Urol Clin North Am, 10:509, 1983.
13. Lowe FC, Jeffs RD: Wound dehiscence in bladder exstrophy: an exam of the etiology and factors for initial failure and subsequent success. J Urol 130:312, 1983.
14. Ansell JS: Surgical treatment of exstrophy of the bladder with emphasis on neonatal primary closure: personal experience with 28 consecutive cases treated at the University of Washington Hospital from 1962 to 1977: techniques and results. J Urol 121:650, 1979.
15. Leadbetter GW Jr: Surgical correction of total urinary incontinence. J Urol 91:261, 1964.
16. Cohen SJ: Ureterozysloneostomie eine neue antirefluxtechnik. Aktuel Urol 6:24, 1975.
17. Marshall VF, Marchetti AA, Krantz KE: The correction of stress incontinence by simple vesicourethral suspension. Surg Gynecol Obset 88:509, 1949.
18. Gearhart JP, Williams KA, Jeffs RD: Intraoperative urethral pressure profilometry as an adjunct to bladder neck reconstruction. J Urol 136:1055, 1986.
19. Gearhart JP, Jeffs RD: Augmentation cystoplasty in the failed exstrophy reconstruction. J Urol 139:790, 1988.
20. Lepor H, Shapiro E, Jeffs RD: Urethral reconstruction in boys with classical bladder exstrophy. J Urol 131:512, 1984.
21. Johnston JH: Lengthening of the congenital or acquired short penis. Br J Urol. 46:685, 1974.
22. Koff SA, Eakins M: The treatment of penile chordee using corporeal rotation. J Urol 131:931, 1984.
23. Schillinger J, Wiley MJ: Bladder exstrophy: penile lengthening procedure. Urology 24:434, 1984.
24. Woodhouse CRJ: Management of erectile deformity in exstrophy and epispadias. Abstr 115. p 1245. American Urological Association. Atlanta, May 1985.
25. Shapiro E, Lepor H, Jeffs RD: The inheritance of classical bladder exstrophy. J Urol 132:308, 1984.
26. Kanzari SJ, Majid A, Ortega AM, et al: Exstrophy of the urinary bladder complicated by adenocarcinoma. Urology 3:496, 1974.
27. Hendren WH: Exstrophy of the bladder: an alternative method of management. J Urol 115:195, 1976.
28. Dixon CF, Weisman RE: Polyps of the sigmoid occurring 30 years after bilateral ureterosigmoidostomy for exstrophy of the bladder. Surgery 24:6, 1948.

COMPLICATIONS OF URETERAL REIMPLANTATION AND MEGAURETER REPAIR

42

W. Hardy Hendren

Reimplantation of the ureter, with or without tapering its caliber, is one of the most important procedures in the urologic surgeon's armamentarium. A high degree of success has been reported by many authors using a variety of techniques.[1–7] Success in such surgery must include the following parameters: (1) anatomic success, i.e., reimplanting the ureter so that there is normal drainage, absence of obstruction, and cure of reflux; (2) successful control of ascending infection, which can cause pyelonephritis; and (3) avoiding risk to the patient's renal function or life in accomplishing these goals.

Ureteral reimplantation is major surgery. It offers great benefit to patients who have ureteral obstruction or reflux. However, great harm can result if the procedure is done poorly. In some types of surgery, such as cardiac or plastic surgery, poor technical performance is apparent immediately. In urologic surgery, however, a less than ideal technical operation may result in late renal failure many years later, less readily identifiable as the aftermath of a poorly performed operation. Thus in urologic reconstructive surgery, which includes ureteral reimplantation, continuing long-term follow-up and monitoring are very important. Complications in this type of surgery seldom just happen. They are usually an operating room occurrence. To be particularly avoided are tension, angulation, loss of blood supply, trauma to the tissues from rough handling intraoperatively, inaccurate anastomoses, and a poor choice of the procedure to be performed. If technical aspects of a procedure look questionable in the operating room, the postoperative result is generally poor.

Ureteral reimplantation is not a single procedure but several, depending on the size of the ureter, the disease, and the state of the bladder. Therefore, we must consider as separate entities (1) straightforward ureteral reimplantation, usually a ureter of normal or near-normal size into a normal bladder; (2) difficult cases in which the ureter is dilated and the bladder can be abnormal; (3) cases of ureterocele; and (4) megaureters.

INDICATIONS FOR URETERAL REIMPLANTATION

Before considering techniques for reimplanting the ureter, the complications that can occur, and how to avoid complications, we must consider when ureteral reimplantation should be performed. Clearly, not every ureter with vesicoureteral reflux needs to be surgically corrected. Some patients, especially children, will cease having vesicoureteral reflux on long-term follow-up.[8–10] Others will not. It is important, therefore, to differentiate which patients can be safely followed on suppressive antimicrobial therapy from those who are at risk for renal deterioration if ureteral reimplantation is not performed. Approximately half the patients with reflux whom I see are followed initially without operation with the expectation and hope that reflux will cease. The other half are treated surgically. I do not refer to the former group as being treated "conservatively," because often surgical correction of reflux is the conservative way to treat the patient if the word "conservative" is used in the sense of preserving renal function. I do not believe that surgeons and physicians should regard nonoperative and operative treatment of reflux as being at opposite ends of the spectrum. Instead, I believe that there should be a consensus as to which patients can be followed, at least for a time, in contrast to those for whom properly performed surgery is the better choice.

The Amount of Reflux. Reflux can vary from minimal to massive. It is recognized that bacteria can enter the bladder easily, particularly in women, in whom the urethra is short. Even modest degrees of reflux can allow bacteria to ascend to the kidney, causing pyelonephritis (Figs. 42–1 and 42–2). Massive reflux poses the additional threat of hydrostatic damage to the renal tubules. This has been shown in laboratory animals[11] as well as by clinical observation. Pyelorenal reflux (Fig. 42–3), when contrast opacifies the renal cortex, is especially prone to result in renal atrophy. Cortical atrophy associated with this degree of reflux is most often seen at the upper pole of the kidney. Massive reflux will seldom resolve spontaneously and usually should be corrected surgically.

The Upper Tract. If evaluation discloses reflux, and if the upper tract shows already significant scarring, it seems foolhardy to elect nonoperative treatment. To risk further scarring by nonoperative management invites late hypertension from cortical atrophy and even renal failure with subsequent transplantation. To me, scarring indicates that reflux is a malignant condition in that patient, and surgical correction should be performed. On the other hand, if the upper tract is completely normal, temporizing with reflux in that patient under antimicrobial cover and regular monitoring of cultures for bacilluria can be a reasonable course.

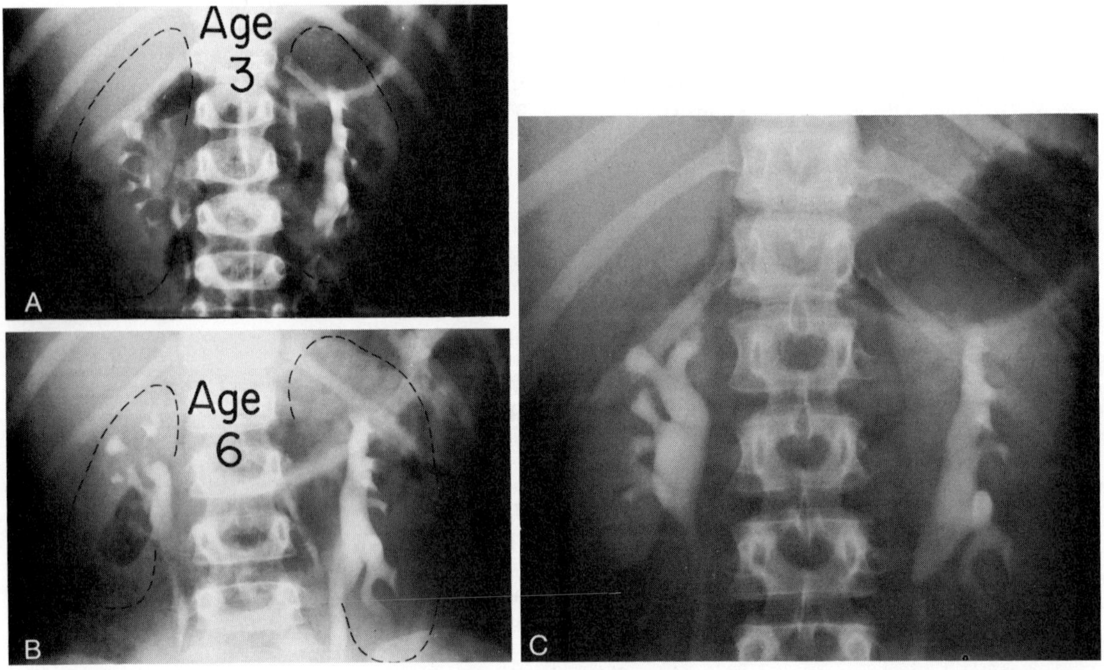

Figure 42–1. Intravenous pyelography (IVP) showing renal damage from reflux with infection.

A, IVP made when the first clinical infection occurred, showing early, minimal change of infection on the right side. Note that the two kidneys were of equal size. The patient had multiple episodes of fever and dysuria. She was treated on each occasion with several weeks of antimicrobial therapy. At age 6 years she was referred belatedly for complete investigation. Cystogram showed bilateral reflux, greater on the right than the left.

B, IVP showing atrophy of the right kidney, especially at the upper pole. This could have been prevented by appropriate antireflux surgery.

C, IVP made when the patient was 14 years of age, 8 years after operation. Note the marked disparity in the size of the two kidneys. The patient was clinically well, with no further episodes of infection. However, this type of patient requires continuing indefinite follow-up, with monitoring of blood pressure to detect late onset of hypertension from reflux-induced renal scarring in childhood. Late nephrectomy or partial nephrectomy has been required in some cases to control hypertension.

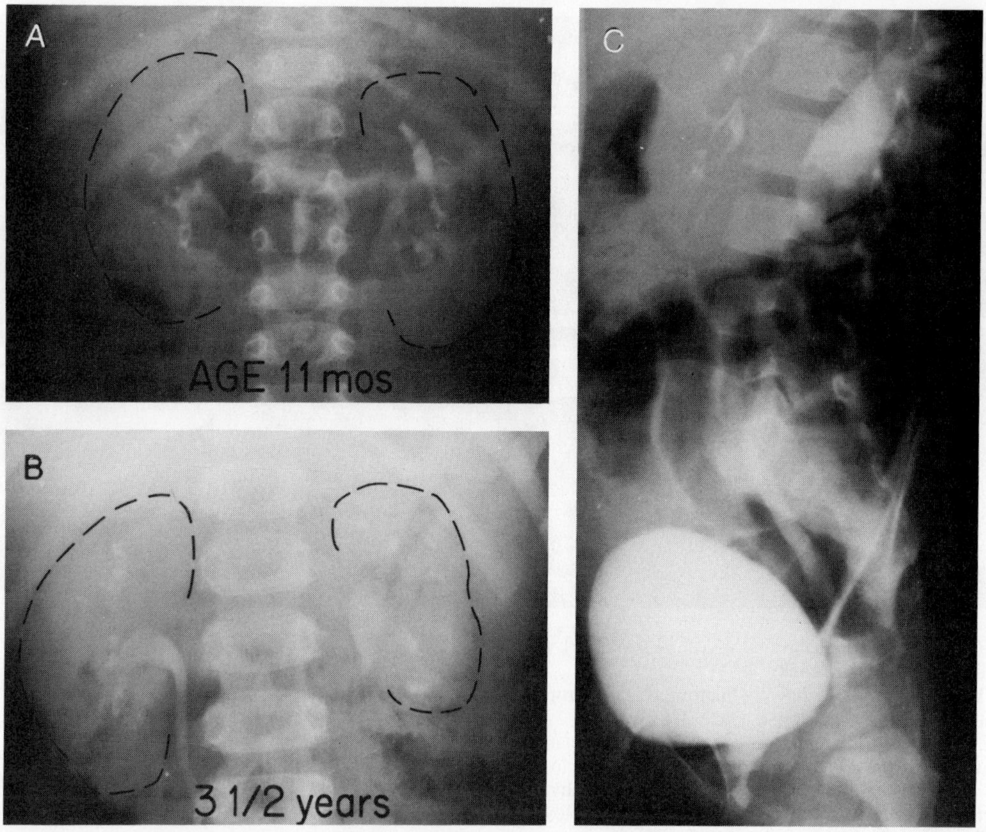

Figure 42–2. The potentially devastating effects of reflux of only moderate degree in the presence of infection.

A, IVP in an 11 month old girl, taken after her first urinary infection. The kidneys are of equal size. Short-term therapy cured the infection. Unfortunately, no cystogram was obtained.

B, IVP at age 3½ years. Note marked atrophy of the left kidney with severe pyelonephritic scarring. This is entirely preventable by appropriate close bacteriologic follow-up of children with urinary infection and correction of vesicoureteral reflux when indications for surgery are present.

C, Cystogram study at age 3½ years, showing only minimal reflux on the right and moderate reflux on the left. Nevertheless, reflux of this degree can ruin a kidney in a short period of time if infection is not controlled. It is interesting that the patient's mother had undergone resection of the left kidney in childhood, presumably the result of reflux.

Outlet Obstruction. This can produce high intravesical voiding pressures, which can cause reflux up a ureterovesical junction that may be competent at normal voiding pressures. For example, in boys with urethral valves, it is common to see voiding pressures three to four times higher than normal. Endoscopic resection of valves can result in a lower voiding pressure with disappearance of reflux in many cases, especially if the ureterovesical junction is not very abnormal. In girls, it is common to see a small amount of reflux with distal urethral stenosis. Opening the distal urethral fibrous ring surgically sometimes will abolish recurrent cystitis and lesser degrees of reflux. A cystogram should not be made until several weeks after acute urinary infection has been controlled, because inflamed and edematous bladder mucosa can shorten and straighten the ureterovesical tunnel, producing reflux. Reflux demonstrated during those conditions can disappear with appropriate antimicrobial therapy that clears infection and edema. Dysfunctional voiding also can mimic anatomic obstruction, producing reflux that can disappear with appropriate therapy.[12]

Ureterovesical Junction Anatomy. Reflux is commonly caused by maldevelopment of the trigone with excessively lateral placement of ureteral orifices (Fig. 42–4). For this reason I believe that cystoscopy is important in a patient with urinary infection and reflux. It allows direct observation to assess the location and appearance of ureteral orifices. A gopher hole orifice through which the surgeon can pass a panendoscope, or look directly up the ureter for several centimeters, will continue to reflux. It

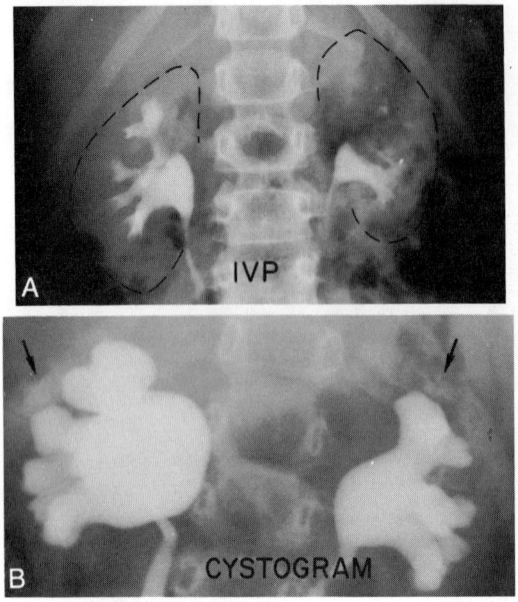

Figure 42–3. Pyelotubular reflux in a 5 year old girl with recurrent infection and reflux.

A, IVP preoperatively, showing bilateral cortical atrophy, most marked at the right upper pole.

B, Cystogram at the same time showing massive bilateral reflux with opacification of some of the renal tubules in the cortex (arrows). This radiographic finding is noteworthy because this type of reflux has a high association with severe cortical damage.

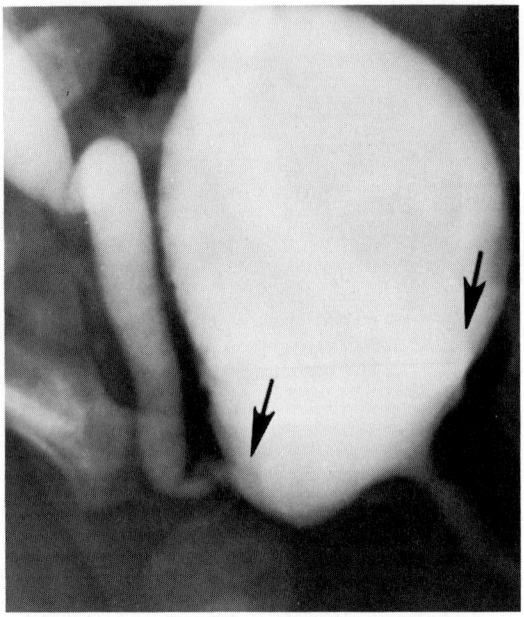

Figure 42–4. Primary vesicoureteral reflux in a 2 year old girl. This is a normal bladder with congenitally abnormal ureterovesical junctions. Note that the ureters enter laterally, with a straight course through the bladder wall (arrows). This abnormal position and lack of obliquity results in massive vesicoureteral reflux, which should be corrected surgically.

should not be treated nonoperatively with the expectation that reflux will cease spontaneously. On the other hand, if the ureteral orifice is almost normal in appearance and if its submucosal tunnel is not short, reflux can disappear. Paraureteral diverticulum is commonly associated with vesicoureteral reflux (Figs. 42–5 and 42–6). At cystoscopy, the ureteral orifice will often be on the lower rim of the diverticulum. At the site of the diverticulum, the bladder mucosa usually will herniate through the ureteral hiatus. After filling the bladder and the diverticulum the lower ureter can be pulled out into the back wall of the diverticulum where there is no muscle backing to the ureter. This allows reflux. Thus the presence of the paraureteral diverticulum often indicates the need for its repair with ureteral reimplantation.

A duplex collecting system is another finding that can be noted cystoscopically. Usually this is evident upon intravenous pyelogram; however, the precise anatomy of the lower ureters may not be evident except by cystoscopy. Most often with a duplex collecting system there is selective reflux to the lower pole of the kidney via the upper orifice in the bladder, which lacks a submucosal tunnel (Figs. 42–7 through 42–9). The most common finding is that the lower orifice in the bladder, which drains the upper pole ureter, has a satisfactory tunnel that prevents reflux. However, the upper ureteral orifice, which drains the lower pole of the kidney, is often dilated and lacks muscular backing, therefore allowing reflux. Sometimes the two orifices lie in a side-to-side arrangement, like the barrels

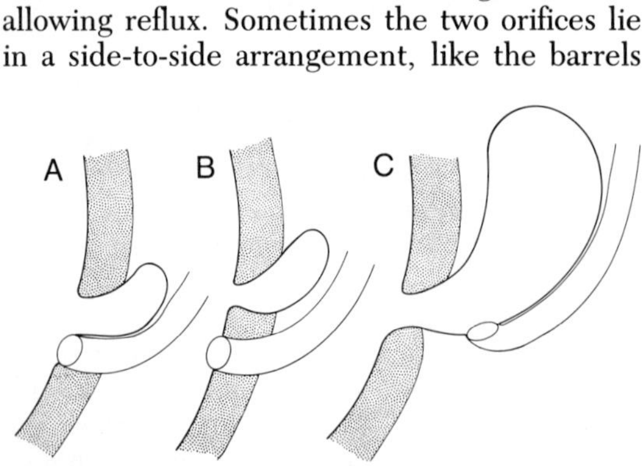

Figure 42–5. Paraureteral diverticula. In many children with reflux, the ureterovesical junction is imperfect, allowing protrusion of bladder mucosa through the hiatus. Most commonly, the diverticulum is just above the ureter (*A*). In some, there is a small bridge of muscle between the ureteral orifice and the mouth of the diverticulum, shown in *B*. In others, the diverticulum is large and pulls the ureteral orifice out into its back wall (*C*) as the diverticulum fills. Reflux is common with paraureteral diverticula, because the ureter lacks muscle backing.

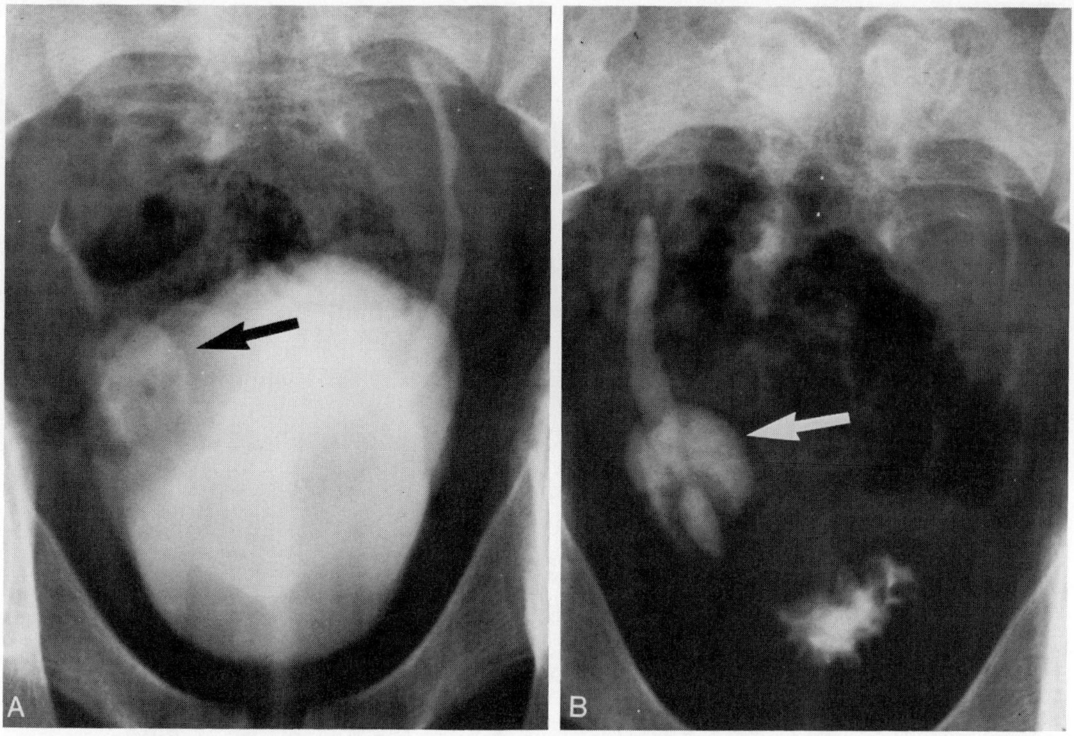

Figure 42–6. Paraureteral diverticula.

A, Cystogram showing a paraureteral diverticulum (arrow) and bilateral reflux.

B, Postvoiding film showing the diverticulum on right side filled and a refluxing ureter located in its back wall. There was a small diverticulum on the left also, not seen on these films.

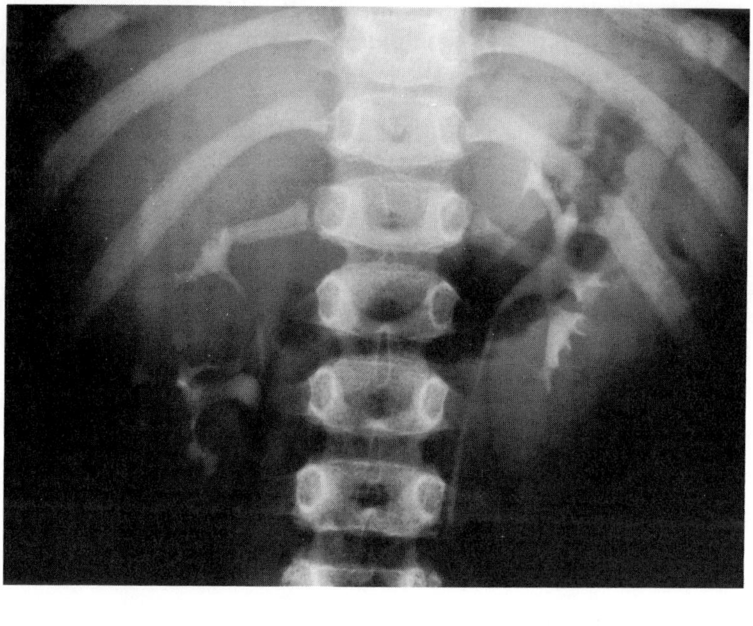

Figure 42–7. Intravenous pyelogram from a 4 year old girl, showing a normal left kidney and a normal upper pole of the right kidney, but a badly damaged calycectatic lower pole of the right kidney is evident. She had massive reflux selectively to that renal unit only. This is the most common pathology seen in patients with ureteral duplication.

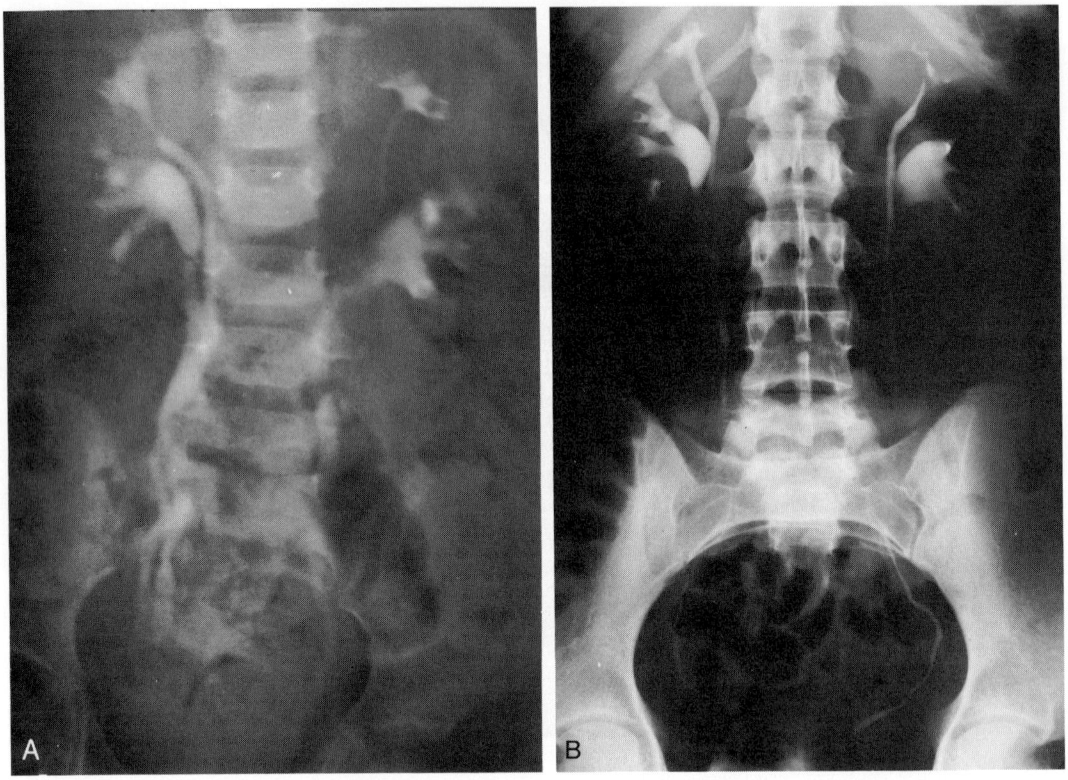

Figure 42–8. Bilateral ureteral duplication, incomplete on the right and complete on the left.

A, IVP at age 3 years. On the right side, the two ureters joined just above the bladder, draining into the bladder by a common lower ureter. There was reflux up this common lower ureter to both upper and lower poles. On the left side, the ureters were duplicated all the way to the bladder. Cystogram showed reflux selectively to the lower pole. Common sheath reimplants were performed for all four ureters, which cured the patient's reflux.

B, IVP at age 17 years, showing delicate upper tracts on both sides. The patient was well.

of a shotgun. There can be reflux into both. Similarly, the two ureters may join a centimeter or two above a common lower ureter that lacks a tunnel, allowing reflux to both ureters. Rarely, in cases with a duplex system, there is selective reflux up the upper pole orifice. This is nearly always the result of its being located ectopically, more caudad than normal, in the bladder neck or urethra, so that it lacks a submucosal tunnel to prevent reflux. An ectopic ureter in the bladder neck or urethra, paradoxically, can show both obstruction and reflux. During micturition, reflux is evident. In the resting state, however, when the bladder neck is closed, the lower ureter can be functionally obstructed. Thus, endoscopic evaluation of the anatomy is important to rule out urethral obstruction and to determine the position and configuration of the ureteral orifices.

Additional Considerations. If reflux and recurrent infection remain despite long-term antimicrobial therapy, it seems reasonable to proceed with ureteral reimplantation. In addition to considering the amount of reflux; whether there is previous scarring; whether there is outlet obstruction, which can be relieved; what the anatomy looks like; and what prior treatment has been given, several other parameters must be considered. One is whether the family will be compliant and faithful about keeping the child on antimicrobial therapy and about getting cultures to be certain that clinically inapparent bacilluria is not causing renal damage. An infant with massive reflux is at great risk. An older child with minimal reflux and normal upper tracts is at much less risk for pyelonephritic scarring. A child with neuropathic bladder can exhibit a change from mild to severe reflux in a short time. This is seldom seen in a child with a basically normal bladder. Thoughtful consideration of all these risk factors and circumstances will usually guide a sensible decision.

TECHNIQUES OF URETERAL REIMPLANTATION

Figure 42–10 shows schematically the comparative anatomy of the normal and the refluxing

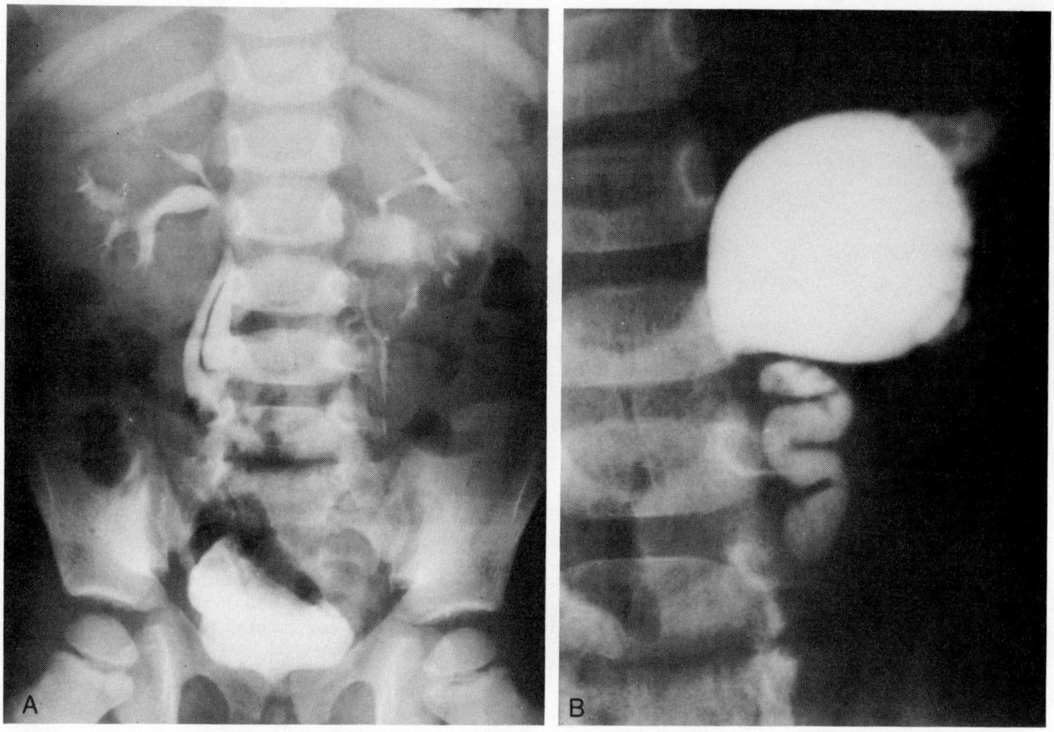

Figure 42–9. Three year old boy with duplex collecting systems.

A, IVP. Note the Y-shaped configuration on the right, where two ureters join halfway between the kidney and the bladder. On the left, ureters were duplicated all the way to the bladder.

B, Selective massive reflux to the lower pole of the left ureter, which had no function by radionuclide scan, obtained with a catheter in the bladder to prevent a false indication of function by reflux of contrast up the ureter during the study. There was reflux on the right side as well. At operation, the right ureter was reimplanted. The nonfunctional lower pole on the left was removed, together with its refluxing ureter. The adjacent upper pole ureter was reimplanted. Alternatively, the lower pole could have been removed, dividing its ureter low next to the bladder, leaving a short stump. However, it was chosen to remove the entire refluxing stump and reimplant the adjacent nonrefluxing upper pole ureter.

ureterovesical junction, and the surgeon's goal in correcting reflux. The task is to create a submucosal tunnel and muscle backing of the ureter so that when the bladder contracts there is a valvelike mechanism to prevent backwash up the ureter. In our early efforts with ureteral reimplantation (1959–1962), we used independently an extravesical procedure (Fig. 42–11). This method was also used by Lich and colleagues[13] and by Grégoir and Van Regemorter.[14] The bladder muscle was incised down to mucosa, laying the ureter in a submucosal position and closing the muscle around the ureter to create a tunnel. The procedure had appeal because of its simplicity; however, we abandoned it because our failure rate was unacceptable.[3,15] We found it to be an unreliable procedure. In some cases both sides were done in an identical fashion but postoperatively there was reflux or obstruction on one side and a good result on the other. An obvious disadvantage of this means for reimplantation is that it does not change the position of the ureteral orifice, which is frequently abnormal at the outset. To endure, a surgical procedure must provide predictably good results. This one did not, in my experience. However, some surgeons today prefer the Lich-Grégoir procedure, because it can be done without entering the bladder and the patient can be discharged just a few days postoperatively. I do not believe those are important considerations for an operation that must give a predictably good result to last a lifetime.

Intravesical Ureteral Reimplantation by the Politano-Leadbetter Technique

Since 1962, for most ureteral reimplantations I have used the technique described by Politano and Leadbetter in 1958,[16] with certain modifications (Fig. 42–12).

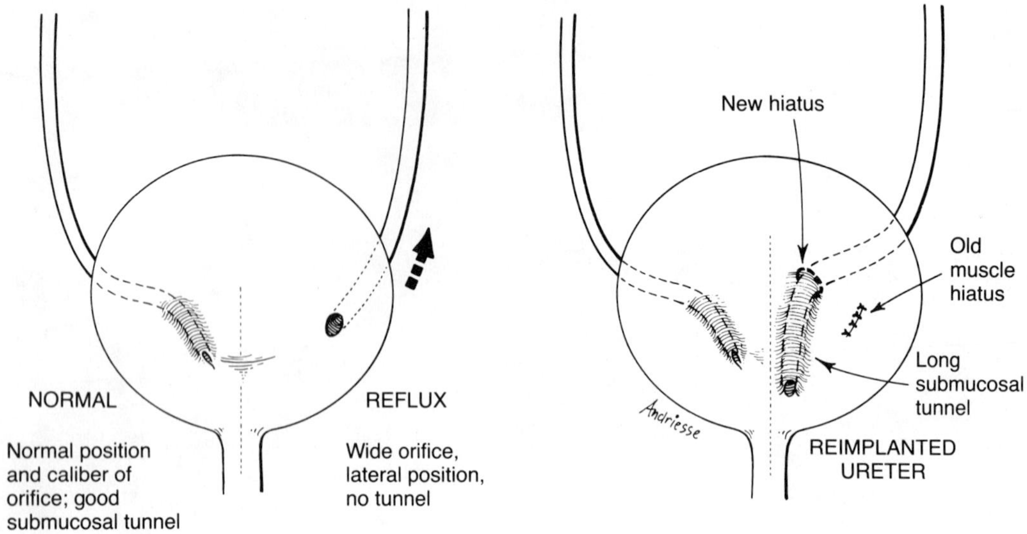

Figure 42–10. Normal versus reflux anatomy when the ureteral orifice is laterally located and the ureter has little or no submucosal tunnel. Ureteral reimplantation involves relocating the ureter more medially and distally in the trigone to give it a long submucosal tunnel and good muscle backing, avoiding angulation at its new point of entry through the bladder wall.

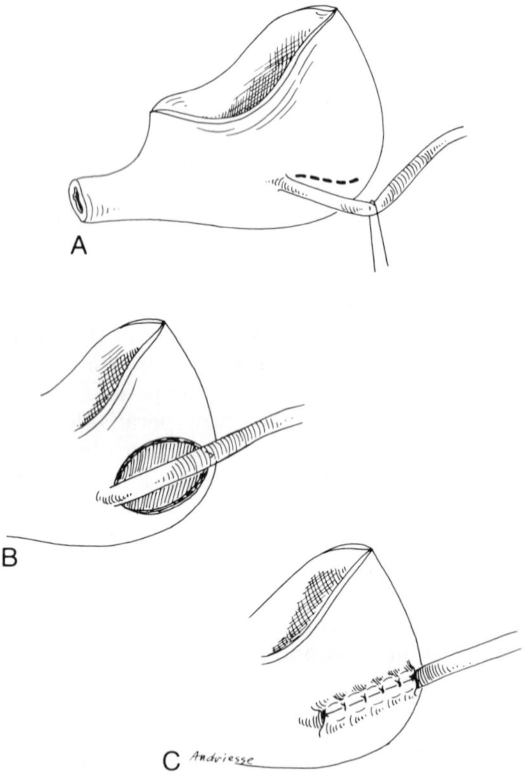

Figure 42–11. Extravesical reimplantation used many years ago. Results were unsatisfactory.

Operative Steps

1. A small plastic catheter is passed up the ureter and sewn to the upper rim of the ureteral hiatus with an atraumatic silk suture. Gentle traction on the catheter obviates handling the tip of the ureter during its mobilization. The ureteral orifice is circumscribed sharply, leaving a generous cuff of mucosa attached. I do not use cautery, for this can cause thermal injury at the tip of the ureter.

2. The ureter is mobilized for 4 to 6 centimeters intravesically, cutting its periureteral adventitial attachments. This adventitia carries the ureteral blood supply. When the ureter is being mobilized, it is important to divide the attachments as far from the ureter as possible to avoid skeletonizing it, which can result in ischemia. The attachment to be divided is picked up with a fine forceps and divided, and then only the end away from the ureter is coagulated. Thus no cautery is applied to the end of the attachment, which remains with the ureter. It is virtually never necessary to grasp a ureter with a forceps during its mobilization.

3. Before the ureter is brought through the bladder at a higher point, any tissue crossing in the peritoneum anterior to the ureter is divided, so that there will be nothing to angulate the ureter when it is brought through the bladder wall at a higher level. There is nearly always a vessel crossing the ureter in the peritoneum. We routinely divide it.

4. A right-angle clamp is passed anterior to the ureter and behind the bladder muscle, incising onto the tip of the right angle to make a new muscle hiatus higher and more medial than the original one. This maneuver should be done under direct vision. It is helpful to have the assistant elevate the bladder forward with the retractor held in the dome of the bladder, to visualize the cul-de-sac peritoneum when passing the right-angle clamp. Otherwise the clamp can go into the pelvic peritoneal cavity, injuring bowel. I have seen two cases in which the ureter was brought through the wall of the adjacent sigmoid colon, resulting in peritonitis.

5. After the new muscle hiatus is created, a ligature is brought through it, pulling a second right-angle clamp back through the hiatus. The second clamp is used to bring the ureter upward through it.

6. While being brought upward, the ureter is held gently with forceps to prevent its twisting during the maneuver. It is helpful to mark the front wall of the ureter with a skin-marking pencil or brilliant green dye applied with a toothpick to be sure that the ureter is not twisted during this maneuver.

7. A submucosal tunnel is created, making the direction of the tunnel craniad, not lateral. The eventual position of the ureter in its new tunnel should be as medial in the trigone as possible. The ureteral orifice will be located distally in the trigone just superior to the bladder neck. In some bladders it is not easy to make this submucosal tunnel. It is best then to incise the mucosa (see megaureter technique), laying back mucosal flaps, placing the ureter next to muscle, and then closing the mucosal flaps over the ureter.

8. It is vital to make the new ureteral hiatus large enough. We routinely incise its lower rim for 3 to 4 mm to avoid sharp angulation where the ureter traverses the bladder muscle and enters its submucosal tunnel. To visualize this rim easily, a forceps is placed next to the ureter, and the spread forceps can be used to display the rim to be incised.

9. After the ureter is placed in its bed and checked to ensure that it is under no tension, the mucosa is incised a few millimeters more distally and medially, advancing the ureter, to give it additional tunnel length.

10. The ureter is sutured into position. The most distal suture passes through not only mucosa but also trigone muscle, for this suture will anchor the ureter distally. The remaining sutures join bladder mucosa to the cuff around the ureteral orifice. These latter sutures are fine chromic catgut. For the anchoring suture, I use polydioxanone suture, which will remain somewhat longer, for I had a case in which the catgut dissolved early, allowing the tip of the ureter to become detached before healing had occurred.

11. The completed ureteral reimplantation tunnel is usually 20 to 35 mm long, depending on the size of the patient. There is good muscle backing behind the ureter. The location of the ureteral orifice is distal and medial in the trigone. Only rarely is a ureteral drainage catheter used. If one is used, it should be a soft plastic tube. Early in our experience, when a stiff catheter was used we observed several fistulas from the ureter to the bladder at the upper end of the tunnel. These eroded the wall of the ureter at the point where it turned to enter the muscle hiatus.

Combined Technique

In some cases of ureteral reimplantation it is better to mobilize the ureter both intravesically and extravesically to accomplish its reimplantation (Fig. 42–13). If intravesical mobilization is proceeding with difficulty, as it does in some cases, we do not hestitate to continue the mobilization extravesically, rather than struggling from an entirely intravesical approach. I use a combined approach for ureters in about 13 percent of initial operations. The indication is usually (1) a moderately dilated ureter, (2) when the intravesical mobilization is proving difficult, or (3) when the bladder wall is hypertrophied. Combined technique is preferred when a previous operation has been performed.

Operative Steps

1. Initial mobilization of the ureter is carried out as with intravesical reimplantation. A catheter is sewn into the ureter and is mobilized with a cuff of mucosa; periureteral adventitial attachments are divided as far as possible from the ureter to preserve its investing adventitia. A scissors is passed parallel to the ureter and through the paravesical web, several centimeters above the level of the bladder. Retraction of the peritoneum upward and medially is facilitated by dividing and ligating the obliterated umbilical artery ligament. Some surgeons mobilize the ureter extravesically by dissecting adjacent to the bladder. I believe this is more likely to injure nerves to the bladder wall than is the

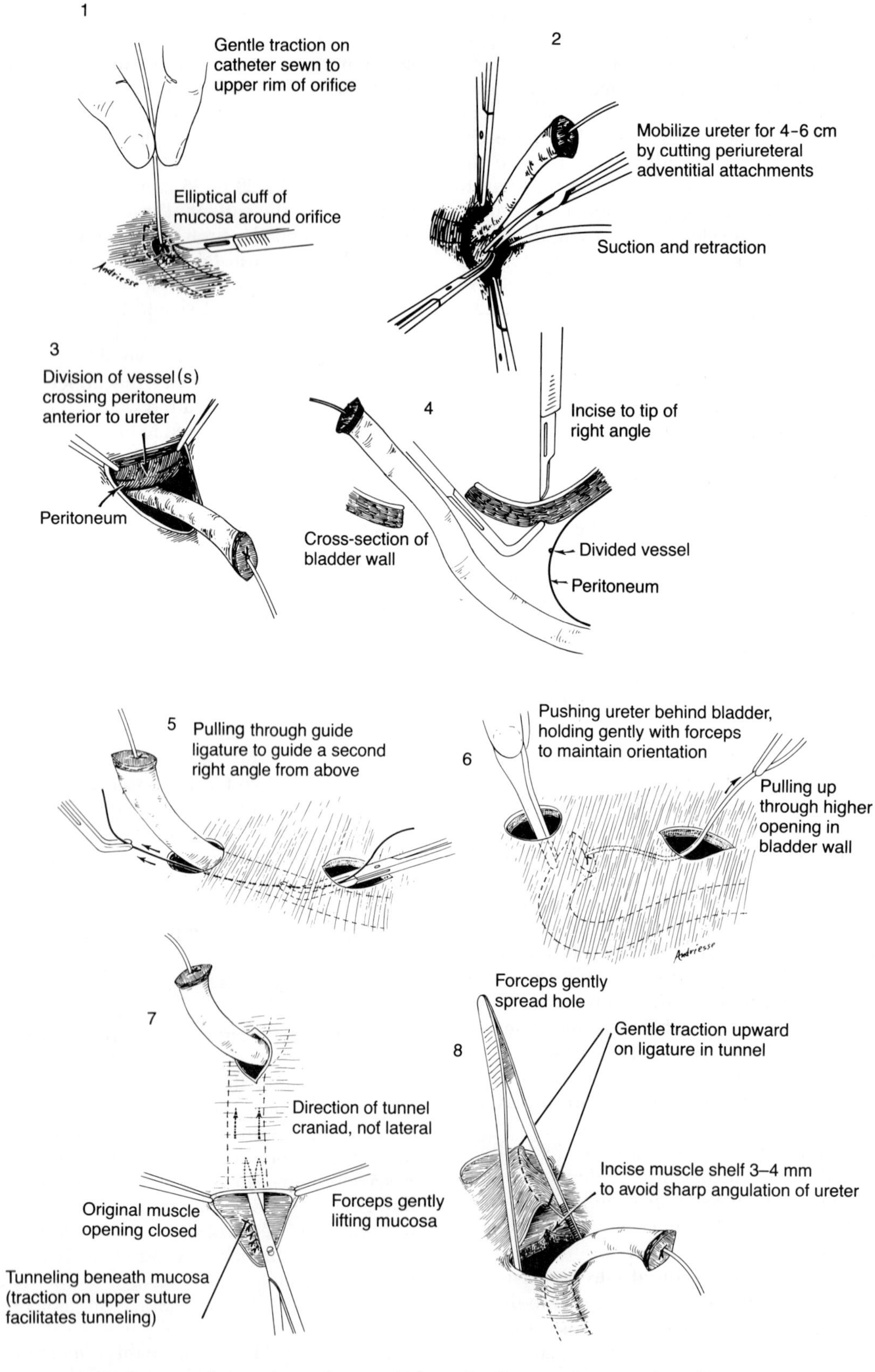

Figure 42–12. Intravesical ureteral reimplantation (Politano-Leadbetter technique with modifications). See text.

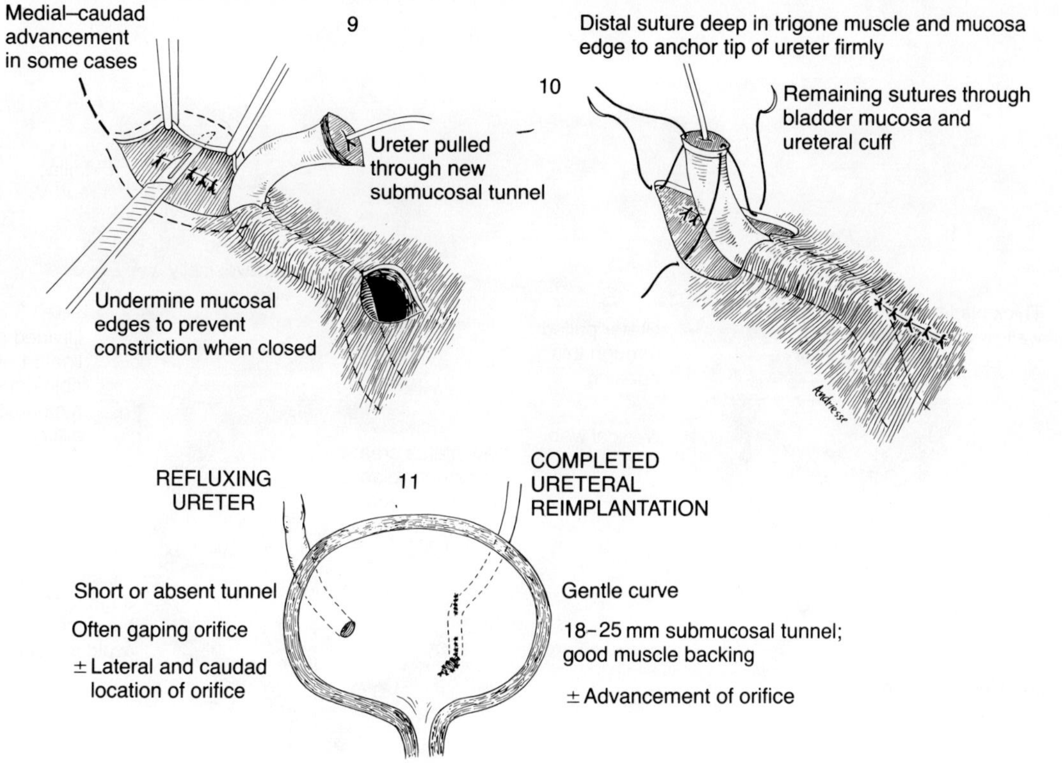

Figure 42–12. *Continued*

method described. I have seen several cases in which the bladder was partially denervated because of bilateral paravesical mobilization of ureters. That complication can be avoided if initial mobilization is done intravesically.

2. The ureter is then pulled through into the posterior gutter and mobilized upward to the level of the iliac vessels. It is important to preserve the ureteral blood supply coming from above, which runs medial to the ureter along its attachment to the peritoneum. When those attachments are divided, the division should be as far as possible from the wall of the ureter to prevent creating ischemia. A new ureteral hiatus is created. As shown, this hiatus should be posterior in the back wall of the bladder. If the ureter is brought through the dome or side wall of the bladder, it is likely to angulate and obstruct when the bladder is filled. The inferior rim of the new muscle hiatus should be incised to enlarge the opening enough to avoid angulation. The original ureteral hiatus should be closed accurately, first mobilizing the adjacent mucosa from it, especially when a paraureteral diverticulum was present preoperatively.

3. The ureter is brought through its new hiatus and adjusted to lie without tension. A submucosal tunnel is made in which to place the ureter. In some bladders this is easy. In hypertrophied bladders, or reoperative cases, it is much better to incise the mucosa, laying back flaps to create a bed for the ureter, and then closing these flaps over the ureter after anchoring the ureter distally.

4. The completed tunnel is usually a little longer than that accomplished by intravesical reimplantation.

Duplex Collecting System

Figure 42–14 shows the most common anatomy with a duplex collecting system. There is selective reflux to the lower pole, drained by the upper ureteral orifice. We have managed this problem by mobilizing the two ureters just as one would a single ureter and reimplanting them together as a single unit. A common sheath surrounds the lower end of the two ureters, which makes it easy to reimplant them as one would a single ureter. This can be done by either intravesical or combined technique, depending on other aspects of the case. Rarely, the two ureters will be far enough apart that they do not lie in

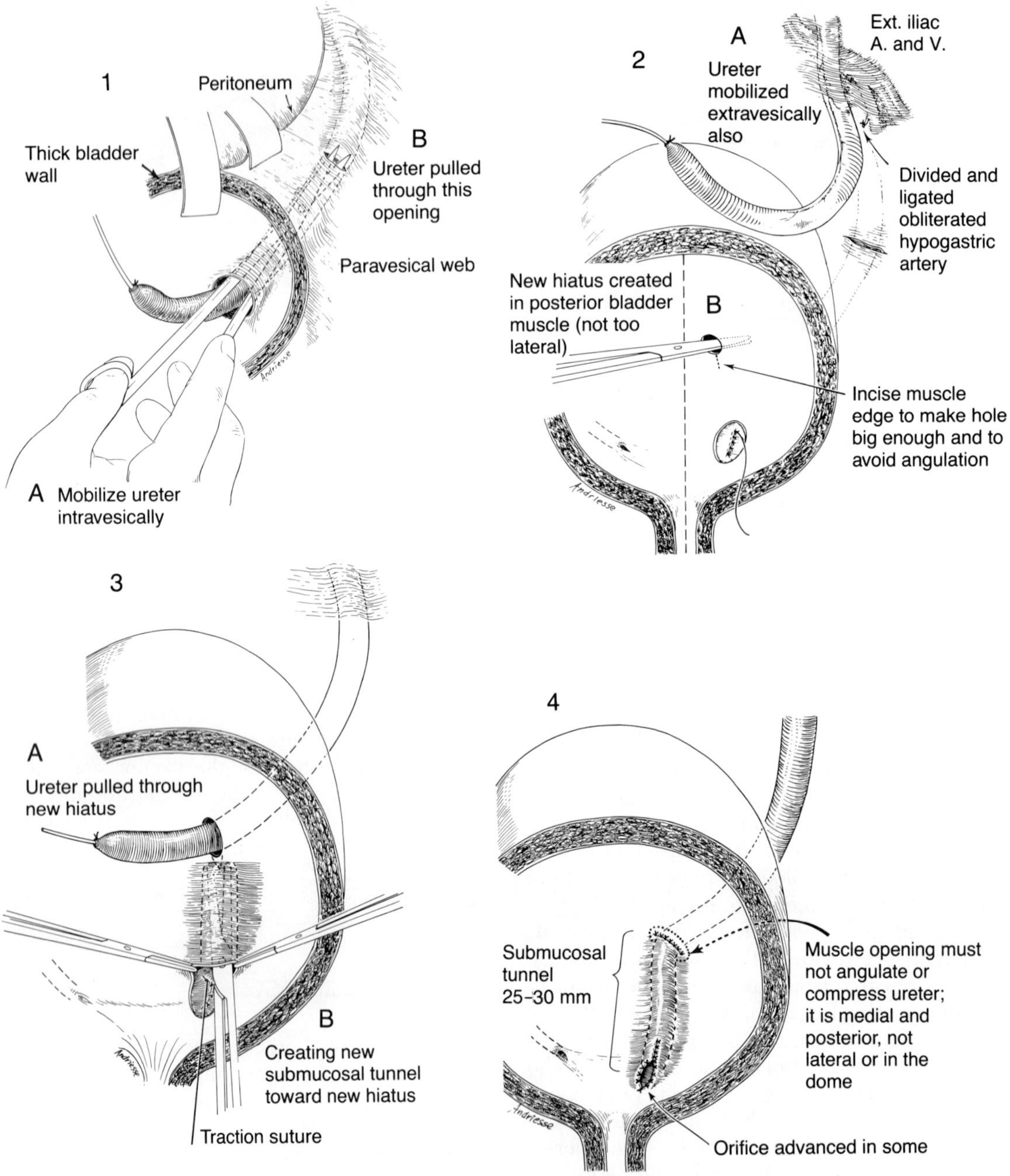

Figure 42–13. Combined intravesical-extravesical reimplantation technique. (See text.)

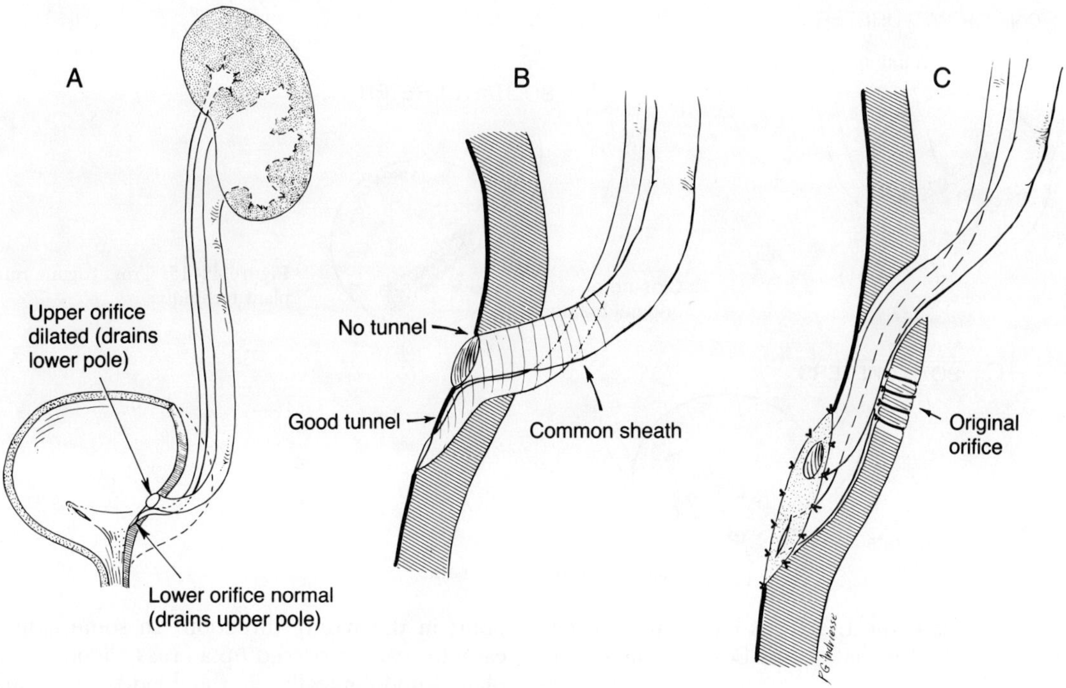

Figure 42–14. The most common anatomy of ureteral duplication.
A, Selective damage to the lower pole of the kidney with slight dilatation of the ureter.
B, The anatomy most frequently seen where there is no tunnel for the upper orifice draining the lower pole.
C, The preferred method of management when the lower pole is salvageable, which it usually is. Both ureters are reimplanted as a single unit.

a common sheath, so that only the refluxing ureter is reimplanted. That is very unusual in my experience. Another approach that has been described is extravesical ureteroureterostomy, anastomosing the refluxing lower pole ureter to the nonrefluxing upper pole ureter.[17] If the two ureters are wider apart than usual, there may be a separate muscle hiatus for each one, particularly if the upper pole ureter is ectopic in the bladder neck. To correct this, the upper pole ureter can be mobilized through its hiatus to the point where it lies adjacent to the lower pole ureter; then they can be mobilized together for a combined reimplantation, discarding the excess length of the upper pole ureter.

Sometimes selective reflux to one pole of the kidney is best treated by heminephrectomy and ureterectomy when there is no significant function in that renal moiety, as shown in Figure 42–9.

Cross Trigone Reimplantation

In some bladders it is impossible to obtain a satisfactory reimplant by the aforementioned methods. Examples include some particularly hypertrophied bladders in children with myelodysplasia or in boys who have had urethral valves. Another instance is the previously exstrophied bladder in which the ureters are located very laterally and caudally, so that simple advancement of the ureter is easier than mobilizing it and bringing it in at a higher point in the trigone, which may be very small. In girls with cloacal malformations, the ureters are sometimes more easily reimplanted by the cross trigone advancement technique described by S. J. Cohen of Manchester, England[18] (Figs. 42–15 and 42–16).

Operative Steps

One or both ureters can be mobilized intravesically or, if necessary, extravesically. If only one ureter is to be reimplanted, it can be done obliquely and upward, using its original hiatus. If there is only one ureter, often a new hiatus will be made, gaining extra tunnel length by crossing the trigone diagonally and downward. When both ureters are to be reimplanted, they can lie parallel to one another, using sep-

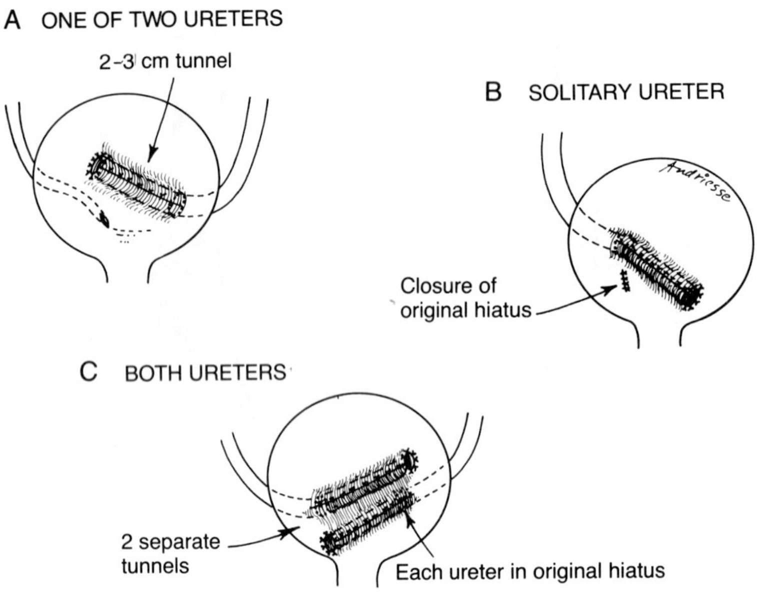

Figure 42–15. Cross trigone reimplant technique.

arate tunnels if the trigone is large enough, or in a single bed if that seems best, as shown in Fig. 42–16.

Cross trigone ureteral reimplantation is more easily accomplished than the other two techniques described. This has led some surgeons to use it routinely. I am opposed to its routine use, however, and reserve this method only for problem cases as described. The reason is that it may be impossible to have access to the ureter with a ureteral catheter by conventional means at cystoscopy, because the ureter simply may point in the wrong direction. In some cases a catheter can be passed up a cross trigone reimplant endoscopically, if the bladder is nearly empty, if a bent wire stylette is in the tip of the ureter, and so on. Placing a percutaneous needle into the bladder from above and threading a ureteral catheter through the needle from a lateral vantage point is another technique that can be used. Although there probably will be no need to catheterize many ureters reimplanted by the cross trigone technique in the future, some of these patients may develop ureteral

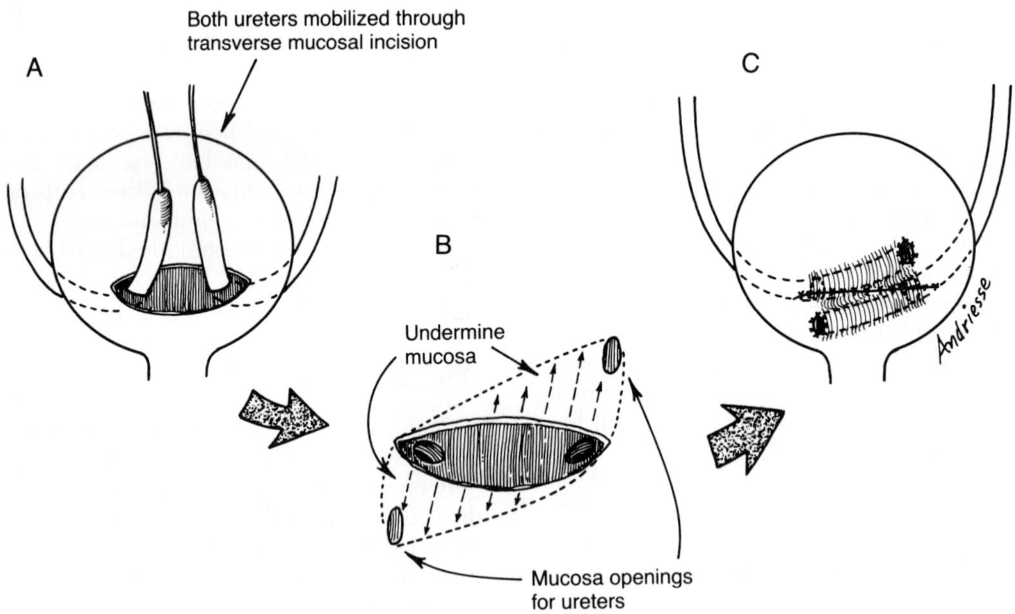

Figure 42–16. Cross trigone reimplant technique.

stones; then management will be more difficult if the ureter has been reimplanted by this technique, which makes endoscopic access difficult or impossible.

Postoperative Care

After ureteral reimplantation, bladder drainage is maintained for 5 or 6 days using a small plastic catheter per urethra. I do not use a Foley catheter, not wishing to have a balloon resting on a recent reimplant. Similarly I seldom use a suprapubic tube, unless there is some special indication, such as performing a bladder neck operation for continence. In those cases a suprapubic tube will be useful until the patient has demonstrated the ability to void or self-catheterize for bladder emptying. An IVP or radionuclide scan is obtained on the 7th postoperative day to be certain that there is satisfactory drainage. As shown in Figure 42–17, there is often periureteral edema, with slight compression of the distal ureter and mild hydronephrosis. This will subside in 2 to 3 weeks. If there is more than mild hydronephrosis, an IVP is repeated in 3 to 4 weeks to make certain that the problem is simply edema rather than actual mechanical obstruction of the distal ureter. If the IVP at 1 week shows poor visualization of the kidney, the child remains in the hospital under close observation to make certain that temporary decompression of the kidney by percutaneous nephrostomy is not needed. Should a bona fide obstruction be evident soon after ureteral reimplantation, renal function should be protected by either passing a soft catheter up from below or percutaneous nephrostomy. Reoperation on the lower ureter should be delayed for several months until the postoperative inflammatory reaction has subsided, so as to improve the chance of accomplishing a satisfactory reoperation, unless it is clear that transureteroureterostomy would be the best method for managing the complication.

Complications of Ureteral Reimplantation

The most common complications we have seen are shown in Figure 42–18. Reflux can persist if the new ureteral orifice is too lateral in the bladder or the submucosal tunnel is too short. We have seen several examples of reflux in a fistula caused by a stiff ureteral catheter-stent. Obstruction of a reimplant most often results from angulation at the new hiatus. Rarely, a diverticulum can form at the new hiatus, com-

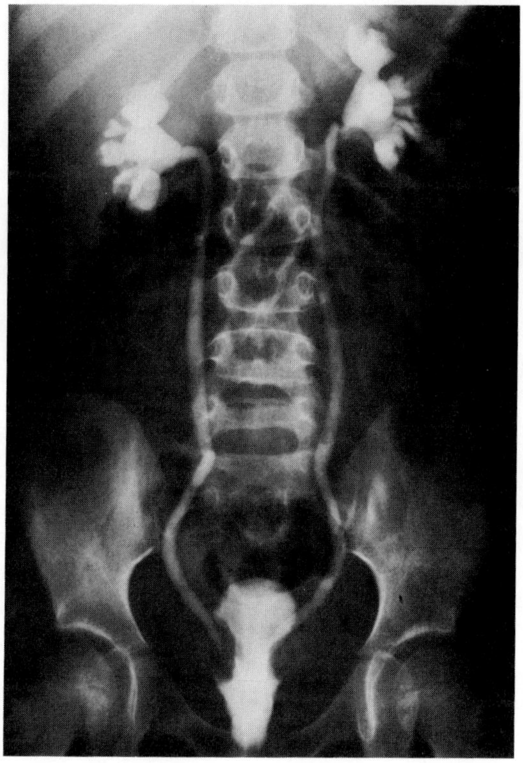

Figure 42–17. IVP 1 week after bilateral ureteral reimplantation in a 5 year old girl. Note postoperative edema surrounding both lower ureters and moderate bilateral hydronephrosis. This is quite usual on early postoperative study. Subsequent examination a few weeks later will be normal, unless there is a postoperative complication.

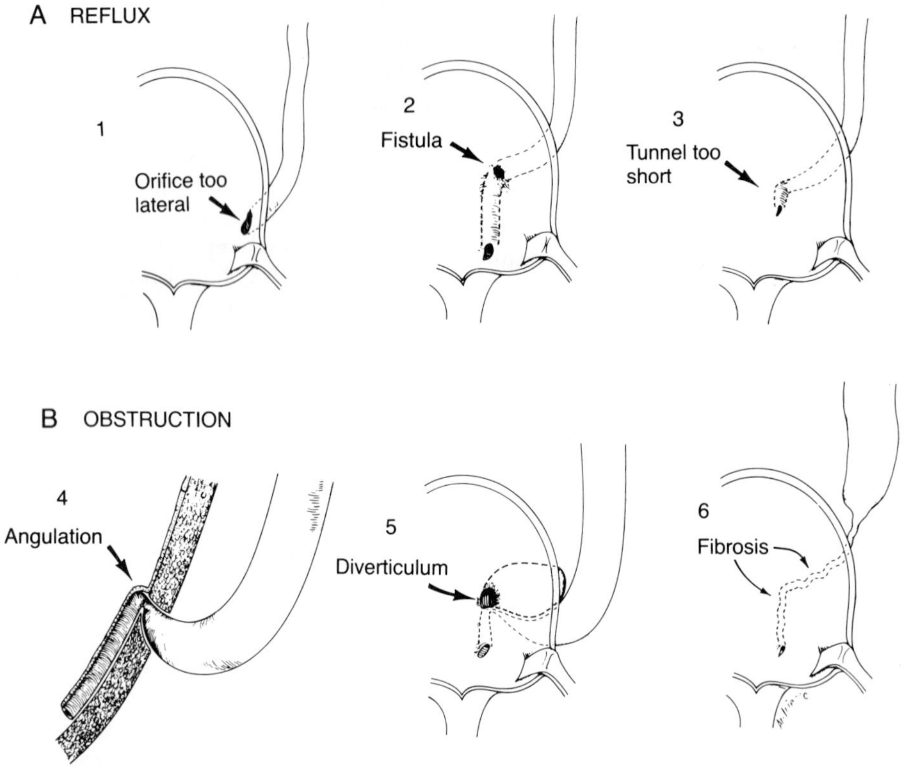

Figure 42–18. The most common reasons for failure of ureteral reimplantation.

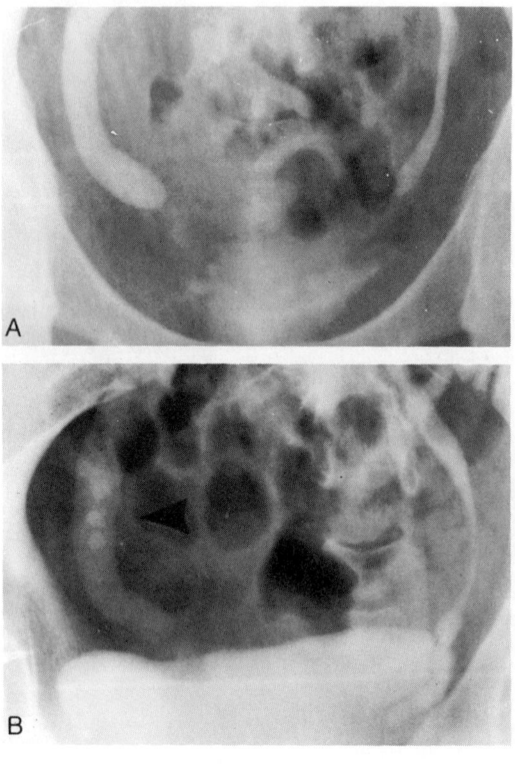

Figure 42–19. Bilateral moderate ureteral obstruction following ureteral reimplantation. On the right side there is angulation at the ureterovesical junction, and on the left side there is fibrosis of the terminal ureter.

A, IVP 1 year after the ureteral reimplantation. The patient was asymptomatic.

B, IVP 2 years postoperatively. The patient had developed infection. Note three small stones visible in the right ureter. Reoperation corrected the problem. The patient is now a 33 year old adult, married, and free from urinary infection; upper tracts are stable.

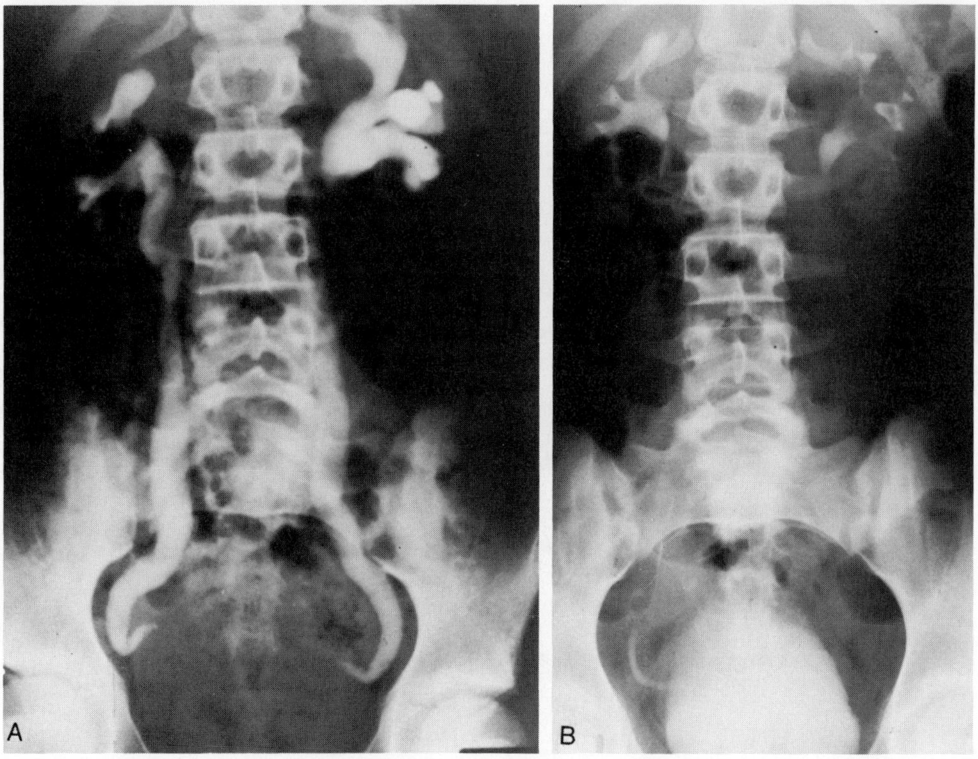

Figure 42–20. Ureteral obstruction in an 8 year old girl referred 1 year after ureteral reimplantation.

A, Note the "fish hook" deformity of both lower ureters, which had been implanted too high and too far to the side in the wall of the bladder. Although reflux had been corrected, both ureters were obstructed.

B, IVP 6 months after reoperation, which consisted of combined repeat reimplantation of both ureters, bringing them through a new hiatus more posteriorly in the trigone. Normal drainage and no reflux. IVP 10 years later was excellent. Patient is well, 20 years after this reoperation.

presssing the adjacent ureter. Fibrosis of the distal ureter can result from loss of blood supply. Figures 42–19 and 42–20 show two typical cases in need of reoperation.

Technique of Operation

Occasionally a simple intravesical procedure can correct a failed reimplant. In the majority of cases, however, I have found it best to do a complete remobilization of the ureter and repeat reimplantation by the combined technique,[15] as shown in Figure 42–21. Mobilizing a previously reimplanted ureter can be difficult. There should be an inlying catheter in the ureter. It should be mobilized with as much of its surrounding tissue as possible to avoid its devascularization.

As discussed later in this chapter, when dealing with two failed reimplants it may be better to reimplant only the better ureter, with a long tunnel and psoas hitch, draining the opposite one by transureteroureterostomy.[19,20]

URETEROCELES

In managing patients with ureteroceles, ureteral reimplantation is generally required.[21–23] Ureteroceles occur in a variety of anatomic types, as shown in Figure 42–22. The small "adult type" of ureterocele is usually seen with a single ureter. It tends to incur less upper tract damage than do large ureteroceles, often termed "infant-type," which present earlier in life with greater obstruction and hydronephrosis. In younger patients, more often girls than boys, there is a duplex collecting system. The ureterocele involves the upper pole ureter of the duplex system. The upper pole of the kidney is usually dysplastic or very hydronephrotic and often does not visualize during intravenous pyelography.

Ureteroceles can do more than merely obstruct the ureter. For example, the ureterocele can prolapse down into the bladder outlet, causing bladder neck obstruction. There is often reflux on the opposite side, as well as reflux up the ipsilateral lower pole ureter that is located

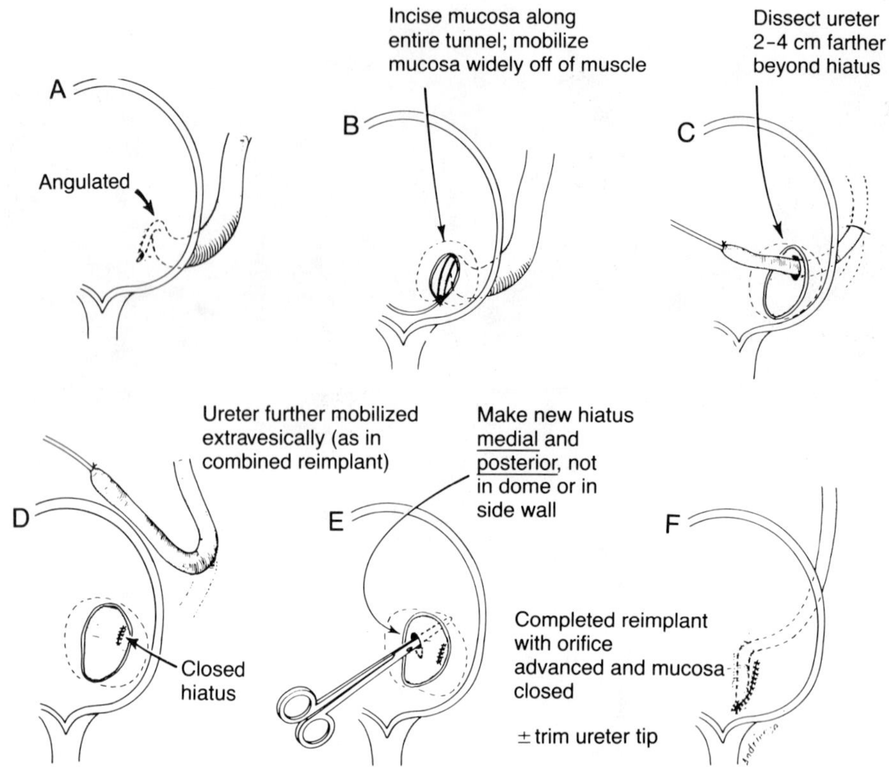

Figure 42–21. The technique of reoperation found most satisfactory in the majority of reoperative cases. Lesser revisions are not usually as successful as a more complete operation, as shown.

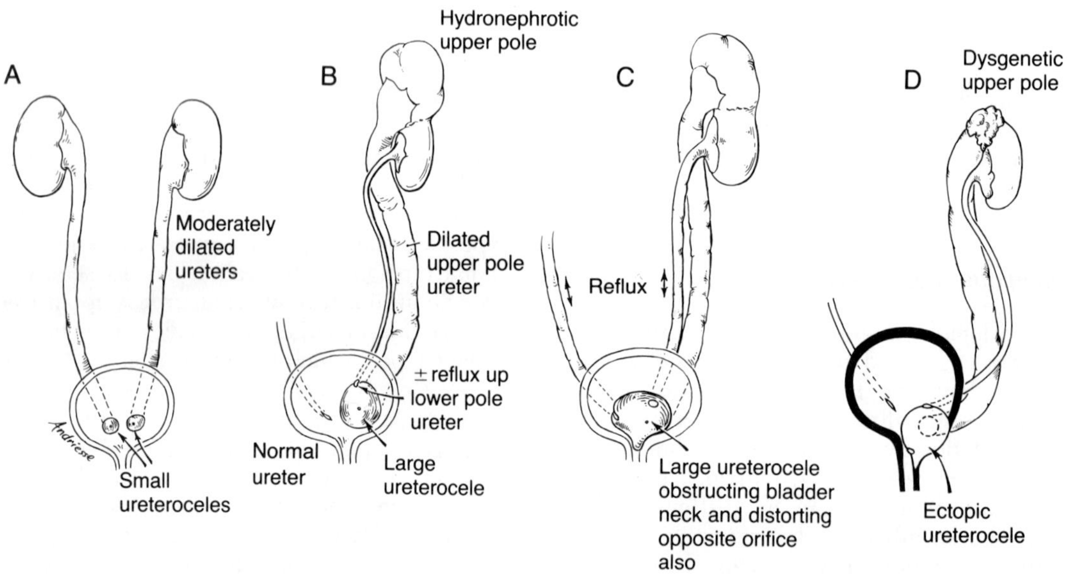

Figure 42–22. Types of ureteroceles.

A, Small "adult-type" ureteroceles with single ureters, minimal upper tract dilatation, and excellent renal function.

B, Large "infant-type" ureterocele with duplex ureters. There is hydronephrosis of the upper pole and often reflux to the ipsilateral lower pole.

C, Large ureterocele extending into the bladder neck and proximal urethra, causing outlet obstruction and encroaching on the opposite renal collecting system, resulting in obstruction or reflux.

D, Ectopic ureterocele in which the orifice enters the posterior urethra, not the trigone. The upper pole is frequently dysplastic. If the ureter enters distal to the external sphincter in the terminal urethra or vestibule, it becomes a different problem: ectopic ureter with incontinence.

on the upper aspect of the ureterocele. "Ectopic ureterocele" is a descriptive term for the ureterocele that extends down beyond the trigone through the bladder neck and into the urethra. In these cases, a muscle defect in the bladder neck and urethra is usually present. This too can cause bladder outlet obstruction if the defect is not repaired.

Operative Technique

Unroofing ureteroceles was considered accepted practice many years ago. There has been a curious resurgence of interest in this method; however, it risks trading reflux for obstruction. In my view, the only need for unroofing a ureterocele today is to allow drainage of a pus-filled ureter by means of a small endoscopic incision in the ureterocele, as a temporizing procedure in a sick infant. I would not use the method for "definitive drainage" of an obstructed renal moiety. Figure 42–23 shows a patient with vesicoureteral reflux following endoscopic incision of a ureterocele of modest size. A small ureterocele is best treated by open resection of the ureterocele and combined reimplantation of the ureter, as shown in Figure 42–24. Occasionally, the "adult" ureterocele will have a ureter dilated enough to require tapering, as will be described under megaureter repair.

For "infant" ureterocele (a large ureterocele with a duplex collecting system), a much more extensive procedure is generally required. A scheme for management is shown in Figure 42–25. The ultimate goal of reconstruction is usually resection of the ureterocele, removal of the dilated upper pole ureter, reimplantation of the ipsilateral lower pole ureter, and upper pole partial nephrectomy. Occasionally the upper pole is worth salvaging, but only rarely. The manner of proceeding with reconstruction can vary according to how sick the patient is, the age of the child, and so on. We have done a complete reconstructive procedure in one sitting in most cases.

There are alternative ways of management, however. For example, in a sick patient with a pus-filled upper pole and ureterocele, endoscopic unroofing to allow drainage for a few days may be useful before definitive repair, meanwhile treating the patient with appropriate antibiotics. In this situation, as shown, it is also reasonable to perform upper pole nephroureterectomy, deferring definitive management of the ureterocele stump and the adjacent ureter until a later time. In dissecting out the large ureterocele, which occupies most of the trigone, it is advisable to preserve enough mucosa to cover the trigone. As shown in Figure 42–26, in ectopic ureterocele it is important to repair the associated muscle defect to avoid having a diverticulum defect that can act as a flap valve and obstruct the bladder outlet. Figure 42–27 illustrates the technique for preserving the better ureter to be reimplanted, while discarding the larger ureter associated with the upper pole, which is usually removed. A typical "infant" ureterocele case is shown in Figure 42–28. A poorly managed case with serious complications is shown in Figure 42–29.

MEGAURETER

Megaureter is a descriptive term for the wide and often tortuous ureter often seen with hydronephrosis. As shown in Figure 42–30, megaureters can be grouped into those with ureteral obstruction and those with reflux. In some, the pathology is primary in the lower ureter. In others, megaureter is the result of distal obstruction from urethral valves, myelodysplasia, ureteral ectopia, ureterocele, the prune belly syndrome, and so on. In most cases needing operation, however, repair involves resection and tapering of the distal ureter and its reimplantation into the bladder so that there is no reflux or obstruction.

Megaureter was once thought to be a problem too complex to repair.[24–27] Bischoff demonstrated the feasibility of shortening, straightening, and tapering widely dilated, tortuous ureters.[28] Soon thereafter, the principle of tunneled reimplantation was applied with a high degree of success.[29–37] In patients with obstructive megaureter, the ureteral orifice is usually normal in appearance, the terminal ureter is small, and cross-section of it shows a fibrous wall with little muscle. Peristalsis is usually active in the dilated ureter above. In general, the prognosis is better for obstructive megaureter because the kidney is relatively better preserved. In refluxing megaureter, the orifice is usually patulous. Often a panendoscope can be inserted into the orifice and passed several inches up the ureter. A periureteral diverticulum is often present. Sometimes the ostium of the diverticulum is mistaken for the ureteral orifice, which in fact lies on the back wall of the diverticulum. Peristalsis can be active with refluxing megaureter, but in some it may be sluggish or absent, especially if there has been considerable urinary

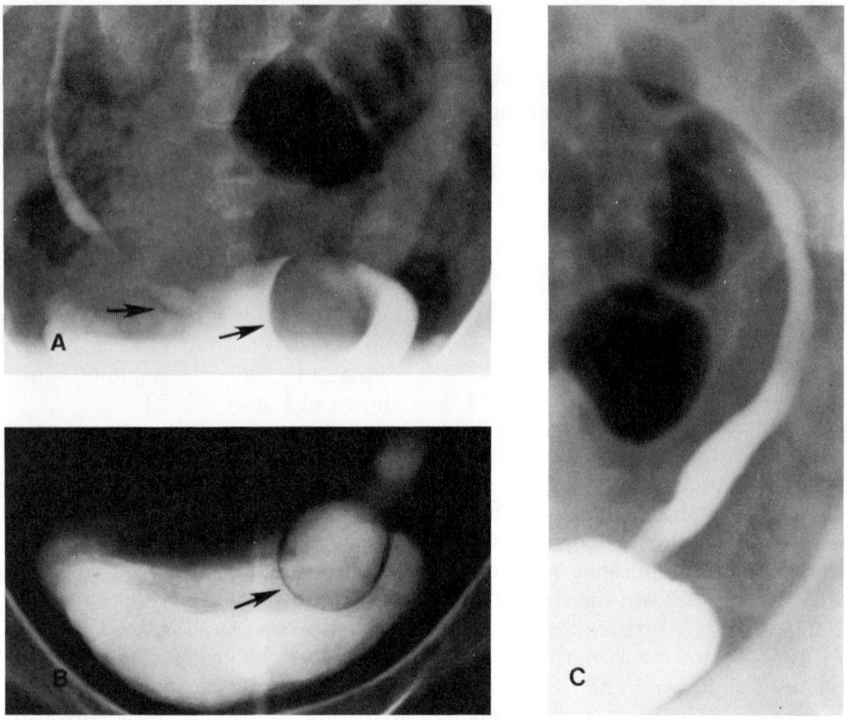

Figure 42–23. "Adult-type" ureteroceles in a 23 year old nurse, treated by endoscopic unroofing. This resulted in reflux, for which she was referred.

A, Preoperative IVP, showing a small ureterocele on the right and a moderate-sized ureterocele on the left, outlined by contrast in the bladder (arrows).

B, Preoperative IVP, delayed film, showing the left ureterocele now filled with contrast (arrow).

C, Cystogram showing left reflux that resulted from unroofing. We believe that unroofing in general is not satisfactory, for it is very apt to exchange reflux for obstruction.

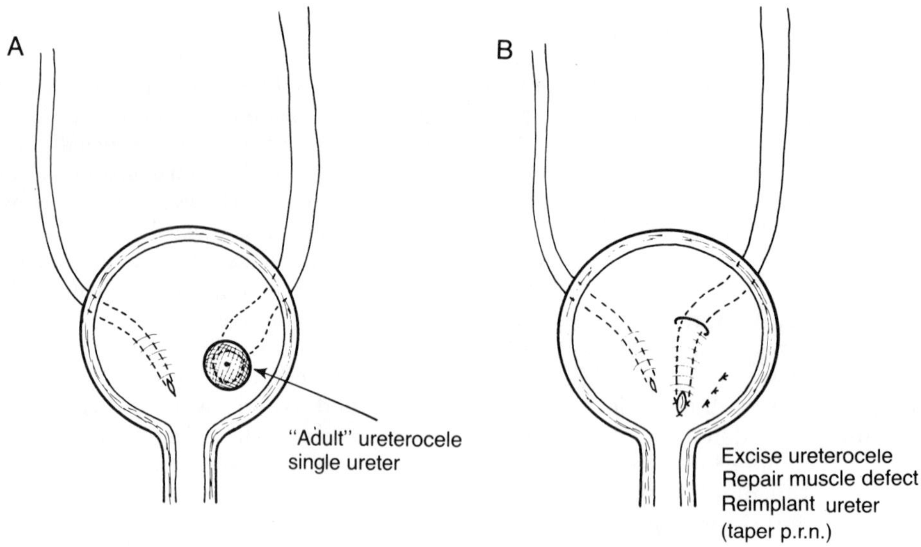

Figure 42–24. Management of a small ureterocele with a single collecting system. With a larger ureterocele and greater dilatation of the ureter, megaureter repair should be performed.

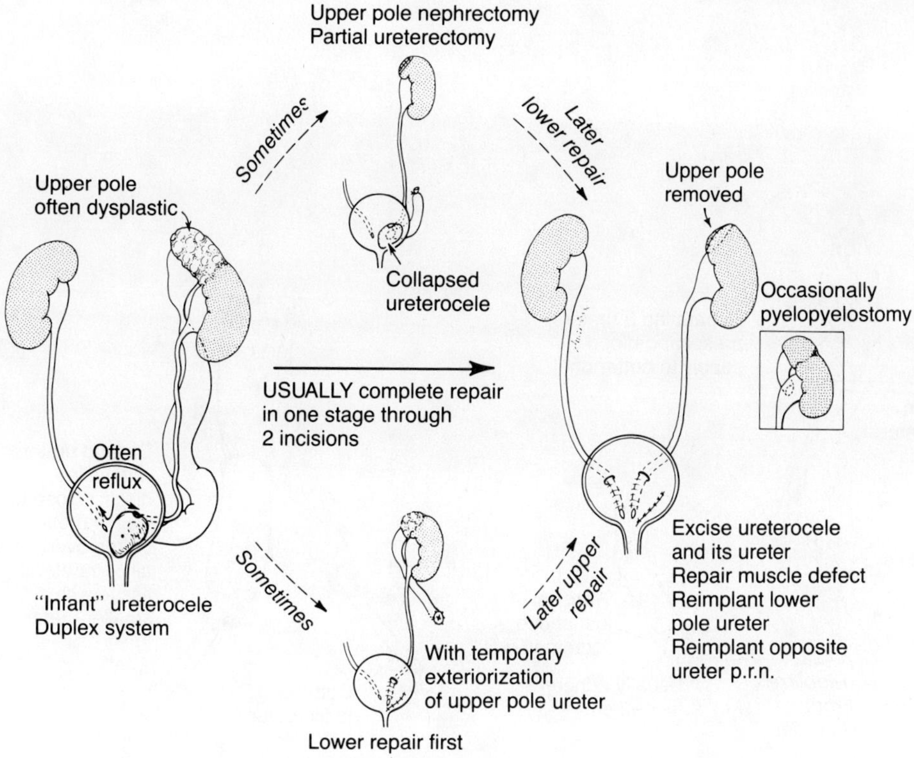

Figure 42–25. Methods of managing a patient with a duplex collecting system and ureterocele.

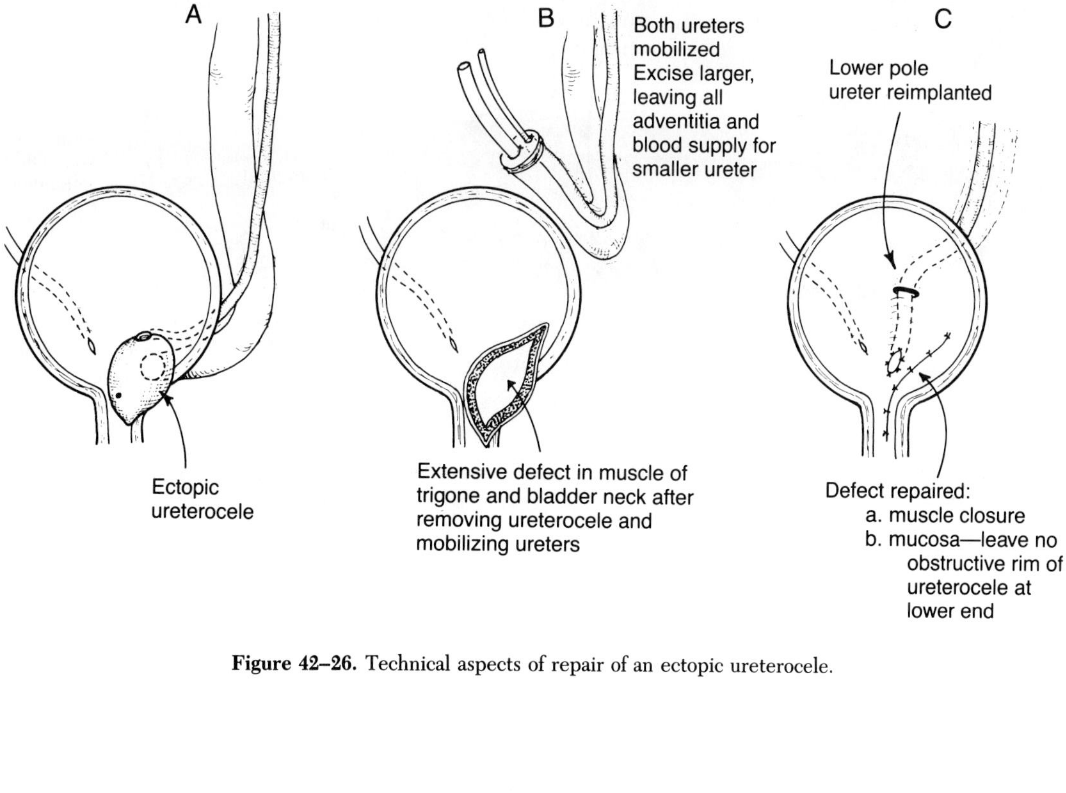

Figure 42–26. Technical aspects of repair of an ectopic ureterocele.

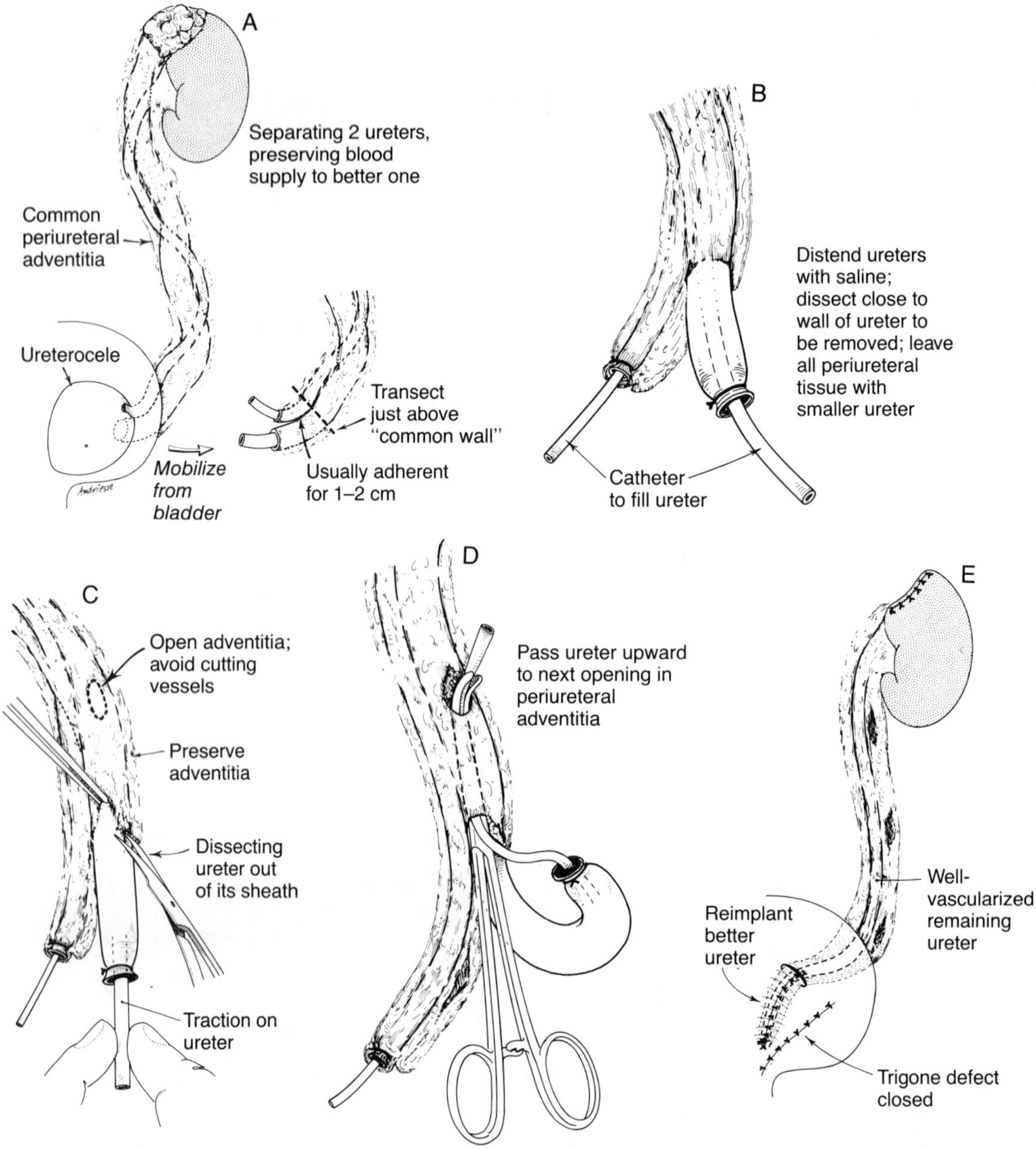

Figure 42–27. Technique for separating two ureters while preserving the blood supply of the lower pole ureter to be spared and reimplanted.

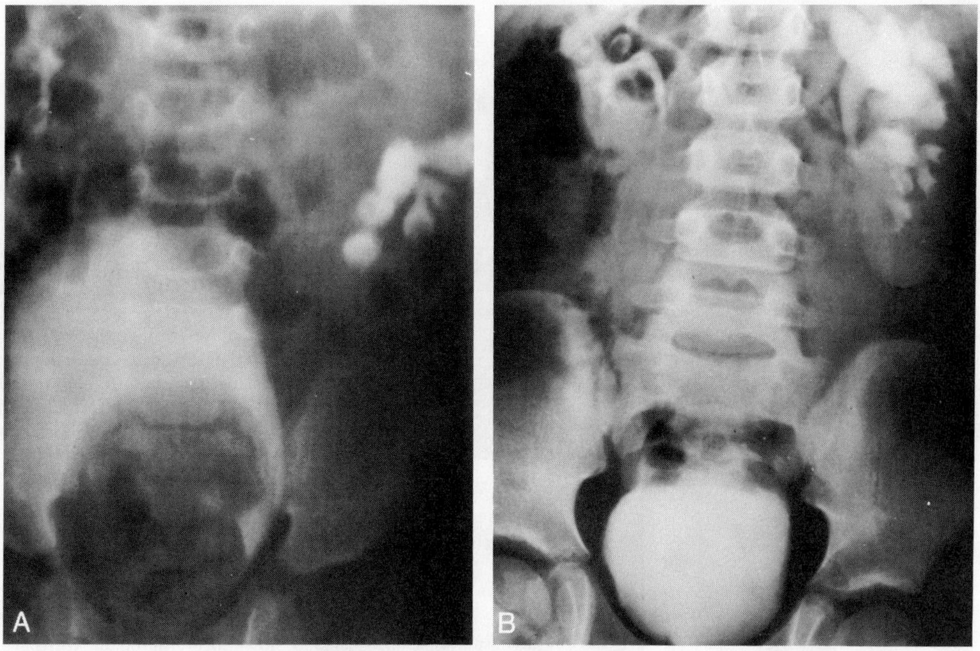

Figure 42–28. Three month old girl with a large ureterocele.

A, Preoperative IVP. Note the large ureterocele in the bladder and displacement of the lower pole of the left kidney inferiorly and laterally by a nonvisualized, hydronephrotic upper pole. Cystogram showed massive reflux to the ipsilateral lower pole. Surgery consisted of a single-stage repair, resection of the ureterocele and its megaureter, reimplantation of the ipsilateral refluxing ureter, advancement and reimplantation of the right ureter, and then exploration of the kidney. The upper pole appeared to have reasonable parenchyma, and it was anastomosed to the adjacent lower pole renal pelvis, rather than removing it.

B, IVP two years later. The patient was well at that time but subsequently began having intermittent episodes of left flank pain and urinary infection. Therefore, a left upper pole nephrectomy was performed at age 8 years. She has subsequently been well. We have seen this situation in several cases when the seemingly good upper pole was spared to avert removing parenchyma, only to have to remove it later.

infection, which can cause fibrosis of the ureteral wall. The renal parenchyma may be less well preserved in cases with reflux, compared with those with obstruction.

Megaureter can occur as an isolated problem on one side only or can be seen on both sides, especially in males with urethral valves. Furthermore, megaureter can be part of an overall uropathy, e.g., the prune belly syndrome. In such cases the kidneys can be dysplastic and the ureters very elongated and tortuous, with a very abnormal bladder. The majority of megaureter cases present in infancy and childhood, although an occasional adult will be seen who had no early symptoms and thus escaped detection during childhood.

Operative Technique

Figure 42–31 illustrates the incisions I prefer for these operations. In a primary case, or one without great tortuosity, a transverse suprapubic skin incision, as for ordinary ureteral reimplantation, will suffice to repair the lower ureters. In a secondary case, or one with great tortuosity, it is much better to use a vertical midline incision, to provide easy access not only paravesically but also up into the gutter on each side to a level above the iliac vessels.

Figure 42–32 shows the operative steps in megaureter repair. The Denis Browne universal retractor is of great help in performing these lower tract reconstructions (Fig. 42–32*A*). Four traction sutures on the edges of the cystostomy aid in the exposure. Surgical gauze is placed in the trigone and retracted upward by one hand-held retractor. An infant feeding catheter is sewn into the ureteral orifice. The orifice is circumscribed, and the ureter is mobilized intravesically for several centimeters (Fig. 42–32*B*). In some very tortuous ureters, 6 to 8 inches of ureter can be delivered through this intravesical mobilization. Some surgeons prefer to mobilize the dilated ureter extravesically. This may require considerable dissection paravesically, which can injure some of the nerve supply of

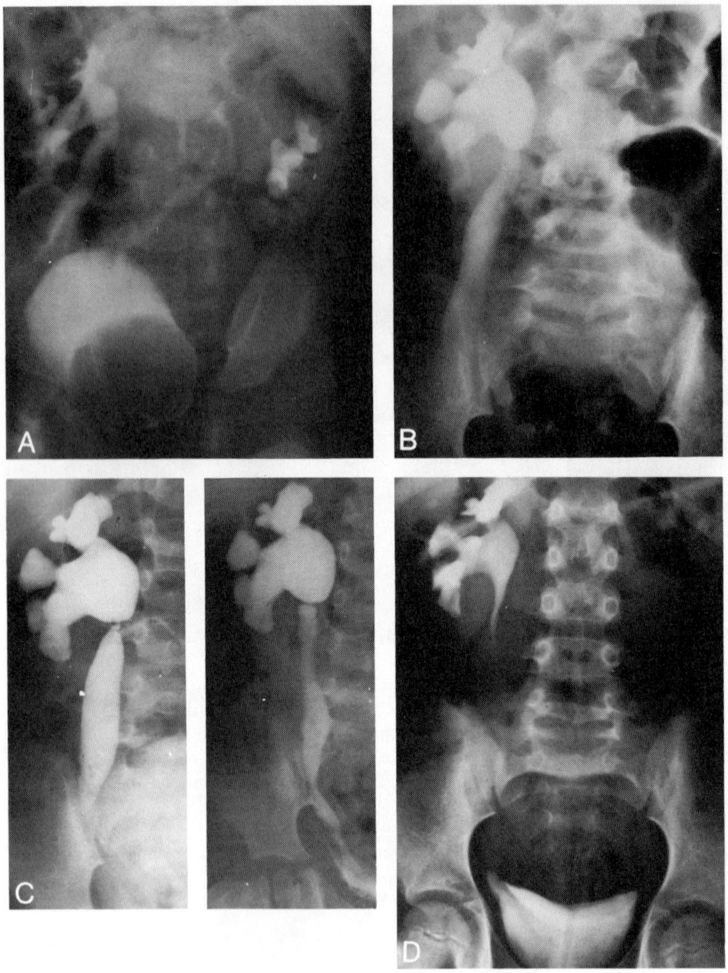

Figure 42–29. Typical "infant-type" ureterocele in a 2 month old girl.

A, IVP of a patient aged 2 months. A large ureterocele fills the bladder. It drained a hydronephrotic upper pole of the left kidney. Note downward displacement of the good lower pole of the left kidney. Unfortunately, total left nephrectomy and ureterectomy were performed, removing a good lower pole. Also, right ureteral reimplantation was done in an unsatisfactory manner, into the dome of the bladder.

B, IVP when the patient, aged 3 years, was referred for recurrent urinary infection. There was massive reflux up the right ureter, which had been improperly reimplanted. The ureter was trimmed and reimplanted.

C, Retrograde study 6 months after lower ureteral repair. Note partial functional obstruction of the ureteropelvic junction. Dismembering pyeloplasty was performed.

D, IVP when the patient was aged 7 years shows a normal ureter and no reflux. The patient is now 23 years of age and is completely well. Renal function and IVP have remained stable.

the bladder. I have seen this result in a partially denervated bladder that emptied poorly.

After the initial intravesical mobilization for as long a length as proceeds easily, the ureter is pulled out of the bladder and the dissection is carried upward outside the bladder. After the obliterated umbilical artery ligament is divided, the peritoneum can be retracted upward and medially to afford access to the extravesical ureter. In males, the vas must be seen and spared. In continuing the extravesical mobilization of the ureter (Fig. 42–32*C*), it is important to preserve its periureteral tissue, which carries a collateral blood supply and lymphatics. A skeletonized ureter may become ischemic. Obviously, some of the small blood vessels to the lower ureter must be divided, but this should be as far from the ureter as possible, so that despite considerable mobilization there is ample adventitia surrounding the ureter. Gonadal vessels can be retained with the ureter being mobilized, as will be discussed and illustrated later (see Fig. 42–41).

The degree of mobilization of the ureter will vary with its degree of tortuosity. Some megaureters are very dilated but not very tortuous. Others are moderately dilated but quite tortuous. The lower mobilization is seldom carried much higher than the external iliac vessels. If the ureter is especially tortuous, dissecting it free at that level may deliver several inches of ureter that had been coiled in the pelvis. As shown in Figure 42–32*D*, the length of ureter to be tapered does not generally need to be extensive. It usually includes that segment of ureter that will be reimplanted in the trigone, plus a few centimeters of that part of the ureter that will lie outside the bladder. If a tortuous lower ureter is being straightened out, particularly important is its blood supply, which runs longitudinally along its medial aspect, close to its attachment with the peritoneum, which can

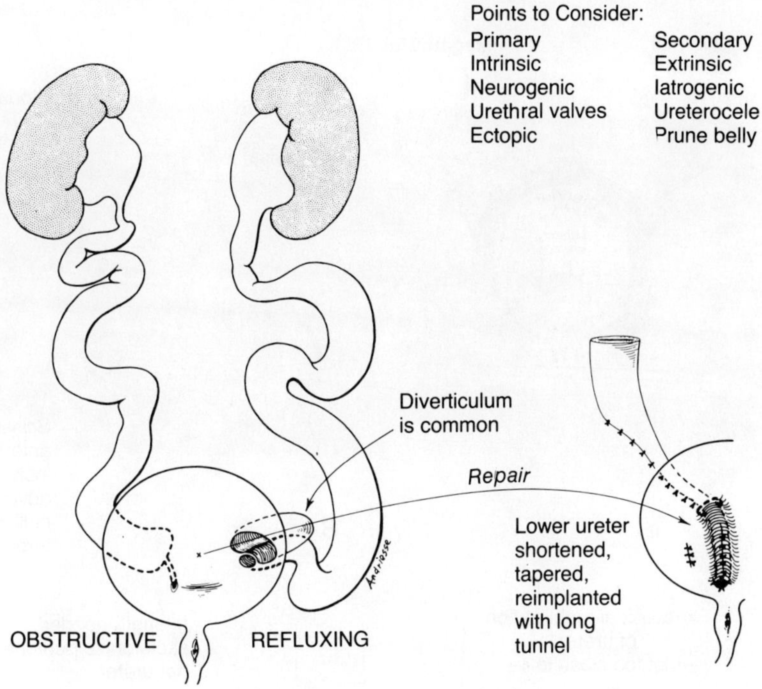

Figure 42–30. The two most common types of megaureter and some of the causes of megaureter.

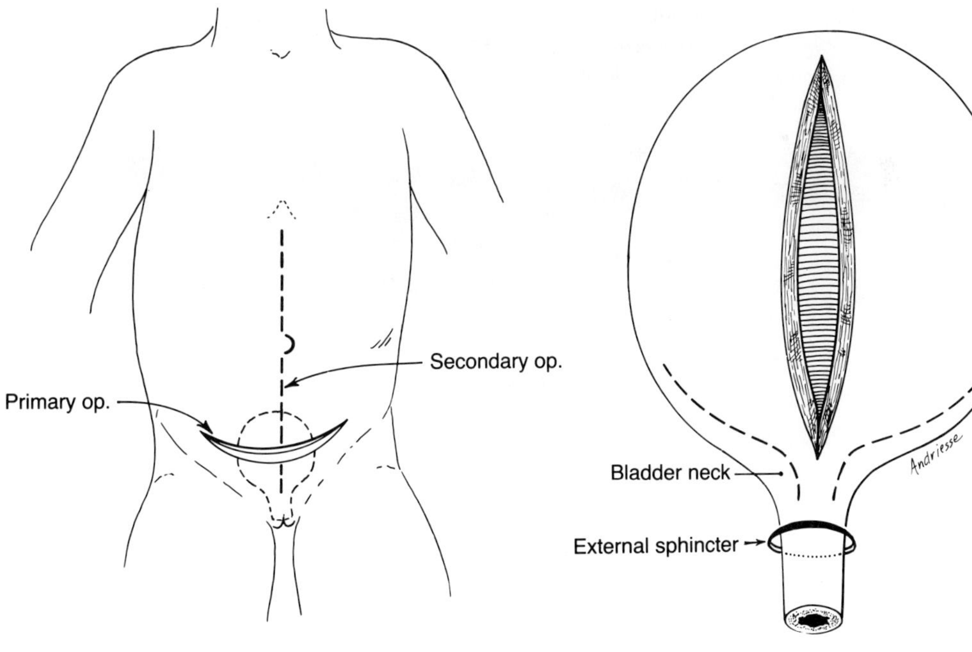

Figure 42–31. Operative exposure for megaureter surgery.

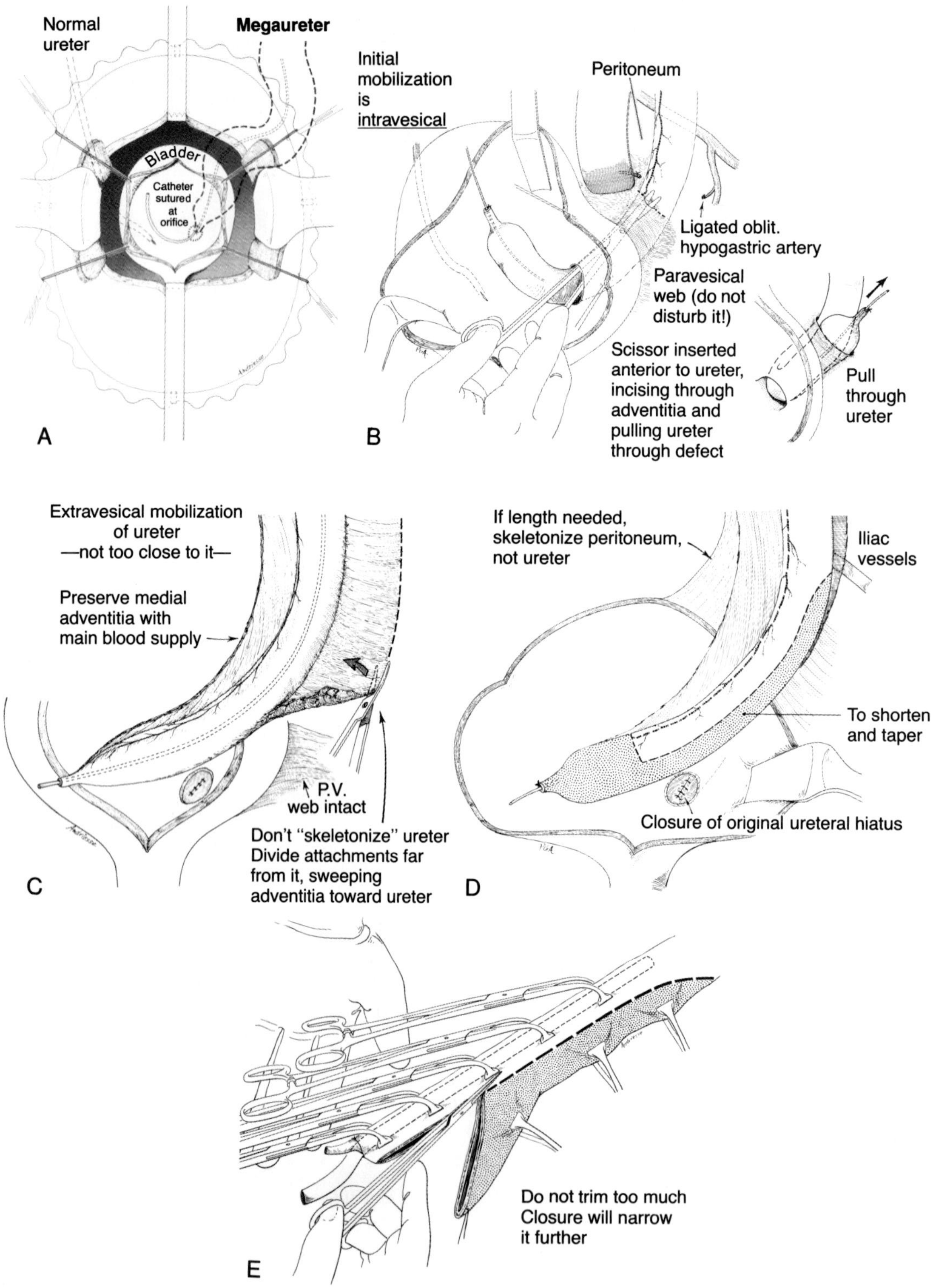

Figure 42–32. Technique for repair of lower ureter. See text.

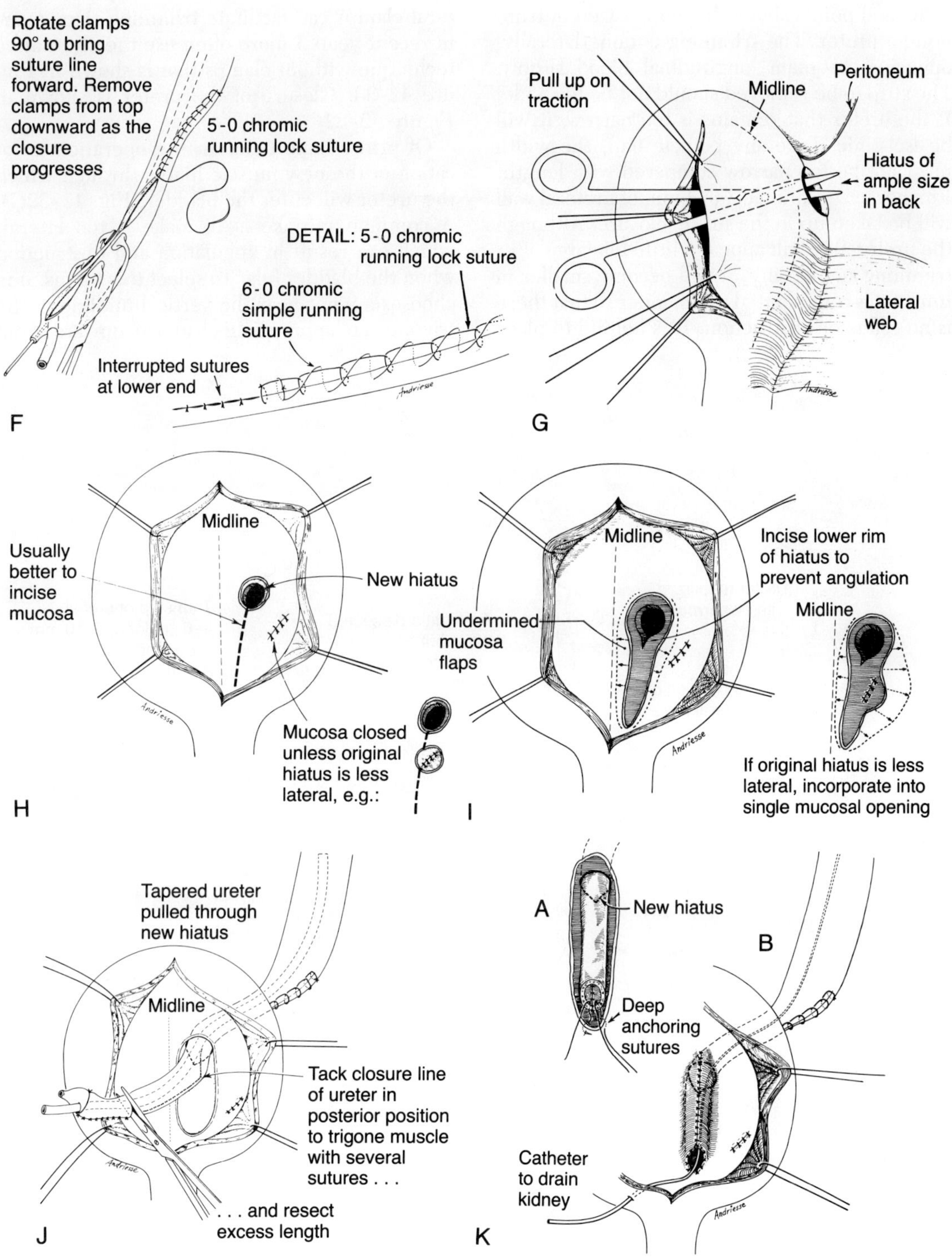

Figure 42–32. *Continued*

restrict straightening of the ureter. The peritoneum can be dissected away from the ureter without injuring the ureter or its adventitia.

Several points should be emphasized in trimming a ureter. The trimming is done laterally, opposite the main longitudinal blood supply. The strip to be removed should not be too wide. If the ureter that remains is too narrow, it will be ischemic. Like any pedicle flap, the width must not be too narrow compared with length. Further, an additional 3 to 4 mm of ureteral wall will be taken up in the suture closure. Although the ureter may still appear a little too large after trimming and closure, it will become smaller in time if it is reimplanted in a manner so that there is no reflux or obstruction. It is helpful to place a catheter in the lumen of the ureter during its trimming; the size will depend on the size of the patient. As shown in Figure 42–32*E*, special ureteral clamps can facilitate trimming. However, in recent years I more often use the alternative technique without clamps that is shown in Figure 42–33. Closure of the ureter is shown in Figure 42–32*F*.

Of prime importance in the operation is location of the new muscle hiatus through which the ureter will enter the bladder (Fig. 42–32*G*). A common mistake is to make it too lateral, which can result in angulation and obstruction when the bladder fills. To select this hiatus, one chooses a point near the vertical midline of the trigone, an appropriate distance upward from

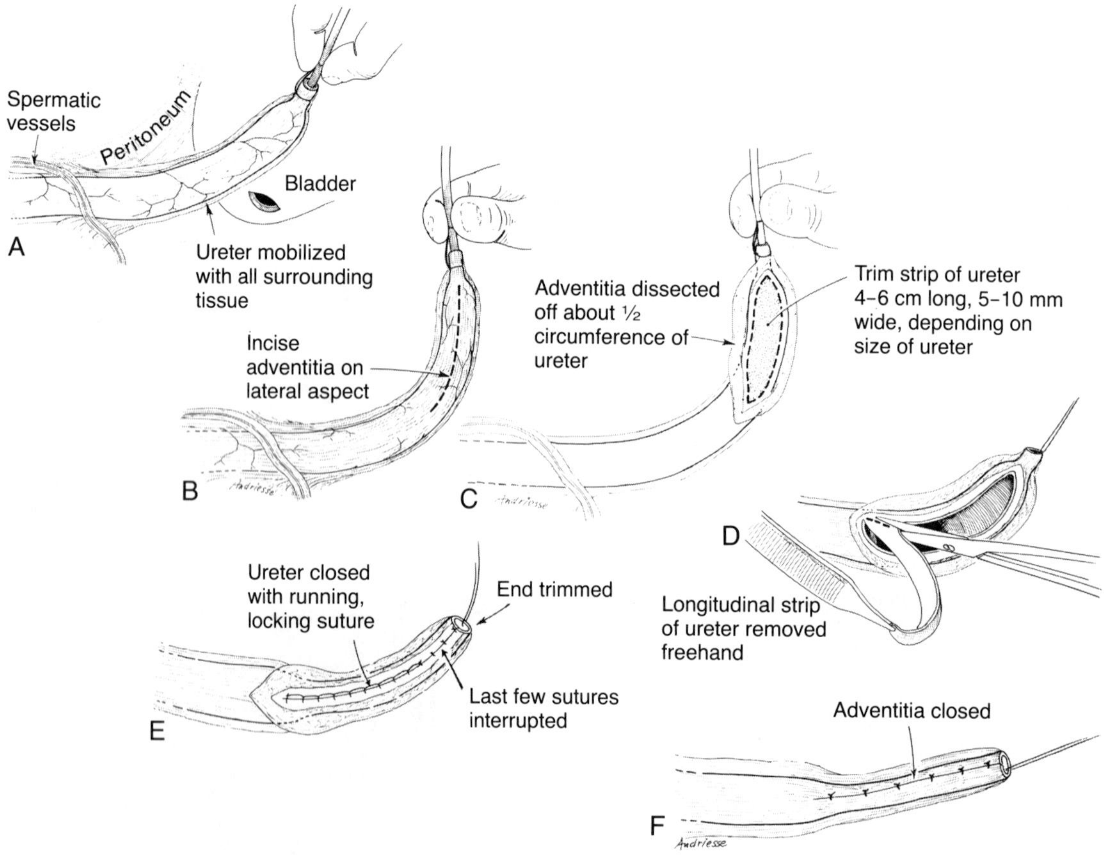

Figure 42–33. Alternative means for tapering a ureter without clamps and preserving all the periureteral tissue for collateral blood supply.

A, Ureter is mobilized with all its periureteral adventitia.

B, While the ureter is distended with saline, the adventitia is mobilized on its lateral aspect. This is done by undermining it with scissors from the distal end of the ureter and then opening it.

C, After laying back the adventitia, the lateral strip to be removed is marked with a skin-marking pencil or brilliant green dye on a toothpick.

D, The strip to be removed is excised using scissors with straight blades. It is important to avoid trimming too much, because closure will use up 3 to 4 more millimeters of ureteral wall.

E, The ureter is closed.

F, The periureteral adventitia, which was saved, is closed as a second layer.

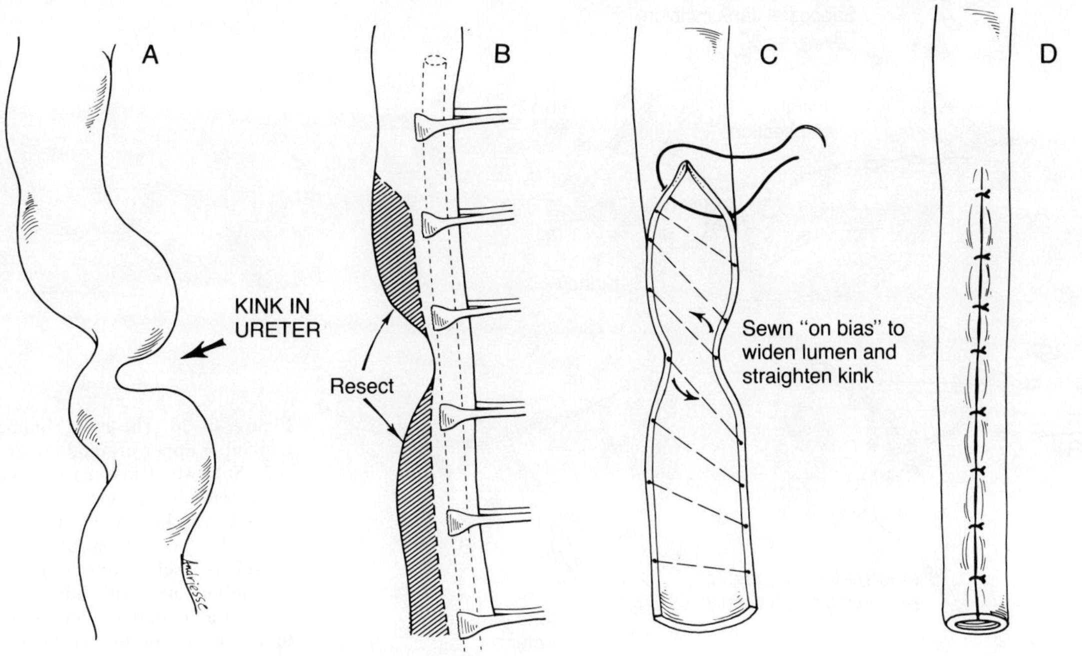

Figure 42–34. Management of kinked ureter.

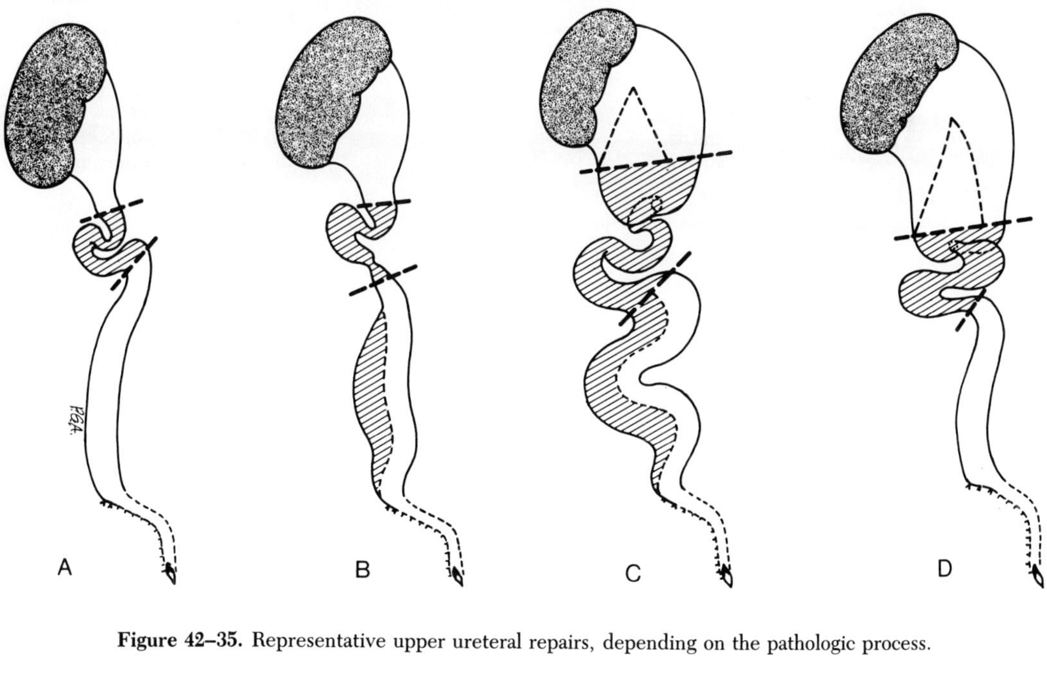

Figure 42–35. Representative upper ureteral repairs, depending on the pathologic process.

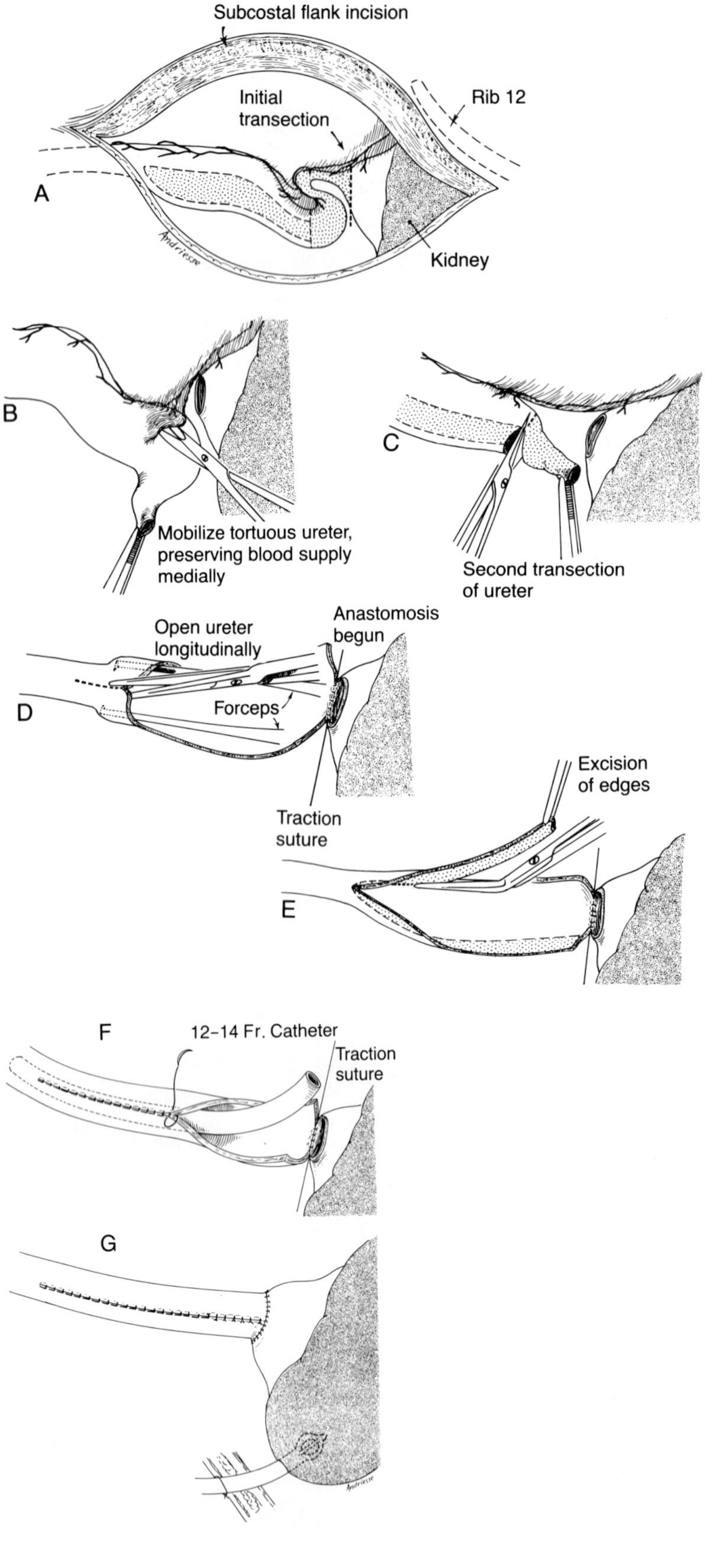

Figure 42–36. The most common method of upper ureteral repair.

A, Subcostal flank incision, with posterolateral exposure of the ureter and lower kidney. The kidney is not mobilized further, nor is the ureter dissected unnecessarily. Peripelvic ureteral adventitia, which is an important blood supply to the upper ureter, is reflected medially. The lower renal pelvis is transected above the tortuous ureteropelvic junction.

B, The ureter is mobilized, reflecting its blood supply medially.

C, The ureter is transected, saving the blood supply.

D, Anastomosis is begun before trimming the ureter.

E, Edges are trimmed with straight-edged, angled scissors. The blood supply is preserved.

F, Running locking closure, over a loose-fitting catheter, which is removed before completing the anastomosis.

G, Completed closure, using interrupted sutures near the T-shaped junction. Nephrostomy drainage of the kidney is used for 10–12 days postoperatively when the kidney is hydronephrotic.

the bladder neck. A hole is made through the mucosa, through the back wall of the bladder, and to the cul de sac peritoneum but not through it. Pulling upward on the traction sutures in the bladder wall, the operator can see the scissors points emerging through the back wall of the bladder, between it and the cul de sac peritoneum. In the male, this is near the vas deferens, which should be spared. In the female, this is just anterior to the upper vagina. This opening should be large enough to avoid constricting the ureter.

Incising the inferior rim will prevent angulation of the ureter where it enters the bladder. This is especially true in hypertrophied bladders, such as in boys with urethral valves in which heavy strands of muscle crossing the ureter can obstruct it. As shown in Figure 42–32*H* and 42–32*I*, we generally incise the mucosa downward, laying back mucosal flaps, to prepare a bed for the ureter. The original hiatus is closed. If a diverticulum is present, the original muscle hiatus must be closed with great care to correct the diverticulum. The trimmed ureter is then brought through the new hiatus in the back wall of the bladder (Fig. 42–32*J*), placed in its bed, and adjusted to lie without tension. Retractors in the bladder and on the peritoneum should be released temporarily to make certain that there is no tension between the bladder in its collapsed state and the ureter as it is to be implanted. The suture line closure of the ureters should be in back next to the bladder muscle, so that a fistula will not occur between it and the bladder.

The ureter is tacked with fine chromic sutures to its bed in the trigone. Excess length is then resected. In anchoring the ureter at its new hiatus (Fig. 42–32*K*), we place the most distal sutures deep in the trigone, taking both mucosa and muscle to anchor the tip of the ureter. The remaining sutures around the circumference of the orifice fasten the bladder mucosa to the full thickness edge of ureter. If the diameter of the orifice is still too large it can be narrowed deliberately a little during closure. The mucosa flaps of trigone are then closed over the ureter. A reimplanted megaureter usually has a tunnel 3 to 4 cm long. The kidney is drained for 10 to 12 days via a plastic catheter brought through the opposite side of the bladder wall and the abdominal wall. Rarely has nephrostomy been necessary.

Figure 42–33 shows an alternative method we have used for the past decade or more in trimming the caliber of the dilated lower ureter by freehand technique instead of using special clamps. This has the advantage of not clamping the lower ureter at all, which is possibly better than applying even a relatively gentle clamp. Also, it preserves all the periureteral tissue, which is so important for its blood supply. In patients with bilateral megaureters, we routinely repair both lower ureters at once. This is a long, tedious procedure. The drainage catheters are removed 10 to 12 days later, always one side at a time, and usually after examination by injecting contrast medium to be certain there is no suture line leak.

A troublesome "kink" in a ureter can be managed as shown in Figure 42–34. This type of plastic closure can widen the lumen at the site of the kink.

Early in our experience with megaureters 3 decades ago, we frequently did a similar procedure at the upper ureter several weeks or months after lower ureter surgery. Greater experience, however, showed that many wide and tortuous ureters will normalize in time after satisfactory repair of the lower ureter. However, some upper ureters remain tortuous, and in some this tortuosity produces partial obstruction. In others, the upper ureter remains dilated. A dilated ureter whose walls cannot produce effective peristaltic waves will not empty properly. If on long-term follow-up the upper ureter remains dilated and tortuous and shows inadequate peristalsis and delayed emptying, upper ureter repair should be performed. Variations of the upper repair are shown in Figure 42–35. Details of this are shown in Figure 42–36. If only a tortuous ureteropelvic junction is to be resected, just the segment to be resected is mobilized; then an oblique anastomosis is performed between the upper ureter and the lower renal pelvis. If it is too large, a dilated renal pelvis may be partially resected, just as in any pyeloplasty. If the upper ureter needs to be trimmed, it is incised longitudinally in situ and an appropriate width of its edge trimmed with straight-blade scissors. A Malecot catheter is placed temporarily in the lower pole of the kidney to drain it after these upper repairs.

Complications

Megaureter repair for an isolated anomaly in a patient with a normal bladder should have a very low complication rate, probably no greater than 2 to 3 percent. However, with abnormal bladders, seen in boys with urethral valves in

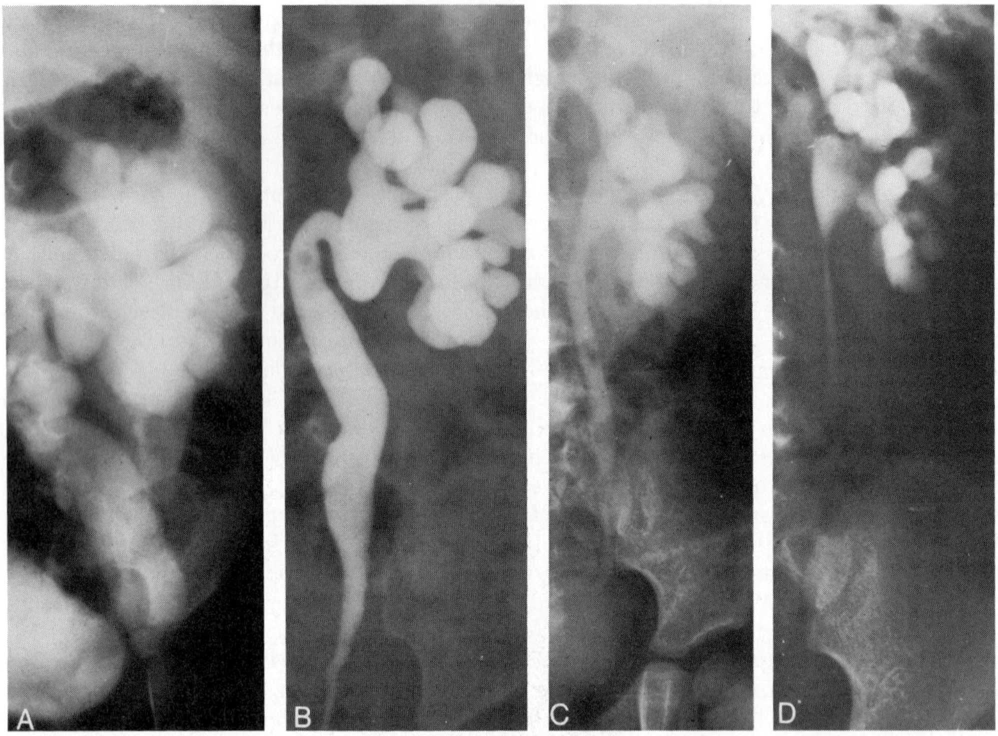

Figure 42–37. (**Case 1**) An infant was referred at 4 months of age with a left flank mass, thought to be a tumor. It proved to be a solitary left kidney with an obstructive megaureter and hydronephrosis.

A, Preoperative IVP. Lower megaureter repair was performed.

B, Retrograde pyelogram 6 months after the lower ureteral repair. An upper repair was deferred to see whether the tortuosity would recede, which it did not. Therefore, the upper ureter was shortened and tapered.

C, IVP 1 year later.

D, IVP when the patient was 4 years of age. It is interesting that preoperatively the blood urea nitrogen (BUN) level was only 16 mg/dl, deceptively normal, and the serum creatinine was 0.6 mg/dl. However, preoperative creatinine clearance was only 15 liters/m^2 of body surface area. It increased to normal levels postoperatively. The patient's original admission weight was in the 3rd percentile. At age 6 years, it was at the 70th percentile. Cinefluorography of the upper ureter showed ineffective peristalsis and poor emptying of the dilated, tortuous upper ureter before its repair. Later, after the upper ureter was shortened and tapered, there were excellent peristaltic waves with normal ureteral emptying. The patient, now age 24 years, is entirely well. She has never had urinary problems. Renal function and IVP have remained stable.

which endoscopic resection alone does not suffice, even meticulous megaureter repair technique will have some failures, in the range of about 5 percent. This is acceptable, however, when compared with the alternative of urinary diversion. Most failures can be repaired by reoperation.[38]

Kalicinski and associates have described a ureteral plication technique[39] to avoid the possible complication of devascularizing the ureter, and others have reported a favorable experience with plicating the ureter instead of trimming it.[40] I believe, however, that devascularization can be avoided in most megaureter repairs if the principles outlined earlier are followed. Selected cases of megaureter repair, with and without complications, are shown in Figures 42–37 through 42–40.

Case 1 (Fig. 42–37). This patient was referred at age 4 months with a flank mass that proved to be a solitary left kidney with obstructive megaureter. The lower ureter was tapered, shortened, and reimplanted. The upper ureter remained tortuous and drained poorly. One year later it was repaired by shortening and tapering it. Creatinine clearance was originally only 15 L/m^2 of body area. It later rose to 104 L, which is normal.

Comment. This case shows the remarkable capacity of a hydronephrotic kidney to improve in childhood, particularly if repair is done early. Although the patient was only 4 months of age,

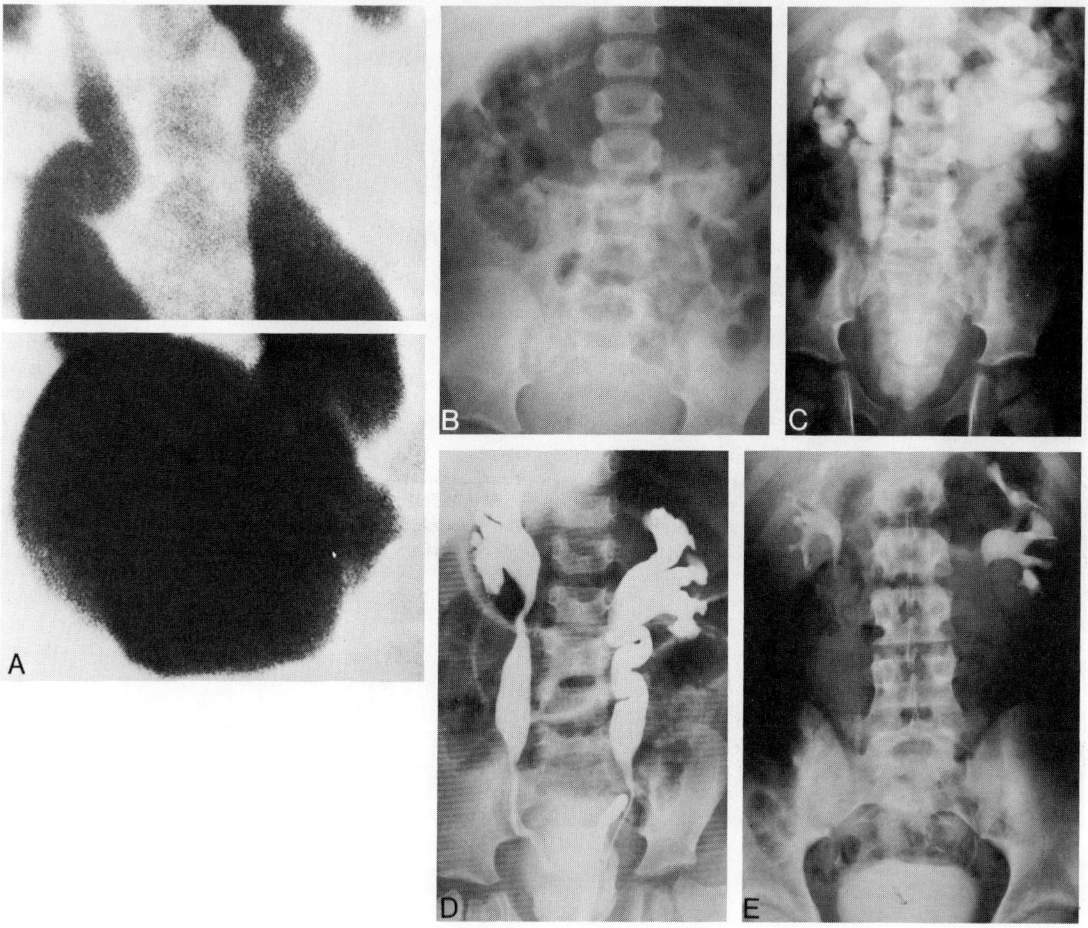

Figure 43–38. **(Case 2)** A 2½ year old boy with massive vesicoureteral reflux causing infection.

A, Frames from a preoperative cystogram, showing massive reflux and dilatation.

B, Preoperative IVP, demonstrating severe hydronephrosis and poor visualization.

C, IVP 2 weeks after lower megaureter repair. Severe hydronephrosis is still evident, as expected.

D, Retrograde study 2 months after lower repair. Note that the right ureter is straight; it emptied well despite dilatation of the upper ureteral segment. The left upper ureter was still tortuous; it emptied poorly. Therefore, left upper ureter repair was performed.

E, IVP 13 years later. The patient, now age 27 years and 25 years postoperative, has had no further urologic difficulties.

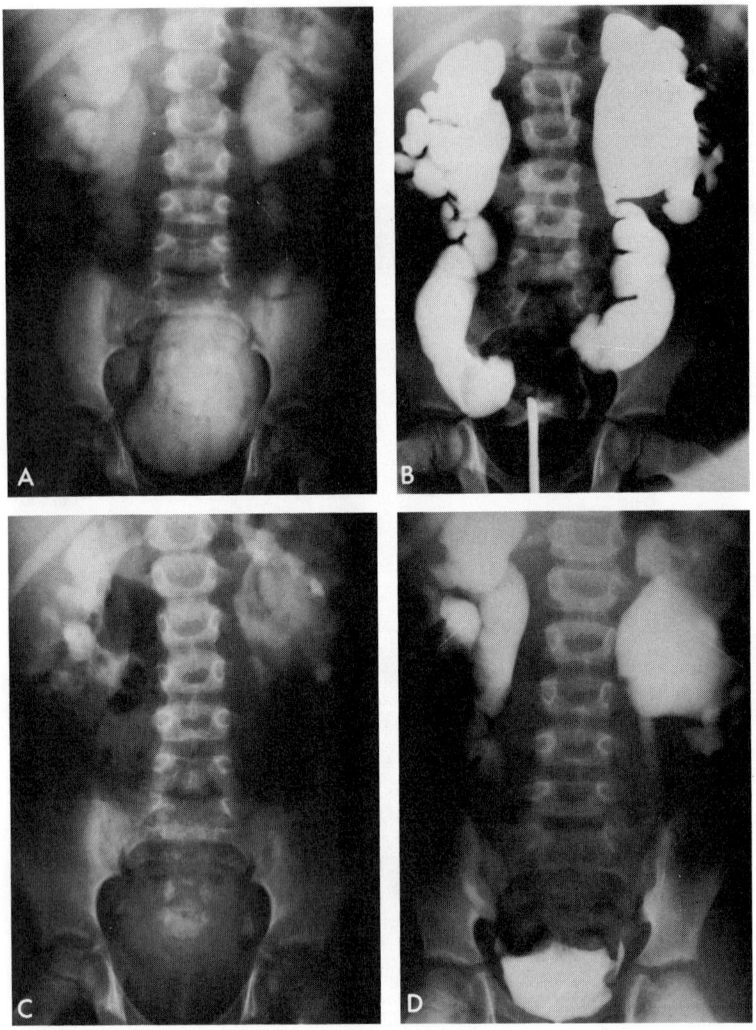

Figure 42–39. **(Case 3)** A 5 year old boy referred after bilateral megaureter repair with complications.

A, IVP showing bilateral hydronephrosis. There was a nephrostomy tube in the left kidney.

B, Preoperative retrograde examination. Both ureters were obstructed at the ureterovesical junction, which had been placed too far laterally, angulating the ureters.

C, IVP 9 months postoperatively.

D, Antegrade percutaneous pyelogram study 9 months after repeat operation on both lower ureters. They drained well, at normal pressures. There was no reflux. Note the spontaneous straightening of the upper ureters, which has continued. Now 15 years later, the patient is well.

direct repair was undertaken without need for ureterostomy, nephrostomy, or other type of preliminary diversion.[41–45] Now age 24 years, the patient has been completely well, with stable creatinine clearance and normal IVP during long-term follow-up.

Case 2 (Fig. 42–38).This patient was referred at age 2½ years, after urinary tract infection prompted urinary tract screening. There was a history of recurring high fevers of unknown etiology with multiple febrile convulsions. A cystogram showed massive reflux and very dilated tortuous ureters (Fig. 42–38*A*). An IVP showed bilateral severe hydronephrosis, megaureters, and a large bladder that emptied poorly (Fig. 42–38*B*). Bilateral lower ureteral tapering and reimplantation were performed. An IVP taken immediately postoperatively showed still severe dilatation of both upper tracts, especially the left side, but the patient was clinically well (Fig. 48–38*C*). A retrograde pyelogram 2 months later (Fig. 48–38*D*) showed satisfactory lower ureters, continued dilatation of the upper tracts, and persisting tortuosity of the left upper ureter, which emptied poorly on radiographic evaluation. Nothing further was done on the right side. The left upper ureter required resection for tortuosity, with tapering of the mid-ureter. A subsequent IVP (Fig. 42–38*E*) showed greatly improved upper tracts and normal ureters. The IVP has remained completely stable during a 25-year follow-up on this patient, who is now age 27 years.

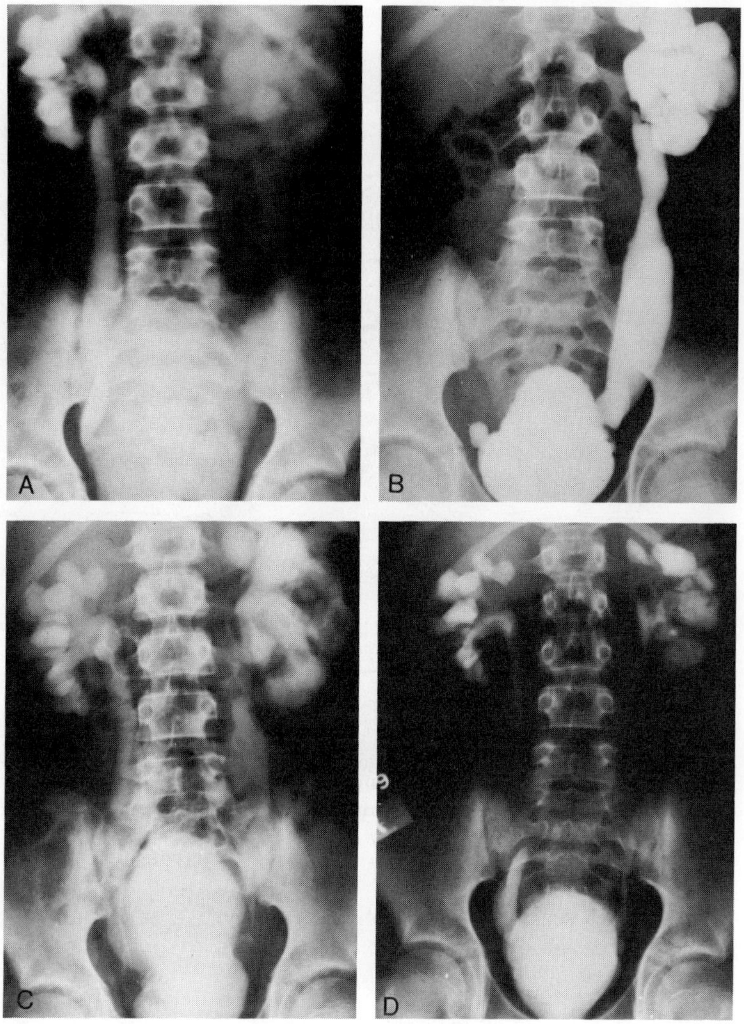

Figure 42–40. **(Case 4)** A 12 year old boy referred for diminishing renal function after unsuccessful bilateral megaureter repair.

A, IVP at age 12 years. Poor function on the left (massive reflux) and partial ureteral obstruction on the right from angulation are seen.

B, Cystogram showing massive left reflux.

C, IVP 2 weeks after bilateral repeat megaureter repair. Note the tapered lower ureters, which are no longer angulated. Hydronephrosis is temporarily greater from postoperative edema around the lower ureters.

D, IVP 4 months later. There is considerable improvement compared with the preoperative state. The cystogram showed no reflux. When last seen at age 21 years, the patient was well.

Comment. Physically this patient has matured and grown in normal fashion and has never had further urinary infection. His parents are convinced, however, that he sustained brain damage from his multiple febrile convulsions resulting from failure to diagnose his severe uropathy before age 2½ years. Before those episodes he had been a bright, alert baby. They think this changed. Although physically well, he did much less well in school than two siblings who are college graduates. It is known that febrile convulsions can cause cortical scarring and alter cognitive ability. Thus, unrecognized and untreated reflux in early infancy may well have profoundly damaged his central nervous system by causing repeated high fevers with convulsions.

Case 3 (Fig. 42–39). A 5 year old boy was referred for secondary megaureter surgery. Fevers of unknown cause dated back to age 9 months. One year previously, hydronephrosis had been discovered. After bilateral nephrostomy, lower megaureter repair had been performed. Neither side drained well. He was referred for reoperation.

Reoperation was performed through a vertical midline incision to gain extensive transabdominal exposure of both ureters. Each had been implanted too laterally, causing obstruction. They were extensively mobilized, preserving their blood supply, shortened, tapered, and reimplanted through a new hiatus medially and closer to the center of the trigone. Now age 21

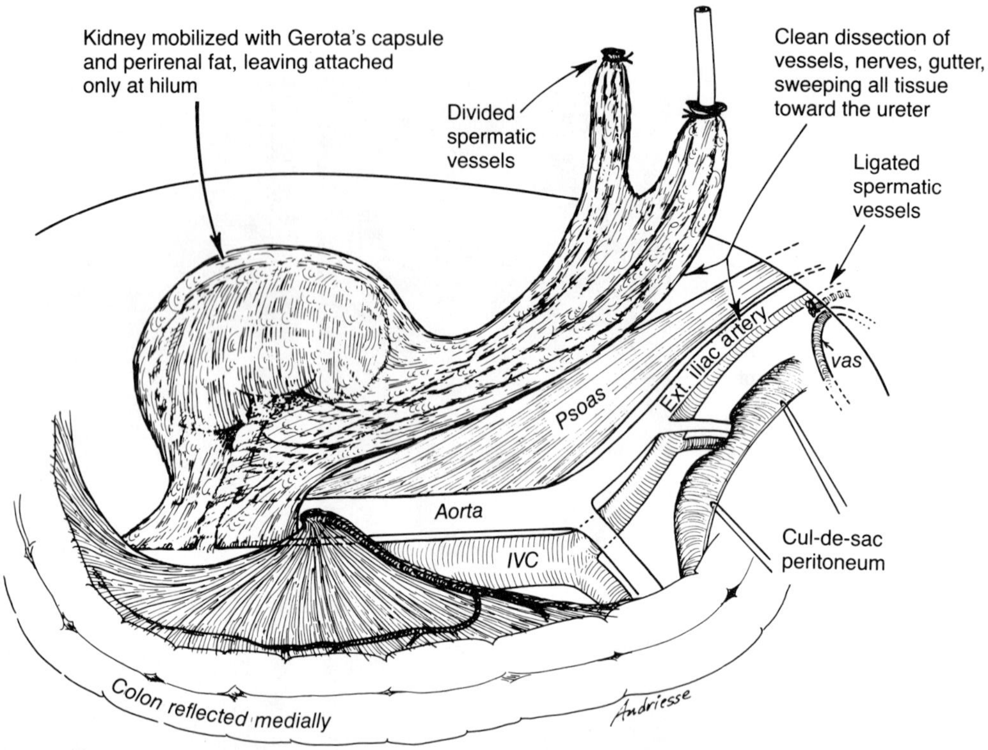

Figure 42–41. Technique for mobilizing the kidney and the ureter to gain additional length. The ureter is mobilized with all its periureteral tissue, including the gonadal vessels, for collateral blood supply. There has been no instance of injury to an ovary or testis from the maneuver. With this meticulous preservation of all periureteral tissue and blood supply, we often have simultaneously tapered and reimplanted the lower ureter, anastomosed a contralateral ureter to its mid-section as a transureteroureterostomy, and resected a tortuous, functionally obstructed ureteropelvic junction. Operating on more than one level of the ureter in an operation requires very careful preservation of its blood supply.

years, and 15 years postoperatively, the patient is well. Creatinine clearance at age 16 years, when he was more than 6 ft tall, measured 86 L/m^2 of body surface area.

Comment. The difficulty of a secondary operation of this sort should not be underestimated. The procedure lasted 8 hours. This case illustrates two important complications: (1) the ureters were obstructed by bringing them to the bladder wall at a point too lateral, and (2) excessive tapering led to ischemic fibrosis of each lower ureter. Permanent urinary diversion had been considered for this boy at one time. Permanent urinary diversion in this type of case has its advocates,[27] but we strongly disagree with that concept.[46] Urinary diversion, particularly with an ileal loop that will have reflux, is often associated with deteriorating renal function.[47–50] Furthermore, there is no question that the quality of life with a bag does not measure up to life without a bag.

Case 4 (Fig. 42–40). This patient was referred at age 12 years for reoperation. At age 3 years, an endoscopic procedure for urethral valves had been done. At age 5 years, both ureters were reimplanted for reflux, together with tapering of the left side. Suprapubic tube drainage had been maintained for 6 months. The patient was referred with deteriorating renal function. An IVP (Fig. 42–40*A*) showed partial obstruction on the right and poor visualization on the left. A cystogram (Fig. 42–40*B*) showed massive left reflux. Cystoscopy revealed that typical type I urethral valves remained, but the top of the verumontanum was missing, evidently resected several years previously. The right ureteral orifice was located high and lateral on the bladder wall, with angulation. The left orifice was also laterally located but had no tunnel. Angulation of the right side was corrected by a combined reimplantation. The left side was treated similarly, but also tapered. An IVP 2 weeks postoperatively (Fig. 42–40*C*) showed edema surrounding both recently reimplanted ureters, but satisfactory upper tract drainage. An IVP 4 months later (Fig. 42–40*D*) showed great improvement. A cystogram showed no reflux. When last seen in 1983, at age 21 years, the

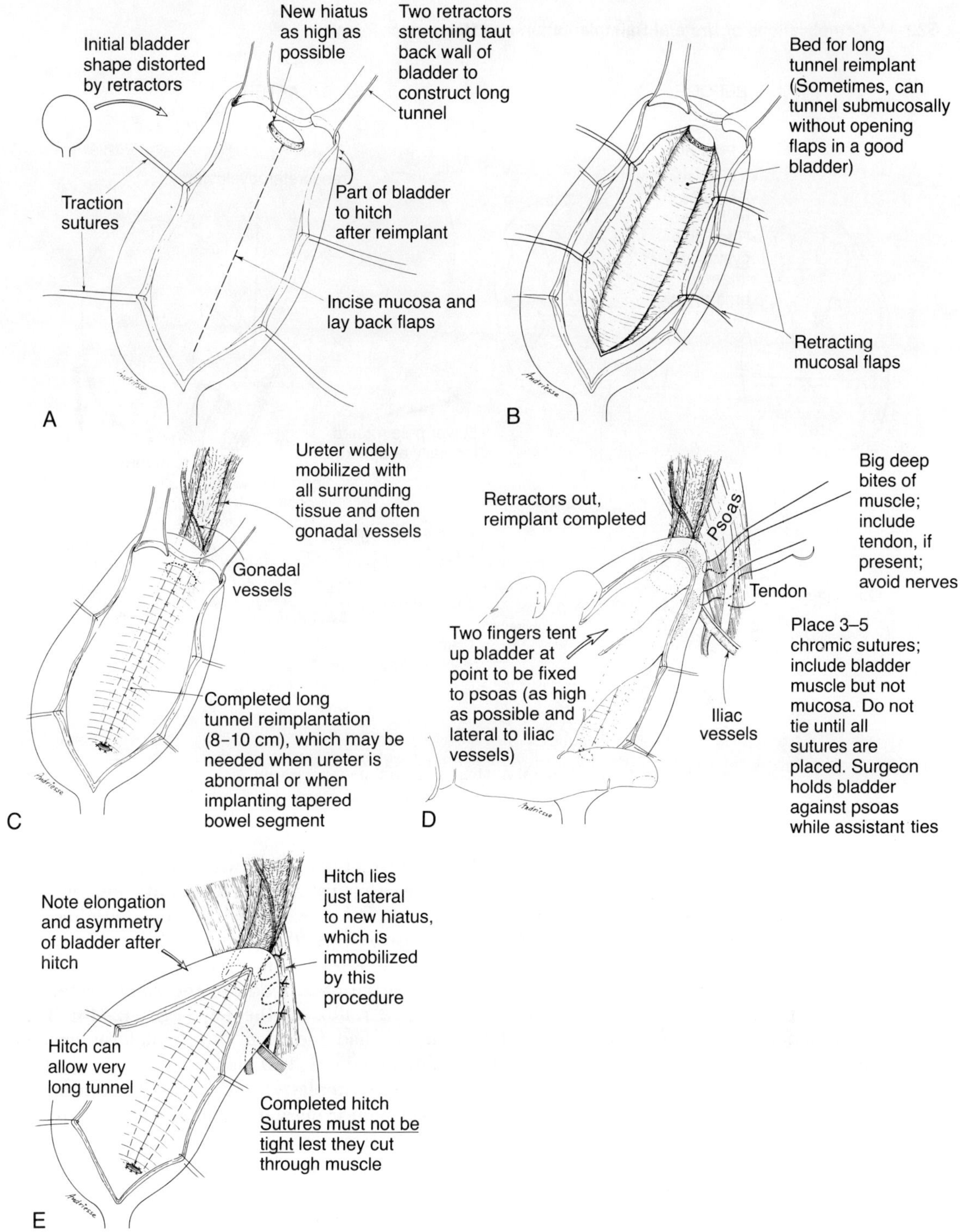

Figure 42–42. Technique for psoas hitch fixation of the bladder. This allows creating a superlong ureteral reimplantation tunnel. It also fixes the point of entry of the ureter into the bladder so that it does not become angulated when the bladder fills.

A, The bladder is stretched upward using two retractors, selecting a point for the new ureteral hiatus as high as possible on the back wall.

B, Dissecting back flaps to expose the bed in which the ureter will be placed. This technique is necessary in most bladders that are scarred and pockmarked with cellules.

C, Placement of the ureter in a tunnel.

D, Placement of fixation sutures. This can be done with chromic catgut; however, monofilament nonabsorbable sutures may be more effective in holding the bladder in position. If nonabsorbable suture material is used, it must not enter the bladder lumen, lest it cause stone formation.

E, Completed hitch. Note that reimplant is done before the hitch is performed.

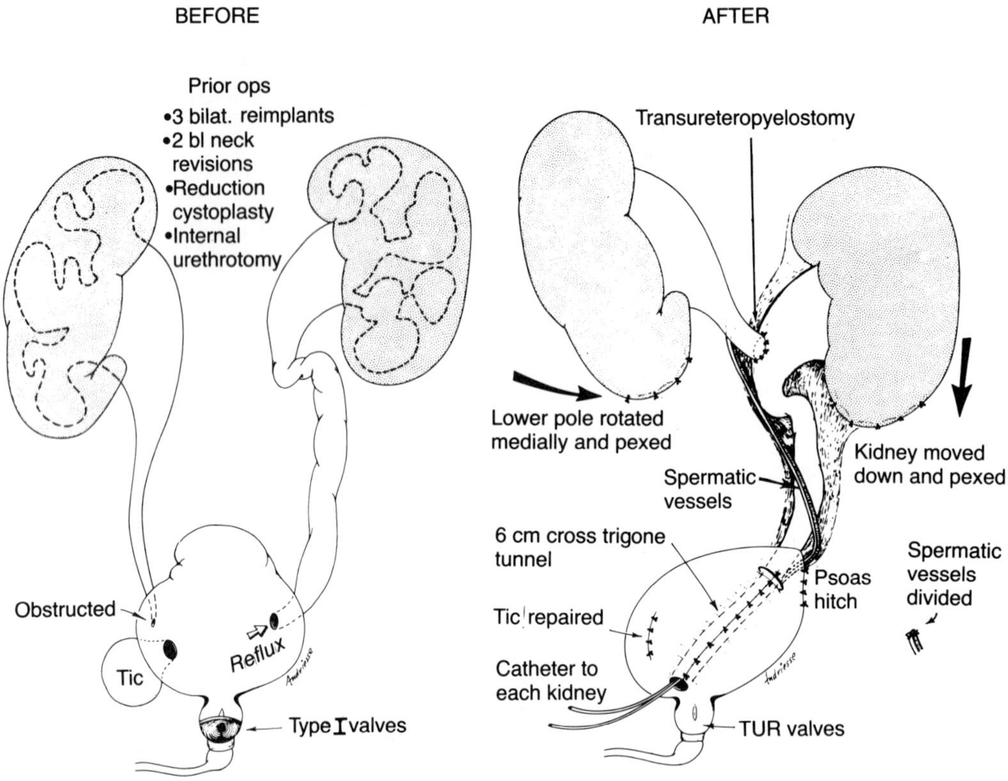

Figure 42–43. (**Case 5**) Anatomy pre- and postoperatively.

patient was asymptomatic and in law school. His blood chemical values included a BUN level of 13 and a creatinine level of 1.4 mg percent.

Comment. This case underscores the following important complications:

(1) Typical urethral valves had been overlooked despite multiple previous endoscopic procedures. Undoubtedly, persisting valves contributed to the problem of reflux.

(2) Both ureters had been improperly located on the side wall of the bladder, creating obstruction on the right and allowing persistent reflux on the left.

Special Cases

Some patients cannot be treated by straightforward repeat ureteral reimplantation. In some, the ureter is deficient; in others, the bladder is thick-walled, scarred, and noncompliant. We have seen many such patients who were treated by urinary diversion and then later referred for undiversion.[51,52] Wide mobilization of the ureter, as shown in Figure 42–41, together with psoas hitch, as shown in Figure 42–42, can make reconstructing such patients possible. The cases to follow will illustrate those methods.

Case 5 (Figs. 42–43 and 42–44). A 15 year old boy was referred in 1977 for reoperation. He had partial obstruction of the right ureter and massive reflux on the left (Fig. 42–43). Prior surgery had included three bilateral ureteral reimplantations, two bladder neck revisions, reduction cystoplasty, and internal urethrotomy. Permanent urinary diversion had been advised. At cystoscopy, previously overlooked type I urethral valves were resected. Both ureters were mobilized widely with all surrounding tissue. The right ureter was unsuited for reimplantation. By sliding down the left kidney and performing a psoas hitch, a satisfactory left ureteral reimplantation was possible. The right kidney was mobilized and fixed medially, and a right-to-left transureteropyelostomy was performed. The procedure lasted 12 hours. Follow-up roentgenogram showed no reflux and less hydronephrosis. Now at age 27 years, 12 years later, the patient has had no further urinary infection. His serum creatinine is 0.8 mg percent. Renal func-

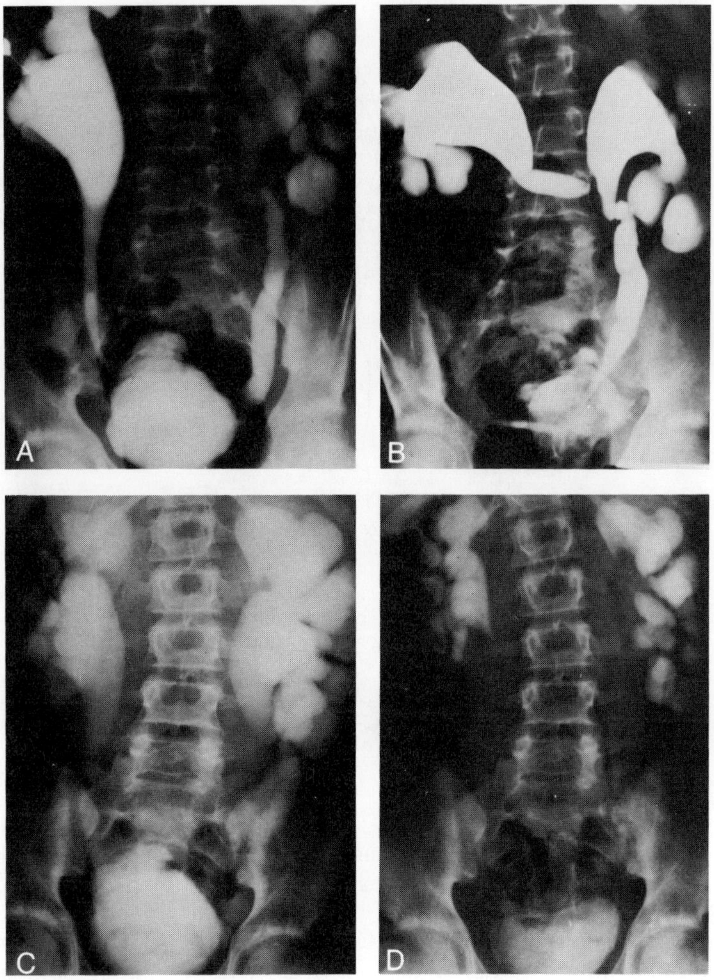

Figure 42–44. Roentgenograms from Case 5.

A, Preoperative antegrade study, right side. Note the narrow right lower ureter and reflux up the left side.

B, Right antegrade study 2 weeks postoperatively. There is edema at the transureteral pyelostomy.

C, IVP 2 weeks postoperatively, showing still massive hydronephrosis bilaterally, as expected.

D, IVP 5 months later, showing marked reduction in hydronephrosis. Now 12 years later, the patient is age 27 years with stable renal function and IVP. There has been no further urinary infection.

tion and intravenous pyelograms have remained stable. Unfortunately, the patient sustained a broken neck from diving into shallow water in 1983, making him a paraplegic. Since then he has required intermittent catheterization to empty the bladder, which had previously been functioning well.

Comment. The techniques described made possible reimplantation of the left ureter for a 4th time with success. It is regrettable that the patient's life has been so altered by preventable trauma, which is the greatest single cause for morbidity and mortality in young men.

Case 6 (Figs. 42–45 and 42–46). A 7 year old girl was referred in 1977 with severe bilateral hydronephrosis and bilateral duplex systems. The original problem had been bilateral ureteroceles. Ureteral reimplantation had been done on the left, but obstruction followed. There was reflux to the lower pole on the right. As shown in Figure 42–45, reconstruction was performed by draining the entire urinary tract via the best of 4 ureters, i.e., the right lower pole ureter. It was reimplanted with a long tunnel and a psoas hitch. The right upper pole was drained into the adjacent lower pole. The left upper pole ureter was the better of the two on the left and was used for transureteroureterostomy. The left lower pole renal pelvis was drained into the adjacent upper pole ureter. Three years later the patient's serum creatinine level was 1.2 mg percent and the BUN, 24 mg percent. Although

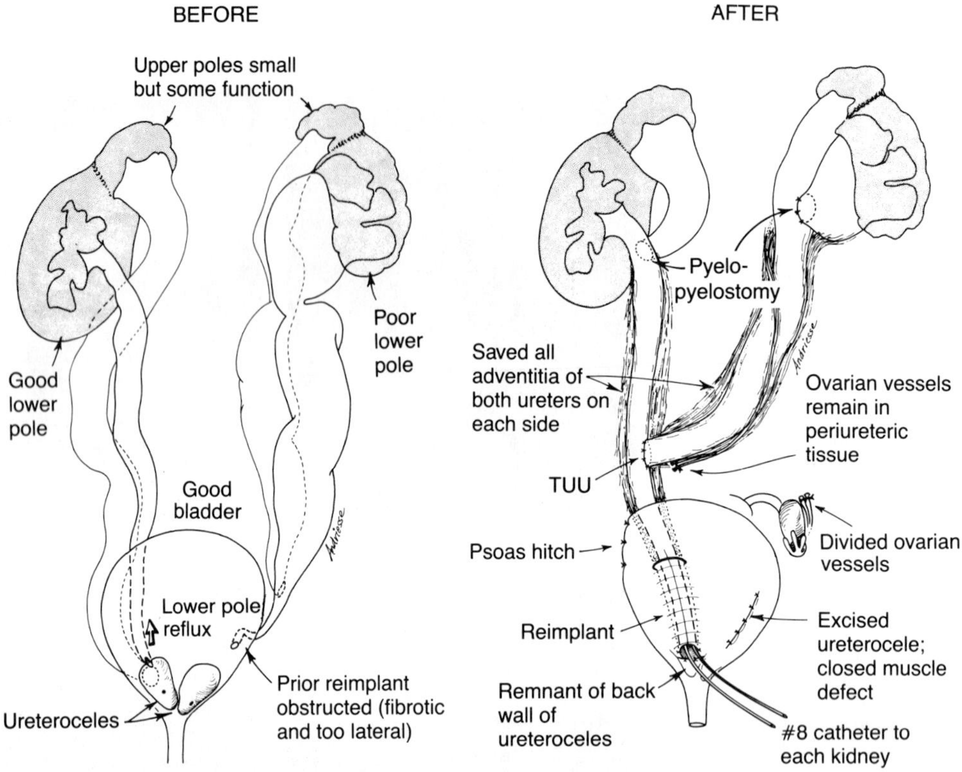

Figure 42–45. **(Case 6)** Anatomy before and after reconstruction.

long-term follow-up was arranged, the family proved unreliable and the patient's current status is unknown.

Comment. When there are two large ureters on one side, it is better to remove one, do a pyelopyelostomy, and rely on the better ureter for drainage of the entire kidney. This is more reliable than reimplanting two big ureters, especially if tapering is necessary. Figure 42–27 shows the techniques by which two ureters can be separated, leaving all the common periureteral adventitia with the one to be preserved. The ureter to be removed is dissected free, close to its wall. It is passed up through a series of "stair-step" incisions in the common periureteral adventitia. This preserves maximal blood supply for the ureter to be saved.

Case 7 (Figs. 42–47 to 42–49). A 17 year old girl was referred for possible urinary reconstruction. A ventriculoperitoneal shunt for hydrocephalus had been performed during her infancy. An ileal loop urinary diversion had been performed because of urinary incontinence and recurrent urinary infection secondary to myelodysplasia. During the next 15 years, she had many episodes of urinary infection. There were progressive dilatations of the upper urinary tract and multiple strictures of the ileal loop (Fig. 42–48). Preoperative bladder cycling was not attempted because the bladder was freely incontinent when filled with saline. Reconstruction was performed as shown in Figure 42–47. Wide mobilization of the two ureters disclosed that the left one was long enough for satisfactory implantation into the back wall of the bladder. Long tunnel reimplantation was performed, with psoas hitch fixation of the bladder to maintain tunnel length and prevent angulation of the ureter during bladder filling. The opposite ureter was drained by transureteroureterostomy. The urethra and bladder neck were narrowed and elongated to provide more outlet resistance. The bladder was augmented with the sigmoid colon applied as a large cap to the patient's own small, noncompliant bladder. Since this 16 hour reconstructive procedure, the patient has done well. Unexpectedly, she is able to empty the bladder almost completely by abdominal pressure and the Credé maneuver. Her upper tracts are greatly improved since getting rid of her

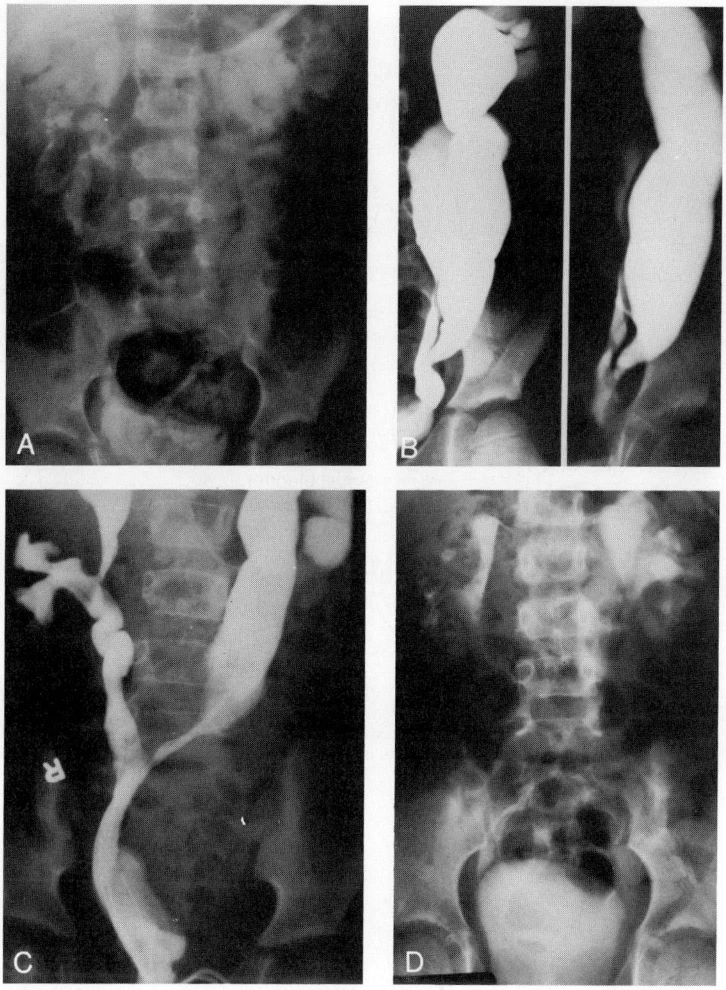

Figure 42–46. Roentgenograms from Case 6.

A, Preoperative IVP showing marked bilateral hydronephrosis and poor visualization of the upper tract.

B, Preoperative left percutaneous antegrade pyelogram showing two large ureters obstructed at the site of reimplantation.

C, Study 10 days postoperatively by injecting contrast medium into drainage catheters. Note the long tunnel implantation of the right lower pole ureter, psoas hitch, transureteroureterostomy, and right pyelopyelostomy.

D, Intravenous pyelogram 2½ years postoperatively reveals excellent function and marked improvement in hydronephrosis. Cystogram showed no reflux.

strictured ileal loop with massive reflux. Although free from urinary infection, she has been maintained on suppressive therapy, to avoid risking infection with her previously compromised upper tracts. Twice daily intermittent catheterization after voiding has been advised to be absolutely certain that she continues to empty the bladder completely.

Comment. This patient was an ideal candidate for undiversion, being an intelligent and highly motivated teenager anxious to get rid of her bag and recurrent episodes of infection. I had thought that intermittent catheterization would be the only method for emptying her bladder. This illustrates that it is impossible to predict for these patients the details of their postoperative management. Happily she can void. Reconstruction as illustrated has improved her long-term outlook from the standpoint of preserving renal function as well as improving her social status.

Urinary diversion was common for this type of patient a decade or two ago. There are many patients like her who can be undiverted.[51,52] To date I have undiverted 175 children and young adults. Each is a special undertaking. This is feasible even in patients with poor renal function who will later need renal transplantation. This series includes one patient who had already undergone renal transplantation into an ileal loop. Another was anephric after two failed transplants into a colon conduit. The bladder was recon-

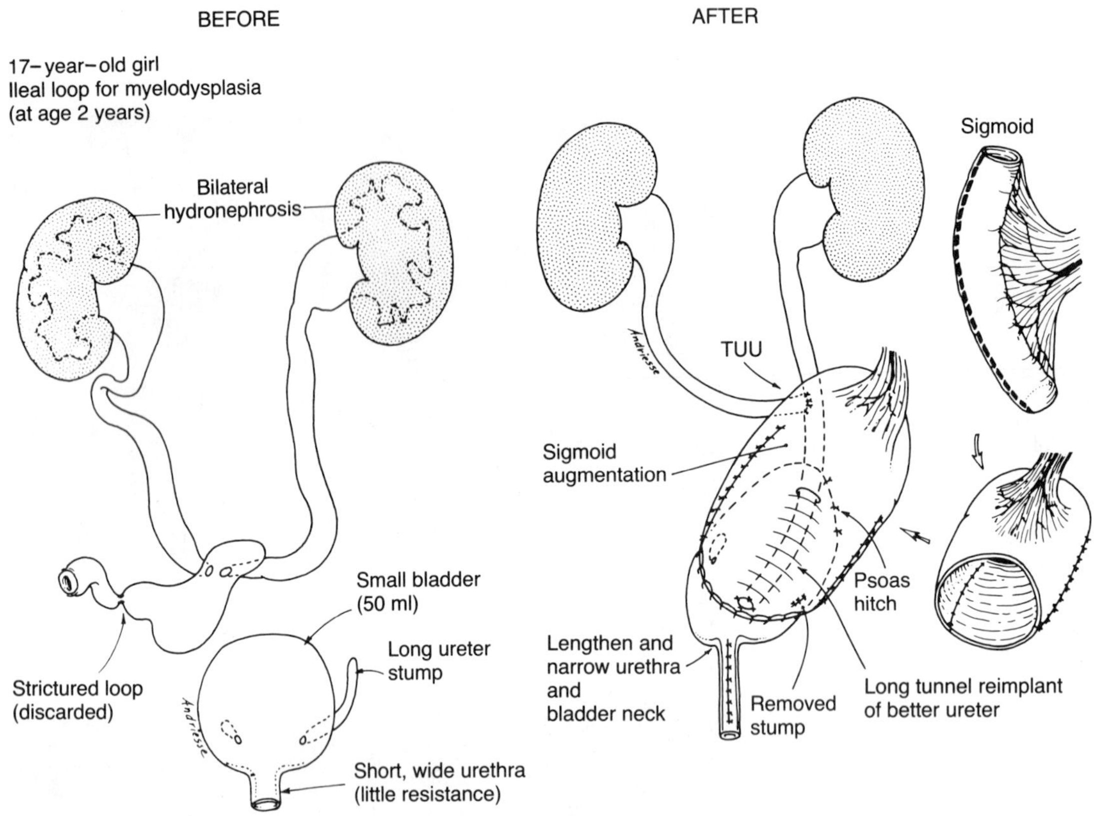

Figure 42–47. (**Case 7**) Pre- and postoperative anatomy.

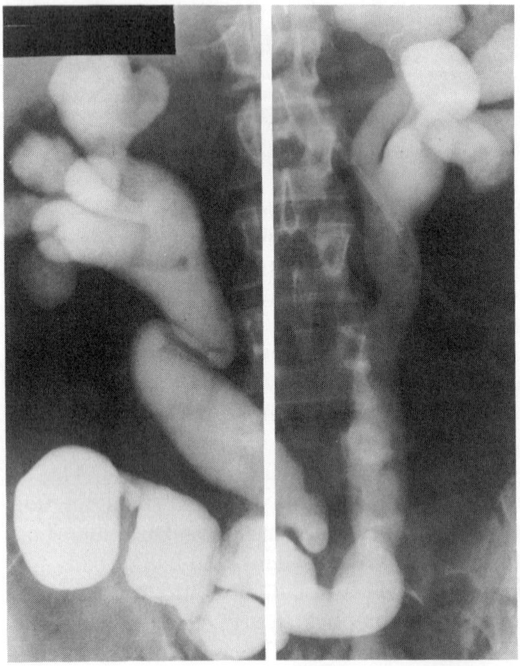

Figure 42–48. (**Case 7**) Preoperative study of urinary tract by instilling contrast through an ileal loop stoma. Note multiple strictures of the ileal loop, massive bilateral reflux, and hydronephrosis.

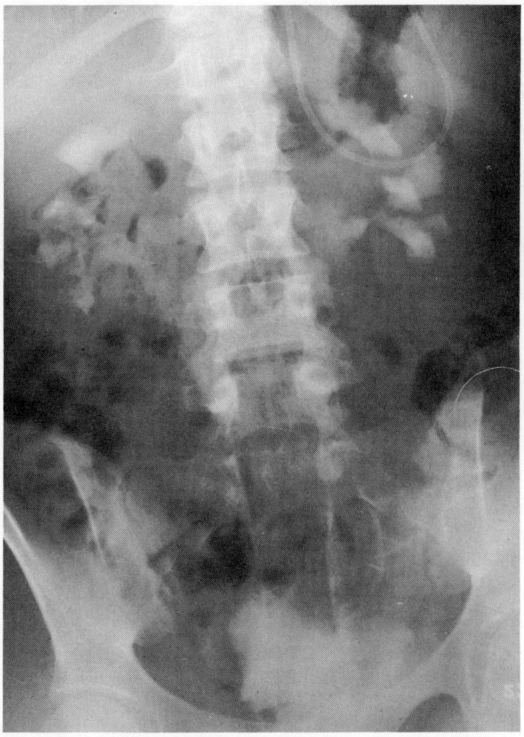

Figure 42–49. (**Case 7**) IVP 6 months following undiversion operation. Note the marked improvement in hydronephrosis. The patient is well, now 2 years postoperatively.

structed, following which a living related transplant was done with success.

Today the problem of myelodysplasia can be managed often by intermittent catheterization of the bladder, ureteral reimplantation to stop reflux, and sometimes narrowing of the bladder outlet and augmentation of the bladder if pressures are high and the bladder wall is noncompliant.

CONCLUSION

Staightforward ureteral reimplantation of normal ureters into a normal bladder should be possible in most hands with a minimal complication rate and a high degree of success. Even the severely decompensated ureter with tortuosity and elongation from obstruction or reflux can be repaired in most instances. However, in many cases, this is a very difficult task. Like many specialized types of surgery, it should be attempted only by those with a suitable background and technical skill. Furthermore, the surgeon should do it often enough to acquire and maintain proficiency. Those who lack this experience should not, in our opinion, perform temporary exteriorization of the upper tracts in the belief that the task will be easier at an older age. Such an approach can be followed by successful subsequent reconstruction, but it can also introduce several additional complications, making ultimate reconstruction more difficult. Attention to the pitfalls enumerated, some judgmental and others technical, can reduce the complication rate after ureteral reimplantation and megaureter repair to an acceptable level.

References

1. Politano VA: One hundred reimplantations and five years. J Urol 90:696, 1963.
2. Williams DI, Eckstein HB: Surgical treatment of reflux in children. Br J Urol 37:13, 1965.
3. Hendren WH: Ureteral reimplantation in children. J Pediatr Surg 3:649, 1968.
4. McGovern JH, Marshall VF: Reimplantation of the ureters into the bladders of children. J Urol 99:572, 1968.
5. Gonzales ET, Glenn JF, Anderson EE: Results of distal tunnel ureteral reimplantation. J Urol 107:572, 1972.
6. Mounger EJ, Scott EVZ: Surgical correction of vesicoureteral reflux. J Urol 108:347, 1972.
7. Woodard JR Jr, Keats G: Ureteral reimplantation: Paquin's procedure after 12 years. J Urol 109:891, 1973.
8. Stamey TA: Urinary Infections. Baltimore, Williams & Wilkins, 1972.
9. Normand C, Smellie J: Vesicoureteric reflux: the case for conservative management. In Hodson J, Kincaid-Smith P, eds: Reflux Nephropathy. New York, Masson Publishing Company, 1979, p 281.
10. Medical versus surgical treatment of primary vesicoureteral reflux: a prospective international reflux study in children. J Urol 125:277, 1981.
11. Hodson CJ, Craven JD, Lewis DG, et al: Experimental obstructive nephropathy in the pig. I. Radiology. Br J Urol *41*:5, 1969.
12. Koff SA: Disordered vesicoureteral function in the pathogenesis of urinary infection and vesicoureteric reflux. Chap. 8 In Johnston JH, ed: International Perspectives in Urology. Baltimore, Williams & Wilkins, 1984.
13. Lich R Jr, Howerton LW, Davis LA: Recurrent urosepsis in children. J Urol 86:554, 1961.
14. Grégoir W, Van Regemorter G: Le reflux vesico-ureteral congenital. Urol Int 18:122, 1964.
15. Hendren WH: Reoperation for the failed ureteral reimplantation. J Urol 111:403, 1974.
16. Politano VA, Leadbetter WF: An operative technique for the correction of vesicoureteral reflux. J Urol 79:932, 1958.
17. Amar AD: Reflux in duplicated ureters. Br J Urol 40:385, 1968.
18. Cohen SJ: Ureterozystoneostomie: eine neue Antirefluxtechnik. Akt Urol 6:1, 1975.
19. Hendren WH: Reoperative ureteral reimplantation—Management of the difficult case. J Pediatr Surg 15:770, 1980.
20. Hendren WH, Hensle TW: Transureteroureterostomy—Experience with 75 cases. J Urol 123:826, 1980.
21. Williams DI, Woodard JR: Problems in the management of ectopic ureteroceles. J Urol 92:635, 1965.
22. Johnston JH, Johnson LM: Experiences with ectopic ureteroceles. Br J Urol 41:61, 1969.

23. Hendren WH, Mitchell ME: Surgical corrections of ureteroceles. J Urol 121:590, 1979.
24. Nesbit RM, Withycombe JF: The problems of primary megaloureter. J Urol 72:162, 1954.
25. Stephens FD: Treatment of megaureters by multiple micturition. Aust NZ J Surg 27:130, 1957.
26. Bergman H: The Ureter. New York, Harper & Row, 1967.
27. Derrick CF Jr: Management of the large, tortuous, adynamic ureter with reflux. J Urol 108:153, 1972.
28. Bischoff P: Operative treatment of megaureter. J Urol 85:268, 1961.
29. Johnston HJ: Reconstructive surgery of mega-ureter in childhood. Br J Urol 39:17, 1967.
30. Hendren WH: Operative repair of megaureter in children. J Urol 101:491, 1969.
31. Tanagho EA: Ureteral tailoring. J Urol 106:194, 1971.
32. Hendren WH: Restoration of function in the severely decompensated ureter. In Johnston HJ, Scholtmeijer RJ, eds: Problems in Pediatric Urology. New York, Excerpta Medica of Elsevier Publishing, 1972.
33. Flatmark AU, Maurseth K, Knutrud O: Lower ureteric obstruction in children. Br J Urol 42:434, 1970.
34. Williams DI, Hulme-Moor I: Primary obstructive megaureter. Br J Urol 42:140, 1970.
35. McLaughlin AP, Leadbetter WF, Pfister RC: Reconstructive surgery of primary megaloureter. J Urol 106:286, 1971.
36. Belman AB: Megaureter classification, etiology, and management. Urol Clin North Am 1:497, 1974.
37. Hendren WH: Megaureter. In Welch KJ, Randolph JG, Ravitch MM, O'Neill JA Jr, Rowe MI, eds: Pediatric Surgery. Chicago, Year Book Medical Publishers, 1986.
38. Hendren WH: Complications of megaureter repair in children. J Urol 113:238, 1975.
39. Kalicinski ZH, Kansy J, Kotarbinska B, et al: Surgery of megaureters: modification of Hendren's operation. J Pediatr Surg 12:183, 1977.
40. Ehrlich RM: Ureteral folding technique for megaureter surgery. Society for Pediatric Urology Newsletter, May 5, 1982.
41. Johnston HJ: Temporary cutaneous ureterostomy in the management of advanced congenital obstruction. Arch Dis Child 38:161, 1963.
42. Wasserman DH, Garrett RA: Cutaneous ureterostomy: indications in children. J Urol 94:380, 1965.
43. Lome LG, Williams DI: Urinary reconstruction following temporary cutaneous ureterostomy diversion in children. J Urol 108:162, 1972.
44. Perlmutter AD, Patil J: Loop cutaneous ureterostomy in infants and young children: late results in 32 cases. J Urol 107:655, 1972.
45. Dwoskin JY: Management of the massively dilated urinary tract in infants by temporary diversion and single-stage reconstruction. Urol Clin North Am 1:515, 1974.
46. Hendren WH: Some alternatives to urinary diversion in children. J Urol 119:652, 1978.
47. Ray, P, DeDomenico I: Intestinal conduit urinary diversion in children. Br J Urol 44:345, 1972.
48. Smith ED: Follow-up studies on 150 ileal conduits in children. J Pediatr Surg 7:1, 1972.
49. Richie JP: Intestinal loop urinary diversion in children. J Urol 111:687, 1974.
50. Middleton AW Jr, Hendren WH: Ileal conduits in children at the Massachusetts General Hospital from 1955 to 1970. J Urol 115:591, 1976.
51. Hendren WH: Urinary tract refunctionalization after prior diversion in children. Ann Surg 180:494, 1974.
52. Hendren WH: Refunctionalization of the previously diverted urinary tract. In Retik AB, Cukier J, eds: Pediatric Urology. Baltimore, Williams & Wilkins, 1987, pp 398–442.

COMPLICATIONS OF LASER SURGERY

43

Joseph A. Smith, Jr.

One of the potential advantages of lasers in a number of clinical settings is that treatment can be performed with less morbidity than with alternative surgical techniques. The unique physics and tissue interactions of laser energy allow relatively precise control over the extent of thermal injury. Despite this, complications can occur and have been observed in association with a variety of applications of lasers in urologic surgery. The fact that complications can, in large part, be anticipated and avoided through proper education, experience, and patient selection is not unique to laser surgery. This chapter reviews the potential complications that can occur during laser treatment in urology. More importantly, it defines controllable factors that may contribute to the incidence of complications. Finally, recognition of complications and appropriate management are discussed.

INJURIES TO PERSONNEL

When used properly and with adequate education, surgical lasers are safe for personnel. However, serious accidents have occurred. Most hospitals with laser capabilities have appointed a Laser Safety Officer (LSO) whose responsibility it is to ensure that proper precautions for safety are maintained in laser treatment areas.[1] Furthermore, the LSO makes certain that surgeons have proper credentials and training before privileges for laser use are granted.

Electrical Safety

Some source of external power is necessary for the process of stimulated emission of radiation to occur within the laser resonator cavity. Most surgical lasers use electricity as a power source. Neodymium:yttrium-aluminum-garnet (Nd:YAG) and argon lasers require three-phase 220-volt electrical power. Most carbon-dioxide lasers use 110-volt outlets. It seems obvious to state that caution should be used in connecting the plug to a high-energy electrical outlet. However, serious electrical injuries have occurred during the simple maneuver of inserting the plug of a laser into an electrical outlet. Cautions in this regard are particularly appropriate in urologic surgery. The irrigant used for cystoscopic examination often leaves the floor wet or with puddles of fluid. As much as possible, the floor should be kept dry around the laser machine, and any persons handling the electrical wiring should make certain that there is no standing water nearby.

Eye Injury

The potential injury to personnel that requires greatest attention during laser surgery is damage to the eye. Both a direct and a reflected laser beam can cause eye injury. A carbon-dioxide laser has a wavelength of 10,600 nm. Light at this wavelength is strongly absorbed by water. Therefore, impact of a CO_2 laser upon the eye results in a corneal burn, but energy rarely is transmitted to the fundus. Although CO_2 laser eye injuries may heal without sequelae, they are painful and initially dangerous. Both argon and Nd:YAG laser energy pass through the anterior chamber of the eye with little absorption. Therefore, they cause damage to the retina, resulting in a scotoma.

The critical distance between the laser head or fiber tip and the eye that must be maintained to avoid a significant injury is uncertain. There is a 5- to 8-degree angle of divergence from most laser fibers, so the greater the distance between the instrument tip and the eye, the less the potential damage. Nevertheless, it is mandatory that all persons within the operating area, including the patient, have adequate eye protection.

Goggles or glasses with appropriate filtering lenses are manufactured for each wavelength laser. If desired, custom-made prescription lenses can be obtained. For the 1060 nm wavelength of an Nd:YAG, a green-tinted lens is used. An argon laser requires an amber lens for proper filtration. Any clear plastic or glass lens, including ordinary eyeglasses, will filter carbon-dioxide laser energy.

Glasses or goggles that completely cover the eye are desirable, and side protection is necessary. Because of this, the wearing of appropriate eye protection during laser surgery is often a nuisance. The lens may fog during surgery, although antifogging cleansers are helpful. In addition, the colored lens used for Nd:YAG or argon treatment decreases visibility somewhat, especially during endoscopic treatment. Because of this, a lens cap has been developed for cystoscopes. Once the fiber is inserted into the cystoscope, the lens cap is applied and glasses or goggles are not mandatory (Fig. 43–1). Caution is still necessary, though, because of the possibility of fiber breakage at a point proximal to the insertion into the cystoscope.

All areas in which laser surgery is performed should conform to established safety standards. Windows should be equipped with blinds or coverings to prevent transmission of the laser beam from the immediate operating area. Doors should be closed at all times when laser treatment is being performed. Controlled access entry is desirable, and a sign should be placed outside the room indicating that a laser procedure is in progress. Finally, the laser itself should be kept in the standby mode whenever treatment is temporarily interrupted.

Thermal Injury to Skin

If the laser beam inadvertently comes in contact with the skin of the operating surgeon or an assistant, a thermal injury can occur. Because of the slight amount of beam divergence, the target tissue must be in relatively close proximity to the end of the fiber or handpiece for the thermal effects to be injurious. Most often, laser burns occur on the fingers or hands of the surgeon. The injuries are not serious but are completely avoidable through careful handling of the laser fiber or handpiece.

TREATMENT COMPLICATIONS

Most often, complications of laser treatment are caused by excessive energy density. The formula for determining energy density is power × duration/cm^2. Thus, a number of factors are important in determining the energy density. Some factors, such as power output and duration, are under relatively precise control of the surgeon.[2] However, the area of tissue being treated is determined by the spot size of the laser beam and is dependent on the distance between the fiber tip and the target tissue, angulation at the point of impact, irregularities in the tissue surface, and fiber damage. For purposes of discussion, complications of laser surgery are grouped by the site of treatment.

External Application

Most external applications of lasers in urologic surgery have involved treatment of carcinoma of the penis or condyloma acuminatum. In both instances, the rationale for treatment is based in large part on the excellent functional and cosmetic results that can be achieved with laser surgery.[3] For the most part, complications are caused by excessive energy density resulting in full-thickness thermal injury with subsequent skin slough.

With a carbon-dioxide laser, precise tissue removal can be accomplished, and the penetration depth is limited. Tissue effects are primarily caused by vaporization rather than by thermal coagulation. Carbon-dioxide lasers are used commonly to treat condyloma acuminatum.[4] The key to avoiding complications is to recognize amounts of tissue vaporization that are adequate for total excision of the condyloma but are not excessive. In general, penetration to the deep layers of the dermis is unnecessary.

The lowest power that will accomplish adequate vaporization—often 3 to 5 watts—should be used. Energy is delivered with a focusing

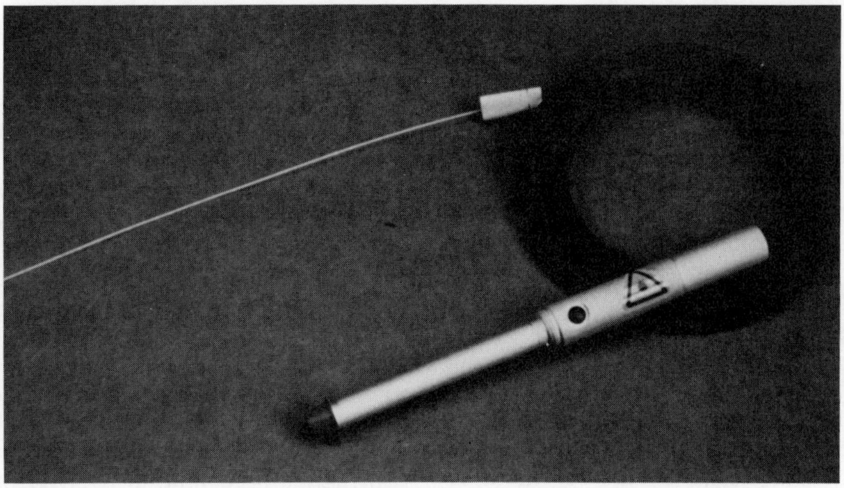

Figure 43–1. Fiber for conduction of Nd:YAG laser energy. Once the fiber is inserted through a cystoscope, a lens cap with appropriate filter can be used for eye protection.

handpiece. The focal length that is used is relatively unimportant and simply should be one with which the surgeon is comfortable. When the base of the lesion is approached, the energy should be defocused to prevent excessive penetration. Bleeding usually is not observed in the epidermis. Bleeding itself should be a sign that further penetration is unnecessary. The coarse, cottony fibers of the dermis are visible under close inspection when the condyloma has been completely vaporized. Further application of energy will result in a full-thickness injury (Fig. 43–2).

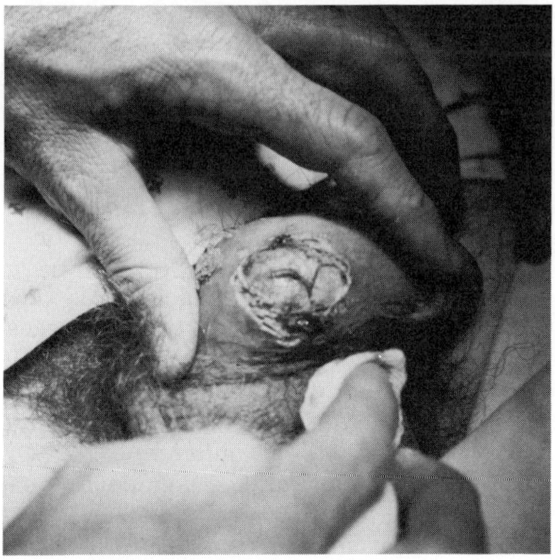

Figure 43–2. Full-thickness dermal injury from CO_2 laser treatment of condyloma acuminatum of penile shaft. Despite the extent of injury, healing by secondary intention resulted in minimal scarring.

An Nd:YAG laser penetrates 3 to 5 mm in tissue, and a full-thickness skin injury is possible. If a broad-based condyloma has been treated, a significant amount of tissue slough may occur over 6 weeks. The lesion sometimes becomes secondarily infected and requires antibiotics. When a carcinoma of the penis is treated, a deep thermal injury is desirable, but up to 3 months may be necessary before epithelialization is complete.

Management of a full-thickness laser injury to the skin of the penis is relatively straightforward. Debridement usually is not necessary because the devitalized tissue will slough spontaneously. Topical antibiotics may be useful, and systemic antibiotics are sometimes indicated. Even when the skin loss is considerable, as much as 3 or 4 cm in diameter, conservative treatment is indicated. Skin grafting or skin flaps are unnecessary. Although several months may elapse before complete healing is observed, the end result is surprisingly good if spontaneous healing is allowed.

Whenever laser surgery is performed in an open surgical field, care should be taken to avoid direct contact between the beam and surgical drapes or sponges. Paper drapes in particular could ignite if heated sufficiently. Retractors and surgical instruments with a dull finish and irregular surface are used by some laser surgeons. This prevents a deflection of coherent light by producing scattering if the laser beam comes in contact with an instrument. For the most part, special instruments are unnecessary if minimal caution is maintained.

Urethra

Endoscopic laser treatment usually is performed using a flexible fiber inserted through a cystoscope or a ureteroscope. Treatment is performed in a fluid medium, and saline or water may be used as the irrigant. A prototype carbon-dioxide laser cystoscope has been developed,[5] but the rapid absorption of CO_2 energy by water requires gaseous distension of the urethra. Unless proper suprapubic venting is carefully maintained, gaseous distension of the urethra during laser therapy can be an extremely dangerous situation. Either intentional or inadvertent laser incisions through the urethral mucosa could allow absorption of the gas by the cavernous or spongy tissue, leading to air embolus. Intraoperative death has been reported in at least two patients undergoing laser treatment of urethral strictures under gaseous distension.[6] Even when more soluble gases such as carbon dioxide are used, the risk of air embolus is real.

When using an Nd:YAG laser, air embolus is not a problem. An Nd:YAG laser has been used to treat urethral condyloma, urethral strictures, and some urethral cancers. Especially in treating benign lesions of the urethra, a potential concern is that strictures could be induced because of the thermal injury. Nevertheless, laser-induced urethral strictures are extremely uncommon, even when circumferential application of laser energy is performed in proximal portions of the urethra (Fig. 43–3).[7] Most often, condyloma acuminatum occurs in the fossa navicularis or at the meatus. We have observed some fossa navicularis strictures after laser treatment, but these have responded readily to dilation and have been seen only in patients with extensive condylomatous growths.

Bladder

The most common laser use in urology is treatment of transitional cell carcinoma of the bladder. A number of benign lesions, including interstitial cystitis and bladder hemangioma, have also been successfully managed with laser therapy. To a great extent, the use of lasers in both benign and malignant diseases of the bladder is predicated upon the low morbidity of the procedure. Nevertheless, complications can occur and each of the potential problems associated with intravesical laser use are addressed individually.

Bleeding

A primary advantage of laser treatment in the bladder is the general absence of bleeding. Most often, an Nd:YAG laser is used, and this provides excellent thermal coagulation up to depths of 3 to 5 mm.[8] During treatment, a white discoloration of the tissue becomes obvious as protein denaturation occurs. Simultaneously, blood vessels are coagulated and no bleeding at all is usually observed. It has been mentioned that treatment should be performed around the periphery of the lesion to seal blood vessels prior to laser treatment.[9] However, this is not necessary and hemostasis is usually excellent even if the laser beam is initially applied directly to the lesion. Furthermore, significant delayed bleeding has not been observed in any patient.

Ureteral Stenosis

Often, bladder tumors are located over the ureteral orifice or extend just inside the intramural tunnel of the ureter. Even when a pure cutting current is used, electrocautery resection sometimes results in stenosis and obstruction of the ureter. A frequent concern during laser treatment of tumors overlying the ureter is that a similar type of stenosis could occur as the laser-treated area heals. However, there have been no reports of ureteral obstruction or stenosis development after laser treatment (Fig. 43–4). As experience is gained and the follow-up period is extended, this could change. Nevertheless, it appears that the risk of inducing ureteral obstruction from laser treatment is less than that associated with electrocautery.[10]

Double-J ureteral stents should be removed prior to laser treatment of tumors near the ureteral orifices because they are damaged by the laser beam.

Bladder Perforation

The thermal damage from an Nd:YAG laser injury extends 3 to 5 mm into tissue. A transmural coagulation of the bladder wall is possible and, in some instances, desirable. However, the bladder maintains its structural and architectural integrity even after a transmural injury.

With an Nd:YAG laser, the therapeutic temperature range is between 60 and 100° C. This produces a coagulation necrosis and protein denaturation. However, tissue vaporization and carbonization are minimal. After a laser injury, the bladder heals by collagen deposition with relative preservation of the elastic fibers.

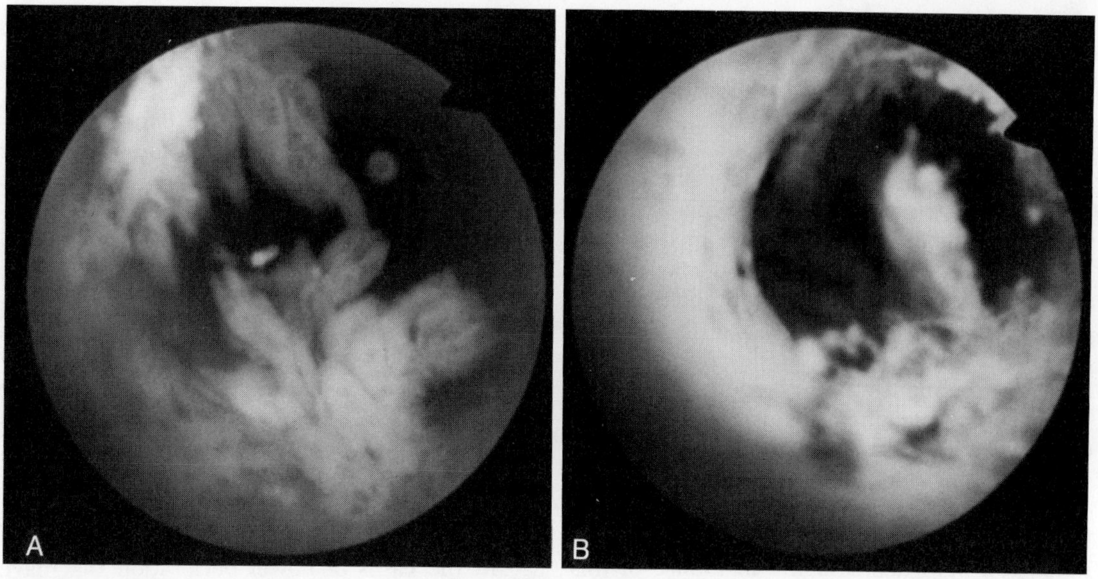

Figure 43–3. Condyloma acuminatum of bulbous urethra. *A*, Before laser treatment. *B*, After Nd:YAG laser therapy. Despite the thermal damage to the urethra that occurs, treatment-induced strictures have not been observed in the pendulous or bulbar urethra.

Because of these properties, clinically evident bladder perforation with extravasation of urine has not been observed after laser therapy. In fact, an intact bladder wall has been documented after intravesical application of laser energy, even in situations in which damage to adjacent organs has occurred. In addition, small amounts of urinary extravasation would likely remain subclinical and undetected. At any rate, bladder perforation with urinary extravasation is not a particular concern after laser therapy and Foley catheter drainage of the bladder for this reason is unnecessary.

Damage to Adjacent Organs

Perhaps the most feared complication of laser urologic surgery is damage to adjacent organs, in particular, the small bowel. A number of factors contribute to the possibility that perforation

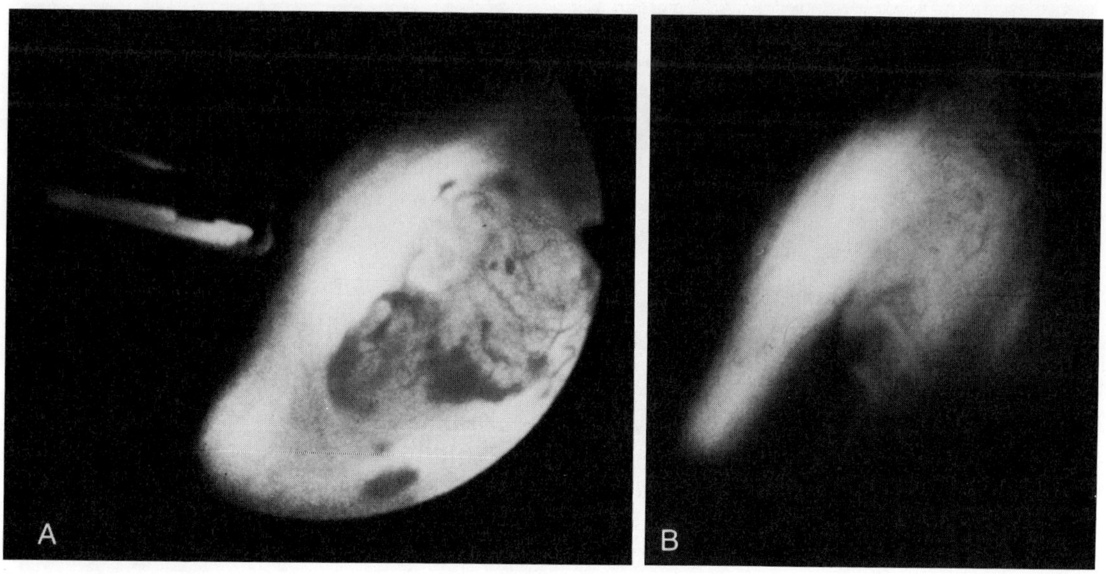

Figure 43–4. *A*, Left ureteral orifice with an overlying papillary bladder tumor. The Nd:YAG laser fiber is seen in position for treatment. *B*, Six weeks after treatment, the orifice has healed without stenosis or residual tumor.

of the small bowel can occur while the bladder itself remains intact. First of all, some 20 to 30% of Nd:YAG laser energy is propagated with forward scatter, with this energy being absorbed primarily by extravesical tissue. In addition, the thick muscular wall of the bladder allows it to maintain its structural integrity with a greater resistance to perforation than the small bowel. Finally, small bladder perforations may remain subclinical, whereas bowel perforation results in peritonitis.

The incidence of small bowel perforation during laser treatment of the bladder is quite low. We have not encountered this complication in over 200 laser treatments. Hofstetter has observed small bowel perforation three times in over 700 treatments.[9] Recognition of several factors that may contribute to small bowel perforation can help decrease the incidence of this complication. The risk is greatest during treatment of lesions of the intraperitoneal portion of the bladder, primarily the bladder dome. The bladder in women often is thinner than that in men. The bladder should not be overdistended during treatment; it should simply be filled to a volume that allows adequate visualization of the lesion. Adhesions of small bowel to the bladder dome after previous pelvic surgery, irradiation, or inflammatory bowel disease may increase the risk.

It is of extreme importance to ensure that the laser is calibrated properly and that excessive energy is not used. The fiber should be calibrated before each treatment and intermittently during therapy if treatment is prolonged. Malloy has seen bowel perforation in one patient because of an unrecognized increase in the power during treatment.[10] After the laser had been calibrated, the power gradually rose as warmer water from the outside water source circulated through the laser machine.

Excessive energy should be avoided and treatment terminated when the desired tissue effects are visible. For superficial bladder tumors, the white discoloration of the tissue is characteristic and indicative of adequate thermal necrosis (Fig. 43–5).[11] Continued treatment beyond this point could result in excessive forward scatter of energy without visible perforation or vaporization.

In the cases of bowel perforation that have occurred, clinical signs of peritonitis most often have been evident within the first 12 to 24 hours. However, clinical signs of peritonitis have been seen as late as 1 week after treatment. Hofstetter has indicated that patients should be observed for 24 hours after laser treatment to rule out bowel perforation.[9] This does not seem necessary as a routine because of the low incidence of bowel perforation. Moreover, clinical evidence of peritonitis may not be obvious within this period of time.

Along with clinical signs of peritonitis, free intra-abdominal air often is noted when a bowel

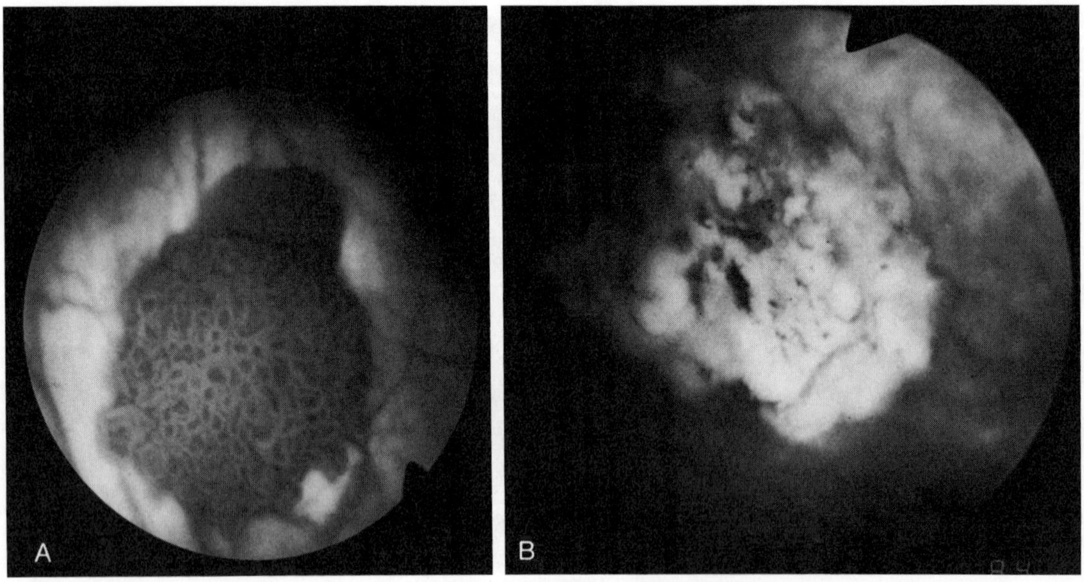

Figure 43–5. *A*, Papillary transitional cell carcinoma of the bladder. *B*, After laser therapy, the tumor underwent a white discoloration indicative of adequate thermal necrosis. Care should be taken to avoid excessive laser energy.

perforation occurs. Immediate laparotomy should be performed. Because the thermal injury may be greater than is apparent, the involved bowel should be resected and a primary anastomosis should be performed rather than a simple oversewing of the perforation.

Photodynamic Therapy

Photodynamic therapy is an investigational form of treatment with potential complications peculiar to this technique. The process involves photosensitization of malignant and dysplastic cells with a drug, usually a hematoporphyrin derivative, with activation of a cytotoxic effect through application of light onto the photosensitized tissue.[12] The tissue effects are nonthermal. Limited clinical experience with photodynamic therapy of bladder cancer is available, so definitive statements regarding the short- and long-term complications of the procedure are not possible. The photoactivating drugs themselves currently in use have an extremely high margin of safety. Bladder contracture, which is possibly treatment-related, has been reported in occasional patients. Of greatest immediate concern is that the photosensitization process not be limited to the bladder because systemic administration of the drug is required. A certain amount of the photoactivating drug accumulates in the skin, making it extremely light-sensitive. After drug delivery, all areas of the skin must be protected from direct sunlight for at least 6 weeks. Longer periods of skin photosensitivity have been seen in some patients. Severe sunburn is possible if skin protection is not used.

SUMMARY

In general, laser surgery in urology is associated with few complications. Indeed, the relative safety of laser surgery is one of the factors that increases the usefulness of the technique. As with any treatment, the key to avoiding complications is proper education and training, recognition of factors that could lead to complications, and appropriate patient selection.

References

1. Lundergan DS: Laser safety. In Smith JA Jr, ed: Lasers in Urologic Surgery. Chicago, Year Book Medical Publishers, 1985, ch 12.
2. Stein BS, Kendall AR: Lasers in urology. Urology 23:411, 1984.
3. Hofstetter A, Frank F: Laser use in urology. In Dixon JA, ed: Surgical Application of Lasers. Chicago, Year Book Medical Publishers, 1983, pp 146–162.
4. Rosemberg SK, Jacobs H, Fuller T: Some guidelines in the treatment of urethral condylomata with carbon dioxide laser. J Urol 127:906, 1982.
5. Willscher MK, Filoso AM, Jako GJ, et al: Development of a carbon dioxide laser cystoscope. J Urol 119:202, 1978.
6. Vourc'h G, Berreti E, Trichet B, et al: Two unusual cases of gas embolism following urethral surgery under laser. Intensive Care Med 8:239, 1982.
7. Smith JA Jr, Dixon JA: Neodymium:YAG laser treatment of benign urethral strictures. J Urol 131:1080, 1984.
8. Pensel J, Hofstetter A, Frank F, et al: Temporal and spatial temperature profile of the bladder serosa in intravesical neodymium:YAG laser irradiation. Eur Urol 7:298, 1981.
9. Hofstetter A, Frank F: Laser treatment of the bladder: experimental and clinical results. In Smith JA Jr, ed: Lasers in Urologic Surgery. Chicago, Year Book Medical Publishers, 1985, pp 63–81.
10. Malloy TR: Personal communications, 1987.
11. Hofstetter A, Frank F, Keiditsch E, et al: Endoscopic Nd:YAG laser application for destroying bladder tumors. Eur Urol 7:278, 1981.
12. Benson RC: Hematoporphyrin phototherapy. In Smith JA Jr, ed: Lasers in Urologic Surgery. Chicago, Year Book Medical Publishers, 1985, ch 11.

Index

Note: Page numbers in *italics* refer to illustrations; page numbers followed by (t) refer to tables.

I

O

P

Q

R

T

V